Ham's
Primary Care Geriatrics
A Case-Based Approach

Ham's
Primary Care Geriatrics
A Case-Based Approach
6TH EDITION

Richard J. Ham, MD
Director, WVU Center on Aging
Professor of Geriatric Medicine and Psychiatry
Robert C. Byrd Health Sciences Center
West Virginia University
Morgantown, West Virginia

Philip D. Sloane, MD, MPH
Elizabeth and Oscar Goodwin Distinguished Professor
Department of Family Medicine
Co-Director, Program on Aging, Disability, and Long-Term Care
Cecil G. Sheps Center for Health Services Research
University of North Carolina at Chapel Hill
Chapel Hill, North Carolina

Gregg A. Warshaw, MD
Martha Betty Semmons Professor of Geriatric Medicine
Professor of Family and Community Medicine
Director, Geriatric Medicine Program
University of Cincinnati College of Medicine
Cincinnati, Ohio

Jane F. Potter, MD
Harris Professor of Geriatric Medicine
Chief, Division of Geriatrics and Gerontology
Department of Internal Medicine
University of Nebraska Medical Center
Home Instead Center for Successful Aging
Omaha, Nebraska

Ellen Flaherty, PhD, APRN, AGSF
Dartmouth Center for Health and Aging
Geisel School of Medicine at Dartmouth
Department of Primary Care-Geriatrics
Dartmouth-Hitchcock Medical Center
Lebanon, New Hampshire

ELSEVIER
SAUNDERS

SAUNDERS

1600 John F. Kennedy Blvd.
Ste 1800
Philadelphia, PA 19103-2899

HAM'S PRIMARY CARE GERIATRICS   ISBN: 978-0-323-08936-4

Notices

Knowledge and best practice in this field are constantly changing. As new research and experience broaden our understanding, changes in research methods, professional practices, or medical treatment may become necessary.

Practitioners and researchers must always rely on their own experience and knowledge in evaluating and using any information, methods, compounds, or experiments described herein. In using such information or methods they should be mindful of their own safety and the safety of others, including parties for whom they have a professional responsibility.

With respect to any drug or pharmaceutical products identified, readers are advised to check the most current information provided (i) on procedures featured or (ii) by the manufacturer of each product to be administered, to verify the recommended dose or formula, the method and duration of administration, and contraindications. It is the responsibility of practitioners, relying on their own experience and knowledge of their patients, to make diagnoses, to determine dosages and the best treatment for each individual patient, and to take all appropriate safety precautions.

To the fullest extent of the law, neither the Publisher nor the authors, contributors, or editors, assume any liability for any injury and/or damage to persons or property as a matter of products liability, negligence or otherwise, or from any use or operation of any methods, products, instructions, or ideas contained in the material herein.

Library of Congress Cataloging-in-Publication Data

Primary care geriatrics.
  Ham's primary care geriatrics : a case-based approach / [edited by] Richard J. Ham, Philip D. Sloane, Gregg A. Warshaw, Jane F. Potter, Ellen Flaherty. — 6.
    pages cm
  Primary care geriatrics
  Preceded by: Primary care geriatrics : a case-based approach / [edited by] Richard J. Ham . . . [et al.]. 5th ed. 2007.
  Includes bibliographical references and index.
  ISBN 978-0-323-08936-4 (pbk. : alk. paper)
  I. Ham, Richard J., editor of compilation. II. Sloane, Philip D., editor of compilation. III. Warshaw, Gregg A., editor of compilation. IV. Potter, Jane F., editor of compilation. V. Flaherty, Ellen, editor of compilation. VI. Title. VII. Title: Primary care geriatrics.
  [DNLM: 1. Geriatrics. 2. Primary Health Care. WT 100]
  RC952.55
  618.97—dc23
                                                        2013034089

Senior Content Strategist: Suzanne Toppy
Content Development Specialist: Julia Rose Roberts
Publishing Services Manager: Patricia Tannian
Senior Project Manager: Sharon Corell
Senior Book Designer: Ellen Zanolle

Printed in the United States of America

Last digit is the print number: 9 8 7 6 5 4 3 2 1

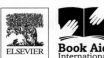

To my patients and their families and friends, whose insights, knowledge, sacrifice, and caring continue to daily rekindle my admiration and awe of the human spirit, and who have taught me most of the really important aspects of growing old and living wisely.

RJH

To those who have taught me the most: my patients, my parents, and my colleagues.

PS

To my University of Cincinnati colleagues in the Geriatric Medicine Program and the Department of Family and Community Medicine for their many years of support and inspiration.

GAW

To my husband, Daniel Francis Schafer, MD, who is endlessly patient and supportive.

JP

To my husband, Mel Aaron, and our amazing children, Eric, Marsha, Megan, and Kelsey, who through their joy and compassion motivate me to reach higher.

EF

My thoughts on old age . . .

A gift for old age is to be able to delight in comfort.
Bed, bath, food, drink. To enjoy the simple and
immediate.

Acknowledge one's disabilities—then try to forget them.
EILEEN M. HAM (1920-2001)

"I feel like my brain is full of tiny drawers, and this
little man is running around opening drawers trying
to find the thing that I'm trying to remember."

"Everybody's in a hurry these days, except old folks."

"Getting old sounds like an accomplishment. But it's
not, because the last few years all you do is sit
around."

"I'm not like I used to be, but then again, who is?"
Quotes from GRACE HEDDESHEIMER
(1911-2009) on aging

Contributors

Omair Abbasi, MD
House Officer
Psychiatry Residency Program
Creighton University–University of Nebraska
  Medical Center
Omaha, Nebraska

Cathy A. Alessi, MD
Director
Geriatric Research, Education, and Clinical Center
  (GRECC)
Chief, Division of Geriatrics
Veterans Administration
Greater Los Angeles Healthcare System
Professor, David Geffen School of Medicine at UCLA
Los Angeles, California

Neil B. Alexander, MD
Mobility Research Center
Division of Geriatric and Palliative Medicine
Department of Internal Medicine
Institute of Gerontology
University of Michigan
Health Care System
Geriatric Research Education and Clinical Center
Ann Arbor, Michigan

Priyal Amin, DO
Clinical Instructor
Immunology, Allergy, and Rheumatology
Department of Internal Medicine
University of Cincinnati
Cincinnati, Ohio

Lodovico Balducci, MD
Professor of Oncology and Medicine
University of South Florida College of Medicine
Program Leader
Senior Adult Oncology Program
H. Lee Moffitt Cancer Center and Research Institute
Tampa, Florida

Judith L. Beizer, PharmD, CGP
Clinical Professor
Clinical Pharmacy Practice Department
St. John's University College of Pharmacy and Health
  Sciences
Queens, New York

Christopher R. Bernheisel, MD
Assistant Professor of Family Medicine
The University of Cincinnati
Program Director
The Christ Hospital/University of Cincinnati
Family Medicine Residency Program
Director of Inpatient Family Medicine
Cincinnati, Ohio

Malaz A. Boustani, MD, MPH
Chief Operating Officer
Indiana University Center for Innovative
  and Implementation Science
Department of Medicine
Indiana University School of Medicine
Indianapolis, Indiana

Susana M. Bowling, MD
Director, Vascular Neurology
Summa Health System
Akron, Ohio

Suzanne F. Bradley, MD
Professor of Internal Medicine
University of Michigan Medical School
Physician Scientist, Geriatric Research Education
  and Clinical Center
Program Director, Infection Control
Veterans Affairs Ann Arbor Healthcare System
Ann Arbor, Michigan

Kenneth Brummel-Smith, MD
Charlotte Edwards Maguire Professor and Chair
Department of Geriatrics
Florida State University College of Medicine
Tallahassee, Florida

Gwendolen T. Buhr, MD, MHS, MEd, CMD
Assistant Professor
Department of Medicine
Geriatrics Division
Duke University
Durham, North Carolina

William J. Burke, MD
Anna O. Stake Professor of Psychiatry
Vice-Chair for Research
Department of Psychiatry
University of Nebraska Medical Center
Omaha, Nebraska

Julie P. W. Bynum, MD, MPH
Associate Professor
The Dartmouth Institute for Health Policy
    and Clinical Practice (TDI)
The Department of Medicine
Geisel School of Medicine at Dartmouth
Lebanon, New Hampshire

James W. Campbell, MD, MS, AGSF
Professor of Family Medicine
Case School of Medicine
Center Director, Geriatrics
The Metro Health System
Cleveland, Ohio

Elizabeth Herskovits Castillo, MD, PhD
Assistant Clinical Professor
Department of Family Medicine
The University of North Carolina at Chapel Hill
Chapel Hill, North Carolina
Medical Director
Asheville Buncombe Institute Parity of Achievement
Asheville, North Carolina

Melissa Christensen, PA-C
Sanford Health Systems
Fargo, North Dakota

Heather B. Congdon, PharmD, BCPS, CDE
Assistant Dean
The Universities at Shady Grove
Rockville, Maryland

Debra A. Danforth, MS, ARNP, FAANP
Associate Professor
Director of The Charlotte E. Maguire and Tallahassee
    Memorial Healthcare Clinical Learning Center
Florida State University College of Medicine
Tallahassee, Florida

Della Dillard, MD, MBA
Assistant Professor
D. W. Reynolds Department of Geriatric Medicine
University of Oklahoma College of Medicine
Oklahoma City, Oklahoma

Catherine E. DuBeau, MD
Professor of Medicine
University of Massachusetts Medical School
Worcester, Massachusetts

Justin O. Endo, MD
Department of Dermatology
University of Wisconsin—Madison
Madison, Wisconsin

Jerome J. Epplin, MD
Clinical Professor
Family Medicine
Southern Illinois University School of Medicine
Springfield, Illinois
Litchfield Family Practice Center
Litchfield, Illinois

Michael P. Feloney, MD
Assistant Professor
Department of Surgery, Urologic Surgery
University of Nebraska Medical Center
Omaha, Nebraska

Ellen Flaherty, PhD, APRN, AGSF
Dartmouth Center for Health and Aging
Geisel School of Medicine at Dartmouth
Department of Primary Care-Geriatrics
Dartmouth-Hitchcock Medical Center
Lebanon, New Hampshire

Craig B. Fowler, DDS
Division of Oral and Maxillofacial Pathology
University of Kentucky College of Dentistry
Lexington, Kentucky

Nisha Gajendra, MD
Resident
SIU Center for Family Medicine
Springfield, Illinois

Aimée D. Garcia, MD, CWS, FACCWS
Associate Professor
Department of Medicine
Section of Geriatrics
Baylor College of Medicine
Michael E. DeBakey VA Medical Center
Houston, Texas

Nathan E. Goldstein, MD
Hertzberg Palliative Care Institute and
    the Brookdale Department of Geriatrics and Adult
    Development
The Mount Sinai School of Medicine
New York, New York
The Bronx–New York Harbor Geriatric Research,
    Education, and Clinical Center
Bronx, New York

Lisa J. Granville, MD, AGSF, FACP
Professor and Associate Chair
Department of Geriatrics
Florida State University College of Medicine.
Tallahassee, Florida

Richard J. Ham, MD
Director, WVU Center on Aging
Professor of Geriatric Medicine and Psychiatry
Professor, Blanchette Rockefeller Neurosciences Institute
Robert C. Byrd Health Sciences Center
West Virginia University
Morgantown, West Virginia

Elizabeth N. Harlow, MD
Assistant Professor
Division of Geriatrics
Home Instead Center for Successful Aging
Department of Internal Medicine
University of Nebraska Medical Center
Omaha, Nebraska

Jennifer Hayashi, MD
Director, Elder House Call Program
Division of Geriatric Medicine and Gerontology
Johns Hopkins University School of Medicine
Baltimore, Maryland

Arthur E. Helfand, DPM
Professor Emeritus
Retired Chair, Department of Community Health,
    Aging, and Health Policy
Temple University School of Podiatric Medicine
Consultant, Temple University Institute on
    Aging—School of Medicine
Treasurer and Past Chair, Board of Directors
Philadelphia Corporation for Aging
Honorary Staff, Temple University Hospital
Honorary Staff, Thomas Jefferson University Hospital
Past President, American Podiatric Medical Association
Philadelphia, Pennsylvania

Margaret Helton, MD
Professor, Family Medicine
University of North Carolina at Chapel Hill
Chapel Hill, North Carolina

Masaya Higuchi, MD
Director of Geriatric Medicine
SIU Center for Family Medicine
Springfield, Illinois
Assistant Professor
Southern Illinois University School of Medicine
Springfield, Illinois

Teresita M. Hogan MD, FACEP
Director, Geriatric Emergency Medicine
University of Chicago
Chicago, Illinois

Peter A. Hollmann, MD
Associate Chief Medical Officer
Blue Cross and Blue Shield of Rhode Island
Providence, Rhode Island

Gregory J. Hughes, PharmD, BCPS, CGP
Assistant Clinical Professor
Clinical Pharmacy Practice Department
St. John's University College of Pharmacy and Health
    Sciences
Queens, New York

Matthew S. Jacobs, MA, RD, LD, NSCA-CPT
Clinical Dietitian
Oklahoma City VA Medical Center
Oklahoma City, Oklahoma

Jason M. Johanning, MD, FACS
Professor
Department of Surgery
Division of General Surgery—Vascular Surgery
University of Nebraska Medical Center
Omaha, Nebraska

Karin Johnson, DO, OD
Jack C. Montgomery VA Medical Center
Muskogee, Oklahoma

Daniel I. Kaufer, MD
Associate Professor and Director
Memory Disorders Program
Department of Neurology
University of North Carolina at Chapel Hill
Chapel Hill, North Carolina

Babar A. Khan, MD, MS
Assistant Professor of Medicine
Indiana University School of Medicine
Center Scientist
Indiana University Center for Aging Research
Research Scientist
Regenstrief Institute, Inc.
Indianapolis, Indiana

Christine Khandelwal, DO
Palliative Care and Hospice Physician
Department of Palliative Care
Hospice of Wake County
Raleigh, North Carolina

Bruce Leff, MD
Professor of Medicine
Division of Geriatric Medicine
Johns Hopkins University School of Medicine
Baltimore, Maryland

Timothy J. Lewis, MD
Medical Director
Geriatric Medicine Inpatient Consult Service
Medical Director
Acute Care for Elders Unit
Division of Post Acute and Senior Services
Summa Health System
Akron, Ohio

Robert J. Luchi, MD
Professor of Medicine
Chief, Geriatric Section
Director, Huffington Center on Aging
Baylor College of Medicine
Associate Chief of Staff for Geriatrics
    and Extended Care
Houston VA Medical Center
Houston, Texas

William L. Lyons, MD
Associate Professor
Division of Geriatrics
Home Instead Center for Successful Aging
Department of Internal Medicine
University of Nebraska Medical Center
Omaha, Nebraska

Alayne D. Markland, DO, MSc
Associate Professor
University of Alabama at Birmingham
Department of Medicine
Division of Gerontology, Geriatrics, and Palliative Care
Department of Veterans Affairs
Birmingham/Atlanta Geriatric Research, Education,
    and Clinical Center
Birmingham VA Medical Center
Birmingham, Alabama

Jennifer L. Martin, PhD
Adjunct Associate Professor/Research Health Scientist
Department of Medicine/Geriatric Research,
    Education, and Clinical Center
University of California Los Angeles
VA Greater Los Angeles Healthcare System
North Hills, California

Migy K. Mathew, MD
Clinical Assistant Professor of Geriatric Medicine
D. W. Reynolds Department of Geriatric Medicine
Associate Professor of Family Medicine
Department of Family Medicine
University of Oklahoma Health Sciences Center
Oklahoma City, Oklahoma
Staff Physician—Ambulatory Care Department
Oklahoma City VA Medical Center
Oklahoma City, Oklahoma

Craig S. Miller, DMD, MS
Division of Oral Medicine
University of Kentucky College of Dentistry
Lexington, Kentucky

John E. Morley, MD
Professor of Internal Medicine
Division Director, Endocrinology
Saint Louis University School of Medicine
St. Louis, Missouri

R. Sean Morrison, MD
Professor
Department of Geriatrics and Adult Development
    and Department of Medicine
The Mount Sinai School of Medicine
New York, New York

Laura Mosqueda, MD
Associate Dean of Primary Care
School of Medicine
University of California—Irvine
Orange, California

Hillary R. Mount, MD
Assistant Professor of Family Medicine
The University of Cincinnati
The Christ Hospital/University of Cincinnati
Family Medicine Residency Program
Cincinnati, Ohio

Nadia Mujahid, MD
Assistant Professor of Medicine
Warren Alpert Medical School of Brown University
Providence, Rhode Island

Thomas Mulligan, MD
Medical Director, Senior Services
St. Bernards Healthcare
Jonesboro, Arkansas

Jean C. Munn, PhD, MSW
John A. Hartford Faculty Scholar
Associate Professor
College of Social Work
Florida State University
Tallahassee, Florida

Soumya Nadella, MD
Geriatric Medicine Fellow
The Christ Hospital/University of Cincinnati
Cincinnati, Ohio

Yuri Nakasato MD, MBA
Sanford Health Systems
Fargo, North Dakota
Associate Clinical Professor
University of North Dakota Medical School
Grand Forks, North Dakota

Aman Nanda, MD, AGSF, CMD
Associate Professor of Medicine
Department of Medicine
Warren Alpert Medical School of Brown University
Division of Geriatrics
Rhode Island Hospital
Providence, Rhode Island

Konrad C. Nau, MD
Associate Vice President HSC
Dean, Eastern Division
Department of Family Medicine—Eastern Division
West Virginia University
Martinsburg, West Virginia

Heidi D. Nelson, MD, MPH
Department of Medical Informatics and Clinical
    Epidemiology and Medicine
Oregon Health and Science University
Providence Health Services
Portland, Oregon

Robert A. Norman, DO, MPH
Dr. Robert A. Norman and Associates
Tampa, Florida

Neil J. Nusbaum, JD, MD
Chief of Staff
VA Central Western Massachusetts Healthcare System
Associate Dean of Veterans Affairs
University of Massachusetts Medical School
Worcester, Massachusetts

Jerry L. Old, MD
Associate Professor and Geriatrics Clerkship Director
Department of Family and Community Medicine
Kansas University School of Medicine—Wichita
Wichita, Kansas

Alice K. Pomidor, MD, MPH
Professor, Department of Geriatrics
Florida State University College of Medicine
Tallahassee, Florida

Jane F. Potter, MD
Harris Professor of Geriatric Medicine
Chief, Division of Geriatrics and Gerontology
Department of Internal Medicine
University of Nebraska Medical Center
Home Instead Center for Successful Aging
Omaha, Nebraska

Imaad Razzaque, MD
Housestaff Resident
Graduate Medical Education
Saint Louis University
St. Louis, Missouri

Stephen W. Record, OD
Director, Low Vision Clinic
University of Virginia
Health Sciences Center
Charlottesville, Virginia

Barbara Resnick, PhD, CRNP, FAAN, FAANP
Professor
Sonya Ziporkin Gershowitz Chair in Gerontology
School of Nursing
University of Maryland
Baltimore, Maryland

Tonatiuh Rios-Alba, MD
Section of Emergency Medicine
University of Chicago
Chicago, Illinois

Jeffrey M. Robbins, DPM
Director, Podiatry Service
Department of Veterans Affairs Central Office
Professor of Podiatric Medicine
Ohio College of Podiatric Medicine
Clinical Assistant Professor
Department of Surgery
Independence, Ohio

Miriam B. Rodin, MD, PhD
Associate Professor of Medicine
Saint Louis University School of Medicine
St. Louis, Missouri

Laurence Z. Rubenstein, MD, MPH
D. W. Reynolds Professor and Chair
D. W. Reynolds Department of Geriatric Medicine
University of Oklahoma College of Medicine
Oklahoma City, Oklahoma

Marcia M. Russell, MD, PhD
Assistant Professor, Surgery
David Geffen School of Medicine at UCLA
Los Angeles, California

Jeffrey D. Schlaudecker, MD
Associate Professor of Family Medicine
University of Cincinnati
Program Director
Geriatric Medicine Fellowship Program
Assistant Director of Inpatient Family Medicine
The Christ Hospital/University of Cincinnati
Family Medicine Residency Program
Cincinnati, Ohio

Lorraine S. Sease, MD, MSPH
Assistant Professor
Department of Community and Family Medicine
Duke University
Durham, North Carolina

Sonia R. Sehgal, MD
Associate Clinical Professor, Geriatrics
Department of Medicine
University of California—Irvine
Irvine, California

Philip D. Sloane, MD, MPH
Elizabeth and Oscar Goodwin Distinguished Professor
Department of Family Medicine
Co-Director, Program on Aging, Disability,
    and Long-Term Care
Cecil G. Sheps Center for Health Services Research
University of North Carolina at Chapel Hill
Chapel Hill, North Carolina

Andrew M. Smith, MD, MS
Assistant Professor of Immunology
University of Cincinnati College of Medicine
Division of Immunology, Allergy and Rheumatology
Cincinnati VA Medical Center
Cincinnati, Ohio

Monica Stallworth-Kolinas, MD
Chief Medical Officer and Chief of Staff
Western Maryland Hospital Center
Washington, District of Columbia

Pamela Sparks Stein, DMD, MPH
Division of Dental Public Health
University of Kentucky College of Dentistry
Lexington, Kentucky

Niharika Suchak, MD, FACP
Department of Geriatrics
Florida State University College of Medicine
Tallahassee, Florida

George E. Taffet, MD
Associate Professor of Medicine
Department of Geriatrics
Baylor College of Medicine
Houston, Texas

James A. Wallace, MD
Clinical Associate of Medicine
The University of Chicago
Chicago, Illinois

Gregg A. Warshaw, MD
Martha Betty Semmons Professor of Geriatric
    Medicine
Professor of Family and Community Medicine
Director, Geriatric Medicine Program
University of Cincinnati College of Medicine
Cincinnati, Ohio

Janice Weinhardt, MSN, RN, GCNS-BC, ANVP
Stroke Coordinator
Summa Akron City Hospital
Akron, Ohio

Heidi K. White, MD, MHS, MEd, CMD
Associate Professor
Department of Medicine, Geriatrics Division
Duke University Medical Center
Durham, North Carolina

E. Foy White-Chu, MD, FAPWCA
Associate Geriatric Fellowship Director
Assistant Professor of Medicine
Department of Hospital and Specialty Medicine,
    Geriatrics
Portland Veterans Affairs Medical Center
Oregon Health and Science University
Portland, Oregon

Tanya M. Wildes, MD, MSCI
Assistant Professor of Medicine
Division of Medical Oncology
Washington University School of Medicine
St. Louis, Missouri

Doug Woolley, MD, MPH
Delos V. Smith, Jr., Professor of Community
    Geriatrics
Vice Chair for Research
Department of Family and Community Medicine
Kansas University School of Medicine—Wichita
Wichita, Kansas

Robert A. Zorowitz, MD, MBA, FACP, AGSF
Medical Director
Evercare New York/OptumHealth
New York, New York

I am excited to be writing, in 2013, the Preface to the *sixth* edition of *Primary Care Geriatrics: A Case-Based Approach*—a book that was first published 30 years ago as a pioneering, case-based textbook on geriatric medicine, which at that time was neither thought of nor defined as a medical specialty.

It was conceived from the outset as a case-based book, developed from a project of the American Geriatrics Society (AGS), with an advisory group chaired by the late Isadore Rossman. The first edition aimed to appeal to and inform any clinician tackling the problems of complex elderly patients and needing pragmatic help in categorizing the chaotic and ambiguous presentations of such patients in a primary care setting in order to produce satisfactory outcomes.

I am pleased and proud that our editors and contributors for this edition have maintained the freshness, style, breadth of scope, expertise, and, perhaps most important, enjoyability of previous editions. We know that our book has been appreciated and has a loyal following, perhaps because every clinician likes a "good" case, and the book's text is driven by the progress of each case. It was after all in this way that we learned the art and science of medicine when we were young apprentices.

Some examples of the types of cases discussed in this edition include patients with the following conditions:

- multiple concurrent problems
- a clinically silent impending medical emergency
- inability to communicate problems or symptoms
- a rich lifetime of social and medical history
- requirement for a surrogate or advocate (often not a family member)
- family or patient in denial about early dementia or imminence of death

This book—although originally designed with the primary care physician (PCP) in mind, and always starting from a primary care site in the community (e.g., office, patient's home, nursing home, urgent care)—is very suitable for the use of any health professional who wishes to learn more about care of the elderly patient. All clinicians with adult patients—even those with focused specialties—see elderly patients, often regularly, and need to be able to "cover" issues that a good general physician would (especially one who has absorbed the essentials of this book!), making sure that some serious problem (e.g., early dementia, possible sleep apnea) observed while the patient is under his or her watch is suitably referred

for diagnosis and management, including informing a family member in many instances.

This sixth edition also includes other updates:

- The following subjects are now covered in separate chapters: Emergency Care, Persistent Pain, Frailty, Arthritis and Related Disorders, Anemia, and Billing and Coding.
- The chapter questions and all the references for each chapter are now included on Expert Consult (see the inside cover for details on how to access this content online). In the book itself, each chapter cites all the references numerically, but only the Key References are listed. In many chapters Web Resources with Suggested Readings or Web guidelines are included just before the Key References. Additionally, a dermatology quiz and a chapter on dizziness are included exclusively on Expert Consult.
- Phil Sloane has coordinated and largely written the vital opening chapter, Principles of Primary Care of Older Adults, covering the range of the prior first three chapters.

An outline of the unchanged basic format of the book follows (this is mainly for new readers):

- Three "Units" are included: Principles and Practice, Geriatric Syndromes and Common Special Problems, and Selected Clinical Problems of the Organ Systems.
- Each clinical chapter (Chapters 10 and 15-53) has core text with the following subheadings to assist readers when using the text for reference: Prevalence and Impact, Risk Factors and Pathophysiology, Differential Diagnosis and Assessment, Management, and Summary.
- In virtually all chapters, cases and discussions of the case (both set in a font that differs from that used in the core text), generally in several numbered parts, are interspersed with the core text at appropriate points. Although the case and its discussion illustrate the text in all chapters and show the text "in action," the text itself does stand alone. With few exceptions, all the core information—as in a conventional textbook—is in the text itself.

I must heartily thank my friend Phil Sloane for his assistance with this book. Without his firm insistence that it would take the two of us to organize and edit a second edition, there would have been no subsequent volumes in this series of *Primary Care Geriatrics*; it has become a very durable book. He has worked with me on every subsequent edition. He is the single most important link in the long chain of authors, editors, and publishers who have worked to continue this book's success over these last 25 years.

Gregg Warshaw, a longtime friend and colleague, joined Phil and me as third co-editor for our third edition in 1997, and the three of us have now continued working together through four editions. For this book, he graciously agreed to lead this initiative and chair the editorial group and oversee the entire project; he has earned the gratitude of all of us for his efficient, considerate, firm, and effective leadership. Thanks, Gregg.

I would be remiss in not thanking our publishers who have not only once again produced a pleasing layout for our rather complicated format but also patiently endured waiting for some very late drafts from this physician, who wished to do clinical care for the remainder of his working life and ended up overcommitted but enjoying the life of a primary care geriatrician and "dementologist" (a word invented by Phil to describe the *really* challenging Lewy and Pick's patients I am following); however, it was regular ward attending in acute medicine (I learned a lot) that took me over the top.

It is a privilege to be a doctor —indeed any health care provider—a privilege won through years of education, training, and a lot of sleep deprivation. Particularly rewarding is the field of primary care geriatrics. Whether your patients are friends or a strangers, they are trusting you with their physical and mental health and, even more, their stories—the history of who they were as well as who they are now, which often are very different pictures.

I hope so much that using this book will help you on your journey of knowledge, empathy, and appreciation of the stories that the old will tell you, in their words, by their symptoms, and in their very faces, and that it will empower you to help our elders to a more dignified, pain-free, and serene last stage of their lives. I also hope that you, the PCP, will experience the joy and satisfaction of knowing that you are responsible for achieving the best outcome for a life entrusted to your care.

Richard J. Ham, MD

Acknowledgments

Without my friends and fellow editors who have worked so hard to make it a reality, this sixth edition would not have existed. My heartfelt thanks to Gregg, Phil, Jane, and Ellen. To everyone at Elsevier, especially Suzanne Toppy, Julia Rose Roberts, and Sharon Corell, for their patience, understanding, and skill, a huge "thank you." And to Joanna, for her wit and wisdom, imagination, and kindness

—*Richard Ham*

To my wife, Sheryl, with whom I hope to experience for many years that about which we together have studied and taught.

—*Philip Sloane*

I wish to acknowledge the wisdom shared with me by my patients and their families during 33 years of clinical practice. I would also like to thank my colleagues at the University of Cincinnati Medical Center for their dedication to educating the next generation of clinicians to care for older adults.

—*Gregg Warshaw*

Thanks to my co-editors who taught me the process, coached and mentored through uncertainties, and taught me new and different insights on care of the aged. Thanks also to my mother and good friend, Marie Weis Potter, who at 97 years of age helps to keep me focused on what is important in later life and the meaning of graceful aging.

—*Jane Potter*

In gratitude for the wisdom bestowed upon me from my patients, their families, and my colleagues over the past 30 years at NYU, Dartmouth, and throughout the world.

—*Ellen Flaherty*

A Note on Level of Evidence Ratings

Where A through D ratings are used, they correspond (as appropriate) to:

A, Evidence from well-designed meta-analysis, or well-done synthesis reports such as those for the Agency for Healthcare Policy and Research or the American Geriatrics Society; B, evidence from well-designed controlled trials, both randomized and non-randomized, with results that consistently support a specific action; C, evidence from observational studies or controlled trials with inconsistent results; D, evidence from expert opinion or multiple case reports.

A, Supported by one or more high-quality randomized clinical trials (RCTs) in an appropriate population, without contradictory evidence from other clinical trials; B, supported by one or more high-quality nonrandomized cohort studies or low-quality RCTs; C, supported by one or more case series and/or poor-quality cohort and/or case-control studies; D, supported by expert opinion and/or extrapolation from studies in other populations and/or settings; X, the preponderance of evidence supports the treatment being ineffective or harmful.

Contents

UNIT 3: Selected Clinical Problems of the Organ Systems

UNIT 1

Principles and Practice

An archeologist is the best husband any woman can have; the older she gets, the more interested he is in her.

AGATHA CHRISTIE, 1890-1976

You know, by the time you reach my age, you've made plenty of mistakes if you've lived your life properly.

RONALD REAGAN, 1911-2004, at 86, in *The Observer*, March 8, 1997

I haven't felt this well since I was 70!!

A 93-year-old patient (of RH), to her daughter, after she had inflicted extra fluids on her mother for 2 complaining weeks.

Oh, to be seventy again!

GEORGES CLEMENCEAU, French statesman, on seeing a pretty young girl on the Champs D'Elysee on his 80th birthday.

Being over seventy is like being engaged in a war. All our friends are going or gone and we survive among the dead and dying as on a battlefield.

DAME MURIEL SPARK, 1918-2006, in *Memento Mori*

It is as natural to die as to be born; and to a little infant, perhaps, the one is as painful as the other.

FRANCIS BACON, 1561-1626, in *Essays*, "Of Death"

It's not that I'm afraid to die. It's just that I don't want to be there when it happens…

WOODY ALLEN, b.1935, in *Without Feathers*, "Death (A Play)"

Old men are dangerous; it doesn't matter to them what is going to happen to the world.

GEORGE BERNARD SHAW, 1856-1950, in *Heartbreak House*

Optimistic lies have such immense therapeutic value that a doctor who cannot tell them convincingly has mistaken his profession.

GEORGE BERNARD SHAW, 1856-1950, in *Misalliance*, Preface

A medical revolution has extended the life of our elder citizens without providing the dignity and security those later years deserve.

JOHN F KENNEDY, 1917-1963, in his Democratic Party nomination acceptance speech, 1960

It is not by muscle, speed or physical dexterity that great things are achieved, but by reflection, force of character, and judgement; in these qualities, old age is not only not poorer, but is even richer.

CICERO, 106-43 BC, Roman statesman and orator, in *On Old Age, V1*

The key to a long friendship or marriage is a great sense of humour—and a weak memory!

JEH, married to RJH for 46 years

Old age is not a disease–it is strength and survivorship, triumph over all kinds of vicissitudes and disappointments, trials and illnesses.

MAGGIE KUHN, 1905-1995, U.S. activist, founder of the Grey Panthers

Now more than ever seems it rich to die,
To cease upon the midnight with no pain….

JOHN KEATS, 1795-1821, in *Ode to a Nightingale*

1

Principles of Primary Care of Older Adults

*Philip D. Sloane, Gregg A. Warshaw,
Jane F. Potter, Ellen Flaherty, and
Richard J. Ham*

OUTLINE

Additional online-only material indicated by icon.

OBJECTIVES

*Upon completion of this chapter, the reader
will be able to:*

- Describe and identify at least one clinical
  implication of each of the following key
  aspects of physiologic aging: the rule of
  fourths, normal physiologic changes,
  functional reserve, reduced stamina and
  fatigue, increased physiologic diversity,
  the relationship between environment and
  function, and immobility in older persons.

- Describe and identify at least one clinical
  implication of each of the following key
  aspects of psychological aging: looking old
  but not feeling or thinking old, ageism,
  life review and adjustment to changes,
  the activity and disengagement theories
  of healthy aging, cognitive impairment,
  and the importance of relationships in
  older age.

- Describe and identify at least one clinical
  implication of each of the following key
  aspects of health care provision involving
  older persons: multiple morbidity, function-
  oriented care, icebergs in geriatric assessment, iatrogenic disease, slow medicine,
  polypharmacy, the U.S. health care system,
  transitions in care, interprofessional care,
  and the value of a generalist in primary
  care geriatrics.

When is a person old? Most people would say 65 years—the age adopted by Germany under landmark legislation introduced by Otto von Bismark in the 1880s. With the passage of the U.S. Social Security Act in 1935, retirement at 65 became national policy and hence the reason why 65 is commonly regarded as the beginning of old age. Ironically, Germany had initially adopted 70 as the retirement age, lowering it to 65 in 1916. Now, with increases in life expectancy, many countries are making efforts to raise the retirement age, and we may eventually come full circle.

Of course, the question of how to define *old* often depends on the age of the person you ask. A recent poll of 1000 adults aged 50 and older found that the majority thought middle age began at 55 and older age at 70.[1] In ironic contrast is the fact that some of these same individuals had earlier in their lives subscribed to the catch phrase "never trust anyone over 30" that was popular among youth in the 1960s.

In fact, for many persons throughout life, *old* is defined as "somewhat older than I am." Indeed, the feeling that "I'm not old yet" can persist long beyond age 65, as many older adults equate "old age" with disability.

Still, over time a variety of changes creep into one's body, one's mind, and one's social circumstances, such that people who are older are different from young adults in many ways. These changes affect health risks, health behavior, and health care decisions. Therefore health professionals who care for older persons need to understand how older persons differ from younger adults. This chapter provides an overview of the most important principles, drawing from the authors' more than 150 years of combined experience in clinical care of aging persons. We begin with physiologic principles, then discuss some psychological factors, and then talk about aging and the health care system.

AGING AND THE BODY

Aging brings about physical and physiologic changes, some of which are universal, and many more of which are unique to the individual person. This section highlights some of the key principles of physiologic aging that have therapeutic implications.

The Rule of Fourths

"Is this a normal part of aging?" Clinicians are asked to answer this question thousands of times a day about a new symptom or sign in an older patient. Perhaps the presenting complaint is a problem with memory, possibly an accidental fall. Maybe it is a sore joint, declining vision, or falling asleep during the day.

In the past, medical providers were much more likely to write off symptoms such as these as normal (Box 1-1). In fact, research during recent decades has taught us that much of the disability that we used to attribute to "normal aging" is not normal at all.

The way we now think about changes in aging is the *rule of fourths* (Figure 1-1). This rule states that, of changes often attributed to normal aging by the general public (and in past decades by the medical profession), about one fourth is due to disease, one fourth to disuse, one fourth to misuse, and only about one fourth to physiologic aging.

THE RULE OF FOURTHS

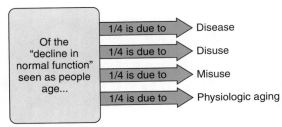

Figure 1-1 The rule of fourths. In the past, all of the decline in function that occurs between young adulthood and old age was called normal aging. We now know that approximately one fourth can be attributed to disease, one fourth to disuse (e.g., sedentary lifestyle, lack of mental stimulation), and one fourth to misuse (e.g., smoking, injuries from contact sports, and adverse effects of prescription and/or recreational drugs). Only about one fourth can be attributed to physiologic aging.

Disease-related disability, for example, could manifest as decreased exercise tolerance in a chronic smoker; *disuse-related disability* as shortness of breath on minimal exertion in a largely sedentary older person; *misuse-related disability* as knee arthritis in a former football player; and *disability related to physiologic aging* as trouble reading fine print in a 50-year-old.

The job of health care providers is to determine whether and to what extent a new symptom is caused by each of these etiologic categories and then develop a treatment plan.

- If the problem is disease, then medical treatment is indicated.
- If the problem is disuse, it can often be cured with an activity regimen.
- If the problem is misuse, prior damage cannot be reversed but steps can be taken to prevent deterioration and to preserve function.
- If the problem is physiologic aging, then steps should be taken to adapt and compensate for the disability.

Normal Physiologic Changes

Whereas much of the change seen with aging results from causes other than physiologic aging, some changes are inevitable. Table 1-1 lists and describes many common physiologic changes noted with aging. Among the many notable changes are the following:

- The age at which reading glasses are needed because of reduced lens elasticity is between 42 and 50.
- Vestibular sensitivity gradually increases until about age 60, which is one of the reasons why adults have increasing trouble on amusement park rides as they age.

BOX 1-1

A POPULAR JOKE ILLUSTRATING WHY DISABILITY IN OLDER AGE CAN RARELY BE ATTRIBUTED TO AGE

Patient: My right knee hurts. What's wrong, doc?
Doctor: You've been using that joint for 86 years; you've got to expect a little arthritis.
Patient: Yeah, but my left knee's 86 years old too, and it doesn't hurt.

TABLE 1-1	Some Common Anatomic and Physiologic Changes with Aging (in the Absence of Identified Disease)
System or Function Affected	**Change Noted**
Body composition:	
Percent body water	Decreased
Percent body fat	Increased
Brain:	
Weight	Decreases by 7%
Anatomy	"Atrophy" commonly noted
Sleep patterns	Markedly reduced stage 3 and 4 sleep
	More frequent awakenings; reduced sleep efficiency
Vision:	
Lens accommodation	Markedly reduced after age 40-50
Amount of light reaching the retina	Diminished by up to 70%
Color perception	Reduced intensity (especially of blues and greens)
Hearing	Acuity declines beginning about age 12, with decline steepest in high pitches (>5000 Hertz [cycles/second])
Taste:	
Number of taste buds	Reduced by 70%
Changes in preferences	Increased tolerance for very sweet and very salty foods (as a result of reduced perception)
Cardiac function:	
Maximum heart rate	Reduced from about 195 to about 155 beats/min
Renal perfusion	Decreased by 50%
Bone mineral content	Diminished by 10%-30%
Prostate gland anatomy	Size increases by 100%
Sexual function:	
Men	Reduced intensity and persistence of erections; decreased ejaculate and ejaculatory flow
Women	Menopause; reduced lubrication; vaginal atrophy

Adapted from Sloane PD. Normal aging. In: Ham RJ, Sloane PD, Warshaw GA, editors. *Primary care geriatrics: A case-based approach.* 4th ed. St. Louis: Mosby-Yearbook; 2002, p. 15-28.

- Fertility in women peaks between 15 and 25 and declines thereafter, with menopause typically occurring about age 50.
- Reaction time tends to increase with age (which explains why teenagers are usually far better at games of speed—including many video games—than older persons).
- The amount of sway a person will experience if asked to stand still with his or her eyes closed is high in early childhood, is minimized between about ages 15 and 16, and then gradually increases beyond age 60.
- Ankle jerk reflexes are increasingly diminished or absent with older age, in the absence of detectable musculoskeletal pathology.
- Bone density plateaus between ages 20 and 50, then gradually declines, with the slope of decline being more rapid in women than in men.

The list of physiologic changes with age is long, and the clinical implications vary from merely interesting to very important. Also, the line between "normal physiology" and changes caused by other factors is frequently blurry.

What is important for the clinician to recognize is that aging does result in real, profound changes. Many of these changes cannot be reversed, and the older person will need to make adjustments. An important role of primary care clinicians is therefore to help provide access to the variety of mechanisms that can help compensate for bodily change and preserve function. In addition, the clinician may need to help the patient successfully make changes in goals and lifestyle that will help him or her successfully adjust to aging.

Functional Reserve

All body systems tend to have functional ability over and above what is used during everyday activities; this is called functional reserve. For example, the average adult's cardiac output is around 5 L/min when sedentary, whereas the heart of a trained athlete is capable of generating 40 to 50 L/min.[2] All other key body systems, such as the kidney, the lungs, the liver, and the brain, have reserve capabilities as well, so significant impairment from disease, disuse, misuse, or physiologic aging is needed to result in impaired function during normal activity.

Clinically significant impairment in function occurs when demands exceed functional reserve. As people age, patterns of disease, disuse, misuse, and physiologic aging combine to decrease functional reserve. Among the losses in functional reserve that have particularly common implications in geriatric care are the following clinical situations:

- Delirium is common in postoperative older persons, because brain functional reserve capacity is overwhelmed by the stress of the surgery and the persistence of anesthetic agents in the central nervous system and the bloodstream.
- Nocturia is almost ubiquitous in older persons, largely because of changes in bladder physiology (decreased capacity and increased residual volume) combined with altered control of fluid excretion (related to low nighttime antidiuretic hormone levels and increased nighttime natriuretic polypeptide levels).
- An older person will often fall when a younger person would not, because neuromuscular mechanisms to reestablish equilibrium from a minor perturbation (e.g., tripping on the edge of a rug) are impaired, often by a combination of disuse and normal aging changes in nerve conduction and vibratory sensation in the feet.

When functional reserve is impaired, the clinician should work with the patient to explore ways to improve this capacity and thereby to improve function. For a patient with chronic obstructive pulmonary disease, for example, solutions include continuous low-flow oxygen and pulmonary rehabilitation exercises. For a patient with impaired brain reserve, minimizing sedating and anticholinergic medications is often the best approach.

Reduced Stamina and Fatigue

One of the inexorable physiologic declines with aging is reduced stamina. An insidious reduction in stamina occurs, beginning in one's 20s and terminating in advanced age (Figure 1-2). Of course, this gradual decline in stamina and fatigue can be accelerated by disease, disuse, and misuse; however, gradual decrease in stamina and need for more frequent rest is a universal phenomenon as one ages. This is why medical interns in their 20s can pull an all-night shift much more easily than they would be able to if asked to follow the same schedule when in their 50s.

When reduced stamina and fatigue are so great that they become the defining feature of one's physiologic status, we refer to this as *frailty*. A commonly accepted, evidence-based definition of frailty is that of Fried et al.; it defines *frailty* as the occurrence of three or more of the following: unintentional weight loss (10 lbs in past year), self-reported exhaustion, weakness (reduced grip strength), slow walking speed, and low physical activity.[3] One can see that all but the first of these criteria are manifestations of reduced stamina

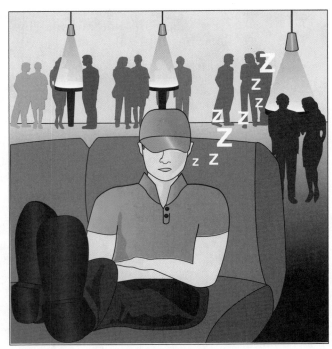

Figure 1-2 Inability to party all night is one of the earliest signs of aging. With increasing age and disability, diminished stamina can progress to the point where the older person no longer has enough energy to complete the necessary activities of daily living. This severe fatigue is the cardinal symptom of the frailty syndrome.

and fatigue. Frailty is a common and important geriatric syndrome (see Chapter 29).

Increased Physiologic Diversity

Another characteristic of aging is that, with advancing age, physiologic diversity increases. Indeed, the range of "normal" (i.e., the range that encompasses the performance of 95% of people) becomes increasingly wide as populations age. When we say, for example, "Jason is a normal 5-year-old," we have a pretty good idea what Jason can and cannot do. The same is true at age 20. However, with each advancing decade the range of normality becomes wider (Figure 1-3), to the point that saying, "George is a normal 75-year-old," tells you practically nothing about George other than how long ago he was born.

This increased diversity with age has many clinical implications. For example, it is easy to develop age-related guidelines for children, because, except in rare cases of chronic or developmental illness, age predicts performance in children. In older adults, however, age is not very helpful in determining health care norms or needs. In geriatrics, however, age-related protocols and guidelines are virtually nonexistent, and the clinician must individualize most aspects of assessment, goal setting, and care planning.

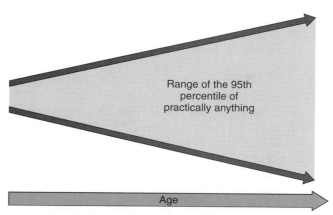

Figure 1-3 As people age they become more diverse. This explains why individualized care rather than protocol-based care is especially important in the geriatric population.

> Because of increasing diversity with age, protocols and guidelines are less useful in geriatric care than for younger ages, and instead care must be individualized.

Environment and Function

An often unappreciated aspect of aging is the importance of the environment in which an older person is asked to live and function. Indeed, the environment within which one lives and functions can make the difference between being independent and being unable to carry out basic everyday activities.

In health care it is useful to think about three distinctive types of environments: the physical environment, the social environment, and the organizational environment.[4] The physical environment refers to the physical setting in which a patient lives; it includes such things as size and decor of spaces, lighting, temperature, acoustic properties, and access to outdoors. The social (caregiving) environment refers to the people who interact directly with the patient—how they approach the person and what they do. The organizational environment refers to rules and regulations that affect a patient's life, such as when they can eat, whether and how they can go outdoors, and what type and amount of services they receive. Needless to say, these environmental characteristics can have a huge impact not only on function but on quality of life for a dependent older person.

How living units are designed can greatly influence an older adult's independence. Fortunately, with the aging of the population has come increased interest in housing design features that make it easier for persons who have a variety of disabilities to function. For example:

- Doorknobs that are levers can markedly improve ease of door use for persons with arthritis.
- Widened doorways can permit entry for persons in wheelchairs.
- Motion sensors that turn on lighting can help prevent falls at night among cognitively or physically impaired older persons.

A movement to improve the usability of housing for seniors and persons with disabilities is called universal design. A simplification of universal design is visitable housing, which is a movement to have all housing units built in such a way that they can be visited by people with disabilities, which includes many older adults. Visitable housing includes these three basic features: at least one no-step entrance, doors and hallways that are wide enough to navigate through in a wheelchair or walker, and a bathroom on the first floor big enough to get into in a wheelchair and close the door.[5]

Immobility

A common case scenario: Grandma has an episode of dizziness, perhaps caused by a transient ischemic attack, and the daughter with whom she lives encourages her to go to bed. The family mobilizes to help her; a bedside commode is brought in, and she is encouraged to "relax and get better." Nearly a week goes by.

After a week the dizziness is gone, and grandma gets up to go to Sunday dinner. When she does, she feels light-headed and weak on her feet and stumbles. Her postural reflexes have been blunted by a week in bed, and her blood pressure drops when she stands up. "Don't hurt yourself," the daughter says. "We'll bring your dinner, and you can eat in bed."

Grandma never walks again.

This scenario happens all too frequently. Older persons need to move it or lose it, but well-meaning caregivers do too much for them and the result is permanent disability.

Numerous studies have verified that immobility is bad for older persons. Among younger adults, a week in bed in the hospital is like adding 10 years to your age. Among older persons extended immobility is often the end of ambulation.

Wheelchairs are part of the problem. They are useful for transportation, making it easier for disabled persons to get around, but they increase the risk for many medical complications and adverse events, which they share with overall sedentary existence. Among these complications are muscle atrophy, increased risk of constipation, increased risk of pressure sores, increased risk of urinary tract infections (caused in part by bladder outlet obstruction from constipation), decreased involvement in activities, and increased risk of radial nerve palsy.[6,7]

In summary, the physiologic changes of aging place older persons at a heightened risk for a permanent loss of function if they are kept in bed or in a wheelchair for as short a time as a week or two. So as soon as an older person can get up, he or she should be cajoled into getting up, and as long as an older person can be cajoled to walk, he or she should walk. For older persons, the well-known statement "Use it or lose it" could be extended to "Use it or lose everything."

AGING AND THE MIND

Psychological aspects of aging are often underappreciated by health professionals, especially younger persons who have little firsthand experience with the emotional aspects of aging. Yet identifying and addressing these factors is often the most important aspect of an encounter with an older person. This section introduces a few key neurologic and psychological issues that are common in geriatric medicine, many of which are discussed in greater detail in subsequent chapters.

Looking Old but Not Feeling or Thinking Old

It is common for older persons to say, "I don't feel old." In doing so, they are reflecting a very prevalent feeling among persons of "geriatric" age—that they have energy and interests that are not different from those of many younger adults.

In fact, the characteristics that health professionals most associate with older adults—aging, disease, and disability—are rarely foremost in the minds of older persons. Instead, they are more often concerned with personal finances, family problems, national politics, world events, issues in the community, the health of a pet, or other areas of personal interest. Furthermore, the common belief that older persons are interested only in themselves is just not true. Older persons are often among the most active and vocal supporters of such issues as environmental preservation, quality education, and help for disadvantaged persons.

For example, in a study of near-retirement physicians about their interest in volunteering during retirement, more than a third (37%) expressed interest in volunteering. However, working with older populations in assisted living, nursing homes, or hospice settings was not what fired them up—fewer than 4% expressed interest in this type of engagement. Instead, they tended to be interested in free clinics, disaster relief, international service, and medical teaching.[8]

Ageism

One reality that confronts older persons repeatedly is the ubiquity of ageism in society. *Ageism* can be defined as the systematic stereotyping of and discrimination against people because they are old. The reasons for societal ageism are numerous and have their origins in older persons as well as younger ones. Studies have verified that older persons often have negative attitudes toward people in their own age group, particularly if they have an aging-related condition or disability such as slow walking speed (or driving speed), impaired hearing, or cognitive impairment.[9] Ageism is not only pervasive, it can lower self-esteem, reduce opportunities, and lead to isolation, loneliness, and depression.

The following are a few of the many examples of how ageism manifests itself in society:

- Older persons who are out of work have greater difficulty reentering the workforce than younger persons, and opportunities for meaningful engagement in part-time work for older persons are limited in today's society.
- Popular ideas about beauty rarely extend to old age. *People* magazine, for example, ends its annual "Beauty at Any Age" pictorial at 59.
- Until recently older persons were rarely portrayed at all on television, and when they were it was typically as an object of pity or ridicule.

In medical practice ageism is also rampant. Although decisions to withhold care based on age have been increasingly challenged in recent years, rates of application of lifesaving interventions such as cardiovascular procedures and organ transplantation continue to decline with increasing age, and when resources are limited, youth is prioritized.[10] Ageism applies to physicians' opportunities as well. One highly ranked medical school, for example, has a policy that faculty cannot engage in direct patient care after age 65.

It is true that behind many ageist notions is more than a grain of truth. As people age, they do change, often insidiously losing capability to optimally perform. A surgeon described his experience with this process in an essay published in *JAMA, The Journal of the American Medical Association*, in 1983. At 67 he thought that he was performing as well as ever, but a couple of small lapses, both easily correctable without any adverse impact on patient care, got him to wondering. "I began to inspect the anesthesiologists' charts," he wrote. "I noticed that my operating times had moved from 50 to 60 minutes, and then over a period of one year to about 70 to 80 minutes—always for the same procedure." Because longer operating times are associated with increased risk of adverse outcomes, he decided that it was time for him to retire.[11]

> Ageism can lower self-esteem, reduce opportunities, and lead to isolation, loneliness, and depression.

Life Review and Adjustment to One's Changing Life Status

The story of the surgeon who decided to retire provides an excellent example of our next principle of aging as well—that the aging process involves active reflection on one's life (life review) and that the changing nature of one's physical state necessitates psychological adjustment. The surgeon we discussed in the previous section had to, as he put it, "kneel at the grave of memories," reflecting on what he had accomplished and what he wished he had accomplished. "All of a sudden you are in an unfamiliar, ill-defined world," he wrote.

Adjusting to losses is a key element of successful aging—loss of one's role as a worker through elective or forced retirement; diminished physical strength and stamina; reductions in vision and hearing; impaired or lost sexual capability; loss of a sense of physical attractiveness; death or disability of a spouse, of siblings, and/or of close friends; the sadness of saying good-bye to the home that houses memories of children; and the loss of vigorous independence. In addition, as one progresses through the decades, the horizon of one's future becomes increasingly limited; hopes and dreams become increasingly replaced by memories.

All this requires continual psychological adjustment, and a key part of this process is life review. This process of adjustment to one's changing life status is gradual; it begins in middle age, with the "midlife crisis" often representing initial awareness of the finiteness of life. During older age, key elements of successful psychological adjustment include developing a sense of satisfaction with one's accomplishments; enjoying the advantages that come with being older, such as time with grandchildren, a slower pace to life, and more ability to choose how one spends time; and developing a new sense of both serenity with and ability to enjoy each day as it comes. This process usually is successful and explains why happiness increases with age and persists throughout most of the geriatric years, only fading if and when chronic illness, disability, and pain take over.[12]

Activity versus Disengagement

In the 1950s and early 1960s, an intellectual battle raged among gerontologists as to which psychological approach to aging was healthier. In one corner were the proponents of the *disengagement theory,* who posited that letting go of the trappings of earlier life was the key to successful aging. The icon of this theory was an old man in a rocking chair on the front porch. In the other corner were advocates of the *activity theory,* who believed that staying active and engaged was the key to healthy aging. Their icons were people who

some referred to as representatives of *exceptional aging,* people like Pablo Casals, who in his 90s was still actively performing as a musician.

As the data came in, it became clear that activity and engagement are healthier for the majority of older persons than disengagement. That is, of course, provided the individual is realistic and makes the needed adjustments to losses and changing life circumstances discussed in the previous section.

Unfortunately, the retirement industry was founded based on the disengagement theory and has been slow to adjust. The developers of Sun City, Arizona—the prototypical retirement community on which thousands of others were subsequently modeled—hired gerontologists who were proponents of disengagement.[13] This led to creation of communities prohibiting adult residents younger than 55 (and children), focused on leisure activities such as golf and shuffleboard, and encouraged the attitude, "You've worked hard; you deserve to relax."

Attitudes are, however, beginning to change, but they still have a long way to go. To promote healthy engagement in late life, more work opportunities need to be created for seniors that are interesting, part-time, and flexible; more older persons need to be engaged as volunteers and entrepreneurs; and seniors need more opportunities to be integrated into the rest of society rather than ghettoized in age-segregated settings. Such developments will be useful to the nation as well, because they will reduce the number of people who are dependent on social welfare and increase national productivity.

Cognitive Impairment and Worry

Cognitive impairment is a central concern of health care providers and older persons. Indeed, dementia or worry about memory is the reason for nearly 50% of consultations to geriatric assessment clinics, and dementia is the most common reason for nursing home placement. Because the prevalence of dementia is strongly correlated with age, the increasing life expectancy of today and tomorrow's seniors means that increasingly more persons are likely to have dementia.

Worry about memory is ubiquitous among older persons. B.F. Skinner, in an address to the American Psychological Association when he was 78 years old, described some of his experiences:

Forgetting is a classical problem. It is most conspicuous in forgetting names because names have so little going for them by way of context. . . . When I have time—and I mean something on the order of half an hour—I can almost always recall a name. . . . But that will not work in introducing your wife to someone whose name you have forgotten. My wife and I use the following strategy:

if there is any conceivable chance that she could have met the person, I simply say to her, "of course, you remember . . .?" and she grasps the outstretched hand and says, "Yes, of course. How are you?" The acquaintance may not remember meeting my wife, but is not sure of his or her memory either.[14]

At the time that Dr. Skinner delivered his address, what he was describing would have been termed "benign senescent forgetfulness" and unequivocally distinguished from "dementia." Over the past couple of decades, however, the lines between normal and abnormal cognition have become increasingly blurred. For one thing, it has become clear that good social skills (as in Dr. Skinner's example) can cover up considerable cognitive impairment (Figure 1-4). More important, recent discoveries have made it clear that measurable reductions in neuronal anatomy and function occur years—often decades—before the onset of dementia. The terms *mild cognitive impairment* and *executive function impairment* have emerged as clinically important entities to define and screen for— the former primarily because it increases the risk of Alzheimer's disease; the latter, because it identifies persons at risk for poor decision making (including susceptibility to scams). As a result, the medical profession is increasingly concerned about early cognitive impairment, and perhaps as a result there is an increasing fear among the older population that they may be "starting to get Alzheimer's."

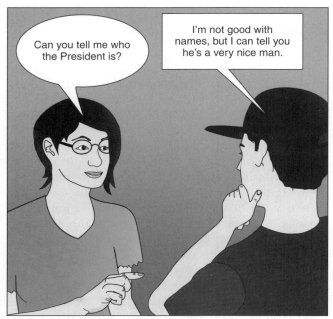

Figure 1-4 Good social skills can cover up a considerable amount of cognitive impairment, as in this example involving a patient with moderate dementia. Therefore formal screening and evaluation of cognitive status is a key element of geriatric practice.

The irony of all this is that enjoying life does not depend on being at one's peak of cognitive function. For example, planning, shopping for, cooking, and cleaning up after a gourmet meal takes a fairly high level of cognitive function and is considered fun by some people. But the majority of people would consider it even more fun to have the same meal prepared for them, eat it leisurely, and then relax with a cup of coffee or a glass of brandy while someone else cleans up—activities that require far less cognitive capability. The trick is for the living environment of a person with cognitive impairment to be structured in a way that maximizes opportunities to enjoy life, to use one's remaining abilities, and to not be stressed by demands that exceed capabilities.

Relationships and Family are Crucial to Health and Survival

Medical students are taught to obtain a family history of illness (e.g., Who had what? Who died of what?). However, in geriatric medicine a family history of illness is not useful, because whatever the patient was going to inherit he or she pretty most likely already has. Instead, the family history that matters is the relationship history (e.g., Who lives with the patient? Who provides support? Who should be consulted if a surrogate decision maker is needed? What are the dynamics within the family unit?). This information is critical because it can be a harsh world for people who are old and limited by disability, and they need help. Things they may need help with can include maintaining a household, managing medications, doing personal care activities such as bathing, navigating the health care system, and deciding what to do when new symptoms develop. Not surprisingly then, the availability of family and/or an established circle of friends has a tremendous impact on health outcomes and overall quality of life. Without such bonds, older persons are at high risk for isolation, depression, and institutionalization (Figure 1-5).

Approaching one's later years in an established long-term relationship (usually marriage), with the intimate knowledge and actual obligations such a relationship implies, provides a built-in caregiving dyad. Ideally each can help the other as problems develop, "in sickness and in health," thereby reducing the actual dangers and limitations of living alone. However, not everyone can be so blessed, and in most partnerships one dies or becomes disabled before the other, so couplehood is only a partial answer. If there is a younger generation, the loyalty of good family bonds can immeasurably enhance the security and quality of the life of an older person. Often it is a daughter or daughter-in-law who steps forward to fulfill this role, although men are increasingly caregivers as well. The caregiver role often subjects the caregiver

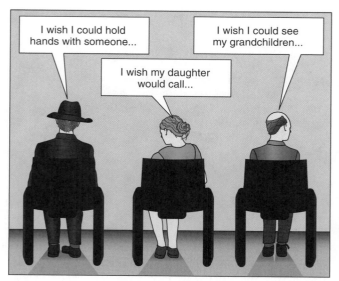

Figure 1-5 Loneliness is profound for many older persons, not just in long-term care (as pictured here) but for many living alone in community settings.

BOX 1-2

SOME OF THE WAYS IN WHICH FAMILY CAREGIVERS CAN ENHANCE HEALTH OF OLDER PERSONS

- Facilitate early diagnosis and treatment of new health problems.
- Ensure that the care recipient receives needed preventive measures (e.g., flu shots), nutrition, and hydration.
- Assist in the maintenance of mobility, balance, continence, and hygiene.
- Simplify ADLs (e.g., by laying out the right clothes for the day, or, if necessary, dressing the person).
- Initiate activities that many elders (because of poor executive function) cannot start but can complete.
- Manage finances or arrange for them to be managed.
- Enhance compliance with medications and all the other medical orders (e.g., physical therapy).
- Minimize behavioral symptoms through application of person-centered care principles.
- Implement stopping driving when the time comes ("You should give it up for now").
- Act as an advocate in hospitals and emergency rooms.
- Make it possible to remain in the familiar environment of "home" for as long as possible.

ADLs, Activities of daily living.

---

to stress and an increased likelihood of illnesses such as acute infections and depression. However, if done well, caregiving, which may continue for years, can be experienced as a profound responsibility that enhances life for both members of the dyad.

Box 1-2 lists some of the areas in which a well-informed, well-supported family caregiver can enhance the health and life of a care recipient. Here the primary care clinician can be invaluable by caring

directly or indirectly for the caregiver's own health and by assisting the caregiver in obtaining access to available resources. If properly educated, backed up by a knowledgeable and available primary care practice, and assisted if necessary in prudent use of the Internet, caregivers can make a world of difference to the life and outcomes of older persons.

DELIVERY OF PRIMARY HEALTH CARE TO OLDER PERSONS

Providing excellent primary care for older persons requires an in-depth knowledge of general clinical medicine. In addition, older persons practically never have one disease, so the approach needs to be functionally oriented and to take into account multiple morbidities. It requires the primary care provider to look for hidden functional problems; to be aware of the potential to interfere with homeostasis, causing unanticipated complications; to treat the patient in the context of his or her values and family; and to understand the many options and pitfalls in today's health care system.

Multiple Morbidity and the Geriatric Syndromes

One way that care of older persons tends to differ from that of younger persons is that multiple problems are the norm rather than the exception. Decline has typically occurred in multiple systems, leading to an insidious increase in the burden of dysfunction and disability with aging. When looked at in isolation the deficits may seem modest, but in aggregate the results can be devastating.

Take, for example, an 82-year-old woman named Hazel. She has developing cataracts, so her vision in one eye is 20/40 and in the other is 20/50. She had an episode of labyrinthitis 20 years ago, which left her with a clinically undetectable but measurable reduction in vestibular function. She has type 2 diabetes, which is well controlled, with a glycosylated hemoglobin (HbA$_{1c}$) of 6.8, but after 25 years of living with diabetes she now has proprioceptive deficits in both lower extremities. Taken individually, none of these sensory deficits would cause functional disability. However, together they make Hazel at very high risk for falls. Furthermore, she exercises little and is a bit overweight at 180 pounds and 5 foot 2 inches.

This accumulation of multisystem deficits is responsible for the existence of geriatric syndromes—problems that are typically multifactorial in etiology and that therefore are rare in younger persons and common in the elderly. Among the most important geriatric syndromes are falls, frailty, dizziness, gait problems, weakness, incontinence, and confusion (see Unit 2).

Function, Not Diagnosis, is What Counts

Another implication of the multiple morbidities in geriatric medicine is that the most important issue is what the patient can and cannot do, not what medical diagnoses the physician can identify. In geriatric medicine, the role of the primary care physician (PCP) should be to identify functional deficits that adversely affect the patient's prognosis and quality of life, to identify what the physician can do something about (i.e., where there is evidence supporting medical intervention), and to identify what cannot be improved with medical treatment but can be helped with rehabilitation, social support, and empathy.

Activities of daily living (ADLs) and instrumental activities of daily living (IADLs) are useful approaches to defining the function of geriatric patients. ADLs are tasks that people need to do every day, often multiple times each day, such as dressing, bathing, eating, changing position, and going to the toilet. People who are dependent in two or more ADLs generally will qualify for nursing home care; if they remain at home, they will require daily assistance to continue to live in the community. IADLs are tasks that are required to maintain a household but do not need to be done every day; examples include talking on the telephone, shopping, and making the bed. People who are dependent in two or more IADLs generally need someone to help them several times a week, and with adequate support these people will be able to continue to live in the community.

The best doctor is not the one who makes the most diagnoses, it's the one who identifies and addresses the patient's most important functional problems.

"Icebergs" are Common

Some key symptoms and functional impairments in older persons are often not reported during routine office visits. Sometimes this is because the older person thinks the problem is part of normal aging; this is especially true about musculoskeletal complaints such as bilateral weakness or joint pain. At other times it is because the older person is embarrassed to report the problem; this is especially true when the issue involves urinary or fecal incontinence, sexual problems, and depressive symptoms (particularly in men). Or the problem may be unreported because the older person is not aware that a problem exists; this is particularly common when the problem is dementia.

These frequently unreported symptoms are referred to as icebergs (Figure 1-6). For the primary care clinician to avoid missing important problems such as these, primary care office visits must be organized to conduct systematic case-finding for common unreported symptoms in older adults. Symptom checklists

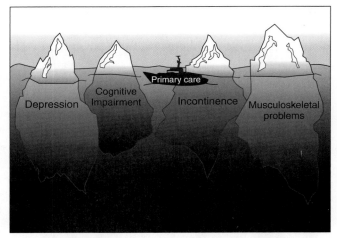

Figure 1-6 Icebergs in geriatric medicine. Some symptoms in geriatrics are commonly undetected by physicians because the older person either thinks the problem is a normal part of aging or is embarrassed to talk about it. Prominent "icebergs" include depression, cognitive impairment, incontinence, and musculoskeletal problems.

help some. In addition, specific screening for cognitive function, depressive symptoms, and physical function (e.g., falls risk) should be routine for all persons older than age 75.

Iatrogenic Disease

Illness caused by medical interventions, known as iatrogenic illness, is one of the most common medical problems of older persons. Increasing age is a risk factor for virtually any medical complication. Older people have more diseases and therefore have more tests and treatments despite their increased risk. Hospitals are particularly hazardous, but no medical venue is safe. The list of possible iatrogenic complications is long and includes many of the geriatric syndromes, such as falls, confusion, dizziness, and urinary incontinence.

Three especially common iatrogenic problems in geriatrics are adverse drug effects, acute kidney injury, and adverse surgical outcomes.

- Adverse drug effects (ADEs). This is an expensive problem for the health care system and all too frequently a morbid (and occasionally fatal) problem for patients. So ubiquitous are adverse drug reactions that one expert suggested that "any symptom in an elderly patient should be considered a drug side effect until proven otherwise."[15] The majority of persons aged 65 and older take at least five medications, and more than a third of them will experience an ADE during a year.[16] Because taking five or more medicines is a potent predictor of ADEs, regular review and discontinuation of unnecessary prescription and over-the-counter drugs is a critical preventive measure (see Chapter 6).

- Acute kidney injury (AKI). At least two thirds of persons older than 65 have a significant decline in renal function, making them vulnerable to AKI. On top of baseline renal dysfunction, risk factors for AKI are multifactorial and include nephrotoxic drugs, sepsis, hypotension, and radiologic contrast media. By some estimates 7% to 10% of hospitalized older people experience AKI.[17] Therefore nephrotoxic drugs and contrast agents should be avoided when possible in hospitalized older patients, and hydration should always be maintained. Also, when considering a study using radiologic contrast, we need to ask whether the test results will lead to an important change in care that would be consistent with the patient's care goals.

- Adverse surgical outcomes. Surgery provides tremendous benefits for many but by no means all geriatric patients. Replacing a painful hip that limits mobility, for example, can improve function and help maintain independence—if the patient is not too frail or unmotivated to do the necessary rehabilitation exercises. The challenge is that older people as a whole are more prone to poor outcomes after surgery; thus many operations leave the patient worse off than before. Frail patients are at especially high risk; therefore surgeons increasingly are interested in frailty measures to assess risk and benefits of surgical interventions.[18] When patients ask if they are "too old" for surgery, the question we should pose is whether they are "too frail," and if they are "kind of frail" whether the potential benefits justify the risks. These are hard decisions, because the patient and/or family members will often grasp at any possibility of improvement, no matter how remote.

> Iatrogenic illnesses are among the most common preventable problems experienced by older people.

Slow Medicine

"Don't just do something, stand there." This is useful advice not only for doctors in training but for the health care system. The reason is that aggressive treatment, when applied to older persons, more often than not leads to adverse consequences than to improvement. If, for example, an older person has florid pulmonary edema, the best treatment is often to give oxygen and a little intravenous furosemide, see what happens, and then decide about the second drug. If a more aggressive regimen were used instead, the patient might experience a drop in blood pressure and possibly even suffer a stroke.

"Start low, go slow." This is another mantra of geriatrics; it refers to the best way to approach pharmacotherapy in older persons. Once again, the issue is that adverse effects are more common in the elderly than in younger persons. Additionally, beneficial effects are often more uncertain in older persons. An example is the use of antidepressants. They do sometimes work in older persons but less reliably than in younger populations and with a greater risk of adverse effects. Concomitantly one should not so underdose older patients that they have no chance of responding to a drug; instead, starting at a low dosage and gradually increasing is the way to proceed.

Slow medicine describes a philosophy and approach that applies the principle of beneficence (i.e., "first do no harm") to the general care of geriatric patients. The idea is to pace care decisions so that both patients and health care providers have a chance to evaluate care options before proceeding, because acting hastily is more likely to do harm than not acting at all. Dennis McCullough elegantly advocates for slow medicine in the book *My Mother, Your Mother*:

> *The practice of Slow Medicine has taught me that it is wise to slow down and moderate the urgent pressures of decision-making that are often pushed prematurely on elders by society, the medical profession, worried friends and family. Well-intentioned, we want to make good and humane choices for ourselves and for those we love.*[19]

> In geriatric medicine acting hastily is more likely to do harm than not acting at all, and a slow medicine approach is often ideal.

Polypharmacy

Older persons take a lot of medicine. As of 2011, persons older than 65 comprised only 13% of the U.S. population but consumed a third of all prescription drugs. In 1 year the average older adult with 5 or more chronic illnesses will see 14 different physicians, make 37 physician office visits, and fill 50 prescriptions (see Chapter 6).[20]

Taking so much medicine has its drawbacks. The risk of adverse drug-drug interactions or drug-disease interactions rises with the number of medications. Considering the number of medications taken by older persons, it should be no surprise that adverse drug events are the primary cause of more than 10% of hospital admissions by older adults.[21]

The term *polypharmacy* was coined to describe persons (most of whom are older) who take a lot of medications. During the past decade and a half, the level of polypharmacy among older persons has risen markedly, despite admonitions that it is dangerous.

The challenge is that, although too many drugs can be bad, so can too few. In fact, much of the rise in prescription drug use over the past decade or two has been because of appropriate use of preventive medications such as beta-blockers after myocardial infarction, warfarin for persons with atrial fibrillation, plus more aggressive treatment of hypertension and congestive heart failure, all of which are supported by evidence-based disease-specific guidelines from professional organizations and expert panels.

However, such disease management guidelines must be applied selectively when the patient is an older adult with multiple chronic illnesses.[22] Disease management guidelines are usually developed from research on patients younger than age 65 without comorbidities, not on patients with multiple and complex problems.

The challenge of applying disease management guidelines in older adults is illustrated by the following example:

A physician's 92-year-old mother was hospitalized with a mild heart attack. Following standard guidelines, her cardiologist prescribed atenolol. Not long after the woman complained of considerable fatigue and a "fuzzy" head. The physician daughter had heard these complaints from her mother six years earlier when she had been prescribed the same medication for her hypertension. At that time, stopping the atenolol had alleviated the symptoms, so the daughter called the cardiologist on behalf of her mother to request that the atenolol be discontinued. The cardiologist's response was that this was impossible, because not using a beta-blocker after a heart attack was tantamount to malpractice! The daughter debated with the cardiologist the potential benefits of this protective medication versus its adverse effect on her mother's quality of life. The daughter won the debate, the medication was discontinued, and her mother felt much better. So far there has been no recurrent heart attack.

The U.S. Health Care Nonsystem

The U.S. health care system for older adults has traditionally had an acute care focus, with access to services largely driven by illness episodes. Thus the major insurers—Medicare, Medicaid, and Veterans Health Administration benefits—tend to provide coverage primarily for active medical treatment. Older adults and the clinicians who care for them experience significant gaps in coverage for primary, preventive care, and proactive interventions. Integration of services is limited between care settings: the hospital, assisted living and the nursing home, home- and community-based services, and the PCP's office. This is a particular problem for older adults who require more time to recover from acute illness and frequently have multiple chronic illnesses. The result is a fragmented system that funds the most intensive and expensive settings while requiring individuals and their families to privately fund less expensive alternatives.

The cost of providing medical care services to older adults is substantial. In 2011 Medicare sending accounted for 15% of total federal spending and 21% of total national health spending.[23] In an effort to contain the rising costs of care, Medicare has created numerous complex rules to control costs. These rules are confusing for providers and for patients and their families. Although the majority of health care funding for older Americans is public, many older adults also have high out-of-pocket expenses. Health care, including insurance premiums, accounted for 15% of household budgets among Medicare recipients in 2009 ($4,620 annually, out of a mean annual household budget of $30,966).[23]

The most significant coverage gaps for older adults involve long-term care. Many older adults believe their Medicare benefits under Part A and B will cover long-term care services; however, Medicare offers only limited skilled nursing benefits at home or in a nursing home and no coverage for assisted living. Furthermore, Medicare benefits are designed to be intermittent and are triggered by hospitalization. As a result, more than 90% of bed days in nursing homes and virtually all assisted-living bed days are paid for either privately or (once private funds are depleted) by Medicaid.

Putting all this together, it is probably most accurate to describe U.S. health care as a nonsystem (Figure 1-7). *System* usually implies not just a series of parts but the concept of working together in some kind of harmony. U.S. health care consists of a variety of separate providers and service types, each of which tends to have its own access requirements, structure, record system, and billing. Having many providers and services leads to duplication, high cost, fragmentation, access barriers, and problems when a patient transitions from one setting or provider to another.

Transitions in Care are Dangerous

Care transitions occur whenever a patient changes level or location of care, and a whole new set of care providers has to get to know a patient. In today's health care, these transitions occur with dizzying frequency. They are especially problematic around hospitalizations, because patient information has to be passed at least twice—and three times if, as usually happens, an emergency room visit is part of the admission. In addition, hospital stays are increasingly short, with patients often being discharged before they are ready to return home. This leads to an additional transition involving a posthospitalization nursing home stay. All these handoffs can lead to misunderstandings of diagnoses and plans, to

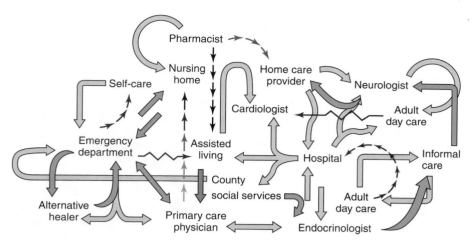

Figure 1-7 The U.S. health care system for older persons is a confusing array of largely independent providers. Anyone with significant cognitive, physical, or sensory impairment—and many persons who are quite intact but are not good at understanding and navigating complex systems—requires assistance to understand and appropriately use the resources that are available.

medication discrepancies, and to confusion on the part of patients and families.

In years past, a primary care provider who knew the patient would oversee hospital care and arrange follow-up, so transitions were more seamless. The advent of hospitalists and other aspects of health care specialization changed all that. Nowadays provider continuity rarely occurs; thus special effort must be undertaken to ensure that accurate information on a patient's history, capabilities, disabilities, care preferences, medications, allergies, and family/social support are communicated across transitions. Failure to address these issues will lead to complications, hospital readmissions, and patient dissatisfaction.

Fortunately, essential elements of safe transitions have been identified and studied. A widely acknowledged program is the Care Transitions Program.[24] Among its key elements are the following indicators of high-quality transitional care (and reduced hospital readmissions):

- Accurate and timely information transfer to the next set of providers
- Patient and family education about the disease process, self-management recommendations, and expectations for the next level of care
- Empowerment of patients to assert their preferences for the type, intensity, and location of services received

Because hospital readmissions are costly, they have been a focus of Medicare health care reform.[25] Under the Affordable Care Act considerable funding has been allocated to foster strategies that will improve care transitions for Medicare beneficiaries. In addition, the Centers for Medicare and Medicaid Services has approved two new transitional care management service codes that reimburse a Medicare patient's primary physician for both non–face-to-face and face-to-face transitional care management services provided within 30 days of discharge. This change will place primary care providers back in the center of

care coordination during transitions out of the hospital (see Chapter 10).

> Transitions from one provider or care setting to another can lead to misunderstanding of diagnoses and plans, medication discrepancies, and confusion on the part of patients and families.

Interprofessional Nature of Geriatric Care

Evidence from numerous studies supports the use of interprofessional teams in the care of older adults. Managing patients as a team leads to better continuity, enhanced care coordination, improved patient safety, better chronic illness care, enhanced medication adherence, fewer adverse drug reactions, preserved function, and decreased hospital readmissions.[26-29]

A number of recent events and new care models, including the following, have led to an increased emphasis on geriatric care teams in primary care:

- The 2008 Institute of Medicine (IOM) report, *Retooling for an Aging America: Building the Health Care Workforce,* emphasized the importance of training all health care professionals in the skills needed to work effectively in teams and calls for the implementation of new geriatric care models that use interprofessional teams.[30]
- The Affordable Care Act, with its encouragement of Accountable Care Organizations (ACOs), in which clinicians and hospitals are held accountable not only for treating patients once they get sick but also for helping to keep them out of the hospital and emergency rooms.
- The Patient Centered Medical Home (PCMH) model of primary care, which focuses on use of interprofessional teams to provide improved continuity, comprehensiveness, and coordination of care. Implementation of the PCMH model

requires additional resources that have not been provided through traditional payment mechanisms; thus payment models that encourage and reward primary care practices for achieving improved outcomes are an essential component necessary to drive this interprofessional team model.

Whereas the importance of teamwork is evident, it can be challenging to implement in an effective yet cost-efficient manner. For years, academic medical centers had "geriatric assessment and management clinics" in which interprofessional teams took several hours or longer to evaluate a patient; however, this model was never feasible in primary care. Instead, primary care geriatricians tend to use virtual, ad hoc interprofessional teams consisting of an office-based core (usually a physician and a nurse) supplemented as needed by consultations or referrals to other professionals who may work for different organizations (e.g., medical offices, home care agencies, hospitals). For less complex patients, the team is often small, whereas for very frail elders managed at home the care team can be large. In addition to a variety of health professionals, interprofessional teams usually include an identified care manager and must always explicitly include the older person and his or her family.

The essential elements of teamwork include coordination of services, shared responsibility, and communication. Because each profession has its own approach to care, differences in values, expectations, and/or language can occur within a team. Therefore a good team requires its members to not only have excellent clinical skills but also be knowledgeable and skillful at working as a team. Good teamwork does not happen by accident but is a function of a well-developed structure that includes mutual respect; clarity about each member's roles and responsibilities; frequent, clear communication; and mechanisms for managing team conflict. Fulfilling these requirements can lead to care goals and care planning that emphasize the particular needs of the older adult (see Chapter 2).

> Interprofessional care is important but challenging to implement in an effective yet cost-efficient manner.

A Generalist is Often the Best Clinician for a Geriatric Patient

Because older persons so often have impairments in multiple organ systems, a generalist clinician is often better able to set priorities and identify the remediable problem than a multitude of specialists. Therefore specialist clinicians should generally be viewed as

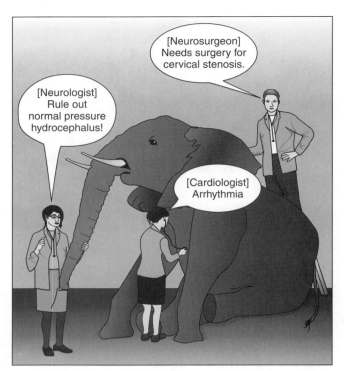

Figure 1-8 Medical specialists often approach geriatric patients in a manner reminiscent of the blind man and the elephant. In this case of a patient with a gait disorder and multiple falls, three specialists viewed the situation through the lens of their own subspecialty and recommended invasive procedures that could have harmed the patient. The actual diagnosis was failure to adhere to a medication regimen because of mild cognitive impairment. See text for details.

consultants, and patient *referrals* should only be made once the primary care provider has weighed the evidence and decided on the best course of action. Often this process of decision making involves not only obtaining specialist opinions but also meeting with the patient and family to identify goals and priorities and putting all available information in the context of the patient's overall health status and prognosis.

The view of specialists as very useful but secondary adjuncts to the primary care process can best be illustrated by the story of the blind men and the elephant (Figure 1-8). As the case study illustrates, specialists view patients through a narrow lens and at times can fail to see the forest because they are accustomed to looking at trees. For these reasons, a good generalist is often the best clinician for an older person.

CASE 1

Frieda (Part 1)

Frieda is a 79-year-old woman who was hospitalized after falling and bruising her face and shoulder. Once a significant orthopedic injury had been ruled out, several subspecialists were consulted to evaluate the patient's recurrent falls (see Figure 1-8). A neurologist ordered a head computed tomography (CT) scan, thought the cerebral ventricles were unusually large for a person with her degree of cerebral atrophy, and wanted further evaluation and possibly shunting for normal pressure hydrocephalus. A neurosurgeon ordered a CT scan of the neck, which was interpreted as showing spinal stenosis, and wanted to operate. A cardiologist noted that the patient had a right bundle branch block and 3 to 5 premature ventricular contractions per minute and, when the echocardiogram showed an ejection fraction of 30%, recommended evaluation for possible pacemaker placement.

Frieda, a stubborn woman, refused all of these.

1. **What other next steps might be possible in Frieda's care?**
2. **Which of the proposed interventions if carried out would be most likely to help Frieda?** ▣

CASE 1

Frieda (Part 2).

Frieda's primary care physician reassessed her status in light of the conflicting specialist recommendations and her own frame of mind. He noted that she had mild short-term memory loss and admitted to not always knowing whether she had taken her medications; thus he recommended that a family member place Frieda's daily medications in a pill dispenser. She took a sleeping pill each night, which he discontinued, advising her to read in bed and consider taking melatonin. He also noted that Frieda was highly deconditioned, with weak leg and hip muscles but intact peripheral nerve function, so he arranged for her to have physical therapy at home three times a week. The frequent falls stopped and, three years later, Frieda continued to do well. ▣

CASE 1

Discussion

Frieda's case history illustrates that, although subspecialists can often be invaluable in clarifying a diagnosis or providing needed therapy, they can at times make recommendations

that are not the best course of action for a particular patient. Because conducting multiple tests on complex older persons always reveals a host of abnormal or questionable findings, it often takes a generalist to identify what is most important and what will be most helpful to the individual patient. ▣

SUMMARY

The unique clinical characteristics of the elderly and the principles of delivering good care for older adults, as described in this chapter, should serve as the foundation for providing optimal primary care for older patients. Our approach to the older patient starts with a careful clinical assessment to identify correctable or manageable acute or chronic medical problems and geriatric syndromes. Next, the management of chronic problems is conducted in the context of the patient's goals of care, always assessing the risk versus benefit of therapy. Finally, we maintain an emphasis toward restoring and maintaining the older adult's function and independence.

Web Resources

www.caretransitions.org. Website of the Care Transitions Program, which aims to support patients and families and increase skills among health care providers around care transitions.

www.youtube.com/watch?v=xdBObrGc1Yw. Short, upbeat video about nursing home residents who go snow tubing. A good illustration of how fun can occur even with significant disabilities.

www.kff.org. Kaiser Family Foundation's website provides a trustworthy resource about health policy, including up-to-date information on Medicare and Medicaid programs.

www.needymeds.org. A nonprofit information resource devoted to helping people in need find assistance programs to help them afford their medications and costs related to health care.

http://hartfordign.org/practice. Hartford Institute for Geriatric Nursing's *Practice* website with resources on geriatric assessment and other key topics, including "Try This" evidence-based assessment tools.

www.americangeriatrics.org. Official website of the American Geriatrics Society provides access to a variety of guidelines and clinical tools.

References available online at expertconsult.com.

2

Interprofessional Team Care

Kenneth Brummel-Smith, Jean C. Munn, and Debra A. Danforth

OBJECTIVES

Upon completion of this chapter, the reader will be able to:

- Describe three traits of effective geriatric care teams.
- Describe two barriers to team care.
- Describe four components of an effective geriatric care team.
- Describe the role of the patient and the family in the team.

Additional online-only material indicated by icon.

Health care teams play a crucial role in geriatric care. Geriatrics is characterized by its complexity and attention to biopsychosocial needs of the patient. It is virtually impossible for the primary care provider (PCP) to provide comprehensive assessment and management of complicated elders without working in a team of professionals. Many older people have several chronic conditions, geriatric syndromes, polypharmacy, perhaps some cognitive problems, functional deficits, and social needs. The best care requires the skills of an interprofessional team. It is important that all members of the geriatric health care team have adequate knowledge and skills and appropriate attitudes regarding team care.

The major organizations involved in physician training have established recommendations regarding team training and core competencies in interprofessional collaborative practice. The Accreditation Council of Graduate Medical Education, in its discussion of the competency "interpersonal and communication skills" requires residents to "demonstrate interpersonal and communication skills that result in effective information exchange and teaming with patients... and professional associates."[1] Residents should be trained to "work effectively with others as a member or leader of a health care team." Training in teamwork is also recommended under the "systems-based practice" competency. The Association of American Medical Colleges has also recognized the importance of team-related training.[2] The core competencies in collaborative practice have been agreed upon by the major organizations in health professional training.[3] (See Box 2-1.)

CASE 1

Rachel Paul (Part 1)

Mrs. Rachel Paul is a 78-year-old who was living independently in an apartment. Earlier this morning, she tripped while going to the bathroom, and landed on her hip. She felt an immediate pain and was unable to get up to walk. She dragged herself to the bedside table, where she was able to reach the phone and call her daughter. You now see her in the emergency room and the emergency physician informs you she has a fractured neck of the left femur.

During Mrs. Paul's treatment and rehabilitation for her femur fracture what are the likely health disciplines she will encounter?

Although much of the discussion of health care teams focuses on the roles of the health professionals, patient-centered care requires that the patient needs always be given priority. In addition, because most care is provided to older persons by their families it is crucial that the patient's caregiver and family be included in the team process. This approach can be difficult for health care professionals. Asking patients for their input, encouraging them to ask questions, and remembering to provide the patient and family with all the information needed to make informed decisions takes time and sensitivity. However, it is through patient involvement that we can achieve the desired outcomes and at the same time reduce errors and iatrogenic disease. ▪

Effective health care teams have certain traits—roles and responsibilities are clear and understood by all, and members are flexible and knowledgeable of the other members' skills. The team has a strong sense of collegiality, trust, and mutual respect. An especially important characteristic of an effective team is the ability to collaborate. Collaboration requires not just respect of other team members, but a mutual dependence. Perhaps the most important trait is the ability to communicate effectively. This ability is not limited to being able to exchange information; team members also must be able to both support and confront one another, especially in situations involving patient safety. Ultimately, the goal of the health care team is to optimize patient-centered outcomes while reducing the risk for error.

Barriers to Effective Team Function

Both external and internal factors can result in barriers to the use of teams in health care. Teams, by their nature, increase complexity. Many teams are formed with members who have received no training in team-based care. To be effective teams must develop communications systems, protocols, and have time to interact. The common, hierarchical model of medicine is antithetical to effective team care. Finding the exact number of team members to provide efficient care is difficult. There may be a U-shaped nature to team member numbers; too few does not allow for improved efficiency, and too many becomes too complicated to manage. One study found that in primary care 6 team members was the ideal number, and teams with greater than 12 members were less effective.[4] Finally, the fee-for-service reimbursement system does not place value on team care. Many of the activities of key team members,

such as social workers, are not reimbursable in standard Medicare billing.

The most important trait of an effective health care team is the ability to communicate effectively.

Teams in Different Geriatric Care Settings

Team care occurs in a variety of health care settings. In its simplest form a physician works with an assistant and sometimes a clerical support person. However, when the demands of care are diverse and require professionals with different skill sets, a formal team structure is necessary. In the well-developed patient-centered medical home primary care practice, every office staff member works together as an integrated team, partnering with the patient, family, and community health workers. Teams are also seen in geriatric assessment clinics, long-term care settings, rehabilitation, hospice care, transplantation units, and surgical settings.

The disciplines participating in a geriatric health care team will vary by setting and the needs of the patients. Regardless of which members are on the team, it is important that all team members are trained not only in their discipline, but also in teamwork. In the care of a frail and complicated older person, the minimum team is comprised of a PCP, a nurse, and a social worker. Table 2-1 lists the skills of a variety of health care disciplines. A more detailed description of the PCP, social work, and nurse roles follows, though it is clear that many others, including pharmacists, rehabilitation therapists, chaplains, music therapists, and others are involved in the patient's care.

CASE 1

Rachel Paul (Part 2)

Mrs. Paul undergoes left hip replacement with no complications and has minimal pain with walking. But she is unsteady and somewhat fearful when ambulating. The physician reviews her past medical history and finds that she has been taking hydrochlorothiazide for hypertension, ibuprofen for osteoarthritis, and diphenhydramine for sleep. Recognizing that the nonsteroidal antiinflammatory drug could be contributing to Mrs. Paul's hypertension, he discusses with the patient using acetaminophen. He discontinues the diphenhydramine and discusses sleep hygiene with the patient. The physician orders evaluations by occupational and physical therapists.

What are the distinct roles of the occupational and physical therapist in the assessment and rehabilitation of Mrs. Paul? ▪

TABLE 2-1	Geriatrics Team—Selected Discipline Participants
Audiology	Evaluates, diagnoses, and treats hearing loss and balance disorders. Recommends and provides hearing aids.
Chaplain	Provides spiritual and emotional support to patients and family.
Dietitian (Registered)	Evaluates the nutritional status of patients; sets nutritional goals; educates patient and family.
Geriatrician	Physician with special training in the care of older adults.
Registered Nurse	Provides direct and indirect patient care; helps to maintain function; coordinates care; provides patient education.
Nurse Practitioner/Advanced Care/Geriatric Medicine	Nurse with advanced training in clinical practice, geriatric medicine, health education, and counseling.
Occupational Therapist	Assists patients with developing independence with ADLs and IADLs, especially upper extremity function; home safety evaluations; adaptive equipment recommendations; extremity splinting.
Pharmacist	Monitors optimal medication therapy; information resource.
Physical Therapist	Assists patient with mobility, balance, strength training, and pain relief; adaptive equipment recommendations.
Physician (Primary Care)	Diagnosis and treatment; prevention, prescribing, manage chronic illness.
Physician Assistant	Practices medicine with supervision of physician.
Psychiatrist	Physician who treats patients with mental, emotional, and behavioral disorders.
Psychologist	Assessment, treatment, and management of mental disorders.
Social Worker (Medical)	Assessment and management of patient and family psychosocial functioning; locating services; counseling.
Speech/Language Pathologist	Evaluate and diagnose speech, language, cognitive. Communication and swallowing disorders.

ADLs, Activities of daily living; *IADLs,* instrumental activities of daily living.

ROLES OF CORE TEAM MEMBERS

Primary Care Provider (Physician, Nurse Practitioner, Physician Assistant)

The primary care provider on the geriatric team usually has the responsibility of assessing and managing the patient's medical problems. In addition, when the team does not have a pharmacist the PCP, along with the nurse, is also responsible for careful monitoring for medication effects. There are some important differences between a primary provider's standard role in a primary care practice versus a primary provider's role as part of a geriatric care team. In traditional primary care the PCP interviews and examines the patient, considers medical recommendations, and then enters into a discussion in which the patient's goals and wishes are clarified, education is provided, and the patient and provider decide on a course of treatment. This is the essence of shared decision making in primary care. In a team environment, the PCP has the additional responsibility to not only inform other team members of the patient's conditions, but also to learn from other team members the patient's needs that were identified in their assessments. Furthermore, because the areas of need are much broader than the standard medical approach, the team and patient (and often family or other caregivers) must determine priorities and decide which problems to address first. This is a more complicated, but also more comprehensive, approach to patient management.

In older adults with multiple medical problems decisions will need to be made about the balance of benefits and risks of simultaneous treatment of multiple conditions. Based on the patient's goals, targets for treatment will be decided. For example, although many guidelines recommend a target of <7.0% for glycosylated hemoglobin (HbA$_{1c}$) in diabetic patients, such a target may not be appropriate for many older patients.[5] Similarly, decisions on the appropriate approach to symptom management and preventive screening tests will be required. The PCP also reviews the patient's medication regimen, assesses the use of over-the-counter medications, and decides on appropriate medications to continue or to stop. The process continues with oversight and adjustments based on the patient's responses.

> In a team environment, the PCP has the responsibility to inform other team members of the patient's conditions, and also to learn from other team members the patient's needs that were identified in their assessments.

A key area of involvement for the PCP is advance care planning. Often this process is initiated by the social worker through a discussion of the patient's goals and wishes. A number of initiatives and techniques are available to facilitate the discussions, such as using the "Go Wish" cards.[6] These are a set of 36 playing cards with statements about common things people value at the end of life. The patient is asked to sort the cards into his or her top-10 prioritized wishes and then use that as a springboard for discussing advance care planning. Although this part of the advance care planning may be led by the social worker, the physician or nurse practitioner is crucial to discussing the medical implications of the patient's wishes and for completing a set of orders if desired. The Physician Orders for Life Sustaining Treatment form is one mechanism for doing that.[7] It is now used in more than 13 states.

The PCP also serves in the important role as a patient advocate within the medical care system. Given the diversity of older persons, each patient will make health care decisions not only on the medical facts, but on their own goals and wishes. Spouses, family members, and even other members of the geriatric care team may have opinions about the proper course of treatment. Sometimes these opinions are in the direction of less intensive care, sometimes more. It is the PCP's role to help patients choose among treatment options, and to help patients understand the risks and benefits of the choices as well as what is likely to happen if no treatment is provided. This is the essence of informed consent. When working with a surrogate (or proxy) decision maker the PCP must be certain that the decisions of the surrogate reflect those choices that would have been made by the patient.

A word of caution is warranted regarding the role of the physician in geriatric care teams. Physicians are socialized through their professional training to be leaders. Many assume the physician will be the team leader. This is often not the case in geriatric care teams. Leadership not only varies by the type of team, but also may vary by the situation. For instance, in Program of All-Inclusive Care of the Elderly sites, the social worker is often the team leader. As nursing homes move toward more homelike settings, nurses are often team leaders. In well-functioning teams with good communication skills, team leadership may shift based on the primary issue being addressed, such as when decisions are being made about transfer of care to a different site. Physicians on geriatric care teams must be facile at changing roles and in providing the support needed by the team to achieve the best patient outcomes.

CASE 1

Rachel Paul (Part 3)

Mrs. Paul is now in rehabilitation for her repaired hip fracture. The physical therapist notices that the patient becomes extremely anxious when she attempts to start gait training. The patient expresses, under her breath, "I don't know that I'll ever be able to go home again . . ." The therapist reports this to the social worker on the team, who decides to conduct a depression screen.

What are the multiple roles of a hospital social worker in ensuring Mrs. Paul's successful recovery from her fracture? ▣

Social Work

Social workers provide both tangible and intangible contributions to the geriatric health care team. Historically, social workers became active in health care settings, especially hospitals, as informants to doctors and nurses regarding the social and psychological impacts of disease upon patients and their families. This remains a critical role of social workers in the geriatric health care teams of today. Furthermore, shorter hospitalizations have resulted in patients requiring more health-related social work services in the community.[8] Indeed, the social worker can become a translator between the patient and the rest of the geriatric care team. Social workers often meet with the patient and/or his or her family and provide critical information for meeting the needs of the whole person (Box 2-2).

> In well-functioning teams with good communication skills, team leadership may shift based on the care topic being addressed.

Advocacy

Essentially, social workers serve as advocates for the patient. This advocacy serves to support the patient's right to self-determination regarding medical decisions. As an advocate, the social worker focuses on the patient, with the patient's needs, wishes, well-being, and interests taking precedence over all else.[9] The social worker consults privately with patients and represents patients who cannot represent themselves (e.g., homeless, cognitively impaired). Therefore, one part of the social work role is to engage parties who might feel ignored.

At times, the prevailing medical model of patient care clashes with the social work profession's model of patient autonomy and self-determination.[10] Team members may become angry with the patient and expect the social worker to force the patient to get "the help she needs." In these instances, the social worker must skillfully model respect for the patient's autonomy as well as educate the patient on the importance of considering all treatment options.

BOX 2-2

SOCIAL WORK ON GERIATRIC TEAMS

Medical social work is a form of practice that:
• Occurs in hospitals and other health care settings.
• Facilitates good health and prevention of illness.
• Aids physically ill clients and their families to resolve the social and psychological problems related to disease and illness.

In some cases, the patient's right to refuse treatment is overridden by concerns regarding patient safety or the safety of others. When there is the possibility of irrefutable, irreversible harm involved and the social worker has made every effort to gain consent, the social worker will work with the team to obtain appropriate treatment for the patient. Constantly, the social worker balances the advocacy role with responsibility to the health care delivery system.

In other cases, the social worker serves as a cultural broker or advocate. In today's diverse world it is essential that the health care team understand how an individual's culture shapes his worldview and how he interprets medical care. Cultural dynamics can require adjustment of medical approaches and the social worker can interview the patient and learn as much as possible about his or her background and cultural and individual traits and beliefs. Social workers also seek help from other members of the patient's family and frequently research the patient's culture and cultural perceptions of aging and medical care. Finally, the social worker brings this information to the team to assist in diagnosis and treatment planning and interprets the culture to the rest of the team.

For example, social workers can provide information regarding the culturally specific systems that affect the patient as well as provide the patient with the names and purposes of tests. In addition, the social worker translates a greater understanding of the health care system and medical terms. Yet, it is also essential that the social worker, as well as the rest of the health care team, avoid losing sight of a patient's individuality by stereotyping the patient on the basis of culture.[11] When appropriately nuanced, this inclusion of the patient's beliefs and rituals affects everyone and leads to the increased comfort of the patient and to greater trust of the medical providers. However, in no case does the social worker interpret the test results or diagnose medical conditions. Rather, the social worker is a translator and communicator.

Assessment

In addition to bringing psychosocial issues to the geriatric medical team, social workers perform both formal and informal psychosocial assessments. Assessment is considered the basis of social work practice,[12] specifically characterizing gerontologic social work.[13] Individualized assessments are essential in developing patient-specific interventions and treatments.[14] Comprehensive assessments, within the purview of social work, encompass physical, functional, financial, social, emotional, spiritual, and psychological resources, supports, and unmet needs.

Ideally, a social worker develops a social history for each patient that provides critical information regarding the patient's past as well as current social, psychological, spiritual, and financial issues. Embedded in this history is the person-in-the-environment perspective,[15] suggesting that understanding the patient's environment influences understanding and enhances care. In addition, social work endorses a strengths-based perspective,[16] that is, looking for both strengths and weaknesses in the personal characteristics of the patient, immediate support systems, and the environment. These perspectives promote empowering patients to be active in medical decision making as well as taking responsibility for their health and wellness. Also, through evaluation of a patient's history and environment, the social worker gains insight into the patient's reasons for his or her decisions. Subsequently, the social worker brings information regarding strengths as well as needs back to the team, offers feedback to the team as to the perceptions of the patient and the family, and assists in incorporating this information into the care planning process.

Formal Assessments

Social workers are trained in completing assessments beyond the social history. They can administer a number of standardized measures typically included in geriatric practice such as the Folstein Mini-Mental State Exam, the Geriatric Depression Scale, and the Patient Health Questionnaire as well as the Lubben Social Networking Scale and the Spiritual Needs Inventory. Furthermore, social worker skills such as interviewing and recording engender competence beyond simple measures to more complex assessments. The assessment process is highly dependent on establishing a rapport with patients that involves open-ended or conversational modes. Indeed, social workers are adept at informal assessments and can serve as another set of eyes when identifying needs and changes in patient status.

Psychological assessments also serve as interventions. When a patient or family is guided by recognizing psychosocial strengths as well as problems, they typically respond by addressing or at least acknowledging opportunities not recognized as unmet needs. Notably, all team members, including the patient and family, benefit from identifying strengths as part of the assessment process. In addition, the interaction between the social worker and the patient establishes trust and lessens the patient's feelings of isolation and helplessness.[17]

> Formal and informal psychosocial assessments are the basis of social gerontologic social work practice.

Case Manager

A more commonly recognized role of social workers is generally referred to as case manager. In this role, social workers link patients or families of patients with resources. For example, social workers frequently make community referrals. Social workers can make phone calls, fill out forms, directly obtain entitlements or facilitate meetings with Medicare and Medicaid professionals, financial advisers, attorneys, hospice care providers, and family members (Box 2-3).

Facilitator

Social workers frequently fill the role of facilitator among the team members as well as with the patient and family and, as such, are extremely significant components of successful collaborative endeavors. This contribution is enhanced by the professional processes of learning to manage their own emotions[18] and unresolved issues, especially those that can interfere with patient care or collaboration among staff. Social workers are often critical in mitigating differences among family members and the patient. In many instances, a geriatric patient's goals for care can be lost in the effort to please family members who are more articulate and take over the decision-making process. The social worker is the ideal team member to advocate for the patient, often mediating the conflicting viewpoints while maintaining the role of patient advocate.

The effective social worker can be characterized as a team player who is open to learning, change, new experiences, and has a high tolerance for ambiguity. The profession also places a high value on trust, respect, and understanding. The National Association of Social Workers provides the Code of Ethics that guides the profession. Clearly stated as the primary goal of social work is to "help people in need . . . address social problems . . . and elevate service to others above self-interest." Other values include "respect for the inherent dignity and worth" of all people while being "mindful of individual differences and cultural and ethnic diversity." Furthermore, the Code "recognizes the central importance of human relationships" and social workers "seek to strengthen relationships among people in a purposeful effort to promote, restore, maintain, and enhance the well-being of individuals, families, social groups, organizations, and communities."[21]

> Social workers are often critical in mitigating differences between family members and the patient.

Nursing

Nurses represent the largest component of the health care workforce and have the most direct contact with patients, ensuring that the patient receives accessible, high-quality care. PCPs and other physician specialists, being the next largest component, have traditionally held the most decision-making authority. Understanding, mutual respect, and close working relationships between nurses, physicians, and other health care providers are essential to providing the patients with quality health care. In 2008 the Robert Wood Johnson Foundation (RWJF) and the Institute of Medicine (IOM) launched a two-year initiative to respond to the need to assess and transform the nursing profession. The IOM appointed the Committee on the RWJF Initiative on the Future of Nursing, at the IOM, with the purpose of producing a report that would make recommendations for an action-oriented blueprint for the future of nursing.[19] Through its deliberations, the committee developed four key messages:
- Nurses should practice to the full extent of their education and training.
- Nurses should achieve higher levels of education and training through an improved education system that promotes seamless academic progression.

- Nurses should be full partners, with physicians and other health care professionals, in redesigning health care in the United States.
- Effective workforce planning and policy making require better data collection and information infrastructure.

Many nurses in practice care for elderly patients; however, not all nurses who care for elderly patients are certified as gerontologic nurses. A gerontologic nurse is a nursing specialty that revolves around the care of older adults; these nurses usually take additional courses focusing on the geriatric population or pursue advanced degrees to become a gerontologic advanced practice nurse or a gerontologic clinical nurse specialist. Gerontologic nursing practice involves assessing the health and functional status of older adults, planning and providing appropriate care, and evaluating the effectiveness of such care. Emphasis is placed on maximizing functional ability in the activities of daily living, and on promoting, maintaining, and restoring health. Nurses may work in a nursing home, residential facility, hospital, or in a patient's home. These nurses work closely with other medical disciplines and with the patient and/or family members, significant other, or caregiver.

The traditional nursing role has focused on bedside care and providing emotional support for the patient and family. Now, more than ever, a nurse's communication skill set must extend beyond traditional interactions with patients to the team context, where nurses are expected to build team morale and relationships, coordinate team tasks to facilitate care, and promote joint decision making.[20] For example, when a physician comes to a nurse on rounds the physician may ask about a patient's status, recent course of events, and/or any unattended patient needs. The nurse will give an SBAR (**S**ituation, **B**ackground, **A**ssessment, **R**ecommendations) (see Box 2-4) of the patient to the physician; however, in today's professional environment nurses will generally ask questions or clarify information if they do not understand what a physician has ordered or stated. In the past, nurses would not question a physician. Nurses also communicate with a social worker when a physician or health care provider has made an order to transfer the patient to another facility. Nurses, physicians, and social workers are examples of a diverse group of clinicians who communicate with each other regularly about the care of a patient and participate in that care to optimize the patient's health.

Nurses are frequently required to act as an advocate for the patient, nursing home resident, or family member. The American Nurses Association Code of Ethics delineates nursing responsibilities in a manner consistent with quality assurance and ethical guidelines for nursing care.[21] The National League for Nursing has elucidated the patients' rights that nurses are expected to follow.[22] Fulfilling these obligations may present ethical dilemmas for nurses at times. The nurse working with a patient or family member has the responsibility to explain and clarify information that the patient may receive from the physician or other health care team members. The nurse must make sure the information is not distorted, that it is well presented, and that the patient and/or family member understand the explanation offered. In addition to providing information to a patient, a nurse may advise, counsel, or assist the patient in making a decision by making appointments and referrals, coordinating care, filling out forms, or helping with negotiation of the health care system. If conflict arises between a health care system and patient the nurse may act as patient advocate. Finally, the nurse can act as a patient advocate by joining local, state, and national organizations engaged in improving health care.

> Nurses working with a patient or family member explain and clarify medical information that the patient may receive from the physician or other health care team members.

CASE 1

Rachel Paul (Part 5)

The nurse, social worker, physician, and other team members have been working to achieve the patient's goal of returning to her home. The plan is for the patient to be transferred to the nursing home for rehabilitation prior to being discharged home. The nurse calls the nursing home and gives an SBAR report about Mrs. Paul's status and physicians' orders. This report will include key nursing topics to be addressed, as well as a functional status report and a list of the patient's goals. The nurse then works with Mrs. Paul and her family on the transfer to the nursing home and answers questions. The nurse also reviews Mrs. Paul's medications with her including what the medications are for, how often they should be taken, and any side effects.

What are the best strategies to ensure that Mrs. Paul's medication list will be accurately communicated to the nursing home staff and eventually to her home care team? ▪

Box 2-4
SBAR COMMUNICATION
Situation: What is happening with the patient? Background: What is the clinical background? Assessment: What do I think is going on? Recommendation: What do I recommend?

EVIDENCE OF TEAM CARE EFFECTIVENESS

There is a large body of evidence that supports the importance of teams in health care.[23] There is also a growing literature on the best methods for developing and training in teamwork.[24] Much of this research has come from other fields, such as defense and aviation. This is not surprising because in both defense and aviation the effective collaboration of multiple team members is critical to successful outcomes and safety. Recently, the Agency for Healthcare Research and Quality, in conjunction with the Department of Defense, developed an evidence-based training program for teams—TeamSTEPPS© (http://teamstepps .ahrq.gov). *STEPPS* stands for *S*trategies and *T*ools to *E*nhance *P*erformance and *P*atient *S*afety. The next section of this chapter provides an overview of TeamSTEPPS training; however, anyone interested in becoming an effective "team player" is encouraged to participate in a formal TeamSTEPPS training program.[25] The critical components of teamwork include team leadership, situation monitoring, mutual support, adaptability, a shared mental model, and communication.

COMPONENTS OF EFFECTIVE GERIATRICS TEAM CARE

Team Leadership

Team leadership refers to the ability to coordinate and direct the activities of other team members. Team leaders assign tasks, help members find their internal motivation to perform successfully, help to plan and organize activities so they are most effectively completed, and contribute to the positive atmosphere a team needs. A team leader may be designated, such as a charge nurse on a medical ward. This type of leader has a clear set of responsibilities and ensures that all members possess the necessary knowledge, skills, and attitudes to function effectively; being the team leader is essentially part of the job description. Alternatively, situational team leaders rise into the role because of changing demands. It is possible that any member of the team may serve as a situational leader at one time or another. An example of a situational leader is the professional who first arrives at an emergency or code.

Effective team leaders must be skillful in organizing the team, establishing clear goals, and promoting good teamwork. To accomplish these goals the leader must be sensitive to the needs of all members, encourage them to speak up, and help to resolve conflict. The most effective team leader rarely makes decisions alone, but rather facilitates the team arriving at the decision based on the input of each member.

One of the key skills of the team leader is delegation. Delegation involves deciding how team members other than the leader can best accomplish tasks. Leaders often fail because they try to manage too many decisions and activities themselves. Delegation not only ensures that the team leader does not become overloaded, but more important, that all team members share in responsibilities and accomplishments. Delegation requires clear assignments, checking back for understanding, monitoring outcomes of the task, and providing feedback.

Team leaders must model and cultivate the behaviors that are desired. This includes not only being an effective communicator but also fostering mutual support and helping to resolve conflicts. It is very important that the leader not form alliances with individuals or subgroups within the team. The challenge in leading a team is remaining a member while carrying the responsibility of effective management.

An important role of the team leader is facilitating communication. In clinical situations communication is often conducted through briefs, huddles, and debriefs. *Briefs* are short (5-minute) planning discussions. These discussions should include roles of the members, clinical status of the team's patients, any goals and problems to be faced, and any other issues affecting the team's duties. For instance, in assessing a new patient referred for evaluation for possible admission to an assisted living facility, the team must decide who will conduct evaluations today, what is known of the patient's status, how and who will communicate the results of the assessment, and any intervening issues, such as family discord.

A *huddle* is a method for reinforcing plans already in place or modifying an existing plan when a change is needed. This is used especially when there is an unexpected increase in the workload of an individual team member resulting from a significant clinical status change. For instance, a patient undergoing rehabilitation may have developed a urinary tract infection, affecting his ability to participate in physical therapy. During the huddle, the team can decide to shift the focus of rehabilitation to planned family training that was to occur later in the patient's course.

Debriefs are useful ways for the team to learn from its mistakes or handling of unexpected events. The principle in quality assurance is that the goal is not to establish blame, but rather for all to learn to spot risky situations and develop better methods for handling them. It is crucial that the team leader conduct these short, 3-minute to 5-minute debriefs with an attitude of inquiry and discovery, not accusation. The team leader can facilitate this discussion by framing it correctly: "Let's take a look at what happened, what we did well and how we can improve on our performance."

Perhaps the most challenging role of the team leader is in helping to resolve conflict. Conflicts can arise because of disagreements over roles, the belief that other team members are not "carrying their weight," and differences in opinions and personalities. Ideally, each team member should try to resolve individual conflicts directly with the other team member. The leader should foster such direct communication. Team members can also be taught techniques for resolving conflict (see later section on Mutual Support).

> One of the key skills of the team leader is delegation.

Situation Monitoring

Clinical care is a dynamic process, where change in the patient's status is to be expected. This is especially true in geriatrics where the patient's health status may fluctuate because of unstable chronic medical conditions, sudden acute problems, emotional reactions to illness, or adverse reactions to medications or other treatments. The team must be adept at monitoring the patient's situation and skillful at communicating any changes to the rest of the team. Most medical encounters team members have with patients occur without another team member present. Communication of changes and rapid development of appropriate interventions is necessary.

Effective situation monitoring requires that all members of the team work in concert—team leadership must be open to reports of change and trusting of others' evaluations, members must be ready to support others when needed, and good communication skills are required. Situation monitoring, and sharing any changes with other team members, is what distinguishes an interprofessional team from a group of individual practitioners taking care of the same patient.

Experienced team members in geriatric care have learned to not only monitor the aspects of care for which they are responsible, but also to "cross monitor," observing and recognizing problems that are the province of another team member.

This process of awareness and notification of the team has been identified using the acronym STEP (*S*tatus of the patient, *T*eam members, *E*nvironment, *P*rogress toward goals). A team member becomes aware of an important feature in the status of the patient (e.g., possible anxiety or depression). He or she then involves other team members as appropriate (e.g., social work). The environment of the situation is analyzed (e.g., therapy brings up worries about future dependence). The team arrives at the best intervention to help the patient achieve his or her goals (e.g., independent ambulation at home) (Box 2-5).

> **BOX 2-5**
>
> **STEP PROCESS**
>
> *S*tatus of the patient
> *T*eam members
> *E*nvironment
> *P*rogress toward goals

Situation monitoring leads to situation awareness. This is the shared perception of the current clinical environment. Interprofessional teams lead to better outcomes because multiple members are observing the same situation but from different viewpoints. Situation awareness is enhanced by team members sharing information with the team, asking for information from others, documenting the clinical situation in concise, accurate reports, and by always involving the patient and the family in the information-sharing process. When each team member is aware of the situation in which he or she is working, patient safety is improved.

> The most challenging role of the team leader is in helping to resolve conflict.

Mutual Support

Mutual support refers to team members providing "backup" to others. This aspect of an effective geriatric care team is closely related to situation monitoring and awareness, because often in the busy clinical environment it is difficult to ask for help. Effective teams are aware, and can even anticipate, when a team member may need some assistance. Mutual support is enhanced in an environment of "no blame," but this concept is made most real with the experience each member has in both receiving and giving support. The ability to provide mutual support is dependent on team members knowing the roles of one another. Again, this factor is one of the differences from traditional medical situations where each discipline operates separately. "It's not my job" is not in the lexicon of an effective geriatric care team.

There are two main types of mutual support: task assistance and feedback. Task assistance refers to the ability to help other team members perform their tasks; this may require recognizing when a team member is stressed or overwhelmed, rescheduling noncritical activities, or shifting workload to others. When situations like this arise it is incumbent on the team leader to evaluate whether the plan needs adjustment or whether resources are available to meet the patient's needs and provide for safe care. Although the experience of feeling overwhelmed may be solely the result of a sudden unexpected increase in clinical needs, it also may signal that the team member is in

BOX 2-6

I'M SAFE ACRONYM

Illness: Am I feeling so bad I can't do my duties?
Medication: Could medications I'm taking be affecting my performance?
Stress: Am I under so much stress that it is affecting my performance?
Alcohol/drugs: Has use of these impaired my abilities?
Fatigue: Have I gotten the sleep and rest I need to function properly?
Eating & Elimination: Have I eaten recently or used the bathroom?

need of help. TeamSTEPPS training advises team members to use the "I'M SAFE" acronym to monitor when help may be needed (Box 2-6).

The other type of mutual support that is crucial is feedback. Even the most experienced clinician should have feedback. Patterns of behavior can develop that become habitual and we may even be unaware of our attitudes or actions. Having feedback allows us to see how we are doing from another person's view. The well-functioning team builds feedback into its team processes, and does not limit feedback-giving opportunities to chance or to annual performance reviews.

Feedback is unfortunately often feared, particularly in clinical situations. We may feel like we received enough feedback when we were in school and now that we are professionals we know what to do. The team leader plays an important role in modeling providing feedback in a considerate manner, setting the expectation that members will provide feedback to others, and celebrating when success in behavior modification is seen. The leader can foster feedback receptivity by being open to receiving feedback regularly.

It is important that feedback be specific to a particular situation or task, and not general, such as, "You're doing a good job." Generally feedback should first include elements of the task that were performed correctly (again specific behaviors should be addressed). Then if behavior change is needed the specific actions that occurred and the alternative actions should be presented. An approach that has been shown to be effective is to ask the person receiving the feedback if he or she can think of an alternative behavior before suggesting one. Following this, the person should again receive commendation for the things done well. This way of providing feedback has been called the feedback sandwich.

Feedback should never be provided in an accusatory manner or in front of others. It also must be timely. When feedback is given immediately following a behavior, the person being addressed is likely to remember the behavior. Given too late feedback increases the risk of the person denying that the behavior occurred.

Because the patient is the center of the team's attention, all team members should advocate for the patient's needs. But each team member is likely to view those needs differently. The physician, for example, may see the need for a diagnostic test, or for a medication adjustment, as the most important next step in care. The nurse may believe that patient training in self-monitoring and self-management should be at the top of the list. The social worker may think the next step is to arrange support services in the community. But the key question is, What is the patient's view of the situation? If the patient is motivated toward a particular goal, the ideal time to assist the patient is when the motivation is high. Hence, a team member may need to advocate for the patient's view, even when the team member has good reasons for his or her own agenda. When there are differences of opinion conflicts can arise between team members. Resolution of such conflict is the responsibility of each team member, not just the team leader. Research has shown that when teams neglect advocacy and avoid conflict resolution patient safety is jeopardized. In these circumstances, malpractice risk is increased and patient goals are less likely to be achieved.[26]

There are a number of ways to lessen conflict between team members. These include being assertive (but not aggressive), being willing to challenge another team member when necessary, and being willing to use other team members' assistance.

Assertiveness involves voicing concerns in a non-threatening, respectful way. The team member can open the discussion by addressing the other team member by name, stating his or her concern and the problem that has arisen from that concern, offering a solution, and then obtaining agreement. Assertiveness is different than aggressiveness in that it is never condescending, demeaning, or abusive. When making assertive comments one tends to use "I" much more than "you." Most questions and disagreements can be resolved with this level of interaction.

Sometimes problems arise that necessitate a higher level of intervention. The TeamSTEPPS training process uses two techniques that can be used to resolve difficult conflicts; these techniques are called the "two challenge" rule and "DESC scripts." The two challenge rule was initially used in aviation to help avoid catastrophic failures in flight. If an initial attempt at an assertive intervention failed to result in agreement, and there is the threat of serious harm to the patient, the team member should attempt a more direct challenge twice. Sometimes the other team member is so preoccupied by concerns about the patient that he or she may simply not respond. The first challenge should be framed as a question with an immediate response desired. If that does not work, then the second challenge should be a focused and direct statement of concern. If there still is no response, or the response does

BOX 2-7

DESC SCRIPT EXAMPLE

*D*escribe: Yesterday, in team meeting you said that I was being overly concerned about the patient's adjustment to his stroke.

*E*xpress: This made me feel uncomfortable in front of the other team members because it seemed to devalue my contribution to the patient's care.

*S*pecify: In the future, I would like you to talk to me in private about any concerns you may have about my assessments.

*C*onsequence: If we are both on the same page about the patient's needs I think we'll feel more comfortable working together, and more important, the patient will have a better outcome.

not address the patient safety issue, then the team member must report the issue to the team leader. If the issue is with the team leader, then the problem should be raised to the team leader's supervisor.

The DESC scripts technique can be used when the issue is more interpersonal. The technique was developed in assertiveness training as a method for conveying concerns about behaviors in a nonjudgmental way. Often team members may get bogged down with worrying about who is "right" and who is "wrong" in a situation. The acronym DESC stands for *D*escribe, *E*xpress, *S*pecify, *C*onsequences. The speaker should first describe, in behavioral terms, the problem. It is very important to describe only behaviors, not attitudes, feelings, or any other emotion that the speaker may believe the other person experienced. One can always deny a thought or feeling, but observed behaviors are facts. Then, the speaker expresses his or her concern. The speaker then specifies an alternative behavior and suggests a positive consequence that is likely if the alternative behavior is used. A second DESC script may be necessary, using a negative consequence, if the positive consequence is not successful in changing the team member's behavior (Box 2-7).

When team members provide mutual support to one another, a collaborative practice is possible. Teams that collaborate have the best chance of helping the patient reach desired goals. It does take time and effort, but in geriatric patients with complicated needs the failure to collaborate to understand patient goals, advocate for patient needs, and work to resolve differences can lead to unnecessary hospitalizations and worsening clinical outcomes for the patient.

> Experienced team members in geriatric care have learned to not only monitor the aspects of care for which they are responsible, but also to "cross monitor," observing and recognizing problems that are the province of other team members.

Communication

Much of the previous discussion about the components of an effective geriatric care team focuses on the importance of communication among team members and the patient and family. Communication is the mechanism by which multiple goals are met. Care of complex older patients is inherently risky. Reliable communication between primary team members, as well as secondary members such as consultants, is required for both patient safety and achieving desired outcomes. Research shows that most medical errors involve failures in communication between team members. Communication is the way that teams can provide mutual support, make one another aware of situations that are developing, and resolve disagreements.

One of the most critical times when effective communication skill is needed is during transitions in care, often referred to as hand offs. Effective communication should be complete, clear, brief, and timely. Although it may seem that written communication is likely to be the most explicit, this is often not the case. Handwriting is a frequent cause of medical errors. Key factors in the patient's care may be left out, or abbreviations used that are misunderstood. Written summaries may be produced too late to be useful in the patient's next stage of care or when seeing a different team member.

The SBAR technique was developed in the Navy as a mechanism for clearly communicating a critical situation. It meets all the elements described above for communicating information to another care provider. First, the team member describes the patient's situation. Then key background information is provided. This step takes skill and experience in deciding how much information is to be provided; enough information to allow the other member to function is needed, but too much information can overwhelm him or her with data. Then, the speaker provides an assessment of the patient's needs. Each team member has his or her own area of expertise and that knowledge and experience is communicated in this step. Finally, a recommendation is made. This type of communication can be used in one-on-one discussions between two team members, in briefs and debriefs, and in huddles. Team leaders can promote the behavior by asking for presentations in team meetings to be organized using the SBAR approach (see Box 2-4).

There are many challenges to good communication in teams. There may be differences in language skills or different team members may use different terminology. Interpersonal conflicts and the workload can create stressors. Each discipline in the team comes with its own culture and training. Information may be unavailable or incorrect, and actions by others not on the team may be unknown. But if all team members are committed to a shared mental model that says information about the patient is each of their responsibility, the patient's safety and desired outcomes are more likely to be assured.

> The well-functioning team builds feedback into its team processes, and does not limit feedback-giving opportunities to chance or to annual performance reviews.

ROLE OF THE PATIENT AND FAMILY IN THE TEAM

Perhaps one of the greatest challenges geriatric health care teams face is including the patient, and his or her family, in the team. Professionals use a common language that is not understood by most laypersons. We operate in an environment that usually demands quick and efficient use of resources. We serve multiple patients at one time whereas the family usually is dedicated solely to their loved one. In spite of these challenges teams must include the patient and his or her family in order to provide patient-centered care. There are a number of stages at which patient involvement is crucial. During assessment it is important to obtain the input of the patient and the caregivers to adequately characterize the problems and the resources. This is especially important when the patient has a cognitive deficit or mental health problem. Even when there are no such problems, patients may overestimate or underestimate problems, especially functional deficits. Obtaining copies of previous evaluations is also facilitated by the involvement of the family. The geriatric team members can gather assessment information from multiple sources and then compare notes to form a more complete picture of the problem.

One of the areas to assess early is the patient's goals and wishes. The geriatric care team can offer a variety of suggested interventions or management pathways. Ultimately the patient, or the surrogate decision maker if the patient is incapacitated, must be the one to choose among them. The geriatric care team must be wary of viewing the patient as having "low motivation" or poor adherence when the actual problem may be that the patient does not completely understand the choices or share the same goals as the care team.

When the patient will experience a transition in care setting, he or she must be fully integrated into the team's decision-making process. Ideally, the transition plan will have been developed through a careful elucidation of the patient's goals and wishes, adjusted through the care process based on observed outcomes, and agreed upon by the patient and family. During transitions, each team member has particular goals.

For instance, the physician or nurse practitioner will be establishing follow-up plans for any outstanding studies or consultations, and reconciling the medication list. The nurse will be checking on home care programs, and patient/family education regarding self-management skills. The social worker may be confirming plans for involvement with community-based services and follow-up on mental health issues. Such plans are complicated and inherently increase the risk of "hand-off" problems. The team will need to make sure that the patient and family are not only educated about the plan, but also that everyone involved agrees to the plan.

The final crucial time for ensuring that the patient and family are integrated into the team is when a significant change in status occurs. Older persons have multiple chronic, and often progressive, problems. High-quality geriatric care involves not only managing today's problems, but also helping the patient anticipate future problems. Most chronic conditions are characterized by long periods of slow decline, punctuated by sudden episodes of serious change. For example, when the geriatric team is caring for a patient with heart failure, the team's initial efforts may focus on educating and training the patient in self-management skills and working with the family to support the patient's diet, exercise, and medication program. However, because heart failure is usually a progressive condition, early discussion of the patient's goals and wishes for future interventions is important. Although many patients early in the course of an illness are desirous of aggressive interventions, after years of decline and multiple hospitalizations, many may change their goals and choose less aggressive care. By involving the patient routinely in team discussions, these types of natural changes can be identified and care plans can be adjusted to meet the patient's desires.

> High-quality geriatric care involves not only managing current problems, but also helping the patient anticipate future problems.

CASE 1

Discussion

Mrs. Paul is transferred to the skilled nursing facility and begins her rehabilitation. The new team of the physician, director of nurses, licensed professional nurses, social worker, occupational therapist, and physical therapist each evaluate her needs and develop a care plan based on the patient's plans to return to her apartment after discharge. The social worker discusses with the patient and her daughter ways to increase social engagement and continued physical activity after discharge. A referral to home care is made for continued in-home rehabilitation and a safety assessment. After two weeks Mrs. Paul returns home. The local Retired Senior Volunteer Program volunteer arrives to install grab bars in her bathroom. A visit with her primary care provider was confirmed before discharge from the skilled facility and her daughter accompanies her to that important follow-up visit. ▪

SUMMARY

Older patients often have multiple, interacting chronic conditions, multiple medications, mental health issues, functional limitations, financial challenges, and family or social stresses. This complex web of conditions is overwhelming to the solo practitioner. A team approach is necessary not only because of the complexity, but because different disciplines are more skillful and knowledgeable than physicians in their area of expertise. The team must make every effort to involve the patient and the caregivers in the team deliberations and decisions.

Through this type of patient-centered and family-centered care, geriatric health care teams can achieve cost-effective outcomes that are desired by the patient.

KEY REFERENCES

3. Interprofessional Education Collaborative Expert Panel (American Association of Colleges of Nursing, American Association of Colleges of Osteopathic Medicine, Association of Schools of Public Health, American Association of Colleges of Pharmacy, American Dental Association, Association of American Medical Colleges). Washington, DC; 2011.
12. Gwyther LP, Altilio T, Blacker S, et al. Social work competencies in palliative and end-of-life care. Journal of Social Work in End-of-Life & Palliative Care 2005;1(1):87-120.
18. Nelson K, Merghi J. Emotional dissonance in medical social work practice. Soc Work Health Care 2003;36(3):63-79.
24. Baker DP, Gustafson S, Beaubien JM, et al. Medical teamwork and patient safety: The evidence-based relation. Washington, DC: American Institutes for Research; 2003.

References available online at expertconsult.com.

3

Assessment

Elizabeth N. Harlow and William L. Lyons

OBJECTIVES

Upon completion of this chapter, the reader will be able to:

- Know that successful care of an older adult requires an individualized approach based on the patient's values and preferences.
- Be aware that geriatric patients with common diseases may have uncommon or ill-defined presenting symptoms.
- Know that a detailed history is the major component of initial geriatric assessment.
- Understand that functional assessment provides a window into a patient's overall well-being and can help in prioritizing treatment plans.
- Know that the geriatric physical examination should focus on systems that affect function.
- Maintain realistic expectations when planning for the encounter; complete geriatric assessment will often take several clinic visits to accomplish.

Geriatric assessment is a challenging process that integrates patient-centered medical care and broad medical knowledge. A special approach is needed to care for older adults given the complexity in this patient population. Older adults often have subtle manifestations of disease and an increased prevalence of chronic illness, which make caring for them a challenge. In addition, many older adults will evolve in their health care priorities, which require an adjustment in the provider's clinical approach. Priorities often change from prolongation of life to prolongation of independence and quality of life. These attributes of older adults necessitate individualized care. Caring for older adults does not tend to follow an algorithm, nor is it "cookie cutter" medicine; rather, it requires attention to specific patient needs. Successful care plans align with patients' individual preferences and values.

Adequate evaluation of this challenging, yet very rewarding, cohort requires both an organized approach and flexibility. Geriatric assessment encompasses four main domains of patient care: mental, physical, functional, and social/economic. Not all elements need to be addressed during the initial assessment for every patient; however, each element should be considered eventually as each significantly contributes to overall patient well-being. Complete geriatric assessment will take planning and organization to accomplish over a series of visits. The physician's goal for the initial assessment is not to cover each domain or all of the topics that are covered in this chapter, but rather, to prioritize and plan for the future. Time is often a limiting factor in assessment of the geriatric patient.

Geriatrics by nature is interprofessional. The clinic nursing staff will play an essential role in data collection and patient assessment. Other professionals, such as home health care providers, physical and occupational therapists, and social workers can provide services that will greatly enhance patient care. Communication with these other team members will provide insights that are otherwise unavailable (see Chapter 2).

One practice model through which geriatric interprofessional care works well is the patient-centered

Additional online-only material indicated by icon.

medical home. This model of patient care emphasizes the team medical approach, with the physician as the leader of a team of professionals focused on providing care that reflects the patient's individual priorities. The physician coordinates and facilitates care provided by different participants in the health care team. Disciplines within the patient-centered medical home may include nursing, pharmacy, social work, physical and occupational therapy, and specialty providers. This care model focuses on shared decision making with the patients.

> An individualized approach based on a patient's preferences and values is needed for successful care of an older patient.

CASE 1

Ms. M (Part 1)

Ms. M is an 84-year-old female who visits a clinic to establish care. She has recently relocated to live closer to her daughter after her husband passed away. She is now living in an independent living apartment as part of a senior living center. She is accompanied by her daughter today in the clinic, but she does state, "I could have come alone if I wanted to." As the nurse takes Ms. M into the examination room you note that her gait is relatively stable with use of a cane. The nurse begins the encounter by obtaining vital signs and reviewing the medications that she has brought with her. You sit down to review your notes from her past medical records.

1. **What are some of the unique things you should think about while preparing to care for an older patient such as Ms. M?**

2. **What preparation should be done prior to the clinic visit with a new patient?** ▣

COMMON BARRIERS TO CARE

Several unique challenges are often encountered when caring for older people. The patient ideally should be able to participate in the creation and negotiation of the plan of care. This can be particularly difficult with older adults for several reasons, the first of which is sensory deficits, specifically hearing and vision loss. Providers will often expect that a patient who may be unable to hear verbal or see written instructions is following along, when, in fact, this may not be the case. It is important to ensure that written and pictorial information is visible to older patients with visual impairment. Similarly, when with a patient who is hard of hearing, ensure that the room is quiet and face the patient to enable lip reading. These simple maneuvers ensure that the patient has the best chance of retaining the information. Undiagnosed sensory deficits can lead to inadequate understanding

of care plans. Beyond sensory impairments, diminished health literacy decreases a patient's ability to process information presented to him or her in either a verbal or written format. (To assess a patient's health literacy, consider using an assessment tool such as the Rapid Estimate of Adult Literacy in Medicine—Short Form [REALM-SF][1] or a similar instrument.) For these reasons, it is crucial that a provider use "teach back" methods to ensure appropriate understanding of the treatment plan. If a patient can explain the medical plan to a family member or friend, chances are improved that she will be able to implement the plan at home.

A second significant challenge is that of cognitive impairment. It becomes significantly more difficult to collaborate with a patient regarding a treatment plan if that patient is unable to articulate symptoms or concerns. A caregiver or family member's corroborative history in such a circumstance is invaluable. However, it is important not to ignore the patient. It remains important to involve patients with cognitive impairment in the decision-making process to the greatest extent possible. Building a treatment plan based on a patient's preferences and priorities (see later discussion of goals of care) enables better adherence to the treatment plan regardless of cognitive abilities. It is also wise to send written instructions with all patients, but especially those with cognitive impairment, for later reference. Their written instructions should be written at an appropriate level given a patient's health literacy, which can be assessed using a straightforward tool developed by the Agency for Healthcare Research and Quality. (See active link in web resources.)

A third barrier to care of older adults is that many in the current cohort are passive in interactions with providers. Some will attribute pathologic change to normal aging and pass off important complaints as "no different than anyone else my age." They do not want to be seen as complainers, or worse, burdensome to their caregivers. Additionally, some older patients will be embarrassed by common symptoms such as urinary incontinence, constipation, or falls. Patients will often not bring up symptoms unless asked directly. For this reason, it is important to conduct a complete review of systems, focused on geriatric syndromes.

ASPECTS OF CARE UNIQUE TO OLDER ADULTS

Several health conditions are peculiar to older adults. Some can be the result of decreased physiologic reserve and functional decline, for example, delirium. Others, including Alzheimer's and Parkinson's diseases, result from neurodegeneration. (See Box 3-1 for a complete list.) Many of these diseases will be co-managed with specialists. This necessitates frequent communication for best patient management.

Furthermore, older adults commonly have multiple chronic diseases, or comorbidities. Patients with multiple comorbidities have poorer self-rated functional status and overall health.[2] They also use health care services to a greater degree than older adults with single diseases. Additionally, with increasing comorbid chronic disease, dependency for activities of daily living (ADLs) is seen to increase.[3]

Certain common conditions in older patient populations have been termed *geriatric syndromes*. Geriatric syndromes typically reflect the loss of a person's physiologic reserve caused by the combination of aging and multiple comorbid pathologies. Examples of geriatric syndromes include delirium (loss of brain reserve), urinary incontinence (loss of bladder reserve), and falls (loss of musculoskeletal reserve). Often, screening for geriatric syndromes is incorporated into the history portion of the patient encounter or by incorporating a review of functions into the review of systems.

Geriatric medicine is made more challenging by the way in which common clinical entities present in an uncommon fashion. Older patients will often have ill-defined presenting symptoms such as fatigue, weakness, dizziness, or simply "not feeling well." Such symptoms are nonspecific and difficult to interpret. However, they are often the only presenting symptoms for serious underlying processes. On the other hand, common disease markers in a younger patient population such as fever, leukocytosis, tachycardia, or chest pain may be absent in the elderly because of medication use or physiologic aging. Atypical disease presentation is made more difficult by the fact that geriatric patients have multiple medical comorbidities, often involving more than one organ system, with many overlapping symptoms. Additionally, an older patient may be unable to effectively communicate as a result of limitations in cognition or language. In the absence of stated symptoms, disease processes may present as new functional deficits, delirium, or other geriatric syndromes. A change in functional status should alert an astute practitioner as a potential sign of a serious condition such as infection or worsening of an underlying preexisting condition such as heart failure.

> Geriatric patients will often experience common diseases in an uncommon fashion with vague symptoms.

CASE 1

Ms. M (Part 2)

On review of the medical record you have learned that Ms. M has a medical history significant for hypertension, diabetes mellitus that is diet controlled, hypothyroidism, osteoarthritis, hyperlipidemia, and a stroke with mild residual left-side weakness. With regard to health care maintenance, she is up to date with her annual flu shot, tetanus, and zoster immunizations. She has not had a pneumococcal vaccine, so you make a note for the nurse to administer it later in the visit. She had a bone density scan showing osteopenia approximately 1 year ago. Her last colonoscopy was 8 years ago, with recommended 10-year follow-up. It is unclear when her last pelvic exam with Papanicolaou smear was done. It is also not evident in the medical records when her last eye and dental exams took place. You make a note to enquire regarding all three screens. ◾

PRE-ENCOUNTER PREPARATION

When preparing for a new patient visit, it is prudent to review the patient's medical record ahead of time for an overall understanding of the patient's past medical history. This preview of the available medical information will guide the visit, allowing the provider to prioritize the pertinent medical issues. It will also aid in efficiency because there is often much to cover in little time at the initial visit. A preview of the medical history allows for identification of gaps in understanding. It is wise to review the record for information regarding health care maintenance including vaccinations and screenings (such as dual-energy x-ray absorptiometry scan if appropriate). It is also important to have annual eye and dental exams, because both can be areas of complication with older patients. Medical record review allows for knowledge regarding any specialists also involved in the patient's care with whom coordination will be needed. On the day of the visit, it is important to ask patients to bring their medications (including over-the-counter preparations, and preferably all medications in their original containers), assistive devices (canes, walkers), glasses, and hearing aids with them. If needed, involve family members and caregivers in the visit. Caregivers may be needed for collateral history if there is a question of cognitive impairment, and their presence provides information regarding available caregiver support.

Ideally, the office design and patient flow should keep older patients in mind. The needs of older individuals vary, but it is often necessary to ensure wheelchair accessibility and close parking. It is also helpful to employ rooms large enough to accommodate the patient as well as family members who may accompany the patient. When possible, scheduling should be done in such a way that allows for adequate time for a new patient encounter (often about 50 to 60 minutes).

HISTORY

A detailed history is often the majority of the initial assessment and remains a crucial part of follow-up visits. Although it is unnecessary (and often not feasible) to discuss all of the following with every visit, it is important to maintain a complete understanding of the full patient history and problem list (Box 3-2). Consider allowing the patient to remain dressed for this portion of your patient encounter. This allows patients to remain comfortable (many older adults do not tolerate temperature extremes) and maintain their dignity. It is wise to ensure that enough chairs are available for all parties to be seated. Sitting down while eliciting the history gives reassurance that you are interested in what the patient has to say. It also minimizes dominance in a provider's body language. Finally, it gives the appearance of being unrushed. At some point during the encounter it is appropriate to ask any accompanying family members to step out of the room. This allows for privacy for the patient to speak about any sensitive issues including, but certainly not limited to, elder abuse or sexual dysfunction. It also presents an opportunity for a member of the clinic staff to obtain a collaborative history from the patient's family member(s).

CASE 1
Ms. M (Part 3)

After initial introduction, Ms. M says that overall she has been doing fairly well since her move to your town. She has been feeling somewhat more fatigued than is normal for her. She has been sleeping well, approximately 7 to 8 hours per night. She states that she simply feels more run down. She does note that she has not yet started water aerobics classes, which had always helped her to stay active in her previous town. ◾

BOX 3-2

COMPONENTS OF GERIATRIC HISTORY

Chief complaint
History of present illness
Past medical history
Medications
Social history
Family history
Functional status
Review of systems

Chief Complaint

It is recommended to start the history with the patient's chief concern. This may be as simple as a bothersome symptom, or potentially involved, such as why the patient is transferring care to a new health care provider. Allowing the patient to set the agenda helps him or her to feel more in control. It also establishes rapport if your focus at the onset of the encounter is that which is most important to the patient. After understanding what is most important to the patient you should proceed with other concerns that are pressing either from previous visits or review of the medical record. When evaluating a new patient, important insight can be gained into a patient's understanding of her health by eliciting her understanding of her medical diagnoses.

CASE 1
Ms. M (Part 4)

Ms. M brings a bag of her medications with her. She has brought in an angiotensin-converting enzyme inhibitor for hypertension, thyroid replacement, a statin for hyperlipidemia, and an aspirin, all of which were anticipated from review of her medical record. In addition, she brings in a calcium/vitamin D supplement, ibuprofen that she takes for pain, and a multivitamin. She uses a pill organizer to help her remember what medications she takes when. She denies any problems with missing medication doses. You notice that her thyroid dose is actually different than what was noted in the last clinic visit chart from her previous provider. She also has remembered to bring in her over-the-counter medications, which is extremely informative. You make a note to discuss with her possible alternatives to nonsteroidal antiinflammatory drugs, given their many risks in older patients, when discussing her pain later in the visit. ◾

Medications

During each encounter it is necessary to document an updated, reconciled medication list. Accurate knowledge of a patient's medications is crucial to appropriate prescribing and for quality medical care. Similar to discerning a patient's understanding of medical diagnoses, checking for a patient's understanding of medications can give important information about adherence and cognitive abilities. Discuss with patients their method of medication administration (pillboxes, for example) to see if education or simplification of the regimen can be used to improve adherence. Medication changes and generic medication names are often not recalled accurately, so asking patients to bring their medications to each clinic visit is very helpful. Having access to the actual medication bottles also provides insight into the number of pharmacies and prescribers involved, and refill dates may also be useful in assessing adherence.

This is important to reduce redundant prescribing (see Chapter 6). On review of a patient's medication list, one should scrutinize for problem medications (medications that may be inappropriate for older adults, medications requiring lab follow-up, etc.). It is also important to ensure that your list of patient allergies is up to date.

Ms. M (Part 5)

Ms. M denies tobacco or recreational drug use. She is taking her medications as prescribed. She does drink one glass of wine each evening with her evening meal. She lives alone in an independent living apartment. She has two daughters, one who lives in town and one who lives out of state. Her local daughter is her health care power of attorney. Ms. M notes that she feels safe in her place of residence, although she does not yet feel like it is home. She is continuing to adjust to life in a new city and without her husband of 62 years. When asked to talk a little more about herself, her interests, and her values she mentions that her family has always been the most important thing in her life. She attends church and finds a great deal of comfort in her faith. She has always been active in her community, volunteering and participating in civic organizations. She also mentions that she enjoys playing cards, and she is hoping to find a bridge group soon. When asked about exercise, Ms. M states that she does water aerobics twice weekly, although her daughter disagrees, noting that she has not done this in 6 months.

1. **Beyond health-related habits, how can obtaining a social history be useful?**

2. **How can the social history be used to obtain information regarding a patient's health care goals?** ▣

Social History

Social history can be an enlightening section of the history. Habits, such as tobacco use, alcohol consumption, and exercise, as well as prescription and nonprescription drug use, should be discussed. Alcohol abuse can masquerade as other conditions common in the older population. Alcohol abuse, for example, can appear as gait instability or functional impairment. A person who has a history as a long time social drinker can get into trouble with continued use of alcohol as he or she ages because of changes in metabolism. Similarly, alcohol abuse can slow cognitive functioning or make underlying cognitive dysfunction significantly worse. Additionally, being aware of a person's alcohol habits can be helpful if the patient is ever admitted to the hospital, because withdrawal can be an occult cause of delirium (see Chapter 16).

Beyond discussing a patient's health-related habits, it is important to inquire about a patient's support system at home. Who lives at home? Are there adult children who live in the area? Is the spouse still living? Does the patient serve in a caregiving role? The overarching goal of this discussion is to determine the strengths and weaknesses of an elder's support system. The majority of older adults will experience a period of dependency in their later life. Knowledge of family resources in such cases is helpful in providing optimal care. Additionally, it is important to evaluate for home safety. Does the person feel safe in his or her own home? Are there any concerns for potential elder abuse (financial abuse, caregiver or self-neglect)? It is also important to note who the patient prefers as a surrogate decision maker and to ensure that this is documented in the medical record.

Consider beginning new patient encounters by expressing a desire to get to know the patients and asking them to tell their story. For example, "Can you tell me a little about yourself?" Followed by, "What are some of the things that I need to know to help me take the best care of you?" In this way it is possible to begin to understand in greater detail what the patient values and what some of his or her priorities are. In this discussion attempt to determine what it is that the patient expects from the health care provider. Discuss what the patient's goals are with regard to health care. For example, does the patient desire a primary emphasis on life prolongation? Or an emphasis on preserving independence and self-care function? Or a focus on comfort and symptom control? If the patient is open to it, this may be an opportunity to discuss goals of care and code status. Many providers prefer to wait to start this more difficult conversation until they know the patient better and have a deeper understanding of the patient's medical conditions (Box 3-3). Regardless, it is important to pursue this topic early in the relationship because it sets the framework for many future health care decisions. It also establishes rapport and ensures the patient that his or her opinions and values are an important part of the decision-making process. This process of listening to a patient tell his or her story enables the physician to practice medicine with empathy and understanding.[4]

Ms. M (Part 6)

When discussing her family, Ms. M says that most of her family has been fairly healthy. Her children are in good health, and she has multiple grandchildren that she is quite proud of. Her mother passed away from "old age" in her late 80s. She describes her mother as a "go-getter" to the end of her life, and states that she died after returning home from a gathering, dressed up, and cocktail in hand. Ms. M's father died in his 70s, she thinks of heart disease, but she is not positive. Her husband, who passed about 3 months ago, died after he fell and broke his hip. He subsequently had pneumonia. Ms. M notes that it was all rather sudden and "at least he didn't suffer; I am glad for that." ▣

Family History

Family history in the traditional sense is relatively less important in an older adult, because hereditary risks have usually declared themselves by old age. A family history of dementia can be informative, especially if it is of early onset. A particular benefit of taking a family history is in learning a patient's perspective on the illnesses and treatments received by his or her family members. Both positive and negative experiences with the health care system bring to light what the patient's preferences may be. Additionally, inquiring into the health of children can provide information regarding their potential as future caregivers for the patient.

CASE 1

Ms. M (Part 7)

Ms. M continues to be able to care for herself. She tells you that she is able to perform all of her own activities of daily living without difficulty. She has had someone come in to help with her cleaning for many years because, she says, it was "never something I was good at." She does make all of her own meals, and states that she eats three meals a day. Her daughter notes, however, that part of what prompted the move from her previous home was that on several occasions expired food was found in the refrigerator, untouched. Ms. M manages her own finances, with some oversight by her son-in-law. She states proudly, "for years I have been perfect in balancing my checkbook to the penny" but later admits to a few mistakes more recently. She has not missed paying bills or had overdrafts on her accounts. She drove her car prior to moving to the new city. Now she notes that she no longer wants to drive for fear of getting lost in her new surroundings. She has never had accidents or moving violations, but had gotten lost once previously when she drove to visit her daughter.

1. **What can a patient's functional status tell you about her overall health?**

2. **What is the most efficient way to determine functional status in an office setting?** ■

Functional Screen

Assessment and understanding of functional ability are critical to caring for older patients. Functional status refers to the ability to perform the tasks necessary to participate in daily life. Function gives the provider a picture of the interaction between medical conditions, physical aging, cognition, and overall health in the setting of the patient's environment. Function is a predictor of mortality[5] and a reflection of a patient's level of independence and, by extension, quality of life.[6,7] Understanding a patient's functional abilities gives a window through which to view and prioritize medical illness. It is important to understand a person's baseline functional abilities because a change in baseline function can represent emerging or worsening illness. Functional loss is often the final pathway for progression of multiple clinical conditions. Despite this fact, health care providers often do not recognize the importance of functional disabilities in their patients. Limited care of diseases is just a portion of the complete care of an older adult. At times, disease management is less important than maximizing a patient's function. In addition, knowing a patient's functional status is the only means by which to assess the patient's resource needs and appropriate level of care. Loss of independence is often a sign of the need for involvement of other members of the care team, such as physical or occupational therapists.

It is important to assess skills ranging from basic activities of daily living to more complex instrumental and advanced activities of daily living. Basic ADLs are self-care skills such as bathing or dressing that are necessary to get ready for the day[8] (Box 3-4). Instrumental activities of daily living (IADLs) require more complex mental processes such as executive function and judgment. Such tasks are needed for independent living such as financial management and meal preparation[9] (see Box 3-5). Advanced activities of daily living are individual occupational, social, and recreational activities; decline in these types of activities typically precedes that of ADLs/IADLs.

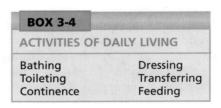

Difficulty in advanced activities of daily living or IADLs may even precede a decline in scoring on cognitive screens. Such a decline should prompt more thorough evaluation.

There are two methods by which to gain information regarding the functional status of a patient: self-report and performance. Self-report is significantly more practical (because it is quicker) but often unreliable. Self-report methods of determining functional status are limited by patients' tendencies to overrepresent or underrepresent their true abilities.[10] Confirmation of function by family members is often necessary, especially in patients with cognitive impairment. There are several easily available questionnaires that can track a patient's status of ADLs and IADLs.[11,12]

Performance-based measurements are more objective assessments of functional status and can be used to confirm a patient's self-report. Several tests that can be performed quickly can give a large volume of information. The "get up and go" test[13] is an assessment of gait and lower leg function. This is done by observing a patient rise from a chair without use of the arms, walk 10 feet, turn around, and return. A wealth of knowledge can be gained by watching this simple maneuver. Gait speed, for example, is a predictor of mortality. The ability to rise from a chair gives information regarding lower extremity strength and the ability to transfer. Similarly, shoulder function can be assessed by having a patient touch the back of his or her head and then placing hands together behind the back to test range of motion. Hand function can be easily tested by having the patient pick up a pencil. Balance can be assessed using a modified Romberg's test, during which the patient stands with the feet together and eyes open. Simple observation of patients' ability to dress and undress themselves and put on socks and shoes provides valuable information regarding independence. Occupational therapy can be usefully consulted for more extensive performance-based functional testing.

One IADL that is particularly important to address is meal preparation. Ask who does the cooking and grocery shopping at home (and who has traditionally done these tasks to see if it has changed). This provides information about the ability to manage a complex task as well as physical stamina. This inquiry may also provide insight into a patient's worrisome nutritional status. Also inquire as to the use of any community resources such as Meals on Wheels or church-delivered food.

Another important aspect to address is patient safety in the home. Is the patient able to navigate any steps required to get in and out quickly in the case of emergency? Are there any firearms in the home? Are there other safety concerns? In this regard, driving status is often a sensitive issue to address. If a patient is driving, it is important to ask not only if he or she has had any driving-related problems, but specific questions such as: Any recent accidents? Moving violations? Passenger complaints? Problems with getting lost in familiar areas? Any of these red flags may indicate a need for further examination and formal driving evaluation by occupational therapy (see Chapter 35).

Assessment of mood and cognition are of particular importance in the older population. Depression can often go unrecognized. It can be a primary condition or associated with comorbid illnesses such as dementia. Screening is easily accomplished through use of a standard instrument such as the Patient Health Questionnaire 2, with more in-depth questioning used as needed. Cognitive assessment (further discussed in Chapter 17) can begin with a screening tool for use with asymptomatic patients. Proven screening tools include the mini-cog (3-item recall and clock drawing) or 3-item recall alone. It is important to know when undertaking a cognitive screen to whom to refer for further cognitive evaluation of persons who screen positively. A full evaluation by neuropsychiatry is often useful in individuals whose cognitive deficits are difficult to tease out with brief testing (such as Montreal Cognitive Assessment or Mini Mental State Exam testing). Screening for cognitive impairment in asymptomatic patients remains controversial and is not universally recommended. One quick screen of attention and concentration that can be used when evaluating for delirium is asking a patient to state the months of the year forward and backward. Inability to complete this task may reflect inattention, which is one criterion for diagnosing delirium. (See chapters regarding specific disease states for more information regarding specific portions of the geriatric examination.)

> **Functional assessment is a crucial piece of the initial assessment because it reflects a patient's overall health status and quality of life.**

CASE 1

Ms. M (Part 8)

On review of systems, Ms. M says multiple times, "I really think I am doing well. I guess I am blessed." She had a recent eye doctor visit with no change in her prescription. She states that her hearing is "not perfect" and that she does have some difficulty in large group settings understanding what people are saying. She does not wear hearing aids. She had a fall approximately 2 weeks ago, just after she moved in to her new apartment. She awoke in the middle of the night to urinate and fell shortly after getting out of bed. She denies any other recent falls. She has not experienced feelings of faintness or palpitations. She does occasionally feel light-headed with standing but denies room-spinning sensations of dizziness. She notes occasional pain in both knees, but adds that it is relieved with ibuprofen. She otherwise has no musculoskeletal complaints. She moves her bowels on a daily basis without difficulty. She does note urinary frequency and urgency symptoms, but no dysuria. She occasionally will leak urine, "but not much" she is quick to add. It does not keep her from participating in her daily activities. She does answer in the affirmative to the question "Have you in the last 2 weeks felt down or depressed," and she states that it started "even before my husband passed." She denies problems with sleeping, but does experience increased fatigue. Her appetite is mildly decreased, but she believes her weight has been stable (her daughter registers surprise on hearing this). When asked about her memory, she says, "Well, I don't remember as well as I used to, but I think that is because of my age." Her daughter has noted her mother to have some difficulty with repetition in conversation and some word-finding problems recently. After you have finished your history, you politely ask the daughter to step out as one of your nurses helps Ms. M get dressed in a gown. You take this opportunity to verify the history you have just obtained. Ms. M's daughter agrees with much of what has been said, but further expresses a concern for her mother's memory. She explains that her mother has always been very bright, but that she has been making more mistakes in her financial management, and has had more difficulty than expected in adjusting to her new environment. She also expresses concern that her mother is not, in fact, eating well. She confides that they have recently had to go shopping for smaller-sized clothes and that she thinks that her mom has lost more than 20 pounds in the last year. You then direct her to the waiting room for the examination portion of the visit, reassuring her that someone will come and get her to wrap up this initial visit.

1. **Why is review of systems of particular importance in the geriatric population?**
2. **What are common symptoms among geriatric patients that are important to screen for?** ▣

Review of Systems

The goal of the review of systems is to ensure that all systems are adequately covered using a method of direct questioning. This is of particular importance in the geriatric population because of their many "hidden symptoms." Patients will often not bring up symptoms owing to embarrassment, normalization, or skepticism that anything can be done. Review of systems typically focuses around geriatric syndromes, many of which patients attribute to normal aging so will not be mentioned without focused questioning. Changes in vision or hearing should be asked about because sensory deficits can exacerbate, or be mistaken for, other common geriatric problems. Ask about falls and feelings of unsteadiness. Has the patient experienced any associated dizziness or presyncope? Make sure to discuss

BOX 3-6	
GERIATRIC REVIEW OF SYSTEMS	
Visual impairment	Hearing impairment
Sleep disturbance	Loss of appetite/weight loss
Depression	Cognitive impairment
Constipation	Urinary incontinence
Falls	Dizziness

any musculoskeletal complaints or pain the patient may be having. Ask about joint mobility because limited range of motion can restrict function. Ask about changes in bladder habits, specifically problems with urinary incontinence, frequency, or urgency. Similarly, bowel habits, such as constipation or diarrhea, can be difficult problems for an elder to bring up but extremely important to their perception of health. A complaint (or admission) of diarrhea should prompt a question about fecal incontinence (see Chapter 24). Screen all patients for depression with the Patient Health Questionnaire 2 (or similar measure). One can quickly uncover symptoms of depression by asking plainly, "In the past 2 weeks how often have you had problems with the following: (1) Little interest or pleasure in doing things? (2) Feeling down, depressed, or hopeless?"[14] A positive screen is appropriately followed up with a more in-depth assessment (see Chapter 18). Questions regarding sleep patterns, appetite, and weight loss are appropriate to pursue after depression screening. The first-line screen for cognitive decline should be the simple question to the patient: "Have you noticed any changes in your memory?" Along the same lines, any patient or family reference to memory decline, behavioral changes, or functional decline may reflect cognitive impairment, depression, or other emerging conditions and require further evaluation. Health care providers can be misled by patients who retain their social skills while masking impairment in executive function, memory, judgment, and orientation.[15] For a full list of important symptoms to cover, see Box 3-6.

A detailed history, including an expanded social history and an in-depth review of systems, is the majority of an initial assessment of a geriatric patient.

CASE 1

Ms. M (Part 9)

On physical exam, Ms. M's vital signs are temperature of 98.2° F, heart rate of 68 beats per minute, respiratory rate of 16 breaths per minute, and blood pressure lying down of 132/86 mmHg. Standing blood pressure after 3 minutes is 126/82 mmHg. Her weight is 142 lbs (which from your review of the medical records is about 20 lbs less than she weighed a year ago, but relatively stable since her last visit with her previous provider 6 weeks ago). Before she leaves the chair, you ask her to cross her arms and attempt to rise unassisted. She is able to do so without difficulty. As she ambulates to the examination table, you observe that she has a narrow-based gait with short strides and a mildly forward-flexed torso. The head, ears, eyes, nose, and throat examination reveals intact vision (acuity of 20/30 in each eye tested individually, with correction). She fails the whisper test bilaterally, but is found to have cerumen blocking her ear canals bilaterally. You make a note to proceed with cerumen removal, and to recheck prior to a referral to audiology. Her oropharynx is mildly dry but otherwise clear. Her dentition and oral hygiene are good. Chest examination reveals regular cardiac rhythm with occasional premature beats and an S4 gallop. No murmurs were heard. Lungs are clear to auscultation bilaterally. Her abdomen is benign. Because she is having symptoms of urinary incontinence, you proceed with a pelvic exam. She has mildly atrophic vaginal mucosa but no other abnormalities. On musculoskeletal exam, she has full range of motion in both hips and shoulders. Her strength is mildly decreased on the left in both upper and lower extremities. Her cranial nerves, with the exception of olfactory, are intact. She demonstrates positive glabellar and snout primitive reflexes, as well as a positive Hoffman's sign on the left. Her neurologic exam is otherwise intact. On cognitive evaluation, she recalls 2 of 3 on the 3-item recall. She draws a clock that is the right shape with accurate numbering; however, the hands are placed incorrectly. Before bringing her daughter back into the room, you confirm that Ms. M feels safe in her home. Finally, you step out as Ms. M redresses to gather all of the information you have collected and to formulate orders for further workup.

1. **What should be the focus of the geriatric physical examination?**

2. **How does a geriatric physical examination vary from that of a younger patient?** ▣

GERIATRIC-SPECIFIC PHYSICAL EXAM

A geriatric-specific physical examination embraces an increased focus on systems that affect function (Box 3-7). Many of the components remain the same as those for a younger individual, but the examination typically includes a more in-depth musculoskeletal and neurologic assessment. A general survey of the patient can provide a wealth of information during the history portion of the exam. It is helpful to take note of the patient's level of alertness and ability to answer questions appropriately. Note also the use of language, in particular, any slurring of speech, word-finding difficulties, or repetitiveness. Evaluate the patient's thought content (is it logical, requiring redirection, or delusional?) and listen for tangential thought patterns. Observe the way the patient is dressed, including grooming and hygiene, as

---

BOX 3-7

IMPORTANT EXAM FINDINGS IN OLDER ADULTS

Eyes:
Cataracts
Decreased visual acuity

Ears:
Decreased hearing
Excess cerumen blocking ear canals

Mouth:
Poor dentition
Dry mucous membranes

Neck:
Elevated jugular venous pressure
Carotid bruits
Limited range of motion in the cervical spine

Chest:
Kyphosis/scoliosis

Cardiovascular:
Irregular heart rhythm
Systolic murmurs and S4 are common

Abdomen:
Palpable aorta
Abdominal bruit

Genitourinary:
Male: prostatic enlargement/nodules
Female: cystocele, rectocele, adnexal masses

Musculoskeletal:
Gait abnormalities
Asymmetry in strength

Neurologic:
Apraxia
Loss of coordination

---

well as the appropriateness of dress for the current weather conditions. This may provide insight into underlying cognitive and functional status. Observe the fit of a patient's clothing, and examine for temporal wasting to determine nutritional status.

Vital signs deserve careful review. Abnormalities such as weight loss, irregular pulse, or tachypnea have important implications. Elevated blood pressure is not unusual with new patients, given an expected level of anxiety, so this should be rechecked, preferably at home. Home blood pressure monitoring has been shown to be an accurate and useful measure of blood pressure.[16] It is helpful to include orthostatic blood pressure and heart rate as part of the routine vital signs taken with older adults. Blood pressure should be taken in the supine position, then at 1 and 3 minutes after standing. The prevalence of orthostatic hypotension (a drop in systolic blood pressure greater than 20 mmHg with standing) significantly increases with age and the finding is common in patients over the age of 85.[17]

This reflects a patient's baroreceptor sensitivity and also provides information about why a patient may be dizzy or unsteady (two common geriatric complaints).[18] A pain scale should be included as part of the vital sign intake because pain, similar to other parts of the review of systems, may be viewed as expected by an elderly patient. Additionally, this provides a way in which to objectify and trend chronic pain.

During the head, ears, eyes, nose and throat examination, visual acuity and visual fields should be checked for deficits. Visual assessment becomes particularly important if the patient has a problem with falls or if there are questions regarding driving abilities. Refer to ophthalmology for further evaluation if visual acuity is 20/40 or worse. There are several methods by which to quickly screen for hearing deficits. When available a handheld audioscope may be most accurate in identifying people most likely to benefit from and use hearing aids. The whisper test and the audioscope, if performed consistently, have been proven to be effective screens for hearing loss (see Chapter 25). If a handheld audioscope is not available, the whisper test is the preferred method because it allows for detection of the specific inability to hear speech. If the patient fails either the whisper or audioscope screening, the next step is evaluation for occluding cerumen. If present, one should retest after removal. If the screen is again failed, the provider should offer referral to audiology for definitive diagnosis and treatment. The oral examination is a useful portion of the geriatric exam because it can give clues to unexplained weight loss (for example, if dentition is poor) or give a potential explanation for falls (if mucous membranes are dry, demonstrating dehydration and possible orthostasis.)

Examination of the chest may reveal dry crackles at the lung bases that do not necessarily imply pathology. Similarly, atrial or ventricular ectopy are also typically benign. A fourth heart sound is common among older adults, even among those without hypertension or heart disease. However, a third heart sound is always pathologic and indicative of heart failure. Systolic heart murmurs are commonly present in many older adults. Many are benign, representing turbulence over a sclerotic aortic valve. If unsure, further evaluation with an echocardiogram may be helpful.

A genitourinary exam is helpful based on patient presentation. With patients who complain of urinary incontinence it is an important part of the evaluation for etiology. Examine for stress incontinence by locating the urethral meatus and asking a patient to cough. Leakage of urine with cough is positive for stress incontinence. Also, one should evaluate for signs of cystocele as possible contributors to urinary incontinence. In addition, vulvar malignancies are not uncommon and palpable ovaries in an older woman are always pathologic. A rectal exam is helpful if there is concern for bowel incontinence (assessment of sphincter tone and perirectal hygiene). Additionally, checking for occult blood can explain anemia, or uncover an impaction that points to the etiology of fecal soiling. In a male with urinary symptoms consistent with benign prostatic hyperplasia (urgency, frequency, nocturia, etc.), a rectal exam can give clues to prostate size and more worrisome symptoms of malignancy such as nodules. Because hyperplasia limited to the vicinity of the urethra (median lobe hypertrophy) can impair urine flow significantly, a gland that feels normal on palpation does not rule out benign prostatic hyperplasia as the cause.

The musculoskeletal and neurologic examinations are particularly important because they provide direct information regarding functional ability. Several of the performance measures of functional ability (discussed earlier) can be incorporated into the flow of the physical exam. Examine any assistive devices needed for ambulation. Check the height of the device to ensure proper fit. With the patient in a standing position, and with their arms fully extended, the top of the cane or walker should be at the break of the wrist (see Chapter 13). Prior to getting on the examination table, ask the patient to perform the "get up and go" test to evaluate leg strength, gait, and balance. Examine the gait for step length, arm swing, and base width. Be sure to note unsteadiness, favoring of one side versus the other, or staggering during a turn. Once the patient is on the examination table, test range of motion, particularly in the hips, shoulders, and hands, because these are most closely related to functional activities. Assess for strength, muscle tone, and bulk. Assess for manual dexterity or clumsiness with rapid alternating movements. Additionally, observe for tremor that may inhibit the ability to perform tasks requiring fine coordination. Finally, with regard to the musculoskeletal system, observe for signs of osteoporosis (for example, kyphosis) and examine specific joints of complaint. When testing cranial nerves, observe for signs of facial droop or tongue deviation that may be indicative of prior stroke. Loss of sense of smell (cranial nerve 1) may occur early in Alzheimer's disease, although this is nonspecific. Primitive reflexes, such as the glabellar, snout, or rooting reflex, indicate evidence of brain dysfunction, although they are not specific to location. Stereognosis and graphesthesia test cortical integration (the ability to integrate multiple areas of input) as well as sensation. Some neurologic changes are commonly seen in older adults (see Box 3-8), and there is debate about the extent to which these changes are pathologic or simply part of normal aging.

Skin examination in older adults can often be overlooked; however, skin is an important source of pathology. Evaluate closely for skin tears and early signs of pressure ulceration in at-risk patients (for example, patients with poor mobility). In particular, examine areas of increased pressure (sacrum and heels) for

BOX 3-8

COMMON NEUROLOGIC CHANGES IN OLDER ADULTS

Cranial Nerve Dysfunction:	**Motor Dysfunction:**
Diminished olfactory sensitivity	Tremor
Unequal pupils	Increased tone in extremities
Diminished pupillary reaction to light	Diminished strength in extremities
Hearing loss	Abnormal gait, decreased arm swing
Diminished Sensation:	**Reflex Abnormalities:**
Decreased vibratory sense in the feet	Absent/diminished ankle jerks

signs of ulceration. Also evaluate for bruising patterns as possible indicators of multiple falls or elder abuse. Monitor lesions for growth, color change, and border irregularity as signs of malignancy.

> **Physical examination of an older adult focuses on systems that directly affect function.**

CASE 1

Ms. M (Part 10)

For further laboratory workup you are interested in Ms. M's kidney function, given her ibuprofen usage. You are also interested in further workup for fatigue and cognitive impairment. Options for further workup are then discussed with Ms. M and her daughter. It is decided to move forward with an expanded workup to gain as much information as possible prior to making decisions regarding treatment. ▣

LABORATORY/IMAGING WORKUP

The primary purpose of laboratory and imaging investigations is to inform clinical decision making in a way that is beneficial for the patient. There is no global evidence-based approach for deciding appropriate laboratory and imaging studies for older adults. To conserve resources and avoid false-positive findings, testing should be based on a patient's presentation and complaints. Overly aggressive testing also runs the risk of finding "incidentalomas," unexpected lesions or results with uncertain significance. Their workup can be costly, risky, and provide ambiguous results. Testing should only be pursued if the result will change the patient's treatment plan and if likely benefits outweigh risks. For example, a screening colonoscopy is an important part of care for a younger patient (see Chapter 4). For an older patient, however, several questions should be

answered prior to proceeding with the study: What are the patient's comorbid conditions? Could the patient tolerate a colonoscopy and its associated anesthesia? What would be done with the knowledge gained by the results? Is the patient an operative candidate, and does surgery fit with the patient's stated goals of care? Is the patient's life expectancy (which reflects age, gender, disease burden, and functional status) great enough that treatment of discovered colonic polyps or cancer would make a difference in her life expectancy? Overall, diagnostic and screening investigations for older patients should be ordered after careful deliberation, with consideration given to procedural risk, "incidentaloma" findings, and patient preferences.

CASE 1

Ms. M (Part 11)

You now feel that you have gotten to know Ms. M fairly well, and you are getting familiar with many of her medical issues. At this point you feel that a strong enough connection has been made for you to broach the topic of goals of care. You start the conversation by saying to Ms. M, "I would like to talk with you about your health care goals. I have patients who tell me that they want me to do everything I can to keep them alive. On the other side, I have patients who request that I make their comfort and quality of life the top priority. Other patients are somewhere in between. What is your thinking on these things?" After much thought, Ms. M comes down somewhere in the middle. She states, "I am not afraid to die, but I just don't think I am ready yet." It is decided that screening procedures will be discussed on a case-by-case basis. She determines that at this time, she would like to remain "full code" (meaning that she wants everything done to prolong her life), but that she would like to "think about this idea more" and talk about it with her daughter.

1. **What is one way to ask a patient about his or her goals of care?**

2. **What is the patient's role in decision making regarding the treatment plan?** ▣

GOALS OF CARE

Discussion regarding goals of care is an important, and ongoing, part of geriatric care. This tends to be a combination of advice and directed decision making based on the information gathered during the social history (the patient's values and treatment preferences). It is helpful to ask the patient, "What are your major health care goals?" Worded differently, this question may be better asked, "What is most important to you at this stage in your life?" This question can be followed up by determining what the patient would want if doing whatever was most important to him or her was no longer possible. Consider subsequent questions to understand the patient's priorities (for example, is life prolongation the priority? remaining independent? symptom control?). It is helpful to understand how the patient wants major health care decisions to be made (if the patient wants to involve family, for example). Finally, given the patient's current quality of life and health care goals, consider discussion regarding resuscitation efforts in the event of cardiac or respiratory arrest. This portion of the discussion may need to be tailored based on a patient's culturally based beliefs and preferences (a good resource from the American Geriatrics Society is available as part of *iGeriatrics* at https://itunes.apple.com/us/app/igeriatrics/id365560773?ls=1&mt=8).

Discussion of goals of care may involve discussion regarding screening and prevention. The importance of screening and prevention in a patient's care is a balance of the patient's preferences and overall prognosis. Additionally, the feasibility of the test to be performed given the functional status of the patient must play a role in the decision-making process. Health promotion, or health and wellness education, should be an important part of this discussion regardless of goals of care. This involves encouragement toward smoking cessation and reduction of alcohol use. Additionally, education should be provided on the benefits of exercise in aging including reduced mortality, balance, cognition, and function (see Chapter 4). This is also an opportunity to encourage patients to be socially active. These topics may be more aptly covered in a "Welcome to Medicare" or annual Medicare wellness examination. This is also an excellent time to ensure vaccinations are up to date.

PATIENT EDUCATION/ SELF-MANAGEMENT

Patient education is a crucial step toward successful patient management outside of the office setting. Assess the ability and willingness of your patient to self-manage his or her medical issues. This can be done by demonstration of understanding of medical problems and the treatments proposed. Self-management can be difficult in older patients given the complexity of medical illness, cognitive deficits, complex drug regimens, and other factors. It may be necessary to involve family members or other supportive individuals in this discussion because they can be helpful in promotion of self-management at home. In discussion with the patient, it is important to set reasonable health care goals. Appropriate goals can include increasing exercise or socialization or setting up a pillbox for medication management. As the clinical encounter comes to a close, it is important to reiterate many of the main points established during the visit and check for understanding. As electronic health records become universal, meaningful use of those

records includes a written after-visit summary that includes any medication changes or important points for the patient to take home for future reference or sharing with caregivers. It is a good idea to ensure that any information provided to the patient is at an appropriate level of health literacy.

CAREGIVER SUPPORT

Caregivers will often accompany an older adult to clinic visits. They can be invaluable sources of collateral history or provide clues as to subtle changes or problems that the patient may be unaware of or unconcerned about. The more dependent a patient is, the more demands are placed on the caregiver. In such situations it becomes important to recognize the importance of the caregiver in the overall well-being of the patient. Although the health of the caregiver of your patient is not your primary concern, caregiver health does, indirectly, affect the health of your patient. Take a few moments to acknowledge the hard work that is being done by the caregiver on behalf of the patient. Emphasize to the caregiver the importance of looking after his or her own health and well-being. Stressed caregivers have been shown to suffer increased mortality.[19] The caregiving role can have negative psychological effects resulting in anger, depression, and anxiety. Maintaining the health of the caregiver, therefore, can be vital in maintaining the stability of an elder's health and preventing institutionalization. It can be helpful to have a list of resources available in the community that may be helpful should a need arise (Alzheimer's Associations [www.alz.org], Area Agencies on Aging [www.n4a.org], www.caregiver.org, driving resources, etc.).

CASE 1

Discussion

With Ms. M's daughter back in the room, you now begin to wrap things up. It is unclear at this time, given her cognitive screening results, how well Ms. M is able to self-manage her health, although she has not shown much difficulty in the past. For this reason, you write down all of your instructions for Ms. M to take home with her. You have arranged for further cognitive evaluation as a result of her cognitive screen. You discuss with Ms. M initiation of a medication for depression; however, she declines. She states that she feels that this is secondary to all of the changes that have recently taken place in her life and that she prefers to wait on medication. You additionally have encouraged her to change from ibuprofen to acetaminophen because it has a more favorable side-effect profile. You will also proceed with cerumen removal between now and her next visit. As they are leaving, you reiterate to both Ms. M and her daughter the importance of follow-up. Much was accomplished in this first visit, but you still feel like there is much to do. You then sit down to construct your to-do list for their next visit in 1 month: (1) Follow up results of cognitive testing and discuss implications. (2) Arrange meeting with social worker for additional support for Ms. M and her daughter. (3) Rescreen hearing in the absence of cerumen; refer to audiology as needed. (4) Query regarding repeat falls; send to physical therapy if needed for balance training and strengthening. (5) Follow up on depression, and if symptoms persist, recommend treatment.

1. **How can you avoid becoming overwhelmed by complicated geriatric patients?**
2. **What can you realistically expect to accomplish on the initial clinic visit?** ▣

FOLLOW-UP VISITS

Commonly, new geriatric patients will require follow-up shortly after their initial visit (typically 4 to 6 weeks) for continued evaluation. It is very likely that much evaluation work has been left undone after the initial visit. Follow-up visits certainly do not need to readdress all aspects of the initial history and physical (Box 3-9). Focus your encounter first on things that have changed since the last visit. Additionally, spend time tying up loose ends from previous visits and any aspects that are most important to patient function (cognition, mobility, hearing and vision in particular). Review medications and functional status with every visit. With complex geriatric patients it can be helpful to cultivate a habit of creating a next-visit to-do list at the end of your clinic notes. This helps provide focus and structure for an otherwise challenging patient population.

> When planning for a geriatric patient encounter, maintain realistic expectations.

BOX 3-9

TIPS TO AVOID FEELING OVERWHELMED

Focus on the patient's priorities (usually function and quality of life).
Do not attempt to do it all in one visit.
Plan for future visits (keep a to-do list).
Delegate tasks to other members of the staff when possible.
Be conservative with testing.

SUMMARY

It is easy to be overwhelmed by the vast needs of a complex geriatric patient. Remember to set realistic goals and plan for the future. Set goals with your clinic encounters as to what has to be done initially, and what can realistically be followed up at a future time. Make sure that your expectations are communicated effectively with the patient and his or her family. It is important to ensure that their expectations align with your own. Realistic goals for the initial patient encounter focus on establishing a relationship with the patient and his or her family. A solid relationship will allow for development of trust and understanding from both parties. Second, establish goals for the care partnership by inquiring as to the patient's expectations and priorities. Third, attempt to maximize medical management of the patient's current medications by simplifying medications and making any changes that are necessary to current treatment regimens. Finally, make any changes possible to improve quality of life and functional status.

Assessment of an older patient is a complex process with several components. Prioritizing before the appointment is crucial to success. Proceed with an organized, patient-centered approach but maintain flexibility. Functional status should be the driving portion of your overall assessment because it is a window to disease progression and quality of life. Use any additional available resources, whether they be nursing, social work, pharmacy, or other professions, because good geriatric care necessitates a team-based approach to medicine.

Web Resources

Rapid Estimate of Adult Literacy in Medicine-Short Form: http://www.ahrq.gov/professionals/quality-patient-safety/quality-resources/tools/literacy/index.html.
iGeriatrics: https://itunes.apple.com/us/app/igeriatrics/id365560773?-ls=1&mt=8).
National Association of Area Agencies on Aging: www.n4a.org.
The Family Caregiver Alliance: www.caregiver.org.

KEY REFERENCES

2. Lee PG, Cigolle C, Blaum C. The co-occurrence of chronic diseases and geriatric syndromes: The health and retirement study. JAGS 2009;57:511-6.
3. Cigolle C, Langa KM, Kabeto MU, et al. Geriatric conditions and disability: The Health and Retirement Study. Ann Intern Med 2007;147:156-64.
4. Charon R. Narrative medicine: A model for empathy, reflection, profession, and trust. JAMA 2001;286:1897-1902.

References available online at expertconsult.com.

4

Wellness and Prevention

Barbara Resnick

OBJECTIVES

Upon completion of this chapter, the reader will be able to:

- Define the purpose of health promotion and disease prevention in older adults.
- Describe an appropriate immunization schedule for older adults.
- Describe three lifestyle modifications that can prevent disease.
- Describe the relevant relationship between nutrition and nutritional status and health.
- Delineate the use of prophylactic medication on cardiovascular, musculoskeletal, and cancer prevention.
- State appropriate cancer screening guidelines for older adults.
- Plan strategies for putting prevention into practice by identifying facilitators and motivational techniques.

ESSENTIALS OF HEALTH PROMOTION FOR AGING ADULTS

Health promotion is the science and art of helping people change their lifestyle to move toward a state of optimal health, defined as a balance of physical, emotional, social, spiritual, and intellectual health.[1] The purpose of health promotion and disease prevention is to reduce the potential years of life lost in premature mortality and to ensure better quality of remaining life. It is the latter focus that is noted to be critically important for older adults. Health promotion activities include the use of immunizations to prevent the occurrence of acute problems such as influenza and pneumonia, risk factor reduction through lifestyle modifications such as smoking cessation or regular physical activity, and the prophylactic use of medication to prevent cardiovascular disease or prevent musculoskeletal disorders.

Additional online-only material indicated by icon.

In addition, health promotion includes screening to facilitate the early identification of disease so that reatment can be initiated. Most important among these is the screening for malignancies.

There are multiple guidelines for health promotion activities available for clinicians as well as patient-specific information to help individuals decide what type of health promotion activities they want to engage in. The decisions about whether or not to adhere to these guidelines are often difficult for the older individual or the individual with health care power of attorney (or proxy) to make. Guidelines for overall health screening decisions[2] can help direct clinicians and the patient or their proxy in this decision process. An individualized approach is critical when working with older individuals in the area of health promotion and should drive the decision process.

CASE 1

Mrs. W

Mrs. W is an 81-year-old white female who is a new patient at your outpatient clinic. She has a history of Parkinson's disease, hypertension, irritable bowel disease with a lactose intolerance, urinary incontinence, hypothyroidism, glaucoma, alcohol abuse (with no alcohol intake for 25 years), and regular nicotine use with a one half pack per day history for 50 years. She currently lives in a senior high-rise and is independent with personal care activities, although she gets help with medication set up into a weekly pillbox. She fixes her own breakfast, but she has her two other meals in the cafeteria or facility dining room. Her weight has been relatively stable, with a consistent body mass index (BMI) of 29.2.

Mrs. W is very concerned about her health and fearful of future health impairments. She participates in regular screenings, including routine colonoscopies, annual mammograms, Pap tests, and dermatologic evaluations, all of which have been negative. She reports that she is unable to tolerate aspirin, calcium, and bisphosphonates because of diarrhea. She has made attempts to cut back and/or stop smoking but has been unsuccessful. She does not exercise regularly. She is, however, very interested in learning about ways to improve her health and prevent problems, although she acknowledges that she does not always follow through with what is suggested. Her medications include dopa/dopadecarboxylase 25/100 mg twice daily, amlodipine 10 mg daily, loperamide up to 12 mg a day as needed, and intermittently tolterodine 4 mg daily.

1. **What interventions might you implement to help Mrs. W's quality of life?**

2. **How would you prioritize your interventions?**

3. **What motivational strategies would you use to help Mrs. W change her behavior in areas such as smoking cessation and exercise?**

PREVENTION OF DISEASE

Immunizations

Table 4-1 provides an overview of recommendations for immunizations for older adults. The U.S. Advisory Committee on Immunization Practices and the Centers for Disease Control currently recommend that all older adults be immunized against influenza annually and that they receive at least one pneumococcal vaccination.[2,3] All older adults 65 years of age and older should receive an additional pneumococcal vaccination 5 years or more after their first immunization, if they were vaccinated with $PPSV_{23}$ before the age of 65. The Food and Drug Administration has approved the zoster vaccine for use in persons age 50 and above; however, the Advisory Committee on Immunization Practices continues to recommend that vaccination begin at age 60.[3] Compliance with recommended immunization guidelines has improved, although the goal set in Healthy People 2010 of 95% adherence to immunization has not been met and adult adherence rates continue to lag behind those seen in children.[4] To facilitate compliance the federal government in 2002 approved standing orders for annual influenza vaccinations and pneumococcal pneumonia vaccination for older adults in institutional settings and home health agencies for all Medicare and Medicaid beneficiaries. Medicare health

TABLE 4-1	Immunizations Indicated for Older Adults
Vaccine	**Indicated for Older Adults**
Influenza	1 dose annually
Tetanus, diphtheria, pertussis (Td/Tdap)	1-time initial dose and a booster every 10 years with Td
Varicella	2 doses are needed if the individual has never had varicella
Zoster	1 dose
Measles, mumps, rubella	1 dose if never had the diseases—adults born before 1957 are assumed, however, to be immune.
Pneumococcal	1 dose unless high risk and then may be revaccinated once in 5 years after initial vaccination.
Hepatitis A	Vaccinate only if at high risk/seeking protection from hepatitis A (behavioral risk factors; occupational risk factors; travel to countries that have high or intermediate endemicity of hepatitis A)
Hepatitis B	Vaccinate only if at high risk as noted above

coverage (Part B) will cover vaccines to prevent influenza and pneumonia and hepatitis B if the patient is at medium to high risk for this disease. No copay is associated with these vaccines. All vaccines, other than those for flu, pneumonia, or hepatitis B, are covered under Medicare Part D; this includes the vaccine for zoster.[5]

Risk Factor Reduction through Lifestyle Behaviors

Smoking Cessation

Even though older adults are less likely to get counseled for smoking cessation, they can successfully quit smoking and have demonstrated quit rates similar to that of younger adults. Despite common assumptions, older adults are not more likely than younger individuals to have nicotine addiction.[6] Unfortunately, however, older adults are less likely to be exposed to smoking cessation interventions.[7]

The most commonly used model to promote individual smoking cessation is Prochaska's transtheoretical model of change.[8] Individuals are evaluated and encouraged to proceed through the following stages: precontemplation, contemplation, preparation, action, and maintenance. The Agency for Healthcare Research and Quality recommends the use of the "4 As" (ask, advise, assist, and arrange follow-up) in patients ages 50 and older, counseling interventions, physician/health care provider advice, buddy support programs, age-tailored self-help materials, telephone counseling, and the nicotine patch as effective interventions to facilitate smoking cessation in adults 50 and older. There is Medicare coverage to implement these interventions for up to eight visits per year.

Pharmacologic interventions for smoking cessation are also an option and are known to augment behavioral interventions. Seven first-line medications (five nicotine and two non-nicotine) reliably increase long-term smoking abstinence rates: Bupropion SR; nicotine gum, inhaler, lozenge, nasal spray, or patch; and varenicline. Nicotine replacement is generally well tolerated; but it may cause a local skin reaction if used in patch formulation, mouth soreness or dyspepsia if gum is used, nasal irritation with nasal spray, or oral irritation if used as an inhaler. Nicotine may also cause some insomnia. Likewise bupropion can cause insomnia and dry mouth, and varenicline can cause nausea and depression.

Prevention of Polypharmacy

Polypharmacy is the use of more medications than are clinically needed or indicated. Older adults are particularly at risk for polypharmacy because of multiple comorbidities and the risk of seeing multiple health care providers. The best way to prevent polypharmacy is to avoid unnecessary medication use and attempt to implement behavioral interventions as a first line of treatment. Specifically, dietary interventions, exercise, stress management, and behavioral management techniques will often be sufficient if implemented and adhered to. Moreover, combining behavioral interventions with medications may allow for lower drug dosages to be used. Clinicians should also make certain to be very clear about drug use instructions and provide both verbal and written accounts of how to use the medication. Drug regimens should be simplified, and medications should be reviewed at each provider–patient interaction (see Chapter 6).

Screening for Alcohol Use/Abuse

> The CAGE questionnaire is well suited to busy primary care settings because it poses four straightforward yes/no questions.

The prevalence of current alcohol use tends to decrease with increasing age, with results in 2010 showing a decrease from 65.3% among 26- to 29-year-olds to 51.6% among 60- to 64-year-olds and 38.2% among people 65 or older.[9] The rate of binge drinking among persons 65 or older in 2010 was 7.6%, and the rate of heavy drinking was 1.6% in this age group.

The most reliable alcoholism-screening instruments are self-report questionnaires. Screening instruments vary in their ability to detect different patterns and levels of drinking and in the degree of their applicability to specific subpopulations and settings. The CAGE (Box 4-1) questionnaire[10] is commonly used among clinicians. When used with older adults, it has reported sensitivities ranging from 43% to 94% for detecting alcohol abuse and alcoholism. The CAGE questionnaire is well suited to busy primary care settings

---

BOX 4-1

CAGE QUESTIONNAIRE

CAGE Questions*
1 Have you ever felt you needed to Cut down on your drinking?
2 Have people Annoyed you by criticizing your drinking?
3 Have you ever felt Guilty about drinking?
4 Have you ever felt you needed a drink in the morning (Eye-opener) to steady your nerves or get rid of a hangover?

From Liskow B, Campbell J, Nickel EJ, Powell BJ. Validity of the CAGE questionnaire in screening for alcohol dependence in a walk-in (triage) clinic. J Stud Alcohol 1995;56:277-81.
*Two or more positive answers is considered to be a positive screen.

because it poses four straightforward yes/no questions. It may fail, however, to detect low but risky levels of drinking and often performs less well among women and minority populations. Other measures include the 25-question Michigan Alcohol Screening Test (MAST),[11] which was revised to be more relevant for older adults,[12] or the Alcohol Use Disorders Identification Test.[13] (See also Chapter 34.)

Health Benefits and Risks of Alcohol Use

The signs and symptoms associated with alcohol abuse in the older adult are numerous and include the same spectrum of physical, behavioral, and psychological problems that can be found in younger individuals. Conversely, however, a number of health benefits have been associated with moderate alcohol consumption.[14] Specifically, there is evidence to suggest that one to two standard drinks has a positive effect on lipid metabolism,[15] results in decreased mortality following a myocardial infarction, decreases risk of developing congestive heart failure, and may lower the risk of ischemic stroke in the young-old (60 to 69 years of age).[16] In several large epidemiologic studies[17,18] an association between alcohol and cognition suggests that moderate alcohol use was not associated with cognitive decline.

PHYSICAL ACTIVITY

> For healthy, asymptomatic adults of any age, the U.S. Preventive Services Task Force (USPSTF) does not recommend any type of cardiac screening before initiating of physical activity. For asymptomatic sedentary older people, low-intensity physical activity can be safely initiated regardless of whether or not an older person has had a recent medical evaluation.

A substantial body of scientific evidence indicates regular physical activity can bring dramatic health benefits to older adults (Table 4-2). Moreover, physical inactivity increases one's risk of dying prematurely, of dying of heart disease, and of developing diabetes, colon cancer, and high blood pressure. Physical activity allows older individuals to increase the likelihood that they will extend years of active independent life, reduce disability, optimize mental health, and improve their quality of life in midlife and beyond.[19-22]

Guidelines for Physical Activity

Older adults need to regularly engage in both aerobic and resistive exercise weekly to optimize health.[23]

TABLE 4-2	Health Benefits of Physical Activity for Older Adults		
Health Issue	**Physical Activity**	**Level of Evidence for Effectiveness***	**Comments**
Cardiovascular health[74-76]	Increasing aerobic activity	A	• Improves myocardial performance • Increases peak diastolic filling • Increases heart muscle contractility • Reduces premature ventricular contractions • Improves blood lipid profile • Increases aerobic capacity • Reduces systolic/diastolic blood pressure • Improves endurance • Improves muscle capillary blood flow
Body composition[77]	Increasing aerobic activity	A	• Decreases abdominal adipose tissue • Increases muscle mass
Metabolism[78]	Increasing aerobic activity	A	• Increases total energy expenditure • Improves protein synthesis rate and amino acid uptake into the skeletal muscle • Reduces cholesterol/very low density/LDL lipoproteins/triglycerides • Increases high-density lipoproteins • Increases glucose tolerance
Bone health[79,80]	Increasing weight-bearing exercise	A	• Slows decline in bone mineral density • Increases total body calcium, nitrogen
Psychological well-being[81,82]	Increasing aerobic activity	A	• Improves perceived well-being and happiness • Decreases stress-related hormones • Improves attention span • Improves cognitive processing speed • Increases slow wave and rapid eye movement sleep • Provides sense of accomplishment • Decreases anxiety and improves mood

*A = supported by one or more high quality randomized trials; B = supported by one or more high quality nonrandomized cohort studies or low-quality RCTs; C = supported by one or more case series and/or poor quality cohort and/or case-control studies; D = supported by expert opinion and/or extrapolation from studies in other populations or settings

Older adults should also do exercises that maintain or improve balance if they are at risk of falling. Specifically, clinicians should recommend that older adults engage in 150 minutes of moderate intensity physical activity weekly. This activity should be done in at least 10-minute spurts and should be spread throughout the week. Moderate intensity of activity is defined as physical activity that is done at 3.0 to 5.9 times the intensity of rest. On a scale relative to an individual's personal capacity, moderate intensity physical activity is usually a 5 or 6 on a scale of 0 to 10.[24] Activities such as brisk walking, dancing, swimming, or biking are considered moderate intensity activities. Resistance training or muscle strengthening should also be done 2 days a week and should include all the major muscle groups (legs, hips, back, abdomen, chest, shoulders, and arms).[23,25] Generally 8 repetitions of each exercise are recommended and the amount of resistance will vary for each individual. The individual should use a weight that can be comfortably lifted for the full 8 repetitions. Balance exercises, such as backward walking, sideways walking, heel walking, toe walking, and standing from a sitting position should be done at least 3 days a week.

Guidelines for Screening before Exercise

Initiation of a moderate intensity exercise program is safe for all older adults.[26,27] Moreover, there is evidence to support that engaging in sedentary lifestyles increases risks to cardiovascular health.[28] If the clinician feels that it will be helpful to the older adults to go through some type of screening, the Exercise and Screening for You screening tool[27] can be completed. This interactive web-based tool can be done by the older adults or the clinician and provides assurance that, given no underlying clinical problems, the individual is safe to exercise. In addition the tool provides guidance for what type of exercises to do given underlying health concerns. There are also numerous resources available at no cost to guide the older adult through resistive exercise programs and aerobic activities such as those from the National Institute of Aging[25] and the Centers for Disease Control.[29]

MAINTAINING OPTIMAL NUTRITIONAL INTAKE

> Evaluating food intake in older adults is important because inadequate intake can result in weight loss, loss of muscle mass, decreased strength and power, decreased walking speed, impaired balance, and a decline in activity.

Age-Relevant Requirements

Nutritional health is important to consider in older adults because it can reflect medical illness, depression, dementia, inability to perform the functional tasks of shopping or cooking, inability to self-feed, financial challenges, or poor oral health, among other problems. In addition, nutrition contributes to frailty. A low body mass index (kg/m^2 ≤20) or an unintentional weight loss of ≥10 lbs in 6 months suggests poor nutrition and should be evaluated.

For older adults there is a general decline in calorie needs resulting from a slowing of metabolism and a decrease in physical activity. Nutritional requirements, however, generally remain the same. MyPlate for older adults addresses the needs of older adults based on the 2010 Dietary Guidelines for Americans.[30] Table 4-3 lists the recommendations in MyPlate. MyPlate for older adults replaces the Modified MyPyramid for older adults. The following foods, fluids, and physical activities are represented on MyPlate for older adults: bright colored vegetables; deep colored fruits; whole, enriched, and fortified grains and cereals; low-fat and nonfat dairy products; dry beans; nuts; fish; poultry; lean meat; eggs; liquid vegetable oils; soft spreads low in saturated and trans fat; spices to replace salt; fluids such as water and fat-free milk; and physical activity including walking, resistance training, and light cleaning. Icons are used to facilitate understanding.

Water

Water is essential for joint lubrication; transport of nutrients and salts; hydration of skin, eyes, nose, and mouth; removal of waste products; regulation of body temperature; and adequate blood volume. Inadequate hydration can result in constipation, fatigue, hypotension, hyperthermia, dizziness, breathing difficulties, and irregular heartbeat. Fluids are best taken in the form of water, juice, or milk; alcohol, caffeinated tea and coffee, and soft drinks have a diuretic effect and raise fluid level more modestly.

Fats

Fat intake should be no more than 20% to 35% of total calorie intake per day.[31] The 2010 Dietary Guidelines[30] recommend that older adults consume less than 10% of calories from saturated fat and that they replace saturated fat with monounsaturated and polyunsaturated fat. In addition, older adults should consume less than 300 mg of dietary cholesterol and keep trans fat consumption as low as possible by limiting partially hydrogenated oils and solid fats. Saturated fats can raise blood cholesterol and increase risk of heart disease. A simple way to determine the allowable grams of fat per day is to divide the individual's ideal weight in half and allow that number of grams of fat. Monounsaturated fats (e.g., olive oil) are best

TABLE 4-3	MyPlate Guidelines for Older Adults	
Foods to Reduce	**Foods to Increase**	**Weight Management**
Reduce daily sodium to less than 2300 mg; further reduce to 1500 mg for those ≥51 years and those at any age who are African American, hypertensive, diabetic, or suffering from chronic kidney disease. Consume <10% of calories from saturated fatty acids and replace them with monounsaturated and poly-unsaturated fatty acids. Consume <300 mg per day of dietary cholesterol. Keep trans fatty acid consumption as low as possible by limiting foods that contain synthetic sources of trans fats, such as partially hydrogenated oils, and by limiting other solid fats. Reduce the intake of calories from solid fats and added sugars. Limit consumption of foods that contain refined grains, especially refined grain foods that contain solid fats, added sugars, and sodium. Keep alcohol intake to one drink per day for women and two drinks per day for men.	Increase vegetables and fruits Consume at least half of total grains consumed as whole grains. Increase intake of fat-free or low-fat milk/milk products. Choose various protein foods (seafood, lean meat, poultry, eggs, beans, peas, soy products, unsalted nuts, seeds). Increase the amount and variety of seafood consumed. Replace protein foods high in solid fats with food lower in solid fats/calories and/or sources of oils. Use oils to replace solid fats. Choose foods high in fiber, potassium, calcium, and vitamin D.	Prevent and/or reduce overweight and obesity through improved eating and physical activity. Control total calorie intake to manage body weight. Increase physical activity and reduce time spent in sedentary behaviors. Maintain appropriate calorie balance during each stage of life.

Adapted from U.S. Department of Agriculture and U.S. Department of Health and Human Services. Dietary guidelines for Americans, 2010. 7th ed. Washington, DC: U.S. Government Printing Office; December 2010.

because they lower low-density lipoprotein (LDL) but leave the high-density lipoprotein (HDL) intact. Poly-unsaturated fats, such as sunflower, corn, and soybean oils, appear to lower LDL and HDL.

Fiber

Fiber, an indigestible residue of food, is a natural laxative, adds bulk to stool, absorbs water, and reduces gut transit time. It is recommended that older adults consume 14 g of dietary fiber per 1000 calories consumed. Ideally fiber intake should include cereal fibers and be consumed with 64 oz of fluid daily.

Protein

Proteins form antibodies that help resist disease and enable growth and repair of cells. Complete proteins contain the eight essential amino acids needed and are found in foods such as fish, dairy products, and eggs. Protein should make up 12% to 20% of the total calories.[31] It is common for acutely ill older adults to become protein deficient (see Chapter 28).

Micronutrients: Vitamins and Minerals

Micronutrients (vitamins and minerals) are important to overall health. Five servings of fruits and vegetables daily optimizes vitamins A, C, and E, and potassium. Vitamin B_{12} intake is generally adequate, although older adults should be encouraged to increase intake of the crystalline vitamin B_{12} found in fortified foods such as whole-grain breakfast cereals. Vitamin D intake is generally below recommendations, which range from 1000 to 2000 IU daily.[30,32] Supplementation is generally needed. Water-soluble vitamins (C and eight of the B vitamins) are excreted in urine, although adverse effects can result from exceeding the upper-level recommendations. The surplus fat-soluble vitamins (A, D, E, and K) are stored in body tissue, and excessive amounts can be toxic.

Assessment of Nutritional Health and Approach to Obesity

Nutritional screening using the Mini Nutritional Assessment[33] identifies individuals who are malnourished or at risk (see Chapter 28). Obesity is a growing problem among older adults and individuals should be evaluated for obesity (BMI ≥30). Obesity puts older adults at risk for decreased physical activity and may actually be indicative of poor diet quality.

The most effective route to weight loss in older adults combines nutrition education, diet, and exercise with behavioral strategies. Studies demonstrate little difference in weight loss between individuals using low-carbohydrate versus low-fat diets.[34,35] For individuals who have hypertension and are overweight, the Joint National Committee on Prevention, Detection, Evaluation, and Treatment of High Blood Pressure[36] suggests counseling patients on adopting a salt-restricted diet, increasing physical activity, and decreasing alcohol consumption. The Dietary Approaches to Stop Hypertension (DASH) eating plan is recommended because it consists of fruits, vegetables, whole grains, low-fat dairy products, poultry, and fish.[37]

PROPHYLACTIC MEDICATION USE
Prevention of Cardiovascular Disease

> Despite evidence that oral anticoagulation with warfarin is the most effective prevention of stroke caused by atrial fibrillation, older adults are less likely to receive this treatment. When addressing anticoagulation, consideration should be given to quality-of-life issues and the need for ongoing monitoring of blood work, as well as underlying disease and lifestyle issues.

Clinical trials remain the cornerstone for guiding providers as to what treatment options are provided to older individuals regarding prevention of cardiovascular disease. The "ABC" format (antiplatelet agents/anticoagulation, blood pressure control, cholesterol management) has been used to best summarize findings and organize recommendations.

Antiplatelet Agents

The latest guidelines for secondary stroke prevention recommend that aspirin monotherapy, aspirin 25 mg plus ER dipyridamole 200 mg twice daily, or clopidogrel monotherapy (75 mg/day) are all acceptable options for initial therapy for patients with noncardioembolic (i.e., atherothrombotic, lacunar, or cryptogenic) ischemic stroke or transient ischemic attack who have no contraindications to the use of an antiplatelet agent.[38,39] Aspirin inhibits the cyclooxygenase enzyme involved in the production of thromboxane, a factor that promotes platelet aggregation. Guidelines for the primary prevention of stroke recommend that aspirin be used in individuals whose risk is high enough for the benefits to outweigh the risks of this antiplatelet therapy (i.e., 10-year risk of coronary heart disease of 6% to 10%).[40] The use of aspirin, according to these recommendations, is associated with a reduction in the risk of a first stroke in women but not in men. As a result, aspirin is not recommended for the prevention of a first stroke in male patients. However, according to the recommendations above, aspirin can be used in at-risk men to reduce the risk of cardiovascular events. In the absence of a contraindication, the use of aspirin is also recommended for all patients with asymptomatic carotid artery stenosis for the primary prevention of stroke.[40,41] Aspirin use is known, however, to increase the risk of gastrointestinal irritation owing to the antiplatelet and gastric mucosal effects, and cotherapy with a proton pump inhibitor is an effective preventive option. Clopidogrel inhibits platelet activation by blocking the binding of adenosine diphosphate to its receptor on the platelet surface. As shown in several randomized trials, clopidogrel should be recommended in place of aspirin in patients who are intolerant or resistant to the effects of aspirin.[38,39]

The use of warfarin or aspirin to prevent stroke in older adults with a known history of atrial fibrillation should likewise be addressed. (See Chapter 6 for an extensive discussion of warfarin management.) As with other health prevention interventions, the patient needs to be aware of the risk versus benefit to treatment and the implications of accepting or rejecting treatment options. Repeatedly, it has been shown that oral anticoagulation with warfarin is the most effective prevention of stroke caused by atrial fibrillation.[42,43] Clinicians, however, are often fearful of anticoagulating older adults because of the risk of falls and associated bleeding. Consideration should certainly be given to the risk/benefit of anticoagulation among older individuals and the individual or proxy should be included in the decision-making process. If a decision to treat with warfarin is made, optimal anticoagulation in the range of 2.0 to 3.0 international ratios (INR) should be the goal. The risk for intracranial hemorrhage was reported to increase for those 85 years of age or older when the INR ranged from 3.5 to 3.9. The risk of intracranial hemorrhage at INRs of less than 2.0, however, was not different from the risk of hemorrhage at INRs of 2.0 to 3.0.[44]

Beta-Blockers

Beta-blocker use has been recommended to prevent first events of nonfatal myocardial infarction in patients with high blood pressure since 1989.[45,46] Beta-blocker use has also been noted to be effective as secondary prevention of a myocardial infarction and can lead to a 19% to 48% decrease in mortality and up to a 28% decrease in reinfarction rates.[46] Older adults may need to be started on a lower dose than recommended in the younger adult population owing to normal physiologic changes that increase the risk of low cardiac output and bradycardia. In patients with type 1 diabetes, nonselective beta-blockers can impair glucose control, leading to hypoglycemia, and blood glucose levels should be monitored regularly in these individuals. In patients with type 2 diabetes, the incidence of hypoglycemia with beta-blockers is much lower. However, hyperglycemia is more common in patients with type 2 diabetes as a result of beta-blocker inhibition of insulin release. Beta-blockers should be avoided in patients with type 1 diabetes if possible, primarily in those prone to developing hypoglycemia. Because glucose regulation is mediated in part by beta-2 receptors, beta-1 selective agents may cause less of an alteration in glucose, insulin, and glucagon concentrations in diabetic patients. The greatest risk when using beta-blockers is the risk of bradycardia, particularly among older adults who have a sinus bradycardia and partial AV block, and are also receiving diltiazem, verapamil, or digoxin. Bronchoconstriction can occur, especially when nonselective beta-blockers are administered to asthmatic patients. Therefore, nonselective beta-blockers are contraindicated in patients with asthma or chronic obstructive pulmonary disease. Abrupt withdrawal may precipitate rebound tachycardia or a myocardial infarction.

Statins

The Adult Treatment Panel III of the National Cholesterol Education Program established current recommendations based on a review of five randomized, controlled clinical trials. Overall, the statins seem to be most helpful in patients who have underlying cardiovascular disease.[47,48] In the meta-analysis by the Cholesterol Treatment Trialists Collaboration, statins prevented 18 major cardiovascular events for every 1000 patients without preexisting coronary heart disease treated. In contrast, 30 major coronary events were prevented for every 1000 patients with existing coronary heart disease treated more than 5 years. This reduction was similar in patients older than 65 years of age.[49] It should be recognized, however, that although there were some older adults in these trials, very few of the participants were older than 70 years of age. In high-risk persons, treatment should be aggressive, and the recommended LDL cholesterol (LDL-C) goal should be less than 100 mg/dl and ideally could drop to an LDL-C goal of less than 70 mg/dl. Moreover, when a high-risk patient has high triglycerides or low HDL cholesterol (HDL-C), consideration can be given to combining a fibrate or nicotinic acid with an LDL-lowering drug. For moderately high-risk persons (two or more risk factors and 10-year risk of 10% to 20%), the recommended LDL-C goal should at least be less than 130 mg/dl. In addition to drug treatment, all individuals at high or moderately high risk for coronary heart disease who have lifestyle-related risk factors (e.g., obesity, physical inactivity, elevated triglycerides, low HDL-C, or metabolic syndrome) should be encouraged to engage in appropriate lifestyle modifications.

Prevention of Musculoskeletal Disorders

> It is never too late to initiate healthy habits that augment musculoskeletal health. This is best done by incorporating exercise into daily activities and getting optimal calcium and vitamin D intake.

Although prevention of musculoskeletal disorders ideally should begin in childhood and young adulthood, it is never too late to initiate healthy habits that will augment musculoskeletal health as one ages. This is particularly true with regard to osteoporosis and degenerative joint disease. Osteoporosis by definition is a bone density that is 2.5 or more standard deviations below the young-adult peak bone density. Osteopenia, defined as 1 to 2.5 standard deviations below the young-adult peak bone density, is a weakening of the bones that, if left untreated, will likely progress to osteoporosis. The USPSTF recommends that routine screening for osteoporosis begin at age 65 for all women.[2] It is not clear, however, how often individuals should go through screenings and/or when such screening should be terminated.

Exercise is central to prevention of osteoporosis and is one of the most effective nonpharmacologic treatments for osteoarthritis.[50,51] (See Chapter 44.) Muscular conditioning can be achieved through long-term walking, isokinetic quadriceps exercise, high- and low-intensity bicycling, aquatic exercise classes, and tai chi.[52-57] In addition to exercise, dietary and pharmaceutical interventions are effective in maintaining and improving bone density.[58] (See Chapter 43.)

Calcium and Vitamin D

The nutritional needs for bone health can be met by a diet high in fruits and vegetables, adequate in protein but moderate in animal protein, and that includes dairy or calcium-fortified foods. When calcium from diet is inadequate, supplements spread out through the day, for a total intake of 1200 to 1500 mg, are recommended. No more than 500 mg should be consumed at a meal to optimize absorption. The upper limit for calcium supplementation is 2500 mg per day. Calcium is difficult to absorb, and foods such as spinach, green beans, peanuts, and summer squash inhibit calcium absorption. In addition, high levels of protein, sodium, or caffeine increase excretion of calcium and should be avoided. Calcium citrate is better absorbed than is calcium carbonate and does not need to be taken with food.

In individuals older than 70 years, vitamin D intake of at least 600 IU per day (up to 1000 IU per day) and an upper limit of 2000 IU per day is recommended to enhance absorption of calcium, strengthen bones, and decrease risk of fracture.[59,60] Dosages of 100,000 IU every 4 months have been reported to decrease the risk of first fracture among older males and females living in the community.

Bisphosphonates

Bisphosphonates are recommended for the prevention and management of osteopenia. Decisions regarding their use should be based on the individual's comorbidities, lifestyle, cognition, and personal preferences. Adherence to the treatment protocol for safe and effective use of bisphosphonates may be challenging for older individuals (see Chapter 43).

Glucosamine and Vitamin D

Glucosamine in dosages of 1.5 g per day and vitamin D are currently recommended to prevent osteoarthritis. It is not clear what dose of vitamin D is needed. It appears that adequate blood levels may help delay onset of hip osteoarthritis and decrease risk of progression of knee osteoarthritis.[61] In addition, glucosamine may help in management of osteoarthritis, but only certain preparations and a subset of patients with more severe disease are likely to respond.[62] (See Chapter 44.)

CANCER SCREENING

> Determining whether an older adult should undergo screening depends on the risk of the disease, the benefit of screening, the implications of not screening, and whether or not treatment is an acceptable option.

There are numerous published recommendations for cancer screening for older adults and specific guidelines for Medicare coverage for the recommended screening tests. Determining whether an older adult should undergo screening depends on several key factors: the risk of the disease, the benefit of screening, the implications of not screening, and whether or not treatment is an acceptable option. Strict adherence to guidelines for all older adults, however, can result in unnecessary stress and burden to the individual. Decisions about screening should be individualized, so that the potential benefit and burden can be assessed by patient or proxy and clinician.

Breast Cancer Screening

Breast cancer screening guidelines from organizations differ on when to stop screening, the frequency of screening, and whether to include clinician or breast self-examination. The USPSTF recommends biennial screening mammography for women aged 50 to 74. In women age 75 and older there is insufficient evidence to determine the benefits versus harm to continued use of screening mammography. There is also insufficient evidence to assess the additional benefit versus risk of clinical breast examination beyond screening mammography in women 40 years of age and older.

Colon Cancer Screening

Consistently the published guidelines recommend that individuals 50 years of age and older undergo annual colon cancer screening. The USPSTF 2 recommends screening for colorectal cancer using fecal occult blood testing, sigmoidoscopy, or colonoscopy in adults, beginning at age 50 years and continuing until age 75 years. The USPSTF recommends against routine screening for colorectal cancer in adults 76 to 85 years of age. There may be considerations that support colorectal cancer screening in an individual patient, although the recommendation is to not ever screen those 86 years and older. Given that 90% of all colon cancer occurs after age 50, all older adults are at risk. Individuals with additional risk factors (i.e., a personal or familial history of adenomatous polyps, colon cancer, or inflammatory bowel disease) should be targeted for screening and follow-up. Screening focuses on identifying premalignant adenomatous polyps. It is believed that this type of polyp will progress to cancer over a 5- to 10-year period. Screening for colon cancer has the advantage in that it is more likely to prevent the occurrence of cancer rather than just identify disease once it is present.

There is no single best test to screen for colon cancer so four options are provided: fecal occult blood test (FOBT), a flexible sigmoidoscopy, colonoscopy, and double-contrast barium enema. New approaches to screening include screening for DNA mutations. DNA is not degraded during passage through the gastrointestinal tract and is excreted in the stool. More research is needed before this type of screening goes into use. Moreover, it may be burdensome for the patient both in terms of the cost ($500 to $700) and the stool collection process. The USPSTF 2 concluded that the evidence is insufficient to assess the benefits and harms of computed tomographic colonography and fecal DNA testing as screening modalities for colorectal cancer. Virtual colonoscopy is another new technique in need of study to determine its cost/benefit over traditional colonoscopy.

Cervical and Prostate Cancer Screening

The USPSTF recommends against screening for cervical cancer in women older than age 65 years who have had adequate prior screening and are not otherwise at high risk for cervical cancer. Older women who have never had a Pap test should be screened until there are two negative tests. There are no consistent recommendations regarding screening for prostate cancer. The USPSTF recommends against prostate-specific antigen (PSA)–based screening for prostate cancer.

PUTTING PREVENTION INTO PRACTICE

Despite evidence to support the benefits to older adults of participating in health promotion activities and cancer screening, adherence to these recommendations remains low.[63] Unfortunately, adherence rates to guideline-based health promotion activities are often equated with the quality of care the individual is receiving. There are, however, some major pitfalls to that assumption. When caring for an older adult, it is possible that the sample audited should not be screened based on patient preferences or clinician judgment. With older adults an individualized approach is essential. Health promotion and disease prevention opportunities should be addressed with each patient or proxy and outcomes geared toward immediate benefit. The health care system in the United States traditionally has not focused on or supported health promotion. Increasingly, however, there are opportunities to provide direct health care services that are focused on disease prevention as well as management (Table 4-4). Medicare now covers a preventive "welcome to Medicare" health care visit for those who are new to Medicare and are within the first 6 months of enrollment. The examination includes education and counseling about preventive services such as depression, cognition, hearing, activities of daily living, falls, and home safety. It should also include a blood pressure measurement, height and weight measurement, electrocardiogram, visual screen, vision, cancer and bone health screenings, and diet education (particularly for those who are at risk for diabetes). Subsequent to that visit, every Medicare enrollee is eligible for an annual wellness visit that includes the following: a comprehensive history with a focus on alcohol, tobacco and illicit drug use, and potential need for additional counseling; discussion of diet and physical activity for health promotion; assessment of mood, function, and safety (functional ability, falls risk, and home safety); an examination that includes assessments of blood pressure, height and weight, vision, BMI, and other relevant factors; end-of-life planning; provision of or referral for education and counseling with a brief written plan given to the beneficiary to obtain screening electrocardiogram if appropriate; and other relevant screening tests. For example, if smoking and alcohol abuse are noted then up to eight counseling sessions are covered throughout a 12-month period. Table 4-5 some assessment tools to use when evaluating the elements recommended in the annual wellness visit.

Facilitators for Implementation of Prevention Practices

Professionals and Resources

Using an interprofessional team and advances in technology can help put prevention-focused activities into practice.

Patient Facilitators

> Maximizing participation in health promotion activities among older adults is best done using a multidimensional framework, as is afforded by social cognitive theory and the theory of self-efficacy.

Working with older adults to have them engage in health promotion activities and, in some cases, to change lifelong behaviors can be challenging. There are many known patient barriers to these activities, including a lack of understanding of the benefits and an assumption that with increased age there is no point to good health behaviors and prevention, lack of resources that generally include money and/or easy access to services, and never being told by their clinician what health promotion activities to consider engaging in.[67,68] Older adults can, however, change behavior. Maximizing participation in health promotion activities among these individuals is best done by using a multidimensional framework, as is afforded by social cognitive theory and the theory of self-efficacy. This theory suggests that the stronger the individual's efficacy expectations, the more likely he or she will be to initiate and persist with a given activity.[69] Efficacy expectations include both self-efficacy, which is the belief in one's ability to organize and execute a course of action, and outcome expectations, which are the beliefs that if a certain behavior is performed there will be a certain outcome. Efficacy expectations are dynamic and are both appraised and enhanced by four mechanisms: (1) performance accomplishment; (2) verbal persuasion; (3) role models, or seeing similar individuals perform a specific activity; and (4) physiologic or affective states such as pain, fatigue, or anxiety associated with a given activity. Motivational interviewing, which incorporates the tenets of self-efficacy theory, has been used with older adults and shows some benefits in changing behavior.[70,71] Motivational interviewing is a directive, client-centered counseling style for eliciting behavior change by helping clients to explore and resolve ambivalence. Compared with nondirective counseling, it is more focused and goal-directed.

Thus motivational interviewing requires that the individual be cognitively intact and able to engage in decision making and dialogue to set goals and establish ways in which to address overall challenges. Conversely, approaches based on self-efficacy can be used to engage all older adults in healthy behaviors, even those with moderate to severe cognitive impairment.[72,73]

TABLE 4-4	Medicare Coverage for Preventive Services		
Service	**Who is Covered**	**Frequency**	**Cost to Beneficiary**
Welcome to Medicare	All beneficiaries with Part B coverage	Once within 6 months of enrollment	None
Annual wellness visit	Part B beneficiaries	Annual	None
Ultrasound screening for abdominal aortic aneurysm	Beneficiaries with risk factors	Once in a lifetime	None
Cardiovascular screening (lipid panel, cholesterol, lipoprotein, triglycerides)	Beneficiaries without known cardiovascular disease	Every 5 years	None
Diabetes screening	Beneficiaries with risk factors	Two/year if "pre-diabetic"; one/year if never tested	None
Diabetes self-management training	Beneficiaries with diabetes	10 hours of initial training and 2 hours annually	Deductible applies
Medical nutrition therapy	Beneficiaries with diabetes, renal disease, or kidney transplant	3 hours counseling in year and 2 hours each year by a nutrition specialist	None
Screening Pap	All female beneficiaries	Annually if at high risk or childbearing age with abnormal Pap within 3 years; or every 24 months. Not provided if >65 and 3 negative tests obtained	None
Screening pelvic	All female beneficiaries	Annually if high risk for cervical or vaginal cancer; or childbearing age with abnormal Pap within 3 years. Not provided if >65 and negative test obtained or no risk factors.	None
Screening mammography	Female beneficiaries aged 35 and older	Annually for those aged 50-74 and then no screening recommended	None
Bone mass measurements	Estrogen-deficient beneficiaries and at risk; vertebral abnormalities; glucocorticoid therapy for >3 months; primary hyperparathyroidism; or on drug therapy for osteoporosis	Biennial	None
Colorectal cancer screening	Beneficiaries aged 50 and above	FOBT annually; flexible sigmoidoscopy every 4 years; colonoscopy every 10 years; barium enema biennial if high risk. No screening if ≥76 years.	None (except for barium enema)
Prostate cancer screening	Male beneficiaries aged ≥50	Not recommended unless risk factors	None for PSA; copay for DRE
Glaucoma	Beneficiaries with diabetes or family history, African Americans ≥50 or Hispanics ≥65 years	Annually	Copay applies
Influenza vaccine	All beneficiaries	Annually	None
Pneumococcal vaccine	All beneficiaries	Once in a lifetime; or repeat after 5 years based on risk	None
Hepatitis B vaccine	Beneficiaries at risk for hepatitis B	Scheduled dosages	None
Tobacco counseling	Tobacco users	Two cessation attempts/year; up to 8 sessions annually	None
Human immunodeficiency virus screening	Beneficiaries at risk	Annually	None

TABLE 4-4	Medicare Coverage for Preventive Services (Continued)		
Service	Who is Covered	Frequency	Cost to Beneficiary
Behavioral therapy for cardiovascular disease	Focus is on lowering cardiovascular risk (i.e., aspirin use); screening for high blood pressure and hyperlipidemia; diet counseling	Annually	None
Screening and counseling for alcohol use	All beneficiaries	Annual screening for misuse; 4 counseling sessions/year	None
Depression	All beneficiaries	Annual	None
Sexually transmitted infections	Sexually active individuals at risk	Annual	None
Behavioral counseling for obesity	Obese (BMI >30) beneficiaries	One visit/week for 1 month; every other week months 2-6; one/ month for months 7-12.	None

BMI, Body mass index; *DRE*, digital rectal examination; *FOBT*, fecal occult blood test; *PSA*, prostate-specific antigen.

TABLE 4-5	Tools for Assessment of Required Elements of the Annual Wellness and Health Promotion Visits
Elements	Recommended Tools (Web Access)
Alcohol use	• The Michigan Alcoholism Screening Test–Geriatric Version (*MAST-G*) (www.ssc.wisc.edu/wlsresearch/pilot/.../Aging_AppB5_MAST-G.pdf) • The CAGE (http://pubs.niaaa.nih.gov/publications/arh28-2/78-79.htm)
Depression	• Centers for Epidemiological Studies Depression Scale (http://patienteducation.stanford.edu/research/cesd.pdf) • Geriatric Depression Scale (http://www.stanford.edu/~yesavage/GDS.html) • Beck Depression Scale (http://www.fpnotebook.com/Psych/Exam/BckDprsnInvntry.htm) • Cornell Scale for Depression in Dementia (http://www.thedoctorwillseeyounow.com/articles/behavior/depressn_12/) • The Patient Health Questionnaire-9 or 2 (PHQ-9 or PHQ-2) http://www.cqaimh.org/pdf/tool_phq2.pdf • Hospital Anxiety and Depression Scale (HADS) http://www.scireproject.com/outcome-measures/hospital-anxiety-and-depression-scale-hads
Diet	• The Mini Nutritional Assessment for Older Adults (http://www.mna-elderly.com/)
Functional ability	• The Barthel Index (www.healthcare.uiowa.edu/igec/tools/function/barthelADLs.pdf) • The Katz Index (http://www.mainehealth.org/workfiles/mh_PFHA/Katz%20ADL_LawtonIADL.pdf)
Smoking	• The Agency for Healthcare Research and Quality recommends the use of the "4 As": ask, advise, assist, and arrange follow-up.
Safety/Falls prevention	• Check for Safety: A Home Fall Prevention Checklist for Older Adults (http://www.cdc.gov/ncipc/pub-res/toolkit/checklistforsafety.htm)
End-of-life counseling and planning	• End-of-Life Care. American Family Physician (http://www.aafp.org/afp/topicModules/viewTopicModule.htm?topicModuleId=57. • The Physician Orders for Life-Sustaining Treatment (http://www.ohsu.edu/polst/)
Cognition	• Mini-Cog (www.bami.us/Neuro/MiniCog.html) • The Brief Interview for Mental Status (BIMS) (dhmh.dfmc.org/longTermCare/.../BIMS_Form_Instructions.pdf)
Physical activity	• The Yale Physical Activity Survey (http://dapa-toolkit.mrc.ac.uk/documents/en/Yal/Yale_Physical_Activity_Survey.pdf) • The CHAMPS Physical Activity Questionnaire (http://sbs.ucsf.edu/iha/champs/resources/qxn/)

Motivating Patients to Engage in Health Promotion Activities: The Seven Step Approach

Based on prior research and using the theory of self-efficacy, a seven-step approach (Box 4-2) was developed to help motivate older adults to engage in health behaviors. The steps include (1) education, (2) assessment of need for health promotion activity, (3) goal identification, (4) elimination of barriers, (5) exposure to role models, (6) verbal encouragement, and (7) ongoing verbal reinforcement and rewards. It is particularly important to define the barriers to engaging in the behavior and working with the individual to eliminate those barriers.

BOX 4-2

SEVEN STEPS TO MOTIVATING OLDER ADULTS TO ENGAGE IN HEALTHY BEHAVIORS

Step 1: Educate
To facilitate learning, give information in multiple formats: an interactive lecture, a written handout, and videotape. Repeat the information and reinforce it both informally in one-on-one conversations with patients and formally in teaching programs.

Step 2: Assess Needs
Evaluate the individual to establish his or her need to participate in a given health promotion/disease prevention activity:
- Conduct physical examination, including health history
- Review prior screenings
- Evaluate barriers to engaging in the behavior (e.g., fear, no access, too old)

Step 3: Identify Goals
Set realistic goals and let the patient know exactly in what behavior to engage:
- Walk daily for 30 minutes
- Decrease to three cigarettes a day
- Avoid all desserts

Step 4: Eliminate Barriers
Aggressively attempt to eliminate the barriers associated with a given activity.

Step 5: Provide Role Models
Provide examples of successful patients who have changed health behaviors and noted benefits.

Step 6: Supply Verbal Encouragement
At the next encounter, make sure to ask the patient about his or her health behaviors, and provide verbal encouragement toward any positive change.

Step 7: Continue Verbal Reinforcement and Rewards
At each visit, continue to address health promotion behaviors and provide the patient with positive reinforcement as well as other rewards of interest to the patient. Rewards may include anything from a hug from a staff member for improved blood pressure or weight, to a prize once a certain weight is achieved, and so on.

CASE 1

Discussion

Mrs. W has some obvious areas of health promotion activities that would be beneficial to improve her physical health and quality of life. The first is to decrease and ultimately to quit smoking. The second area is to increase physical activity. She is worried about her bone health and unable to take medication for bone strengthening. You use this information as motivation to have her consider changing her behavior and improve her bone health without medication. You employ a self-efficacy approach and together identify goals and review the benefits of changing these behaviors and the outcomes she could expect. The goals are specific in what you expect her to do in terms of smoking and physical activity. Together you set a plan for her to decrease to 3 cigarettes a day for 2 weeks and then you will revisit her goal and work toward complete cessation. She will try replacing the cigarette break with a favorite treat. This would be up to 4 times a day as she normally smoked 10 cigarettes in a day. With regard to physical activity, she does not like group exercise so she will exercise in a facility that is supervised by a trainer during daytime hours. Her goal was to start with 5 minutes a day at least 3 days a week. You reinforce that you believe that she can achieve both these goals. At your 2-week follow-up she has achieved the set behaviors and you respond enthusiastically. New goals are established and the process continued until she has ceased smoking completely and is exercising routinely. Knowing that there are challenges to long-term adherence to health behaviors, you set up a motivational inoculation plan and at her regular 3-month follow-up visits and any acute visits you review her goals and she receives reinforcement for adherence to smoking cessation and exercise. Moreover, you relate healthy behaviors to positive health outcomes such as improvements in her blood pressure and improved gait speed and ability to get up from a chair. ■

SUMMARY

Older adults vary in their willingness to engage in health-promoting activities. With age there seems to be less interest in engaging in health promotion activities for the purpose of lengthening life, and greater interest in engaging in these activities only if they improve current quality of life. It is important, therefore, to approach health promotion activities with older adults by using an individualized approach. The goal of each professional engaged in health care of older individuals is to provide these individuals with information about each health promotion activity and the risks and benefits associated with each, and to help them engage in activities that will optimize health and overall quality of life.

Web Resources

www.cms.gov/MLNProducts/downloads/MPS_QuickReference
Chart_1.pdf. The Center for Medicare Services list of the Medicare-covered preventive services.

https://www.cms.gov/Outreach-and-Education/Medicare-Learning-Network-MLN/MLNProducts/downloads/MPS_QRI_IPPE001a.pdf. Medicare ABC Guide for Wellness Visit.

www.mna-elderly.com. The Mini Nutrition Assessment.

http://lpi.oregonstate.edu/infocenter/olderadultnut.html. Detailed recommendations for micronutrients for older adults.

www.choosemyplate.gov/information-healthcare-professionals.html. Information and tools for health care providers about MyPlate.

www.ahrq.gov/path/tobacco.htm. Treating tobacco use and dependence: An update on effective interventions.

www.cdc.gov/nccdphp/dnpa/physical/pdf/PA_Fact_Sheet_Older
Adults.pdf. Centers for Disease Control guidelines for physical activity for older adults.

www.cdc.gov/physicalactivity/growingstronger/exercises/index.html. Centers for Disease Control exercise resources for older adults.

www.easyforyou.info. Exercise and Screening for You website for older adults and providers.

KEY REFERENCES

5. Medicare interactive. Medicare coverage of vaccines and immunizations. http://wwwmedicareinteractiveorg/page2php?topic=counselor&page=script&slide_id=1519. Accessed July 2012.

22. Chodzko-Zajko WJ, Proctor DN, Singh MAF, et al. American College of Sports Medicine position stand: Exercise and physical activity for older adults. Med Sci Sport Exer 2009;41:1510-30.

32. Houston C, Tooze JA, Davis CC, et al. Serum 25-hydroxyvitamin D and physical function in older adults: The cardiovascular health study all stars. J Amer Geriatr Soc 2011;59:1793-801.

38. Furie KL, Kasner SE, Adams RJ, et al. Guidelines for the prevention of stroke in patients with stroke or transient ischemic attack: A guideline for healthcare professionals from the American Heart Association/American Stroke Association. Stroke 2011;42:227-76.

40. Goldstein LB, Bushnell CD, Adams RJ, et al. Guidelines for the primary prevention of stroke: A guideline for healthcare professionals from the American Heart Association/American Stroke Association. Stroke 2011;42:517-24.

References available online at expertconsult.com.

OBJECTIVES

Upon completion of this chapter, the reader will be able to:

- Describe the core attitudes/skills/knowledge of advanced cultural competency (ACC).
- Consider how the experience of dementia is shaped by each subculture's concept of what makes a person a person.
- Recognize that acknowledging and exploring the nature of health care disparities is necessary to achieve ACC, and that seeking to understand one's own internal biases is an integral part of this effort.

- Discuss the model of offering truth, and possible scripts for sharing end-of-life information respectfully.
- Realize that health beliefs may shed some light on but are never sufficient to explain patient preferences and behavior, and that it is critical to consider the patient and his or her community's personal and historical experience and perception of health care.

DEFINING CULTURAL COMPETENCY

CASE 1

Dr. Thaddeus Overman

Dr. Overman is a white male gay doctor, born, raised, and trained in Alabama. He moved to California for his residency in internal medicine. While caring for a patient with end-stage chronic obstructive pulmonary disease (COPD), he walked into the intensive care unit waiting room to discuss code status with the patient's family and discovered more than 20 family members. When Dr. Overman asked who was the patient's next of kin, he was told, "We are all kin." He asked who had power of attorney and was met with silence. When he clarified, all the women in the room identified themselves as the patient's sisters, and all the men as his brothers, and he started to feel that he needed to identify the patient's cultural group; "I had been taught that if only I could figure out what culture the patient was, then I could find the right article or textbook chapter to read," Dr. Overman explained later. Upon further discussion he realized that the patient was a Gypsy and he learned that the Gypsy definition of family centered around clan; this was not the same type of family or clan Dr. Overman had grown up with in Alabama. Many years have passed, but Dr. Overman vividly recalls the intensity of what he feels was his seminal clinical encounter with the necessity of understanding a patient's cultural context.

What patient encounters come to mind in your own experience that have made you feel that you were out of your cultural element? ▣

The importance of cultural competency is widely accepted as fundamental to quality care[1,2] and increasingly is seen as essential to combating health care disparities and in providing high-quality health care to all.[3-7] However, at the same time, there are few rigorous studies regarding the efficacy of cultural competency training,[8,9] and there are many critiques of cultural competency as it is often defined and taught.[10-15]

Additional online-only material indicated by icon.
Special Thanks to Sharon Kaufman, Mary Jo Del Vecchio Good, Lawrence Cohen and Paul Farmer, who have been tremendous mentors and allies throughout my journey as a clinician-anthropologist.

Conventional cultural competency training implies that one can master a body of knowledge to become culturally competent.[16,17] However, competency as a goal is inherently flawed because cultures are complex and varied. Assuming that a clinician can be competent in understanding other cultures is naive and implicitly leads to oversimplification and stereotyping, objectification of the patient, and failure to develop valuable, generalizable skills.

> Conventional cultural competency has often led to oversimplification and stereotyping, objectification of the patient, and failure to develop valuable, generalizable skills.

Advanced cultural competency involves learning and applying Attitudes, Skills, and Knowledge that will allow the clinician to function empathically and therapeutically. Note that this turns around the traditional medical hierarchy (Knowledge, Skills, and Attitudes), and thereby acknowledges that *Attitude* is the key to developing *Skills*, which then allow you to gain *Knowledge* of the individual patient and his or her cultural contexts. The resulting acronym—ASK—indicates the primary posture of advanced cultural competency.

> Advanced cultural competency acknowledges that attitude is the key to developing skills, which then enables you to gain knowledge of the individual patient and his or her cultural contexts.

Table 5-1 identifies the key attitudes, skills, and knowledge of advanced cultural competency. The remainder of this chapter presents case scenarios that demonstrate how these factors interact and can be applied in common geriatric situations.

TABLE 5-1	Key Elements of Advanced Cultural Competency
Attitudes	• Cultural humility • Self-awareness • The primacy of the relational aspects of health
Skills	Development of Communication and Relational Skills: • The right questions to ask • The ability to listen well • Collaboration with the patient and family
Knowledge	• Awareness of the history and shared life experience of the local patient population • Knowledge of where (and how) to turn to seek further information and guidance

DEMENTIA, PERSONHOOD, AND CULTURE

CASE 2

Ms. Nettie Mae (Part 1)

Ms. Nettie Mae is 78 years old. She lives with her grandson and his wife and their three small children. Her own children live nearby and join for meals on a weekly basis. The family knows that Ms. Nettie Mae is forgetful, and they do not like to leave her alone. She started a small fire in the kitchen last year, and her family no longer lets her cook. In a joking but firm way they took her car keys and stopped allowing her to drive. For the past 3 years she has helped out when the children come home from elementary school. She sits with them while they watch TV or do their homework. She helps out with dinner by cutting things up, setting the table, and mixing things together under the direction of her granddaughter-in-law.

Although she has lost the ability to converse, dress herself, and toilet herself, Ms. Nettie Mae has remained a part of the family. She is often honored at family occasions, as the matriarch. For example, at the church and community center events, when prizes are given away with doorway raffle tickets, several are always reserved and given to the elders in the room. The stories of days gone by that Ms. Nettie Mae has told for decades are now told by others on her behalf, while she sits and politely smiles. It is not clear that she follows or understands the stories, nor is it clear that she does *not* understand them. She smiles and laughs at the socially appropriate times.

As her disease progresses, she loses the ability to dress herself and toilet herself, causing increased physical stress on her caregivers. One day the granddaughter-in-law sees you for a back strain she got helping Ms. Nettie Mae off the commode. Seeing this stress, you encourage her family to visit assisted living and nursing home settings, to explore the possibility of placing her. The family politely and repeatedly declines the need for any assistance.

If you had a parent or grandparent who needed assistance at the level of Ms. Nettie Mae, what criteria would you use to determine whether you could maintain her in your home or whether you would begin to look for a long-term care facility? To what extent do these criteria reflect your culture and/or family of origin? ▫

> The dominant U.S. cultural definition of personhood in terms of independence and achievement leads to excess disability and suffering.

The dominant cultural approach to dementia in the United States reflects the cultural definition of an intact person as a person with value; the focus of achieving full personhood is on independence and achievement.[18-21] In contrast, other cultures may value more highly such qualities as interdependence, spiritual connection, embodied activity, or social relationships and role.[22-25] In the above case, we see that Ms. Nettie Mae is still valued as a full person because she still is the family matriarch. The role as a surviving elder is honored as an embodiment of the community's history and the community's ability to survive in a fairly hostile environment (e.g., slavery, Jim Crow, Civil Rights struggles, ongoing structural and institutional racism in the contemporary United States). Finally, her personhood endures because she still is able to participate interpersonally and emotionally with family and community members. Indeed, we increasingly recognize that emotional and relational abilities persist far into the progression of Alzheimer's disease and other dementias. Therefore, when personhood is defined as the ability to relate to others appropriately, dementia is less of a threat to the patient's personhood. In contrast, by narrowly defining full personhood as independence and cognitive achievement, the dominant U.S. cultural approach to personhood leads to excess disability and suffering.[26]

> It is a valuable moment when a physician realizes what a truly odd subculture we belong to. In this respect, almost every clinical encounter is cross-cultural.

CASE 2

Ms. Nettie Mae (Part 2)

Ms. Nettie Mae has fallen, breaking her hip. Before the fracture she was not walking more than a few steps at a time, and it was not uncommon for family members to carry her about. When the orthopedist suggests that a reasonable option is to not do surgery, given her minimal preinjury ambulatory status, the family disagrees. The choice to not have surgical repair is not considered a real option. "Of course we want the surgery," the grandson says. "Just like I would have it, if I broke that bone!"

Do you agree with Ms. Nettie Mae's grandson? Why or why not? ▣

Discussion

As already discussed, Ms. Nettie Mae is considered by the family to be a full person, just like everyone else in the community, with the same value as everyone else in the family/community. Her dementia and its increasingly significant deficits have not diminished her value and status as a full person.

HEALTH CARE DISPARITIES

CASE 2

Ms. Nettie Mae (Part 3)

During her hospitalization, the family is quite concerned that Ms. Nettie Mae's pain is not well controlled. They frequently complain that the nurse won't bring enough medication and that she does not answer the call button soon enough.

Which do you feel is more likely: (a) that Ms. Nettie Mae is being treated differently from other patients, or (b) that these complaints reflect differential family expectations? ▣

Disparities are a significant and persistent issue in our health care world. The evidence base documenting the pervasive reality of health care disparity is voluminous and spans every organ system and medical subspecialty.[27] For example, the undertreatment of pain in patients of color is well documented. Latinos with long bone fractures in a Los Angeles emergency department, for example, did not receive the same pain medication given to Caucasians with the same fractures.[28] A similar study in Atlanta confirmed that African Americans with long bone fractures received less pain medication than Caucasians.[29]

Increasingly, we recognize that clinical thinking and decision making are influenced by clinical biases.[30-33] When studies control for insurance, economic class, socioeconomic status, and education, a stubborn persistence of health care disparities remains, most strikingly along axes of race and ethnicity, but also along axes of gender and age.[27] Advanced cultural competency, by recognizing equity as essential to quality care, always seeks to address the complex processes that lead to health care disparities.

Palliative Care and "Giving Up"

CASE 2

Ms. Nettie Mae (Part 4)

Ms. Nettie Mae is no longer talking and is nonambulatory. She is incontinent of urine and stool and wears disposable undergarments. The family is enthusiastic and open to regular family meetings. They confirm and appreciate the opportunity to discuss the experiences they have had in health care, where they at times have felt disrespected or treated poorly because they are black. They have, over time, come to recognize their physician as an ally working to protect Ms. Nettie Mae from possible medical bias against elder and/or African American and/or female patients. Also, like most U.S.-born American patients, they are comfortable talking about avoiding futile care and they repeatedly confirm that they want to focus on quality of life. At the same time they consistently confirm full code* status.

What cultural factors about this family's background might be responsible for this inconsistency? ◧

There are many reasons that U.S.-born African Americans tend to elect full code status, even in terminal or end-stage disease processes. As already stated, personhood may not be thought to be lost when someone has significant functional deficits. Furthermore, the preservation of life for its own value is elevated in the African American community, in part for spiritual/religious reasons,[34-36] but also because the "will to live" carries value in the context of the challenges it takes to survive and thrive in the relatively hostile context of the historical and contemporary United States.

What do I mean by the will to live? Consider this: As a geriatrician, several years ago I was invited to speak to a community group of Holocaust survivors. These were all individuals who had survived concentration camps in large part because of their strong will to live (e.g., their personal willingness to endure a great degree of suffering and discomfort, in order to remain alive). They were not particularly interested in exploring with me the option of choosing to come to the end of their life. They had already surmounted tremendous odds against life and this served as a meaningful reference point for them when new life challenges appeared. Similarly, many African Americans have faced, and continue to face, tremendous obstacles in the United States, and those who survive into their elder years often have done so because of a tremendous will to live. The option of "giving up" is not considered acceptable, and a growing body of ethnographic research indicates that for most patients, the decision to implement a do not resuscitate (DNR) order or engage Hospice care is generally perceived as symbolic of giving up and choosing death.[37,38]

Finally, as will be discussed further later in the chapter, the African American historical and contemporary experience of health care results in a logical mistrust, a feeling that the health care system is very likely to not provide the best possible care to them, solely because they are African American.[39-41]

Talking about Dying

CASE 3

Professor Han

Professor Han is a retired molecular biologist from Beijing with hepatitis B and newly diagnosed hepatocellular carcinoma. He speaks only Mandarin, so you generally communicate with his adult son, who is bilingual and is also a scientist. When you notify the son about the diagnosis and the general contours

of the prognosis, he makes the strong request that you *not* inform his father of the cancer diagnosis and focus instead on the "liver infection." He also tells you, "I know Father would wish to have a DNR put in place, but please do it without discussing this with him directly. Can we do that now?"

When you suggest that you are uncomfortable with establishing a DNR order without including Professor Han in the discussion, and especially uncomfortable doing so without discussing the diagnosis and prognosis, the son suggests that it would be best just to "forget the whole issue then." When you press for a family meeting to really open the topic with the patient, he becomes more firm, saying quietly and politely that "I am very sorry, but no, this is *absolutely* not appropriate."

What cultural factors about this patient's background might explain this behavior? ◧

In contemporary U.S. culture and medical practice, we assume that it is appropriate and even beneficial for individuals to consider their own future death, to discuss and then make choices about possible options for care in the setting of terminal diagnoses. In fact, we have begun to assume that it is necessary to do this, and as health care providers we become uncomfortable when we skip this step.

The U.S. attitude, however, is an unusual anomalous cultural approach to the relationship of individuals to their own death. Even though all involved may be tacitly aware that death appears imminent, the vast majority of cultures and subcultures in the world consider it far more appropriate and beneficial to focus on living, on hope, and to avoid the topic of the individual's death.[42-44] Professor Han is, therefore, more typical of the world's populations; many if not most communities believe that discussing someone's potential death is dangerous and does the person harm.[45,46]

If, as in Professor Han's case, the patient and family consider that talking about death is dangerous and pathogenic, you might do well to recognize and consider the nocebo effect (Box 5-1). A nocebo effect occurs when, because of pessimistic beliefs and expectations, a patient has an adverse reaction to an inert or innocuous treatment (i.e., the inverse of the placebo effect).[47-49] In this case, a well-intentioned action on the part of the health care team can lead to patient harm.[50]

On the other hand, it may be acceptable to discuss with any patient and family the theoretical situation of someone (not the patient) who is very sick, and the doctor believes is approaching the end of his or her life. One could then ask the patient/family what they think that other person should do, that is, what they think is the right thing to do when a person is so sick that he or she is approaching the end of life. This approach can help identify the patient's personal values regarding goals of care. A similar approach is described in the literature with regard to working with contemporary Navajo patients in the United States.[51]

---

*The wish to have aggressive resuscitation with CPR, electrical shocks, and medications, in the event of cardiopulmonary arrest.

BEWARE OF THE NOCEBO EFFECT

- Nocebo refers to the patient's expectation that something bad will result from an intervention.
- An example is the apocryphal story of the patient with a viral gastroenteritis who overheard the team of physicians discussing the imminent cardiac demise of the patient in the next bed. He became alarmed and asked if he were dying. Despite multiple reassurances, he could not shake his belief that the doctors were simply trying to shield him from the truth, and he did, in fact, die that night. Though this tale is a bit of an urban legend, there is literature indicating the validity of the nocebo effect (although medical ethics precludes any contemporary research on the phenomenon).
- The bottom line is that if a patient believes that talking about his or her potential death will be harmful, it may be reasonable, in the context of the nocebo effect, to regard such discussion as harmful to that patient.

Discussing Prognosis: Offering Truth

> Offering truth is a reasonable way to honor the physician's need to provide frank, unvarnished medical information, while recognizing that the patient and/or family may not want to talk about the patient's potential death.

"Offering truth" has emerged as a reasonable way to honor the physician's need to provide frank, unvarnished medical information, while recognizing that the patient and/or family may not want to talk about the patient's potential death.[52-54] Offering truth is the practice of giving the patient and the family an opportunity to describe how much information they wish to know. This approach is a way to honor patient autonomy, because the patient tells the doctor to what degree he or she wishes to be informed. Here is a possible mini-script to accomplish this:

> *Some of my patients would like to know quite a lot about their disease, all the details and information about what might be going to happen. Some even want to know the specific numbers or statistics. Some patients wish to know general information but not numbers and statistics. Other patients want to know very little, sometimes almost nothing in detail. What sounds about right to you?*

Although dominant U.S. culture values the individual as the primary unit of being and designates the individual as the default autonomous decision maker,

one can best preserve patient autonomy by inviting the patient to designate the appropriate decision maker. Once documented appropriately, all members of the health care team will be aware of the patient's preference, and therefore will be able to honor it. It should be no surprise that many patients will tell you that someone else is the appropriate decision maker (not substitute decision maker, as we often define the healthcare power of attorney, but simply the primary decision maker), given that the contemporary United States is culturally unusual in the primacy it places on individual autonomy and self-determination.[55,56]

This process of offering truth should continue throughout your interactions with the patient. For example, at each clinical encounter in which you have information to offer, you should pause and ask, "Would you like to know more information about what is going on?" The patient will let you know how much information and detail is wanted, if you provide the opportunity to do so.

Advanced culturally competent physicians are aware of the need to offer truth and be cautious about the nocebo potential of truth telling, but balance this with the need, as a physician, to acknowledge when a patient is likely approaching the end of his or her life. The following is a script reflecting how I seek to accomplish this balance, to inform patients, without requiring them to discuss their own death and dying:

> *It is important to me as your physician to make sure you know that you are very sick and that you are closer toward the end of your life. (Note: I have elected to never use the words death or dying, unless the patient first uses them.) I do not know if you have a shorter or longer period of time until the end of your life. It may well be [days/weeks/months] or longer than that. And a lot of patients ask me, "Why do I even feel it is important to say this?!" It's not an easy thing to say or to hear. But the main reason I think it's important to draw any attention to it, is because I want to make sure you have the opportunity to spend "whatever amount of time that you have" doing whatever you feel is important for you to do. For some people, they want to make sure they do some legal or financial things before the end of their lives, or to make a specific trip, have specific conversations with people, or address some specific spiritual or emotional concerns. Whatever they want to do during the time they have left is always very individual to the person and their family. But I don't want you to miss the opportunity for those things. That's why I felt it was so important for me to let you know, that although it may be a longer time or a shorter time, in my experience as a physician, I am concerned that you are coming closer to the end of your life.*

THE COHORT EFFECT: SUBCULTURES ARE LOCAL IN TIME

CASE 4

Dr. Walter Daniel

Dr. Daniel is a 96-year-old retired psychiatrist living in a nursing home at a continuing care retirement community. His wife lives in an apartment in the same community and visits him daily. Their daughter, a gerontologist, has been urging them to discuss death and dying.

The wife comes to you with some anguish. "Do we *have* to talk about this?" she asks. "Our daughter is telling me that we do have to, but I just know he doesn't want to! It is not what we would do. It is not what *he* would want to do. We've been married over 60 years, I have no doubt about how he feels about this!"

What cultural factors about this patient's background might explain this behavior? ▣

Dr. Daniel is not a patient from an exotic culture. He is a white, Anglo-Saxon Presbyterian whose family has been here in the United States for at least three generations. In fact, he is a retired physician. Not only a physician; he is a retired psychiatrist, a person who we might expect to be particularly comfortable with the presumed psychological benefits of discussing and preparing for his impending death. Nonetheless his "native culture" still is not congruent with the contemporary U.S. medical-health professional cultural approach to death and dying. That's because 70-plus years ago when his cultural values were formed, talking about death was much less open. Dr. Daniel's experience of U.S. health care culture is at least two generations removed from our current health care cultural norms.

> The patient and his or her community's expectations arise from their shared life experience regarding doctors and the medical system.

This cohort effect makes many older persons behave differently than younger health care professionals expect. Because Dr. Daniel is a white mainstream American and a retired physician, our prevailing assumption is that he will share the culture of current white American physicians. Will he?

Sharon Kaufman's ethnographic work suggests that most of our patients, not just those from exotic "other" cultures, do not share our medical cultural approach to death and dying. For many older patients and their families, the decision about DNR and Hospice is symbolically understood to be a matter of choosing life or choosing death, and further, that "choosing death" is unacceptable to almost all of

them.[36] To paraphrase the words of Dr. Kaufman's informants: "I know I am very sick and might be dying, and I don't want the rest of my life to be about that. I want to live; I don't want to choose death. The visit from Hospice workers is just a reminder that 'You are dying.' I don't want that reminder. I would rather focus on thinking about living now, and not turn my attention away from life."

In contemporary U.S. health care culture, we have a specific approach to death and dying that rests on several assumptions:

- We feel it is important and valuable to consider, think about, and talk about our own personal future deaths, perhaps even necessary/healthy to do so.
- We feel that this is generally an autonomous individual experience and process, and should be individual, although family and friends play an important role.
- We feel that we can have a certain degree of personal control over the process leading to our death.
- We feel that to achieve that individual control is to make decisions/choices about our own death/dying process. Personal choice and decision making are integral to the process.

All this seems self-evident and commonsensical to those of us within the culture of medicine. However, in fact, this approach is not the norm. It is a valuable moment when a physician realizes what a truly odd subculture members of the medical profession belong to, and that "mainstream" patients in the United States are not inside our subcultural approach. In this respect, almost every clinical encounter is cross-cultural.

EXPERIENCE AND EXPECTATIONS SHAPE DOCTOR-PATIENT INTERACTIONS

The patient and his or her community's expectations of doctors and the medical system arise from their shared life experience, and shape their future interactions with the medical system.

CASE 5

Don Jorge Rodriguez

Don Jorge Rodriguez has end-stage congestive heart failure, an ejection fraction of 15%. He has consistently stated his desire to avoid futile care. He is a devout man, and talks about being at peace with dying, about looking forward to his place in heaven. Each time he is offered aggressive care—a biventricular pacemaker, for example, or a dobutamine drip—he enthusiastically chooses these options. At the same time Mr. Rodriguez also consistently states his desire to avoid treatments that will not help him, "I only want things that will help," he says. The team is confused about why he continues to choose aggressive care in the face of a death that he seems, in some respects, to be welcoming.

What factors about California Latino culture might help us understand this apparent inconsistency? ◙

Mr. Rodriguez's apparent contradictions have been characterized by ethnographic research[57] in which the majority of southern California Latino informants expressed the desire to avoid "futile" care while at the same time consistently opting for all care offered by their physicians. Open-ended interviews allowed informants to explain what it meant to them to express these two apparently conflicting wishes, and here is what emerged: Physicians and the health care system were perceived by the informants to be at their primary essence benevolent; they could be trusted to always seek the best interests of the patient. Therefore, it was understood that physicians would offer only helpful options, only beneficial options. In other words, anything the physician offered was perceived to be beneficial. It was believed to be impossible for a doctor to offer a treatment that would be bad for the patient.

CASE 6

Katrina Lublavitz

The family of Mrs. Katerina Lublavitz struck terror in the hearts of the medical team. Mrs. Lublavitz had end-stage dementia and was wheelchair-bound. She was minimally verbal and required hand feeding. The staff of the nursing home sought an thics consultation because they felt that the daily care of Mrs. Lublavitz was increasing her suffering. When the patient was hospitalized for acute cholecystitis, every interaction with the daughter to discuss treatment options and alternatives was fraught with conflict and argument. One resident asked whether there was something to know about Jewish culture, or Russian culture, that would help.

What cultural factors about this patient's background might explain this behavior? ◙

Immigrants from the former Soviet Union often have a shared life experience in which their interactions with physicians and the health care system have been laced with conflict. Medical care was an agent of the state in ways more direct than found in most countries. (In the United States, the government is also involved with the provision of health care, but in a much more indirect way than was found in the former Soviet Union.) Access to appropriate care was obstructed by the physician and the medical system, so the usually correct expectation held by patients and their families was that strong battle with the physician/medical team was necessary to obtain the appropriate medical care.[58,59] It is not some essence of Jewishness nor of Russianness that clarifies the experience the medical team had with Mrs. Lublavitz's family. Rather, when one understands the specific shared life experience of immigrants from the former Soviet Union and their consequent perceptions and expectations of physicians and health care, the adversarial stance begins to make sense.

CASE 2

Ms. Nettie Mae (Part 5)

Nettie Mae is now in a nursing facility. The family visits daily. The patient is mute, immobile, and incontinent of urine and stool. The family continues to participate in regular family meetings, and they recognize that Nettie Mae has little quality of life. However, each meeting, when they come to the moment of electing DNR or comfort-oriented care, they confirm their desire to remain full code. In the context of all their other statements, the doctor becomes a bit surprised and confused.

If you were Nettie Mae's physician, would you be surprised and confused? Why or why not? ◙

The shared life experience of the African-American individual and community has consistently confirmed that physicians and health care do not provide the highest quality medical care to them, and that medicine is not a primarily benevolent institution. Unfortunately, hundreds of studies from the Tuskegee study onward confirm the historical and contemporary accuracy of this perception.[27] U.S.-born African Americans and U.S.-born white Americans appear to share many common values: that quality of life is more important than quantity, that the individual is and should remain autonomous, that the individual can be master of his or her own destiny. However, the perceptions and expectations of U.S.-born African Americans regarding doctors and health care are quite different than those of U.S.-born white Americans. U.S.-born white Americans trust physicians and health care to act in the patient's best interest, whereas U.S.-born African Americans often do not.[60-62] The historical and contemporary record indicates that this is an accurate perception.[63,64,41] If we wish to change these perceptions, we will need to change the reality of health care disparities.

> If we wish to change the appropriate mistrust of African-American patients for doctors and medical care, we will need to change the reality of health care disparities.

The patient and his or her community's expectations of doctors arise from their shared life experience regarding doctors, and shape their future interactions with doctors and the medical system. The above three cases capture the very important theme that the patient and the community have a shared life experience of what doctors and the medical system are like, and consequently the patient has learned an expectation and perception of doctors and the medical system, and therefore how best to interact with them. Based on their shared life experience, some Latino immigrant patients have an expectation that the doctor will be always benevolent and can be trusted, so one should always say "yes" to the doctor. Based on their shared life experience, many former Soviet Union patients have an expectation that the doctor is an agent of the state and an obstacle to good care, so one should always anticipate and engage in battle with the doctor. Based on their shared life experience, many U.S.-born African-American patients have the expectation that the doctor and medical system are often malevolent and cannot be trusted, so one should always be wary and seek to protect oneself and one's loved ones in this hostile environment.

WHEN THE PATIENT'S EXPLANATORY MODEL AND ACTIONS APPEAR TO BE IN CONFLICT

CASE 7

Mr. E. Kim

Mr. E. Kim has end-stage pulmonary hypertension and is on home oxygen and long-acting nitrates. He ambulates with a walker and is increasingly dependent on assistance for bathing, toileting, and dressing, so he now lives with his eldest son and his family. He has been hospitalized for pneumonia each winter for 3 years in a row. The medical student on the team has spent a lot of time with Mr. Kim during the hospitalization and is confused about what he is hearing. On several occasions, Mr. Kim has said that he wishes to never be intubated, and would prefer to never return to the intensive care unit. At other times, however, Mr. Kim acknowledges that he will be intubated in the future and that this is "as it should be."

Could this behavior have a cultural explanation? ◉

A rigorous mixed-methods study of 800 informants revealed confusing results about Korean-Americans living in greater Los Angeles.[57] Informants indicated their preference to avoid life-sustaining treatment, such as intubation and mechanical ventilation, but also indicated that they knew they would be intubated. Open-ended interviews clarified the contradiction.[65] The elders stated that their children would never permit a DNR and would do anything possible to keep their parent alive longer, in accord with their understanding of filial piety, and that although they personally did not wish to be kept alive on machines, the family obligations of filial piety were more important than their personal preferences.

> We cannot expect a patient's explanatory model to always explain his or her medical decisions.

This is a terrific example of the complex factors involved when people make medical decisions. It seems logical that a patient's beliefs about the body, illness, and healing—what has sometimes been termed the patient's explanatory model[66,67]—should guide the patient's health—related decisions. And yet the notion that people make rational choices about their health, based on the internal logic of their beliefs about the body and illness, is well-recognized as incorrect.[68,69] Certainly beliefs about the body and illness (such as our own medical model, for example) are important factors, and it demonstrates respect and collaboration when a physician seeks to elicit the explanatory model of the patient and the family. Nonetheless, the majority of medical anthropologic studies demonstrate that a variety of factors influence how people make decisions about their health care. For example, Libbet Crandon-Malamud's work in rural Bolivia demonstrated that villagers' choices about whether they wished to receive care from a doctor in the missionary clinic, a shaman in a local religious service, or a *curandero* (healer) trained in the local herbal traditions were reflections of the villager's self-identify, who they wished to have in their personal relationships, and what local resources they wished to mobilize.[70] Similarly, when upper middle class white women in the urban United States choose to see an acupuncturist, it appears to be an expression of the individual's personal values and self-identity, rather than of a deeply held explanatory model of how the body works.[71-73]

What, then, is Advanced Cultural Competency?

Advanced culturally competent physicians recognize that physicians treat illness primarily, not disease primarily. In medical school, in textbooks and articles, we learn about disease, but when we practice medicine, we encounter illness (i.e., disease located in the human experience). Patients suffer from illness, not from disease,[74-76] and if we wish to maximize clinical efficacy, we will need to focus on treating illness. If a physician wants to treat illness, then the physician needs to relate well to people who have illness, communicate effectively with them, and come to know them.

There is no set of textbooks and articles to read in order to master the body of knowledge for advanced cultural competency. Just as we practice medicine, rather than master it, we practice advanced cultural competency, and if we are attentive and learn from our patients, we get better at it over time; yet we never master it.

> Just as we practice medicine, rather than master it, we practice advanced cultural competency. If we are attentive and learn from our patients, we get better at it over time, but we never master it.

Recall that the patient and his or her community's shared life experiences of doctors and the medical system shape their perceptions and predispositions. In this respect, cultures are always local phenomena. There simply is no essential "Chineseness" to be discovered and "mastered," but there are many Chinese (sub)cultures located in space (the Chinese subculture in Toronto versus the West Indies versus urban Beijing versus rural Guizhou province) and time (the Chinese subculture in contemporary Beijing versus the Cultural Revolution Beijing versus 1920s Beijing). Whatever subcultures are represented by your patients—immigrants from Guatemala who are undocumented and, for example, or U.S.-born African Americans with ancestors who were enslaved and/or who lived through Jim Crow, or rural Appalachians who consider themselves Scots-Irish mountain folk who have been repeatedly exploited by other white outsiders or recent Ukrainian immigrants from the former Soviet Union—then those are the specific histories you must learn to be an effective physician for the patients you serve. You may accomplish this by reading or watching movies, but always you will learn by asking and listening to the stories told by your patients and their families.

SUMMARY

To practice advanced cultural competency (ACC), you must always demonstrate the characteristics represented by the acronym ASK:

- Attitude—a focus on the development of cultural humility,[16,77] self-awareness,[78] and the primacy of the relational aspects of health care.[79]
- Skills—a focus on communication, with a mastery of the right questions to ask and the ability to listen well and to negotiate/collaborate well with the patient and family.

- Knowledge—a focus on developing awareness of the history and shared life experience of the local patient population, and the knowledge of where (and how) to turn to seek further information and guidance.

Advanced culturally competent physicians seek, by definition, to provide high-quality care to all patients. We will achieve this only if we include ourselves in the local phenomena to be understood. As we recognize our own internal biases and assumptions, including those arising from the culture of health care, we become better equipped to achieve the goals of quality and equality.

ACKNOWLEDGMENTS

Special thanks to Sharon Kaufman, Mary Jo Del Vecchio Good, Lawrence Cohen, and Paul Farmer, who have been tremendous mentors and allies throughout my journey as a clinician-anthropologist.

Elizabeth Herskovits Castillo

Web Resources

https://implicit.harvard.edu/implicit. The Implicit Assessment Test, a web-based resource to explore one's own internal preferences and unconscious biases.

www.case.edu/med/ccrhd/education_videos.html. Case Western Reserve University's Center for Reducing Health Disparities; video archive of Health Disparity Class lectures

www.stanford.edu/group/ethnoger. A core curriculum in ethnogeriatrics, as well as ethnic-specific modules, developed by the Collaborative of Ethnogeriatric Education of the Geriatric Education Centers.

KEY REFERENCES

26. Castillo EH. Doing dementia better: Anthropological insights. Clin Geriatr Med 2011;27(2): 273-89.
27. Smedley BD, Stith AY. Unequal treatment: Confronting racial and ethnic disparities in health care. Washington, DC: National Academy Press; 2003.
31. Green AR, Carney DR, Pallin DJ, et al. Implicit bias among physicians and its prediction of thrombolysis decisions for black and white patients. J Gen Intern Med 2007;22(9):1231-8.
37. Kaufman, S. And a time to die: How American hospitals shape the end of life. New York, NY: Scribner; 2005.
52. Freedman B. Offering truth: One ethical approach to the uninformed cancer patient. Arch Intern Med 1993;153(5):572.
57. Blackhall LJ, Frank G, Murphy ST, et al. Ethnicity and attitudes towards life sustaining technology Soc Sci Med 1999;48(12): 1779-1789.

References available online at expertconsult.com.

6

Appropriate Prescribing

Gregory J. Hughes and Judith L. Beizer

OBJECTIVES

Upon completion of this chapter, the reader will be able to:

● Describe physiologic changes that may impact how medications should be used in older patients.

● Outline a prescribing strategy to maximize benefit and minimize harm.

● Explain how prescription drug coverage impacts use of medication in geriatric patients.

● Explain how pharmacists add value to the geriatric health care team.

The older population is prescribed more medications than any other age group.[1] With initiation of Medicare Part D in 2006, all 43 million Medicare beneficiaries had immediate access to outpatient prescription drug plans. By June 2006, 90% of beneficiaries were enrolled in Medicare D or a creditable drug coverage plan.[2] The Agency for Healthcare Research and Quality (AHRQ) reports that older people fill 31.6 prescriptions annually,[1] as well as having more unique prescriptions and more refills than the younger population. In 2009, the New England Healthcare Institute addressed the issue of medication nonadherence for chronic diseases. Chronic diseases account for 75% of health care spending in the United States, and the cost of medication nonadherence reached $100 billion in terms of excess hospital admissions alone.[3]

Over the past two decades, the cost of prescriptions has increased more rapidly than increases in the gross domestic product. In 2009, it was estimated that total expenditures for prescriptions in noninstitutionalized patients over 65 years was $86.5 billion in the United States.[4] This figure does not include any over-the-counter medications or medications given in a physician's office, in a clinic, or in the inpatient setting.

CASE 1

LM (Part 1)

LM is a 76-year-old female with a past medical history of atrial fibrillation, systolic heart failure, hyperlipidemia, and migraines. She visits you, her primary care physician, complaining of intermittent palpitations. She denies chest pain, shortness of breath, pain, unusual bleeding, swollen extremities, weight gain, or headache. Her chronic medications include warfarin 3 mg daily, metoprolol tartrate 100 mg twice daily, digoxin 0.125 mg daily, lisinopril 20 mg daily, and simvastatin 40 mg daily. She is also taking amitriptyline 150 mg at bedtime for migraine prophylaxis. Her vital signs reveal a blood pressure of 120/75 mmHg, which is near baseline, and an irregularly irregular heart rate of 130 to 150. You perform an electrocardiogram that reveals atrial fibrillation with a rapid ventricular rate. A recent serum digoxin concentration was reported to be 0.9 mcg/L (upper limit considering atrial fibrillation with concomitant systolic heart failure). You decide to initiate LM on amiodarone as her metoprolol and digoxin are at the maximum recommended doses.

What pharmacokinetic and pharmacodynamic age-associated changes will affect LM's medications? ▣

PHARMACOKINETIC CHANGES IN THE ELDERLY

Clinical pharmacokinetics is the discipline describing drug behavior with regard to absorption, distribution,

---

Additional online-only material indicated by icon.

metabolism, and elimination with the intent to use medications effectively while limiting adverse effects. Aging brings physiologic changes that affect these four characteristics in a clinically meaningful and relevant way. With age, organ function and physiologic reserve both decline, resulting in enhanced susceptibility to adverse effects of medications.[5-7] See Table 6-1.

Absorption

Medications (except those given parenterally) are subject to variations in absorption. Bioavailability of oral medications may fluctuate with changes that are common in older patients such as reduced acidity of the stomach, gastric motility, and first-pass metabolism. Medications that require an acidic environment for optimal absorption (e.g., calcium carbonate or ketoconazole) have reduced absorption in patients with hypochlorhydria (whether physiologic or acid suppressant–induced). Fortunately, most medications do not require active transport to be absorbed and passive diffusion remains relatively unchanged in most older patients. Absorption of topical medications (e.g., creams, ointments, or patches) may fluctuate because of changes in the skin such as atrophy and reduced blood flow to the dermal layer. Although some medications may have reduced absorption, this is frequently counterbalanced by a decreased first-pass effect. For medications that have a low bioavailability in average adults, such as propranolol or morphine, a small decrease in the initial first-pass effect may drastically impact drug serum concentrations. Although absorption may be the pharmacokinetic factor least impacted by age, alterations in absorption should be considered when the patient response varies from what is expected.

Distribution

A medication's distribution describes the extent to which a drug passes into different body compartments. Depending on drug characteristics such as size, solubility, and plasma-binding affinity, a medication may be more likely to achieve higher concentrations in hydrophilic or lipophilic compartments or to pass through the blood-brain barrier. Older patients have lower total body water and higher body fat. Therefore lipophilic medications have a larger volume of distribution. This leads to a longer elimination phase and prolonged therapeutic or toxic effect because drugs are typically not efficiently eliminated from the lipid compartment. Examples of lipophilic medications include phenytoin, valproic acid, diazepam, olanzapine, amiodarone, and lidocaine.

Medications reach equilibrium between compartments and also between bound and free forms. As patients age, albumin and alpha-1-acid glycoprotein may decrease or increase, resulting in higher or lower free fractions of medication. Alterations to concentrations of these proteins are not caused by aging but rather by chronic conditions. For example, serum albumin decreases with prolonged illness, raising the free fraction of highly bound acidic drugs such as naproxen, phenytoin, and warfarin. With illness, patients may develop adverse events or side effects from a medication that was previously well tolerated. This is particularly true for medications needing a closely maintained therapeutic range, such as warfarin and phenytoin. Serum drug concentrations of the total (bound and free fractions) should be monitored because the free fraction may be in a toxic range, while the bound level is therapeutic.

TABLE 6-1	Pharmacokinetic Changes of Aging and Disease	
Changes of Age and Disease	**Pharmacokinetic Effect**	**Examples of Some Drugs Affected**
↓ First-pass metabolism	↑ Drug serum concentration	Oral nitrates, beta-blockers, calcium channel blockers, estrogens
↓ Rate of absorption	↓ Clinical effect	Furosemide
↓ Lean mass and total body water	↓ Volume of distribution	Digoxin, lithium
↑ Fat content	↑ Volume of distribution	Diazepam, chlordiazepoxide, flurazepam, alprazolam
↓ Food intake/catabolic disease states	↓ Serum protein concentration with ↓ binding	Warfarin, phenytoin
↓ Approximately one half of CYP 450 metabolic pathways (Phase I reactions)	↓ Reduction, oxidation, hydroxylation, demethylation →↑ half-life	Diazepam, chlordiazepoxide, flurazepam, alprazolam
↓ Renal elimination	↓ Clearance →↑ half-life	Aminoglycosides, vancomycin, digoxin, salicylates

From Stratton MA, Gutierres S, Salinas R. Drug therapy in the elderly: Tips for avoiding adverse effects and interactions. Consultant 2004;44:461-7.

Metabolism

Metabolism is the body's process of altering a medication in some way. In the liver, the result of metabolism may be a product that is more or less active in the body or one more easily eliminated by the kidneys or biliary tree. Aging decreases liver size and blood perfusion, but quantitative changes in liver function and histology are minimal. Metabolism of medications usually occurs via reactions that are classified into one of two phases. Phase I metabolism occurs via cytochrome P450 isoenzymes, which have a high interpatient variability even in young adults. Studies of changes in specific isoenzymes with age are plagued by small sample sizes, confounders such as effects of smoking and genetic polymorphism, and the potential to interpret cohort effects as age-related effects. However, studies suggest a decrease in elimination of substrates of 1A2 and 2C19, a decrease or no change in elimination of substrates of 3A4 and 2C9, and no change in elimination of substrates of 2D6.[5,7] These phase I reactions result in an oxidized, reduced, or hydrolyzed form of the parent drug but not all medications must pass through this step. Interindividual variability and confounders (listed earlier) affect phase I metabolism more than aging does. However, attention must be paid to medications with a high hepatic extraction ratio such as lidocaine, morphine, labetalol, propranolol, verapamil, and imipramine.

Many medications, such as lorazepam and oxazepam, are metabolized only through the phase II reactions glucoronidation, acetylation, or sulfation, resulting in larger, more water soluble, more easily eliminated metabolites. Evidence thus far suggests that phase II is unaffected by aging.

Elimination

Elimination of medications generally occurs via conversion to inactive metabolites in the liver, excretion in bile, or elimination through the kidneys. The rate at which medications are excreted in the urine is determined by a combination of glomerular filtration, tubular secretion, and reabsorption. With age most patients experience a decline in glomerular filtration rate. Nomograms and algorithms have been developed and validated to estimate glomerular filtration by calculating the estimated creatinine clearance. Creatinine is cleared by glomerular filtration and active tubular secretion. These equations were typically determined using healthy adults. With this in mind, validity of these equations in patients at extremes of age and with active disease is less reliable. Given these limitations, the Cockcroft-Gault equation is the recommended equation for most scenarios. Other equations, such as the modification of diet in renal disease (MDRD)

equation, may automatically calculate the estimated glomerular filtration rate in some electronic medical records and results may vary substantially from those of the Cockcroft-Gault equation. As with any patient encounter, the entire scenario needs to be considered in addition to the calculated creatinine clearance (CrCl). The Cockcroft-Gault equation uses the following formula to determine CrCl:

Creatinine clearance (CrCl) mL/min = $(140 - age) \times weight/(72 \times serum\ creatinine\ concentration)$, multiply by 0.85 for females

> About two thirds of all older people experience a decline in creatinine clearance (CrCl). Despite limitations, estimated CrCl is a useful tool for estimating appropriate drug doses.

This equation uses serum creatinine concentration, which decreases in older patients because of their decreased muscle mass. This may result in a higher calculated CrCl, especially in underweight or malnourished older patients. To correct for these possibilities, many clinicians round the serum creatinine concentration up to 1 mg/dL, which may in turn underestimate CrCl. The estimated CrCl may vary drastically with extremes in weight. It has been suggested to use lean body weight when calculating CrCl in patients who are significantly obese. It is also important to appreciate that drug dosages and recommended dose adjustments for patients with renal impairment are based on estimated CrCl rather than on the often reported laboratory estimate of glomerular filtration, the MDRD.

It is important as a clinician to pay particular attention to dosages for medications that are eliminated unchanged in the urine or that have active metabolites that are eliminated in the urine because these drugs will accumulate in most older people.

Because of the variables discussed in this section, predicting a medication's serum concentration or clinical effects may be difficult in a geriatric patient. The starting dose for most renally excreted drugs should be based on the estimated CrCl, but patients must be monitored for both overdosing and underdosing. For medications with a narrow therapeutic range or low ceiling for toxic effects, measuring serum drug concentrations is prudent, particularly when a patient is acutely ill.

In summary, the clinical impact of age-related changes in pharmacokinetics is difficult to predict. Vigilance to adverse effects of medications caused by altered drug pharmacokinetics is necessary in elderly patients and a thorough medication history is warranted in the presence of any new complaints. The adage to "start low and go slow" applies when initiating medications with potentially adverse effects.

In patients with significant renal impairment (creatinine clearance approaching 30 mL/min), refer to medication monographs for appropriate dosages for renally excreted drugs.

PHARMACODYNAMIC CHANGES IN THE ELDERLY

Although numerous studies and reviews[8-11] describe the pharmacokinetic changes in geriatric patients, there are limited data on age-related pharmacodynamic changes. Pharmacodynamics refers to the response of the body to a drug. Geriatric patients may have altered pharmacodynamics because of changes in receptor affinity or number, postreceptor alterations, and/or impairment of homeostatic mechanisms. Unfortunately, it is difficult to generalize age-related changes because studies have shown patients to have a higher "sensitivity" to some medications and a lower "sensitivity" to others. One example of higher sensitivity is increased central nervous system effects with benzodiazepines. One small study found that geriatric patients had a higher sensitivity index and a more profound central nervous system depressant effect, even when receiving a lower dose of midazolam.[12] The opposite is found with beta-agonists/antagonists where patients tend to be less responsive to these agents. Some generalizations that can be made are that geriatric patients will frequently have a greater responsiveness to the central nervous system depressant effects of benzodiazepines, to the analgesic effects of opioids, and to the anticoagulant effects of warfarin and heparin.

CASE 1

LM (Part 2)

LM's presentation is not uncommon and several pharmacokinetic/pharmacodynamic issues should be considered. The addition of amiodarone to the current medication regimen poses numerous issues. Amiodarone is a highly lipophilic medication with a large volume of distribution and a half-life of weeks to months. In LM, who likely has increased body fat because of her age, a steady state concentration will not be reached for several months. Likewise, if she were to experience an adverse event from this medication, it may take months for the medication to be eliminated and the reaction to resolve. Amiodarone is metabolized to an active metabolite in the liver via the cytochrome P450 complexes and also inhibits the activity of these enzymes including 3A4, 2D6, 2C9, and 1A2. Amiodarone interferes with the metabolism of warfarin, an anticoagulant that older patients are frequently sensitive to. LM will require frequent monitoring of her international normalized ratio (INR) and her warfarin dose should be carefully adjusted over the next few months

until a new steady state therapeutic dose of warfarin is reached. Inhibition of multiple cytochrome P450 enzymes and p-glycoprotein by amiodarone also interferes with the clearance of digoxin, simvastatin, and amitriptyline. Because LM's serum digoxin concentration is already at the upper therapeutic limit for heart failure, addition of amiodarone is likely to increase her digoxin concentration to a potentially harmful level. Digoxin clearance is dependent on renal elimination and the dose may need to be decreased to every other day to avoid toxicity. Amiodarone itself has some beta-blockade activity and through its inhibition of the metabolism of metoprolol via 2D6, the extent that the heart rate will decrease in LM is difficult to estimate. This interaction could benefit the patient by reducing the rapid ventricular rate, or it could cause bradycardia. Simvastatin use at the current dose may also become problematic with the addition of amiodarone. The U.S. Food and Drug Administration issued a statement in 2011 that warned of muscle injury with HMG-CoA reductase inhibitors and recommended certain dose restrictions when using these drugs with certain medication classes.[13] Geriatric patients are at an increased risk of statin-induced myopathy and increased exercise fatigue even prior to the inhibition of simvastatin metabolism by amiodarone.[14,15] In this patient, the dose of simvastatin should be reduced to no more than 10 mg daily to minimize the risk of myopathy. Amiodarone also interferes with amitriptyline metabolism, will lead to increased concentrations, and will increase the risk of QTc prolongation. With all of these issues at hand, amiodarone is still an option though adjustment of other medications will be necessary to avoid toxicities. ■

GENERAL GUIDELINES FOR SAFE PRESCRIBING

This section describes strategies to avoid side effects and drug interactions, to minimize the prescribing cascade, to promote medication adherence, and to understand benefits and harms of medications. Writing prescriptions is the most common intervention performed by health professionals in many settings. Older patients, with multiple comorbidities, frailty, and use of more medications, are particularly at risk for adverse drug events. Drug-adverse effects and nonadherence may account for 28.2% of hospital admissions of elderly patients.[16] The Institute for Safe Medication Practices reported 19,551 drug-related deaths in the United States in 2009.[17] This is greater than the 17,520 deaths attributed to homicides in the same year. Creating a therapeutic drug regimen that benefits patients while minimizing ill effects is paramount and requires deliberate planning and careful attention.

A principle in geriatric care is that the law of parsimony often does not apply. Problems, especially the geriatric syndromes (see Unit 2), often have more than one cause. Geriatric patients frequently have atypical signs and symptoms and new complaints or increasing dysfunction are frequently related to medication adverse events. The problem of mistakenly identifying adverse medication effects as new medical conditions may lead to a drug-related problem known as the prescribing cascade. This effect occurs when a new complaint is assumed to be from a disease state rather than from a drug, which leads to addition of new medications, further increasing the risk of adverse events. Common examples[18] include the use of nonsteroidal antiinflammatory drugs leading to antihypertensive therapy, the use of thiazide diuretics leading to treatment for gout, and the use of metoclopramide leading to treatment for Parkinson's disease. Another example would be a patient taking a benzodiazepine for anxiety who experiences central nervous system depression that leads to a diagnosis of dementia and prescription of an acetylcholinesterase inhibitor. Acetylcholinesterase inhibitors are known to cause (or exacerbate) urinary incontinence, which could spark the initiation of an anticholinergic medication, further causing cognitive dysfunction. This chain of events demonstrates how with any new complaint, an adverse medication reaction should be in the differential diagnosis. The need for continued use of possibly offending agents must be questioned and a dose reduction or discontinuation should occur. If treatment is needed for a new condition, nonpharmacologic treatment should be considered.

> The differential diagnosis of any geriatric problem should include an adverse drug effect.

Creating individualized patient care plans in the face of a growing number of treatment guidelines and diminishing time to spend with each patient is a daunting task. Treatment guidelines rarely have recommendations on when to discontinue therapies in later life. Also, older patients are susceptible to medication adverse effects (such as anticholinergic burden).

Four criteria have been suggested to assist prescribers in deciding when to start or continue medications in their patients.[19] These criteria are (1) a patient's life expectancy, (2) the time until benefit from medication, (3) goals of care, and (4) treatment targets. Life expectancy can be estimated based on comorbidities, functional status, and disease markers of poor prognosis. Time until benefit of a given medication can vary drastically. For example, the use of HMG-CoA reductase inhibitors for primary prevention of coronary artery disease will take many years to benefit and have a large number needed to treat whereas opioids for acute pain control will have a short time to benefit and low number needed to treat. Determining goals of care is challenging because the health care provider,

the patient, and the patient's family all have input on the goals. Setting treatment targets follows the goals of care discussion. For example, a patient may value a more symptom-targeted approach rather than a disease-modifying approach that may have untoward effects. These decisions are on a spectrum that ranges from a curative to a palliative stance. An optimal plan would consider all of these factors. For example, if life expectancy is likely a few months, and goals of therapy are palliative, then targeting symptoms, rather than prescribing a drug with a long time to benefit, would be appropriate.

EXPLICIT CRITERIA FOR PRESCRIBING

Tools are available to guide clinicians in the choice of medications for older adults. A review by Levy et al. compared nine sets of explicit criteria developed by various groups around the world.[20] The best-known criteria in the United States are the Beers Criteria for Potentially Inappropriate Medication Use in Older Adults, which were developed in 1991.[21] There have been three revisions of the Beers Criteria, most recently in 2012 led by the American Geriatrics Society.[22] This version is evidence-based and intended for use in all care settings. The Beers Criteria (Figure 6-1) are used as quality measures by the Centers for Medicare and Medicaid Services (CMS) and the National Committee for Quality Assurance (NCQA). Medications on the Beers list either have limited effectiveness in older adults or have risk of serious adverse events and safer alternatives are available. Medications are organized by pharmacologic class and listed in tables as drugs to avoid, drugs to avoid in older adults with specific disease states, and drugs to use with caution.

The other well-known sets of criteria are the STOPP and START (Screening Tool of Older Persons Potentially Inappropriate Prescriptions, and Screening Tool to Alert Doctors to the Right Treatment), which were developed in Ireland.[23,24] Both sets of criteria are organized by pharmacological class. The START focuses on prescribing omissions and consists of 22 evidence-based criteria for use of medications in particular disease states (example: use of angiotensin-converting enzyme [ACE] inhibitors following an acute myocardial infarction). The STOPP, similar to the Beers Criteria, consists of 65 medications that are potentially inappropriate for use in the elderly. There is some overlap between the Beers and STOPP, but both tools are useful in clinical practice.

Another set of prescribing guidelines is the ACOVE (Assessing Care of Vulnerable Elders).[25] This set of indicators provides guidance in choice of medications, monitoring parameters, and overall pharmacologic care, such as keeping up-to-date medications lists and doing periodic drug regimen reviews.

AGS BEERS CRITERIA

FOR POTENTIALLY INAPPROPRIATE MEDICATION USE IN OLDER ADULTS

FROM THE AMERICAN GERIATRICS SOCIETY

This clinical tool, based on The AGS 2012 Updated Beers Criteria for Potentially Inappropriate Medication Use in Older Adults (AGS 2012 Beers Criteria), has been developed to assist healthcare providers in improving medication safety in older adults. Our purpose is to inform clinical decision-making concerning the prescribing of medications for older adults in order to improve safety and quality of care.

Originally conceived of in 1991 by the late Mark Beers, MD, a geriatrician, the Beers Criteria catalogues medications that cause adverse drug events in older adults due to their pharmacologic properties and the physiologic changes of aging. In 2011, the AGS undertook an update of the criteria, assembling a team of experts and funding the develop-ment of the AGS 2012 Beers Criteria using an enhanced, evidence-based methodology. Each criterion is rated (qual-ity of evidence and strength of evidence) using the American College of Physicians' Guideline Grading System, which is based on the GRADE scheme developed by Guyatt et al.

The full document together with accompanying resources can be viewed online at ***www.americangeriatrics.org***.

INTENDED USE
The goal of this clinical tool is to improve care of older adults by reducing their exposure to Potentially Inappropri-ate Medications (PIMs).

- This should be viewed as a guide for identifying medications for which the risks of use in older adults outweigh the benefits.
- These criteria are not meant to be applied in a punitive manner.
- This list is not meant to supersede clinical judgment or an individual patient's values and needs. Prescribing and managing disease conditions should be individualized and involve shared decision-making.
- These criteria also underscore the importance of using a team approach to prescribing and the use of non-pharmacological approaches and of having economic and organizational incentives for this type of model.
- Implicit criteria such as the STOPP/START criteria and Medication Appropriateness Index should be used in a complementary manner with the 2012 AGS Beers Criteria to guide clinicians in making decisions about safe medication use in older adults.

The criteria are not applicable in all circumstances (eg, patient's receiving palliative and hospice care). If a clinician is not able to find an alternative and chooses to continue to use a drug on this list in an individual patient, designationof the medication as potentially inappropriate can serve as a reminder for close monitoring so that the potential for an adverse drug effect can be incorporated into the medical record and prevented or detected early.

TABLE 1: 2012 AGS Beers Criteria for Potentially Inappropriate Medication Use in Older Adults

Organ System/ Therapeutic Category/Drug(s)	**Recommendation,** Rationale, *Quality of Evidence (QE) & Strength of Recommendation (SR)*
Anticholinergics (excludes TCAs)	
First-generation antihistamines (as single agent or as part of combination products) • Brompheniramine • Carbinoxamine • Chlorpheniramine • Clemastine • Cyproheptadine • Dexbrompheniramine • Dexchlorpheniramine • Diphenhydramine (oral) • Doxylamine • Hydroxyzine • Promethazine • Triprolidine	**Avoid.** Highly anticholinergic; clearance reduced with advanced age, and tolerance develops when used as hypnotic; increased risk of confusion, dry mouth, constipation, and other anticholinergic effects/toxicity. Use of diphenhydramine in special situations such as acute treatment of severe allergic reaction may be appropriate. *QE = High (Hydroxyzine and Promethazine), Moderate (All others); SR = Strong*
Antiparkinson agents • Benztropine (oral) • Trihexyphenidyl	**Avoid.** Not recommended for prevention of extrapyramidal symptoms with antipsychotics; more effective agents available for treatment of Parkinson disease. *QE = Moderate; SR = Strong*

PAGE 1 Table 1 *(continued on page 2)*

Table 1 *(continued from page 1)*

TABLE 1: 2012 AGS Beers Criteria for Potentially Inappropriate Medication Use in Older Adults

Organ System/ Therapeutic Category/Drug(s)	**Recommendation,** Rationale, *Quality of Evidence (QE) & Strength of Recommendation (SR)*
Antispasmodics • Belladonna alkaloids • Clidinium-chlordiazepoxide • Dicyclomine • Hyoscyamine • Propantheline • Scopolamine	**Avoid except in short-term palliative care to decrease oral secretions.** Highly anticholinergic, uncertain effectiveness. *QE = Moderate; SR = Strong*
Antithrombotics	
Dipyridamole, oral short-acting* (does not apply to the extended-release combination with aspirin)	**Avoid.** May cause orthostatic hypotension; more effective alternatives available; IV form acceptable for use in cardiac stress testing. *QE = Moderate; SR = Strong*
Ticlopidine*	**Avoid.** Safer, effective alternatives available. *QE = Moderate; SR = Strong*
Anti-infective	
Nitrofurantoin	**Avoid for long-term suppression; avoid in patients with CrCl <60 mL/min.** Potential for pulmonary toxicity; safer alternatives available; lack of efficacy in patients with CrCl <60 mL/min due to inadequate drug concentration in the urine. *QE = Moderate; SR = Strong*
Cardiovascular	
Alpha$_1$ blockers • Doxazosin • Prazosin • Terazosin	**Avoid use as an antihypertensive.** High risk of orthostatic hypotension; not recommended as routine treatment for hypertension; alternative agents have superior risk/benefit profile. *QE = Moderate; SR = Strong*
Alpha agonists • Clonidine • Guanabenz* • Guanfacine* • Methyldopa* • Reserpine (>0.1 mg/day)*	**Avoid clonidine as a first-line antihypertensive. Avoid others as listed.** High risk of adverse CNS effects; may cause bradycardia and orthostatic hypotension; not recommended as routine treatment for hypertension. *QE = Low; SR = Strong*
Antiarrhythmic drugs (Class Ia, Ic, III) • Amiodarone • Dofetilide • Dronedarone • Flecainide • Ibutilide • Procainamide • Propafenone • Quinidine • Sotalol	**Avoid antiarrhythmic drugs as first-line treatment of atrial fibrillation.** Data suggest that rate control yields better balance of benefits and harms than rhythm control for most older adults. Amiodarone is associated with multiple toxicities, including thyroid disease, pulmonary disorders, and QT interval prolongation. *QE = High; SR = Strong*
Disopyramide*	**Avoid.** Disopyramide is a potent negative inotrope and therefore may induce heart failure in older adults; strongly anticholinergic; other antiarrhythmic drugs preferred. *QE = Low; SR = Strong*
Dronedarone	**Avoid in patients with permanent atrial fibrillation or heart failure.** Worse outcomes have been reported in patients taking dronedarone who have permanent atrial fibrillation or heart failure. In general, rate control is preferred over rhythm control for atrial fibrillation. *QE = Moderate; SR = Strong*
Digoxin >0.125 mg/day	**Avoid.** In heart failure, higher dosages associated with no additional benefit and may increase risk of toxicity; decreased renal clearance may increase risk of toxicity. *QE = Moderate; SR = Strong*

PAGE 2 Table 1 *(continued on page 3)*

Table 1 *(continued from page 2)*

TABLE 1: 2012 AGS Beers Criteria for Potentially Inappropriate Medication Use in Older Adults

Organ System/ Therapeutic Category/Drug(s)	**Recommendation,** Rationale, *Quality of Evidence (QE) & Strength of Recommendation (SR)*
Nifedipine, immediate release*	**Avoid.** Potential for hypotension; risk of precipitating myocardial ischemia. *QE = High; SR = Strong*
Spironolactone >25 mg/day	Avoid in patients with heart failure or with a CrCl <30 mL/min. In heart failure, the risk of hyperkalemia is higher in older adults if taking >25 mg/day. *QE = Moderate; SR = Strong*
Central Nervous System	
Tertiary TCAs, alone or in combination: • Amitriptyline • Chlordiazepoxide-amitriptyline • Clomipramine • Doxepin >6 mg/day • Imipramine • Perphenazine-amitriptyline • Trimipramine	**Avoid.** Highly anticholinergic, sedating, and cause orthostatic hypotension; the safety profile of low-dose doxepin (≤6 mg/day) is comparable to that of placebo. *QE = High; SR = Strong*
Antipsychotics, first- (conventional) and second- (atypical) generation *(see online for full list)*	Avoid use for behavioral problems of dementia unless non-pharmacologic options have failed and patient is threat to self or others. Increased risk of cerebrovascular accident (stroke) and mortality in persons with dementia. *QE = Moderate; SR = Strong*
Thioridazine Mesoridazine	**Avoid.** Highly anticholinergic and greater risk of QT-interval prolongation. *QE = Moderate; SR = Strong*
Barbiturates • Amobarbital* • Butabarbital* • Butalbital • Mephobarbital* • Pentobarbital* • Phenobarbital • Secobarbital*	**Avoid.** High rate of physical dependence; tolerance to sleep benefits; greater risk of overdose at low dosages. *QE = High; SR = Strong*
Benzodiazepines *Short- and intermediate-acting:* • Alprazolam • Estazolam • Lorazepam • Oxazepam • Temazepam • Triazolam *Long-acting:* • Chlorazepate • Chlordiazepoxide • Chlordiazepoxide-amitriptyline • Clidinium-chlordiazepoxide • Clonazepam • Diazepam • Flurazepam • Quazepam	**Avoid benzodiazepines (any type) for treatment of insomnia, agitation, or delirium.** Older adults have increased sensitivity to benzodiazepines and decreased metabolism of long-acting agents. In general, all benzodiazepines increase risk of cognitive impairment, delirium, falls, fractures, and motor vehicle accidents in older adults. May be appropriate for seizure disorders, rapid eye movement sleep disorders, benzodiazepine withdrawal, ethanol withdrawal, severe generalized anxiety disorder, periprocedural anesthesia, end-of-life care. *QE = High; SR = Strong*
Chloral hydrate*	**Avoid.** Tolerance occurs within 10 days and risk outweighs the benefits in light of overdose with doses only 3 times the recommended dose. *QE = Low; SR = Strong*
Meprobamate	**Avoid.** High rate of physical dependence; very sedating. *QE = Moderate; SR = Strong*

PAGE 3 Table 1 *(continued on page 4)*

Table 1 *(continued from page 3)*

TABLE 1: 2012 AGS Beers Criteria for Potentially Inappropriate Medication Use in Older Adults

Organ System/ Therapeutic Category/Drug(s)	**Recommendation,** Rationale, *Quality of Evidence (QE) & Strength of Recommendation (SR)*
Nonbenzodiazepine hypnotics • Eszopiclone • Zolpidem • Zaleplon	**Avoid chronic use (>90 days)** Benzodiazepine-receptor agonists that have adverse events similar to those of benzodiazepines in older adults (e.g., delirium, falls, fractures); minimal improvement in sleep latency and duration. *QE = Moderate; SR = Strong*
Ergot mesylates* Isoxsuprine*	Avoid. Lack of efficacy. *QE = High; SR = Strong*
Endocrine	
Androgens • Methyltestosterone* • Testosterone	**Avoid unless indicated for moderate to severe hypogonadism.** Potential for cardiac problems and contraindicated in men with prostate cancer. *QE = Moderate; SR = Weak*
Desiccated thyroid	**Avoid.** Concerns about cardiac effects; safer alternatives available. *QE = Low; SR = Strong*
Estrogens with or without progestins	**Avoid oral and topical patch. Topical vaginal cream: Acceptable to use low-dose intravaginal estrogen for the management of dyspareunia, lower urinary tract infec tions, and other vaginal symptoms.** Evidence of carcinogenic potential (breast and endometrium); lack of cardioprotective effect and cognitive protection in older women. Evidence that vaginal estrogens for treatment of vaginal dryness is safe and effective in women with breast cancer, especially at dos-ages of estradiol <25 mcg twice weekly. *QE = High (Oral and Patch); Moderate (Topical); SR = Strong (Oral and Patch), Weak (Topical)*
Growth hormone	**Avoid, except as hormone replacement following pituitary gland removal.** Effect on body composition is small and associated with edema, arthralgia, carpal tunnel syndrome, gynecomastia, impaired fasting glucose. *QE = High; SR = Strong*
Insulin, sliding scale	**Avoid.** Higher risk of hypoglycemia without improvement in hyperglyce -mia management regardless of care setting. *QE = Moderate; SR = Strong*
Megestrol	**Avoid.** Minimal effect on weight; increases risk of thrombotic events and possibly death in older adults. *QE = Moderate; SR = Strong*
Sulfonylureas, long-duration • Chlorpropamide • Glyburide	**Avoid.** Chlorpropamide: prolonged half-life in older adults; can cause prolonged hypoglycemia; causes SIADH Glyburide: higher risk of severe prolonged hypoglycemia in older adults. *QE = High; SR = Strong*
Gastrointestinal	
Metoclopramide	**Avoid, unless for gastroparesis.** Can cause extrapyramidal effects including tardive dyskinesia; risk may be further increased in frail older adults. *QE = Moderate; SR = Strong*
Mineral oil, given orally	**Avoid.** Potential for aspiration and adverse effects; safer alternatives available. *QE = Moderate; SR = Strong*
Trimethobenzamide	**Avoid.** One of the least effective antiemetic drugs; can cause extrapyramidal adverse effects. *QE = Moderate; SR = Strong*

PAGE 4 Table 1 *(continued on page 5)*

Figure 6-1 2012 Beers Criteria pocket card. (From www.americangeriatrics.org/search/?cx=008664580565903273424%3Auo2vk7ffzna&cof=FORID%3A10&ie=UTF-8&q=Beers&sa=%C2%A0.)

Table 1 *(continued from page 4)*

TABLE 1: 2012 AGS Beers Criteria for Potentially Inappropriate Medication Use in Older Adults

Organ System/ Therapeutic Category/Drug(s)	Recommendation, Rationale, *Quality of Evidence (QE) & Strength of Recommendation (SR)*
Pain Medications	
Meperidine	**Avoid.** Not an effective oral analgesic in dosages commonly used; may cause neurotoxicity; safer alternatives available. *QE = High; SR = Strong*
Non-COX-selective NSAIDs, oral • Aspirin >325 mg/day • Diclofenac • Diflunisal • Etodolac • Fenoprofen • Ibuprofen • Ketoprofen • Meclofenamate • Mefenamic acid • Meloxicam • Nabumetone • Naproxen • Oxaprozin • Piroxicam • Sulindac • Tolmetin	**Avoid chronic use unless other alternatives are not effective and patient can take gastroprotective agent (proton-pump inhibitor or misoprostol).** Increases risk of GI bleeding/peptic ulcer disease in high-risk groups, including those ≥75 years old or taking oral or parenteral corticosteroids, anticoagulants, or antiplatelet agents. Use of proton pump inhibitor or misoprostol reduces but does not eliminate risk. Upper GI ulcers, gross bleeding, or perforation caused by NSAIDs occur in approximately 1% of patients treated for 3–6 months, and in about 2%–4% of patients treated for 1 year. These trends continue with longer duration of use. *QE = Moderate; SR = Strong*
Indomethacin Ketorolac, includes parenteral	**Avoid.** Increases risk of GI bleeding/peptic ulcer disease in high-risk groups (See Non-COX selective NSAIDs)Of all the NSAIDs, indomethacin has most adverse effects. *QE = Moderate (Indomethacin); High (Ketorolac); SR = Strong*
Pentazocine*	**Avoid.** Opioid analgesic that causes CNS adverse effects, including confusion and hallucinations, more commonly than other narcotic drugs; is also a mixed agonist and antagonist; safer alternatives available. *QE = Low; SR = Strong*
Skeletal muscle relaxants • Carisoprodol • Chlorzoxazone • Cyclobenzaprine • Metaxalone • Methocarbamol • Orphenadrine	**Avoid.** Most muscle relaxants poorly tolerated by older adults, because of anticholinergic adverse effects, sedation, increased risk of fractures; effectiveness at dosages tolerated by older adults is questionable. *QE = Moderate; SR = Strong*

*Infrequently used drugs. Table 1 Abbreviations: ACEI, angiotensin converting-enzyme inhibitors; ARB, angiotensin receptor blockers; CNS, central nervous system; COX, cyclooxygenase; CrCl, creatinine clearance; GI, gastrointestinal; NSAIDs, nonsteroidal anti-inflammatory drugs; SIADH, syndrome of inappropriate antidiuretic hormone secretion; SR, Strength of Recommendation; TCAs, tricyclic antidepressants; QE, Quality of Evidence

TABLE 2: 2012 AGS Beers Criteria for Potentially Inappropriate Medication Use in Older Adults Due to Drug-Disease or Drug-Syndrome Interactions That May Exacerbate the Disease or Syndrome

Disease or Syndrome	Drug(s)	Recommendation, Rationale, *Quality of Evidence (QE) & Strength of Recommendation (SR)*
Cardiovascular		
Heart failure	NSAIDs and COX-2 inhibitors Nondihydropyridine CCBs (avoid only for systolic heart failure) • Diltiazem • Verapamil Pioglitazone, rosiglitazone Cilostazol Dronedarone	**Avoid.** Potential to promote fluid retention and/or exacerbate heart failure. *QE = Moderate (NSAIDs, CCBs, Dronedarone), High (Thiazolidinediones (glitazones)), Low (Cilostazol); SR = Strong*

Table 2 *(continued on page 6)*

Table 2 *(continued from page 5)*

TABLE 2: 2012 AGS Beers Criteria for Potentially Inappropriate Medication Use in Older Adults Due to Drug-Disease or Drug-Syndrome Interactions That May Exacerbate the Disease or Syndrome

Disease or Syndrome	Drug(s)	Recommendation, Rationale, *Quality of Evidence (QE) & Strength of Recommendation (SR)*
Syncope	Acetylcholinesterase inhibitors (AChEIs) Peripheral alpha blockers • Doxazosin • Prazosin • Terazosin Tertiary TCAs Chlorpromazine, thioridazine, and olanzapine	**Avoid.** Increases risk of orthostatic hypotension or bradycardia. *QE = High (Alpha blockers), Moderate (AchEIs, TCAs and antipsychotics); SR = Strong (AChEIs and TCAs), Weak (alpha blockers and antipsychotics)*
Central Nervous System		
Chronic seizures or epilepsy	Bupropion Chlorpromazine Clozapine Maprotiline Olanzapine Thioridazine Thiothixene Tramadol	**Avoid.** Lowers seizure threshold; may be acceptable in patients with well-controlled seizures in whom alternative agents have not been effective. *QE = Moderate; SR = Strong*
Delirium	All TCAs Anticholinergics (see online for full list) Benzodiazepines Chlorpromazine Corticosteroids H_2-receptor antagonist Meperidine Sedative hypnotics Thioridazine	**Avoid.** Avoid in older adults with or at high risk of delirium because of inducing or worsening delirium in older adults; if discontinuing drugs used chronically, taper to avoid withdrawal symptoms. *QE = Moderate; SR = Strong*
Dementia & cognitive impairment	Anticholinergics (see online for full list) Benzodiazepines H_2-receptor antagonists Zolpidem Antipsychotics, chronic and as-needed use	**Avoid.** Avoid due to adverse CNS effects.Avoid antipsychotics for behavioral problems of dementia unless non-pharmacologic options have failed and patient is a threat to themselves or others. Antipsychotics are associated with an increased risk of cerebrovascular accident (stroke) and mortality in persons with dementia. *QE = High; SR = Strong*
History of falls or fractures	Anticonvulsants Antipsychotics Benzodiazepines Nonbenzodiazepine hypnotics • Eszopiclone • Zaleplon • Zolpidem TCAs/SSRIs	**Avoid unless safer alternatives are not available; avoid anticonvulsants except for seizure.** Ability to produce ataxia, impaired psychomotor function, syncope, and additional falls; shorter-acting benzodiazepines are not safer than long-acting ones. *QE = High; SR = Strong*
Insomnia	Oral decongestants • Pseudoephedrine • Phenylephrine Stimulants • Amphetamine • Methylphenidate • Pemoline Theobromines • Theophylline • Caffeine	**Avoid.** CNS stimulant effects. *QE = Moderate; SR = Strong*
Parkinson's disease	All antipsychotics (see online publication for full list, except for quetiapine and clozapine) Antiemetics • Metoclopramide • Prochlorperazine • Promethazine	**Avoid.** Dopamine receptor antagonists with potential to worsen parkinsonian symptoms. Quetiapine and clozapine appear to be less likely to precipitate worsening of Parkinson disease. *QE = Moderate; SR = Strong*

Table 2 *(continued on page 7)*

Table 2 *(continued from page 6)*

TABLE 2: 2012 AGS Beers Criteria for Potentially Inappropriate Medication Use in Older Adults Due to Drug-Disease or Drug-Syndrome Interactions That May Exacerbate the Disease or Syndrome

Disease or Syndrome	Drug(s)	Recommendation, Rationale, *Quality of Evidence (QE) & Strength of Recommendation (SR)*
Gastrointestinal		
Chronic constipation	Oral antimuscarinics for urinary incontinence • Darifenacin • Fesoterodine • Oxybutynin (oral) • Solifenacin • Tolterodine • Trospium Nondihydropyridine CCB • Diltiazem • Verapamil First-generation antihistamines as single agent or part of combination products • Brompheniramine (various) • Carbinoxamine • Chlorpheniramine • Clemastine (various) • Cyproheptadine • Dexbrompheniramine • Dexchlorpheniramine (various) • Diphenhydramine • Doxylamine • Hydroxyzine • Promethazine • Triprolidine Anticholinergics/antispasmodics (see online for full list of drugs with strong anticholinergic properties) • Antipsychotics • Belladonna alkaloids • Clidinium-chlordiazepoxide • Dicyclomine • Hyoscyamine • Propantheline • Scopolamine • Tertiary TCAs (amitriptyline, clomipramine, doxepin, imipramine, and trimipramine)	**Avoid unless no other alternatives.** Can worsen constipation; agents for urinary incontinence: antimuscarinics overall differ in incidence of constipation; response variable; consider alternative agent if constipation develops. *QE = High (For Urinary Incontinence), Moderate/ Low (All Others); SR = Strong*
History of gastric or duodenal ulcers	Aspirin (>325 mg/day) Non–COX-2 selective NSAIDs	**Avoid unless other alternatives are not effective and patient can take gastroprotective agent (proton-pump inhibitor or misoprostol).** May exacerbate existing ulcers or cause new/ additional ulcers. *QE = Moderate; SR = Strong*
Kidney/Urinary Tract		
Chronic kidney disease stages IV and V	NSAIDs Triamterene (alone or in combination)	**Avoid.** May increase risk of kidney injury. May increase risk of acute kidney injury. QE = Moderate (NSAIDs), Low (Triamterene); SR = Strong (NSAIDs), Weak (Triamterene)
Urinary incontinence (all types) in women	Estrogen oral and transdermal (excludes intravaginal estrogen)	Avoid in women. Aggravation of incontinence. *QE = High; SR = Strong*

Table 2 *(continued on page 8)*

Table 2 *(continued from page 7)*

TABLE 2: 2012 AGS Beers Criteria for Potentially Inappropriate Medication Use in Older Adults Due to Drug-Disease or Drug-Syndrome Interactions That May Exacerbate the Disease or Syndrome

Disease or Syndrome	Drug(s)	Recommendation, Rationale, *Quality of Evidence (QE) & Strength of Recommendation (SR)*
Lower urinary tract symptoms, benign prostatic hyperplasia	Inhaled anticholinergic agents Strongly anticholinergic drugs, except antimuscarinics for urinary incontinence *(see Table 9 for complete list).*	**Avoid in men.** May decrease urinary flow and cause urinary retention. QE = Moderate; SR = Strong (Inhaled agents), Weak (All others)
Stress or mixed urinary in-continence	Alpha-blockers • Doxazosin • Prazosin • Terazosin	**Avoid in women.** Aggravation of incontinence. QE = Moderate; SR = Strong

Table 2 Abbreviations: CCBs, calcium channel blockers; AChEIs, acetylcholinesterase inhibitors; CNS, central nervous system; COX, cycooxygenase; NSAIDs, nonsteroidal anti-inflammatory drugs; SR, Strength of Recommendation; SSRIs, selective serotonin reuptake inhibitors; TCAs, tricyclic antidepressants; QE, Quality of Evidence

TABLE 3: 2012 AGS Beers Criteria for Potentially Inappropriate Medications to Be Used with Caution in Older Adults

Drug(s)	Recommendation, Rationale, *Quality of Evidence (QE) & Strength of Recommendation (SR)*
Aspirin for primary prevention of cardiac events	Use with caution in adults ≥80 years old. Lack of evidence of benefit versus risk in individuals ≥80 years old. *QE = Low; SR = Weak*
Dabigatran	Use with caution in adults ≥75 years old or if CrCl <30 mL/min. Increased risk of bleeding compared with warfarin in adults ≥75 years old; lack of evidence for efficacy and safety in patients with CrCl <30 mL/min *QE = Moderate; SR = Weak*
Prasugrel	Use with caution in adults ≥75 years old. Greater risk of bleeding in older adults; risk may be offset by benefit in highest-risk older patients (eg, those with prior myocardial infarction or diabetes). *QE = Moderate; SR = Weak*
Antipsychotics Carbamazepine Carboplatin Cisplatin Mirtazapine SNRIs SSRIs TCAs Vincristine	Use with caution. May exacerbate or cause SIADH or hyponatremia; need to monitor sodium level closely when starting or changing dosages in older adults due to increased risk. *QE = Moderate; SR = Strong*
Vasodilators	Use with caution. May exacerbate episodes of syncope in individuals with history of syncope. *QE = Moderate; SR = Weak*

Table 3 Abbreviations: CrCl, creatinine clearance; SIADH, syndrome of inappropriate antidiuretic hormone secretion; SSRIs, selective serotonin reuptake inhibitors; SNRIs, serotonin–norepinephrine reuptake inhibitors; SR, Strength of Recommendation; TCAs, tricyclic antidepressants; QE, Quality of Evidence

The American Geriatrics Society gratefully acknowledges the support of the John A. Hartford Foundation, Retirement Research Foundation and Robert Wood Johnson Foundation.

AGS THE AMERICAN GERIATRICS SOCIETY
Geriatrics Health Professionals.
Leading change. Improving care for older adults.

40 Fulton Street, 18th Floor
New York, NY 10038
800-247-4779 ot 212-308-1414
www.americangeriatrics.org

Figure 6-1, cont'd

Older adults are more likely to experience anticholinergic side effects from medication (e.g., sedation, confusion, urinary retention, constipation). There are many medications with strong anticholinergic effects, but there are also medications that have subtle anticholinergic effects. The combination of two or more medications with even subtle anticholinergic effects can cause significant adverse effects in older adults. Hilmer et al. described a "drug burden index" that is based on anticholinergics, sedatives, and total medications used.[26] They found that increased exposure to medications with anticholinergic and sedative effects was associated with poorer physical and cognitive performance.

MEDICATION ADHERENCE

Terms used to describe the ability of a patient to use his or her medications as instructed include adherence, compliance, and persistence. Compliance implies a sense of one-sidedness where the patient is dealing with or adapting to a situation. Persistence refers only to the duration that a patient will continue with a medication treatment, not addressing the issue that an estimated 24% of prescriptions are never even filled.[27] Adherence has a broader, more team-based definition of "the extent to which a person's behavior—taking medication, following a diet, and/or executing lifestyle changes, corresponds with agreed recommendations from a health care provider."[28] The World Health Organization defines adherence to account for more than just the use of medications. Adherence is a dynamic process that requires individual patient strategies and follow-up and a multidisciplinary approach (Box 6-1). It is not entirely in the hands of a patient to be adherent and many determining factors for adherence lie with providers and the health system. It is estimated that adherence to long-term therapy for chronic illnesses averages 50%.[28]

> The first step in ensuring appropriate prescribing is obtaining an accurate and complete medication history.

> Decreasing complexity of a medication regimen will improve adherence.
> - When selecting a regimen, choose a medication requiring fewer doses per day.
> - Use combination tablets to reduce pill burden.

ADHERENCE AIDS

Adherence aids are available to help patients organize and remember to take their medications. The simplest method is to design a schedule for medications and the time of day to take them. Medication boxes that hold one day's or one week's worth of medication are commercially available in a variety of styles, with some boxes having two to four boxes for each day of the week to accommodate different dosing times. There are electronic aids that beep or light up when a dose is due, with some devices connected to the phone line to alert a family member or call center if a dose is not taken on time.

There are other products available to assist with the administration of medications. Tablet splitters and crushers may help patients who have difficulty swallowing tablets. Eyedrop guides, fit on the eyedrop bottle, help steady the hand and direct the drop into the eye (Figure 6-2). For patients using any type of inhaled medication, their ability to use the device correctly should be assessed. For metered-dose inhalers, spacer devices (e.g., Aerochamber) are available. Transdermal patches can be difficult for older patients to apply if they have decreased vision or diminished manual dexterity. Child-resistant caps, which have been required on prescription medications in the United States since 1970, can be barriers to adherence in older patients. The pharmacist and the prescriber should ask patients if they need a non–child-resistant cap. The prescriber can note it on the prescription or the patient can tell the pharmacist.

BOX 6-1

TIPS FOR ASSESSING MEDICATION ADHERENCE

Ask about medication/supplement/over-the-counter use in different ways throughout an encounter.
Have patient demonstrate inhaler/eyedrop/topical medication use.
Request that patient bring all medications (preferred) or at least a medication list to all appointments.
Explicitly inquire about missing doses and difficulties with adherence using open-ended questions.

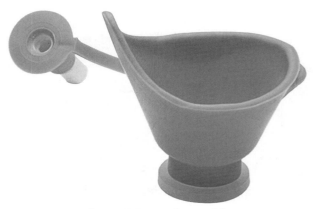

Figure 6-2 Eyedrop guide.

LM (Part 3)

Because of LM's new complaints, a seventh medication is now being added to her medication list. Adherence should be assessed to ensure that the new findings are not caused by missed doses of her beta-blocker. If uncontrolled heart rate is a result of nonadherence to beta-blocker therapy, adding another agent (amiodarone) may not fix the problem and may only increase the medication burden. Because the complexity of a regimen may affect adherence, efforts should be made to simplify the regimen if possible. LM is currently taking metoprolol tartrate twice daily for heart failure. This could easily be switched to the long-acting once daily metoprolol succinate at a dose of 200 mg daily. Also, there is better evidence for efficacy with the succinate salt in patients with heart failure. If amiodarone is initiated, its interaction with warfarin will require increased frequency of monitoring the INR for several months. Switching warfarin to dabigatran would eliminate the need for more frequent lab work but would increase pill burden because dabigatran is taken twice daily. Patient preference as to which is more convenient should be strongly considered in making such therapeutic decisions. ◾

MEDICARE PART D

The Medicare Prescription Drug, Improvement, and Modernization Act of 2003 included a new outpatient prescription drug benefit, known as Medicare Part D. This benefit began in January 2006 as a voluntary component of the Medicare program. All participants in Medicare A and/or B are eligible to enroll in a Part D Prescription Drug Plan (PDP). Although the guidelines for Part D are developed by the Centers for Medicare and Medicaid Services (CMS), PDPs are offered by private companies and vary from state to state. Each plan has a distinct formulary and restrictions on prior authorization, quantity limits, and step therapy. Prescribers must be familiar with the program to help patients receive the most cost-effective regimens.

The Part D benefit includes a deductible ($325 in 2013), and then the beneficiary pays 25% of the cost of medications until a predetermined amount ($2970 in 2013). At this point there is a coverage gap ("the doughnut hole"). When Part D was implemented in 2006, the coverage gap was a true gap—patients paid 100% of the cost of the medications until they hit catastrophic coverage. With the passage of the Patient Protection and Affordable Care Act in 2010, the coverage gap will gradually be phased out by 2020. The intent of Part D was to make medications more accessible to older adults, and studies evaluating the use of medications by patients with Part D coverage have found an increase in the number of prescriptions filled during the initial coverage period.[29-31] However, during the coverage gap an increase in nonadherence was seen.[32]

As an alternative to the 25% copayment, many Part D plans have a tiered copayment system. The difference in copayment between a Tier 1 medication (preferred generic) and Tier 3 (nonpreferred brand) can be substantial. This added economic burden on the patient may impact adherence, so it is important that prescribers be familiar with the formularies of commonly used PDPs in their patient population. Pharmacists can assist patients in reviewing their medications and the various plans available to them during the annual Medicare open enrollment period using the Plan Finder tool on the Medicare website. It is recommended that patients review their plan annually because costs and formularies change with each calendar year.

> Prescription of generic medications under Medicare D keeps patients out of the "doughnut hole" and improves adherence.

An important component of Medicare Part D is medication therapy management (MTM). CMS requires that each PDP have an MTM program for enrollees. Patients who have multiple chronic disease states, are on multiple medications, and are projected to use >$3000 of medications per year are eligible for MTM services. MTM consists of a comprehensive evaluation of the patient's medication regimen by a pharmacist or other qualified provider; the goals are to decrease adverse drug events and improve patient outcomes by promoting appropriate medication use. Starting in 2013, each patient receiving MTM will receive a Medication Action Plan and Personal Medication List from their MTM provider. The action plan is a summary of the MTM session reminding patients of what was discussed and what they need to do with their medications. In one study of the influence of an MTM program, there was a 47% acceptance rate of the MTM recommendations, mainly in the areas of guideline adherence, cost savings, and safety concerns.[33] Another study found that MTM resolved significantly more medication and health-related problems as compared to a control group.[34] As MTM programs continue to develop, more studies of their impact on patient outcomes are needed.

> Learn more about Medicare Part D at www.medicare.gov and www.Q1medicare.com.

Discussion

Because LM is having problems keeping her INR within the therapeutic range, you decide to switch her to dabigatran

75 mg twice daily. On her next visit, LM reluctantly admits to you that she is having trouble paying the copayment for the medication because it is a Tier 3 medication in her Part D prescription plan. LM likes the fact that she does not have to get her INR monitored, but she worries about the expense. You call LM's pharmacist to ask for suggestions and find out that the open enrollment period is soon and that if LM can stay in the plan for a few more months, she could then switch into a plan that has dabigatran as a Tier 2 and a minimal copayment for all of her generic drugs. In the meantime, the pharmacist suggests looking into the manufacturer's assistance plan. In reviewing LM's drug regimen, the pharmacist notes that LM is on several Beers Criteria medications and suggests that amitriptyline for migraine prophylaxis be discontinued. This will minimize the risks of anticholinergic effects, orthostatic hypotension, and sedation, all of which can increase her risk of falls. The pharmacist notes that metoprolol may also be effective as migraine prophylaxis. ▪

ROLE OF THE PHARMACIST IN GERIATRIC CARE

Since 1997, pharmacists have had the opportunity to become a Certified Geriatric Pharmacist (CGP) through an examination conducted by the Commission for Certification in Geriatric Pharmacy. More information about this program and how to locate a CGP is available at www.ccgp.org.

The role of the pharmacist in geriatric care has traditionally been in nursing facilities. The federal government has mandated monthly drug regimen reviews in skilled nursing facilities for 40 years. The medication regimen review is "a thorough evaluation of the medication regimen of a resident with the goal of promoting positive outcomes and minimizing adverse consequences associated with medications."[35] For more information, the reader is referred to the American Society of Consultant Pharmacists (www.ascp.com).

Given the benefits and risks of pharmaceuticals, there is an important and evolving role for the pharmacist in geriatric care. There are pharmacists in private practices assisting patients with adherence and disease management. Others operate anticoagulation and hypertension clinics, serve as consultants in hospitals, with hospice agencies, and in Program of All-Inclusive Care of the Elderly (PACE) programs. Pharmacists assist in designing appropriate medication regimens, including choice of medication, dose, dosage form, and monitoring parameters. Pharmacists provide information on adverse events and drug interactions, assess adherence, and advise about cost issues. Medication reconciliation is a patient safety goal and is particularly important in geriatrics because of the number of medications used, multiple prescribers, and multiple sites of care. Pharmacists are the ideal team member to accurately reconcile patients' medications during transitions in care.

Although specific regulations vary by state, community pharmacists are required to counsel patients on all new prescriptions; patients should be encouraged to ask their pharmacist about over-the-counter medications and other health-related products. Most important, patients should use only one computer profile. This allows the pharmacist to monitor for drug interactions, duplications, and potential adverse effects. The pharmacist can also track adherence through refill records and provide advice on adherence and reminder aids.

SUMMARY

Because of the complexity of physiologic, social, and financial issues that older patients experience, care needs to be taken to ensure a logical, pragmatic, and efficient pharmacotherapeutic plan. Aging per se does not explain all or even most of the complexity of prescribing. The most reliable physiologic change is a decline in renal excretion. However, comorbid disease and drug interactions expand the complexity for this population. More and more powerful medications present advantages and also risks. Providers for patients with complex needs will find pharmacists their allies in provision of safe, reliable, and cost-effective patient care. The aids and resources outlined in this chapter can provide valuable assistance in caring for older people.

Web Resources

www.medicare.gov or www.Q1medicare.com. Information on Medicare D plans.

www.ccgp.org. The Commission for Certification in Geriatric Pharmacy.

www.americangeriatrics.org/search/?cx=00866458056590327 3424 %3Auo2vk7ffzna&cof=FORID%3A10&ie=UTF-8&q=Beers&sa= %C2%A02012. Beers Criteria, available as printable pocket guide or mobile app.

www.epill.com. Examples of medication adherence aids for patients.

KEY REFERENCES

5. Delafuente JC. Pharmacokinetic and pharmacodynamic alterations in the geriatric patient. Consult Pharm 2008;23(4):324-34.

7. Cusack BJ. Pharmacokinetics in older persons. Am J Geriatr Pharmacother 2004;2(4):274-302.

19. Holmes HM, Hayley DC, Alexander GC, et al. Reconsidering medication appropriateness for patients late in life. Arch Intern Med 2006;166:605-9.

22. The American Geriatrics Society 2012 Beers Criteria Update Expert Panel. AGS updated Beers Criteria for potentially inappropriate medication use in older adults. J Am Geriatr Soc 2012;60:616-31.

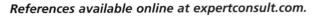

References available online at expertconsult.com.

7

Ethics

Robert A. Zorowitz

- Understand the use of the term *futility* as it applies to medical decision making.
- Discuss ethical concerns regarding assisted suicide and what's known as the double effect.
- Discuss the unique issues involving provision of food and fluid.

OBJECTIVES

Upon completion of this chapter, the reader will be able to:

- Discuss the most commonly cited principles of ethical decision making in medical care.
- Understand how to systematically elucidate and resolve ethical dilemmas.
- Discuss the requirements of informed consent and the criteria for decisional capacity.
- Discuss the role and use of different types of advance directives, including do-not-resuscitate (DNR) orders.

Additional online-only material indicated by icon.

The rapid advancements in medical technology, the growing population of the elderly, and the increasing awareness of the legal and moral issues confronting the elderly, their families, and their caregivers have resulted in the need for a methodology to evaluate and resolve moral conflicts that may confront clinicians who care for older patients.

Ethics is the field that systematically studies morality, which is defined as the rightness and wrongness of human acts. Medical ethics is the discipline that studies morality in health care, generally using a process that attempts to recognize and seek solutions to moral questions or dilemmas that arise in the care and treatment of patients. As a branch of moral philosophy, medical ethics is responsive to shifts in philosophical opinion and fashion. It is also a field that is a fusion of theory and practice.[1]

Moral dilemmas arise when the rights and wishes of patients conflict with the obligations of clinicians or when there are competing obligations among clinicians. These rights and obligations may be informed by philosophic, cultural, religious, or personal principles, beliefs, and values. In geriatric medicine, rights and obligations are often influenced and complicated by factors such as limited life expectancy, cognitive impairment, impaired decision-making capacity, insufficient social and economic resources, and the complexity of multiple concomitant medical problems and functional disorders.[2]

Over the past 20 years, there has been a growing awareness of the need to institute clinical ethics as a required discipline in medical training and in health care organizations. Ethics courses are becoming more common in medical schools, and ethics committees and similar venues for the resolution of ethical conflicts have become a required and expected presence in hospitals, nursing homes (NHs), and other health care organizations. The rise of medical consumerism has resulted in a population of patients and caregivers who are increasingly well-informed about their rights and choices in the health care market. As a result, it is vital that clinicians develop a shared language of ethical decision making.

This chapter introduces the basic principles of ethical decision making and examines common ethical issues encountered in the care of older patients.

Alice Oliver (Part 1)

Mrs. Alice Oliver is an 83-year-old woman, an active swimmer and gardener, who suffered a right-sided stroke with mild left hemiparesis and dysphagia. During hospitalization, her motor deficits were improving but the dysphagia persisted. A swallow evaluation indicated that she was able to tolerate a chopped or pureed diet with nectar-thick liquids, but she experienced asymptomatic aspiration with thin liquids. The speech therapist recommended thickening all liquids, and you enter this order on the chart. Mrs. Oliver, however, refuses thickened liquids, insisting that she would rather take her chances with thin liquids. The nurses and the dietician tell you they do not want to provide her with thin liquids; they believe that by doing so, they will be contributing to the risk they were trying to ameliorate.

You are confronted with an ethical dilemma. On one hand, you think the patient should have the right to take risks and eat what she wants. On the other hand, you can sympathize with the other health care professionals' discomfort in abetting risky behavior. Medical ethics provides a means for articulating and analyzing such dilemmas.

1. **What ethical principles are in conflict in this case?**
2. **Is there an ethical principle that takes priority over others?** ◪

PRINCIPLES OF MEDICAL ETHICS

Traditional principles of medical ethics derived largely from the works of Greek philosophers such as Hippocrates[3] and Pythagorus.[4] During the second half of the twentieth century, increasing pressure on the medical establishment from technological change, cultural upheaval, and the increasing complexity of medical care and the issues it raised resulted in the need to more explicitly frame the principles of medical ethics.

Although there are a number of alternative theories of medical ethics—such as the virtue-based theories favored by the Greek philosophers, the ethics of caring,[5] and casuistry[6]—there remain four prima facie principles that are most often cited as the bedrock of clinical ethics. These are autonomy, beneficence, nonmaleficence, and justice.[7]

Autonomy

The principle of autonomy refers to the duty to respect a patient's right to self-determination. This has been legally enshrined in the judicial ruling of *Schloendorff v. Society of New York Hospital* (NY 1914), in which Justice Cardozo found that, "Every human being of adult years and of sound mind has a right to determine what shall be done with his body."[8]

Traditionally, clinicians have assumed a strongly authoritarian and paternalistic role in the medical decision-making process. With the increase in consumerism and the availability of medical information, patients have been more likely to assert their autonomy. Health care providers have been increasingly recognizing autonomy as a fundamental ethical principle.

Integral to the principle of autonomy is the right to receive sufficient factual information to allow self-determination. This is the basis of informed consent, established in the Nuremberg code, which states, "The voluntary consent of the human subject is absolutely essential."[9] In *Nathanson v. Kline* (KS 1960), a case that centered on the failure to inform a patient of potential surgical risks, the ruling found that, "It follows that each man is considered to be master of his own body, and he may, if he be of sound mind, prohibit the performance of life-saving surgery or other medical treatment."[10]

In addition to establishing the right of an autonomous patient to refuse treatment, these rulings also introduce the "of sound mind" concept, which is indicative of a patient's capacity to understand what has been explained, appreciate the situation and its consequences, rationally manipulate information, and communicate choices.[11] Decision-making capacity is a critical requirement for providing informed consent and, therefore, for exercising autonomy.

Effective clinician–patient communication is an integral part of providing informed consent throughout the process of reaching an autonomous decision. The clinician has a duty to tell the truth and provide fact-based, objective information to the patient. Such discussions must be free of personal, subjective biases. The information must be fair and lawful and must not be swayed by any financial or personal gain. This does not preclude the clinician from providing advice as to what would be the clinician's own preference, but the clinician should avoid labeling that choice as the "right" decision and assure the patient of support, regardless of the patient's own decision.

Truth-telling is an essential component of the exercise of autonomy. The recognition that there is an obligation to provide truthful information to patients about potentially life-threatening conditions is a relatively recent phenomenon. A 1961 survey of physicians in the United States reported that 90% would not reveal a diagnosis of cancer to their patients.[12] A 1979 survey reported that 97% of physicians would reveal a diagnosis of cancer to their patients.[13] A recent survey of hospitalized patients reported that a large majority would prefer to be told of a diagnosis of cancer or Alzheimer's disease. Among those who were unsure or who did not want to be told, a majority would want to be told if it was essential to treatment. Preferences did not differ by age.[14]

Age is not, by itself, an obstacle to the full exercise of autonomy. In one study, even very old hospitalized patients were able to express their health values, underscoring the need to elicit such choices directly from the patient, unless that patient lacks decision-making capacity.[15]

Beneficence

The principle of beneficence refers to the clinician's responsibility to provide benefit or help the patient (i.e., "to do good"). Beneficence is the essence of the patient–doctor relationship. Promotion of good health, curing disease, and relieving pain and suffering are all key elements in the principle of beneficence. Conversely, medical interventions that provide no benefit should be avoided.

Nonmaleficence

The principle of nonmaleficence states that throughout the physician–patient relationship, the physician shall "at the least, do no harm." It is incumbent upon all clinicians to determine the goals of the intervention and to weigh these goals against the potential risk of an adverse outcome. Factors such as advanced age, concurrent disease states, comorbidities, and expected prognosis must be considered in the equation. When available, the clinician may use formal algorithms to assess risk. For instance, preoperative cardiac risk stratification can help the clinician determine the risk of an adverse cardiac event from surgery. A short life expectancy may suggest that a particular screening test or procedure is not likely to have its expected benefit. In essence, the duty of nonmaleficence is balanced against the duty of beneficence when weighing risks and benefits.

Justice

Justice refers to the duty to treat patients fairly. Justice can be viewed along two dimensions: access and allocation.[16] Access refers to whether those who are entitled to health care resources can obtain them. Allocation refers to the determination of how resources are distributed. The distribution of rights and responsibilities among the members of a society in a manner governed by consistent moral norms is often referred to as distributive justice.

The principle of justice can apply to either the macroenvironment, such as the decisions made to ration health care within Oregon's Medicaid program,[17] or the microenvironment, such as decisions made to allocate money and other resources within a hospital, nursing home, or office practice.

In a hospital or nursing home, conflicts involving the principle of justice may revolve around the use of scarce, expensive, or labor-intensive medical interventions in frail, elderly patients with limited life

expectancies. On a national scale, justice may be the central principle in determining whether Medicare should cover a particular procedure or in determining who should have control over allocation decisions in managed care organizations.[18]

Other Principles

In addition to the principles outlined in the previous sections, there are other ethical principles that are common in geriatrics, particularly in communal settings such as assisted-living facilities or nursing homes, in which elderly residents not only obtain medical care but consider the facility their home. The principle of community, which refers to the duty to balance individual need with communal need, takes on great importance in such settings. Not only is personal autonomy important, but also individual dignity, a closely related but distinct value, is greatly valued. Also closely related to autonomy, the principle of authenticity refers to the ability to choose a lifestyle consistent with one's own values, beliefs, and habits.[19] These ethical principles largely underlie the advocacy of culture change in the nursing home industry. The culture change movement has as its goals to provide residents more homelike environments and choice over their lives, and to provide staff members the authority and empowerment to facilitate those choices.[20,21]

> In Western society, the principle of autonomy has come to dominate other ethical principles, but this may not be true of all cultures.

CASE 1

Alice Oliver (Part 2)

The case of Mrs. Oliver represents a classic conflict between the duty to respect the patient's autonomy and the duty to do good (beneficence) and avoid harm (nonmaleficence). Mrs. Oliver is unable to exercise her autonomy without the cooperation of the care team in providing her food, but the team feels that supplying her choice of diet would violate the duty to avoid harm. Having identified the ethical principles that are at odds with each other, you must now systematically evaluate alternatives for resolution.

1. **How would you go about devising a methodology for examining the ethical dilemma(s) in this case?**

2. **Is there a morally right and a morally wrong decision?** ▣

STRUCTURE FOR DELIBERATING ETHICAL DILEMMAS

There are several models for systematically evaluating and analyzing dilemmas in medical ethics. One of the most commonly used models is the "four topics" model devised by Jonsen et al.[22] This is a case-based approach that allows an organized review of the facts and issues in a given case, according to four topics: medical indications, patient preferences, quality of life, and contextual features (Figure 7-1).

Each topic represents a systematic means of organizing the questions related to the corresponding ethical principles. Under the topic "medical indications" are questions that determine how the facts of the case determine what is beneficence and nonmaleficence. The topic "patient preferences" contains questions that establish the patient's autonomy and how that autonomy fits into the ethical problem at hand. "Quality of life" contains questions that further elucidate what is considered beneficence and what is considered nonmaleficence, according to the patient's own values. "Contextual features" contains grouped questions that tease out other influences on the case and incorporate principles such as loyalty and fairness.

Once the facts of the case are organized, it is important to identify the ethical dilemma(s), if any. Only when the ethical questions are framed is it possible to formulate potential solutions. Frequently, ethical dilemmas have more than one morally permissible alternative. If the ethics consultant or ethics committee has been asked to participate, it may be their role to outline these alternatives. Nonetheless, it generally falls to the health care team and patient to determine which alternative will be followed.

> An ethical conflict may have more than one morally acceptable solution.

What appears at first to be an ethical dilemma may ultimately emerge as an interpersonal dispute among family members or between staff and family members.[23] In geriatrics, patients may have several family members, usually children, who may disagree with each other or with the health care team over decisions, large and small, sometimes making medical management time-consuming and difficult. In these cases, typical ethical deliberation may not always be useful or sufficient. Alternate techniques such as mediation,[24] negotiation,[25] or a combination of these and other methods of conflict resolution may be necessary.

> It is sometimes difficult to differentiate an ethical dilemma from an interpersonal conflict, and one may accompany the other.

MEDICAL INDICATIONS **The Principles of Beneficence and Nonmaleficence** 1. What is the patient's medical problem? History? Diagnosis? Prognosis? 2. Is the problem acute? Chronic? Critical? Emergent? Reversible? 3. What are the goals of treatment? 4. What are the probabilities of success? 5. What are the plans in case of therapeutic failure? 6. In sum, how can this patient be benefited by medical and nursing care, and how can harm be avoided?	**PATIENT PREFERENCES** **The Principle of Respect for Autonomy** 1. Is the patient mentally capable and legally competent? Is there evidence of incapacity? 2. If competent, what is the patient stating about preferences for treatment? 3. Has the patient been informed of benefits and risks, understood this information, and given consent? 4. If incapacitated, who is the appropriate surrogate? Is the surrogate using appropriate standards for decision making? 5. Has the patient expressed prior preferences, e.g., Advance Directives? 6. Is the patient unwilling or unable to cooperate with medical treatment? If so why? In sum, is the patient's right to choose being respected to the extent possible in ethics and law?
QUALITY OF LIFE **The Principles of Beneficence and Nonmaleficence and Respect for Autonomy** 1. What are the prospects, with or without treatment, for a return to normal life? 2. What physical, mental and social deficits is the patient likely to experience if treatment succeeds? 3. Are there biases that might prejudice the provider's evaluation of the patient's quality of life? 4. Is the patient's present or future condition such that his or her continued life might be judged undesirable? 5. Is there any plan and rationale to forgo treatment? 6. Are there plans for comfort and palliative care?	**CONTEXTUAL FEATURES** **The Principles of Loyalty and Fairness** 1. Are there family issues that might influence treatment decisions? 2. Are there provider (physicians and nurses) issues that might influence treatment decisions? 3. Are there financial and economic factors? 4. Are there religious or cultural factors? 5. Are there limits on confidentiality? 6. Are there problems of allocation of resources? 7. How does the law affect treatment decisions? 8. Is clinical research or teaching involved? 9. Is there any conflict of interest on the part of the providers or the institution?

Figure 7-1 Four topics for ethical analysis. (From Jonsen AR, Siegler M, Winslade WJ. Clinical ethics: A practical approach to ethical decisions in clinical medicine. 5th ed. New York: McGraw-Hill; 2002.)

CASE 1

Alice Oliver (Part 3)

Mrs. Oliver's nutrition may be viewed in a dual manner. Because nutrition is considered basic to life and comfort, the team has an obligation defined by the principle of beneficence to provide it. There is, however, a therapeutic component as well, because the food must be provided in a form and texture suitable to Mrs. Oliver's swallowing disorder. You tell the team that although Mrs. Oliver is refusing the recommended therapeutic form of the nutrition, they are still fulfilling the duty of beneficence and respecting her autonomy by providing her thin liquids, although the risk may be greater. In other words, the duties of autonomy and beneficence outweigh the duty of nonmaleficence. So long as Mrs. Oliver understands the increased risk she is assuming, it is ethically permissible to provide her with thin liquids. It is your responsibility, in conjunction with the care team, to establish that Mrs. Oliver has adequate information to make this decision.

Is there another morally acceptable alternative to this case? ◘

INFORMED CONSENT

Informed consent is the foundation for the exercise of autonomy. It has become increasingly central to both the ethical and legal regulation of American medicine and the clinician–patient relationship since the concept was first used in 1957.[26] Informed consent is more than simply the required signing of permission forms before surgery or other medical procedures. In representing the means by which the principles of autonomy, beneficence, and nonmaleficence are balanced and incorporated into medical decision making,[27] informed consent requires disclosure and comprehension of information as well as voluntary and competent decision making[28] (Box 7-1).

Disclosure

The requirement for disclosure is not an obligation for the clinician to impart everything about a proposed intervention to the patient. Some states measure the adequacy of disclosure according to the standard determined by what a reasonable clinician would disclose, whereas others measure adequacy by what information a reasonable patient would need to make the decision.[29] Although this may appear at first glance to be vague, "reasonable" generally means that disclosure should provide information about the goals of the procedure, the probability of success, and the most probable adverse effects. In addition, disclosure should include information about alternative options, including foregoing of any procedure.

Disclosure should allow the patient to weigh not only the risks and benefits of the proposed intervention but also the comparative risks and comparative benefits of alternatives, including the status quo or doing nothing. The information should be provided in a form the patient can understand, in terms of both the language itself and educational level.

Voluntariness

When patients are sick, they are often vulnerable as well. There may be conflicting values, not only among

BOX 7-1

THE ELEMENTS OF INFORMED CONSENT

Disclosing Information

Steps for disclosure: Before launching into a long narrative about the decision at hand, find out what the patient knows: "Can you tell me what you know about Alzheimer's disease?" The answer will reveal the extent of the patient's understanding and appreciation. This information is a useful guide for further discussion and disclosure. After disclosing information ask, "what else?" and then wait at least 10 seconds before speaking again.

> Doctor means teacher, and consent means to feel together. A good physician is an empathetic teacher.

Assuring Voluntariness

Steps to ensure voluntariness: An environment such as a nursing home or assisted-living facility can affect a person's sense of freedom and choice. Most people do not recognize the subtle effect their day-to-day environment has on their voluntariness. Open-ended questions can elicit whether this is a problem: "Do you feel like you have a choice?" Give the person time to make a decision (unless it is an emergency).

> Remind a person that he or she is free to choose, and give time to choose.

Assessing Competency

Steps to assess competency: In situations in which a patient is refusing what a physician considers "standard of care," a competency assessment is essential, but it can be the source of discord. Reassure the patient that the final choice is his or hers: "I am not here to argue. My duty as a doctor is to be a good teacher for you about your health and the options you have. I just want to make sure I've done an adequate job teaching you." Then assess the patient's understanding, appreciation, and reasoning by using the format of the open-ended questions described in Box 7-2.

> Competency derives from the ability to make a decision. Evidence of impaired decision-making capacity may be the first sign of clinically significant cognitive impairment.

From Karlawish JHT. Getting competent at assessing competency. Presented at the 2003 Annual Meeting of the American Geriatrics Society.

the patient's own values but also among the patient's, family's, and other caregivers' values. It is important, therefore, that the clinician ascertain that the decision is not coerced, that it truly represents the free will of the patient.

Simply asking patients whether they feel they have a choice or asking how much time they will need to make a choice may ensure voluntariness. Sometimes family members and friends may need to be excluded from the discussion to allow patients to freely express themselves. Overt threats from family are an obvious impediment to the free expression of choice, but subtle coercion or abuse may also occur.

The clinician may also exert undue pressure on the patient, interfering with the patient's perceived ability to express his or her free will. A patient may be afraid of disappointing the clinician or, worse, of being abandoned by the clinician if he or she does not consent. In some instances, perception by the patient of abandonment may not mean the complete exit of the clinician from the clinician–patient relationship but the fear that the clinician may not be fully committed to all the patient's needs should the patient choose to pursue a course contrary to the clinician's recommendation.[30] Therefore, part of the disclosure process should include information regarding the management of the patient and an assurance of support should he or she refuse the proposed intervention.

Capacity

Although disclosure of information and voluntariness are necessary for informed consent, the patient must also be able to use the information meaningfully to render an informed decision. The ability to cognitively process the provided information appropriately and render a decision is generally referred to as decision-making capacity.

Most authors tend to use the term *competence* as a legal term, referring to the individual's soundness of mind to make most routine decisions. When a court rules that an individual is incompetent, that individual is determined to lack sufficient cognitive function to make most routine decisions. This is usually accompanied by the appointment of a guardian and results in limitations in the individual's exercise of basic rights. The term *capacity* is used clinically on a case-by-case basis to denote the capability to render a specific decision. A patient may have the capacity to make one decision but not another. In everyday practice the distinctions between these terms often break down, leading to the use of the terms *capacity* and *competence* interchangeably.

In geriatric medicine, the prevalence of cognitive impairment owing to dementia or delirium raises difficult questions about the patient's capacity to participate in the process of informed consent. It is important to distinguish between cognitive impairment and impaired decision-making capacity. The presence of cognitive impairment does not necessarily rule out the ability to render all medical decisions, nor is an abnormal Folstein mini-mental state score,[31] by itself, an indication of incapacity.[32]

The determination of capacity should ideally be made on a case-by-case basis as part of the process of obtaining informed consent. A patient, who, because of dementia, is unable to participate in rendering a decision about a lower extremity vascular procedure, may nevertheless be able to clearly express a decision about resuscitation. Thus the inability to provide informed consent for one intervention should not necessarily imply a presumption of incapacity for other interventions. Likewise, the presence of mental illness, such as depression, should not lead to the conclusion that the patient cannot participate in decision making,[33] although there is evidence that the judgment of acutely ill adults may be sufficiently impaired in many cases to interfere with decision making.[34] This underscores the importance of using a systematic assessment of decision making specific to the decision at hand.

> The presence of dementia does not, by itself, indicate that the patient lacks decision-making capacity.

The set of standards that has evolved for assessing decision-making capacity includes the following components: (1) understanding of information that is disclosed in the informed consent process, (2) appreciation of the information for one's own circumstances, (3) reasoning with the information, and (4) expressing a choice[35,36] (Box 7-2).

Understanding represents the ability to comprehend the information provided and to be able to restate it in terms that make this evident. Thus it is helpful to ask the patient to repeat, in his or her own words, the information the clinician has provided, so it is clear that the patient fully comprehends the information.

Appreciation represents the ability to recognize that the information applies to oneself. For instance, a patient may clearly articulate information about a proposed procedure, but if the patient then asserts the procedure is not needed because of an erroneous belief that he or she does not have the condition that indicates the procedure, the patient's appreciation would be questionable.

Reasoning involves the ability to use and apply logic to information. This refers to the patient's ability to infer the consequences of a choice and to weigh the respective merits of various choices. The ability to consider the risks and benefits of a procedure or to compare the risks of two or more procedures is an example of reasoning.

Expressing a choice is self-explanatory and refers to the ability of the patient to make and state a decision.

MODEL QUESTIONS FOR ASSESSING CAPACITY

Ability to Choose

1. Have you made a decision about the treatment options we discussed?

Ability to Understand Relevant Information

2. Please tell me in your own words what I've told you about
   - The nature of your condition
   - The treatment or diagnostic test recommended
   - The possible benefits from the treatment/diagnostic test
   - The possible risks (or discomforts) of the treatment/diagnostic test
   - Any other possible treatments that could be used, as well as their benefits and risks
   - The possible benefits and risks of no treatment at all
3. We've talked about the chance that [X] might happen with this treatment? In your own words, can you tell me how likely do you think it is that [X] will happen?
4. What do you think will happen if you decide not to have treatment?

Ability to Appreciate the Situation and its Consequences

5. What do you believe is wrong with your health now?
6. Do you believe it's possible that this treatment/diagnostic test could benefit you?
7. Do you believe it's possible that this treatment/diagnostic test could harm you?
8. We talked about other possible treatments for you—can you tell me, in your own words, what they are?
9. What do you believe would happen to you if you decided you didn't want to have this treatment/diagnostic test?

Ability to Reason

10. Tell me how you reached the decision to have [not have] the treatment/diagnostic test?
11. What things were important to you in making the decision you did?
12. How would you balance those things?

Adapted from Ganzini L, Volicer L, Nelson WA, et al. Ten myths about decision-making capacity. J Am Med Dir Assoc 2004;5:263-67. Also from Appelbaum PS, Grisso T, unpublished.

The inability to express a choice renders assessment of the other criteria for competency unnecessary, but the ability to express a choice is, by itself, inadequate to judge competency. The inability to express a choice should not be confused with the refusal to make a choice when understanding, appreciation, and reasoning have been demonstrated to be intact. The latter essentially represents an endorsement of the status quo. For instance, a patient who has carefully considered a discussion about do-not-resuscitate (DNR) orders but asks that the clinician return for further discussion in a week has implicitly consented to resuscitative efforts and declined to authorize a DNR order.

How rigorously one applies these criteria to the decision-making process depends on the characteristics of the proposed intervention and the concordance between the patient's decision and the clinician's advice. For instance, few would argue that these criteria should be extensively applied to the question of drawing blood to determine basic electrolytes. In contrast, high-risk procedures or interventions with complex benefit/risk equations might require a more strict application of these criteria. Moreover, when a patient disagrees with the clinician's advice, particularly when the risk/benefit ratio of treatment is clearly favorable, a higher standard may be applied.[37]

> The process of obtaining informed consent for a given procedure is the appropriate means of determining decision-making capacity.

CASE 1

Alice Oliver (Part 4)

To respect Mrs. Oliver's autonomy, it is the responsibility of you and the care team to establish that she has adequate information to make this decision, that she is making the decision of her own free will, and that she is competent to make the decision. Once the criteria for informed consent are met, it is ethically permissible to provide thin liquids despite her increased risk of aspiration.

Although it is not necessary, some institutions may require the patient to sign a written "refusal to consent" form, indicating in writing that the patient is adequately informed about the risks of deviating from the team's recommendations.

1. **Is it ever morally acceptable to override a patient's wishes?**

2. **What can be done if a health care provider continues to have personal moral objections to a patient's autonomously derived decision?** ◻

DISCLOSURE OF MEDICAL ERROR

Studies suggest that there may be 44,000 to 98,000 deaths in the United States each year as a result of medical error.[38] A medical error may be defined as a commission or omission with potentially negative consequences for the patient that would have been judged wrong by skilled and knowledgeable peers at the time it occurred, independent of whether there were any negative consequences.[39] Preventable adverse errors may be more common in elderly patients owing to the clinical complexity of their care, the number of medications prescribed, and their increased use of health care.[40] This may be particularly true in nursing homes.[41] The release of the Institute of Medicine's report on medical error, *To Err Is Human*, focused attention on the problem of medical error and resulted in calls for increased transparency in health care.[42] In 2001 the Joint Commission on Accreditation of Health Care Organizations introduced patient safety standards that included a requirement to disclose all unanticipated outcomes of care.[43] A national survey of risk managers conducted in 2002 revealed that more than half of respondents would disclose a death or serious injury, but respondents were less likely to disclose preventable harms than nonpreventable harms.[44]

Disclosure of unanticipated outcomes of care, including medical error, is widely accepted as an ethical obligation of both physicians and nurses.[45-47] The ethical basis for disclosure involves not only respect for the patient but also support for patient autonomy and maintenance of the confidence and trust in the relationship with the clinician. There is little empirical support for the optimal means of disclosing error,[48] but there is some agreement that disclosure should be accompanied by an apology to the injured patient, emotional support of the patient,[49] an explanation of how the error occurred, and assurance that it will be fully investigated. Although it may seem counterintuitive, there is some evidence that a policy of open communication and disclosure of medical error may reduce liability payments.[50]

EXTRAORDINARY VERSUS ORDINARY CARE

When working with a patient to make medical decisions, clinicians should be cautious about the use of terms such as extraordinary or heroic. The term extraordinary may have originated in the writings of Roman Catholic theologians and refers to treatments that are very expensive, are possibly painful or uncomfortable, may provide an equivocal chance of success, and are not routinely used.[51] This is hardly a rigorous definition, and it is inadequately informative to allow for moral decision making. Treatments, such as dialysis, that were once considered extraordinary are now routine. Conversely, treatments that may be considered routine under usual circumstances, such as antibiotics for pneumonia, may be considered extraordinary in some terminally ill patients. Because the distinction between extraordinary or heroic versus ordinary is not well demarcated, it is best to avoid the terms altogether. It is better to discuss the benefits, risks, and burdens of the possible treatments and to thereby assist the patient in making rational and informed medical decisions. In such conversations, it is critical that words have precise meanings.[52]

> When discussing advance directives with patients, it is better to discuss specific life-sustaining treatments rather than globally referring to "heroic" or "extraordinary" measures.

CASE 1
Alice Oliver (Part 5)

Several days later, Mrs. Oliver suffers a second stroke. This time, the hemiparesis appears to be denser. She is now confused. The dysphagia worsens, and she is unable to take food by mouth without coughing. As you try to explain possible therapeutic options to her, you realize that she may not be able to understand what you are saying. The social worker tells you that she has three children outside in the waiting room. You wonder who will now make decisions.

1. **How do you determine who is the decision maker when a patient loses decision-making capacity?**

2. **How do you weigh competing wishes among multiple family members?** ▣

ADVANCE DIRECTIVES

Advance directives are verbal or written directions provided by an individual outlining what medical decisions are to be made on that individual's behalf when that person no longer possesses decisional capacity. When it has been determined that a patient lacks the capacity to make decisions about medical interventions, health care providers, family, and caregivers often struggle to determine who should make the decision and what is the right decision. The process of making medical decisions on behalf of a patient is known as substituted judgment. Many states have laws governing who is entitled to exercise substituted judgment when the patient no longer possesses decision-making capacity. For instance, the State of New York recently passed the Family Health Care Decisions Act, which allows designated close family members to render substituted judgment on behalf of a patient who has lost decisional capacity, but had not previously executed a health care proxy or appointed a health care agent.[53]

The United States Supreme Court decision *Cruzan v. Director, Missouri Department of Health*[54] established a federal right to withdraw or withhold life-sustaining treatment and established that a state can set a standard of evidence for the previously expressed wishes of patients who lack decision-making capacity that is "clear and convincing," a standard sitting between preponderance of the evidence and beyond a shadow of a doubt.[55] This does not have to be written, but it is far more prudent to create a written record of such wishes than to rely on the memory of family members or caregivers during a time of crisis. These advance directives ensure that the voice of the patient will be heard when the patient is no longer able to participate in making critical medical decisions.

Because it is left to the states to set the standards for advance directives, it is important to understand the laws governing such documents and how they are used. In New York State, for instance, an individual without decision-making capacity retains the right to have life-sustaining treatment withheld or withdrawn, but the evidence of such intent must be clear and convincing. In contrast, Georgia and many other states have legislation allowing family members to withhold or withdraw life-sustaining treatment for incapacitated patients under less exacting standards.

There are two commonly used categories of written advance directives. One document appoints a surrogate or agent to make medical decisions should the individual lose decision-making capacity. This may be known variously as a health care proxy, a durable power of attorney for health care, a designation of health care surrogate, or an appointment of a health care representative. The second, the living will, is a written statement of preferences for care when decision-making capacity is lost. Some advance directives may combine features of both types of documents.

The drawback of the living will is that the patient's actionable preferences are limited to the situations delineated in the document. It is difficult, if not impossible, to anticipate the variety of medical situations that might confront the incapacitated patient in the future. This risks throwing doubt on whether the stipulations in the living will might be applicable to the circumstances at hand. Some have even suggested that the concept of the living will should be abandoned in favor of the durable power of attorney for health care.[56] Such documents may include language indicating future preferences, but by appointing an agent who is familiar with the patient's values, the patient allows greater flexibility for the surrogate to make medical decisions when unanticipated circumstances arise.

Although different state legislatures have adopted different variations of these forms, a statutory form or other statement of preferences completed in one state will generally be recognized in another. The Federal Patient Self-Determination Act[57] requires health care organizations to ask patients whether they possess advance directives, to provide written information regarding the individual's rights under state law, and to educate the staff and community about advance directives.

Although hospital admission may be used as an opportunity to elicit health care preferences and complete advance directives, the stressful period at the onset of an acute illness is not the optimal time to discuss potentially difficult choices. It is more advisable to complete advance directives in a period of good or stable health. Questions about advance directives and an offer to help the patient complete them should be incorporated into a comprehensive geriatric assessment or the periodic examination.

A more recently developed advance directive is the physician order for life-sustaining treatment, or POLST.[58] POLST is a document summarizing the patient's wishes for life-sustaining treatment and combines preferences that may have been expressed separately on a DNR form, living will, health care proxy, or other advance directives. It is specifically designed to be transferred from one setting to another, a transitional period when patients are often vulnerable to errors resulting from inaccurate transmittal of information about medications, therapies, and advance directives[59] (Figure 7-2). Other states have adopted similar forms. New York has adopted Medical Orders for Life-Sustaining Treatment (MOLST), North Carolina has adopted Medical Orders for Scope of Treatment (MOST), and Montana has adopted Provider Orders for Life-Sustaining Treatment (POLST), to name just a few.

> Because patients' experiences and values may change, it is advisable to periodically review advance directives to ascertain concordance with patients' current wishes, thus allowing for revision when necessary.

CASE 1

Discussion

One of Mrs. Oliver's daughters presents to you a health care proxy naming her as agent. You tell her that Mrs. Oliver is unable to swallow a regular diet and thin liquids without coughing, a sure sign that she is aspirating. The daughter, invoking her authority as health care proxy, tells you that her mother had already refused thickened liquids and would not want them now. She requests that her mother be given thin liquids because "that was what she wanted."

Although Mrs. Oliver had previously refused thickened liquids, circumstances have changed. In addition to placing her at higher risk for aspiration, she appears to be experiencing frank discomfort when taking thin liquids. Her previous refusal of thickened liquids was based on the knowledge of asymptomatic aspiration when thin liquids were swallowed and, implicitly, on the notion that this would not be uncomfortable. Autonomy is now being exercised through substituted judgment and is conflicting to a much greater degree with the duty of nonmaleficence. After explaining to the daughter that you cannot in good conscience support her wishes if it is to cause frank discomfort, the daughter agrees to the administration of thickened liquids, expressing her understanding that the avoidance of discomfort overrides whatever pleasure Mrs. Oliver might have obtained from thin liquids. There are clearly trade-offs in achieving this resolution, which was made possible by the careful consideration of the relative benefits and burdens of different nutritional options.[60] ▪

	Physician Orders for Life-Sustaining Treatment (POLST) First follow these orders, then contact physician or NP. **This is a Physician Order Sheet based on the person's medical condition and wishes. Any section not completed implies full treatment for that section. Everyone shall be treated with dignity and respect.**	Last Name First Name/Middle Initial Date of Birth

A *Check one*	**Cardiopulmonary Resuscitation (CPR): Person has no pulse and is not breathing.** ❑ Resuscitate/CPR ❑ Do Not Attempt Resuscitation (DNR/no CPR) When not in cardiopulmonary arrest, follow orders in **B**, **C** and **D**.
B *Check one*	**Medical Interventions: Person has pulse and/or is breathing.** ❑ **Comfort Measures Only** Use medication by any route, positioning, wound care and other measures to relieve pain and suffering. Use oxygen, suction and manual treatment of airway obstruction as needed for comfort. ***Do not transfer*** to hospital for life-sustaining treatment. ***Transfer*** *if comfort needs cannot be met in current location.* ❑ **Limited Additional Interventions** Includes care described above. Use medical treatment, IV fluids and cardiac monitor as indicated. Do not use intubation, advanced airway interventions, or mechanical ventilation. ***Transfer*** *to hospital if indicated. Avoid intensive care.* ❑ **Full Treatment** Includes care described above. Use intubation, advanced airway interventions, mechanical ventilation, and cardioversion as indicated. ***Transfer*** *to hospital if indicated. Includes intensive care.* *Additional Orders:*_____ _____
C *Check one*	**Antibiotics** ❑ No antibiotics. Use other measures to relieve symptoms. ❑ Determine use or limitation of antibiotics when infection occurs. ❑ Use antibiotics if life can be prolonged. *Additional Orders:*_____
D *Check one*	**Artificially Administered Nutrition: Always offer food by mouth if feasible.** ❑ No artificial nutrition by tube. ❑ Defined trial period of artificial nutrition by tube. ❑ Long-term artificial nutrition by tube. *Additional Orders:*_____
E	**Summary of Medical Condition and Signatures**

Discussed with: ❑ Patient ❑ Parent of Minor ❑ Health Care Representative ❑ Court-Appointed Guardian ❑ Other:_____	**Summary of Medical Condition**	
Print Physician/Nurse Practioner Name	MD/DO/NP Phone Number	Office Use Only
Physician/NP Signature (mandatory)	Date	

Figure 7-2 Physician Orders for Life-Sustaining Treatment (POLST). (© Center for Ethics in Health Care, Oregon Health & Science University, Portland, Oregon.)

CASE 2

Carl Peterson (Part 1)

Mr. Carl Peterson is a 79-year-old man with diabetes who was brought by ambulance to the emergency department after experiencing severe substernal chest pain. After developing congestive heart failure and respiratory failure, he required intubation and mechanical ventilation. You have diagnosed a massive anterior wall myocardial infarction. Upon being brought to the coronary care unit, Mr. Peterson's blood pressure started to drop and he became delirious. Despite mechanical ventilation and maximum dosage of pressors, his blood pressure continued to drop.

You have explained the situation to his distraught wife and suggested that she sign a DNR order, explaining that this would apply only if his heart ceased to beat. She replies, "My husband has been through much worse and will make it through this. I want everything done to save him."

The blood pressure continues to fall, and Mr. Peterson sustains a cardiac arrest. You must decide whether to initiate cardiopulmonary resuscitation (CPR).

1. **Does the absence of an order not to resuscitate obligate the clinician to initiate resuscitative efforts in every case?**

2. **Because the process of authorizing an order not to resuscitate is governed by varying state laws, how would the clinician reconcile state laws that he or she considered to be at variance with his or her own moral beliefs?** ▣

FUTILITY

Futility is often invoked when a proposed treatment is unlikely to provide benefit or is clearly pointless. Others have proposed that the uses of the term *futility* in clinical medicine are too varied and diverse to allow for a precise definition.[61,62] It is more useful, perhaps, to examine the origin of the term, its possible uses in geriatric medicine, and the underlying need for its use.

The *Oxford English Dictionary* provides one definition of the term *futility* as "the quality of being futile; triflingness, want of weight or importance; esp. inadequacy to produce a result or bring about a required end, ineffectiveness, uselessness." The term derives from the Latin *futtilis*, an adjective meaning "that easily pours out, leaky, hence untrustworthy, vain, useless." The imagery conjures up a picture of bailing out a leaking boat with a sieve. It is an action that not only will fail to accomplish its intended goal but also can reasonably be predicted to fail.

The principle of beneficence, the obligation to do good, infers that actions that have a reasonable likelihood of providing no good should not be initiated or even offered. Alternately expressed, an intervention that is unlikely to achieve its intended outcome should not be undertaken.

Defining the intended outcomes of interventions in geriatric medicine is not straightforward. Within the literature of comprehensive geriatric assessment are studies that demonstrate improved diagnostic accuracy, improved functional status, improved affect or cognition, reduced prescribed medications, decreased nursing home use, increased use of home health services, reduced hospital admission, reduced medical care costs, prolonged survival, or provided comfort.[63,64] The meaning of the term *futile* therefore depends on the intended outcome of a given action.

Another definition of the term *futile* "refers to an expectation of success that is either predictably or empirically so unlikely that its exact probability is often incalculable."[65] To accurately define futility, one must include a component of probability or chance. Similarly, to appropriately use the term *success*, one must couch it in terms of the intended outcomes. Determination of futility involves two types of value judgments. The first is the judgment that the treatment will not provide positive benefit to the patient. The second is that the likelihood of benefit is too small to justify its undertaking.[66]

If a feeding tube is inserted with the goal to prolong the life of a severely demented patient who is no longer able to eat, there may be a chance, however small, of achieving that goal. If, however, a feeding tube is inserted to provide comfort or improve the quality of life of such a patient, then it is highly unlikely to succeed. The clinician must define the intended outcomes and estimate the chances of achieving these outcomes. The purpose of evidence-based medicine is to establish treatment guidelines based on the probabilities defined in well-designed medical studies. Unfortunately, such data do not always provide guidance in an individual situation. Clinicians may have difficulty assigning a statistical probability that denotes futility. One suggestion is that futility can be presumed if a treatment has not worked in the past 100 cases and will "almost certainly" not work if it is tried again.[67] There is no consensus about this definition, and there is evidence that as an expression of probability, *futility* means different things to different doctors.[68] Other studies have shown that clinicians assign a wide variety of probabilities to define *futile*.[69]

Because futility may refer to a multitude of goals, sometimes perceived differently by patient, provider, and family, there is the risk that wielding the term inevitably results in the introduction of value judgments. Jecker and Schneiderman[70] suggest that even quantitative expressions of probability cannot escape value judgments, such as the worth of taking particular chances and the quality of a patient's life.

When a patient asks for "everything to be done," it is important to explore what this means. Surely, a patient with end-stage heart failure would not request an appendectomy under the rubric "everything." Rather, the clinician must explore with the patient what are realistic goals, what interventions are possible, and what interventions are unlikely to provide benefit.

There are certainly situations in which futility is obvious. Initiating resuscitative efforts on a nursing home resident found in bed in the morning, pulseless and cold, with the beginnings of rigor mortis is clearly futile if restoring cardiac function is the goal. Repairing a fractured hip in a bed-ridden, severely demented elderly woman may also be viewed as futile if the proposed goal is ambulation. Other situations are not so clear. For instance, the literature on the efficacy of acetylcholinesterase inhibitors for treating dementia is mixed and controversial, with clinicians staking out both sides of the treat/don't treat divide.[71,72] A clinician, who is unconvinced of the efficacy of these drugs, may, indeed, consider treatment with them to be futile, whereas others may consider these drugs to be the current standard of care.

Using futility as the basis for withholding treatments or the discussion of treatments must be done with great caution. Age alone, rarely, if ever, provides a rationale for determining that an intervention is futile, although it may be factored into calculations of risk and longevity at times. Until potential goals of treatment are articulated and understood, preferably early in the course of illness, introducing futility into the conversation is unlikely to be productive.[73]

CASE 2

Carl Peterson (Part 2)

Mr. Peterson had already been on mechanical ventilation and the maximum dosage of pressor agents at the time of the cardiac arrest. This is already much of what advanced cardiac life support would have provided, absent the chest compressions. Adding chest compressions when life support has otherwise failed would be highly unlikely to restore a heartbeat, let alone blood pressure. Therefore the initiation of CPR could be considered a futile intervention that the clinician is not ethically obligated to provide. You opt not to initiate CPR and inform Mrs. Peterson that her husband has died. ■

DO-NOT-RESUSCITATE ORDERS

The use of closed chest cardiac massage to resuscitate an individual experiencing cardiac arrest was originally described in 1960.[74] Originally restricted to acute care facilities under specific circumstances, it is now widely accepted as a method for preventing death from cardiac arrest.

In 1974, the National Conference on CPR and Emergency Cardiac Care wrote, "The purpose of CPR is the prevention of sudden, unexpected death. CPR is not indicated in certain situations, such as in cases of terminal, irreversible illness." Discussion with the patient or family was not mentioned in the document. In 1980, the conference reiterated the purpose of CPR but noted, "The patient's family should understand and agree with the decision, although the family's opinion should not be controlling." This time, despite the comments about the family, there were no comments about the patient's wishes.[75]

Much has evolved since the original description of CPR in 1960. Because of the success of the procedure in treating sudden cardiac arrest, many cities, most notably Seattle, have promoted training the general population in techniques of basic CPR. Many office buildings and airports now maintain automatic external defibrillators. Far from being reserved for only "sudden, expected death," the initiation of CPR is almost inevitable in health care institutions if specific orders to withhold CPR have not been entered. Most states have passed legislation specifying how orders to withhold CPR can be authorized. In the absence of a DNR order, it is presumed that the individual consents to CPR. Moreover, in many institutions it is presumed that in the absence of a DNR order, a resuscitative attempt will be initiated.

Studies examining the efficacy of CPR are often flawed, resulting from insufficient elderly subjects, differing endpoints, and differing reports on postresuscitation neurologic status. Nonetheless, age alone has been shown to be a poor predictor of response to attempted CPR and should not be used as the lone determinant.[76]

In one study of out-of-hospital arrests, CPR in the elderly was found to be effective only in witnessed arrests that were not associated with asystole or electromechanical dissociation (now known as pulseless electrical activity).[77] A more recent study confirmed this, demonstrating that despite a reduction in success with increasing age, survival was greater for both octogenarians and nonagenarians whose presenting systems were pulseless ventricular tachycardia or ventricular fibrillation rather than asystole.[78]

In in-hospital cardiac arrests, age has also not been shown to be a determining factor of success by itself. One study conducted in an intensive care unit (ICU) demonstrated survival to discharge in 7% of those suffering arrests, but only 5% survived more than 6 months. No patient who had asystole survived, but of those surviving 6 months, mental status remained unchanged. Interestingly, of the survivors, most stated they would decline future CPR.[79] Another study demonstrated that only 9 out of 52 elderly patients who survived a cardiac arrest by 1 week went on to survive a full month, and only 5 out of 37 previously independent patients remained independent after surviving cardiac arrest. Success was correlated with proper selection, presenting rhythm, and shorter response time, rather than age alone.[80] A subsequent study revealed poor outcomes in elderly patients with hypotension, pneumonia, renal failure, cancer, coma, intubation, pressors, and previous home-bound status. All survivors experienced a decrease in functional status.[81]

Survival after cardiac arrest in the nursing home has been found to be rare,[82,83] leading one study to conclude, "We favor a more radical proposal: that CPR not be offered to NH residents."[84] Another study, although conceding that survival after cardiac arrest in nursing homes was unlikely, found that with appropriate selection and effective response, the survival of certain groups was comparable to that of elderly persons suffering out-of-hospital cardiac arrest. The study recommended that resuscitative efforts be withheld for unwitnessed arrests or arrests in which the presenting rhythm is asystole or electromechanical dissociation.[85]

When discussing DNR orders with the elderly patient, it is important to differentiate resuscitation from a resuscitative effort. Because most attempts at CPR are unsuccessful, it may be misleading to discuss "resuscitation," which implies that the effort will be successful. Using the term resuscitative effort or attempted resuscitation may be more accurate. It is also important to differentiate the DNR orders from the remainder of the care plan. A DNR order applies only to a cardiac arrest and is not equivalent to "do not treat."

A DNR order is unusual in that it is a procedure that requires informed consent to preclude its use. This presents a potential ethical problem. Although consent to resuscitation is generally presumed in the absence of a DNR order, does this mean that it is also presumed that CPR will always be initiated in the absence of a DNR order? Does offering a DNR order equate to offering resuscitation under all other circumstances? Opinions vary on this point, but it is our opinion that the decision to initiate a resuscitative effort remains a medical decision that should be undertaken only if clinically indicated. It would make little sense to attempt resuscitation on a nursing home resident with end-stage dementia who experiences an unwitnessed cardiac arrest and presents with asystole. Likewise, it would not seem logical to initiate CPR on a ventilator-dependent ICU patient whose cardiac arrest was preceded by a gradual drop in blood pressure and vital signs, despite maximum doses of pressor agents and other supportive measures. Such actions must be consistent with state law and institutional policies and procedures. Furthermore, clinicians in training and nurses may feel uncomfortable making such decisions and opt instead for initiating resuscitation, despite its apparent futility.

When a patient with a DNR order undergoes surgery, additional issues must be considered. In the controlled environment of an operating room, cardiac arrest is more likely to occur, but it is also more likely to be reversible, because it would be witnessed and managed by a team experienced with such events. Because the likelihood of a successful resuscitation may be higher, it may be reasonable to offer a temporary suspension of a DNR order during the period in the operating room.[86] Some surgeons and anesthesiologists may even refuse to operate unless such contingencies are made.

CASE 2

Discussion

After Mr. Peterson's death, the nurses express their discomfort to you for withholding CPR in the absence of a DNR order. They ask whether they have breached hospital policy or state law in doing so.

From a purely pragmatic standpoint, it might be difficult for a nurse at the bedside or a first-year intern to make the decision to withhold CPR in the absence of a DNR order. Furthermore, state law or hospital policy might mandate the initiation of CPR in the absence of a valid DNR order, despite its apparent futility. Consequently, although it may be ethically permissible to withhold CPR when clearly futile, the legal obligation may be otherwise. ■

ASSISTED SUICIDE AND THE DOUBLE EFFECT

Assisted suicide remains controversial and polarizing. In January 2006, the U.S. Supreme Court blocked federal efforts to reverse Oregon's legalization of physician-assisted suicide. The 1997 Oregon Death with Dignity Act provides legal guidelines allowing physicians to provide lethal doses of medications to terminally ill patients who request them.[87] A qualitative study of physicians in Oregon revealed that many of them felt unprepared for such requests and were uncomfortable with issues such as pain management and symptom relief, understanding patient preferences, and concern about abandoning patients.[88] This suggests that few clinicians are prepared to confront this terribly difficult issue, and certainly medical students and medical residents are inadequately trained to make such decisions. Where there is consensus, however, is that clinicians must do a better job in providing palliative care to patients experiencing physical or psychological suffering to reduce the possibility that a patient might have to consider such a difficult question.

In providing appropriate pain and symptom management to the dying patient, it is common to worry about whether dosages of narcotics that will successfully relieve pain and discomfort might also hasten death. In fact, there is little in the medical literature to support the notion that narcotics, when properly used, will hasten death in the vast majority of terminal patients suffering pain.[89] However, in a small subset of patients who experience accelerating pain just before death despite conventional dosing of narcotics, it is possible that adequate doses of narcotics to relieve pain may also hasten death, even if by only a small time interval. Under these unusual circumstances, the double effect must be approached like other circumstances requiring informed consent and should not be presumed to be ethically acceptable in the absence of consent.[90] The following questions should be considered: (1) is the patient's suffering proportionately severe to warrant the risks of intervention; (2) has the patient or legal surrogate been fully informed of all likely outcomes of the intervention, both intended and expected, and is he or she aware of all the alternatives; and (3) is the intervention the least harmful one available given the patient's clinical circumstances and personal values?[91]

NUTRITION AND HYDRATION

Whether nutrition and hydration are the obligatory fulfillment of basic human needs or purely medical interventions at the end of life has been debated vigorously in the ethics literature over the past two decades.[92,93] The matter is not settled, and the clinician must take care to understand state laws and explore the patient's values regarding these issues. Most important, when discussing the possibility of withdrawal or withholding of food and fluids with patients, the clinician should have some knowledge of the medical consequences of the decision. For instance, there is little evidence that tube feeding in advanced dementia improves outcomes such as aspiration pneumonia, survival, pressure sores, infections, or comfort.[94,95] There is also evidence that food and fluid beyond that requested by terminally ill cancer patients may provide only a minimal role in providing comfort.[96] Nonetheless, the quality of informed consent for placement of gastrostomy tubes has been shown to be inadequate,[97] and using terminology such as "starvation" is unjustified and unnecessarily provocative.[98] Whether interventions such as a feeding tube or intravenous fluids should be offered when the clinician believes they will provide little benefit remains a thorny issue. It may be more appropriate to focus on those palliative interventions that will provide comfort to the patient and prepare the patient and family for the end of life rather than offer false hope.

CASE 3

Edward Gilliam (Part 1)

Mr. Gilliam is an 86-year-old widower who visits your office for a routine checkup. He apologizes for his lateness, explaining that he got lost driving to the office, a route he has driven for many years. His past medical history is significant for hypertension, diabetes, and osteoarthritis. You have received a consultation report from his ophthalmologist indicating a diagnosis of age-related macular degeneration. On mini-mental state examination, he scores 25/30, a decline of three points since the previous year's examination. A report from a neuropsychological examination is equivocal, indicating the presence of significant but mild deficits in memory and executive function. You recommend to Mr. Gilliam that he cease driving. He responds that he has been driving for almost 70 years and insists he drives safely. He mentions that driving affords the freedom to "come and go as I please."

Case Analysis

When assessing a patient's ability to drive when possibly suffering from dementia, the ethical principle of autonomy conflicts with a potentially broader obligation to ensure reasonable safety, not only of the patient but of the public. There is evidence that self-report is an unreliable indicator of driver safety owing to denial and limited insight,[99] thus throwing into question the patient's capacity to exercise his autonomy. Although the clinician may not have a direct duty of nonmaleficence to the community, it has become increasingly evident that visits such as this may provide an opportunity for the clinician to prevent injuries or fatalities to the public. There is also evidence that although clinicians may be able to identify potentially hazardous drivers, the clinical assessment may be inadequate to accurately identify such drivers.[100] Although laws may vary from state to state, it is ethically permissible and, arguably, obligatory for the clinician to take the necessary steps to establish driver safety or, by appropriate reporting, allow relevant state agencies to make such determination. ▪

CULTURAL AND RELIGIOUS CONSIDERATIONS

Western medical ethical principles are based largely on the perceived rights of individuals, such as privacy, liberty, and self-determination. These underlie the principle of autonomy and, implicitly, its primacy among medical ethical principles. Some religious and cultural traditions may, however, present alternate social norms. Either patient or clinician may come from a non-Western cultural tradition, possibly leading to ethical conflicts stemming from different ethical principles. This may make resolution particularly challenging, given that the usual methodology for analyzing, deliberating, and resolving ethical conflicts assumes agreement on underlying principles. It must be remembered that the extent to which a patient chooses to exercise or cede autonomy is, itself, an autonomous decision. It is important that the clinician keep an open mind to alternative values stemming from unfamiliar cultural and religious traditions and incorporate these into the process of ethical deliberation.[101]

> Do not make assumptions about the patient's moral preferences based only on the religion stamped on the chart.

CLINICAL PRACTICE GUIDELINES: ETHICAL CONSIDERATION

Over the last few years an increasing number of clinical practice guidelines (CPGs) have been published by major medical societies and organizations. The scientific foundations of these guidelines are scrutinized to establish their validity and applicability to the intended target populations. Concurrently, questions have arisen as to the impact on clinical practice guidelines of participating experts who may have a financial interest in the outcomes of the guideline or who may receive significant income from businesses and other entities affected by the guideline. Although this may not be directly pertinent to most health care providers who do not participate in guideline development, it is relevant to clinicians who look to clinical practice guidelines as an objective and unbiased authority of the standard of care.

In 2011 the Institute of Medicine published a consensus report titled *Clinical Practice Guidelines We Can Trust*.[102] The report contained eight categories of standards considered important for quality clinical practice guidelines. The most extensive standards involved the management of conflicts of interest. The thrust of the standards was to eliminate any potential conflict of interest to the extent possible prior to CPG development and foster a culture of disclosure and transparency for any remaining potential conflicts of interest.

A study examining the prevalence of financial conflicts of interest among members of CPG groups that released guidelines on hyperlipidemia and diabetes revealed a high prevalence and underreporting of financial conflicts of interest.[103] Another study examined conflict-of-interest policies for organizations producing a significant number of CPGs and demonstrated that no single organization adhered to the Institute of Medicine standards.[104]

Clearly, organizations need to improve their disclosure and conflict-of-interest policies. As the number of clinical practice guidelines proliferate, clinicians need to carefully examine clinical practice guidelines for conflicts of interest before implementing their recommendations into their practices.

SUMMARY

Medical ethics provides a moral structure for assessing the propriety of clinical decisions, particularly when patients' and clinicians' values conflict. Most health care institutions now have ethics consultants or ethics committees to assist patients and clinicians in resolving difficult ethical dilemmas. By understanding basic principles of medical ethics and the structure for methodical analysis of ethical dilemmas, the clinician can resolve the majority of common dilemmas that often arise in the care of the older patient.

Web Resources

1. www.polst.org. Physician Orders for Life-Sustaining Treatment Program.
2. www.caringinfo.org. Caring Connections, a national hospice and palliative care organization. Provides resources for end-of-life planning, including advance directives from each state.
3. http://www.rihlp.org/pubs/Your_life_your_choices.pdf. *Your Life, Your Choices*—a workbook for advance care planning that includes a combined durable power of attorney for health care (DPAHC) and living will.
4. www.compassionandsupport.org. Website of the organization Compassion and Support at the End of Life contains resources for end-of-life and palliative care with extensive documents for Medical Orders for Life-Sustaining Treatment (MOLST).

KEY REFERENCES

7. Beauchamp TL, Childress JF. Principles of biomedical ethics. 5th ed. New York: Oxford University Press; 2001.
22. Jonsen AR, Siegler M, Winslade WJ. Clinical ethics: A practical approach to ethical decisions in clinical medicine. 5th ed. New York: McGraw-Hill; 2002.
35. Grisso T, Appelbaum PS. Assessing competence to consent to treatment: A guide for physicians and other health professionals. New York: Oxford University Press; 1998.
36. Sessums LL, Zumbrzuska H, Jackson JL. Does this patient have medical decision-making capacity? JAMA 2011;306(4):420-7.
87. Oregon Health Authority. Death with Dignity Act. http://www.oregon.gov/DHS/ph/pas/docs/statute.pdf. Accessed May 16, 2013.
102. Committee on Standards for Developing Trustworthy Clinical Practice Guidelines, Institute of Medicine. Clinical practice guidelines we can trust. Washington, DC: The National Academies Press; 2011.

References available online at expertconsult.com.

8

Financing and Organization of Health Care

Julie P. W. Bynum

OBJECTIVES

Upon completion of this chapter, the reader will be able to:

- Understand the nature and spectrum of publicly funded social services available to older adults in the community.
- Describe the major public sources of funding for health services for older adults: Medicare, Medicaid, Older Americans Act, Title XX of the Social Security Act, and the Department of Veterans Affairs.
- Describe the out-of-pocket expenses older adults can expect to pay for both acute and long-term care.
- Understand the transitions in payer as a person moves from independent to assisted living and nursing home care.
- Describe the basic coverage provided by Medicare's Parts A, B, C, and D and by secondary insurance.
- Describe the range, limitations, and proportions of long-term care costs paid by four sources: patient and family personal funds, Medicare, Medicaid, and private insurance.
- Understand changes that are occurring in the health care market that affect older adults.

OVERVIEW OF SYSTEM OF CARE FOR OLDER ADULTS

The American health care system is complex and expensive; older adults and the clinicians serving them may struggle to understand the available services and how they are paid. One important role for primary care providers is to help older adults access the resources they need at a cost they can afford. The goal of this chapter is to provide the basic knowledge of the organization and funding of health care that will enable primary care providers to play this critical role for patients.

CASE 1

Joseph Marks (Part 1)

Joseph Marks is an 82-year-old man who lives by himself in a two-story home and has high blood pressure and gout. He does not drive so he gets out only a limited amount but can manage public transport. His daughter lives out of town and wonders what they can do to make him safer in his home.

Would Mr. Marks be eligible for any home-based services and what would you suggest? ▫

Unique Financial Challenges of Older Adults

Although not true of all older patients, one characteristic typically associated with older age is that the person has left the workforce and is therefore relying on savings, pensions, or other fixed sources of income. Governmental efforts in 1965 to institute the entitlement program of Social Security followed by

---
Additional online-only material indicated by icon.

Medicare led to an enormous drop in the percentage of elderly people living in poverty.[1] However, this population still faces financial challenges; the median annual income for older persons in 2010 was $25,704 for males and $15,072 for females.[2] In 2010, 13.2% of older adults' total expenditures went to purchase medical care, more than twice the proportion (6.6%) spent by all consumers, according to the Administration on Aging.[2]

In addition to living on a fixed income, older adults, over time, may accumulate chronic medical conditions and functional impairments that are leading drivers of health care costs. Seventy-five cents out of every dollar spent on health care goes toward treating chronic conditions.[3] The costs are even greater when a person has more than one chronic condition. In the United States, per capita spending for people with three chronic conditions is three times greater than for those with one condition ($6178 vs. $2241 in 2001)[4] and two thirds of the people over 65 have two or more chronic conditions.[5] One in four Americans who have chronic conditions also have limitations in activities of daily living (ADL) related to health.[6] These functional impairments lead to older adults requiring not only medical care but also other types of long-term services and support. The health care system on which older populations rely therefore includes not only medical services, but also social services that address long-term functional needs.

Fundamentals of Public Funding of Health Care for Older Adults

Beginning in the 1930s and through the 1960s, the financial challenges facing older adults and their access to medical care were important policy issues. After several prior efforts and lengthy national debate, the Social Security Act with Titles XVII and XIX were passed in 1965, which established the Medicare and Medicaid programs. Another less well known 1965 legislation established the Older Americans Act (OAA) whose objective is to be the vehicle of organizing, coordinating, and providing community-based services for older adults. The OAA led to the creation of the Administration on Aging (AoA). Subsequently, in 1975, Title XX of the Social Security Act was enacted as a mechanism for block grants to states to support social services, including social justice programs for children and elders. Subsequently several laws have made revisions to the health care and social service system for older adults. Most recently, the Patient Protection and Affordable Care Act (PPACA) signed into law in 2010 aims to improve coverage of the uninsured, contain costs, and stimulate health delivery system reform (Table 8-1).

TABLE 8-1	Patient Protection and Affordable Care Act of 2010 Features Important for Older Adults	
Provision	**Description**	**Potential Impact for Older Adults**
Medicare Payment Changes		
Preventive Care Payments	Eliminate cost sharing for preventive services rated A or B by the U.S. Preventive Services Task Force.	Lower copayment burden
Part D Changes	Gradually reduce the doughnut hole patient obligation from 100% to 25%.	Lower copayment burden
Restructure Medicare Advantage Payments	Restructure payments to MA plans.	MA options may change
New Center for Medicare & Medicaid Innovation		
Example Programs:	New center to test, evaluate, and disseminate payment and health system reforms.	
Accountable Care Organizations	Allows providers who are held accountable for total costs of care to share in cost savings if quality thresholds are met.	Greater provider attention to quality and coordination of care
Value-Based Purchasing	Payment to providers will be based on quality, not just quantity of services.	Greater provider attention to quality of care
Bundled Payments	Groups payment for an episode of care such as a hospitalization and post-acute rehabilitation.	Greater provider attention to risk of readmission; enhanced care coordination
Primary Care & Medical Home Initiatives		
Independence at Home	Demonstration program to provide high-need patients primary care in their homes.	Home-based primary care available
Community-Based Care Transitions Program	Tests models to improve transitions from hospital to other settings.	Strengthen community-based organization to assist in medical care

Continued on following page

TABLE 8-1	Patient Protection and Affordable Care Act of 2010 Features Important for Older Adults (Continued)	
Provision	**Description**	**Potential Impact for Older Adults**
Long-Term Care		
CLASS Act	New voluntary insurance program for purchasing community-based services (implementation deferred).	Improve access to long-term care insurance
Dual-Eligible Initiatives	Create new office, the Federal Coordinated Health Care Office, to improve coordination of service and quality of care.	Opportunity to have better acute & long-term care coordination
Research		
New Patient-Centered Outcomes Research Institute	New institute to identify priorities and fund comparative effectiveness research.	One focus will be to increase knowledge about therapies for people not typically in clinical trials, such as the frail elderly

MA, Medicare Advantage.
Adapted from Henry J. Kaiser Family Foundation's Focus on Health Reform. Summary of new health reform law. Available at www.kff.org/healthreform/upload/8061.pdf.

The PPACA does not make changes to the underlying structures of Medicare and Medicaid.

These funding streams as set by law define how we typically categorize services for older adults. Federal, state, and local governments provide the funding and infrastructure for community resources that make housing, food, and transportation accessible and affordable. Acute medical services are primarily covered by Medicare, with some older adults also having private insurance, Medicaid, or Veterans Health Administration benefits. Long-term care is a broad array of services that is not covered by Medicare. Long-term care is funded through various sources, although mostly out-of-pocket unless the individual has purchased private long-term care insurance or is Medicaid eligible, because Medicaid covers both acute and long-term care.

> The Older Americans Act and the Social Services Block Grant program are the two leading federal sources of funding for social or community-based programs that facilitate older adults' ability to remain in the community and in their homes for as long as possible.

FINANCING THE HEALTH CARE SYSTEM

Community-Based Services

In addition to medical care, many other services are available to support the health and well-being of older adults. First among these are the services to make housing, food, and transportation accessible and affordable and to protect vulnerable populations from exploitation or abuse. The OAA and the Social Services Block Grant program are the two leading federal sources of funding for these programs. In the Social Services Block Grant program (Title XX), states are given discretion for using the funds for social programs that prevent, reduce, or eliminate dependency, neglect, or abuse and assure appropriate referral to institutional or home-based services. The OAA has a number of different provisions that are implemented mostly through the AoA.

The AoA funding spans four areas—health and independence, caregiving services, protection of vulnerable older adults, and consumer information access and outreach. In 2012 the AoA budget was $1.9 billion, 40% of which went to nutrition programs and 30% to community-based services.

Operationally, AoA has created a network of Area Agencies on Aging (AAA), and state or tribal agencies that organize and deliver the services locally. These agency programs include meals-on-wheels, congregate meals, adult day service, and adult protective services as well as legal and elder abuse services. The common denominator among the programs is that they facilitate older adults' ability to remain in the community and in their homes for as long as possible by providing social supports, while avoiding exploitation. Locating these services can be daunting but online resources such as the Eldercare Locator maintained by the Department of Health and Human Services (www.eldercare.gov) are helpful (Figure 8-1).

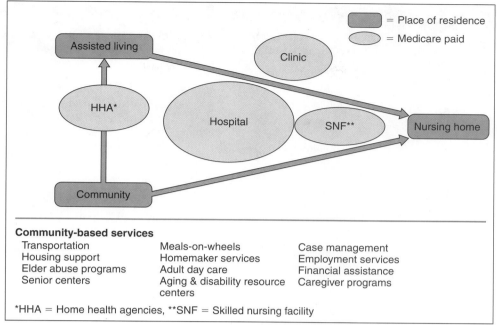

Figure 8-1 Overview of acute care, residential, and community-based services that make up the health care system for older adults.

Joseph Marks (Part 2)

Unfortunately, Mr. Marks falls in the bathroom in spite of the current efforts to keep him safe at home. You learn that he has been evaluated in the emergency room and sent home with narcotics for back pain. Now that he is home, he is afraid of falling again and because of pain is not able to get out of the house on his own. His daughter brings him to your office for follow-up. Investigating the cause of the fall, you find out that Mr. Marks has been feeling dizzy lately and his blood pressure while sitting is 120/80 but drops to 110/65 with symptoms of dizziness when he stands. After a complete medical evaluation, you decide that he needs to have his blood pressure medications changed and the narcotics will have to be reduced as his pain improves.

What additional services can Mr. Marks receive in this new situation? ◼

Federal Insurance Coverage for Older Americans

Federal spending on health care for older adults includes funding from Medicare, Medicaid, the Administration on Aging, the Social Services Block Grant program, and the Veterans Health Administration (Table 8-2).

Since enactment in 1965, Medicare and Medicaid have undergone continual changes to the details of the programs but their fundamental structures have remained the same. Medicare is an entitlement program established to cover the acute care needs of people who have reached the age of 65 (or have end-stage renal disease or are on Social Security Disability Insurance [SSDI]). As an entitlement, Medicare is available to everyone who has paid payroll tax in his or her lifetime (or whose spouse has) regardless of income or ability to pay. Medicaid, in contrast, was established to provide coverage for people who have insufficient income to pay for services whether because of poverty or a disabling condition that limits ability to work.

The funding sources of Medicare and Medicaid are quite different. Medicare is paid for through two trust funds: The Hospital Insurance Trust (HI) fund pays for Part A services and covers all Medicare beneficiaries out of the payroll taxes collected by the federal government. Part A services include inpatient hospital care, skilled nursing facility care, home health care, Hospice, and durable medical equipment. The Supplemental Medical Insurance (SMI) Trust Fund pays for Medicare Part B and Part D services; this fund is supported through general federal tax revenues and by beneficiaries who pay a monthly premium. Part B services cover physician services, outpatient hospital care, some home health care, preventive services and lab tests; Part D is the prescription drug benefit. There is also Medicare Part C, called Medicare Advantage, which comprises the optional private insurance company managed care Medicare programs and for which payment is split between the two trust funds. In summary, Medicare is paid by federal payroll taxes, general federal revenues, and premiums, deductibles, and copayments from patients.

TABLE 8-2	Summary of Federal Spending and Eligibility on Health Care for Older Adults	
Program	**2012 Budget (Dollars) (percent of HHS total)**	**Eligible Elderly Population (percent of total users elderly)**
Dept. of Health & Human Services (HHS)	871.9 billion (100%)	
Medicare	479.6 billion (56%)	Age >65 & paid payroll tax 10 yrs/or disabled receiving Social Security Disability support, ESRD (62%)
Medicaid	255.3 billion (30%)	Low-income & certain populations (children, pregnant women, disabled, aged) (10%)
Administration on Aging	1.9 billion (0.2%)	Age >65 (100%)
Social Services Block Grants	1.9 billion (0.2%)	Determined by state
Veterans Health Administration	51 billion (36% of Dept. of Veterans Affairs budget)	Veterans (43%)

ESRD, end-stage renal disease.

> Medicare is an entitlement program that is available to everyone over the age of 65 who has paid payroll tax in his or her lifetime (or whose spouse has).

Medicaid is jointly funded by the federal and state governments to provide acute and long-term care to low-income Americans. Because Medicaid was created to cover low-income individuals, the contributions made by patients are much lower, although there are some copayments. Federal law stipulates some populations with incomes below specified cutoffs that must be covered (elderly or disabled SSDI beneficiaries, children, pregnant women, some parents, and working disabled). The federal government pays a specified percentage of program expenditures to the states for these designated beneficiaries. States may opt to cover additional populations and receive matching funds from the federal government. Many of the policy debates that arise with Medicaid revolve around state budgetary constraints and efforts to control costs through changes in coverage rules. Medicaid is particularly important for primary care geriatrics because so many elderly nursing home residents ultimately spend-down their assets and transition to dependence on Medicaid for payment of their long-term care services. In fact, 32% of Medicaid's spending is directed toward long-term care and although the aged and disabled make up only 25% of beneficiaries, they account for 70% of total Medicaid spending.

> Medicaid was established to provide health insurance coverage for people who have insufficient income to pay for services, whether because of poverty or a disabling condition that limits ability to work.

Veterans Health Administration

The Veterans Health Administration (VHA) is a large integrated health system that provides acute care, social services, and long-term care to more than 8 million veterans a year (with 21 million eligible) with a budget of nearly $50 billion per year funded by the Department of Veterans Affairs.[7] In 2009 approximately 43% of VHA beneficiaries were older than age 65.[8] The VHA has been a leader in developing the geriatrics workforce and conducting aging-related clinical research. Their centers offer acute care, geriatric assessment, home-based primary care, caregiver support, and nursing and community-based care options. Eligibility for many of these services is determined by whether the individual has service-connected disabilities.

> The Veterans Health Administration offers elderly veterans geriatric assessment, home-based primary care, caregiver support, and nursing and community-based care options in addition to acute care.

PATIENT'S PERSPECTIVE ON PAYMENT FOR HEALTH CARE

From the perspective of the patients, the array of funding streams does not necessarily align with their experience of health care, which may lead to confusion. For example, a single home care agency may provide a physical therapist in the home after a hip fracture but also provide a long-term homemaker. The therapy is paid by Medicare as an acute service but a long-term homemaker would be an out-of-pocket expense or covered by Medicaid (if the patient is eligible). Similarly, a nursing home may provide on the same hallway both acute rehabilitation services (skilled nursing facility level of care) paid by Medicare and long-term residence for those with chronic, severe impairment, which may be paid by Medicaid. Understanding that these services are paid for differently is important for advance care and financial planning (Figure 8-2).

Older adults who are still working at age 65 years need to clarify how their employer's insurance works with Medicare. Most older adults, even those that are employed, start Medicare Part A when they turn age 65 years because it is usually premium free. However, if the employer's coverage meets Medicare standards, delaying Part B and Part D enrollment may be possible, saving the costs of these premiums. Although there are financial penalties for delaying enrollment in Part B and Part D after age 65 years, these are waived if the employer's coverage meets Medicare standards.

Acute Care

Medicare Part A

Hospitalization. Medicare covers any medically necessary hospitalizations, with the hospital receiving a payment based on a prospective determination of the average expected cost of the stay (called a Diagnosis-Related Group [DRG]), and a $1184 deductible that the patient pays. Note that any physician visit made to

the patient while he or she is in the hospital is billed under Part B, so the patient pays 20% of each physician visit. Test, labs, and medications are included in the DRG. There are other types of inpatient facilities, such as critical access hospitals, long-term care hospitals, and inpatient rehabilitation hospitals, that follow similar rules. Some hospitals use "observation" status to keep a patient as an inpatient while determining if full hospitalization is needed. These stays are billed under Part B and the patient pays 20% of the stay and will not be eligible for a posthospitalization skilled nursing facility stay.

Post-Acute Rehabilitation. After hospitalization, many patients benefit from a period of rehabilitation before going home. Inpatient rehabilitation hospitals accept patients with certain diagnoses who are able to participate in 3 hours of rehabilitation per day. These stays are funded similarly to acute hospital stays. Skilled nursing facilities (SNFs) also deliver post-acute rehabilitation as a separate service line in a facility that also delivers long-term care, and accommodate people who are not well enough to do 3 hours of rehabilitation per day. SNFs are also paid on a prospective payment system (the Resource Utilization Group system); patients do not have a deductible for the first 20 days, but they pay a daily rate ($148) for days 21-100, after which the Medicare benefit expires. The covered length of stay in a

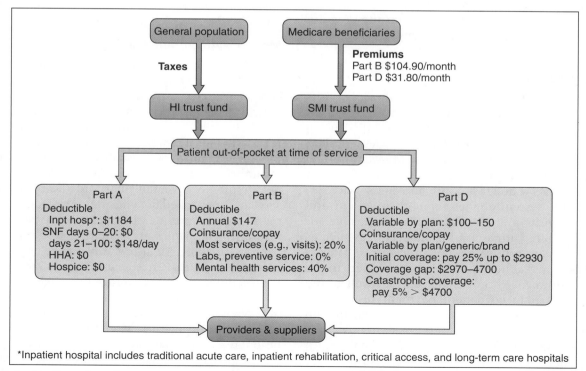

Figure 8-2 Medicare beneficiary out-of-pocket expenditures for Medicare services in 2013. HHA, home health agencies; HI, hospital insurance; SMI, supplemental medical insurance; SNF, skilled nursing facility.

SNF is dependent on the patient's medical stability and progress in rehabilitation therapies. A stable patient whose therapy progress has reached a plateau will no longer receive Medicare coverage in an SNF, even if he or she has not reached the 100-day limit.

Home Care. Medicare-reimbursed home care agencies provide nursing visits; physical, occupational, or speech therapy; social work; and homemaker services for up to 20 days without any out-of-pocket charge to patients who are homebound. These services must be ordered by a clinician to serve a medically necessary need such as rehabilitation after a hospitalization, monitoring blood pressure or pain response with new medications, or to provide home safety evaluation or therapy after a fall.

Hospice. The Hospice benefit is also provided at no cost to the patient except for a small copayment for prescriptions and a 5% coinsurance for inpatient respite stays. When enrolling in Hospice, two clinicians certify that life expectancy is less than 6 months and the patient agrees to forgo curative treatment for his or her terminal illness, but retains coverage for nonterminal conditions.

Durable Medical Equipment (DME). Many health conditions or impaired-function states require supplies, devices, or equipment for management. Medicare covers these DME products with a 20% coinsurance. Diabetic supplies are obtained through this benefit as well as wheelchairs and mobility devices but they require certification by a clinician that they are medically necessary.

Medicare Part B

Medicare Part B covers professional fees (visits to clinicians) as well as services that occur on an outpatient basis. Physician services are billed using Common Procedural Terminology codes familiar to all practicing clinicians and paid according to the Resource-Based Relative Value Scale (RBRVS), which attaches a dollar amount to each service delivered. This system applies for both inpatient and outpatient visits and the patient is responsible for 20% of the bill. Outpatient hospital services such as ambulatory surgery, same-day procedures, laboratory tests, and diagnostic tests are also subject to the 20% coinsurance. Recent changes as a result of the PPACA have reduced patient payment responsibility: preventive services (such as the welcome to Medicare visit, annual wellness visit, and screenings) are now free to patients. And mental health services that previously had a 40% coinsurance are gradually being reduced to 20%, similar to other physician services.

> Medicare Part B provides coverage of professional fees (such as visits to physicians) as well as services that occur on an outpatient basis and requires older adults to pay a monthly premium plus a 20% copayment.

Medicare Part D

Beginning in 2006 under the Medicare Modernization Act, a prescription benefit was added to Medicare. Individuals have the option of enrolling with independent prescription drug plans (PDPs) to which they pay premiums, coinsurance, and copayments. Although the federal government pays for Part D, the administration of each PDP is separate, leading to many plan options and choices for patients; this complexity has led to a great deal of confusion. Part D was designed to provide coverage up to a limit of drug spending ($2970 in 2013) but then started covering again once the drug cost reached what is called a catastrophic level ($4700 in 2013). The gap in coverage between $2970 and $4700 became known as the doughnut hole and is controversial. Provisions in the PPACA aim to close the doughnut hole over time. Prior to the existence of Part D, Medicaid beneficiaries received prescription medication coverage through Medicaid. Those benefits have been transferred to Part D with added low-income subsidies to protect low-income individuals from high out-of-pocket costs. A challenge for patients that arose in this transition was differences in coverage between Medicaid and Part D because Part D does not cover benzodiazepines or over-the-counter medications.

Medicare Advantage (Part C)

In 1981 Medicare created an alternative to the traditional fee-for-service Parts A and B plans to allow beneficiaries to participate voluntarily in managed care, a program later renamed Medicare Advantage (MA). In these plans Medicare pays an organization (e.g., a health maintenance organization, a preferred provider organization), usually organized by a private insurance company, a risk-adjusted sum per member per month to cover all of the Medicare-reimbursed services for enrolled beneficiaries. The federal government current per-member per-month payments to insurance companies are generous, resulting in good benefits, making Medicare Advantage popular with many older adults. These plans usually integrate Part D prescription benefit coverage into their benefits. By 2011 about 26% of Medicare beneficiaries were in MA plans. MA plans are organized in specific geographic areas by county. More than one MA plan may be offered in a single area, resulting in competition among plans. Plans may not be available in all areas, especially in rural counties. Evaluation of the MA payment mechanisms demonstrated that plans were being paid disproportionately higher than the cost of providing similar services under traditional Medicare. Reducing this differential is one of the cost saving mechanisms in the PPACA.

Secondary Payers

Even with Medicare coverage, patient deductibles, coinsurance, and copayments can become significant costs for older adults. Many people choose to buy additional coverage through private insurance called Medigap plans that pay those additional fees and may offer additional coverage. There are 14 standardized plan options and a multitude of vendors from which to choose. For low-income older adults, Medicaid also serves the purpose of Medigap, covering what Medicare does not. Also, some large employers provide Medigap coverage to their retirees.

CASE 1

Joseph Marks (Part 3)

Mr. Marks, like many people older than 80, lives alone and likely could benefit from socialization and the intermittent monitoring that attending a senior center can bring. You can advise that the daughter contact the local area agency on aging to find out what local senior centers and transportation are available. In addition, you can order a home safety evaluation under the Medicare home health benefit at no cost to him. A one-time home safety evaluation is available to all Medicare beneficiaries whether they are homebound or not.

After the fall, however, he would meet the criteria of being homebound and can receive nursing (for medication management) and physical therapy (for gait management) in the home. At this point, it would be advisable also to have a social work evaluation to determine if other types of services such as meals-on-wheels are now indicated to keep him in his home. ▣

LONG-TERM CARE SERVICES AND SUPPORT

Unfortunately for some individuals, community supports are not sufficient and they require daily supervision or assistance with their ADLs. Today, these patients have more options of what type of facility provides that care. Approximately 5% of the elderly population resides in nursing homes and a similar percentage in assisted living.[9,10] These services, however, are not covered by Medicare or traditional insurance plans. Medicaid does cover long-term care, but only low-income older adults are eligible for Medicaid. Families and clinicians are sometimes caught unaware that they will be responsible for these costs, which are high. Some people believe that in-home caregiving would be less expensive but when 24-hour care or nursing care is needed the costs are equivalent. Table 8-3 shows the median costs of various long-term care services.

CASE 1

Joseph Marks (Part 4)

You meet with Mr. Marks 4 years later. He did quite well with in-home services for several years. Lately, however, he has been declining, with continued falls, weight loss, and seeming to make multiple medication errors. Your thorough evaluation reveals that he has developed dementia. He was planning to move in with his daughter but unfortunately he had a stroke before the move could occur. He is now in the hospital with significant functional impairments including an inability to swallow and cognition difficulties. His caring daughter asks for your advice about the options for rehabilitation and long-term care. She is particularly concerned because she works full-time and cannot provide the ADL care needed, and after several years of in-home care the finances are very tight.

1. **What type of post-acute rehabilitation (home-based, inpatient rehabilitation, or skilled nursing facility) would Mr. Marks be eligible for and what would the cost implications be of each of these?**

2. **How many days of coverage would he receive under his Medicare benefit for rehabilitation?**

3. **At the end of the Medicare coverage, what is the likely course for Mr. Marks's long-term care?** ▣

Residential Services

Nursing Home

Residence in a nursing home is an experience faced nearly entirely by older adults. Eighty-eight percent of nursing home residents are older than 65 and 45% are older than 85.[11] Nursing homes provide 24-hour supervision and nursing care for people who have impairments in the ADLs, such as bathing, dressing, feeding, and toileting, or have behavioral or cognitive issues that preclude safe community residence. Traditional nursing homes are organized like hospitals but innovative efforts such as the Greenhouse Model attempt to bring in homelike features.

Many people enter nursing homes after a 3-day hospital stay so that Medicare will pay up to the first 100 days for acute rehabilitation. If the person stays beyond eligibility for Medicare post-acute services, however, payment becomes the individual's responsibility. When an older adult stays long enough to use nearly all of his or her own assets (a home can be protected if a spouse is still living in it), then the person can apply for Medicaid.

Assisted Living

For people who are less impaired and can still live in their own space given adequate supervision, assisted living is an option. Assisted living facilities are highly variable in the services provided (and variable in

TABLE 8-3	Median Cost for Long-Term Care Services in the United States in 2012	
Service	**Description**	**Estimated Annual Expense**
Home		
Homemaker Services (licensed)—provides "hands-off" care such as helping with cooking and errands. Also called personal care or companions	National median hourly rate: $18	15 hr/week × 52 weeks per year = $14,040
Home Health Aide Services (licensed)—provides "hands-on" personal care but not medical care in home such as help with bathing, dressing, and transferring	National median hourly rate: $19	15hr/week × 52 weeks per year = $14,820
Community		
Adult Day Health Care—provides social and other support services in a community-based protective setting during a part of the day	National median daily rate $61	250 business days per year = $15,250
Facility		
Assisted Living (one-bedroom, single occupancy)—provides "hands-on" personal care and some medical care for people who cannot live alone but do not need a nursing home	National median monthly rate $3,300	12 months per year = $39,600
Nursing Home (semiprivate room)—provides 24-hour skilled nursing support	National median daily rate $200	365 days per year = $73,000
Nursing Home (private room)—provides 24-hour skilled nursing support	National median daily rate $220	365 days per year = $80,300

(Adapted from Genworth Companies. Genworth 2012 cost of care survey. Available at www.genworth.com/content/etc/medialib/genworth_v2/pdf/ltc_cost_of_care.Par.40001.File.dat/2012%20Cost%20of%20Care%20Survey%20Full%20Report.pdf.)

state-level regulation) but typically have at least one nurse on duty for 24 hours a day, provide housekeeping, meals, medication dispensing, and for extra fees assistance with ADLs. Forty-one states provide some Medicaid funding for assisted living.

Continuing Care Retirement Community (CCRC)

CCRCs are a newer option that offers older adults residential care over their remaining life span as they move from independent living to assisted living and to nursing home care within a single community. Typically members pay large entrance fees followed by monthly fees, although financing models vary widely. Entrance fees can range from $250,000 to $400,000, with monthly fees ranging from $3,500 to $6000 for a couple.[12]

Other Types of Residential Care

There are residential care alternatives such as board and care homes and some states have adult foster care programs. These types of residential care programs should not be confused with senior housing, which is subsidized but does not necessarily include any additional medical or social service support.

Home-Based Services

Privately Hired Services

Many people who stay in their homes privately hire homemakers, nursing assistants, and even nursing care in the home. These services are typically charged on an hourly basis so the cost depends on the needs of the individual. Companies have emerged that manage a staff of caregivers so that individuals can access trained and vetted caregivers by the hour. These companies are separate from the home health agencies that provide Medicare and Medicaid home care services. As previously noted, for short periods Medicare does pay for these home care services but not as a long-term care management strategy.

Medicaid Waiver Programs

States are increasingly investing their Medicaid dollars into home- and community-based care programs that allow Medicaid recipients to receive long-term care services outside of institutional settings. Being in the community is usually preferable to patients and is less expensive for the states. Many examples and innovative programs are developing in the United States. The Program for All Inclusive Care (PACE) began as a waiver program and is now available across the country. In PACE, people who are eligible for nursing home level of care can opt to enter a PACE program that combines their Medicare and Medicaid benefits to provide care that is centered on a day-hospital model with robust community support and care coordination. The PACE provider takes on the financial risk for both the acute and long-term care of the participant.[13]

CASE 1

Joseph Marks (Discussion)

Mr. Marks was already fairly impaired prior to the stroke and is unlikely to be able to participate in 3 hours of rehabilitation a day. If he could tolerate it, he could go to an inpatient rehabilitation hospital where he would be responsible for a $1000 deductible and 20% of any physician fees (he only has traditional Medicare Part A and B coverage). It is more likely, however, that he would receive his rehabilitation in a skilled nursing facility where he would have no cost sharing for days 0-20 but then he would pay $144 per day until day 100 when his Medicare coverage would end. At that point if he still requires 24-hour skilled nursing, he would stay in the nursing home and would spend down his assets until he became eligible for Medicaid. ■

CHANGING LANDSCAPE OF ORGANIZATION AND FINANCE OF HEALTH CARE

The most sweeping changes in the PPACA are those that serve to broaden coverage of the uninsured through an expansion of Medicaid and those that preclude use of preexisting condition clauses for insurance policies. These efforts to cover the uninsured will have little direct impact on Medicare beneficiaries. However, there are several key elements of the law that affect older adults (see Table 8-1).

There are two main themes that cut across most of the new payment models being rolled out after PPACA: a focus on reimbursing providers for quality not just quantity of services, and developing reimbursement strategies that encourage care coordination. In traditional fee-for-service (FFS), health care providers are paid for a service whether performed well or not.

A common example is the high number of hospital readmissions within 30-days of a hospital discharge under the Medicare program. Under FFS, the hospital would simply be paid for both hospitalizations, limiting the financial incentive to prevent readmission. One innovation to address this issue is to pay with a "bundle" that includes the entire episode (the hospitalization and a period after). Hospitals will have higher margins if the readmission rate is low. And there are also several initiatives to improve providers' ability to manage care transitions clinically.

Better care coordination is seen as an opportunity to improve management of the complex, chronically ill patients who account for a large portion of spending. The primary care initiatives are finding new ways to pay primary care providers for the out-of-visit work that care coordination requires. The accountable care organization (ACO) combines both themes by rewarding providers who hit thresholds of quality while reducing their costs, but the accountable care organization can do so only if the clinicians work together across all settings because the ACOs are accountable for the total costs of care, not only those in one setting.

SUMMARY

The United States has a complex array of federal, state, and local programs to support the medical care and social needs of older adults. Although navigating these programs is challenging for patients, their families, and providers, the services currently available for older adults are comprehensive and provide a strong safety net. As the population ages, new legislation to address the long-term costs of Medicare and Medicaid is expected in the coming years.

Web Resources

www.eldercare.gov. Administration on Aging, Eldercare Locator.
www.kff.org. Kaiser Family Foundation.
www.medicare.gov/pubs/pdf/10050.pdf. Medicare & You 2013.
www.medpac.gov/payment_basics.cfm. Medpac: Medicare and Payment Basics.

KEY REFERENCES
References available online at expertconsult.com.

9

Billing and Coding

Peter A. Hollmann

OBJECTIVES

Upon completion of this chapter, the reader will be able to:

- Understand the relevant coding systems for billing: ICD, CPT, HCPCS Level II.
- Understand that coding and billing rules may vary based on benefits and payer.
- Understand the structure of evaluation and management codes in CPT and the Centers for Medicare and Medicaid Services (CMS) documentation guidelines.

Whether you are in solo practice, pay all your own practice expenses, and earn only what you bill, or whether you are an employee of a large group or institution, you are generating income based on billing. Although there are some payment methods that are not fee-for-service systems, most medical care provided by professionals in the United States is paid for using a fee-for-service payment methodology. This means you, or someone on your behalf, is submitting a bill to the patient or insurance company for the services you perform. Because it is a fee-for-service system, you will need to state the name of the service you performed and your charge for that service. An orderly payment system requires a set of rules so that you are aware of your required behavior and the payers are aware of their requirements. The first rule of order is that there is a nomenclature system for every service. Use of this system is referred to as "coding."

The rules of coverage, payment, coding, and billing can seem daunting. Further stress is added by the knowledge that your livelihood may be on the line or that billing performed incorrectly can have adverse legal and financial repercussions. If you do not bill personally, you are still responsible for the work of your agents. Try to remember that if you are able to care effectively for the complex geriatric patient, you have more than adequate brain power to handle billing and coding processes. As with patient care, a team approach is useful. When available, seek out the expertise of people who regularly perform billing functions.

This chapter is not intended to be a treatise on all important aspects of practice management and does not include topics such as when to refer patients to a collections agent for unpaid bills, accounting methods for tracking accounts receivables, or claims appeals. Nor will the chapter explain details of payment systems and delivery systems such as capitation and accountable care organizations, even though the type of system will affect coding and billing practices. However, the chapter is intended to provide a solid foundation and educational resources for issues related to billing and coding.

CODING SYSTEMS

There are three key coding systems. The first is the diagnostic classification system known as International Classification of Diseases, Clinical Modification (commonly called ICD-9). This system will be replaced in the United States with ICD-10 on October 1, 2014. The World Health Organization creates ICD versions, but the clinical modifications are from the U.S. National Center for Health Statistics; thus ICD-CM versions do vary by country. ICD also includes ICD-PCS, a procedural

---

Additional online-only material indicated by icon.

code set. Hospitals use ICD-PCS for inpatient procedure coding but professionals use the American Medical Association's Current Procedural Terminology (CPT) and the Centers for Medicare and Medicaid's Healthcare Common Procedure Coding System, Level II (known as HCPCS). Hospitals also use CPT and HCPCS for outpatient procedure reporting.

CPT is the backbone of professional procedure reporting, but HCPCS is used to supplement CPT because CPT does not maintain a drug or device (e.g., durable medical equipment) classification system; also, Medicare may need codes that are very specific to its benefits as defined in law. Unfortunately, none of the systems use the terminology that clinicians use when communicating with each other in conversation. With the advent of electronic records, problem lists are now in "ICD speak" and finding the official term for a condition can be frustrating at times. Fortunately, few medical professionals will need to memorize the entire coding lexicon; the key is to understand and be familiar with high-volume codes.

ICD is organized by types of diseases (e.g., infection, cancer, cardiovascular) and has codes for symptoms or reasons for an encounter that are not diagnoses (e.g., V70.0 is the diagnosis code for a routine general medical examination, and 786.0 is the code for dyspnea). CPT is arranged by major categories and then subdivided by body system and anatomically. Major sections are evaluation and management (the office and facility visits often called cognitive services), anesthesia, surgery, radiology, pathology and laboratory, and medicine. The last category actually is a broad mix of services and includes diagnostic tests such as electrocardiograms and codes for immunization administration and the vaccine itself. Evaluation and management services, commonly referred to as E and M (or E/M), are usually the bulk of services performed by geriatric providers who may report them. Physicians, nurse practitioners, clinical nurse specialists, and physician's assistants may use E/M, but physical therapists and nutritionists have their own evaluation and treatment codes in the medicine section. The medicine section also includes the procedures used by mental health professionals, whether physician or nonphysician, and includes psychological testing codes.

All sections are relevant to professionals and it is important to gain familiarity with the range of codes. For example, although a bladder volume scan is not technically imaging and is certainly not surgery it is in the urodynamics subsection of CPT, which is within the surgery/urinary system section. If a code for a common service cannot be located, one should not conclude that a code does not exist; it is more likely that it simply has not been found yet. However, there are some important exceptions. For example, removing sutures that were placed by a clinician from another practice would be considered E/M; there is no suture removal code. A mental status exam is part of E/M, and not in the neuropsychologic testing sections. HCPCS codes are used for drugs administered, such as a steroid injection. Medicare also uses HCPCS codes for specific benefits. For example, a flu shot administration has CPT codes, but Medicare requires that HCPCS G code G0008 is reported. This is because the CPT administration code is agnostic to the vaccine given and not all vaccines are covered by Medicare (outside of a Medicare Part D drug benefit). It is strongly advised that all medical professionals maintain access to current editions of these coding resources. CPT changes annually and HCPCS changes quarterly.

> Keep up to date with annual changes to procedure coding and Medicare benefits.

KNOWING PAYER, BENEFITS, MEDICARE CONTRACTOR, SPECIALTY/LICENSURE, AND GROUP RULES

Geriatrics professionals tend to think Medicare. However, there are Medicare Advantage plans (Medicare Part C) and many retirees have commercial insurance. These payers may cover more than Medicare or require participating providers to report services differently. This is usually because of benefits differences (i.e., what is covered by the plan). Generally speaking all payers follow the same basic coding rules. The most common example of variation can be seen with the "annual physical." Even with the Medicare Wellness Visit benefit, there is no annual physical per se and for years a major point of differentiation for Part C plans was coverage of preventive services that Medicare did not cover. A Medicare Advantage or commercial plan will typically require use of the CPT Comprehensive Preventive Medicine services codes such as 99397. This code will be denied when submitted to traditional Medicare. However, this service is in fact covered, almost entirely, when reported using the correct HCPCS II G codes; thus, practically speaking, it is not truly a noncovered service. Therefore one cannot charge the beneficiary.

Medicare Part B, the part that covers professional services, is administered by multiple contractors (companies Medicare pays to process claims and enforce rules). The rules of different contractors tend to be consistent, but in some cases where national rules have not been promulgated or there is potential for variable interpretation, there can be differences. Even if the policies are the same, enforcement may be divergent. These disparities can occur in some high-volume services. A contractor may define E/M medical decision-making level of complexity as requiring a change in the medication regimen, whereas another may not have such a requirement. The contractor's website is a good source of information concerning these issues.

A health care professional's specialty or license type will dictate both coding and coverage rules. For example, physical therapists and physicians in most cases will not be using the same codes. One may specify E/M whereas the other uses 97001 for assessments. However, a physician who performs a timed "get up and go" test may meet criteria to report it as a physical performance test 97750 if it takes at least 8 minutes and a separate report is created; otherwise the test is considered to be part of a physical examination. In mental health coding there is a great deal of overlap between the various professions. At times very similar services are reported differently by different professions. Physicians do not report the CPT medical nutrition therapy services when counseling a patient on obesity; they report E/M as specified in CPT guidelines, and for certain patients in Medicare, physicians may use G codes for intensive behavioral therapy for obesity. Specialty type as well as license type is relevant. In E/M, a new patient is one who has not received a reported face-to-face service from a professional in the exact same specialty and subspecialty within the same group. Therefore, if an internist refers a patient to a geriatrician within his or her group for an opinion or assistance in management and a joint medical record is used, the patient is nonetheless a new patient to that geriatrician; this means that a new patient code E/M is used as compared to the established patient code. However, if the geriatrician sees the internist's patient in the role as covering physician in the office, the geriatrician is acting on behalf of his or her colleague and the patient is therefore considered an established patient. It is important to be aware of specialty classification listings by payer and also to be aware of Tax Payer Identification numbers and National Provider Identification (NPI) numbers that define groups.

CLAIMS, CLAIMS EDITS, AND MODIFIERS

Billing usually means submitting a claim to a payer. The claims-processing systems use edits, though not all payers use the same edits. Some edits are in place to prevent coding errors. For example, if two skin lesions are removed and the same code is reported twice, it will be assumed this was an erroneous duplicate entry unless a modifier code is appended to the second procedure code to designate that two separate services were performed. The most common modifier relevant to geriatrics professionals is modifier 25, which indicates that the E/M was distinct and not part of a simultaneous surgical service. For example,

if a patient with osteoarthritis is seen for an intraarticular steroid injection and no significant separate assessment was performed, no E/M should be reported. However, if another condition was treated, or the patient required a distinct history and examination to determine the condition and to determine if the injection was warranted, modifier 25 is appended to the E/M code.

Edits also exist for a medical necessity match for services such as laboratory tests. A claim for a thyroid-stimulating hormone test may be paid if the diagnosis is hypothyroidism, but denied for a diagnosis of migraine. The edit may determine the benefit. A diagnosis code that designates a service as preventive may result in no patient cost sharing, whereas the same service with a different diagnosis may have cost sharing such as with lipid testing in Medicare. These claims-processing rules/edits have greater variability among payers and are often the source of a bill not being paid as expected.

EVALUATION AND MANAGEMENT SERVICES

These are the most commonly performed services by geriatric physicians, advanced practice nurses (registered nurse practitioners [RNPs] and clinical nurse specialists [CNSs]) and physician's assistants (PAs). The codes are divided by place of service with separate categories for office/clinic, hospital inpatient, hospital observation, nursing facility, emergency department, home, and domiciliary care facility. The last category is potentially a point of confusion because the designation of type of facility or home varies by state regulation. In some places an assisted living facility is a facility; in other places an assisted living facility is classified as a person's home by regulation. It is important to note that the place of service is where the patient was seen, so if a patient was brought from a nursing facility to the physician's office, the office visit codes are used. Some services are further divided by "new" or "established" patients. A new patient is one who has not had a face-to-face service with the provider, or with a member of the provider's group in the same subspecialty, within the past 3 years, even if the provider has a record on the patient and saw him or her 4 years earlier. This concept does not apply to certain types of E/M, such as inpatient and nursing facility services. In these locations, the applicable concepts are "admission" and "follow-up."

E/M codes have levels. Some types of services have 5 levels (e.g., office), whereas other sites of care (e.g., hospital inpatient) may have only 3 levels. The level of E/M service is tied to how much one gets paid for the service. For example, a level-3 established patient office visit in Medicare in 2012 paid just under $71, and a level-4 visit paid just over $104. If a physician saw

15 level-4 patients a day but billed 15 level-3 visits, and did that every day for a year of practice, the physician would have underbilled by more than $100,000. The physician's overhead would not have changed; therefore, his or her take-home pay is reduced by the underbilled amount.

Getting the level correct presents the largest source of coding consternation. Levels in CPT E/M are determined by three key components: history, examination, and medical decision making. CPT has introductory guidelines helping to define these components and the levels within each component. Some services, such as a new patient office visit, require that all three components be at a minimum level, whereas others, such as an established patient visit, require that two of three components be at a minimum level. CMS created documentation guidelines (DGs) to clarify its interpretation of CPT's key components. The DGs are structured in a manner to make an audit tool possible. Electronic record systems designers have picked up on this and have embedded these rules into some templates, so that the record system will suggest the code to report. Letting the record system, or even a professional coder, do the E/M coding should be avoided. Having others in a compliance program review your coding is helpful.

> The clinician that treats the patient best understands decision making and the code level to report.

Only the treating clinician knows what history and examination elements were required for the patient's problem, and only the clinician understands the true level of medical decision making. An absurd example of incorrect coding by DGs or by using a literal interpretation of CPT relates to the 2/3 requirement for an established patient. For example, if a physician did a careful and complete history and examination and documented it like a medical student would, then the 2/3 requirement is met. Why even consider the differential diagnoses, treatment options, and patient/caregiver counseling? The coding requirement has been met.

However, the DGs do offer some guidance and education on correct coding. CPT also has clinical examples in an appendix and notes typical times of E/M services. This can be very helpful. To some degree, E/M services are all relative (i.e., a physician can have his or her median visit in mind as a standard, code it carefully using DGs, and then code up or down from there depending on how the other visits measure against the standard). This works with one major caveat—what is a median service for a geriatrician may be a rare high level of complexity service for another practice type. Compare evaluating minor complaints that really do not even require a physician's care all day in a walk-in treatment center with a frail elderly practice. The "set point" for the walk-in clinic may be a level 2 office and for the geriatrician a level 4. Physicians also need to remember to code based on the service performed. Even complicated patients can have simple visits. There are three major problems for geriatrics with E/M: a ceiling effect, all services are face to face with the patient, and the code structure reflects the single problem acute care orientation that plagues too much of medical training and care delivery.

DOCUMENTATION GUIDELINES AND CURRENT PROCEDURAL TERMINOLOGY (CPT) DEFINITIONS

CPT defines history and examinations with levels labeled "problem focused," "expanded problem focused," "detailed," and "comprehensive." Medical decision making is "straightforward," "low-complexity," "medium-complexity," or "high complexity." Medical decision making is composed of three components: (1) number of diagnoses or treatment options, (2) amount and/or complexity of data to be reviewed, and (3) risk of complications and/or morbidity or mortality. There is additional detail in the E/M guidelines section of CPT. The history and examination descriptions do lend themselves to quantification based on the traditional parts of the history and examination; medical decision making does not lend itself to such quantification. Simply put, straightforward decision making is the type of decision making that is largely irrelevant; the problem required reassurance at most. The CMS DGs were written in 1995 and modified in 1997 to allow for single system (specialty oriented) examinations. CMS provides educational resources on DGs at www.cms.gov/Outreach-and-Education/Medicare-Learning-Network-MLN/MLNEdWebGuide/EMDOC.html. A common service in geriatrics is 99214, an office visit for moderately complicated care of an established patient. Table 9-1 gives a summary of the 1997 rules for two levels of a history ("detailed" applies to 99214). Table 9-2 gives CMS examples of quantifying risk. Table 9-3 puts together the DGs into a cheat sheet to help one remember the components in a 99214. An example of the type of patient that would warrant a 99214 is an 82-year-female brought to the office by a family member. The patient has hypertension, is on an ACE inhibitor, has chronic pain from osteoarthritis as well as mild dementia, and was recently prescribed a nonsteroidal antiinflammatory drug by another physician. She now is experiencing confusion. (Note: The actual findings may require a higher level of service.) These guidelines can create a ceiling effect given that many patients are at the next to highest level based on complexity, but coding at the highest level, unless time based, may require a fundamentally irrelevant review of systems or a physical

TABLE 9-1	CMS 1997 Documentation Guidelines for History		
History Extent	**HPI**	**PFSH**	**ROS**
Expanded Problem Focused	*Brief*	*n/a*	*Problem Pertinent*
Detailed	*Extended*	*Pertinent*	*Extended*

- ROS and PFSH may be noted in HPI
- ROS and PFSH can be noted as "no changes"
- ROS and PFSH can be obtained on patient form if confirmed

Brief HPI:	1-3 elements*
Extended HPI:	4 or more elements
Pertinent ROS:	the system directly related to the HPI
Extended ROS:	direct and limited number of additional systems (2-9)

Data from Centers for Medicare and Medicaid Services. 1997 Documentation Guidelines for Evaluation and Management Services. Available at www.cms.gov/Outreach-and-Education/Medicare-Learning-Network-MLN/MLNEdWebGuide/Downloads/97Docguidelines.pdf.
*Elements: location, quality, severity, duration, timing, context, modifying factors, associated signs/symptoms.
HPI, history of present illness; *PFSH*, past, family, and social history; *ROS*, review of systems.

TABLE 9-2	CMS Documentation Guidelines for Risk
Risk Level	**Examples**
Low	2 or more self-limited 1 stable (e.g., HTN) minor acute (e.g., UTI)
Moderate	1 illness w/exacerbation 2 chronic stable 1 acute with systemic risk (e.g., pyelonephritis)

Adapted from Data from Centers for Medicare and Medicaid Services. 1997 Documentation Guidelines for Evaluation and Management Services. Available at www.cms.gov/Outreach-and-Education/Medicare-Learning-Network-MLN/MLNEdWebGuide/Downloads/97Docguidelines.pdf.
HTN, Hypertension; *UTI*, urinary tract infection.

examination that is not required to be comprehensive by patient care needs. There is inadequate differentiation within the levels in which geriatricians normally operate.

> When addressing multiple conditions the number of conditions creates additive and interactive complexity to decision making.

Medical Necessity

The array of scoring points and rules in the DGs can easily obscure the fact that all services reported must be necessary. CPT introduces the level of the key components with an important phrase: "which requires." Copied and pasted notes, excessive history or examination findings, or other verbiage not relevant to the problem(s) treated at that encounter do not fulfill any documentation requirement.

> All services must first be medically necessary.

Time and Face-to-Face Services

Time is money and although some codes are based on time, most are not. E/M gives typical times for each code, but time is used as the basis of E/M code selection only when counseling and care coordination dominate the service, meaning it takes up more than 50% of the time spent face to face with the patient. A lot of time is not face to face. Each E/M service accounts for some time doing things such as reviewing a laboratory test, but a lengthy phone call with a family member caregiver is not accounted for and may not be charged to the family member except in limited cases. In the hospital and nursing facility, time does include unit time, not just time in the patient's room. Even though CPT discusses time with respect to the "patient and/or family," payers require that the patient be present for the service. Therefore, a family conference in the physician's office about care planning for a

TABLE 9-3	Summary of Elements for 99214			
History	Detailed:	4 HPI	2-9 ROS	1/3 PFSH
Exam	Detailed:	6 systems with 2 elements each to 2 systems with 6 elements each (12 total)		
MDM	Moderate:	Multiple Diagnoses	Mod Data	Mod risk
TIME				25 minutes
KEY Components				2/3 required

Data from Centers for Medicare and Medicaid Services. 1997 Documentation Guidelines for Evaluation and Management Services. Available at www.cms.gov/Outreach-and-Education/Medicare-Learning-Network-MLN/MLNEdWebGuide/Downloads/97Docguidelines.pdf.
HPI, history of present illness; KEY Components: history, exam, medical decision making; *MDM*, medical decision making; *PFSH*, past, family, and social history; *ROS*, review of systems.

nursing facility patient is reported neither as an E/M office visit nor as a nursing facility visit. However, if the same conference occurs on the patient's unit, the patient was seen for a portion of the service, and the parties are the surrogate decision makers, the visit does count as a covered visit. If a patient with dementia is seen and then sits quietly in the examination area while the discussion with the family takes place, that time also counts; however, if the patient stays home, that time does not count.

> **Consider using time to determine E/M level when counseling and coordination dominate.**

There are some services that completely lack any face-to-face contact with the patient; these include care plan oversight (e.g., CPT 99375 or G code G0181), certifying a home care plan (G0180), and family therapy without the patient present (90846), although the last example does require face-to-face time with the family members. Prolonged services codes 99354-99357 are reportable when the time of the E/M service greatly exceeds the typical time. These are important services to understand given the high amount of extra time related to care coordination and counseling inherent in geriatric care.

Medicare Coding Compared to CPT Codes and Guidelines

> **Report *all* services.**

There are some key areas where CMS/Medicare does not align with CPT. The issue of annual physicals is described in a previous section. There are many preventive services that are commonly performed that have HCPCS codes and when added up are very significant to the economic health of a practice. They include the annual wellness visits, alcohol misuse screening and counseling, depression screening, tobacco cessation services, obesity services, and cardiovascular risk reduction counseling. These all are G code services and the CMS website has descriptions of each service and rules related to them. The other most significant difference between CMS/Medicare and CPT is the recognition of CPT consultation codes. These codes are invalid for Medicare, which instead requires use of the codes that would be reported per CPT if the service was not by referral. A particularly odd result of this policy is that a hospital inpatient consult of a high level (e.g., 99254) is to be reported with a code that CPT intends for use only for the admitting physician or professional (e.g., 99222). Also odd is the required use by consultants of an office code (99201-99215) for patients in a hospital on observation status.

> **Medicare considers CPT consultation codes invalid.**

CHARGES AND CHARGING FOR ALL SERVICES PERFORMED

As mentioned, it is important to know more than a few E/M codes. A nurse visit to check blood pressure is a 99211, as is an anticoagulation clinic visit. Prolonged services may occur with regularity. Critical care is not restricted to any specialty and can occur even in the office or nursing facility. If a discharge takes more than 30 minutes, the lower-paying, less intensive service should not be reported. A private payer may allow reporting of warfarin management (99364), even if CMS does not. There are laboratory test, surgical procedure, machine test, and drug codes. It pays to learn about the Medicare and other payer rules. Pay attention to charges. The physician is usually paid the lesser of the charge or the allowance, so if the physician charges $50 for a service for which Medicare or another payer will pay the physician $75, the physician will get $50. The Medicare fee schedule is updated annually and many payers will pay a percentage (higher or lower) than Medicare; therefore the Medicare fee schedule is a useful reference point. The physician's charges are what he or she actually charges, so when there is patient cost-sharing the physician is expected, generally, to attempt collection up to the allowed amount. This does not preclude writing off charges selectively, when the patient truly cannot pay. It does mean billing Medicaid as a secondary payer, even if no additional payment is expected.

> **Not all payers follow Medicare and may pay for more than CMS does.**

WORKING AS A TEAM— "INCIDENT TO," SHARED VISITS, AND TEACHING

A nurse visit (99211) is allowed to be billed by a physician because it is incident to that physician's care. There was a time when RNP, CNS, and PA services had to be reported by the physician, but now these professionals are given provider status of their own, depending on state scope-of-practice laws. However, when these professionals are providing care for an established patient under an established treatment plan and are employed by the physician or by the party that employs the physician and the physician is in the office suite, the physician may report the service in Medicare, even if the physician had no face-to-face time with the patient for that encounter. Because the other professionals are paid 85% of the physician fee schedule, correct use of this mechanism is like a 18%

raise for these professionals. Not all services are allowed to be reported this way; for example, nursing facility visits cannot be "incident to." There is also "shared visit" reporting. This is when a physician and the other professional both see the patient and the physician reports a single service for the combined services of the two (e.g., in a hospitalized patient cared for by a hospitalist team of physicians and RNPs). It does require physician involvement, not just a countersignature. A similar concept is applied for teaching physicians who may use portions of the work of the trainee or student, so long as the physician independently verifies or is present for the key portions of the service.

> "Incident to" reporting, when allowed, is equivalent to a nearly 20% raise.

CHARGING THE PATIENT OR FAMILY

Not everything is covered by insurance, including Medicare. Special caution is required if billing a Medicaid beneficiary. It is clear that patient-responsibility balances for copayments or deductibles should be collected, but what about noncovered services? It was common practice until Medicare's inclusion of annual wellness visits to charge Medicare beneficiaries for noncovered annual physicals. Now there is not much left in such a visit that is not covered, even if the physician does not bill the annual wellness visit because a required element was not performed. However, if a family requests a conference in the physician's office to discuss whether mother needs a nursing home and mother is not present, that is not covered, is not part of the usual follow-up of a past visit, and can be charged to the family. It is important to inform the family of this fact, why it is the case, and what you will charge. It is always advisable to use a CMS approved Advance Beneficiary Notice (ABN) form (available on the CMS website), even though it is really intended for services that are covered based on circumstance, such as removing a benign skin lesion for cosmetic reasons as compared to removal because the lesion was getting traumatized. It is advisable for recurrent issues to be reviewed with the local payer, Medicare contractor, or billing experts because the billing process is not always as straightforward as it may seem. Completing certain forms, copying charges, and consultations with an attorney related to guardianship are all issues sometimes faced by practices that are not covered. However, if the form is a certification for durable medical equipment, the patient cannot be charged for its completion.

GLOBAL PERIODS AND PER-DAY SERVICES

Geriatricians may perform some services with a global period longer than the date of service. For example, a lesion excision has a 10-day global period and payment includes any related E/M over those days and suture removal. If a rural geriatrician or hospitalist provides all the postoperative care for a patient, the correct code to report is the surgical procedure code. The surgeon uses a modifier designating that the care did not include postoperative care and the geriatrician uses a modifier indicating only postoperative care was provided. Some codes are per visit and some are per day. Two visits to a hospitalized patient in one day are reported with a single hospital inpatient code. The work of both visits is added up, and the single best hospital visit code and possibly a prolonged service code is used. Be sure to record unit time for all visits if using prolonged services codes. All services related to an admission are reported by the admission code. If a physician sends a patient to the hospital from the office and admits the patient that day, reporting the initial hospital care service, then the office visit is not reported. An exception is transfers from the hospital to a nursing facility. A hospital discharge service and an initial nursing facility service may both be reported on the same day if two separate visits occur.

PAYMENT MODIFICATIONS (eRX, PQRS, PRIMARY CARE BONUS, AND MEANINGFUL USE) AND MIGRATION AWAY FROM FEE FOR SERVICE

Participation in federal programs such as eRx, Physician Quality Reporting System (PQRS), primary care bonus, and meaningful use is associated with bonus payments or penalty avoidance. These programs do have elements related to the services reported (e.g., codes must be reported indicating an electronic prescription was used or that a quality measure was addressed). The primary care bonus eligibility relates to what portion of services are primary care procedure codes as determined by CMS and Congress. The impact of these programs is growing steadily. Newer programs will shift payment away from volume-based fee for service to value-based payments and mechanisms that will recognize systems of care. It is difficult to anticipate what coding and billing issues will arise. It is advisable to be aware of these trends and stay informed.

PARTICIPATION STATUS

Upon getting a provider number, and annually, Medicare allows physicians to address their participation status. Being nonparticipating is not as simple as billing and collecting charges from the patient. If a physician elects to not participate but accepts assignments (i.e., lets Medicare pay the physician directly on a claim in return for the physician not billing the beneficiary a balance), the physician receives 95% of the allowance. If the physician does not accept assignments he or she may not attempt to collect more than 109.25% of Medicare's maximal allowed charge for the service. If the physician opts out of Medicare the contract is between the physician and the patient, but if the physician has opted out for all Medicare patients and the patient cannot get reimbursed by Medicare for the physician's services, though the patient may receive Medicare-covered services from others.

Resources

This chapter gives an overview of important aspects of coding and billing. Each year, or more often, new codes, rules, and programs are created. It is important to keep up to date. For Medicare, the CMS website has a great deal of information. One can even subscribe to update notices from MedLearn Matters. The Medicare Part B contractor website will have important information. Having a current CPT code set publication is advised and CPT has other useful educational publications. Specialty societies and professional organizations will often educate members on new issues and have basic coding courses at annual meetings. Billing companies and other practice management professionals are potential sources of information.

SUMMARY

Coding and billing require knowledge of terms and rules. There is some variation by payer or program, but there are many basic principles, such as correct use of CPT, that are general. These rules can be sufficiently understood by clinicians, but do warrant some educational efforts so as to allow professionals to be properly paid for their services.

Web Resources

www.cms.gov/Center/Provider-Type/Physician-Center.html. Physician Center—starting point for many links, including MedLearn Matters educational products.

www.cms.gov/Outreach-and-Education/Medicare-Learning-Network-MLN/MLNProducts/PreventiveServices.html. Medicare Learning Network Preventive Services.

www.cms.gov/Medicare/Quality-Initiatives-Patient-Assessment-Instruments/PQRS/index.html?redirect=/pqri. Centers for Medicare and Medicaid Services' Physician Quality Reporting System.

www.cms.gov/Medicare/Medicare-General-Information/BNI/ABN.html. Centers for Medicare and Medicaid Services Advance Beneficiary Notices.

www.cms.gov/Outreach-and-Education/Medicare-Learning-Network-MLN/MLNProducts/downloads/gdelinesteachgresfctsht.pdf. Centers for Medicare and Medicaid Services' Guidelines for Teaching Physicians, Interns, and Residents.

www.ama-assn.org/ama/pub/physician-resources/solutions-managing-your-practice/coding-billing-insurance.page? American Medical Association—CPT Medical Billing, Coding and Insurance.

10

Hospital Care

Jeffrey D. Schlaudecker, Christopher R. Bernheisel, and Hillary R. Mount

OBJECTIVES

Upon completion of this chapter, the reader will be able to:

- Understand ways in which the admission process to the hospital can be an opportunity for a review of health status for older adults.

- Describe ways that perioperative care of older adults in the hospital is different from the care of younger patients.

- Know how to apply preventative measures in the hospital to reduce risks to hospitalized older patients.

- Describe how to apply selective interventions to improve hospital outcomes and decrease unplanned readmissions and adverse patient outcomes.

Nosocomial infections, loss of independence, functional status decline, medication interactions, polypharmacy, overtreatment, falls, cognitive loss, delirium, misinformed handoffs, and poor care transitions are just some of the complications that can occur during the hospitalization of an older adult. Although advances in medical and surgical care have decreased the morbidity and mortality of many diseases, the hospital has remained a dangerous place for older patients. Care provided to older adults in the hospital should strive to limit exposure to iatrogenic complications, maintain functional status, and provide patient- and family-centered care that is evidence based and disease focused.

Additional online-only material indicated by icon.

The risk of an older adult developing a new activity of daily living (ADL) disability during a hospitalization is estimated to be at least 30%, and about half of all older adults' disabilities develop during a hospitalization.[1] Frail elders with limited functional reserves fare even worse. Unfortunately, one year after hospital discharge, less than half of older adults have returned to their prehospitalization level of functioning.[2] Certainly, hospitalization may be necessary to provide treatment to older adults. Knowledge of the many causes of functional decline in the hospital and actions aimed at functional status preservation are paramount for any practitioner caring for hospitalized older patients. It has been estimated that 7% to 15% of the 1 million older adults with Medicare who are hospitalized each year experience a preventable adverse event.

> Because of severe physiologic stressors and nosocomial exposures, hospitalization is best thought of as a resource to use carefully in the care of older adults.

CASE 1

Robert Johnson (Part 1)

You are called by a local emergency department about your 81-year-old patient, Mr. Johnson, who has suffered a mild stroke and fractured his hip during a related fall. Mr. Johnson has been your patient for about 7 years, since relocating to be near his adult children. Since losing his wife 3 years ago, Mr. Johnson's visits to your office have been sporadic, and he is under the care of several subspecialists for his macular degeneration, presbycusis, hypertension, and mild diastolic congestive heart failure. Cognitive testing was borderline during a visit 1 year ago, and a geriatric depression screen was positive, but he declined pharmacologic interventions and counseling at that time. The decision is made to admit Mr. Johnson to the hospitalists and obtain a consultation from the orthopedic service.

What factors in his history need to be relayed to the team that will be caring for him in the hospital? ▣

COMMUNICATION IS ESSENTIAL IN THE HOSPITAL

Caring for older adults in the hospital should involve an interprofessional group of care providers. Optimal geriatric hospital care is provided by nursing case managers and geriatric social workers to assist in coordinating discharge needs, dieticians working to find food that is the correct caloric density and texture, nurses and nursing assistants providing direct patient care who are often the first to notice a patient change, consulting physicians, hospitalists, pharmacists, physical therapists, occupational therapists, and speech and language pathologists all working together to bring optimal care to older adults and their families. This large number of team members all must communicate with each other and with the patient and family during the hospitalization. This gathered information must additionally be communicated in an efficient and accurate way to the receiving facility that will take over care once the patient has left the hospital. This can include a rehabilitation facility, a skilled nursing facility, a long-term acute care hospital, a family member's home, or the patient's own residence (see Chapter 2.

Since the term *hospitalist* was first used in 1996 to describe the growing number of physicians whose primary site of practice was within the hospital, the field has expanded rapidly.[3] In urban areas today, hospitalists provide the majority of nonsurgical care to hospitalized adults in the United States.[3] The hospitalist often is the primary care coordinator and communicator among the many team members involved in the care of an older adult in the hospital.

Outcomes for hospitalists are generally at least as efficient and effective as nonhospitalist providers, but the field has highlighted the critical need for excellent communication within all members of the health care team, including the family. With the increased percentage of patients being cared for by hospitalists, the importance of communication across locations of care has increased. It is critically important for the hospitalist to communicate at the time of admission and discharge with both primary care providers and with accepting physicians at skilled nursing facilities or rehabilitation units.

> Primary care physicians, hospitalists, caregivers, and all members of the health care team caring for a hospitalized geriatric patient need to ensure maximal communication.

HOSPITAL DESIGN AND SYSTEMS CHANGE TO BENEFIT OLDER ADULTS

Much as pediatric hospitals underwent changes in design to better reflect the unique needs of their young patients, specific areas in many hospitals today are designed to optimally meet the needs of older adults. NICHE and ACE units are two specific programs that are aimed to improve the care of older adults in the hospital.

In 1992, with funds from the John A. Hartford Foundation, New York University began broadly field-testing nursing care models including the geriatric resource nurse (GRN) program. This project became known as Nurses Improving Care for Health System Elders (NICHE) and aimed to create a better care environment for the hospitalized elderly patient by improving nursing practice.[4] Nursing leadership is integral to good care of older adults, and the NICHE program provides resources, project management support/mentoring for NICHE-based hospital initiatives, evidence-based clinical protocols that address "never events," and shared information, knowledge, and expertise to more than 300 participating hospitals.[5]

Acute care for the elderly (ACE) units have demonstrated improved functional outcomes without increased costs or length of stay.[6] This model of comprehensive inpatient geriatric care incorporates (1) hospital environment modifications, (2) minimization of adverse effects of hospitalization, (3) early discharge planning, and (4) patient-centered care protocols.[7]

The benefit of ACE units is also being expanded hospitalwide. The concept of a mobile acute care for the elderly (MACE) unit has also been described. The main goals of the MACE unit are to bring the interdisciplinary, patient-centered team approach to hospitalized older adult patients throughout a hospital, rather than having the team located solely on one geographically based unit. A 2010 study found that among more than 8000 older adults, those being treated via MACE service (compared to those admitted to an ACE or a traditional unit) had lower length of stay and lower costs with no change in in-hospital mortality or 7- or 30-day readmission rates.[6]

> Stressors in the hospital are summative and include the inciting medical or surgical event, and also sleep deprivation, medication side effects, sensory deprivation, and caloric deficiencies resulting from restrictive diets, nothing-by-mouth status, or general illness.

Hospital Physical Design

In addition to a redesign of care processes and procedures for caring for older hospitalized adults, the physical environments of hospitals are additionally being designed to allow for improved care.[8] Hospital design that focuses on the needs of older adults and their families has improved the hospital campus, the unit, the room, and the amenities available. Design features can include reserved or valet parking and benches along long walkways; handrails; matte floor finishing or low-pile carpeting; low-color-contrast floors with clear contrast with walls; sound-absorbing materials in rooms with available assistive listening devices; choice of chairs with armrests; automatic faucets and doors; and easy-to-see and easy-to-activate call systems.[8]

Patient- and Family-Centered Geriatric Hospital Care

Because many older adults rely on additional support for successful aging, geriatric hospital care must embrace the principles of patient- and family-centered care. As defined by the Institute for Patient- and Family-Centered Care, the core principles include respect and dignity, collaboration, participation, and meaningful information sharing.[9] Family is defined as broadly as possible to include any person that an older adult may rely on for support, whether emotional, physical, or financial.[9] Partnership with family during the hospitalization of older adults is paramount to a successful admission, and every attempt to involve family at the highest level desired by the patient should be sought. Minimizing barriers to family participation in health care should always be a paramount goal of excellent care.

> The use of specialized acute care for the elderly (ACE) units can improve outcomes by modifying the hospital environment to be less disruptive to older adults.

THE ADMISSION PROCESS: OPPORTUNITIES FOR HEALTH STATUS UPDATES

When an older adult requires admission to the hospital, communication among providers inside and outside the hospital is critically important. The primary care physician and/or the nursing home physician and the family must all be involved to ensure a meaningful admission. For patients living in long-term care settings, often the nurses and/or patient care attendants/nursing assistants have valuable information about symptom development, and attempts to contact these care providers should be undertaken. Because older adults vary widely in their functional and health status, critical decisions about treatment should never be based solely on the patient's age. The in-hospital medical team will need guidance from community-based providers to accurately assess the older patient's baseline functional status.

At the time of admission, the hospital provider should perform a review of systems that focuses on geriatric syndromes and other issues common to older adults, including cognition and functional independence in ADLs and instrumental activities of daily living (IADLs). Vaccine status, especially about pneumococcal, seasonal influenza, and herpes zoster should also be ascertained. The time of admission to the hospital is also an excellent time for a medication review for both accuracy and necessity of all medications, both prescribed and over-the-counter. The presence of advance directives and documentation of a surrogate decision maker is also among information that should be incorporated into the admission record. Advance directives should also be discussed and documented.

> The admission process provides an opportunity to review medications and ensure appropriate indications for all prescriptions, as well as ascertain vaccine status, code status, alcohol use, and elder abuse risk factors.

Elder Abuse

Screening for elder mistreatment among asymptomatic populations has not been evaluated, but the presence of elder abuse has been estimated to be between 2% and 10%.[10] Elder abuse can broadly be defined as physical, psychological, or sexual abuse, material exploitation of money or property, or neglect and failure to meet a dependent older person's needs. The possibility of nonaccidental trauma or neglect of an older adult admitted to the hospital should be entertained by the clinician based on a high index of suspicion.[10] Identification of social support and appropriate referral to area Adult Protective Services agencies should be made whenever elder abuse is suspected (see Chapter 33).

Alcohol Abuse

During the admission to the hospital, a discussion on alcohol use should be completed. The prevalence of older adults with alcohol-related problems has been reported to be between 2% and 22%, depending on the definition used.[11] With the aging population, even with a constant prevalence, the number of older adults with alcohol use problems will increase dramatically. Screening tools for younger adults usually focus on work or legal difficulties that arise from drinking, and these consequences are rarer in older adults with harmful drinking patterns.[11] Unfortunately there are currently no appropriate screening questionnaires validated for older adults to detect harmful or hazardous drinking patterns (see Chapter 34).

Frailty as a Risk for Poor Hospital Outcomes

Frailty is a geriatric syndrome defined as a state of increased vulnerability to both acute and chronic stressors as a consequence of reduced physiologic reserve.[12] Frailty is associated with functional decline, loss of independence, and mortality. The identification of this syndrome should be readily considered for any older adult being admitted to the hospital (see Chapter 29). The concept of frailty is relevant for providers of geriatric hospital care, because it provides a ready explanation for the different stress tolerances of older adults. Stressors in the hospital are summative and can include not only the inciting medical or surgical event, but also sleep deprivation, medication side effects, sensory deprivation, and caloric deficiencies resulting from restrictive diets, nothing-by-mouth status, or general illness.[12-14] For men and women older than age 60, ten days of bed rest results in a similar loss of muscle mass as a decade of normal aging.[13] To help lessen the impact of hospitalization on older adults, physical activity (especially resistance training), nutritional consultations and supplementation, and vitamin D supplementation when appropriate should be strongly considered.[13]

PERIOPERATIVE CARE OF THE ELDERLY PATIENT IN THE HOSPITAL

Nearly half of all patients undergoing a surgical procedure are now older than age 65, with the percentage expected to increase further over the next 15 years as the population continues to age.[15] Studies have shown 21% of elderly patients will suffer from at least one perioperative complication following a nonthoracic surgery, potentially leading to prolonged hospitalization, increased mortality, and long-term morbidity.[16,17] Because of the heterogeneity of elderly patients, a patient-centered approach in close conjunction with the surgical team is required to reduce the risk of complications and adverse outcomes.

CASE 1

Robert Johnson (Part 2)

Mr. Johnson was admitted to the hospital yesterday for his focal weakness and hip fracture. He was seen by a neurologist, who expects continued recovery of left leg weakness that is the result of a small ischemic stroke. He was put on nothing-by-mouth status at the time of admission and the orthopedic surgeon is planning on taking him for operative repair later this afternoon.

In what ways can his care be optimized at this point in the hospitalization? ▣

Establishing Goals of Care

The preoperative evaluation of elderly patients begins with a frank discussion on goals of care (Figure 10-1).

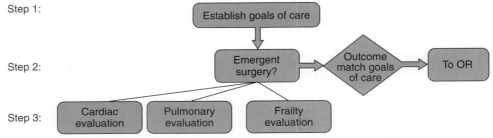

Figure 10-1 Preoperative evaluation. (Adapted from Fleisher LA, Beckman JA, Brown KA, et al. 2009 ACCF/AHA focused update on perioperative beta blockade incorporated into the ACC/AHA 2007 guidelines on perioperative cardiovascular evaluation and care for noncardiac surgery: A report of the American College of Cardiology Foundation/American Heart Association Task Force on Practice Guidelines. Circulation 2009;120(21):e169-e276.)

Survival and longevity may be the most important outcomes for a younger population but it may not be the primary goals for every elderly patient. A more important outcome may be related to the patient's functional status following the surgery. A full discussion of all the potential outcomes is necessary, with an honest discussion of prognosis of recovery related to functional status and the potential loss of independence. Elderly patients may elect to forgo emergent interventions if the outcome would likely lead to loss of independence and functional status, and instead may elect for only comfort care measures. The role of the medical clinician in the preoperative evaluation is to help review all of the options for the patient including the option for palliative care. The preoperative evaluation provides an excellent opportunity to better define end-of-life decision making for the patient, especially for those surgical interventions that carry significant risks for the elderly patient. Patients should be encouraged to discuss their decisions with family members and their health care power of attorney to prevent undesired interventions in the future.

Emergent Surgery

Generally, patients who have acute surgical emergencies may proceed to the operating room with the assumption that any potential risk would be less than the potential benefit of the surgery. This may not be as true for elderly patients, and goals of care still must be addressed even in the emergent situation. A lifesaving surgical intervention that leads to loss of independence may not match the goals of care for an elderly patient, and palliative care is an important option to provide the patient. The emergent evaluation includes a brief discussion on preoperative functional status to help assess functional reserve along with the goals of care for the individual patient. Elderly patients who undergo emergent surgeries have a higher risk of adverse outcomes and long-term morbidity that may lead to loss of independence especially in those with low preoperative functional status.

> Perioperative care in the hospital must be based on goals of care and should strive to ensure evidence-based use of risk stratification, medications, and early mobilization to prevent prolonged hospitalizations and nosocomial infections.

CARDIAC EVALUATION

Active Cardiac Conditions

For nonemergent surgeries, the clinician must inquire about any active cardiac conditions. Active cardiac conditions include all of those conditions that would warrant urgent treatment whether the patient was planning a surgical intervention or not: acute coronary syndrome, myocardial infarction within 30 days, significant arrhythmias, and severe valvular disease.[24] The time frame for delaying the surgical intervention depends on the cardiac event and the intervention. There is a paucity of evidence for the correct timing of surgery following medical intervention. Decisions are based on best available evidence and consensus statements (Figure 10-2).

A vital component of the perioperative care of patients with a history of a recent cardiac event is the management of antiplatelet therapy. Dual therapy with aspirin and clopidogrel is required for 3 to 6 months following acute myocardial infarction, 2 weeks following angioplasty, 6 weeks following a bare metal stent, and 1 year following a drug-eluting stent.[18] All nonemergent surgeries that require discontinuing clopidogrel must be delayed until these time frames are met. Then the surgery can be performed with the patient taking aspirin alone.

Primary care doctors must work closely with their surgical colleagues to weigh the risk of bleeding against the risk of coronary artery disease, with strong consideration to continue aspirin for secondary prevention of coronary heart disease in the perioperative period. The procoagulant, proinflammatory state following

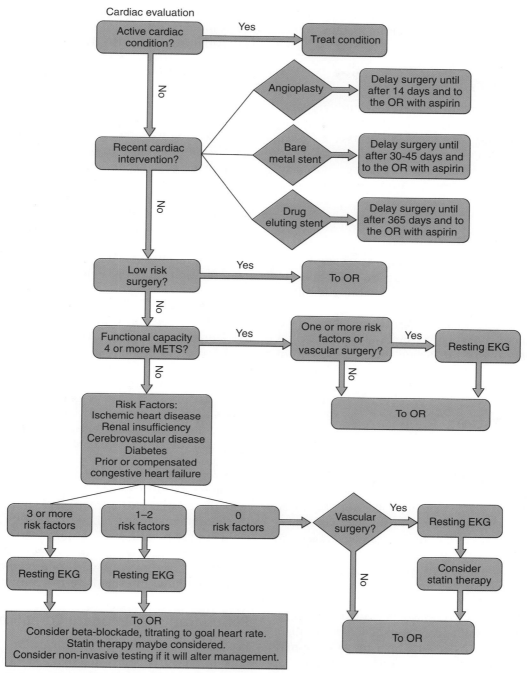

Figure 10-2 **Preoperative cardiac evaluation.** *EKG,* Electrocardiogram; *METs,* metabolic equivalents of a task. (Adapted from Fleisher LA, Beckman JA, Brown KA, et al. 2009 ACCF/AHA focused update on perioperative beta blockade incorporated into the ACC/AHA 2007 guidelines on perioperative cardiovascular evaluation and care for noncardiac surgery: A report of the American College of Cardiology Foundation/American Heart Association Task Force on Practice Guidelines. Circulation 2009;120(21):e169-e276.)

surgery places patients at a significantly higher risk for cardiac in-stent stenosis with potential catastrophic results, with an odds ratio of 3.1 peaking 10 days after surgery.[19] Restenosis has been reported with withdrawal of aspirin even after 2 years from stent placement, which emphasizes the absolute importance of

continuation of aspirin.[20,21] Evidence on the risk of continuation of aspirin in the perioperative period has not been well studied, but a meta-analysis did not demonstrate increased mortality or postoperative complications when aspirin was continued.[22] In addition, outside of neurosurgical interventions, there is no evidence to demonstrate that the increased risk of bleeding with continuation of aspirin therapy translates to an increase in mortality.[23]

Low-Risk Surgery

Patients undergoing low-risk ambulatory surgical procedures (e.g., endoscopic procedures or cataract, simple breast, or ambulatory surgeries) do not have a higher 30-day risk of cardiac events compared to peers.[24] With the lack of apparent increased cardiac risk, patients may proceed to the operating room (OR) without any additional evaluation for low-risk surgeries.

Functional Assessment

Functional assessment is of vital importance, especially in the elderly population who can have a broad range of activity and functional levels. Functional capacity can be estimated by history using published charts or having the patient perform a treadmill test using standard protocol. Patients who are able to perform physical activities at or higher than 4 METS (metabolic equivalents of a task) may proceed to the planned procedure without additional evaluation.[25]

Cardiac Risk Factors

For patients who are unable to achieve 4 METs or if functional capacity is unknown, an evaluation of risk factors for perioperative events (e.g., ischemic heart disease, renal insufficiency, cerebrovascular disease, diabetes, or history of congestive heart failure) should be pursued.[24] Patients who have no risk factors may proceed to the OR without any further cardiac evaluation. Patients with one to two risk factors may proceed to OR with beta-blockade, or noninvasive coronary evaluation can be considered. Patients with three or more risk factors undergoing an intermediate-risk surgery may also proceed to OR with beta-blockade or may undergo noninvasive coronary evaluation. Those patients with three or more risk factors undergoing high-risk surgery may proceed to the OR with beta-blockade and a statin, or noninvasive coronary evaluation should be considered if those results have the potential to alter decision making and change management.

Cardiac Risk Reduction through Medical Interventions

Beta-Blockade

There have been multiple studies looking at beta-blockade in the perioperative period, with conflicting results.[25-28] Early studies showed significant promise for the prevention of acute myocardial infarction; unfortunately, follow-up studies have not consistently demonstrated this benefit. Two studies in 2007 and 2009 led to an update of the American College of Cardiology Foundation/American Heart Association (ACCF/AHA) Perioperative Guidelines in 2009, and provide guidance for applying the conflicting data in practice.[25]

More recent studies confirmed the cardioprotective benefit of perioperative beta-blockade but demonstrated the increased risk of stroke and death. The differences between the studies provide insight into the mechanism of risk for perioperative beta-blockade and provide guidance for initiating beta-blockade. *The avoidance of hypotension and bradycardia appears vital to reduce the risk of ischemic stroke.* Beta-blockade should be initiated at a low dose and titrated slowly up to goal prior to surgery. The exact timing for initiating beta-blockade has not been established, but based on the results of available data, same-day initiation with rapid titration should be avoided.[27]

HMG-CoA Reductase Inhibitors (Statin Therapy)

The only prospective randomized trial on perioperative statin use was a small study of 100 patients investigating the perioperative use of atorvastatin for vascular surgery.[29] Patients were placed on 20 mg atorvastatin for a total of 45 days and a minimum of 2 weeks prior to the surgery with a composite outcome of death from stroke and acute coronary syndrome. A statistically significant difference in composite outcome was reached in the atorvastatin arm versus placebo at 6 months (8% vs. 26%). Multiple retrospective studies have also shown reduced perioperative cardiac events with the use of statins in both vascular and nonvascular studies. Based on the limited evidence available, the 2009 ACCF/AHA Guidelines find the use of statins "reasonable" for patients undergoing vascular surgery and "may be considered" for patients with one or more risk factors undergoing intermediate-risk surgery.[25]

Perioperative Pulmonary Complications

Perioperative pulmonary complications (PPCs) are encountered frequently following noncardiothoracic surgeries and contribute significantly to perioperative and long-term morbidity and mortality. The American College of Chest Physicians includes atelectasis, pneumonia, respiratory failure, and exacerbation of underlying chronic lung disease as PPCs. An incidence of 5.5% to 6.8% is found when using rigorous methods to define PPC.[17,31] PPCs are an even stronger predictor than perioperative cardiac complications for longer term perioperative mortality in the elderly, with a hazard ratio of 2.41.[30] Despite being a stronger predictor for adverse outcomes and having a similar frequency as perioperative cardiac events, perioperative pulmonary evaluation and PPCs prevention are often placed at a lower priority by clinicians and patients. Because advanced age is a risk factor for PPCs, clinicians who care for the elderly need to have increased awareness and diligence in evaluating and preventing PPCs.

Preoperative Pulmonary Evaluation

The preoperative pulmonary evaluation starts with identification of risk factors for developing PPCs (Box 10-1). Of the risk factors listed, a history of chronic obstructive pulmonary disease (COPD) and age older than 60 are the two highest predictors of the development of PPCs. The risk for PPCs increases with each decade, with odds ratios of 2.09 for patients 60 to 69 and 3.04 for patients 70 to 79.[32] Another important risk factor is functional status, which predicts both overall mortality and risk for PPCs with an odds ratio of 2.51 for developing PPCs if patients are unable to perform any ADLs and 1.65 if they require assistance for some of their ADLs. Those patients who are identified as having any risk factors for PPCs should proceed to additional evaluation and undergo preoperative and postoperative interventions to reduce risk.

Pulmonary function tests (PFTs) have an important role in the evaluation and risk analysis for patients undergoing cardiothoracic surgery, but evidence has not demonstrated benefit for non-cardiothoracic surgeries. A PFT threshold level used to decide when to withhold surgery has not been demonstrated in non-cardiothoracic surgeries. Patients who meet criteria for PFTs for alternative reasons, such as initial evaluation of COPD, should have PFTs ordered. There is not a separate indication for non-cardiothoracic perioperative PFT evaluation, even in the setting of stable COPD, because the test results do not add any additional value past what is obtained in the history and examination.[32]

The routine use of chest x-ray examinations also does not provide additional data past what can be identified with a history and physical. Although abnormalities may be identified, rarely do they lead to a change in management for the patient. Based on the available evidence, the American College of Physicians does not recommend the routine use of chest x-ray studies for a preoperative pulmonary evaluation.[32]

Low albumin is a very powerful predictor of perioperative mortality and long-term morbidity in addition to a predictor of PPCs. Patients with an albumin lower than 3.5 g/dL had an incidence of 27.6% of PPCs compared to an incidence of 7.0% in patients with normal albumin.[32] Unfortunately, nutritional support strategies such as total parenteral nutrition (TPN) in the perioperative period have not demonstrated any benefit over regular diet.[33] Patients who have one or more risk factor for PPCs or are undergoing a high-risk surgery should have a preoperative albumin level test so they can be better counseled about the potential risk of the surgery.

Interventions to Reduce Pulmonary Complications

Evidence-based interventions to reduce PPCs are limited, with studies either not rigorously designed or not demonstrating any significant benefit. The best evidence for the prevention of PPCs has been seen with deep breathing exercises or incentive spirometry (IS) in the perioperative period. IS has been compared to deep breathing exercises, with both modalities appearing to have similar results. PPCs are cut in half with either of these techniques.[34] The results seem to be superior if the patient receives education prior to the surgery and even greater if the patient begins inspiratory training exercises several weeks prior to surgery.[35] For patients who are unable to participate in breathing exercises, continuous positive airway pressure (CPAP) may be an option and has been demonstrated to reduce PPCs.[36]

Smoking cessation has also been investigated as a method to reduce PPCs, with some evidence showing benefit. The best evidence is in the setting of cardiothoracic surgery, with a greater benefit if the patient quits more than 2 months before the surgery.[37] Based on the overall benefits, it would be appropriate to provide counseling to patients on smoking cessation as part of the routine perioperative evaluation.

BOX 10-1

PULMONARY RISK FACTORS

Age >60 years old
Chronic Lung Disease
   COPD
   Restrictive Lung Disease
   Pulmonary Arterial Hypertension
Smoking
Congestive Heart Failure
Poor Functional Status
ASA Classification of 2 or Greater
Perioperative Delirium
Surgery Longer than 3 Hours
Abdominal Surgery, Thoracic Surgery, Neurosurgery, Head and Neck Surgery, Vascular Surgery, Aortic Aneurysm Repair, Emergency Surgery
General Anesthesia
Albumin <3.5 g/dL

ASA, American Society of Anesthesiologists; *COPD*, Chronic obstructive pulmonary disease.
Source: Owens WD, Felts JA, Spitznagel EL Jr. ASA physical status classifications: A study of consistency of ratings. Anesthesiology 1978;49:239-43.

Delirium is an additional significant risk factor for both PPCs and poor outcomes for the hospitalized elderly patient. Following surgical interventions, patients are at very high risk for delirium with one study showing an incidence of 50%.[38] Clinicians should monitor for signs of delirium and implement strategies during the perioperative period to reduce risk (see Chapter 16).

Postoperative Considerations

Venous Thromboembolism Prevention

Venous thromboembolism (VTE) is considered the top preventable etiology for hospital death, with the postoperative state placing patients at even higher risk than hospitalized general medical patients. Table 10-1 summarizes the most recent guidelines from the American College of Chest Physicians.[39] Frequent and clear dialogue with surgical colleagues to balance postoperative bleeding risk with thromboembolism risk is essential (see further discussion in the following section on Preventative Measures in the Hospital).

Postoperative Anemia

There are very few studies that evaluate transfusions for patients in the postoperative period. Recently, a study comparing a liberal transfusion cutoff of a hemoglobin of 10 g/dL to a restrictive transfusion cutoff hemoglobin of 8 g/dL was performed on patients following hip replacement surgery.[40] In this trial, patients were transfused at the randomized predefined transfusion cutoffs or if they demonstrated symptomatic anemia (such as orthostatic hypotension, chest pain believed to be cardiac in origin, tachycardia that did not respond to fluids, or signs of congestive heart failure). At 30 days, the groups did not differ in mortality, functional status, cardiac events, infectious events, VTE, stroke, or congestive heart failure. Based on this trial, the American Association of Blood Banks (AABB) recommends a transfusion cutoff of 8 g/dL hemoglobin unless signs and symptoms of anemia are present.[41]

TABLE 10-1	Venous Thromboembolism Prophylaxis	
Patient Category	**Method of VTE Prophylaxis**	**Duration**
Hospitalized Patients	High risk for VTE (Padua Prediction Score ≥4): LMWH or UFH or fondaparinux High risk for VTE and bleeding or high risk for major bleed: Mechanical thromboprophylaxis with GCS Low risk (Padua Prediction Score <4): No pharmacological or mechanical prophylaxis	Duration of hospitalization
Critically Ill Hospitalized Patients	Routine use of LMWH or UFH. If bleeding or high risk for major bleed: Mechanical thromboprophylaxis with GCS	Duration of hospitalization
Major Orthopedic Surgery (Elective Hip Replacement, Hip Fracture Repair, Elective Knee Replacement)	LMWH—start 12 hr prior to surgery or 12 or more hours postoperative. Administer with IPC.	10-35 days (aim for 35 days when possible)
Knee Arthroscopy	No risk factors: Early and frequent ambulation Additional risk factors: LMWH	Until ambulatory
Elective Spine Surgery	No risk factors: IPC and early and frequent ambulation Risk factors (high-risk VTE, cancer): UFH, LMWH once hemostasis established or IPC with GCS	Until ambulatory
Major GYN Surgery (any non-laparoscopic)	If for *benign* disease: Very low risk (<0.5%; Rogers Score <7; Caprini Score 0): Ambulation Low risk (1.5%; Rogers Score 7-10; Caprini Score 1-2): IPC Moderate risk (3.0%; Rogers >10; Caprini 2-4) and not at high risk for bleed: LMWH, UFH, or IPC High risk (6.0%; Caprini Score 5 or higher): LMWH or UHF with IPC Malignancy: LMWH or UFH TID and IPC	Until hospital discharge For *high-risk* patients (major cancer surgery or prior VTE)—Continue prophylaxis for 28 days post–hospital discharge
Minor or Entirely Laparoscopic GYN Surgery	Low-risk patient: Early ambulation High-risk patient: LMWH, UFH or IPCs w/GCS	Until hospital discharge

TABLE 10-1	Venous Thromboembolism Prophylaxis (Continued)	
Patient Category	**Method of VTE Prophylaxis**	**Duration**
General Abdominal-Pelvic Surgery	Very low risk for VTE (Rogers Score <7; Caprini Score 0): No intervention other than ambulation Low risk (Rogers Score >20; Caprini Score 1-2) not at high risk for bleeding complications: LMWH or UH or mechanical prophylaxis by IPC Low risk for VTE (Rogers Score >20; Caprini Score 1-2) with a high risk for bleeding complications: Mechanical prophylaxis by IPC Moderate risk for VTE (Rogers Score >10; Caprini score 3-4) not at high risk for bleeding complications: LMWH or UFH or mechanical prophylaxis by IPC Moderate risk for VTE (Rogers Score >10; Caprini score 3-4) at high risk for bleeding complications: Mechanical prophylaxis by IPC High Risk for VTE (Caprini score ≥5) not at high risk for major bleeding complication: LMWH or UFH with mechanical prophylaxis by IPC High risk for VTE (Caprini score ≥5) at high risk for major bleeding complication: Mechanical prophylaxis by IPC	General: Hospitalization High VTE-risk undergoing surgery for cancer: 4 week duration with LMWH

VTE, Venous thromboembolism; *LMWH*, low molecular weight heparin; *UFH*, unfractionated heparin; *GCS*, graduated compression stockings; *IPC*, intermittent pneumatic compression.

Source: Gutterman D, Akl E, Guyatt G, Schuünemann HJ, Crowther M, and the American College of Chest Physicians Antithrombotic Therapy and Prevention of Thrombosis Panel. Executive summary: Antithrombotic therapy and prevention of thrombosis (9th ed). American College of Chest Physicians evidence-based clinical practice guidelines. Chest 2012;141;7S-47S.

PREVENTATIVE MEASURES IN THE HOSPITAL

Assuring patient safety in the hospital setting is a nationwide challenge. The geriatric population is at a higher risk of complications in the hospital for multiple reasons including longer length of stays, more frequent hospitalizations, higher numbers of medical problems, and more severe illness at presentation.[42-45] Greater than 50% of elderly patients will experience at least one complication related to their hospitalization.[46] These complications lead to longer length of stay per hospitalization, higher costs, and higher rates of institutionalization at discharge.[43,46,47] Older adults account for 43.6% of all hospital charges—nearly $329 billion (2003).[43] A proactive approach to the problem should include preventative measures targeted at common complications.

CASE 1

Robert Johnson (Part 3)

Mr. Johnson underwent successful hip replacement 9 days ago. His neurologic deficits from the acute stroke have almost totally resolved, but his son calls your office to report that Mr. Johnson is extremely confused and has been very agitated in the evenings, requiring restraints to keep him from removing his own Foley catheter and intravenous lines.

He has not been eating well at all, and the son also reports that his father is being treated for a deep venous thrombosis in his leg, a urinary tract infection, and pneumonia.

> **What things might have been done to prevent Mr. Johnson's postoperative delirium and other illnesses?**

Delirium Prevention

Delirium affects 8% to 30% of hospitalized patients older than 65 years, leading to longer hospital stays and almost $4 billion in Medicare expenditures (2004).[48] Patients with delirium have a higher mortality rate, higher rate of institutionalization, and a higher incidence of dementia.[49] Prevention begins with a thorough history and physical examination to identify risk factors for delirium. Once the at-risk patient is identified, all available preventative measures should be implemented (see Chapter 16).

Studies evaluating actionable steps to prevent delirium are few, but a 2006 Cochrane review identified the need for further studies because of the large scope of the problem.[50-53] It is clear that a multidisciplinary approach is effective[54] and that education of all patient-care team members is key to implementing preventative measures.[50,52] When available, specialized acute care for elders units (ACE units) should be used because they have been shown to decrease hospital stays, reduce costs, and maintain functional status with no change in overall outcomes or readmission rates.[55] Despite studies showing that ACE units may decrease length of stay and improve outcomes in patients with delirium, small studies are inconclusive on the ability of ACE units to prevent delirium in high-risk patients.[56,57]

Preventative measures must address a range of risk factors. Interventions include addressing and minimizing environmental risk factors, avoiding medicines that may predispose to delirium, and ensuring optimal pain control (see Chapter 16). A useful patient-centered tool is recruiting family members or other visitors to aid in cognitive stimulation (reorienting, reminiscence, etc). Family members may also be able to help in bringing any of the patient's sensory aids (glasses, hearing aids, dentures, etc.) to the hospital.

Fall Prevention

Patient falls in the hospital are a serious concern, leading to injuries, longer hospital stays, decreased functional status, higher rates of institutionalization, more malpractice claims, and increased medical costs.[58,59] On average, patients who fell stayed 12 days longer and had charges $4,233 higher than controls, after adjustment for potential clinical and nonclinical confounders.[59] Efforts to prevent falls intensified in most hospitals after a change in Medicare reimbursement policy in 2008. At that time, the Centers for Medicare and Medicaid Services included hospital falls in a group of eight hospital-acquired diagnoses that were deemed preventable. Now hospitals are not reimbursed for a higher-paying diagnosis-related group (DRG) after a fall in the hospital.[58]

Fall prevention begins with a thorough assessment of the patient on admission. Risk factors for falls can be divided into four main categories: mechanical, physical, cognitive, and environmental (see Chapter 20). An action plan for fall prevention may benefit all patients, but the cost-effectiveness of this in hospitalized patients is unknown.[60] Ideally, prevention should target the patient's specific risk factors (see Chapter 20).[61-63] Vitamin D supplementation may decrease the risk of falls by as much as 20%[64,65] and the American Geriatrics Society's guidelines for fall prevention give a strong recommendation for at least 800 IU of vitamin D per day in deficient or high-risk patients.[66] A more recent (2010) randomized controlled trial evaluating a preventative health information technology tool (fall prevention tool kit [FPTK]) developed by a Massachusetts group showed a significant decrease in falls in the intervention group.[67]

It is important to balance the desire to decrease fall rates with the need for continued mobility.[58,68,69] Provider and patient fears of falling have the potential to cause more harm if preventative measures are too restrictive and safe mobility is not encouraged.

> Delirium, falls, venous thromboembolism, skin breakdown, respiratory illnesses, and many other infectious diseases have modifiable risk factors that should be targeted in the hospital.

Sensory Deprivation

The hospitalized elderly patient is particularly vulnerable to complications related to sensory deficits. At baseline the elderly are more likely to have auditory, visual, taste, or balance problems. Without the necessary sensory aids these patients are at a higher risk of delirium, falls, medication administration errors, hospital-acquired disability, institutionalization, and readmission. Visual deficits in particular have a greater effect on balance in the elderly than in younger patients.[70] It is important to assess the elderly patient on admission for these deficits and request that family or friends bring any necessary aids to the hospital. Glasses, hearing aids, and ambulatory aids help the patient stay mobile and cognitively engaged in their care.

Venous Thromboembolism Prophylaxis

Venous thromboembolism (VTE) prophylaxis should be a priority in all hospitalized patients because VTE is responsible for 10% of U.S. hospital deaths each year.[71] The risk of VTE is increased in the hospitalized patient as a result of infections, immobility, and procedures. The Institute of Medicine (IOM) defines failure to provide adequate VTE prophylaxis to hospitalized patients when indicated as a medical error.[72]

All patients should be assessed for risk of VTE on admission.[73] No single risk assessment tool has been prospectively validated for use in deciding on appropriate prophylaxis. Hospitalization for acute medical illness is a risk factor for VTE and in the presence of other risk factors (Table 10-2) should prompt initiation of appropriate prophylaxis (see Table 10-1).[73,74] Pharmacologic prophylaxis should not be used if the risk of bleeding outweighs the risk of thrombosis.[73] Mechanical prophylaxis is a reasonable alternative or adjunct, but may limit activity and increase risk for falls and skin breakdown.

Skin Care

Appropriate skin care in the hospital is an important part of caring for the elderly because they are more

TABLE 10-2	Risk Factors for Venous Thromboembolism
Stasis	Age >40
	Immobility >3 days
	Congestive heart failure
	Stroke
	Paralysis
	Spinal cord injury
	Hyperviscosity
	Polycythemia
	Severe chronic obstructive pulmonary disease
	Anesthesia
	Obesity
	Varicose veins
Hypercoagulable state	Cancer and cancer therapy
	High estrogen states (including HRT)
	Inflammatory bowel
	Nephrotic syndrome
	Sepsis
	Smoking
	Pregnancy and postpartum period
	Inherited or acquired thrombophilia
Endothelial damage	Surgery
	Prior VTE
	Central venous catheterization
	Trauma
Venous compression	Tumor
	Hematoma
	Arterial abnormalities

HRT, hormone replacement therapy; *VTE*, Venous thromboembolism.

Adapted from Anderson FA Jr, Wheeler HB. Venous thromboembolism: Risk factors and prophylaxis. Clin Chest Med 1995;16:235; and Bergqvist D, Pineo GF, Geerts WH, et al., and the American College of Chest Physicians Prevention of Venous Thromboembolism Panel. American College of Chest Physicians evidence-based clinical practice guidelines (8th ed). Chest 2008;133(6 Suppl):381S.

susceptible to skin injury.[75] Proactive care includes providing adequate skin moisturization with avoidance of maceration, shearing, tearing, or pressure damage. It is important to identify skin lesions or breakdown on admission and to include appropriate skin care in the treatment plan (see Chapter 30).

Activity should be encouraged with the appropriate level of supervision or aid as needed. Bed-bound or immobile patients should have pressure-reducing support products applied to cushion bony prominences (sacrum, heels, etc.). These patients should be repositioned at least every 2 hours to decrease risk of pressure ulcers. Staff education on skin care and appropriate repositioning techniques is important to minimize damage. Use of proper protective dressings to prevent infection and minimize pressure damage, as well as wound care specialist consultation, may be appropriate to tailor treatment.

Optimal nutrition and hydration are key to skin health and healing. Avoiding overly restrictive diet orders when possible, encouraging between-meal supplements, and avoiding medicines that impair taste or smell can help maximize nutrition.

> Maintaining optimal nutrition and mobility in the hospital are hallmarks of excellent geriatric hospital care.

Respiratory Illness Prevention

Hospitalized patients are susceptible to respiratory problems because of decreased mobility, exposure to other infected patients, prolonged supine positioning, pain, and other factors. Preventative measures include use of lung expansion maneuvers (incentive spirometry and deep breathing exercises) and encouraging appropriate mobility. Continue home inhalers when possible to maintain baseline control of preexisting pulmonary disease. It is important to achieve adequate pain control to facilitate good lung expansion and mobility.

The elderly are particularly prone to aspiration events that can lead to pulmonary complications such as pneumonitis or pneumonia.[76] To minimize risk for aspiration, encourage the patient to get up to a chair for meals, monitor for signs of oral motor dysfunction (cough, excessive throat-clearing, etc.), encourage mobility, and avoid psychoactive medications. Providing good oral care, avoiding unnecessary acid-blocking medications, and removing nasogastric tubes as soon as possible leads to decreased pulmonary complications.[76,77]

Preventing Infections in the Hospital

Infections are a major source of hospital complications in the elderly. Two out of three infected hospital patients in 2005 were elderly.[78] Patients older than 70 were 10 times more likely to get a hospital-acquired infection than those younger than 50.[79] Possible contributing factors to this susceptibility include poor functional status, malnutrition, greater severity of illness, and decreased reserve.

Decreasing hospital-acquired infections starts with strict adherence to standard precautions and hand washing.[80] When additional isolation protocols (contact, droplet, etc.) are needed these should always be followed. Judicious use of intravenous catheters, urinary catheters, and other invasive monitoring devices decreases risk of infection. It is also important to follow guidelines for length of antibiotic use to avoid excess dosing, which increases the risk for *Clostridium difficile* infection.[81] Probiotics have been used to prevent antibiotic-associated diarrhea and *C. difficile* colitis with mixed results and controversial conclusions.[82,83] The use of probiotics for prevention of *C. difficile* colitis may be of benefit in the high-risk patient, but further studies are needed before this can be universally recommended[82] (see Chapter 49). It is important to remember that alcohol-based hand hygiene products are not as effective against the spores of *C. difficile*; therefore the Centers for Disease Control recommends use of soap and water with this patient population.[80,84,85]

Recognizing infection in the elderly can also be challenging. Infection may be present without fever or leukocytosis. Subtle changes in behavior, alertness, or mood may be the only warning that an infection has set in, requiring a higher level of awareness when working with the hospitalized elder.

Preventing Alcohol Withdrawal

Alcohol withdrawal in the hospital is a potentially life-threatening problem. At least a third of elderly patients exhibit high-risk drinking habits.[86] It is important to ask about alcohol use on admission and anticipate the effects of withdrawal to prevent serious complications.[87] The revised Clinical Institute Withdrawal Assessment Scale (CIWAS-Ar) should be used to monitor these patients. Orders for oral chlordiazepoxide or lorazepam should be scheduled for the high-risk patient (Box 10-2) or as needed for low-risk individuals. A score of 8 or greater is used as a cutoff for administering more medication.[88] Since multiple problems may mimic withdrawal symptoms it is important to rule out other possible explanations, such as infection or delirium.

BOX 10-2

RISK FACTORS FOR MODERATE-SEVERE ALCOHOL WITHDRAWAL

- History of delirium tremens or severe alcohol withdrawal
- Age >30
- Concurrent illness
- History of heavy, sustained drinking (>60 grams, >1 pint liquor, >96 oz beer/day)
- Presentation with withdrawal symptoms >2 days since last drink
- History of seizures

SELECTIVE INTERVENTIONS TO IMPROVE OUTCOMES

Maintaining Nutrition

Nutritional status affects healing time, immune system function, energy levels, and strength, all of which are vital to recovering from hospitalization. Baseline malnutrition leads to higher complication rates, increased mortality, longer hospital stays, and a greater than 300% increase in hospital costs.[89] It is important to identify poor nutritional status and actively manage nutrition in the hospitalized elderly patient (see Chapter 4).

Risk factors for malnutrition prior to becoming hospitalized include age older than 60, poor access (if living alone and inadequate social or financial support), lower education level, fatigue, depression, pain, dysgeusia, dysphagia, lack of teeth or ill-fitting dentures, malignancy, polypharmacy, and medication side effects.[90-94]

Assessment of nutritional status involves a detailed physical examination and, in some situations, laboratory investigation. Multiple screening tools exist with variable utility.[95] Sarcopenia is defined as having a muscle mass greater than two standard deviations below the mean for a healthy young adult as assessed by imaging (dual-energy x-ray absorptiometry or bioelectrical impedence), but is often estimated by physical exam when data are not available.[96] Laboratory evaluation is not necessary in most settings because a thorough history and physical examination identifies most malnourished patients. If indicated, laboratory evaluation can include serum albumin (half-life 20 days), prealbumin (half-life 2 days), transferrin (half-life 10 days), cholesterol panel, and electrolytes.[97,98] In certain settings, such as preoperative monitoring, the albumin level or prealbumin (also known as transthyretin) may be measured serially to aid in identifying improved nutrition prior to scheduling surgery.[98,99]

All hospitalized patients benefit from maximizing nutrition, but this is particularly important for the malnourished elderly patient, and interventions to boost nutrition should be tailored to the needs of the patient. These include assistance with meals, getting up to a chair for meals, avoiding diet restrictions unless imperative to the patient's treatment, and offering nutritional supplements.[100-103] If the patient has any swallowing difficulties, a diet with the appropriate consistency of solids and liquids should be provided. If the patient has new oropharyngeal dysfunction, a speech therapy consultation may be beneficial. Offering supplements between meals is superior to merely adding cans to meal trays. Nutrition consultation may be of benefit in malnourished patients requiring restricted diets or requiring other routes of feeding (nasogastric tube, J-tube, TPN, etc.). Eliminating restrictive diets (low salt, low fat, etc.) except for when use is clearly clinically necessary is also important. For example, despite a past history of coronary artery disease, a 90-year-old woman hospitalized for pneumonia and eating only 50% of meals should be on a regular diet to maximize food choice and caloric density.

Pharmacologic interventions to improve nutrition status include avoiding medicines that alter taste or smell (Box 10-3).[104,105] Appetite-stimulating medicines may be tried, but strong evidence supporting their efficacy is lacking. Mirtazapine has been used for dual-indications in depression and poor appetite.[106] Megestrol acetate (Megase) shows benefit in cachectic or cancer patients, but side effects include increased edema, congestive heart failure, deep vein thrombosis, and adrenal insufficiency.[107,108] There was no demonstrated increase in muscle mass with megestrol acetate in a small study of veterans older than 65 and its use should be avoided in hospitalized elders.[109] Dronabinol and medical marijuana are used primarily in patients with AIDS or cancer to boost appetite, but the elderly patient may be more susceptible to side effects including altered mental status; thus the use of dronabinol and medical marijuana should be avoided.[110]

Mobility

Hospital-associated disability refers to multiple deficits induced or accelerated by hospitalization. This disability leads to greater institutionalization, increased mortality, and greater overall health care costs.[111,112] Greater than 30% of hospitalized elderly older than 70 years leave the hospital with the loss of at least one ADL.[113] Using aggressive preventative measures can avoid or slow decline related to hospitalization. It is important to assess and document the patient's ability to perform ADLs as well as IADLs on admission. Those with dependence in any of these are at marked increased risk for hospital-associated disability.[114-116]

Preventative measures include encouragement of early mobilization, providing ambulation-assist devices as needed, staff education, and environmental modifications. Barriers to mobility such as restricted activity orders and hospital equipment (intravenous lines, urinary catheters, etc.) should be removed if not absolutely necessary. Including family members in the care plan to help encourage ambulation and assist the patient throughout the day is a patient-centered approach and should be undertaken. Early referral to physical therapy and occupational therapy helps ensure structured daily activity. Staff in all locations should be educated on the importance of encouraging ambulation, identification of functional decline, and ways to avoid hospital-associated disability (see Chapter 13).

Glycemic Control in the Hospital

Hospitalized diabetic patients are frequently switched from oral agents to insulin therapy on admission to the hospital. Multiple hospital system policies endorse tight glycemic control using a basal-bolus insulin regimen, a recommendation that followed studies showing improved outcomes in hospitalized patients with strict glucose management.[117] A subsequent meta-analysis of these trials showed a decreased risk of infection with tight glycemic control mainly in surgical patients, but a higher risk of hypoglycemia.[117] Target glucose levels recommended by the American Diabetes Association and American Association of Clinical Endocrinologists are <140 mg/dL (7.8 mmol/L) for fasting levels in general hospitalized patients, with all random glucoses <180 mg/dL (10.0 mmol/L).[118,119]

The elderly patient is more vulnerable to complications with tight glycemic control (see Chapter 41).[120-122] Nutritionists recommend a nutrient-dense, low-glycemic-index, and high-fiber diet to optimize care in elderly diabetic patients.[123] Hypoglycemia puts the patient at risk of falls, delirium, cognitive decline, and fatigue leading to decreased mobility and should be avoided.

BOX 10-3
MEDICINES IMPAIRING TASTE AND SMELL

Allopurinol
Alcohol
Angiotensin-converting enzyme (ACE) inhibitors
β-Lactam antibiotics
β-Adrenergic blocking agents
Calcium channel blockers (except diltiazem)
Chemotherapeutic drugs
Hydrochlorothiazide
Levodopa
Losartan
Lovastatin
Metronidazole
Nicotine skin patches
Nifedipine
Nitroglycerin
Nonsteroidal antiinflammatory drugs (NSAIDs)
Opiates
Spironolactone
Terbinafine
Tetracycline

Adapted from Ackerman BH, Kasbekar N. Disturbances of taste and smell induced by drugs. Pharmacotherapy 1997;17(3):482-96; and Ciancio SG. Medications' impact on oral health. J Am Dent Assoc 2004;135(10):1440-8.

Tight glucose control in the hospital offers few, if any, benefits for older hospitalized adults, is based on extremely limited evidence, and is fraught with potential devastating side effects.

CARE TRANSITION INITIATIVES AND UNPLANNED HOSPITAL READMISSIONS

Care transitions refer to the movement of patients between health care providers or settings. Transitions including outpatient visits, office visits between medical subspecialists, and the movement into and out of the hospital during the admission and discharge processes are particularly fraught with potential errors and dangers. Confusing medication lists, discharge instructions unclearly written or written at inappropriately high health literacy levels, and a lack of connection to receiving providers in the primary care office or skilled nursing facility all have potential to adversely affect the patient's health and trigger an unplanned readmission.

Almost one in five Medicare beneficiaries is readmitted to the hospital within 30 days, and almost one third are readmitted within 90 days. These associated costs to the health care system are immense, estimated to be $17.4 billion in 2004.[124] Readmitted individuals are likely to have multiple medical comorbidities and a longer initial length of stay. Among older adults readmitted within 30 days, age greater than 80 years, depression, and poor patient education on discharge are all linked to higher rates of unplanned readmission.[125] Community-dwelling elderly Medicare beneficiaries readmitted within 30 days also had significantly increased 1-year mortality rates (39% vs. 12%).[125] Decreasing unplanned readmissions is crucial for both improving patient care and reducing unnecessary cost expenditures, and several care transition initiatives are currently active and building evidence of effectiveness.

Project BOOST

The Society of Hospital Medicine (SHM) created Project BOOST (Better Outcomes by Optimizing Safe Transitions) as a year-long mentorship program that aims to improve hospital discharges and reduce unplanned readmissions. Created with input from national leaders on care transitions, hospitalist leaders, payers, and regulatory agencies, Project BOOST also targets improved patient satisfaction and improved information flow between outpatient and hospitalist providers to identify particularly high risk patients and to improve the preparation of patients and families for discharge.[126] Initial pilot data from the mentoring program with expert coaching to implement the program yielded a 21% reduction in unplanned readmissions. Currently in place in over 100 sites across 31 states, Project BOOST has five main elements:

1. Comprehensive evidence-based intervention.
2. Implementation guide to help interdisciplinary teams redesign workflow.
3. Longitudinal technical assistance for 1 year, including train-the-trainer materials for nurses, case managers, physicians, and social workers.
4. BOOST collaboration of site webinars and teleconferences.
5. An online resource center with benchmark data.

The Naylor Transitional Care Model

Whereas SHM's Project BOOST aims to alter the health care system at large and primarily targets physicians and providers, the Naylor Transitional Care Model and the Coleman Care Transitions Intervention (see following section) both focus more on the patient's role in enhanced self-management. The Naylor Transitional Care Model involves interdisciplinary care coordination of master's degree–equipped advanced practice nurses (APNs) working with discharging physicians to provide up to 8 weeks of discharge support to medically complex and high-cost patients.[127] Following in-hospital visits by the APN, the program includes comprehensive discharge planning as well as weekly home-visit follow-up and frequent phone support. The Naylor model has been shown to significantly improve physical function, enhance patient quality of life, and reduce rehospitalizations.[127]

The Coleman Care Transitions Intervention

Similar to the Naylor Model, the Coleman Care Transitions Intervention seeks to empower patients through one hospital visit and one home visit by a "transition coach." An empowered patient is encouraged to have increased knowledge of medication management, follow-up plans, knowledge of disease-specific "red flags" that suggest worsening conditions, and enhanced personal record keeping. The designated Coleman transition coach, who is usually a nurse, social worker, or community health worker with added training, works with patients to prevent unplanned readmissions of medically complex older adults and improve care transitions.[128] The following components make up the Coleman Care Transitions Intervention:

1. A patient-centered personal health record that facilitates interdisciplinary communication during care transitions.
2. A discharge preparation checklist of activities designed to empower patients and caregivers prior to hospital discharge.
3. In-hospital transition coach meeting to assist patients and caregivers in asserting their role in managing care transitions.
4. Transition coach follow-up at skilled nursing facility or home and phone calls to enhance continuity.

A study of 158 community-dwelling older adults found that the Coleman model of a transitions coach to empower patients and caregivers to make their preferences known significantly reduced readmission at 30, 60, and 90 days, and also increased patient understanding of health condition and medication regimen.[128]

> Optimal care transitions and safe discharges to prevent unplanned readmission and adverse patient outcomes are critical for good geriatric hospital care.

THE IDEAL DISCHARGE FOR THE ELDERLY PATIENT

One critical element of a successful hospitalization for an older adult is a safe care transition and an accurate discharge summary. SHM has identified several key elements of an ideal discharge that must be included (Table 10-3). The ideal hospital discharge for the elderly patient focuses on patient education about follow-up, medication changes, patient instructions on activity, code status, and an accurate discharge summary for providers.[129]

CASE 1

Discussion

Mr. Johnson's postoperative delirium and nosocomial complications are unfortunately a common occurrence during hospitalization of older adults. At the time of admission there were a multitude of risk factors for a prolonged and complicated hospitalization, including potential cognitive impairment, vision and hearing impairment, medical comorbidities, and social isolation. Limited primary care supervision with multiple subspecialist physicians raises

TABLE 10-3	Ideal Discharge for the Elderly Patient		
Element	**Particulars**	**Required**	**Optional**
Patient-centered Medication Education	• Written schedule (new, modified, unchanged, and discontinued medications)	X	
	• Purpose and cautions for all medications	X	
	• Clinical pharmacist consultation (if cognitive impairment or >3 medication changes)		X
	• Close follow-up plan for hazardous medications (warfarin, diuretics, corticosteroids, hypoglycemic medications, narcotics, cardiovascular medications)	X	
Cognition	• Description of mentation (lucid, forgetful, significant dementia)	X	
Patient Instructions	• Written at 6th-grade level	X	
	• 24/7 call-back number	X	
	• Teach-back to confirm patient understanding	X	
Provider Identification	• Identify referring and receiving provider	X	
	• Communicate immediate follow-up issues	X	
Follow-up Plan	• 2 weeks or sooner for hazardous medications or fragile clinical condition	X	
	• Testing or provider appointments	X	
Code Status	• Code status and other pertinent end-of-life issue stipulations		X
Discharge Summary	• Presenting problem	X	
	• Primary/secondary diagnosis	X	
	• Key findings/test results	X	
	• Brief hospital course	X	
	• Discharge medicine reconciliation	X	
	• Condition at discharge, including functional and cognitive status	X	
	• Discharge destination and rationale	X	
	• Anticipated problems and suggested interventions	X	
	• Follow-up appointments		X
	• Pending lab testing	X	
	• Recommendations of any subspecialty consultants	X	
	• Documentation of patient education and confirmation of patient/caregiver understanding	X	

Developed by the Society of Hospital Medicine HQPS Committee, 2005. Available at www.hospitalmedicine.org/AM/Template.cfm?Section=QI_Clinical_Tools&Template=/CM/ContentDisplay.cfm&ContentID=10303.

the likelihood of polypharmacy. Certainly operative intervention was warranted on Mr. Johnson's fracture, but his prolonged time not eating before surgery certainly could have increased his already frail health status. These limitations in physiologic reserves, combined with delirium, restraints, decreased mobility from a stroke, and poor nutritional intake all set the stage for nosocomial infections and a prolonged hospital stay. Mr. Johnson would benefit from a seamless transition to his next location of care, likely a skilled nursing facility, through the assistance of an evidence-based care transition program that can ensure a smooth handoff between providers and an accurate and timely discharge summary. ■

SUMMARY

Hospitalization of older adults should be appropriately thought of as a challenging proposition. The need for disease-specific interventions targeting the incident illness must be balanced with the potential hazards lurking in hospitals. Potentially preventable unplanned readmissions are related to increased mortality and loss of functional independence. An interdisciplinary approach to geriatric hospital care that involves social workers, nurses, case managers, collaborating physicians, patients, and families/caregivers is essential. Safer care transitions through evidence-based interventions and accurate medical records should be the goal of all involved in the care of elderly patients in the hospital.

Web Resources

www.hospitalmedicine.org/BOOST. Society of Hospital Medicine Project BOOST (Better Outcomes by Optimizing Safe Transitions).

http://nicheprogram.org/program_overview. Nurses Improving Care for Healthsystem Elders.

www.jhartfound.org. The John A. Hartford Foundation—"dedicated to improving health care for older Americans."

KEY REFERENCES

7. Landefeld CS, Palmer RM, Kresevic DM, et al. A randomized trial of care in a hospital medical unit especially designed to improve the functional outcomes of acutely ill older patients. N Engl J Med 1995;332:1338-44.

25. Fleisher LA, Beckman JA, Brown KA, et al. 2009 ACCF/AHA focused update on perioperative beta blockade incorporated into the ACC/AHA 2007 guidelines on perioperative cardiovascular evaluation and care for noncardiac surgery: A report of the American College of Cardiology Foundation/American Heart Association Task Force on Practice Guidelines. Circulation 2009;120(21):e169-e276.

31. Qaseem A, Snow V, Fitterman N, et al. for the Clinical Efficacy Assessment Subcommittee of the American College of Physicians. Risk assessment for and strategies to reduce perioperative pulmonary complications for patients undergoing noncardiothoracic surgery: A guideline from the American College of Physicians. Ann Intern Med 2006;144:575-80.

39. Guyatt GH, Akl EA, Crowther M, et al. Executive Summary: Antithrombotic Therapy and Prevention of Thrombosis, 9th ed: American College of Chest Physicians Evidence-Based Clinical Practice Guidelines. Chest 2012;141;7S-47S.

48. Inouye SK. Delirium in older persons. N Engl J Med 2006;354:1157-65.

66. The American Geriatrics Society Clinical Practice Guideline. Prevention of falls in older persons. http://www.americangeriatrics.org/health_care_professionals/clinical_practice/clinical_guidelines_recommendations/2010/. Accessed August 30, 2012.

113. Covinsky KE, Pierluissi E, Johnston CB. Hospitalization associated disability: "She was probably able to ambulate, but I'm not sure." JAMA 2011;306(16):1782-93.

124. Jencks SF, Williams MV, Coleman EA. Rehospitalizations among patients in the Medicare fee-for-service program. N Engl J Med 2009;360:1418-28.

References available online at **expertconsult.com.**

11

Long-Term Care

Gwendolen T. Buhr and Heidi K. White

OBJECTIVES

Upon completion of this chapter, the reader will be able to:

- Identify the most common post-acute care and long-term care (LTC) options and list the services provided by each.
- Accurately assess and recommend level of care needs, incorporating information from family, caregivers, therapists, and other members of the interprofessional team.
- Describe the various LTC medical practice models and the role of physicians, nurse practitioners, and physician assistants in each.
- Summarize the role of the medical director in the nursing home.
- Identify and explain five common clinical challenges in LTC medicine.
- Describe the process of evaluating decision-making capacity in older adults and apply shared decision making to clinical situations in LTC.
- Describe how principles of quality improvement and individualized care can be applied in LTC.

CASE 1

Mary Lewis (Part 1)

Mary Lewis is a 91-year-old female with hypertension, osteoarthritis manifested as low back pain, depression, and anxiety who has been your patient for more than 5 years. She has never allowed you to treat her with medications, but her daughter brings her faithfully for appointments. Recently her son died, which has worsened her depression. She lives in her own home but her back pain no longer allows her to tend her garden, which she previously enjoyed. Recently she gave up driving because her depression and anxiety made this more difficult. Her daughter thinks it may be time for her mother to move out of the house but is not sure what alternative setting would be best.

1. **What suggestions do you have for the daughter?**

2. **What questions should you ask to assess Mrs. Lewis's needs?**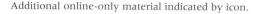

Additional online-only material indicated by icon.

THE GROWING NEED FOR LONG-TERM CARE

The United States is an aging society. The population older than age 65 is expected to grow at a rate of 107% from 2012 to 2050, much faster than the population as a whole.[1] The population older than age 85, which is the group that most frequently uses long-term care (LTC), is projected to grow by 224% during the same time period.[1]

Older persons face a number of challenges that place them at risk for needing LTC:

- Functional disability increases exponentially as people age. Thirty-seven percent of persons older than age 65, and up to 53% of those older than 85 years, have a functional limitation,[1,2] and the presence of functional limitations is a major reason for needing LTC services.
- The prevalence of dementia rises steeply with age, and having dementia is another major risk factor for needing LTC. The prevalence of Alzheimer's disease (AD) and other dementias is 13% among all persons aged 65 and older and 45% among those aged 85 and older.[3] In fact 75% of people with AD will be living in a nursing home by age 80 compared to only 4% for the general population.[3] Furthermore, two thirds of older adults dying of dementia do so in a nursing home, a much higher figure than for other chronic diseases.[3] Behavioral symptoms are a major reason that caregivers of older adults with dementia choose to place them in a nursing home.[4]
- Older persons are more likely to live alone than younger persons and, therefore, lack a potential live-in caregiver. Currently, one third of people older than age 75 live alone[1] and 60% of women older than age 85 live alone.[5]
- Adult children often do not live near enough to their parents to enable them to provide the daily or weekly hands-on care needed. A recent study found that among current older adults with children, only one half had a child within 10 miles.[5] Future older generations will have even fewer children who might care for them, as a consequence of lower fertility rates.
- Poor caregiver health is another reason for entry into LTC.[4] Sixty-one percent of family caregivers of people with AD report high or very high levels of emotional stress; 33% report symptoms of depression; and 43% report high to very high physical stress.[3]

TYPES OF LONG-TERM CARE

LTC has become a critically important area of patient care for the nation because many of the frailest and most vulnerable elders use LTC options to help meet health or personal needs. LTC can be defined broadly as medical or nonmedical care that is provided in the community, congregate housing, residential care facilities (e.g., assisted living), and nursing homes.

> Long-term care can be defined broadly to include medical or nonmedical care that is provided in the community, congregate housing, residential care facilities (e.g., assisted living), and nursing homes.

Table 11-1 summarizes the most common types of LTC. As is evident from Table 11-1, LTC serves many older adults in a variety of settings. Indicators of the breadth of LTC services are these statistics from 2010:

- There were 1.4 million occupied beds in 16,071 nursing homes across the United States.[1] All told, 3.8 million persons were served by nursing homes, because many had short facility stays for post-acute care.[6]
- An additional 1.23 million older adults were living in residential care or assisted living facilities.[1]
- An estimated 42 million family caregivers were providing unpaid care.[1]
- A total of 3.4 million Medicare beneficiaries received home health care,[7] and 2.5 million Medicaid participants received home- and community-based services or home health services.[1]

Nursing Homes

Nursing homes house two types of residents: (1) short-stay, post–acute care residents, who were admitted for rehabilitation, usually after a hospitalization, and (2) long-stay residents who are receiving chronic disease care or palliative care. About 4% of Medicare enrollees older than age 65 had a nursing home stay in 2009, with the rate highest among persons aged 85 and older (14%).[2] Nursing home residents are mostly white (88%), female (66%), and elderly (median age 82.6).[8] The racial make-up of the nursing home population should become more diverse in the future as the population of older adults changes in the United States.[2] Nursing home residents commonly have multiple chronic illnesses; dementia is one of the most prevalent at 46%.[1] Depressive symptoms, sensory impairment, pain, and functional impairment are also common. In addition, most LTC residents have functional limitations. For example, in 2009, 68% of all nursing home residents had three or more activity of daily living (ADL) limitations (bathing, dressing, eating, getting in/out of chairs, toileting) and 95% had at least one instrumental activities of daily living (IADL) limitation (using the telephone, housework, meal preparation, shopping, managing money).[2]

		Approximate Number of Providers and Patients Served	Average Cost / Predominant Source of Payment
Type	Definition and Description		
Short-Term (Post-Acute) Settings			
Inpatient rehabilitation facilities	• Provide intensive rehabilitation using an interdisciplinary team approach in an inpatient hospital environment. • Patients must receive multiple therapy disciplines (PT, OT, SLP, or prosthetics/orthotics), one of which must be PT or OT for at least 15 hours per week and make measurable improvement. • Physician involvement: high (≥3 visits per week).	359,000 cases/year; 1,165 facilities	Inpatient Rehabilitation Facility Prospective Payment System Case-Mix Group $17,085 per case/Medicare
Skilled nursing facilities	• Medicare certified to provide RN, LPN, PT or OT, and /or SLP services essential to the maintenance or restoration of health. • Admission requires a 3-night hospital stay within the last 30 days. • Physician involvement: moderate (required visit every 30 days, but often more frequent as medically necessary).	2,418,442 Medicare covered stays/year; 15,161 SNFs	$398 per day[1]/ Medicare
Chronic care hospitals	• Medicare-certified care for patients with complex care needs (ventilator and weaning) discharged from hospitals. • Physician involvement: high (on-site availability on a daily basis).	134,683 cases/year; 436 long-term care hospitals	Long-term care hospital Prospective Payment System $38,582 per case/Medicare
Home health care	• Medicare-certified care for patients who are confined to home and require intermittent skilled nursing care, PT, SLP, or OT. • Physician involvement: low (as medically necessary when identified by the home health care team).	3.4 million Medicare beneficiaries per year; 12,026 home health agencies	$154 per visit[1]; $2,839 average payment per episode/Medicare
Outpatient rehabilitation programs	• Medicare-certified care for patients who can travel to a rehabilitation location. • Physician involvement: minimal (as problems are identified by the rehabilitation specialist).	4.9 million users/year	$1,173 mean/user; yearly cap of $1,880 for PT and SLP combined and $1,880 for OT/Medicare
Longer-Term Settings			
Nursing homes	• Federally regulated. • Provide room, meals, personal care, 24-hour nursing care, medication management, social and recreational activities, and medical care to residents with chronic conditions. • Physician involvement: moderate (required visit every 60 days and as medically necessary).	1,408,886 residents; 1,696,721 beds	$222 per day (semi-private) $248 per day (private)/ Medicaid (52%), private pay (41%), LTC insurance or other (7%)
Residential care/ assisted living communities	• Regulated by the states under a variety of names (including personal care homes, group homes, board and care homes, and others). • Provide room, meals, supervision, assistance with medications, some personal care, and may include some nursing oversight. • Many charge a base rate with added fees for additional services. • Physician involvement: low (required yearly and as medically necessary).	1,233,690 units; 58,938 facilities	$3,550 per month/ private pay

TABLE 11-1   Types of Long-Term Care[1,7,8,37-40]

Continued on following page

TABLE 11-1	Types of Long-Term Care (Continued)		
Type	Definition and Description	Approximate Number of Providers and Patients Served	Average Cost / Predominant Source of Payment
Adult day care or adult day health centers	• Provide meals, recreation, health-related services (e.g., medication management; weight, blood pressure, and diabetes monitoring), transportation, assistance with ADLs, and exercise in a group environment for individuals with cognitive and/or functional impairments. • Physician involvement: minimal (often initial medical summary required).	Generally licensed or certified by states; 150,000 recipients; 5,000 centers	$70 per day/private pay
Program of All-Inclusive Care for the Elderly (PACE)	• Provides comprehensive long-term services and supports to individuals age 55 or older who live in a PACE service area, are eligible for nursing home care, and are able to live safely in the community. • Care coordinated by an interdisciplinary team composed of a primary care physician, RN, MSW, PT, OT, RT, dietician, PACE center supervisor, home care liaison, personal care attendants, and a driver at a day health center. • Physician involvement: variable according to the needs of the participant but a physician is often on site and may visit people in their homes.	25,653 participants in 86 programs in 29 states	Average monthly payment between $1,700 and $2,600; Medicare and Medicaid risk adjusted capitation payments
Specialized dementia units	• Either RC/AL or NH that provides specialized care for people with dementia—often a separate secured unit, trained staffing, special programming, a modified physical environment, and family involvement. • Physician involvement: variable depending on whether it is RC/AL or nursing home.	38% of RC/AL communities and 31% of NHs have specialized dementia units. No good data on the number of individuals served.	$4,807 per month (RC/AL) $261 per day (private room) (NH)/ Medicaid and private pay
Home care/ personal care	• Home health aide or homemaker/companion that provides nonmedical care (help with ADLs, cooking, shopping, laundry) to enable older adults with chronic illnesses to remain at home. • Physician involvement: minimal.	686,030 personal and home care aides in the US. No data available on the number of individuals served	$10-$21 per hour/ private pay
Hospice	• Benefit under Medicare part A; for individuals certified as having a life expectancy of 6 months or less. Focus on comfort and quality of life rather than curative treatments. • Physician involvement: variable depending on the acuity and setting (hospice medical director and primary care physician often share some responsibility).	3,555 hospice agencies served 1,159,000 patients	$151 per day (routine home care)/Medicare

ADLs, Activities of daily living; LPN, licensed practical nurse; MSW, master's level social worker; NH, nursing home; OT, occupational therapy; PT, physical therapy; RN, registered nurse; RT, recreational therapist; SLP, speech-language pathology; SNFs, skilled nursing facilities; RC/AL, residential care/assisted living communities.

Residential Care / Assisted Living (RC/AL) Communities

Residential care and assisted living communities have a variety of names, depending on state regulations, including assisted living residences, board and care homes, congregate care, enriched housing, homes for the aged, personal care homes, and shared housing. In 2010 there were 1,233,690 units in 58,938 RC/AL residences, most of which were private, for-profit settings.[1,9] Half were small (4-10 beds), but these facilities served only 10% of the overall RC/AL population. The majority of residents (52%) lived in large (26-100 bed) or (29%) in extra-large (>100 beds) facilities.[9] Nearly all RC/AL communities provide basic health monitoring, incontinence care, social and recreational activities, special diets, and personal laundry services.[9] Most also offer transportation to medical appointments and case management, whereas social services, counseling, and physical and occupational therapy tend to be offered only by large RC/AL communities or indirectly through home care agencies.[9]

Residents are typically white (91%), female (70%), age 75 and older (81%), and have a median length of stay of 22 months.[10] Over a third (38%) of residents receive assistance with three or more activities of daily living, of which bathing and dressing were the most common; and another 36% receive assistance with one to two ADLs.[10] These demographic descriptors indicate that considerable overlap exists between the population of RC/AL communities and nursing homes.

Albert Thompson (Part 1)

Albert Thompson is an 89-year-old nursing home resident with advanced Parkinson's disease and mild dementia. A nurse calls you because she noticed that he hardly ate or drank anything for dinner. She reports that a certified nursing assistant (CNA) obtained Mr. Thompson's vital signs, and that his temperature was 100.4, blood pressure 110/60, pulse 80, and respirations 18. When you try to ask further questions, the nurse is unprepared. She has not assessed the patient herself. She does not have his current medication or problem list. She seems to be frazzled and mentions she has only been working in the building for 3 weeks. She suggests strongly that you send the patient to the emergency department (ED).

1. **What additional information would you most like to have? What steps can be taken short of sending this patient to the ED for evaluation?**

2. **Because you are also the medical director of this facility, what steps can you suggest to better prepare nurses to assess and manage patients with physicians over the telephone?** ◾

MEDICAL CARE PROVIDER PRACTICE PATTERNS LONG-TERM CARE

Because exposure to LTC remains limited in medical school and residency programs, expertise in LTC medical practice is typically obtained through experience, a geriatric fellowship program, or through courses offered by the American Medical Directors Association (AMDA). AMDA has a certification program that uses an experiential model in which practicing physicians who are providing LTC and medical director duties can be certified by completing educational requirements through participation in a geriatric fellowship program, continuing medical education, AMDA-sponsored courses in medical direction, and/or other continuing education programs.

Nursing homes are required by law to have a medical director; RC/AL communities are not, but a few do have them. The medical director is a physician who oversees and guides care in a LTC facility.[11] The primary functions are summarized in Table 11-2.

TABLE 11-2	Functions and Duties of a Nursing Home Medical Director
Function	**Duties**
Administrative	• Communicate regularly with the administrator and DON. • Participate in administrative decision making. • Recommend, approve, and inform medical staff about relevant policies and procedures. • Participate in licensure and compliance surveys.
Professional Service	• Organize and coordinate physician services and the services provided by other professionals as they relate to patient care to ensure the quality and appropriateness of services.
Quality Assurance and Performance Improvement	• Participate in monitoring and improving the quality of medical care in the facility, so as to ensure that it is effective, efficient, safe, timely, patient-centered, and equitable. • Participate in the QAPI program, assuring that it encourages self-evaluation, anticipates and plans for change, and meets regulatory requirements. • Help the facility use QAPI results, as appropriate, to update and improve policies, procedures, and practices.
Staff and Personal Education	• Participate in education of facility staff. • Sustain his/her own professional development through continuing education.
Employee Health	• Participate in the surveillance and promotion of employee health, safety, and welfare, specifically regarding infectious disease issues.
Community Relations	• Help articulate the facility's mission to the community.
Resident Rights	• Participate in establishing policies and procedures to assure that resident rights are respected. This includes their right to request practitioners to limit, withhold, or withdraw treatment(s).
Contextual Factors	• Acquire and apply knowledge of social, regulatory, political, and economic factors that relate to patient care and related services.
Person-Directed Care	• Support and promote person-directed care.

Adapted from AMDA. The nursing home medical director: Leader and manager (White Paper A11). Columbia, MD: AMDA; 2011. Available at http://www.amda.com/governance/whitepapers/A11.cfm.
DON, Director of nursing; *QAPI*, quality assessment and performance improvement.

> The American Medical Directors Association has a certification program that uses an experiential model in which practicing physicians who are providing LTC and medical director duties can be certified.

Physicians who practice in nursing homes do so within a variety of practice models. The traditional model has been as an adjunct to an office-based practice. In the last decade new practice models have arisen: the LTC-only practice and the house-call practice. With these, there has been a call to recognize that nursing home medicine is emerging as a specialty in its own right, similar to the hospitalist.[12] Physicians working in this specialty have been referred to as SNFists, nursing home physician specialists, or LTC specialists. The nursing home physician specialist spends a substantial portion of time in the delivery of nursing home care and is proficient in nursing home regulations and the medical management of common syndromes faced by nursing home residents.

> The nursing home physician specialist spends a substantial portion of time in the delivery of nursing home care and is proficient in nursing home regulations and the medical management of common syndromes faced by nursing home residents.

Nurse practitioners (NPs) provide primary care to nursing home residents as nursing home employees, as members of primary care practices, or as employees of health maintenance organizations. NPs are registered nurses who have a master's degree and obtain certification through a national certifying examination or through state certification mechanisms. The NP scope of practice varies by state. In 10 states no physician involvement is required; however, 40 states give NPs the authority to prescribe only with physician oversight.[13] Federal nursing home regulations require collaboration with a physician in all states.

Physician assistants (PAs) function in much the same way as NPs in nursing homes. They are non-nurse providers whose training typically consists of 1 year of basic science classes and 1 year of clinical rotations. PAs must practice under the supervision of a physician, but they have the authority to prescribe in all 50 states and the District of Columbia.[14] The PA scope of practice varies by state and is largely determined by the physician; most commonly, a physician can delegate to PAs anything that is within the physician's scope of practice and the PA's training and experience.[14]

Evercare is a Medicare Advantage program specifically for long-stay nursing home residents that extensively uses NPs or PAs. The NPs or PAs work as employees of the managed care company and provide more intensive primary care than is typical. They are assigned to work in specific nursing homes, usually one or two, carrying a caseload of approximately 100 residents.[15] The nursing home residents continue to have their primary care physician, which Evercare pays on a fee-for-service basis, including payment for time spent in family or care-planning conferences (which is not ordinarily reimbursed under Medicare). The NP also educates the nursing home staff through formal and informal in-service training. Because the NP or PA is present in the nursing home frequently under the Evercare model, they monitor residents closely and develop relationships with the staff, which facilitates early identification of acute illnesses. Because they are salaried employees of the managed care company, Evercare NPs and PAs can spend more time in preventive and early intervention direct care that might not otherwise be reimbursed by Medicare. In addition, Evercare can pay the nursing home for "intensive service days," when an ill resident might otherwise need to be hospitalized. As a result, Evercare sites have fewer hospitalizations and emergency department visits than traditional care models, and Evercare enrollees have higher patient and family satisfaction with the care.[15]

Federal regulations require that nursing home residents be seen by the physician for the initial comprehensive visit and then every 30 days for the first 90 days. Thereafter patients must be seen every 60 days and when medically necessary. Other than the initial comprehensive visit, the routine (regulatory) visits can usually be alternated between the MD and NP or PA. Patients in the nursing home are generally seen by their primary care providers in their residence. This is in contrast to the RC/AL communities, in which the practice norm is for the resident to be transported to his or her provider's office (though models of care where providers come to the RC/AL are growing). Because RC/AL communities are regulated by the states, regulations differ depending on the state of residence, but most commonly only a yearly physician visit is required.

Much of the care delivery in LTC occurs via telephone—more so than in other clinical settings. Many of the telephone calls occur after hours and on weekends to on-call providers who may not be familiar with the patient or the facility. Most telephone calls report a clinical problem. For example, in one study of a typical nursing home, the problems that were most frequently reported by phone were falls, pain, agitation, abnormal blood glucose, and fever, with the calls typically prompting a clinical action, such as ordering a medication or treatment, clinical observation by the nursing staff, or diagnostic studies.[16]

Nursing Homes

Nurses are the foundation of care in the nursing home. Most nurses employed in nursing homes are licensed practical or licensed vocational nurses (LPNs or LVNs). Their work largely consists of administering medications, collecting data on patients, determining the need for interventions, implementing care plans, supervising nursing assistants, and communicating with medical care providers. The LPNs/LVNs work under the direction and supervision of registered nurses (RNs) and physicians in a limited and focused scope of practice. RNs commonly fill administrative or supervisory roles in the nursing home such as charge nurse or director of nursing.

Interdisciplinary team care is a key component of nursing home practice. The interdisciplinary team is made up of nurses, medical providers (physicians, NPs, and PAs), social workers, the nursing home administrator, dietician, activities coordinator, consultant pharmacist, certified nursing assistants (CNAs), environmental service workers, and therapists (occupational, speech, and physical). These individuals pool their expertise and collaborate so that patients receive better care. Every nursing home resident is required to have an assessment that identifies his or her abilities and needs and a comprehensive, individualized care plan developed by the interdisciplinary team that maximizes the patient's abilities and meets his or her needs. Care planning conferences are held with the patient and/or family and the interdisciplinary team soon after admission and at least every 90 days to design and update the care plan.

> The interdisciplinary team is the cornerstone of care in the nursing home.

CNAs fill a critical role in the nursing home, providing most of the basic patient care. They assist residents with ADLs, provide skin care, take vital signs, answer calls for help, and are expected to monitor residents' well-being and report significant changes to nurses. The 2004 National Nursing Assistant Survey (NNAS) found that the majority (92%) of CNAs were female with a high school or less education (74.4%) and a family income of less than $30,000.[17] There was also considerable racial diversity, with 53% of CNAs being white, 38.7% African American, and 9.3% Hispanic or Latino in origin. Average age was 39 years, and 34% were 45 years or older. The average hourly pay rate was $10.36; 75% who were not covered by another source were enrolled in their employer health insurance plan. Most became CNAs because they like helping people, and only 10% said they would not become a CNA again; but 45% revealed that they might leave the facility in the next year because of poor pay or because they found a better job. Being a CNA is hard work; 56% had been injured at work in the previous year.

Staff turnover is a major challenge facing nursing homes in the United States and is costly and a major factor contributing to quality problems. The average U.S. nursing facility staffing turnover rate was 40% in 2010, although in some states it was as high as 70%.[1] Recommendations for increasing staff recruitment and retention include increased training, increased pay, the provision of health insurance benefits, and improving the work environment by nurturing positive relationships between CNAs and their supervisors, fostering respect among the workforce, and providing opportunities for advancement.[18]

Residential Care Communities

The large RC/AL care model grew out of the hospitality industry rather than the health industry. Consequently, the goals of RC/AL communities are to provide a home-like environment emphasizing privacy and freedom and to foster independence and autonomy. RC/AL requirements differ depending on the state, but in general they are considered nonmedical facilities and are not required to have nurses, CNAs, or medical directors.

A key feature of RC/AL practice is that wider variation exists in services offered, amount of staffing available, range of patients served, and cost of care than in nursing homes, which tend to be more tightly regulated. Small RC/ALs (≤10 beds) tend to have a licensed nurse who does assessments and provides care oversight but may be on site as little as 8 hours a week; larger RC/ALs often have at least one full-time nurse. In most states, certified medication aides rather than nurses pass medications, with regulations varying as to whether they "administer" the medications or "assist residents with self-administration"—a process that often bears a strong similarity to administration. When RC/AL residents need skilled nursing or rehabilitative services, these typically are provided either by home health agencies or by temporary transfer to a skilled nursing facility, though some larger facilities have begun offering some rehabilitative services in-house.

CASE 2

Albert Thompson (Part 2)

Later that week you are again called about Mr. Thompson by a different nurse. This nurse indicates that Mr. Thompson rolled out of bed and hit his head on a side table. He has a bruise on his forehead. An ice pack has been applied. His vital signs are normal. They heard the fall and went immediately to the room. There was no loss of consciousness. He is moving all extremities. With help he was able to get up, walk to the bathroom with his walker, and then return to bed. He is complaining of a mild headache. Because he is on warfarin you suggest that he be sent to the ED for evaluation and a computed tomography (CT) scan of his head. However, the nurse says that the patient has discussed with his doctor his desire not to return to the hospital and this is documented.

1. **Describe an appropriate course of management.**

2. **What should be done to assess and manage this patient's future risk for falling?** ◙

COMMON CLINICAL CHALLENGES

The main focus in LTC settings is on maintaining function and quality of life rather than on the diagnosis and treatment of individual medical conditions. The variable capacities of the patients to make decisions, as well as the congregate living situation, create distinctive considerations. What follows are a few medical conditions unique to the LTC environment, or especially prevalent in LTC residents.

> LTC is a unique environment and patient population where the main focus is on maintaining function and quality of life rather than on the diagnosis and treatment of individual medical conditions.

Distinguishing between Dementia, Subacute Delirium, and Depression

Residents in LTC facilities are especially at risk for delirium. The essential features of delirium are inattention, acute onset and fluctuating course, and a change in cognition with associated features of disturbances in the sleep-wake cycle, mood swings, and disturbed psychomotor behavior (e.g., hyperactive, hypoactive, mixed or unclassifiable). In contrast, dementia is a chronic slowly progressive disorder of memory impairment. Hypoactive delirium can appear very much like depression, emphasizing the importance of conducting a structured bedside evaluation. For more on delirium, see Chapter 16.

Delirium that began during a hospitalization can persist for weeks or months in LTC and predispose to geriatric syndromes such as dehydration, pressure ulcers, urinary retention, malnutrition, aspiration, and falls.[19] Often it is unrecognized—one study of long-stay LTC residents found that 21.3% developed delirium over a 6-month period, but the nurses identified only half of cases.[20]

The Minimum Data Set (MDS) version 3.0 uses the following three validated, objective instruments to assess LTC residents for delirium, dementia, and depression:

- The PHQ-9, a valid, simple tool for identifying and following patients with depression over time

- The Brief Interview for Mental Status (BIMS), a valid screen for cognitive impairment
- The Confusion Assessment Method (CAM), a widely-used screening instrument for delirium based on the *Diagnostic and Statistical Manual of Mental Disorders, Fourth Edition* (DSM-IV) criteria

Physical and Pharmacologic Restraints

Physical restraints include anything designed to restrict a resident's movements or prevent a person from getting up from a bed or chair. Pharmacologic restraints are any medication used to manage challenging behaviors. Physical restraints impair mobility and increase risk of injury and of mortality; over the past 25 years, their use has been markedly reduced such that, as of the third quarter of 2012, only 2.2% of residents were physically restrained. In contrast, pharmacologic restraints have proven much more difficult to reduce: as of 2012, 23.7% of long-stay nursing home patients received an antipsychotic medication.

Although it is true that antipsychotic drugs are an important treatment for patients with certain mental health conditions, the Food and Drug Administration has warned that antipsychotic medications are associated with an increased risk of death when used in elderly patients with dementia. Therefore, these medications must be used judiciously and only if the resident's behavioral symptoms constitute a danger to the resident or others. One appropriate use would be the short-term application to treat hyperactive delirium.

To treat challenging behaviors, interventions that do not involve medications or physical restraints should be used first, unless the resident is an immediate threat to himself/herself or others. Nonpharmacologic strategies to treat behavioral and psychological symptoms of dementia should be individualized and based on the patient's level of cognition and physical function and long-standing personality and interests. Alternative strategies that have shown benefit include the patient's preferred music or classical music if the preference is not known, aromatherapy with lavender or lemon balm, massage, pet therapy, physical exercise, light therapy, Snoezelen multisensory therapy, recordings of family members (stimulated presence therapy), and person-centered bathing solutions (www.bathingwithoutabattle.unc.edu). If physical or pharmacologic restraints are employed, they must be carefully monitored.

Infections and Infection Control

The hallmarks of infection in younger people may not be apparent in LTC residents. For example, typically defined fever is absent in more than half of LTC residents with a serious infection, prompting the Infectious Diseases Society of America to define fever in LTC as a single oral temperature >100° F (37.8° C); or repeated oral temperatures >99 F° (37.2° C) or rectal temperatures >99.5° F (>37.5° C); or an increase in temperature of >2° F (or >1.1° C) over the patient's baseline temperature.[21] Infection should be suspected in residents with a decline in functional status defined as new or increasing confusion, new incontinence, falling or deteriorating mobility, reduced food intake, or failure to cooperate with staff. However, restraint should be used with respect to antibiotic prescribing because inappropriate antibiotic use in the nursing home contributes to high rates of antibiotic-resistant pathogens such as methicillin-resistant *Staphylococcus aureus* and vancomycin-resistant *Enterococcus*, and to antibiotic-induced *Clostridium difficile* colitis. In addition, before treating a suspected infection, the resident's advance directives should be reviewed because some LTC residents elect not to treat infections near the end of their lives.

LTC facility residents with infections may become dehydrated. Hypodermoclysis ("clysis") is the infusion of 1 mL/min of intravenous (IV) fluid into the subcutaneous tissue of the leg, abdomen, or chest. It should be considered as an alternative to IV rehydration for treating mild/moderate dehydration because it causes no more complications than IV fluid administration and is cheaper, more comfortable, can be easily done in people with poor veins, and requires less nursing time.[22]

Federal regulations require all LTC facilities to have a program to investigate, control, and prevent infections within the facility. Some of the most common infections in LTC include the following:

Urinary tract infection (UTI)

This is the most common infection in LTC residents. However, UTI is often overdiagnosed because asymptomatic bacteriuria is common in LTC residents and should not be treated because treatment results in antibiotic resistance, drug side effects, increased cost, and no improvement in morbidity or mortality.[23] It is often difficult, however, to differentiate in LTC between symptomatic and asymptomatic bacteriuria because of the high prevalence of communication barriers, chronic genitourinary symptoms, and behavioral symptoms in these settings. Pyuria does not distinguish between symptomatic UTI and asymptomatic bacteriuria either, because it is present in 90% of cases of asymptomatic bacteriuria and 34% of persons without bacteriuria. Thus the absence of pyuria can rule out a UTI but the presence of pyuria lacks specificity.

Norovirus

Responsible for more than half of all reported outbreaks of acute gastroenteritis (AGE) in LTC settings, norovirus infection typically presents with watery diarrhea and vomiting. Norovirus occurs year-round, but most outbreaks occur between the months of November and April. Noroviruses are highly contagious and transmission occurs with person-to-person contact, contact with contaminated food or water, or contact with contaminated objects. During a norovirus outbreak, on average 45% of residents and 42% of staff develop vomiting and/or diarrhea,[24] often leading to dehydration.

C. difficile colitis

Another less common but more serious cause of AGE in LTC settings, and the leading cause of AGE-associated death, is *C. difficile* colitis. Risk for *C. difficile* colitis increases with antibiotic exposure, proton pump inhibitors, staying in health care settings, and advanced age. To prevent and control *C. difficile*, the Centers for Disease Control and Prevention (CDC) recommends that clinicians prescribe antibiotics judiciously, test for *C. difficile* when patients have diarrhea while on antibiotics or within several months of taking them, isolate patients with *C. difficile* immediately, wear gloves and gowns when caring for patients with *C. difficile*, and clean room surfaces with bleach or another Environmental Protection Agency–approved, spore-killing disinfectant after a patient with *C. difficile* has been treated.

Influenza

Outbreaks of influenza in LTC occur sporadically, even when high levels of resident immunization have been achieved. During an outbreak on average 33% of residents and 23% of staff develop influenza-like illnesses. Among infected residents 14% are hospitalized and 6% die.[24] Therefore, influenza vaccination is recommended annually for all residents and staff. Staff vaccination is the most effective way to reduce the risk of influenza outbreaks and mortality of LTC residents; however, only 52% of health care personnel in LTC received an influenza vaccine for the 2011-2012 season,[25] well below the CDC goal of 90% by 2020. A nasopharyngeal swab should be obtained at the onset of a suspected respiratory viral infection outbreak, from which identification of influenza A virus or other common viruses will confirm an outbreak.

Pneumonia

This is the most common infection leading to hospitalization and mortality among LTC residents. Poor mouth care causes up to half of the cases of pneumonia in LTC, and control of gingivitis and dental plaques will reduce incidence rates.

Pressure Ulcers

Pressure ulcers are caused by unrelieved pressure on the skin, usually over bony prominences such as the ischium, sacrum, trochanter, and heel. In 2012 the prevalence of pressure ulcers was 6.8% in U.S. nursing home patients at high risk for pressure ulcers because of malnutrition or mobility limitations prohibiting them from changing position on their own. This rate has been slowly decreasing since 1999 when 14% of these high-risk patients had pressure ulcers.[26] For additional information on pressure ulcers, see Chapter 30.

Pain Management

Pain is common in patients in LTC and is often unrecognized and untreated.[27] Dementia can be a significant barrier to recognizing and appropriately treating pain. There is no evidence that persons with dementia have less pain. They are less likely to report it, but with careful observation pain can be detected by listening to the patient's verbal expression and/or watching for evidence of inflammation or nonverbal signs such as facial grimacing. Treating pain in patients with moderate to severe dementia has been shown to reduce behavioral and psychological symptoms of dementia.[28]

Falls and Fall Risk

Falls are a common cause of loss of independence, injury (e.g., hip fracture and head injury), and death among older adults residing in LTC. Conditions contributing to increased risk include impairment of gait, balance, or vision; sedating medications such as benzodiazepines, selective serotonin reuptake inhibitors, and antipsychotics; orthostatic hypotension; arthritis; Parkinson's disease; and cognitive impairment. A history of falls is a strong predictor of future falls. The most common types of interventions include environmental adaptations and assistive technology (e.g., lighting, hand rails, raised toilet seats, assistive devices), medication review and targeted modification, increasing the number of staff, providing staff training, and exercise. A caveat to the exercise interventions is that programs may increase falls in the frailest residents but reduce falls in less frail residents.[29] For more information on falls, see Chapter 26.

After a patient has fallen, a nurse will record the vital signs and evaluate the patient for possible injury and notify the patient's physician. If a decision is made to not evaluate the patient with a provider visit or a trip to an ED, the patient should be observed for about 48 hours for delayed signs or symptoms of injury, and for complications such as a subdural hematoma. The physician should assess the patient (1) to identify and address risk factors and treat the underlying medical conditions contributing to falls, (2) to determine if the patient sustained an injury, and (3) to determine if medications that may increase fall risk can be decreased or eliminated. Although all falls and injuries resulting from falls cannot be prevented, an interdisciplinary effort and multifactorial approach toward managing falls and fall risk can reduce incidence rates.

CASE 1

Mary Lewis (Part 2)

Before Mrs. Lewis's daughter could make any alternative care arrangements, Mrs. Lewis became ill with Rocky Mountain spotted fever and required hospitalization. After her hospital stay she went to a local nursing facility for rehabilitation. During this stay the daughter was able to consult with the facility social worker and arranged transfer to a senior apartment complex that provides two meals a day in a dining room, transportation services, and housekeeping.

Mrs. Lewis has been living in this setting for 3 years; now she has developed vascular dementia and her mobility has declined. With the help of a case manager the daughter has secured care through a home care agency for 10 hours each day, but her mother is alone at night.

The daughter called you a few days ago because her mother fell and spent 6 hours on the floor because she was not wearing her alert button around her neck. Thankfully she was not injured but the daughter is concerned that it is time again for more care. Her mother keeps "firing" the home care workers and the agency is running out of people to send. The daughter is concerned that her mother will not understand or accept her need for more care and another move.

1. **Does Mrs. Lewis have the capacity to decide whether or not she should move to a higher level of care?**

2. **If she is not capable of making this decision herself, how should you talk to her and her daughter about the need for a change?** ▪

COMMON ETHICAL DILEMMAS

Providers are constantly balancing the principles of autonomy and beneficence for their LTC patients. Generally speaking, older adults want to maintain independence and personal control. Unfortunately, when assistance is needed to maintain optimal function, the limited availability of financial resources and family caregivers may mean that the best care option limits autonomy in an effort to achieve beneficence.

When patients who are unable to function safely where they live are reluctant to move, the physician may be called upon to determine their capacity to make a decision, especially when the patient's preferred decision does not appear to be in his or her best interest. *Capacity* includes the ability to express a choice, understand and make a decision, appreciate one's own situation and the consequences of the decision, and to rationally manipulate information to make comparisons and weigh options. Capacity is decision-specific and exists on a continuum such that it depends on the complexity and degree of risk involved in the particular decision at hand. Individuals may be perfectly able to make simple decisions but lack capacity to make more complicated decisions.

> *Capacity* is decision-specific and includes the ability to express a choice, understand and make a decision, appreciate one's own situation and the consequences of the decision, and to rationally manipulate information to make comparisons and weigh options.

Allowing as much decision-making capacity as possible is important in the LTC setting. In order for patients to make informed decisions, they must have capacity to make the decision in question, be provided with adequate information and alternatives, and be free from coercion. Shared decision making values mutual participation in decision making by the patient, family members, and the physician. The clinician should provide information that includes the burden of treatment, possible outcomes, and likelihood of outcomes. Additionally the clinician can facilitate the process by helping the patient to identify her or his own goals and values.

In the LTC setting, medical providers are often interacting with substitute decision makers chosen by the patient through advance directives (and referred to as a health care proxy or power of attorney) or appointed by a court (and referred to as a guardian). When a patient has not appointed a decision maker, one or more family members serve in this capacity. Each state determines the order in which decision making should proceed based on the proximity of relationships, but in practice this can become complicated. Physicians should encourage families to designate one person as the primary spokesperson and decision maker. However, it is ideal for all family members to be on board when a key decision is made; thus family meetings are often helpful when serious decisions need to be made. Physicians can also help families to understand substituted judgment, the process of making a decision according to what the patient would have decided if he or she were capable. However, when the decision makers do not know the wishes of the patient they can be directed to make decisions in the best interest of the patient.

Sexual expression is another common ethical dilemma in LTC, especially when the cognitive and physical limitations of residents make them vulnerable to sexual advances that are unsolicited and unwanted. Furthermore, patients with cognitive impairment may lose normal inhibitions and express their sexuality to staff or other patients in an inappropriate manner. On the other hand, a lack of privacy and ageist attitudes may inhibit normal and desired intimacy between long-standing partners or the development of new relationships that enhance life satisfaction and quality for mutually consenting LTC residents. Thus sexual expression is often an issue that needs to be frankly discussed and included in care planning.

MEASURING AND PROMOTING QUALITY OF CARE AND QUALITY OF LIFE

Federal Structures That Promote Nursing Home Quality

Nursing homes are required by federal law to collect clinical assessment data on each resident on admission, with any significant change in status, and at quarterly intervals. These assessments are gathered and reported using the MDS, now in version 3.0, from which quality indicators are derived that measure and monitor the care.[30] The data are transmitted to state and federal regulators in a national database called the Online Survey, Certification and Reporting (OSCAR), which has made it possible to compare nursing home performance across the country.

Selected quality indicators for every Medicare- and Medicaid-certified nursing home in the country are available to consumers through the Nursing Home Compare section of the Centers for Medicare and Medicaid Services (CMS) website (www.medicare.gov/NursingHomeCompare). Table 11-3 provides a list of currently published quality indicators. The assumption is that the availability of this public data will foster consumer-driven pressure to improve and maintain quality within nursing homes.

The CMS contracts with a Quality Improvement Organization (QIO) in each state to provide nursing homes, as well as hospitals and other health care providers, with expertise and tools to enact quality improvement initiatives that use quality indicators derived from MDS data. For example, QIOs have worked with nursing homes to reduce pressure ulcer occurrence, reduce the use of physical restraints, and improve transitions between hospitals and nursing homes.

State government entities are responsible for surveying nursing homes annually to ensure compliance with state and federal regulations. They use these data to determine how to apply their efforts during the survey process within a given facility. The review process relies heavily on the interpretation and enforcement of federal regulations often referred to as F-tags. For example F-tag 501 is the federal regulation that codifies the functions of a medical director. CMS provides guidelines to help surveyors interpret the code and apply it in meaningful ways to individual nursing homes. Survey results are available publicly through Nursing Home Compare and provide another means of measuring quality.

Currently federal Quality Assessment and Assurance requirements (483.75(o)) mandate that facilities maintain a Quality Assessment and Assurance committee that meets at least quarterly to address quality-related concerns and deficiencies. In addition, Section

TABLE 11-3	Nursing Home Compare Quality Measures of the U.S. Centers for Medicare and Medicaid Services (CMS)

Measures Applied to Short-Stay (Post-Acute Care) Residents

Percent who self-report moderate to severe pain.
Percent with new or worsened Stage II-IV pressure ulcers.
Percent assessed and given, appropriately, the influenza vaccination during the current or most recent influenza season.
Percent assessed and given, appropriately, the pneumococcal vaccine.
Percent who newly received an antipsychotic medication, but do not have evidence of a psychotic or related condition, such as schizophrenia, bipolar disorder, Tourette's syndrome, Huntington's disease, hallucinations, or delusions.

Measures Applied to Long-Stay Residents

Percent experiencing one or more falls with major injury.
Percent with a urinary tract infection.
Percent who self-report moderate to severe pain.
Percent of long-stay, high-risk residents with stage II-IV pressure ulcers.
Percent of long-stay, low-risk residents who are regularly incontinent of bowel or bladder.
Percent who have had a catheter inserted and left in their bladder.
Percent who are physically restrained on a daily basis.
Percent whose need for help with daily activities has increased.
Percent who had a weight loss of 5% or more in the last month or 10% or more in the last two quarters.
Percent who have depressive symptoms.
Percent assessed and given, appropriately, the influenza vaccination during the current or most recent influenza season.
Percent assessed and given, appropriately, the pneumococcal vaccine.
Percent who newly received an antipsychotic medication, but do not have evidence of a psychotic or related condition, such as schizophrenia, bipolar disorder, Tourette's syndrome, Huntington's disease, hallucinations, or delusions.

Data from Centers for Medicare & Medicaid Services. MDS 3.0 quality measures user's manual. Available at www.cms.gov/Medicare/Quality-Initiatives-Patient-Assessment-Instruments/NursingHomeQualityInits/Downloads/MDS-30-QM-Users-Manual-V60.pdf.

6102(c) of the Affordable Care Act requires CMS to establish Quality Assessment and Performance Improvement (QAPI) standards and provide technical assistance to nursing homes on best practices to meet these standards. This marks an additional step moving nursing homes toward using process improvement procedures as an ongoing methodology to assess needs, implement change, and measure outcomes.

Quality of Life

Promoting quality of care is an important aspect of what needs to be accomplished in nursing homes, but it cannot overshadow another equally important goal, enhancing quality of life. Quality of life encompasses both staff and residents. Measuring quality of life can be a challenge, but the measurement should incorporate issues such as choice and control over ADLs, access to outdoor environments, the quality of interpersonal interactions, privacy, the promotion of function/physical activity, and participation in care planning. In many instances the application of available research has served to promote quality of life in nursing homes; for example, the use of physical restraints has declined and is no longer accepted as an effective means of preventing injury.[31] Similarly, restrictive diets (to control diabetes, cholesterol levels, and salt intake) are being abandoned because they have been associated with poor nutritional intake.[32] Not surprisingly, many residents and their families will choose quality of life over length of life by refusing treatments that are restrictive, unpleasant, or of dubious benefit, such as dialysis for declining renal function or statins for hypercholesterolemia.

Enhancing Quality of Care and Quality of Life through Individualized ("Person-Centered") Care

A growing area of the health care industry involves organizations that focus on providing resources that will assist nursing homes to improve the quality of care and the quality of life experienced by their residents. Advancing Excellence in America's Nursing Homes (www.nhqualitycampaign.org) is a national coalition of nursing home stakeholders working together to help nursing homes improve care. The organization has established statewide stakeholder coalitions called Local Area Networks for Excellence (LANEs). They recruit nursing homes to participate in the Advancing Excellence Campaign in which they select goals of quality improvement. The organization provides online resources for quality assessment and program improvement. Goals the organization has supported include improving staff stability, use of consistent assignment, person-centered care planning and decision making, reduction of hospitalizations, using medications appropriately, increasing resident mobility, prevention and management of infections, reduction of pressure ulcers, and decreasing symptoms of pain.

The Pioneer Network (www.pioneernetwork.net) is a coalition of stakeholders that promotes a movement away from institutional provider-driven models of care to more consumer-driven models that embrace flexibility and self-determination. This shift in focus has been characterized as culture change. Core values include treatment flexibility, consumer choice, dignity, respect, self-determination, and purposeful living.

Early recognition of changes in condition can improve care outcomes. INTERACT (Interventions to Reduce Acute Care Transfers; interact2.net) is a quality improvement program that focuses on the management of acute change in residents' condition. It includes clinical and educational tools and strategies for use in everyday practice in LTC facilities. The program was evaluated in a 6-month collaborative quality-improvement project and resulted in a significant reduction in hospitalizations.[33]

A key area of recent emphasis has been improving transitions between LTC facilities and the acute care hospital. Patients who have been hospitalized or assessed in the ED should return to the LTC setting with the following: (1) appropriate information on the problem that prompted the transfer; (2) contact information for the nursing home, primary care physician, and the resident's legal health care representative; (3) updated medication and allergy lists; (4) functional status; (5) advance directives; and (6) the goals/expectations of patient, family, and provider. Within hospitals, readmission rates are being closely scrutinized, which means nursing homes and LTC physician providers have a growing opportunity to work in collaboration with their hospital colleagues to identify and solve transition problems.

Providing quality individualized care is heavily dependent on communication not only with the patient but with the family as well. Nursing home admission is the best time to make initial contact with the responsible family member, including those of patients who are cognitively intact and in full capacity to make decisions. Another time when communication is crucial is when a patient's condition changes—ideally *before* the situation becomes urgent. Patients are generally appreciative when asked if the physician can speak with a family member regarding their care. Hearing the family concerns, understanding of diagnoses and prognosis, and expectations for personal involvement in care can help to direct the care plan.

> Hearing the patient and family concerns, their understanding of diagnoses and prognosis, and expectations for personal involvement in care can help to direct the care plan.

Goals of care and advanced directives should be established or reviewed as soon as possible after admission to a LTC setting. It is important to address advance directives at the time of admission and when the resident's condition deteriorates. Tools have been developed to assist clinicians in identifying residents appropriate for palliative and hospice care (www.eprognosis.org). Enhancing the role of palliative care in nursing homes will also help align decisions about hospitalization with the individual's overall goals of care.

INNOVATIVE MODELS

A substantial number of stakeholders are advocating for wholesale change within nursing homes and the broader arena of LTC services. As a result of this groundswell of interest in change, a variety of new models have evolved.

The Green House Model

The Green House model involves constructing small homes that offer the full range of nursing home services.[34] Core elements include a 10-person home, private bath and bedroom for each elder with a personal (locked) medicine cabinet, hearth area with open living room, dining room and kitchen, dining table that seats all elders and caregivers, ceiling lifts, fenced outdoor space, and lots of windows. Although hugely popular, the movement is growing slowly because of the need for new construction rather than remodeling of existing institutions, and concerns about cost.

Wellspring

The Wellspring Program, first organized as an alliance of nursing homes in Wisconsin in 1994, offers education, guidance, and tools to nursing homes to assist in culture change. Wellspring primarily focuses on strengthening clinical and managerial skills of staff, empowering residents and frontline staff, and creating a high quality of life for residents. One of the strengths of Wellspring is that it enables nursing homes to implement culture change within an existing physical plant and in a stepwise, incremental manner. Through the Wellspring Program, frontline staff receive quality education and are coached on how to collect relevant data, critically evaluate information, and implement processes that improve care. Nurse consultants serve as clinical experts to oversee the program and provide implementation guidance and support. Networking among participating nursing homes provides a dynamic experience of sharing and encouragement. Research has demonstrated that Wellspring improves the quality of care, resident satisfaction, and employee satisfaction.[35]

Eden Alternative

Originating in the early 1990s, the Eden Alternative (www.edenalt.org) is an international not-for-profit organization dedicated to transforming care environments into habitats for human beings that promote quality of life for all involved. This program is known for bringing plants and animals into the nursing home environment, along with an appreciation for a home-like community that takes into account both residents and caregivers.

Continuing Care Retirement Communities (CCRCs)

An attractive option for LTC available to middle- and upper-income Americans is the continuing care retirement community (CCRC). The CCRC contains independent living units, assisted living, and nursing home care on the same campus, and guarantees access to LTC services in exchange for substantial admission and monthly fees. The CCRC provides 24-hour security, social and recreational activities, a common dining room with some meals provided, housekeeping, transportation, and fitness programs. The reasons for joining are most often in line with the services offered and include access to and insurance for medical care, maintaining independence, and not being a burden on family. The vast majority of residents are satisfied with their choice. Research shows that CCRCs enhance social integration. Disadvantages of CCRCs include the high cost, concentrating the experience of disability and death into a small age-segregated community, and an expectation that residents will move to a higher level of care when the CCRC deems it necessary.

Program of All-Inclusive Care for the Elderly (PACE)

The Program of All-Inclusive Care for the Elderly (PACE) is a community-based model of care that seeks to maintain at home with services persons who are age 55 or older, certified by their state to need nursing home care, desire to remain at home, and can live safely in the community.[36] Support is provided by an interdisciplinary team of health professionals, who provide individualized, coordinated care, much of which is carried out in a medical day care setting. For the vast majority of PACE participants, the comprehensive service package enables them to receive care at home rather than receive care in a nursing home. Financing is through capitated monthly payments from Medicare and Medicaid (or, for persons who do not qualify for Medicaid, from private sources). PACE operates as both a provider and an insurer, and is obligated to pay for whatever health care services its participants need—including hospitalization, nursing home care, and other costs by non-PACE providers. Thus the program has a strong incentive to prevent hospitalizations and maintain participant health.

CASE 1

Discussion

It is common for family physicians to be asked to make recommendations for level of care needs. As Mrs. Lewis's physician, you can help her daughter determine an appropriate level of care by asking questions regarding IADL and ADL performance, financial resources, and personal preferences. Geriatric case managers may be helpful to the daughter in assessing the needs of her mother and determining what settings may be appropriate given the available financial resources. Alternatively, the local Area Agency on Aging may also have resources that would help the daughter to identify appropriate care.

Mrs. Lewis is capable of expressing an opinion about where she wants to live. However, your interview reveals that she does not appreciate the potential dangerous outcomes she narrowly avoided during her recent falls or the extent of her cognitive and physical limitations. She remains resistant even to the help she now has in her home and does not want anyone "watching" her at night. You explain that it is your opinion that she needs to be in an environment with around-the-clock supervision, that you recommend assisted living, and that you are instructing her daughter to begin searching for appropriate options. You would like for Mrs. Lewis to visit the facilities with her daughter to participate in the decision making.

Even though Mrs. Lewis is not able to make this decision on her own, it is important to gain her assent to this transition and offer as much autonomy as is reasonable after the daughter has identified financially feasible options that are close to the daughter's residence. It is also very helpful for you as the physician to take responsibility for this decision so that Mrs. Lewis does not blame the daughter for making the decision against her wishes. ▣

CASE 2

Discussion

Patience and kindness are always the best professional approach, whether face to face or on the telephone. Calmly and with appropriate explanation ask Mr. Thompson's nurse to call you back with the following information: Has the patient been coughing? Does the patient have any dysuria, or changes in urinary frequency, urgency, or incontinence? What allergies does he have? What medications is he taking currently? What do the recent physician notes indicate about this patient? What are his care directives?

When she calls you back she tells you that he has been having dysuria, and a urine sample was sent to the lab earlier that day. The urinalysis is positive for nitrites, leukocyte esterase, with many white blood cells and bacteria. He was successfully treated with ciprofloxacin 3 months ago and has no allergies. You decide to start ciprofloxacin while waiting for culture results.

The next morning you meet with the director of nursing to discuss implementing a program to better prepare new nurses to assess and communicate about problems and concerns. You mention that AMDA has Know-It-All-Before-You-Call cards that can be purchased and made available on each nursing unit. The training will include key data to gather on common problems before calling the provider, and where to find information such as advance directives.

Falls require both an immediate assessment and management plan and a subsequent evaluation process aimed at minimizing risk and preventing future falls. Over the phone, you decide to ask the nurse to perform neurologic checks every 15 minutes for the first hour, then hourly for 3 hours, then every 3 hours for 48 hours. She should call you if she notices any change in alertness, worsening confusion, worsening headache, or asymmetry to Mr. Thompson's strength or coordination. She will give him acetaminophen 650 mg now for the headache and obtain an international normalized ratio in the morning.

Each nursing home has a formal process for reviewing falls, assessing patients, and implementing interventions to prevent falls. It is important that the physician also participate in the evaluation and intervention plan. The nurse tells you the patient is afraid he will no longer be allowed to enjoy half a beer as he usually does each night. In fact, the next day the care team would like your colleague, his usual physician, to discontinue the order that allows him to have alcohol. The physician objects because this will adversely affect his quality of life. You encourage the nurses to check positional blood pressures, and he is documented to be orthostatic. The nurse encourages fluids, and on recheck the following week he is no longer orthostatic. In response to this information, as medical director you suggest that the care team discuss with Mr. Thompson the possibility of abstaining from alcohol when he is ill, in an attempt to limit his risk for falls. Mr. Thompson agrees and so does his primary physician. ▪

SUMMARY

LTC is a rewarding field of practice for a primary care physician that incorporates a complex skill set including an understanding of the health system, care processes, and medical knowledge. Partnership is a key professional quality for successful LTC practice, both within the LTC organization and with other professionals in hospital, hospice, home health, and ambulatory settings, so that care is optimal and transitions are not plagued by unintended consequences. In addition, LTC practitioners must partner with the residents for whom they care and their families, helping them to understand the complexities of the environment and to have the optimal experience possible given the challenges of their health problems and prognosis.

Web Resources

www.amda.com. The American Medical Directors Association is the professional association of medical directors, attending physicians, and others practicing in the LTC continuum.

www.bathingwithoutabattle.unc.eduA significant portion of LTC residents exhibit aggressive behaviors during bathing. This website contains information on a CD and video package that teaches individualized approaches for bathing.

www.interact2.net. INTERACT (Interventions to Reduce Acute Care Transfers) is a quality improvement program that focuses on the management of acute change in resident condition in order to reduce the frequency of transfers to the hospital.

www.medicare.gov/NursingHomeCompare. Nursing Home Compare contains quality of care information on every Medicare and Medicaid-certified nursing home in the country.

www.nhqualitycampaign.org. The Advancing Excellence in America's Nursing Homes Campaign helps nursing homes improve care by focusing on nine goals. The website contains free, practical, and evidence-based resources to support quality improvement efforts in LTC.

www.pioneernetwork.net. The Pioneer Network is the leading advocacy organization of the culture change movement.

KEY REFERENCES

1. Houser A, Fox-Grage W, Ujvari K. Across the states: Profiles of long-term services and supports. Washington, DC: AARP Public Policy Institute; 2012. Available at www.aarp.org/home-garden/livable-communities/info-09-2012/across-the-states-2012-profiles-of-long-term-services-supports-AARP-ppi-ltc.html. Accessed May 26, 2013.
4. Buhr GT, Kuchibhatla M, Clipp EC. Caregivers' reasons for nursing home placement: Clues for improving discussions with families prior to the transition. Gerontologist 2006;46(1):52-61.
11. AMDA. The nursing home medical director: Leader and manager. Columbia, MD: AMDA; 2011. Available at www.amda.com/governance/whitepapers/A11.cfm. Accessed May 26, 2013.
21. High KP, Bradley SF, Gravenstein S, et al. Clinical practice guideline for the evaluation of fever and infection in older adult residents of long-term care facilities: 2008 update by the Infectious Diseases Society of America. Clin Infect Dis 2009;48(2):149-71.
25. Buhr GT, Genao L, White HK. Urinary tract infections in long-term care residents. Clin Geriatr Med 2011;27(2):229-39.
33. Ouslander JG, Lamb G, Tappen R, et al. Interventions to reduce hospitalizations from nursing homes: Evaluation of the INTERACT II collaborative quality improvement project. J Am Geriatr Soc 2011;59(4):745-53.

References available online at expertconsult.com.

12

Home Care

Jennifer Hayashi and Bruce Leff

OBJECTIVES

Upon completion of this chapter, the reader will be able to:

- Describe the types of health care services available to older adults at home.
- Understand the basic payment mechanisms for these services.
- List evidence-based outcomes of home care for older adults.
- Recognize the limitations of the existing evidence base on home care.
- Identify key elements of recent legislation affecting medical home care.

CASE 1

Mrs. K (Part 1)

Mrs. K is an 83-year-old woman with hypertension, type 2 diabetes mellitus, congestive heart failure, and osteoarthritis who lives alone and has missed two clinic appointments with you in the last 6 months. She comes to your office today with her daughter Linda, who is visiting from California. Linda is concerned because Mrs. K seems to be "letting things go" around the house lately and has not filled her

Additional online-only material indicated by icon.

medication prescriptions for the last few months. Mrs. K denies any recent acute illness or injury, but says she has been afraid to leave the house "for a while now" since she tripped on a garden hose and almost fell 8 months ago. Medications include aspirin, metformin, lisinopril, furosemide, and acetaminophen. Physical examination is remarkable for a blood pressure of 156/87 without postural change and symmetric 2+ pitting edema of both legs to mid-shin, which is new since her last visit with you. Lungs are clear to auscultation. Her gait is slow with a wide base and unsteady turning radius. She is unable to rise from the chair without using her arms to push herself up. Cognitive testing reveals mild short-term memory impairment but preserved judgment and executive function. Laboratory studies show a serum creatinine of 1.3 mg/dL, potassium 4.2 mg/dL, and HbA_{1C} of 10.2%. Thyroid function tests are normal. You are concerned about her poorly controlled hypertension and diabetes, as well as her gait and memory impairment, so you decide to refer her to a Medicare-certified skilled home care agency for services.

What home care services do you request for Mrs. K? ▣

WHAT IS HOME CARE?

Home care in its most general sense refers to any diagnostic, therapeutic, or social support service provided to patients in their homes.[1] These services may range from a visiting nurse checking vital signs and counting pills in prescription bottles, a physician or nurse practitioner evaluating and treating pulmonary edema, a speech therapist providing language rehabilitation, an aide bathing a terminally ill patient in home hospice, or a medical social worker helping caregivers identify and coordinate community services to help keep a patient in his or her home instead of moving into institutional long-term care. Table 12-1 shows the array of home care services available.

Medicare, the major insurer for older Americans, makes an important distinction among the services listed in Table 12-1 and defines "skilled" care as care that is "reasonable and necessary" and required on an intermittent basis. Furthermore, Medicare pays for skilled home care only if a patient is homebound (i.e., leaving the home requires considerable and taxing effort, and absences from home are infrequent or of brief duration).[2] It is important to note that Medicare does not cover personal care unless it is in the context of skilled care. Therefore, a patient who requires assistance only for activities of daily living, and does not have a need for skilled care, must find some other way to obtain and/or pay for these services. Medicaid covers personal care at home, usually for a few hours per day, several days per week, but has strict financial eligibility criteria that exclude many older adults who are not impoverished.

TABLE 12-1	What is Home Care?	
Skilled Home Care	Medical/Other House Calls	Personal Care
Nursing	Primary care home visits	Bathing
Therapy	Podiatry	Dressing
Physical	Dentistry	Feeding
Occupational	Optometry	Toileting
Speech	Hospital at Home	
Medical social work	Home hospice	

In addition to these formal services that are directly funded by various insurance payors, informal unreimbursed care provided by family and friends is crucial to keeping patients at home, and represents a silent but enormous economic force in the U.S. health care system.[3] In this chapter, we describe the two most common types of formal home care: Medicare skilled home care and medical house calls. We also briefly describe Hospital at Home, an emerging model of acute care in which intensive home-based medical management substitutes for a hospital inpatient admission, and the Independence at Home demonstration project included in the Patient Protection and Affordable Care Act of 2010.

Figure 12-1 depicts the continuum and overlap of the various major types of home care. The light gray circle on the left represents the population of older adults who receive primary care services from physicians and other medical providers. Most of these patients are seen in the office, but some of them receive primary care visits at home (dark gray circle), and are sometimes referred for skilled home care (gold bar) for additional home-based rehabilitation or medical management and monitoring. Some patients experience acute illness (gold circle) which is managed at home through medical house calls or Hospital at Home, often in conjunction with skilled care (intersection of gold bar with light gray, dark gray, and gold circles).

> Medicare does not cover personal care (bathing, toileting, dressing) at home unless it is in the context of skilled care; informal care to meet these needs is crucial to keeping patients at home, and has tremendous economic implications for caregivers and society in general.

CASE 1

Mrs. K (Part 2)

Mrs. K is referred to skilled home care and is visited by a nurse and a physical therapist at home. The nurse monitors her blood pressure and reports it back to you weekly so that you can adjust her medications. She helps Mrs. K and her daughter organize a pillbox that Mrs. K can fill weekly with telephone prompting as needed from her daughter. She also provides written materials and "refresher" teaching on diabetes self-management and monitoring. Meanwhile, the therapist evaluates Mrs. K's home and suggests several practical options for minimizing safety risks, such as installing grab bars in the bathroom (not paid for by Medicare) and securing some loose carpeting at the base of the stairs. The therapist also works with Mrs. K twice a week to increase her lower extremity strength, balance, and steadiness, and teaches her a home exercise program with written materials that she can use to continue exercises on her own. After about 5 weeks of this level of home care, Mrs. K is ambulating more safely and confidently, and her A_{1c} (drawn by the nurse during a visit for blood pressure monitoring) returns at 9.2%. She is discharged from skilled care, but misses another office appointment with you because she remains fearful of walking outside her home and forgets that she has a medical appointment.

What options are available for ongoing medical primary care for Mrs. K? ◻

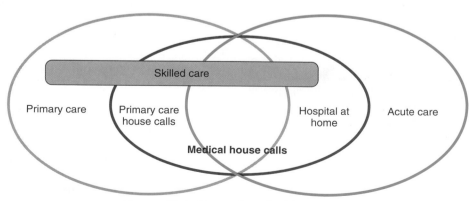

Figure 12-1 Types of medical home care.

WHO NEEDS HOME CARE?

Homebound patients who have a skilled need may receive home care from a Medicare-certified home health agency. These patients generally have medical or functional conditions that are likely to improve with treatment over a short period (1 to 2 months), and have difficulty leaving their homes to access office-based treatment for these conditions. Examples of such skilled needs include nursing care of wounds (surgical, venous stasis, or pressure), physical and occupational therapy after hip fracture, speech therapy after a stroke, or monitoring of blood pressure and renal function during adjustment of medications for uncontrolled medical conditions (diabetes, hypertension, heart failure). Importantly, nursing visits solely for the purpose of drawing blood are not considered a skilled need. While a patient is receiving skilled care, Medicare also covers personal care services, including assistance with bathing and dressing.

Another important group of patients who can benefit from home care may not be homebound by Medicare's skilled home care definition, but are medically complex or have medical conditions refractory to the usual office-based management. Although these patients may not be eligible for skilled home care, a targeted medical house call by a physician or nurse practitioner to assess adherence, functional conditions, caregiver/patient dynamics, and other barriers to effective care can provide invaluable context for the medical provider, and open up new opportunities to work with the patient to optimize care. In fact, one study comparing office-based medical and psychiatric evaluations with in-home assessments showed that a substantial minority of patients had important problems that were discovered only on the home visit, and almost all patients had problems identified at home that increased the risk of morbidity or significant functional decline.[4]

Finally, a subset of older adults are frail, medically complex patients who do not have a need that qualifies for skilled home care, but are unable to access office-based primary care because of functional impairment. This population is particularly appropriate for medical house calls provided by physicians, nurse practitioners, or physician assistants for ongoing management of their chronic diseases.

> Medical house calls by physicians, physician assistants, or nurse practitioners can be useful as an adjunct to office-based care or as primary care for appropriate patients.

HOW IS HOME CARE DELIVERED?

A physician must certify that a patient is homebound and has a skilled need in order for a Medicare-certified agency to receive reimbursement for skilled services. Since 2011, Medicare has required a face-to-face medical visit at the time of initial certification to confirm the necessity of skilled home care. The face-to-face visit may occur in any setting, and must occur in the 90 days before or 30 days after the initiation of skilled home care services. A nurse practitioner, physician assistant, or trainee physician may perform the visit on behalf of the certifying physician, but the certifying physician must personally sign a document confirming the face-to-face visit. Nurse practitioners and physician assistants may not sign home care certification orders, although they can sign orders for durable medical equipment such as canes, walkers, and bedside commodes.

The typical certification period for Medicare skilled home care is 60 days. If a patient receiving speech, physical, or occupational therapy is making progress at the end of this time and still has significant potential for rehabilitation, the physician can recertify that the patient is still homebound and still has a skilled need requiring home care. Similarly, if a skilled nursing need remains active, nursing services can also be reordered. There is no requirement for a face-to-face visit for recertification, and there is no limit on the number of times that a patient may be recertified, as long as these two fundamental conditions (skilled need and homebound) are met. In fact, there are two notable exceptions to the usual expectation that skilled services will be short-term: chronic urinary catheters and pernicious anemia requiring vitamin B_{12} injections. For these two conditions, Medicare will cover ongoing skilled care including monthly nursing visits for injections or catheter changes, as well as personal care and "as-needed" nursing visits.

A related but distinct form of home care is medical home visits, or house calls. Medical house calls comprise a small but growing proportion of provider visits. A landmark 1997 publication showed that <1% of Medicare beneficiaries in 1988 received at least one medical home visit by a physician per year,[5] and a 2005 analysis of Medicare data demonstrated an increase in house calls from 0.78% to 0.90% of outpatient evaluation and management services, or a 43% increase in the absolute number of home visits.[6] These medical house calls occur in a variety of practice structures. Some office-based medical providers make occasional routine or urgent home visits to selected patients, whereas other providers have dedicated house call sessions integrated into their regular office schedule. Still others have mobile practices that exclusively make house calls, either as private practice models or as part of larger academic or institutional practices.[7]

Finally, Hospital at Home is an intensive form of home care in which physicians, nurses, other providers, and home caregivers collaborate to provide hospital-level care in a patient's home for common, uncomplicated acute illnesses that can be diagnosed and treated safely, efficiently, and effectively in the home. Conditions that have been demonstrated to be appropriate for Hospital at Home treatment include community-acquired pneumonia, exacerbations of chronic obstructive pulmonary disease or congestive heart failure, cellulitis, deep venous thrombosis, pulmonary embolism, volume depletion, dehydration, urinary tract infection, and urosepsis.[8] A 2009 meta-analysis showed that patients receiving Hospital at Home care were more satisfied with care than those receiving inpatient care, and that Hospital at Home care was less expensive than usual acute inpatient care. Additionally, there was a remarkable 38% reduction in the risk of death at 6 months for Hospital at Home patients compared with controls at 6 months.[9] Although much of the literature on Hospital at Home was originally generated in nations with robust single-payer health care systems, a successful Hospital at Home program has been developed over the past two decades in the United States, and several related dissemination projects are under way in Veterans Affairs (VA) hospitals and Medicare managed care settings.[10]

> Although not yet widely available outside of select VA and managed care systems, Hospital at Home improves health outcomes at lower costs than usual inpatient care for appropriate patients with targeted conditions.

Mrs. K (Part 3)

You decide to start making primary care medical house calls to Mrs. K as a result of her difficulty getting to her appointments with you because of her gait and memory impairment.

How are home care providers reimbursed? ■

WHO PAYS FOR HOME CARE?

In 2011 Medicare spent $19.6 billion on skilled home care services and $12 billion on home hospice, representing 45% of the total national health care expenditure on home health care.[11] Medicaid, which includes but is not limited to elderly patients, paid for an additional $26 billion (37%), and the remaining 18% was covered by a combination of commercial insurers, social services block grants, Veterans Administration programs, and out-of-pocket payments by patients. Again, the economic contribution of the informal caregiver cannot be overstated: in a comprehensive

1997 analysis, the estimated cost of informal caregiving was $196 billion, or more than 6 times the national health expenditure ($32 billion) on formal home care services during the same year.[3]

On a smaller scale, clinicians should know that Medicare reimburses home health agencies for skilled care based on the amount and intensity of services that are provided in accordance with a plan of care developed and certified by a physician who is overseeing the patient's medical care. Additionally, the physician who signs the skilled care certification can be reimbursed specifically for these activities (certification, code G0180, or recertification, code G0179), as long as the patient has seen that physician at least once in the 6 months before the episode of home care. Physicians and other medical providers may also bill for care plan oversight (CPO; code G0181) if the time spent communicating with other health care professionals (nurses, therapists, consultants, etc.) in a calendar month during an episode of skilled home care adds up to at least 30 minutes. CPO does not include time spent in the presence of the patient communicating with other professionals, but does include the time it takes to document data collection and medical decision making.

Medical house calls are reimbursed by Medicare and most commercial insurers based on the medical necessity of the home visit. Providers must document a medical reason for seeing the patient in a house call instead of an office visit. Inconvenience or lack of transportation is not a medical justification for a home visit. Furthermore, Medicare does not reimburse provider expenses incidental to the provision of house calls, such as mileage or public transportation fares. Although reimbursement rates vary with geographic region, they are generally slightly higher for home visits than for office visits of comparable evaluation and management (E&M) complexity. Table 12-2 lists the codes and typical visit duration expected for various levels of home visits.

> Certification or recertification of home care orders and care plan oversight are reimbursable activities.

DOES HOME CARE WORK?

Because the term *home care* is used to describe a broad range of services, it is challenging to synthesize the evidence that peppers the medical literature. However, several relevant studies of home-based preventive care and medical home visits in the United States and Europe throughout the 1990s and early 2000s demonstrated improvements in health care use (particularly emergency department visits[12]

TABLE 12-2	Health Care Common Procedure Coding System (HCPCS) Codes for Home Visits				
Home Visit, New Patient	Domiciliary Care, New Patient	Typical Time for Code (min)	Home Visit, Established Patient	Domiciliary Care, Established Patient	Typical Time for Code (min)
99341	99324	20	—	—	—
99342	99325	30	99347	99334	15
99343	99326	45	99348	99335	25
99344	99327	60	99349	99336	40
99345	99328	75	99350	99337	60

and nursing home placement;[13,14] satisfaction of patients, caregivers, and physicians;[15-19] quality of life;[15,16] and end-of-life care,[20] particularly when the interventions were longitudinal, multidimensional, and/or targeted to an appropriate population. Notably, the funding mechanisms for most of these interventions did not rely primarily on traditional fee-for-service reimbursement, because such reimbursement is typically insufficient to establish or maintain the home-based primary care services.

HEALTH CARE REFORM AND HOME CARE

In March 2012 the Independence at Home (IAH) Act, section 3024 of the Patient Protection and Affordable Care Act of 2010, became law. The IAH Act mandated a demonstration study of an innovative payment methodology for medical house calls that marked a major change in Medicare reimbursement of care for the frail, medically complex older adults that spend the greatest amount of the Medicare budget. Mobile multidisciplinary teams of primary care providers must demonstrate improved outcomes for these patients by providing or coordinating care across different settings, including hospitals and nursing homes. Each team will work with existing community networks of pharmacies, medical supply companies, home care agencies, and hospices to provide patient-centered care to people at home. Health care technology that supports effective and secure communication about patients among providers and facilities is a fundamental part of the IAH infrastructure, as is around-the-clock access to skilled telephone triage and urgent visits as needed to prevent unnecessary hospital use. The following characteristics define IAH teams selected for the 3-year demonstration project:

1. They will provide home-based comprehensive care to functionally disabled Medicare beneficiaries with multiple chronic illnesses and prior high health care costs.
2. They must show a 5% minimum annual savings for Medicare, compared with predicted costs based on the target population's historical utilization.

3. They will share in any savings to Medicare above this first 5%, to use for program development including technology or other clinical services.
4. They must meet three minimum performance standards (patient and family satisfaction, patient care quality measures to be established by the Centers for Medicare and Medicaid Services, and the 5% savings noted above).
5. They will retain all current traditional Medicare coverage and will be completely voluntary on the part of the patient.

In April 2012, 15 individual medical practices in 12 states were named as IAH demonstration sites, and 3 regional consortia were added in August 2012. More information is available at www.innovations.cms.gov/initiatives/Independence-at-Home/index.html.

The "shared savings" payment model limits the financial risk to Medicare, and unlike previous managed care capitation models, provides incentives for IAH practices to seek out high-cost beneficiaries who have the most potential for cost savings.

> Interdisciplinary teams providing coordinated, around-the-clock patient-centered care have the opportunity to change the face of Medicare for the type of community-dwelling, frail, medically complex older adults who expend the majority of the Medicare budget.

SUMMARY

For the aging population of the United States, home care remains an important form of health care that can complement or replace office or hospital-based care. The current reimbursement system allows many older adults to benefit from both medical home visits and skilled home care services provided by allied health professionals, but economic and demographic projections suggest that recent innovations in home health care delivery and reimbursement are sorely needed. Careful evaluation of patient care and economic outcomes over time should lead to the patient-centered, safe, efficacious, timely, equitable, and cost-effective care that all patients want and deserve.

Web Resources

www.medpac.gov/documents/Jun12DataBookEntireReport.pdf. *Health Care Spending and the Medicare Program*—Medicare Payment Advisory Commission Data Book, June 2012.

www.cms.gov/Research-Statistics-Data-and-Systems/Statistics-Trends-and-Reports/NationalHealthExpendData/Downloads/highlights.pdf. National Health Expenditures 2011 Highlights Fact Sheet.

www.nahc.org. National Association of Home Care and Hospice.

KEY REFERENCES

1. Levine SA, Boal J, Boling PA. Home care. JAMA 2003; 290(9):1203-7.
5. Meyer GS, Gibbons RV. House calls to the elderly—a vanishing practice among physicians. N Engl J Med 1997;337(25):1815-20.
8. Leff B, Burton L, Mader SL, et al. Hospital at home: Feasibility and outcomes of a program to provide hospital-level care at home for acutely ill older patients. Ann Int Med 2005;143:798-808.
14. Stuck AE, Egger M, Hammer A, et al. Home visits to prevent nursing home admission and functional decline in elderly people: Systematic review and meta-regression analysis. JAMA 2002;287(8):1022-8.
16. Hughes SL, Weaver FM, Giobbie-Hurder A, et al. Effectiveness of team-managed home-based primary care: A randomized multicenter trial. JAMA 2000;284(22):2877-85.

References available online at www.expertconsult.com.

Rehabilitation

Neil J. Nusbaum

OBJECTIVES

Upon completion of this chapter, the reader will be able to:

- Understand the burden of functional impairment in the older individual.
- Appreciate how level of function may fluctuate over time in an individual.
- Appreciate the role of rehabilitation in common diseases of the older individual.
- Understand how to support the rehabilitative needs of the patient within the primary care setting.

REHABILITATION AND THE OLDER INDIVIDUAL

The goal of rehabilitative care of older individuals is the prevention or delay of the onset of disability, and there is accordingly great attraction to the idea of directing rehabilitation efforts to the frail elderly.[1] Although there is a modest role of genetic factors in the risk for functional impairment in old age, environmental factors appear to be far more important.[2] Rehabilitative care is one strategy for improving the mix of environmental factors to promote best function. Rehabilitation efforts for frail elders may be directed to avoid loss of function, to help promote return of lost function, or both.[3]

One of the most important concepts to appreciate in evaluating the rehabilitation needs of the older patient is that an individual's level of disability may vary strikingly over time. An episode of acute medical illness, of whatever etiology, raises the risk that the individual's functional status may decline acutely. The decline is likely to be multifactorial, with components ranging from loss of skeletal muscle mass making physical tasks more difficult, to onset of delirium that can make it more difficult for the patient to conduct his or her activities of daily living (ADLs) safely.

Some patients may have a sudden obvious event, such as a stroke or a hip fracture, that is expected to produce an immediate severe functional decline that would benefit from rehabilitation. Many frail older individuals, however, may suffer progressive limitation from a gradual decline in function, and they may have gradually reduced their habitual level of activity to compensate for their decreased functional abilities. Fear of falling may have led patients to restrict walking and other activity even more severely than functional limitations might require, so that their abilities further decline from deconditioning. Many of these patients may benefit from rehabilitative regimens to help them regain their prior level of function.

CASE 1

Alan Baker (Part 1)

Your patient Alan Baker is a 75-year-old man with a 20-year history of diabetes who has developed peripheral neuropathy, and in recent years has had recurrent foot ulcers. He has hypertension, but his blood pressure control varies depending on whether he remembers to take his medication. His wife had driven the family car for the past 2 years, until her

---

Additional online-only material indicated by icon.

death 2 months ago. The patient is brought to your office by his neighbor who reports that, starting a month ago, the patient was noticeably short of breath after walking the one block distance that separates their residences. When you question the patient, he says everything is going "okay." He has a few scattered rales on pulmonary exam, and bilateral pretibial edema. His electrocardiogram (ECG) today shows septal Q waves not present on his ECG a year ago.

1. **What are the patient's current rehabilitative needs?**

2. **What additional rehabilitation issues are likely to arise in the succeeding year?** ▣

Determining if an older adult is a candidate for rehabilitation is not always clear. Among older individuals, there are many who do not have obvious disability, but in fact have already made subtle alterations in their activity pattern in response to a mild decline in function.[4] Many of these individuals may benefit from early preventive rehabilitation efforts, sometimes referred to as "prehabilitation." Such efforts may be directed to improve present function and potentially could also decrease the risk of progression to more frank disability. In some cases this may involve encouraging compliance with general healthy lifestyle recommendations about physical activity. This kind of early rehabilitation may provide a physiologic reserve that can help the individual better tolerate a future loss of function during a future illness. In one meta-analysis, interventions to improve function, and avert nursing home placement, were moderately effective. The absolute benefit of rehabilitation in this regard appeared to be greatest in the patients at the highest baseline risk for future nursing home placement, with a number needed to treat (NNT) of 39 to see this benefit.[5]

Many older individuals will cycle over time between being disabled and having no disability,[6] rather than simply showing a linear course of relentlessly increasing disability. Seen in that light, it is reasonable to regard the hospitalization for an acute medical illness as an event that increases the risk that the patient may transition from no disability to disability.[7,8] Similarly, rehabilitation interventions in the acute medical setting can be considered as an effort to foster rapid transition back from the disabled state to the prior higher level of function. On the other hand, if patients following their acute medical illness later reach a level of disability where they require nursing home admission, the prognosis for a full reversal of their disability is much more guarded. In one study,[9] following such a nursing home admission, only 32% of the nursing home admittees made a full recovery of function. In light of these several studies, a strong case can be made for the use of postacute rehabilitation as a strategy to decrease the risk for future nursing home placement and the risk for later progression of disability.

> Rehabilitation efforts for frail elders may be directed to avoid loss of function, to help promote return of lost function, or both.

An individual's level of disability is determined not just by physical and mental function. This broader view is embodied in the International Classification of Functioning, Disability and Health: "Functioning and disability are viewed as a complex interaction between the health condition of the individual and the contextual factors of the environment as well as personal factors. The picture produced by this combination of factors and dimensions is of 'the person in his or her world.' The classification treats these dimensions as interactive and dynamic rather than linear or static."[10]

Functional impairment is common among older persons, not just the small minority (5% of those aged 65 years and older) who reside in nursing homes. Of all Medicare enrollees aged 65 and older, 14% of the men and 23% of the women are unable to walk two to three blocks. There is evidence that some measures of age-adjusted rates of disability in the United States have declined, although with the growth in the total population older than age 65, the absolute number of chronically disabled older individuals has modestly increased[11] (Figure 13-1).

In the older patient, there is often more than one condition that can contribute to disability. A 1996 survey found that, of Medicare patients aged 65 years and older, 64% had at least one potentially disabling condition (blindness or low vision, deafness or hard of hearing, difficulties walking, difficulties reaching overhead, difficulties grasping and writing), and 30% had more than one of these conditions.[12]

The two most common areas of reported difficulty are in hearing and walking, both of which can benefit from medical attention, but for which the rehabilitative strategies are substantially different. Significant hearing deficits are likely to require provision of a hearing aid, and support by the clinician to encourage the patient to obtain it and to use it once prescribed.[13] Difficulties with gait may reflect one or a combination of deficits (muscle weakness, postural instability, poor vision, peripheral neuropathy), for which the appropriate choice of management will depend in large part on the clinician's evaluation of the relevant contributory factors for the patient.

Rehabilitative strategies for older patients with weakness can be successfully linked to skills necessary to perform ADLs, rather than simply focused on increasing strength.[14] This may make it easier to design regimens that can directly improve functional ability, and which can be readily reinforced during physical activity while performing daily tasks.

How well or poorly an older person may be able to participate in society reflects the influence of both individual and environmental factors, and this broad

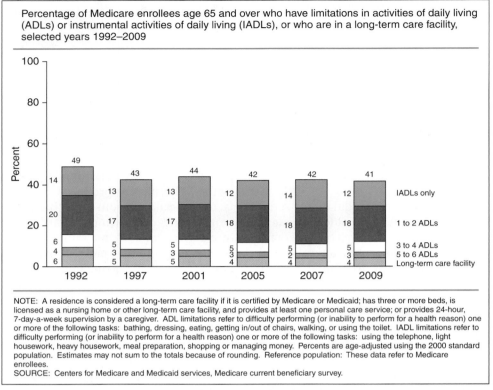

Figure 13-1 Percentage of Medicare enrollees aged 65 and older who have limitations in activities of daily living (ADLs) or instrumental activities of daily living (IADLs), or who are in a long-term care facility, selected years 1992-2009. (Courtesy of the Federal Interagency Forum on Aging-Related Statistics. *Older Americans 2012: Key indicators of well-being.* Washington, DC: U.S. Government Printing Office; June 2012. Available at www.agingstats.gov/Main_Site/Data/2012_Documents/docs/EntireChartbook.pdf.)

view should guide rehabilitation planning. Rehabilitative measures may be directed to improve the person's own intrinsic performance. They may also involve provision of assistive devices that can compensate for the person's intrinsic impairments, as well as modifications of the wider physical environment to better fit the patient's impairments. All these approaches may fruitfully be combined; a patient with diabetic retinopathy may benefit from laser therapy of the retina, from the provision of eyeglasses for refractive correction, and from the use of large print on signs.

The evaluation of function should be tailored to the individual patient's situation, and may incorporate consideration of both objective and subjective information. It can include assessment of motor strength on the neurologic examination, as well as evaluation of the patient's ability to perform ADLs (e.g., getting out of bed to go to the bathroom) and instrumental ADLs (e.g., grocery shopping). The degree to which patients are disabled by a loss of function depends in part on what they consider normal, as well as by their level of social supports. Even if they can still accomplish a task such as walking to go grocery shopping, they may have noted that it involves more pain from knee osteoarthritis, that they have to do it differently such as buying smaller numbers of bags at each trip, and/or that it takes more time to walk to and from the grocery store.[15] These early

complaints may foreshadow the risk of being unable to accomplish the task of grocery shopping at all.

Ideally, rehabilitation can aid in pain management but also simultaneously support other health goals such as maintaining physical fitness. A Cochrane review[16] examined the database in support of the use of aquatic therapy for patients with osteoarthritis of the knee or hip. This review suggests that there may be some short-term benefit in terms of pain control, but it concludes that the evidence base is quite weak regarding the role of aquatic therapy for osteoarthritis. Certainly aquatic therapy is widely recommended in daily practice, often to promote a wider variety of therapeutic aims than just pain management. Other therapeutic objectives may include maintaining coordination and balance, avoiding deconditioning, and promoting social interaction in a group activity.

REHABILITATION SETTINGS

Rehabilitation of older adults can take place in an acute hospital medical or rehabilitation unit,[17] the nursing home, an outpatient area, or the patient's home. The ability to provide in-hospital rehabilitative care to Medicare beneficiaries has been influenced by changes in reimbursement formulas. Between 1994 and 2001, the median length of stay for inpatient rehabilitation fell from 20 days to 12 days.[18,19] Skilled nursing facilities (SNFs) may also deliver rehabilitation services to many of their residents, typically at a lower level of intensity than patients would receive in a hospital facility, and such services may enable the resident to regain enough function to leave the nursing facility and return to the community.[20] Changes pursuant to the Balanced Budget Amendment of 1997, however, not only have affected the reimbursement structure for rehabilitation hospitals,[21] but also have made it less financially attractive for SNFs[22] to offer their residents rehabilitation services. The ongoing changes in the Medicare program[23] are likely to have a significant impact on the availability of rehabilitation services across a variety of care settings. The pressure of the Prospective Payment System on inpatient rehabilitation facilities for prompt discharge may have contributed to a pattern of discharges from inpatient rehabilitation often being directed not to discharge home, but rather to an SNF.[24] The payment schema in turn places strong incentives on the SNFs to control the intensity of the care they provide; Medicare provides reimbursement to the SNF for rehabilitative care to a certain point, but therapy beyond 720 minutes per week offers no marginal reimbursement.[25] Yet another Prospective Payment System methodology has been adopted in the home health setting, creating a financial incentive for the home health provider to limit overall home visitors.[26,27]

In an era when brief hospital stays limit the ability for inpatient rehabilitation, unmet rehabilitative need is a common occurrence. Over the last decade, the federal government through its Medicare statutes and regulations has tried to control the growth of postacute rehabilitation services, but with only limited success. In some cases, the effect of the Medicare reimbursement rules appears to have been less to discourage the provision of postacute rehabilitation than to create incentives to shift the care site where rehabilitation is offered (e.g., for the postacute care to be offered in an SNF rather than in the home setting with home health care).[28] Medicare is estimated to have paid $42.1 billion for postacute rehabilitation services in 2005.[29]

At the same time, there is also Medicare data to suggest that many older individuals do not receive any rehabilitative services at all even though their diagnosis suggests that they might likely have benefited from such services.[30] Inpatient rehabilitation facilities in particular are under fiscal pressure from Medicare to assure that 75% of their admissions fall in one of 13 diagnostic categories, including entities such as stroke or hip fracture, in order to maintain their status as an inpatient rehabilitation facility.[31] This Medicare funding restriction may make it more difficult to obtain postacute inpatient rehabilitation for older patients who have hospital-associated deconditioning but who do not fall within one of the 13 diagnostic categories. Further changes in the medical economic milieu for rehabilitation are likely to occur as the implementation of the Affordable Care Act proceeds.[32] (See Chapter 8.)

A report on Canadian stroke care[33] has documented the need to better integrate stroke rehabilitation into the process of stroke care in Canada, and from a perspective in the United States it is noteworthy how similar the issues and challenges are in the Canadian setting. For example, a Canadian study of hemodialysis patients scheduled their rehabilitation to fit with their 6-times-per-week hemodialysis schedule. This integration of medical and rehabilitative care aids in addressing goals relevant to both interventions (protein intake, mobility, patient fatigue) as part of the patient's overall care.[34] Coordination of the various aspects of care for the patient can significantly help to minimize the cost of care, such as reducing the need for transportation services. Another economical strategy, particularly for patients with less severe levels of impairment, may be to deliver therapy in a group treatment setting.[35]

In the case of patients residing in a nursing home, the impairments are likely to be substantial and multiple;[36] they may be relatively easier to recognize but the process of rehabilitating them may be relatively more complex. Among nursing home residents, for example, those with new impairment in voluntary movement or in range of motion are at particular risk for a decrease in their ability to perform the ADLs.[37] The rehabilitation goals for the long-term nursing home resident are likely to be different and more modest, and a successful outcome may be to maintain level of function rather than to achieve full independence.

Rehabilitation regimens will often need tailoring to the abilities of the frail older individual. Even for those individuals in the nursing home setting, there is reason to suspect that many could benefit from an increased level of therapy, both that delivered formally by therapists and that received from the bedside nursing staff. A study of patients in SNFs demonstrated that patients had a more rapid increase in their functional status, and a greater chance of leaving the nursing home to return to the community, if they were in a facility where the average resident received at least 1.5 hours of therapy per day. Likewise, both the rate of increase in functional status and the chance of returning to the community were higher for patients who were in SNFs that provided higher levels of nurse staffing.[38]

Older medical inpatients may often be discharged from the hospital at a time when they are stable from the point of view of their recent acute medical illness, such as a stroke, but when they have not yet completed their process of rehabilitation from the acute medical event. In this situation, it is important to plan for the postdischarge component of their overall rehabilitation pathway. Otherwise, the risk is that the momentum of their rehabilitation may be lost.[39,40] The transition to home-based rehabilitation postdischarge allows the opportunity for the therapy to be more precisely tailored to the specific home environment, and for the patient and caregivers to be more active participants in that tailoring process.[41]

A particular concern in the discharge planning process is to make sure that the course of rehabilitation is not delayed (or prematurely interrupted) by the transition from the acute hospital setting to the postdischarge setting (such as home or nursing facility). Delayed rehabilitation efforts may not be nearly as effective as efforts begun more promptly. For a stroke patient, even a 1-month delay in beginning poststroke rehabilitation has been associated with a poorer rehabilitation outcome.[42]

The postdischarge course of rehabilitation may be adversely affected by medical complications following discharge, such as aspiration pneumonia in the stroke patient when he or she eats at home. The course of the stroke patient at home in the postacute period may be further complicated by psychological factors, including anxiety or depression.[43] In frail older patients, particularly if they are homebound, their postacute needs for rehabilitative and emotional support may often go unrecognized and so unaddressed. A comprehensive approach to meeting postacute care needs for the patient who returns home may include provision of assistive devices such as wheelchairs, incorporation of family caregivers into the home care plan, and/or modification of the bathroom or other architectural components of the patient's home.[44]

In general, one can best think about rehabilitative needs of the patient across the continuum of care, not just in a particular care setting. The less opportunity there is for rehabilitation in one setting, the more likely it is that the patient will require rehabilitation interventions at another point in the care continuum. Rehabilitative needs that are not fully addressed during the patient's acute inpatient hospitalization are likely to require increased rehabilitation interventions in the patient's postacute care. Likewise, patients with major medical illnesses such as cancer[45] may receive rehabilitative interventions in a rehabilitation setting, but they are often liable to need transfer back to the acute medical inpatient setting if their medical condition worsens.[46]

REHABILITATION TEAM

Rehabilitation is an approach to care provided by a team of professionals. Although physicians specializing in physical medicine and rehabilitation, physical therapists, and occupational therapists are most closely identified with rehabilitation practice, the rehabilitation approach is applicable to older patients being cared for by geriatricians, primary care physicians, orthopedists, neurologists, nurses, psychologists, social workers, and most other health care professionals. In a given case, all rehabilitation disciplines involved will have a discipline-specific focus to their portion of the comprehensive assessment. Table 13-1 lists and briefly describes the roles of various rehabilitation professionals.

> An important preventive measure in primary care is to encourage physical activity to help patients achieve a higher level of baseline function, so that they will have more functional reserve during an illness.

TABLE 13-1	Roles of Rehabilitation Team Professionals
Physiatrist (physical medicine–trained MD)	Evaluates patient, integrates assessment data, determines potential, coordinates rehabilitation plan
Primary Care Physician	Manages acute and chronic medical care
Rehabilitation Nurse	Integrates medical, nursing, rehabilitation plan
Physical Therapist	Addresses mobility, strength, range of motion
Occupational Therapist	Addresses activities of daily living and self-care
Speech Pathologist	Addresses communication, swallowing
Psychologist and Neuropsychologist	Diagnosis/treatment of mood, behavioral, and cognitive conditions
Social Worker	Works with family, patient, financial counseling, discharge planning
Nutritionist	Assesses nutrition status, diet plan
Pharmacist	Reviews medication use
Audiologist	Provides hearing assessment and treatment
Vocational Counselor	Evaluates work potential, provides training
Recreational Therapist	Assists with hobbies, leisure activities, motivation
Orthotist/Prosthetist	Makes and fits orthopedic aids

Adapted from Warshaw GA. Rehabilitation and the aged. In: Gallo JJ, Busby-Whitehead J, Rabins PV, et al, editors. Care of the elderly: Clinical aspects of aging. 5th ed. Philadelphia: Lippincott Williams & Wilkins; 1999, p. 275.

PREVENTION OF FUNCTIONAL DECLINE AND ANTICIPATORY PLANNING

In planning for the primary care of an older individual, even one without current functional limitations, it is useful to consider with the patient the possibility that he or she may become frail in the future. Individuals may vary over time in their degree of disability[47] and in their needs for rehabilitation. Intermittent episodes of disability may be a marker for underlying frailty, and they may contribute to worsening frailty by leading to inactivity and deconditioning. Among the community-dwelling elderly, a commonly reported pattern is to spend occasional brief (one to several days) episodes at bed rest because of illness, injury, or other complaints. Patients with a history of episodic bed rest are at increased risk for functional decline.[48]

Advance planning for the possibility of functional decline may help ameliorate the degree of disability produced by future functional limitations. This may involve such seemingly nonmedical issues as the choice of housing in middle age, that is, an environment that will meet potential future needs. The degree of disability produced in later life by a hip fracture, and the patient's concomitant rehabilitation needs, may differ if the patient lives in a building with access only by staircase than in one with elevator or ramp accessibility. Reassessment of the patient's need for rehabilitation services, and for other services such as social services, may be particularly useful at times when the patient's overall medical condition changes. It may also be of value at times when the patient's system of social supports is altered, such as by the death of a spouse.

Various clinical interventions have been evaluated to test their impact on preventing disability. A detailed multispecialty evaluation of each older patient's functional status may be difficult to accomplish in routine primary care practice, and the yield may be relatively small.[49] One strategy for increasing the yield of rehabilitative care is to focus on situations of highest risk. Clinical situations that pose a particular risk for the onset of disability are hospitalizations (particularly after a fall) and episodes of restricted physical activity.[50] These clinical situations may be particularly fruitful settings for a focus on measures to decrease the risk for incident disability.

One of the important preventive measures in primary care is to encourage physical activity, to help patients achieve a higher level of baseline function, so that they will have more functional reserve. Patients who later experience a functional decline may regain some or all of their functional loss, but they are at high risk for losing function again in the near future. They are more likely to recover their independence of function, and to maintain their regained independence of function for a longer period of time, if they have a baseline pattern of habitual physical activity.[51]

Low-cost rehabilitative strategies may be most feasible for community-dwelling patients in generally stable condition.[52] These may be as straightforward as group exercise programs. In many cases, these strategies will be able to establish a higher functional status for the patient, so that if the patient has a subsequent decline in functional status it will not produce as severe a degree of functional deficit.

CASE 1

Alan Baker (Part 2)

After his last visit to you, you arranged for Mr. Baker to attend a local senior center 3 days a week (Monday, Wednesday, Friday). His son has also been coming to check on him each Sunday. His son says that he also phones his father every Tuesday, Thursday, and Saturday mornings.

You receive a call Monday morning that Mr. Baker is in the emergency room. He slipped on the ice when he went to pick up his morning newspaper. The emergency room physician reports that your patient has a foul-smelling ulcer of his left heel, with bone exposed. He has no focal neurologic deficits, but he thinks he is at home. Mr. Baker's ECG is unchanged from when you recently saw him in your office.

1. **What are Mr. Baker's current rehabilitative needs?**

2. **What additional rehabilitation issues are likely to arise in the succeeding year?** ▣

PREVENTION OF DECONDITIONING DURING ACUTE ILLNESS

Deconditioning is a common occurrence in the hospital setting during an acute medical illness.[53] The temporal association raises the concern that deconditioning may result not only from the medical illness that led to the hospitalization, but also from the hospitalization itself. In order to maintain mobility independence, adequate lower extremity strength and speed are important, as is balance.[54] Even a brief hospitalization tends to produce declines in mobility, limb strength, and even of respiratory muscle strength. A study of brain-dead organ donors who were maintained on a ventilator for 18 to 69 hours demonstrated that, even in that brief interval on a ventilator, diaphragmatic muscle atrophy occurred of both slow and fast muscle fibers.[55]

Some lack of activity may be inherent to the patient's medical condition, but there is considerable evidence to suggest that much of the loss of mobility in the hospital exceeds any medical necessity. In a study of patients who had long stays in the intensive care unit (minimum of 2 weeks, mean of 3.1 weeks), more than a third of the patients developed at least one functionally significant joint contracture, and such contractures usually were still present at the time of hospital discharge. Even if patients have limited ability for active movement, and so are at high risk for further deconditioning, they may well benefit from passive range-of-motion exercises to decrease their risk for developing contractures.

Unnecessarily restricting the patient to bed rest is certainly a strategy to be avoided, but functional declines can be anticipated to occur even if the hospitalized patient has not been ordered to stay in bed.[56] Rehabilitative strategies to prevent or treat deconditioning, therefore, must consider not just the acute medical illness but also the hospital environment, with active consideration of how to integrate rehabilitation into the overall pattern of care.

One strategy that has been employed to prevent deconditioning is a multidisciplinary intervention to promote early mobilization, including involvement by a physiotherapist early in the hospitalization and exercises at least twice a day. This kind of approach did not aim merely to get the patient up from bed to chair, but rather was able to get the patient to spend substantial amounts of time standing and walking.[57]

An important tactic to maintain function in the acute medical patient is to minimize the risk factors for functional decline. One goal of inpatient rehabilitative interventions will often be to prevent further medical complications. In the stroke patient with dysphagia, for example, swallowing rehabilitation potentially can decrease the risk for aspiration pneumonia. Aspiration pneumonia in the stroke patient conversely may be associated with a poorer rehabilitative outcome from his or her poststroke rehabilitation.[58] Worsening of acute medical condition is a common cause for interruption of rehabilitation efforts, with the risk that the efforts may never be resumed.[59]

The multiple demands placed on the patient by inpatient procedural care, delivered on the institution's schedule, may often conflict with the patient's typical rhythm for sleep and for meals. Of note, the hospitalized patient's normal pattern of sleep architecture can also be significantly disrupted, even if the total amount of sleep in a 24-hour cycle is maintained by multiple short fragments of sleep time throughout the night and day.[60,61] In combination, the resultant sleep pattern disruption and negative nutritional impact can leave the fragile older patient poorly equipped to maintain his or her functional status. Patient who have had disrupted sleep may also have impaired daytime alertness, which can affect their ability to participate in rehabilitation and other aspects of their care.

GAIT REHABILITATION, HIP REPLACEMENTS, AND FRACTURES

Patients may attempt to adjust to their gait problems by using strategies such as walking more slowly. Slower walking speed by itself may prove a good compensatory strategy when walking on difficult terrain for older individuals in good health,[62] and even for those with exercise limitations from mild chronic stable angina, but is much less likely to compensate for the effects of diabetic peripheral neuropathy on proprioception.[63] One component of therapy for patients with gait limitation is likely to be physical activity tailored to patient abilities. Frail older patients who engage in even very modest amounts of informal exercise (walking more than one block per day) are likely to preserve their residual mobility better than patients who are more sedentary.[64] Patient selection for rehabilitation should not be restricted by chronologic age, as appropriate patients even in their 90s have been shown to derive benefit from a rehabilitation program.[65,66]

Primary clinicians are in an excellent position to encourage increased physical activity by their patients. One strategy to do so is to identify particularly those patients who are already in the contemplative phase of considering an exercise program, and then to target them with motivational advice and educational materials on the benefit to them of exercise.[67] Printed patient educational materials are far less likely to be useful, however, in meeting the rehabilitation needs of patients who are more acutely ill,[68] particularly if they may suffer from delirium or dementia.

Patients with gait problems may benefit from use of a cane (used in the hand contralateral to the weak leg) or a walker, and there are a variety of each type of device available. A cane, and even more so a walker, permits the upper body muscles to support part of the person's weight. Assistive devices can also widen the patient's base of support, and can offer tactile feedback via the cane to one hand or via the walker to both hands.

These mobility aids can also be associated with falls. The very reason that individuals were prescribed a cane or walker may have been that their gait was unsteady and they were diagnosed as a fall risk. Use of an assistive device can interfere with the patient's ability to use a stairway banister or a wall for stability. The patient can potentially trip over the device itself. Further, use of a cane or walker requires the person to change his or her customary way of walking, a task that may be difficult to master, particularly in the older patient with cognitive impairment.[69] Rehabilitation efforts are likely to be even more challenging if the older patient has required an amputation,[70] such as for diabetic complications.

Rehabilitation therapy can be of benefit to older individuals with a variety of musculoskeletal conditions,[71] including those with lower extremity fractures or following joint replacement surgery. A rehabilitation program is often an important part of the postoperative course of the older patient. The patient may often derive great benefit if the rehabilitation is begun in the early postoperative period in the hospital, rather than being delayed until the patient is discharged from the acute care setting. In one small study of patients who had unilateral hip replacement, early postoperative rehabilitation shortened the mean length of stay in hospital by 6 days.[72] Unfortunately many older individuals will fail to adhere to recommendations for postoperative exercise in the months after they return home.[73]

A concern that sometimes arises in the inpatient rehabilitation setting is that the patient may fall during rehabilitation. Fear of falling by the patient or family can limit the effectiveness of efforts to mobilize the patient. It is noteworthy in that regard that falls in fact are less likely to be injurious when patients are being supervised during therapy sessions, and the improvement in gait with therapy is designed to increase their safety when they may later walk unsupervised.

One study of inpatient falls in a rehabilitation center found that almost 19% of the residents fell at least once, some more than once, but that fractures were uncommon. In this series of 1472 total patients, 140 patients fell at least once; there were 171 falls in total, but only two fractures resulted from the 171 falls. The falls generally did not occur during therapy sessions, but rather mostly occurred when patients were alone unobserved in their room (typically when they were attempting to transit to the bathroom).[74] The important point is that gait rehabilitation should be regarded as a beneficial rather than risky activity.

> **A patient who has a hip fracture may still be ambulatory. Early recognition of the fracture is important for appropriate management.**

Hip fractures are classified into three major categories according to anatomic location: femoral neck (subcapital or intracapsular), intertrochanteric, and subtrochanteric.[75] Hip fractures are an important cause of functional decline in the older individual.[76] The presentation is often clear in a patient with inability to walk and with pain and limb deformity after a fall, but some patients will have much less striking findings.[77] Early recognition of the fracture facilitates prompt management, which is usually surgical in nature, to achieve the best outcome in subsequent rehabilitation. The particular surgical approach to a fracture will vary according to the surgeon's technical

preference, the patient's comorbidities, as well as the site of the fracture[78] and whether it is displaced.

Efforts to avoid medical complications in the immediate postoperative period are imperative. Deep venous thrombosis is a particular risk with and after hip surgery, and it has been recommended that patients receive antithrombotic therapy.[79] Attention to removing bladder catheters postoperatively will help avoid urinary tract infections. Delirium is also a potential concern in the older individual with recent hip fracture, who has undergone the stresses both of a hip fracture and of the orthopedic surgical procedure for repair of the fracture.

Pressure ulcers may result from a combination of factors—sustained high local pressures such as at the site of a bony prominence, shear forces on the underlying tissue, frictional damage to the skin, moisture of the skin—all of which may be present in the patient undergoing rehabilitation.[80] Medications that cause decreased level of consciousness, and devices and lines that restrict patient mobility, may increase the risk for pressure ulcers. Adequate skin care requires exemplary nursing care, including repeated repositioning of those patients with impaired mobility.

> **Better functional outcomes for frail, older hip fracture patients may occur if (following their routine postoperative physical therapy) they undergo an additional 6 months of supervised outpatient rehabilitation.**

Even in frail older patients, prompt surgical intervention is commonly required for hip fracture to achieve the best functional result. Early mobilization postoperatively is also an important part of the patient's care, and the recent trend has been to be more liberal in allowing weight bearing by the patient postoperatively.[81] The older patient with a preexisting cognitive deficit may be unable to participate in any therapy that involves degrees of weight bearing. As a practical matter, it is much easier for the physical therapist to administer postoperative rehabilitation if the doctor's orders allow weight bearing.

A randomized controlled trial has demonstrated better functional outcomes for older hip fracture patients if (following their routine postoperative physical therapy) they undergo an additional 6 months of supervised outpatient rehabilitation, rather than the control condition of simply being discharged from postoperative therapy with advice on home exercise.[82] Attention during rehabilitation to factors that may have placed the patient at risk for his or her first hip fracture (osteoporosis, gait unsteadiness) is important because the older patient with a hip fracture remains at risk for a second hip fracture.[83]

Osteoarthritis of the hip or knee can produce significant limitation of function, and the primary therapy for long-term treatment of severe osteoarthritis is surgical in nature. Rehabilitation therapy[84] has a role in some patients with milder disease as a component of nonsurgical management; in other cases it helps delay the need for surgery, and in still others to assist in postoperative recovery after orthopedic surgery.[85,86]

STROKE REHABILITATION

An important setting where rehabilitation is often needed is in the older patient following a stroke. The nature of rehabilitation services required will reflect the array of neurologic deficits following the event. Patient participation in a rehabilitation program may require emotional support for the patient who is suffering from depression after a stroke. Communication difficulties between patient and therapist, such as in the patient who has a receptive aphasia following a stroke, may also require special attention in order to work effectively with the patient on rehabilitation of various neurologic deficits.

Rehabilitation efforts can begin even during the stroke hospitalization. In particular, efforts should be made to avoid or minimize deconditioning while in the hospital, using measures consistent with the patient's overall condition. Even if the patient is not capable of walking, periods of standing up or even sitting in a chair can help to minimize the deconditioning from bed rest in the hospital.[87] The interdisciplinary rehabilitation approach should include not only the therapy disciplines themselves, but also other caregivers including the nursing staff and family.[88]

Given the risk for episodic disability, important goals of a rehabilitative program may be to try to decrease the risk for recurrent episodes of disability, as well as to help diminish the length and severity of episodes of present and potential future episodes of disability. In a study of hospitalized ischemic stroke patients, those who achieved higher levels of physical function after their stroke were less likely to require hospital readmission in the succeeding 12 months.[89]

Rehabilitation treatment for the stroke patient derives from an ongoing team assessment. The physical therapist's focus is on strength, endurance, and mobility. Motor recovery may display a sequence of patterns. The stroke patient initially may have a flaccid paralysis, which may be followed by phase(s) where groups of muscles act in synergy, before the patient finally regains ability to move individual joints. Only some recovering stroke patients go through such a sequence, and it is often associated with limb spasticity.[90] Although this sequence can vary from case to case, it is helpful to recognize that certain patterns can be capitalized on to assist with particular activities (e.g., extensor synergy and walking).[91] Treatment begins with bed mobility and progresses to balance training and sitting. Ambulation requires adequate strength and trunk stability. Patients with severe impairments may begin walking in parallel bars and then be advanced to walkers or canes. If weakness in the lower leg is present, an ankle-foot orthosis (short leg brace) can promote more efficient ambulation by ensuring fixed dorsiflexion at the ankle and minimizing toe dragging in the swing phase of gait.

The occupational therapist addresses upper extremity function and the ability to perform ADLs and instrumental activities of daily living (IADLs), and visual-spatial perception deficits. Maintenance of range of motion in the affected upper extremity is essential to avoid the development of a painful shoulder or contractures. When distal upper extremity spasm is present, wrist splints are prescribed. To avoid shoulder subluxation, transfers are managed without additional stress on the shoulder joint, and pillows and arm boards are used to support the affected arm. These positioning techniques maintain the humeral head in its proper position when the muscles usually responsible for this alignment are flaccid. Dressing aids, such as clothes reachers, button hooks, sock donners, and Velcro closures may be prescribed. Feeding aids, such as rocker knives and plate guards, can be helpful.

Impairment of language function can be the most frustrating consequence of stroke. Dysarthria and aphasia require assessment by a speech pathologist. Communication boards can be provided to help patients with expressive aphasia make their wishes known. The speech pathologist can also help rehabilitation team members communicate with the patient. The patient's ability to swallow should be assessed before oral fluids and food are started.

Often the most important goal for rehabilitative efforts after stroke is to enable the patient to return home. Depending on the patient's rehabilitative needs, and on the level of support available in the home environment, the process may involve a stay in a subacute unit or an SNF after discharge from the acute hospital setting. Many rehabilitative services can be delivered in the home (or other outpatient) setting, and rehabilitative care begun in the hospital may often be continued at home after discharge. An important primary care goal in such cases is to make sure that there is continuity of the rehabilitative plan across changes in the care setting.

A home rehabilitation process can decrease overall length of stay compared to a program that delivers all the rehabilitation as an inpatient in one or a mix of facilities (e.g., acute care hospital, subacute unit, SNF).[92] The therapist in the home setting can ensure that patients can transfer the rehabilitation skills learned in the hospital and apply them in the environment where they are residing, to help them maintain their ability to live independently.[93] It also provides an opportunity

BOX 13-1

ASSESSMENT OF DISCHARGE ENVIRONMENT

Functional needs
Motivation and preferences
Intensity of tolerable treatment
   Equipment
   Duration
Availability and eligibility
Transportation
Home assessment for safety

Source: U.S. Department of Veterans Affairs. VA/DoD clinical practice guideline for the management of stroke rehabilitation in the primary care setting. Available at www.oqp.med.va.gov/cpg /STR/STR_base.htm.

to directly evaluate the home setting across a variety of dimensions[94] (Box 13-1). These evaluations will determine, for example, if the level of home lighting and the arrangement of furniture will help the patient to maneuver safely in the home.

The use of earlier hospital discharge, coupled with postdischarge rehabilitation services at home, has been demonstrated to decrease health care costs and improve functional outcomes.[95] A Swedish randomized study of poststroke rehabilitation suggests durable benefit for stroke patients if one supplemented their inpatient stroke unit rehabilitation, by adding the use following discharge home of a course of home rehabilitation. Although this intervention involved only a mean of 12 home visits delivered over a mean of 4 months, the patients receiving the home rehabilitation showed benefit on functional outcomes assessed 5 years later.[96]

> Common poststroke medical complications include depression, shoulder pain, falls, and urinary tract infection.

Rehabilitative efforts may often be designed to meet goals of particular relevance to patient quality of life. A focus of rehabilitation may often be to increase the individual's ability to participate in society, such as to leave his or her home, and even modest interventions may have significant effects. An occupational therapy intervention for stroke patients, for example, significantly improved patients' outdoor mobility even though it involved a mean of only 230 minutes total contact time (spread over several visits) of the patient with the therapist.[97]

In patients recovering from a stroke, functional impairment may result not just from muscle weakness alone, but also from its combination with other neurologic deficits. The goals of rehabilitation efforts typically are designed around improving function, rather than around improving a specific neurologic parameter, such as the degree of spasticity. Spasticity after a stroke can further interfere with function. Spasticity, however, can also be used as part of a compensatory strategy for poststroke weakness in the same muscle group.[98]

In the ongoing care of the patient, of particular concern are the complications that may follow a stroke or other disabling event and can potentially interfere with successful rehabilitation. In a Canadian study of a group of stroke patients admitted for inpatient stroke rehabilitation, during their rehabilitation stay (mean length of stay 40 days) two thirds had at least one event characterized by the study author as a medical complication, and a quarter of the patients had multiple such complications. The four most common complications noted were depression, shoulder pain, falls, and urinary tract infection.[99]

The propensity for falls is of special concern because many elderly stroke patients may have baseline osteoporosis, a condition that will likely worsen over time (particularly if they have poor mobility after their stroke).[100] The combination of fall risk and osteoporosis places these patients at risk for hip fracture when they walk or transfer. Interventions to preserve bone mass (bisphosphonate therapy, dietary and/or supplemental calcium and vitamin D) will commonly be useful as part of their management.

CARDIAC REHABILITATION

A common area where rehabilitation may be underused is across the spectrum of patients with cardiac disease,[101-103] and the patient may benefit from clinician encouragement to enter and then to remain with a rehabilitation program. A patient who has just undergone hospitalization for a cardiac event may be particularly motivated to begin a cardiac rehabilitation program.

Patient participation in rehabilitation may be compromised particularly if the patient does not drive and lacks ready access to other transportation to the rehabilitation setting.[104] Cardiac rehabilitation may successfully be delivered in the home setting if resources to do so are available.[105]

A cardiac rehabilitation program can appropriately incorporate an individualized exercise program, as part of the effort to prevent a recurrent cardiac event, and in order to improve the patient's capability to perform daily activities. Occasional cardiac events have been reported during the exercise component of cardiac rehabilitation, and a subset of patients may benefit from more intensive monitoring of their cardiac status during exercise. The long-term benefits in general far outweigh the very small risk of engaging in a supervised cardiac exercise program.

The American Heart Association has strongly endorsed the benefits of a coordinated approach to cardiac rehabilitation, including exercise training, modification of cardiac risk factors, and attention to psychological and social function.[106] A cardiac rehabilitation program may include simultaneous attention to both increasing physical activity and to a variety of other lifestyle changes, such as smoking cessation. A regular exercise program may complement a smoking-cessation program, particularly in patients who have been advised to stop smoking and are concerned about attendant weight gain.

Rehabilitation has been broadly recommended as appropriate for a variety of cardiac conditions, including for patients who have suffered a myocardial infarction (MI). However, only 35% of Americans who experience an MI actually receive cardiac rehabilitation. Women are particularly unlikely to receive cardiac rehabilitation after an MI, echoing a common theme of gender disparity in cardiac care.[107]

Both younger and older patients can benefit from cardiac rehabilitation. Cardiac patients in general, and in some studies the older cardiac patients in particular, are often either not receiving referrals to cardiac rehabilitation or are failing to participate after being referred.[108] The clinician in the primary care setting is in an excellent position to reinforce at outpatient office visits the need for cardiac rehabilitation[109] and to encourage continuing adherence to rehabilitation attendance and lifestyle changes. One innovative strategy that has been suggested to increase referrals for cardiac rehabilitation is to use a system of automated referrals of eligible patients, as triggered by the electronic medical record, but still coupled with a personalized letter to the patient.[110]

> There is evidence for the benefit of starting a program of pulmonary rehabilitation within 10 days following hospital discharge following an exacerbation of chronic obstructive pulmonary disease.

PULMONARY REHABILITATION

Rehabilitation including exercise training may be of particular value for patients with chronic obstructive pulmonary disease (COPD), in order to improve exercise tolerance, reduce dyspnea, and improve quality of life.[111] There is evidence for benefit from starting a program of pulmonary rehabilitation within 10 days following hospital discharge following an exacerbation of COPD.[112] Much of the benefit of pulmonary rehabilitation by exercise training, such as lower extremity exercise (e.g., stationary bicycle riding), comes from the improvement of peripheral muscle function rather than from an effect on the ventilatory muscles.[113,114] Home pulmonary rehabilitation has also been delivered in a program using telephone follow-up by the therapist,[115]

but such minimally supervised exercise strategies require a cognitively intact, motivated patient.

REHABILITATION IN CANCER PATIENTS

Older patients with incurable malignancy may derive significant benefit from a brief and focused rehabilitation program.[116] Rehabilitation may help the patient cope with functional deficits related to the effects of the cancer itself or the therapy received for the cancer. A cancer patient, for example, may have gait difficulty and associated rehabilitative needs for a variety of reasons, ranging from pathologic lower extremity fracture from metastatic cancer, to stroke from brain metastases, to postoperative deficits following surgical excision of a lower extremity sarcoma. Therapy in the cancer setting may also often appropriately consider strategies to help the patient cope with potential future deficits if the cancer progresses.

A particular challenge may be how to integrate a rehabilitation program with a program of cancer treatment, particularly in a patient who may be experiencing fatigue and cachexia related to cancer. However, various studies have been done of exercise programs for cancer, with some evidence that exercise in the setting of cancer can promote a decrease rather than an increase in patient fatigue.[117]

Pain control may often be the primary quality-of-life goal for the patient especially if life expectancy is limited, whether by cancer or otherwise. Even patients with a poor prognosis may benefit from appropriately structured rehabilitation efforts focused on pain prevention. Inadequately treated pain is not only a problem in itself; it can also interfere with the achievement of rehabilitation goals for the patient.[118] Rehabilitation physical modalities such as ultrasound, massage, and local application of heat or cold can contribute to the pain-control regimen, and may be used in conjunction with pharmacologic means of pain control.[119] (See Chapter 27.)

AGING WITH A LONG-STANDING DISABILITY

One of the most challenging areas in geriatric rehabilitative care is the treatment of older patients who have long-standing disabilities from early in life. They may lose some of the physical strength and other reserves they had drawn upon earlier to cope with their baseline disability. The ongoing challenge of coping with their disability may lead to complaints including sleep disorders, pain, or fatigue even in late middle age. Patients may perceive this as aging more rapidly and/or with more complications. In the patient with spinal cord injury,[120] for example, even young patients may have issues of skin breakdown from immobility, and these issues may become even more pressing as the patient ages and becomes less mobile. Individuals with spinal cord injury are at high risk for functional decline if they suffer medical complications such as pressure ulcers.[121]

The care of aging adults with disability may be especially complicated when their parents provide the patient's care, and then the parents themselves become disabled or die. The patients and their families in the past may have given more consideration to their medical needs in the short to medium term, and less to the issues of aging that have become important as patients have prolonged survival despite their disability.[122] Rehabilitation efforts should consider how to address the patient's long-term disability, and how those efforts may need to be reshaped as the patient ages and as their network of social supports may change.

Declines in functional reserve may affect the patient's use of compensatory strategies. A person with baseline paraplegia, for example, may achieve mobility by wheelchair. If the patient later loses upper extremity strength, for example, the patient may lose some of the ability to accomplish wheelchair ambulation. In some cases, these functional declines can be addressed by a change in the rehabilitative regimen, such as from a manually operated wheelchair to an electrically powered wheelchair.

REHABILITATION IN SETTING OF MULTIPLE COMORBIDITIES

Older individuals with a functional limitation may have a combination of other acute and chronic illnesses, many of which can also influence their rehabilitation. Meeting the rehabilitative needs of these complex patients is likely to require a high degree of communication and individualized planning of care. Care planning requires a thorough understanding of the full range of the patient's medical problems, and this task may be particularly complex in the oldest old. Rehabilitative needs should be addressed in the context of other medical issues; rehabilitation following a stroke is important, but even more valuable is stroke-risk reduction by more effective treatment of hypertension.

Rehabilitation for the typical older patient with an acute illness is likely to raise some challenges relative to rehabilitation for the typical younger patient. On average, older patients are more likely to have had significant comorbidities even before their acute illness, and to have entered their acute illness at a lower functional baseline. A particular challenge in the rehabilitation of the older patient is not just achieving functional improvement, but then of maintaining the rehabilitation gains.[123] Nevertheless, the older patient with acute medical illness often can derive great benefit from rehabilitative care.

Much of the support for postacute rehabilitation rests on expert opinion and nonrandomized experience rather than on randomized clinical trials. The dose of rehabilitation received by a patient reflects not only this evidence base, but also the dictates of regulatory bodies such as Medicare. One review suggests that multidisciplinary therapy is particularly beneficial for rehabilitation of the stroke patient.[124]

Therapy for older patients commonly includes the efforts of more than one clinical discipline (PT, OT, speech therapy, nursing, physician) and it can be difficult to sort out which components of the interdisciplinary mix were of the most rehabilitative benefit. A further complicating factor is that a patient who receives therapy from multiple disciplines is likely to get more total rehabilitative effort per day, and so it may be difficult to identify whether the more effective source of therapeutic gain is the interdisciplinary nature of the therapy or if it is instead the total combined amount of therapy.

There is some evidence of a dose response to rehabilitation, with those patients receiving longer treatment sessions improving more than those patients receiving shorter treatment sessions.[125] Not all patients, however, may tolerate lengthy treatment sessions, especially if they were quite sedentary and deconditioned at baseline, so both the length and the content of the rehabilitation session may require modification. Prophylactic analgesia prior to rehabilitation sessions may aid tolerance in those with osteoarthritis. Diabetic patients may need downward adjustment of their insulin regimen if they increase their physical activity substantially with a rehabilitation program.

REHABILITATION AND COGNITIVE PROBLEMS

An issue that commonly arises in rehabilitative geriatric care is the role of rehabilitation in the patient with cognitive impairment.[126,127] Cognitive impairment may tend to lessen the benefit an individual may derive from a rehabilitation program.[128] This may be particularly the case if the rehabilitative program calls on the patient to perform cognitive tasks that are beyond his or her ability. Even mild degrees of cognitive impairment may impede the recovery of more intellectually challenging abilities, such as those represented by the instrumental acitvities of daily living (IADLs).[128a 128b]

Rehabilitative efforts in patients with traumatic brain injury, stroke, or other neurologic insults may be particularly difficult if the insult itself has impaired the patient's self-awareness of a deficit. This lack of self-awareness may manifest itself as a marked difference in how the patient sees the severity of his or her condition compared to how the family members view the deficit's severity.[129] There is evidence from a study of postmenopausal women with stroke that patients' own assessment of their level of function frequently differs from that shown on standardized tests, and this disparity was particularly common in women in certain subgroups, such as those with multiple comorbidities and those with cognitive impairment. For those women for whom self-assessment of function and objective assessment of function were discordant, it was overwhelmingly the case that the patients overestimated their level of function compared to that seen on objective testing. In the setting of reduced self-awareness of one's own deficits, it may be particularly challenging to simultaneously promote patient independence while managing the risk to the patient from injudicious choices.[130]

Learning strategies may work better if tailored to meet the cognitive abilities and learning style of the patient.[131,132] In the patient with dementia, for example, rehabilitation strategies need to be tailored to the patient's cognitive abilities. This may involve use of very specific prompts for each of the components of a task.[133] Even patients with substantial cognitive impairment can benefit from appropriately designed rehabilitation.[134] Appropriate rehabilitative exercise interventions can benefit patients with cognitive impairment, not only in terms of physical endpoints such as strength and flexibility, but also in terms of helping to preserve ability to perform ADLs.[135,136]

In general, delivery of rehabilitation interventions may need to be tailored to fit not just the acute medical condition but also the patient's chronic level of function. Even healthy cognitively intact elders demonstrate a deterioration in their ambulation skills if they are asked to perform cognitive tasks (such as mental arithmetic)[137] that make it more difficult for them to concentrate on their walking. It is prudent, therefore, to provide a rehabilitation environment that enables the patient to focus his or her attention on the rehabilitation process.

> Even minor depression may be associated with a poorer degree of short-term functional improvement during a course of subacute rehabilitation.

REHABILITATION AND DEPRESSION

The older patient's mental state may affect his or her ability to obtain a good rehabilitation outcome. Depression may have been present as a chronic condition or may begin with an acute illness such as a stroke.[138] Delirium (whether as the full blown syndrome or as a subsyndromal variant) can begin coincident with hospitalization for an acute medical illness, but it can persist for many weeks after discharge and impede functional recovery.[139]

Depression is common in the rehabilitation setting and can be exacerbated by the patient having experienced the functional loss that precipitated the need for rehabilitation. Depression is commonly seen in the older stroke patient but can also be present in the patient with disabilities arising from a variety of causes. There is evidence that even minor depression may be associated with a poorer degree of short-term functional improvement by the patient from a course of subacute rehabilitation.[140] Depression also is a risk factor for early rehospitalization following a course of inpatient medical rehabilitation.[141]

REHABILITATION AND NUTRITION

One factor that may complicate the patient's hospital course[142] and make rehabilitation more difficult is inadequate nutrition. The older hospitalized patient may often have inadequate nutritional intake.[143,144] In the case of patients after stroke, depending not only on the patient population investigated but also on the criterion used, malnutrition has been argued to affect anywhere from 6.1% to 62% of patients.[145] An older patient after a stroke may have difficulty consuming adequate calories because of dysphagia, inability to handle eating utensils, or even depression.[146,147]

Malnutrition may limit the patient's ability to cooperate in a poststroke rehabilitation program or to gain muscle mass. In the patient with malnutrition, rigid restrictions on the dietary content (e.g., salt, saturated fats) may often be counterproductive, because increasing caloric intake and protein intake may be the overriding nutritional goals.

Dietary modifications may include changes in the consistency or the caloric density of the food. The patient may benefit from assistance during meals, including reminders to eat, and may need an extended time for meals. Clinical monitoring of the patient's hydration status is also important to avoid dehydration, particularly in older patients who may have a decreased sense of thirst and/or a decreased ability to communicate to caregivers that they are thirsty (see Chapter 28).

ASSISTIVE DEVICES

Assistive devices are used to relieve pain and maintain or restore function. Patients with functional losses who perceive a need for an assistive device need help choosing appropriate equipment. Assistive devices that address problems with hearing, vision, mobility, and most ADLs and IADLs are available. Most require patient education and training for proper use. Physical and occupational therapists can assist the physician, patient, and family in the selection and proper use of available products. Table 13-2 is a summary of selected assistive devices.

TABLE 13-2	Selected Assistive Devices	
Functional Problem	**Device**	**Comments**
Bathing	"Soap on a rope"	Will help when reaching is impaired. These aids will require adequate grip.
	Long-handle back sponge	Helps with strength and range of motion.
	Tub seat or bench	Allows for safe sitting in the bathtub.
	Grab bars	Reducing the risk of falls during transfers is crucial.
	Tub transfer bench	Bridges the tub side with two legs in the tub and two legs beside the tub.
	Hand-held shower hose	
Toileting	Raised toilet seat	Handrails can be attached to the wall or a free-standing frame. Versa frames can be used.
	Bedside commode	
Oral care	Toothbrush grip	
Dressing	Reaching device	Aids in picking things off the floor.
	Button hook	Helps with hand weakness or loss of agility.
	Sock donners	Sock aid helps if hip flexion is limited.
	Velcro closures	Velcro substitutes for buttons or shoelaces.
	Elastic shoelaces	Aid in dressing.
	Clothes hook	
	Long shoehorns	
Grooming	Electric razor	
	Tilt mirror	
	Built-up grips on handles	
Eating	Built-up grips	Grips help with arthritis or decreased strength.
	High-edged plates and nonskid pads	Keep food on plate and plate on table.
	Rocker knives	Allow one-handed food cutting.
	Cups with lids	Useful to prevent spilling that occurs with intention tremor.
Mobility	Orthoses	Foot-modified shoes and lifts.
	Ankle-foot (AFO)	Plastic shell or metal brace used for mild limb weakness (foot drop) after knee-ankle-foot (KAFO) stroke. Aids weight bearing or alignment.
	Cane (hemi-cane or hemi-walker)	Aids knee support. With or without hinge.
	Tri- or quad-cane	A four-point frame that provides considerable support to the hemiplegic standard cane patient. All canes held on the side opposite involved leg. More support than single-point cane. Comes with wide or narrow base. Pistol grip is best. With tip positioned on ground, elbow is flexed 25 degrees.
	Walker (standard rubber tips)	Need to lift when moving. Helps with weakness or imbalance if grip strength is poor, but can be fitted with platform grip attached to forearm if proximal strength is adequate.
	Walker (roller front, three- or four-wheel models)	Can have brakes and cargo baskets. Provides help with balance, but less support than standard walker. Can help patients with Parkinson's disease, unstable gait, or person with limited cardiorespiratory reserve for whom lifting would intolerably increase work (e.g., COPD, CHF).
	Wheelchairs (standard)	Provided if limited endurance or inability to walk. Need to be carefully fitted: seat width, arm height, seat cushion, foot rests. Folding models available.
	Scooter (powered)	A three-wheeled, electric scooter can help with mobility over long distances.

Adapted from Brummel-Smith K. Rehabilitation. In: Ham R, Sloane P, editors. Primary care geriatrics. 2nd ed. St. Louis: Mosby Yearbook; 1992, p. 137-61; Friedmann LW, Capulong ES. Specific assistive aids. In: Williams TF, editor. Rehabilitation in the aging. New York: Raven Press; 1984, p. 315-44; Wasson JH, Gall V, MacDonald R, Liang MH. The prescription of assistive devices for the elderly: Practical considerations. J Gen Intern Med 1990;5:46-54; and Wilson GB. Progressive mobilization. In: Sine RD, Liss SE, Roush RE, et al, editors. Basic rehabilitation techniques. 3rd ed. Rockville, MD: Aspen Publishers; 1988, p. 132-6.
CHF, congestive heart failure; *COPD,* Chronic obstructive pulmonary disease.

Deciding which is the most appropriate device and teaching the patient its appropriate use are probably beyond the scope of the average primary care physician. However, many older persons use self-purchased canes for which they were never properly evaluated and so may be using entirely the wrong type of gait assistive device for their needs, be using the cane improperly, or have an improperly sized cane. Thus, the primary care physician who sees a patient with a cane should ascertain that the cane is in good repair (e.g., rubber tip intact, no cracks), that it is the right size (commonly measured to reach the height of the greater trochanter), and that the patient uses it properly (e.g. for patients with unilateral lower extremity osteoarthritis, he or she generally holds the cane with the contralateral arm).[147a 147b]

A common fate of rehabilitative equipment is for it to go unused by the patient. This may result if the equipment is not a good fit for the patient's cognitive abilities. It may occur if use of the equipment requires more physical strength or coordination than the patient possesses. It may also occur if the patient has unrealistic expectations of what the equipment will accomplish, and is disappointed when these expectations are not fulfilled. Or it may be that the patient does not wish to display in public that he or she has a need for adaptive equipment.

> The use of an assistive device can interfere with the patient's ability to use a stairway banister or a wall for stability and actually increase the risk for a fall.

Figure 13-2[148] displays a checklist that can be helpful in planning with patient and caregivers whether to issue a particular device to the patient. As part of the primary care follow-up of patients who have recently been issued a device such as a wheelchair, it is helpful to ask them about their experience using it, and also to note whether they in fact use it when they come to their follow-up primary care appointment.

MAKE SURE THE MEDICAL DEVICE YOU CHOOSE IS DESIGNED FOR YOU

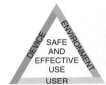

This checklist is designed for health care professionals and patients to use when choosing a medical device that is best for the patient. It is intended to be modified by health professionals to focus on particular devices for certain target populations (e.g., arthritics, diabetics, heart patients).

1. **Do _you_ have limitations that can affect your use of the device?**
   - ☐ Could your health (stress, tired, medication effects, disease) affect the way you use the device?
   - ☐ Do you have the physical size and strength (hand strength, lifting ability, and endurance) to use the device?
   - ☐ Will you be able to see the display, hear the alarm, and feel the controls (knobs, buttons, switches, and keypads)?
   - ☐ Do you have the coordination (manual dexterity, balance) to adjust the controls?
   - ☐ Will you be able to understand and use the device?
   - ☐ Do you need to remember complex instructions to use the device?

2. **Is the device right for the _environment_ where you plan to use it?**
   - ☐ Does the device have safety features to prevent it from harming your children or pets, and to prevent them from harming the device?
   - ☐ Will you be able to hear the device's alarm in a noisy environment?
   - ☐ Will the light levels (low or bright) in your environment affect your ability to use the device?
   - ☐ Are you using other devices at the same time?
   - ☐ Will sources of electromagnetic interference (e.g., ham radio, AM FM TV broadcast antenna, electrical machinery, hand-held transmitters) affect the device?
   - ☐ What things about your home will affect your use of the device (e.g., high heat and humidity, very dry air in the winter, too few electrical outlets, narrow doorways, wood stove heating)?
   - ☐ What happens if you put the device in an inappropriate environment?

3. **Are there _device characteristics_ that can affect its use?**
   - ☐ Is the device simple to set up, operate, clean, maintain, and dispose of, and what happens if you don't do these things properly?
   - ☐ What replacement parts or batteries are required, how frequently are they needed, how expensive are they, and are there special instructions for safely disposing of the device or its parts?
   - ☐ What reading or training is required of you?
   - ☐ Are there things about this device that are different from other similar devices you have operated?

Figure 13-2 Checklist to use when choosing a medical device for a patient. (U.S. Food and Drug Administration. Make Sure the Medical Device You Choose is Designed For You. Available at: http://www.fda.gov/MedicalDevices/DeviceRegulationandGuidance/HumanFactors/ucm128199.htm. Accessibility verified August 23, 2013.)

CASE 1

Discussion

Mr. Baker is a man with two chronic illnesses, both poorly controlled. His history of erratic compliance with his anti-hypertensive regimen suggests that noncompliance may also be a factor in his diabetes management. His history suggests that this patient with diabetes suffered a silent myocardial infarction a month ago, with resultant congestive heart failure.

He is a candidate for cardiac rehabilitation, but he is also likely to have additional rehabilitative needs now or in the future. He has recently lost his wife, who was important in meeting his transportation needs. The fact that he was brought in by a neighbor rather than a family member may suggest that his other family supports are limited. Further history is necessary to determine whether he has functional limitations that impair his ability to care for himself in other ways as well, and which would require rehabilitation.

An assessment for cognitive impairment is indicated, because this may have contributed to his giving up driving and to his forgetfulness about taking his medicines. He is also at risk for depression in the wake of the death of his wife. His cardiac event may be related to the stress of that loss.

Findings and Goals

Mr. Baker had been managing at home with a social support system consisting of both family and institutional supports. He had developed a lower extremity ulcer, which he either did not notice or ignored, and his physical findings suggest that the ulcer has likely progressed to osteomyelitis.

His neurologic findings are more consistent with delirium rather than a stroke. Control of his foot infection may help with his confusion, but Mr. Baker clearly cannot manage for now living alone at home.

An immediate rehabilitation goal is to avoid deconditioning while he begins therapy (debridement, systemic antibiotic treatment) for his infection. Preserving his muscle strength is important to preserve his ability to walk, whether or not he ultimately requires surgery. If he responds to conservative measures, he will benefit from shoes designed to avoid pressure on the healing area. He is at high risk for needing an amputation if he does not quickly respond to more conservative measures. If he does undergo amputation, he will need rehabilitation to walk with a prosthesis, a process that may be complicated by his cardiac disease and resultant impaired exercise tolerance. ▣

SUMMARY

Many older individuals have difficulty with gait or other areas of function that interfere with their ability to accomplish the activities of daily living. The level of function can fluctuate over time, and rehabilitation efforts can be directed to preserve current function and to seek to recover lost function. Many older individuals have a variety of comorbidities rather than just an isolated functional deficit. An important goal of primary care is to ensure that these multiple medical and rehabilitative needs are addressed in a coordinated and comprehensive fashion

ACKNOWLEDGMENT

The author is a federal employee but the personal opinions are those of the author and do not necessarily represent the view of the Department of Veterans Affairs.

Web Resources

www.aapmr.org. American Academy of Physical Medicine and Rehabilitation.

www.rehab.research.va.gov/jrrd. U.S. Department of Veterans Affairs' *Journal of Rehabilitation Research and Development.*

www.ah.ouhsc.edu/geriatric_resources/walkers.htm. University of Oklahoma, Geriatric Rehabilitation Resource for Oklahoma: "Using Walkers."

www.ah.ouhsc.edu/geriatric_resources/canes.htm. University of Oklahoma, Geriatric Rehabilitation Resource for Oklahoma: "Using Canes."

KEY REFERENCES

7. Covinsky KE, Pierluissi E, Johnston CB. Hospitalization-associated disability: "She was probably able to ambulate, but I'm not sure." JAMA 2011;306(16):1782.

8. Ettinger WH. Can hospitalization-associated disability be prevented? JAMA 2011;306(16):1800.

9. Gill TM, Gahbauer EA, Han L, Allore HG. Functional trajectories in older persons admitted to a nursing home with disability after an acute hospitalization. J Am Geriatr Soc 2009;57:195.

32. Boninger JW, Gans BM, Chan L. Patient protection and affordable care act: Potential effects on physical medicine and rehabilitation. Arch Phys Med Rehabil 2012;93(6):929-34.

44. Dudgeon BJ, Hoffman JM, Ciol MA, et al. Managing activity difficulties at home: A survey of Medicare beneficiaries. Arch Phys Med Rehabil 2008;89:1256.

References available online at expertconsult.com.

14

Palliative Care

Nathan E. Goldstein and R. Sean Morrison

OBJECTIVES

Upon completion of this chapter, the reader will be able to:

- Understand the difference between palliative care and hospice.
- Be familiar with the basics of pain management, including pain assessment and treatment.
- Be familiar with the most common nonpain symptoms encountered in palliative care.
- Create a basic framework for structuring conversations with patients and families for both breaking bad news and negotiating goals of care.

CASE 1

Holly Johnson (Part 1)

Holly Johnson is a 70-year-old woman who was diagnosed with stage III ovarian cancer 3 years ago. At that time, she received a total abdominal hysterectomy and bilateral salpingo-oophorectomy along with adjuvant chemotherapy. Six months ago on a routine follow-up appointment with her gynecologic oncologist, her lab results showed a rise in her CA 125 level, and she was diagnosed with a recurrence. Despite chemotherapy, her disease showed continued progression on a follow-up imaging study. She currently lives with her husband who is in good health. Although she was independent 8 months ago, her functional status has now deteriorated and she currently needs assistance with her activities of daily living. Her physicians no longer believe that she would benefit from further chemotherapy. ◼

CASE 2

Pam Rodriguez (Part 1)

Pam Rodriguez is a 70-year-old woman with a medical history significant for osteoarthritis, advanced heart failure, mild cognitive impairment, and diabetes, who has been hospitalized for 6 days with pneumonia. This is her third hospitalization in the past year; the other two were for exacerbations of her heart failure. She is currently debilitated and cannot return to her home. Prior to this hospitalization, she was living in the community with her partner (who is also in failing health). She requires assistance with shopping, cleaning, and cooking. They have two adult sons who live in neighboring towns.

1. **As a member of your hospital's inpatient palliative care consult service, how would you approach the care of this patient and the patient from Case 1, Ms. Johnson?**

2. **How does palliative care for Ms. Johnson differ from that for Ms. Rodriguez?** ◼

WHAT IS PALLIATIVE CARE?

At the turn of the twentieth century, the average life expectancy was 47,[1] and people usually died suddenly as the result of trauma or infection. Over the last 100 years, however, advances in medicine such as antibiotics, improvements in nutrition, and developments in public health and safety have led to a greatly increased longevity such that the average life expectancy in 2001 was 77 years.[1] As a consequence, the typical death is no longer a sudden or unexpected event. Rather, death today usually follows a lengthy period of chronic illness and functional dependency, such that chronic disease has become the leading cause of death. Evidence across all health care settings and disease categories demonstrates a high prevalence of physical, psychosocial, and financial suffering associated with serious illness and chronic disease.

Partly in response to these changes, the field of palliative care has arisen to address the needs of patients and families that have not been well met by traditional medical care. Erroneously, the phrase *palliative care* is sometimes conceived as care that should be provided at the end of life when treatments directed

---

Additional online-only material indicated by icon.

at life prolongation are no longer effective and death is imminent. In actuality, palliative care is interdisciplinary care focused on improving quality of life for patients with serious illness and their family caregivers.[2] It involves formal symptom assessment and treatment, aid with decision making regarding the benefits and burdens of various therapies, help in establishing goals of care, and collaborative and seamless transitions between models of care (hospital, home, nursing homes, and hospice) so as to provide an added layer of support to families and health care providers. Palliative care should be offered simultaneously with life-prolonging and curative therapies for persons living with serious illness (Figure 14-1).

In this sense, the field of palliative care attempts to overcome the artificial dichotomy of cure versus comfort that has been established. A key contributor to this division of health care is the Medicare hospice benefit, which requires that patients forgo life-sustaining care to be able to receive hospice and must have a predictable prognosis of 6 months or less to live. This ignores the fact that the overwhelming majority of older adults living with serious illness require both life-prolonging and palliative treatments at the same time.

With this distinction in mind, it becomes clear that both patients presented in the opening case studies of this chapter can benefit from palliative care, but in different ways. Palliative care for Holly Johnson, with her advanced ovarian cancer and poor functional status, involves treating her symptoms (e.g., nausea, pain, depression), addressing her psychological and spiritual concerns, supporting her husband, and helping to arrange for her increasing care needs. The majority of this patient's care occurs at home (with or without hospice) or in the hospital, and the period of functional debility is relatively brief (months). This differs from the care that Pam Rodriguez needs. Palliative care for this patient involves treating the primary disease process (her advanced heart failure); managing her multiple chronic medical conditions and comorbidities (diabetes, arthritis) and geriatric syndromes (cognitive impairment); assessing and treating the physical and psychological symptom distress associated with all of these medical issues; and establishing goals of care and treatment plans in the setting of an unpredictable prognosis. Additionally, the needs of her caregiver(s) are different from the needs of Holly Johnson's caregiver(s). Ms. Johnson may have only a few months to live. The individuals caring for Ms. Rodriguez will most likely be her adult children who have their own families, work responsibilities, and medical conditions; these roles must be balanced with the months to years of personal care that they must provide to their aging parent. Like most elderly patients, both Ms. Johnson and Ms. Rodriguez can be expected to make multiple transitions across care settings (home, hospital, rehabilitation, long-term care),[3] especially in the last months of life, and palliative care programs for older adults must ensure that care plans and patient goals are maintained from one setting to another.

In this sense, palliative care in the elderly is most appropriately centered on the identification and amelioration of functional and cognitive impairment, intervening to lessen caregiver burnout, and reducing the burden of symptoms. This is in contrast to typical care for patients in a hospice setting, for example, where management is focused on advanced terminal illness and its immediate manifestations. In response to the unique needs of older adults, palliative care is an integral part of geriatric medicine.

> Palliative care is interdisciplinary care focused on the relief of suffering and achieving the best possible quality of life for patients with serious illness and their family caregivers. It is offered simultaneously with other treatments for persons with serious illness, as opposed to hospice, which is focused only on those who are actively dying and which requires patients to agree to forgo life-sustaining treatments.

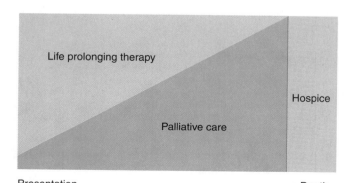

Figure 14-1 Palliative care is offered simultaneously with life-prolonging and curative therapies for persons living with serious, complex, and advanced illness.

CASE 1

Holly Johnson (Part 2)

On your initial visit with Holly Johnson, she describes pain that is not well controlled. You are able to elicit that her pain is a dull ache throughout her abdomen, which is occasionally punctuated by periods of sharp pain when she turns in bed or tries to transfer from the bed to chair. She rates her pain as a 7 out of 10, and the nurse on your interdisciplinary team informs you that she is no longer getting out of bed because of the pain. She is currently on a regimen of Tylenol #3 (acetaminophen 300 mg/codeine 30 mg) by mouth every 6 hours as needed. On review of her medication records, you note that she has consistently asked for it every 6 hours since admission. When you ask if she finds the current regimen acceptable, she states that she does not want anything stronger because she wants to save the "stronger medications for when I will really need them later."

1. **How would you change Ms. Johnson's pain medications?**

2. **How would you address her concern about waiting to take pain medications until she "really" needs them?** ▣

CASE 2

Pam Rodriguez (Part 2)

On your initial visit with Pam Rodriguez, you ask if she has pain. She states that while she does not actually have pain, she does have an intermittent diffuse ache throughout her body. When you ask her to further characterize this discomfort, she cannot further elaborate on it but is able to rate it as mild to moderate. In addition, she complains of an electric, tingling sensation in both of her feet that she has had for several years. On review of her hospital medications, you see that she currently has an order for ibuprofen 400 mg by mouth every 4 hours as needed.

1. **What types of pain is Ms. Rodriguez describing?**

2. **What changes would you suggest to her pain regimen?** ▣

ASSESSING AND TREATING PAIN IN OLDER ADULTS

Pain is an unpleasant sensory and emotional experience associated with actual or potential tissue damage.[4] Nearly 50% of severely ill hospitalized patients report that they have pain.[5,6] Pain in older patients may be poorly controlled because they may underreport pain or may have difficulty communicating, and physicians may undertreat pain because of concerns about side effects in older patients.[7]

Neuropathic pain results from injury to actual nerve fibers as a result of compression, infiltration, or degeneration of neurons in either the peripheral or central nervous system.[8] Patients often describe this pain as burning, tingling, stabbing, or electrical, and they tend to experience it as severe and constant. Examples of neuropathic pain include diabetic neuropathy, pain related to spinal stenosis, and pain resulting from trigeminal neuralgia.

It is important to distinguish between the various types of pain because each is treated differently. Nociceptive pain is treated with, and often responds well to, traditional medications such as acetaminophen, nonsteroidal antiinflammatory drugs (NSAIDs), and opioids. Although neuropathic pain may respond to traditional analgesic agents, with this type of pain it is often necessary to use adjuvant agents such as tricyclic antidepressants, anticonvulsants, corticosteroids, or local anesthetic agents.[9-12]

Pain Assessment

The treatment of pain begins with a thorough and complete assessment. The guiding principle of pain assessment is to ask patients about their pain and then believe their complaints. Several studies have shown that providers' estimates of a patient's pain severity are often lower than the patient's self-report.[13,14] Assessment of pain involves multiple components, and practitioners must consider each in order to best understand the nature and character of a patient's symptoms.

The first step of assessment is to inquire about the location of the pain as well as whether it radiates to any other part of the patient's body. A description of the pain to determine if its origin is nociceptive, neuropathic, or some combination of both should be obtained as well as questions as to when the patient's pain began; this information is required because chronic pain is often treated differently than acute pain. Additionally, it is important to ask what treatments (pharmacologic or otherwise) the patient has tried to relieve the pain as well as any factors that may exacerbate the pain. Temporal patterns of the patient's pain should be understood. For example, joint pain that is relieved shortly after awakening is more likely to be from osteoarthritis than from rheumatoid arthritis. If patients do not freely offer information about these characteristics, then it is important to continue probing until the physician has a complete understanding of the nature of the patient's pain and its associated factors. For a useful mnemonic device for assessing pain, see Box 14-1.

Patients should be asked to rate their pain to better understand its severity as well as to give a baseline assessment to determine changes in the level of pain after treatment.[7] The same scale should be used over time in each patient, so as to best be able to reliably track changes in pain over time. Patients can be asked

---

BOX 14-1

MNEMONIC DEVICE FOR ASSESSING PAIN

O = Onset—When did the pain begin?
P = Provokes/Palliates—What makes the pain worse or better?
Q = Quality—What is the nature of the pain?
R = Radiation—Does the pain go to any other portion of the body?
S = Severity—How bad is the pain? (0 to 10 scale; mild, moderate, severe)
T = Temporal—Is there a certain time of day when the pain is better or worse?

to rate their pain in either words (none, mild, moderate, severe) or using a numeric scale (0 to 10 where 0 is no pain and 10 is the worst pain experienced). They can also be shown a visual analog scale, where patients place a mark indicating their level of discomfort on a horizontal line representing a spectrum of pain (the leftmost portion of the line represents no pain, the rightmost, severe pain). Another visual scale often used includes a series of faces representing various states of emotion relating to the patient's current level of pain.

In addition to the assessment principles outlined above, a crucial component of pain in older adults relates to its impact on function. The presence of symptoms that limit patients' activities of daily living (ADLs)[15] should trigger physicians to focus on the home environment and may signal the need for additional home care services. In cases where the patient cannot provide a thorough history because of conditions such as dementia or aphasia, this information can be obtained from nursing staff and the patient's family.[7] The clinician's physical examination should be used to confirm any suspicion generated during the history taking. Conditions to note include muscle spasm, gait impairment, abnormal joint alignments, and changes in skin color or integrity—to name just a few.[16]

Physicians may have particular difficulty in assessing pain in older individuals for several reasons. Patients may have physiologic barriers to reporting pain such as difficulties with hearing or vision as well as cognitive impairment. These difficulties are not insurmountable, however. Assistive listening devices or visual scales can be used to facilitate pain assessment in patients with hearing loss. Patients with poor vision should be encouraged to express their pain using either a numerical or verbal scale. For patients with both visual and hearing impairments, techniques such as pointing and gesturing are often effective.

Clinicians may assume that they cannot assess pain in individuals with cognitive impairment, but this is often not the case.[17] Patients with cognitive impairment or aphasia are often able to give basic information if questions are asked in a yes/no format. In addition, physicians can use signs such as facial expressions (grimacing or frowning), diaphoresis, and changes in vocal patterns (e.g., increased moaning or changes in pitch) as signs that a patient may be in distress. Clinicians can also ask family members and paid caregivers to report their impressions of the patient's pain as well. Unfortunately, clinical studies have shown that patients' and family members' ratings of pain are not always well correlated, with family members often underestimating the patient's pain intensity.[18-20] With this in mind, however, clinicians may be able to begin with the family's assessment of the cognitively impaired patient and add to this the other visual and diagnostic clues discussed above to better estimate a patient's level of pain.

Older patients' fear of addiction has also been shown to be one of many barriers to effective pain management.[16,21] One way to counteract this barrier is to educate patients and their families about addiction and how it differs from tolerance and dependence.

Tolerance is a pharmacologic phenomenon that refers to diminished analgesic effect of a constant dose of a medication after exposure over time.[16] Tolerance routinely develops after patients receive opioid medications, and relates both to the analgesic properties of the medication (i.e., patients may need more of a medication over time to obtain the same analgesic effect) and to its side effects (e.g., patients will develop tolerance to the sedative effect after a short period of time). Typically when patients with cancer or other systemic diseases begin to need increasing doses of a medication, it is a result of progression of the underlying disease rather than the development of tolerance.

Dependence refers to a biological phenomenon whereupon patients may develop withdrawal symptoms once the medication is discontinued.[7] For example, patients who have been on chronic opioid therapy may experience diarrhea and a dramatic increase in their level of pain if the medication is abruptly halted. Addiction refers to continued use and seeking of a medication despite harm to self and others. This phenomenon is rarely seen in patients who are treated for chronic pain, and is seen no more often in patients with cancer than in the general population.[22] One way to avoid this confusion is to avoid the use of terms such as narcotics and drugs because these words may be associated with societal stigmas. Clinicians must differentiate addiction from pseudoaddiction, a phenomenon in which patients exhibit drug-seeking behavior because of undertreatment of their pain. This is an iatrogenic phenomenon, and it will resolve itself when patients are given an adequate medication regimen with appropriate dosing intervals.[23]

Treatment of Pain

The basic and most widely used approach to management of pain is illustrated by the World Health Organization's "pain ladder"[24] (Figure 14-2). Although originally developed to assist clinicians with assessing and managing pain in patients with cancer, the model can be extended to nonmalignant painful conditions in elderly individuals such as osteoarthritis or pathologic fractures resulting from osteoporosis. The first step, for patients with mild pain, encourages the use of nonopioid medications such as acetaminophen or NSAIDs with or without an adjuvant agent (see following section).[25] If a patient's pain increases to

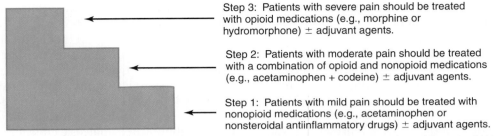

Step 3: Patients with severe pain should be treated with opioid medications (e.g., morphine or hydromorphone) ± adjuvant agents.

Step 2: Patients with moderate pain should be treated with a combination of opioid and nonopioid medications (e.g., acetaminophen + codeine) ± adjuvant agents.

Step 1: Patients with mild pain should be treated with nonopioid medications (e.g., acetaminophen or nonsteroidal antiinflammatory drugs) ± adjuvant agents.

Figure 14-2   Schematic of levels of pain and appropriate medications to use at each step. (Adapted from World Health Organization (WHO). Cancer pain relief. Geneva: WHO; 1986, with permission.)

a moderate level or remains poorly controlled, the next step involves adding a weak opioid medication alone or in combination with the nonopioid (e.g., acetaminophen with oxycodone) with or without the use of an adjuvant agent. The third step, for patients with severe pain, advises the use of a strong opioid (e.g., morphine, hydromorphone) with or without an adjuvant. Recent evidence suggests that patients with moderate or severe pain, especially that related to cancer, may receive faster pain relief by being started on a strong opioid regimen immediately rather than progressing in such a stepwise fashion or employing weak opioids (e.g., codeine) or combination products.[26,27]

Adjuvant agents are medications that can be combined with opioid therapies to either decrease the dose of medication needed or to avoid dose-related side effects. The term *adjuvant* refers to the fact that these medications are drugs with a primary indication other than pain, but they have analgesic properties in some painful conditions.[12] Adjuvant analgesics include antidepressants, corticosteroids, local anesthetics, anticonvulsants, muscle relaxants, osteoclast inhibitors, N-methyl-D-aspartate (NMDA) receptor blockers, alpha-2 adrenergic agents, and radiopharmaceuticals, to name only a few.[28] Some experience is helpful in the use of these medications, however. For example, some of the tricyclic antidepressants (e.g., nortriptyline), selective serotonin reuptake inhibitors (SSRIs) (e.g., paroxetine, citalopram), and anticonvulsants (e.g., gabapentin) are used routinely by primary care physicians as adjuvants, but at doses far below the threshold of being effective for pain management.[12] Recent evidence suggests that combination treatment with an opioid and gabapentin is superior to either agent alone.[29]

When prescribing medications for older patients, the issue of cost and accessibility must be taken into account. Analgesic medications can be expensive, particularly for patients on fixed incomes. Clinicians should inquire how patients pay for their prescriptions to ensure that they have the means to obtain the necessary medications. In addition, certain medications may be difficult to obtain because of local concerns about stocking controlled substances.[30]

Although a thorough discussion of individual pain medications is beyond the scope of this discussion, what follows is a general discussion of the various classes of analgesics and some important points that clinicians should consider when prescribing these agents.

Nonopioid Medications

This category consists mostly of acetaminophen and NSAIDs. Acetaminophen is primarily metabolized by the liver, so patients should not take doses greater than 4 g per day because of hepatotoxicity. NSAIDs are limited owing to the potential side effects of gastric irritation and bleeding, inhibition of platelet function, and worsening of renal function. Of note, the analgesic ceiling dose for NSAIDs is often below that of the manufacturer's recommended dose, so approaching or exceeding the maximum dose often does not result in an increase in analgesic effect.[31] The use of cyclooxygenase (COX)-2 selective agents, while once thought of as an alternative to traditional NSAIDs in older patients because of the lower incidence of gastrointestinal and antiplatelet effects, has come under considerable scrutiny recently owing to cardiovascular complications; thus these medications should be reserved for patients with clear indications after a discussion of the risks and benefits of these medications.[32]

Opioid Medications

Medications in the opioid class mimic the action of naturally occurring opioid peptides and bind to receptors in both the brain and the spinal cord. Unlike acetaminophen and NSAIDs, these medications exhibit no ceiling effect and can produce profound analgesia by gradual dose escalation. In addition, opioids have no long-term toxicity and can be used for years without concerns about organ damage. In the case of Holly Johnson, simply explaining this to her may help to assuage her fears about taking these medications before she "really" needs them.

Opioids can be administered through both enteral and parenteral routes. Morphine, for example, comes in pill, liquid, and suppository form, and can be swallowed or absorbed through the rectal mucosa. In addition, there are both short-acting (i.e., immediate release) and long-acting (i.e., sustained) preparations. Opioids can also be given intravenously, subcutaneously, intramuscularly (although this form is not preferred because of both the pain associated with the injection and the erratic absorption), and absorbed transcutaneously. Rates of onset of analgesic effect differ among these various routes, however. Opioids given intravenously often have an onset within minutes; when taken orally these medications have a longer time to onset, at approximately 1 hour. Subcutaneous injections have a time to onset of approximately 30 minutes. The transdermal fentanyl patch may take from 12 to 24 hours after first application before maximum effect is achieved.

In addition to choosing the route of medication administration, it is important to pay special attention to the dosing interval. Analgesic medications may be given either episodically (i.e., prn—on an as-needed basis) or at regular intervals (i.e., around the clock).[8] Pain that occurs intermittently is best treated with episodic dosing, but pain that is expected to last for an extended period (e.g., postsurgical pain that is expected to last several days, or chronic pain) should be treated with both a regular dosing schedule and a backup additional medication given as needed to relieve breakthrough pain. In these cases, all patients should receive a standing dose of medication with a rescue dose that is approximately 10% of the total daily dose. For example, a regimen of sustained-release morphine 30 mg by mouth every 12 hours would be a total daily dose of 60 mg; thus an appropriate dosing regimen would be written as sustained release morphine 30 mg by mouth every 12 hours along with immediate-release morphine 6 mg by mouth every 1 hour as needed for breakthrough pain.

In prescribing medications on an as-needed basis, one must be sure that the dosing interval is shorter than the duration that the medication is expected to last. For example, dosing acetaminophen with codeine every 6 hours is inappropriate given that the analgesic effect of codeine lasts for approximately 4 hours. In this regimen, Holly Johnson may be in pain for 2 hours before she receives the next dose. In addition, it is important to pay attention to the maximum dose of combination medications. If a patient takes the combination above (specifically acetaminophen 300 mg combined with 30 mg of codeine, also known as Tylenol #3) as one tablet every 4 hours, the patient will receive a total of 1800 mg of acetaminophen—two tablets dosed in this manner will have a patient receive nearly the maximum daily dose of 4 g.

A complete explanation of starting dosages and titration of medications is beyond the scope of this discussion, but there are certain important points that should be stressed. Dosing of opioid medications is based on the half-life of the particular medication and its formulation. As noted earlier, morphine and its related compounds come in short-, intermediate-, and long-acting forms. These medications should be dosed according to manufacturer instructions, but clinicians should remember that metabolism in older individuals is affected not only by age but also by the simultaneous ingestion of other medications (both prescription and nonprescription). Methadone is particularly difficult to dose because of its extremely long half-life, and its use should be reserved only for those individuals familiar with its pharmacokinetics that change over a range of doses.

No discussion of opioid medications would be complete without a discussion of common side effects. The most common side effect of this class of medications is constipation. This is so common that clinicians should start a prophylactic bowel regimen at the same time as beginning opioids,[32] unless contraindicated, especially given that many elderly patients suffer from chronic constipation. Bowel regimens should include a stool softener in addition to either one or a combination of the following laxatives: fiber/bulk-forming, stimulant, and osmotic agents. Nausea and vomiting can also be seen in patients started on opioid medications, but before starting an antiemetic, one must rule out fecal impaction. Diarrhea in the setting of opioid use should alert the clinician to the possibility of overflow incontinence, where a patient may be so obstructed by fecal material that the only matter allowed to pass around the obstruction is of a liquid nature. Other common side effects of opioids include sweating, dry mouth, and urinary retention. Physicians are often most concerned about respiratory depression, but if patients are started on appropriate opioid doses with a gradual escalation over time, this phenomenon is rare. In addition, respiratory depression rarely occurs without a forewarning change in the patient's mental status. The other worrisome but rare side effect of opioid medications is clonus and, in rare cases, seizures. This class of medications is metabolized in the liver and then excreted by the kidney, so caution must be used in giving patients with renal failure certain opioids. For example, the metabolite of meperidine—normeperidine—can accumulate and lead to seizures in patients with decreased glomerular filtration, such as is the case in older adults. For this and other reasons, it is recommended that meperidine not be used.

In the cases discussed earlier, Holly Johnson's pain regimen is currently inappropriate. Codeine is a weak opioid agonist, and the dosing interval of 6 hours is longer than the analgesic half-life of 4 hours. An as-needed dosing schedule is inappropriate given Ms. Johnson's level of pain. A better regimen would be to start morphine elixir 5 mg via mouth every 4 hours, with a rescue dose of 3 mg (5 mg/dose × 6 doses/day = 30 mg total daily dose; 10% [3 mg] is the as-needed dose) every 1 hour as needed. Even without a history of constipation, she should be started on a bowel regimen at the same time. In terms of Pam Rodriguez's pain, ibuprofen is an inappropriate medication given her underlying cardiac disease and concerns with potentially worsening her renal failure. Given that her pain is mild and intermittent, a more appropriate starting medication for her would be acetaminophen 650 mg every 4 hours as needed for pain. Ms. Rodriguez also is complaining of neuropathic pain in her feet, most likely from her underlying diabetes, and she should be started on a medication such as gabapentin for this pain.

CASE 1

Holly Johnson (Part 3)

The next day, you go to see Holly Johnson. She now states that her pain is well controlled, and she has only needed one of the rescue doses of morphine. However, she does note that she has vomited twice in the last 12 hours. This morning she is tearful and does not make eye contact when you speak with her.

1. **What medications would you consider using for Ms. Johnson's nausea?**
2. **Is she depressed, and if so how would you treat her depression given her life expectancy?** ◘

CASE 2

Pam Rodriguez (Part 3)

When you go to see Pam Rodriguez the next day, she states that she had a "rough night." She was feeling extremely short of breath for most of the evening, and it took several doses of parenteral furosemide to relieve her dyspnea. Although she is now comfortable, she is anxious that her shortness of breath may return. On further questioning, she admits that she has occasional problems with anxiety and has a prescription for lorazepam at home that she takes on an as-needed basis.

1. **What recommendations would you have for the team to help treat Ms. Rodriguez's dyspnea?**
2. **How would you treat her anxiety?** ◘

MANAGEMENT OF NONPAIN SYMPTOMS

Patients with chronic illness may have multiple nonpain symptoms over the course of their illness; some of the more common nonpain symptoms that may accompany chronic illness are nausea, dyspnea, depression, anxiety, anorexia/cachexia, fatigue, and pruritis. Discussion of all of these topics is beyond the scope of this chapter, so instead we will focus on the first four.

Multiple physiologic processes underlie the sensation of nausea, so therapy is best directed at the mechanism behind the symptom. The three main areas related to the sensation of nausea are the brain's chemoreceptor trigger zone (located in the area postrema at the base of the fourth ventricle, where the fenestrated capillary walls allow a breakdown of the blood–brain barrier, thus exposing the dopamine, serotonin, acetylcholine, and opioid receptors in this area to the levels of these substances in the bloodstream), the vomiting center (located in the medulla, this area integrates information from the cortex, limbic and vestibular systems, chemoreceptor trigger zone, and vagal input, and it is rich in dopamine, acetylcholine, serotonin, opioid, and histamine receptors), and the gastrointestinal (GI) tract (abdominal organs are rich in serotonin receptors as well as substance P).[33,34] The main classes of medications used for nausea and vomiting are the dopaminergic antagonists, anticholinergics, antihistamines, and serotonin antagonists. The dopaminergic agents such as prochlorperazine, chlorpromazine, and metoclopramide antagonize dopamine receptors in the chemoreceptor trigger zone, but metoclopramide also increases GI motility by binding to cholinergic receptors in the GI tract, so it is contraindicated in patients with bowel obstruction. Anticholinergic agents such as scopolamine work in the vestibular system and in the vomiting center, but these agents should be used with caution in older patients because of their numerous side effects. Serotonin agents such as ondansetron and granisetron are particularly good for patients with chemotherapy-induced nausea. Other agents used in the treatment of nausea are steroids (which act by reducing edema in the bowel wall and brain), aprepitant (which inhibits substance P in the GI tract), octreotide (which reduces GI secretions by reducing blood flow), and benzodiazepines (especially useful in anticipatory vomiting from chemotherapy). Holly Johnson should be started on prochlorperazine, and then other agents can be added that work via alternate pathways as necessary.

Although depression in patients near the end of life may be difficult to diagnose, it is never normal and should always be treated to enable patients to have the highest quality of life in their remaining time. Characteristics of depression such as insomnia, weight loss, and anorexia may not be reliable in patients near the end of life because they may be symptoms of the underlying disease. Two more reliable questions may be, "Do you feel sad or depressed?" and "Have you recently dropped many of your interests and activities?" If patients answer yes to both of these questions, then there is a high likelihood that they are depressed.[35] Although a prevailing fallacy among clinical staff is often that "the patient has cancer; of course they are depressed and do not need to be treated," there are effective medications which should be tried. The SSRIs are usually a good place to begin therapy for depression, but some of these medications may take 3 to 6 weeks before an effect is seen. If a patient has a shorter life expectancy, it may be advisable to begin a stimulant, such as methylphenidate, which should improve patients' mood and increase their energy level within days. Of note, this medication may cause anorexia, so it should be used with caution in patients who may already have this symptom. In general, anorexia can be effectively treated; numerous studies have shown that patients with cancer treated with steroids or megestrol exhibit an increased appetite, which improves their quality of life, but these medications have not been shown to have an effect on survival.[36]

One of the most distressing symptoms for patients and their families is that of dyspnea. The pathophysiology of dyspnea is complex, and it involves sensory input from the chest wall muscles, lung parenchyma receptors, and carotid bodies, as well as output from the brain respiratory center and higher input from the cerebral cortex.[34] The sensation of dyspnea is subjective. It is not correlated with oxygen saturation or partial pressures of oxygen or carbon dioxide in the blood, and thus treating it with oxygen may not always ameliorate the symptom. The most effective way to improve dyspnea is to determine its underlying cause and then treat it. The differential diagnosis for breathlessness is broad, and includes heart failure/ pulmonary edema, anemia, bronchospasm, bronchial obstruction, anxiety, pulmonary embolism, pneumonia, and inability to clear or increased thickness of airway secretions. Treating dyspnea is an ongoing process, and small doses of morphine (2 to 4 mg by mouth in an opioid-naive patient) can be very effective. There is a large body of evidence to show that morphine is effective in treating dyspnea,[37-39] and mechanisms for this action include its ability to decrease respiratory drive in the brainstem, its binding to opioid receptors in the lung itself,[7] and its central ability to decrease the sensation of breathlessness.[40] Although there is not as much evidence supporting the use of benzodiazepines in the treatment of dyspnea, this class of medications may certainly relieve the anxiety associated with breathlessness, and they may decrease central respiratory drive as well. Opioids and benzodiazepines should be used with caution, however, to ensure that they are used to decrease the sensation of dyspnea but not at doses to inhibit the respiratory drive completely so as to cause oversedation and apnea. Finally, nonpharmacologic therapies such as reducing room temperature, repositioning

the patient, introducing humidity, and educating patients and families may also help to reduce the sensation of dyspnea. A fan blowing air across the face of a patient is thought to stimulate the V_2 branch of the trigeminal nerve, thus inhibiting respiratory drive and decreasing the sensation of breathlessness.

Anxiety in patients with chronic disease can be distressing to patients and families, and it can interfere with care. Although anxiety itself causes patients to suffer, it can also lead to insomnia, depression, fatigue, and withdrawal from social supports.[34] Patients should be asked routinely about anxiety; too often it is ignored, trivialized, or accepted as inevitable. Like dyspnea, it is important to determine other factors that may be adding to the patient's anxiety. For example, pain that is not well controlled, dyspnea, and side effects of other medications (e.g., steroids, albuterol, or withdrawal from alcohol, opioids, and sedatives) may all contribute to anxiety. Anxiety that is incapacitating, induces behavioral changes, or that is continuous and ongoing should be treated pharmacologically. In the case of Pam Rodriguez, she has a long-standing history of anxiety and has been treated for it as an outpatient, two factors that indicate that she should be treated with medications in the inpatient setting as well. Although there is not a great deal of evidence comparing benzodiazepines, lorazepam is the most commonly used agent. Other benzodiazepines may have half-lives that are either too long or too short (e.g., clonazepam and alprazolam, respectively) to be effective, especially at the end of life.[41] Neuroleptic medications may be useful in certain conditions. If a patient's anxiety is not treated by benzodiazepines, or if delirium or psychotic symptoms are present, haloperidol may be effective.[34] To date, there are no data to suggest that newer, more expensive, atypical antipsychotic agents (e.g., olanzapine, risperidone, quetiapine) are more effective than haloperidol for this condition, although some patients (e.g., those with Parkinson's disease) may benefit from their different side-effect profile (quetiapine in particular is thought to have a more favorable side-effect profile, although the evidence for this is mostly anecdotal). Given recent data demonstrating a possible relationship between antipsychotic agents and increased mortality, these medications should be used with caution in older adults. Thioridazine may be a useful agent if sedation is desired, especially if a patient has insomnia or agitation.[34] Agents such as buspirone may be effective for patients who have anxiety associated with depression, but antidepressants can take weeks to become effective and as such are not efficacious in treating patients with acute anxiety. Education can be an important component in the treatment of anxiety. For Pam Rodriguez, education about the cause of her dyspnea and the medication that can be used to help relieve it (e.g., morphine, furosemide) may be as effective as a benzodiazepine.

> Patients with chronic disease, regardless of etiology, have multiple symptoms—both pain and nonpain (e.g., nausea, dyspnea, depression, anxiety). There are effective treatments for these, and no patient should be left feeling uncomfortable or with uncontrolled symptoms.

CASE 1

Discussion

Now that Holly Johnson's symptoms are well controlled, you arrange a family meeting to talk with her, her husband, and her adult children. The gynecologic oncologist is unable to attend, but has made it clear that there are no other surgical, radiologic, or chemotherapeutic options. Before you are even able to sit down in the room for the family meeting, the patient asks, "What other options are there for treating my cancer?"

How would you go about answering Ms. Johnson's question about other medical interventions? ◪

CASE 2

Discussion

By the end of the week, Pam Rodriguez is greatly improved, and the primary team has asked you to help arrange a safe discharge plan for the patient. All parties involved, including the patient and her partner, are in agreement that subacute rehabilitation is the next appropriate step. The patient seems to understand the plan, but she asks, "How long will I have to keep coming back and forth to the hospital?"

What more would you want to know about Ms. Rodriguez before you were able to come up with a plan for her care? ◪

COMMUNICATING WITH PATIENTS AND FAMILIES

One of the most important components of palliative care is communication skills, particularly when it comes to breaking bad news. Although there is no substitute for observing a skilled physician having these conversations or being observed while delivering bad news and then subsequently receiving feedback on one's performance, experts in patient–physician communication have developed a six-step protocol for breaking bad news[42] that can be used as a guide to communication (Box 14-2).

> **BOX 14-2**
>
> **SIX-STEP PROTOCOL FOR COMMUNICATING BAD NEWS**
>
> - Getting started.
>   - Create an environment conducive to effective communication.
> - What does the patient know?
>   - Find out what the patient and the family know about the illness and their current understanding of the medical facts.
> - How much does the patient want to know?
>   - Determine what quantity and quality of information the patient and family want to know.
> - Sharing the information.
>   - Deliver the information in a straightforward and sensitive manner.
> - Respond to feelings.
> - Plan and follow up.
>
> *Adapted from Buckman R. How to break bad news: A guide for health care professionals. Baltimore: Johns Hopkins University Press; 1992; and American Medical Association's Institute for Ethics. Education for physicians on end-of-life care (EPEC): Trainer's guide. Chicago: American Medical Association; 1999, with permission.*

The first step begins with deciding who the meeting's key participants are, obtaining necessary background information, and arranging for an appropriate time and place for the meeting. In the case of Holly Johnson, as the gynecologic oncologist is unable to attend the meeting, it is critical for the meeting leader to understand from the oncologist the options and treatments that have already been explored and what information has already been communicated to the family. This step also involves finding a setting that ensures privacy and that will be free of interruptions, and determining whom the patient would like to have present for the discussion (e.g., family, clergy, durable power of attorney for health care).

The second step involves determining what the patient already knows, remembering that although information may have been presented to the patient, it may not have been well understood. This inquiry should begin with open-ended questions, such as "what do you understand about your illness?" or "tell me what your doctors have told you about what has happened here in the hospital." This helps to determine the patient's and family's level of understanding, and can ascertain whether they will be able to comprehend the bad news.

Next, determine how much the patient wants to know. Patients have the right to know as much—or as little—as they want about their medical illness and their prognosis. Questions such as "how much do you want to know about your illness?" or "whom should I talk to about what is going on with your health?" are open-ended question that can help the medical team determine how much detail to give patients about their illness.

The fourth step involves communicating the results. It is useful to deliver a "warning shot" so that patients will be prepared. Phrases such as "I'm afraid I have bad news" or "the results are not what we would like them to be" can alert patients and families that they are about to receive difficult information. The information itself should be delivered clearly and succinctly, without the use of jargon. In the case of Holly Johnson, an appropriate phrase might be "there are no other medical interventions left to try to cure your cancer at this point." Well-intentioned efforts to soften the blow may lead to vagueness and confusion. It is also important to avoid phrases such as "there is nothing else we can do" (patients may interpret this as abandonment) and "I'm sorry" (may be interpreted as the medical team is responsible for the situation or as pity).

Responding to feelings is an important next step in the process of communicating unfortunate information. Patients and families have a variety of ways in which they react to bad news, from anger to denial to sorrow to acceptance. Outbursts of emotion may make the clinician uncomfortable, so it is important to anticipate these feelings so that the clinician will not be surprised when they are expressed. Allowing the patient and/or family to express these feelings is an important step in building the patient–clinician relationship.

The final step involves making a plan for follow-up. Patients and families have a basic need for education, and guiding them by explaining what the next steps will be is important at this point. The clinician must walk a line between being too vague (e.g., "we need to do some tests") and too specific (e.g., "chemotherapy consists of taxol and vincristine"). For example, a phrase such as "we need to image your stomach before we can decide which chemotherapy is most appropriate for you" gives the patient both an idea of what is to come without providing too much information that might overwhelm the patient. Establish when the next visit will be, and begin that session by repeating the news and asking how the patient is coping with it.

Although Pam Rodriguez's question about coming back and forth to the hospital does not actually involve a need to deliver bad news, it is clearly a way of asking for more information about her medical care. Does she mean that she no longer wants life-sustaining treatment if it means having to return to the hospital? Or is she merely asking what her future holds? Responding with a more open-ended question will help clarify the motivation for her question (e.g., "What do you mean when you ask that?"). Regardless of the motivation, given her frequent rehospitalizations, this would seem an appropriate point to renegotiate the overall goals of care.

What is meant by the phrase *goals of care*? Although patients have a fundamental right to choose what forms of care they do and do not want, they may not always be well informed enough to be able to make these decisions. Physicians can help patients make decisions by understanding what is important to the patient, and then after eliciting these preferences, tailor treatments to these goals. For example, instead of asking a patient, "Do you want us to try to restart your heart?" when asking about the option of a do-not-resuscitate order, the clinician might better serve the patient by helping her or him understand what factors are important in her or his overall medical care (e.g., avoidance of pain, quality of life, ability to interact with family) and then suggest which treatments are aligned with those goals.

Although conversations about goals of care can be difficult, having a basic structure (Box 14-3) upon which to base these discussions can be helpful.[43] The first steps are similar to those used for breaking bad news. First, create the right setting, which includes getting all information that may be necessary from other providers in order to be able to understand the patient's illness and available treatment. Second, determine what the patient and family know. Next, explore what they hope for and desire in terms of their overall goal. These may not always be appropriate or possible, so the next step for the physician is to suggest more realistic goals. Phrases such as "we can't cure your illness, but perhaps we can instead focus on keeping you at home, pain free, and able to meaningfully interact with your family for as long as possible" are ways to redirect conversations if patients have unrealistic goals. These two steps are often done in combination, and depending on the patient's and family's level of understanding, can be the most difficult portion of these conversations. As in breaking bad news, it is important to respond empathetically to the emotions and reactions that may arise, and then create a plan for care based on the goals that have

---

BOX 14-3

ASSESSMENT OF DISCHARGE ENVIRONMENT

Seven-Step Protocol to Negotiate Goals of Care
Create the right setting.
Determine what the patient/family know.
Explore what the patient/family hope for or want.
As necessary, suggest realistic goals of the patient's care.
Respond appropriately to emotions that are expressed.
Create a plan of care based on the goals established.
Review the plan over time and revise it as appropriate.

Adapted from American Medical Association's Institute for Ethics. Education for physicians on end-of-life care (EPEC): Trainer's guide. Chicago: American Medical Association; 1999, with permission.

been established. Finally, it is important that these goals be written clearly in the medical record, and these goals must be reviewed and revised periodically as appropriate.

> When communicating bad news or having conversations to negotiate goals of care, it is important to have a method of approach for these often difficult conversations.

SUMMARY

Palliative care for older adults differs from the traditional hospice model in that it is offered simultaneously with life-sustaining treatments. It consists of managing pain and other symptoms, clarifying goals of care, and ensuring continuity across systems of care. Pain management in palliative care involves clear assessment and then establishing a regimen that meets the patient's overall pain needs. Treating nonpain symptoms such as nausea, dyspnea, depression, and anxiety is a cornerstone of palliative care, and this treatment is best served by having a clear understanding of the underlying pathology. When communicating bad news or having conversations to negotiate goals of care, it is important to have a method of approach for these often difficult conversations.

ACKNOWLEDGMENT

Portions of this chapter are adapted from Goldstein and Morrison.[44,45]

Web Resources

www.aahpm.org. Website of the American Academy of Hospice and Palliative Medicine, one of the largest groups representing and providing educational resources for clinicians who practice palliative medicine.

www.epec.net and www.aacn.nche.edu/elnec. Websites for the Education in Palliative and End-of-Life Care (EPEC) and End-of-Life Nursing Education Consortium (ELNEC), two national education projects dedicated to educating clinicians on improving end-of-life care.

www.palliativedrugs.com. Provides information on the medications most commonly used in palliative care.

www.capc.org. The Center to Advance Palliative Care, funded by the Robert Wood Johnson Foundation, is dedicated to increasing the availability of quality palliative care services in hospitals and other health care settings.

http://www.eperc.mcw.edu/EPERC. The End of Life/Palliative Education Resource Center is an online community for sharing resource materials among clinicians involved in palliative care education.

KEY REFERENCES

33. Lipman HI, Meier D. Treatment of nausea and vomiting in the older palliative care patient. Geriatr Aging 2004;7(10):62-7.

References available online at expertconsult.com.

UNIT 2

Geriatric Syndromes and Common Special Problems

What does it matter if he can't remember them, as long as they remember him?
Wife of 94-year-old patient (of RH), about their great-grandchildren's visits

Body and mind, like man and wife, do not always agree to die together.
CHARLES C COLTON, c 1780-1832, churchman and writer,
in *Lacon 1, 324*

Perhaps being old is having lighted rooms inside your head, and people in them, acting.
People you know, yet can't quite name.
PHILIP LARKIN, 1922-1985, English author, in *The Old Fools*

Better by far you should forget and smile
Than that you should remember and be sad.
CHRISTINA ROSSETTI, 1830-1874, in *Remember*

Memory is history recorded in our brain; memory is a painter, it paints pictures of the past and of the day.
GRANDMA MOSES, 1860-1961, Painter, in *My Life's*
History, ed. Aotto Kallir

The humor of the dementia clinic:
(RH to patient) "..and what State are we in?"
(Patient) "Confusion!?"

…AND…Wife of patient with dementia to RH, who has started to discuss medication to calm her husband:
She: "Are you going to zap him? Make a zombie of him?"
RH: "No, no—of course not."
She (interrupting): "Well you need to zap him—he's awful, blows his nose on the table cloth, drinks out of the saucer, and the language—no, doc, you need to zap him!!!"

When I meet a man whose name I can't remember, I give myself two minutes; then, if it is a hopeless case, I always say, "And how is the old complaint?"
BENJAMIN DISRAELI, 1804-1881, Queen Victoria's favorite
prime minister

I am a very foolish, fond old man,
Fourscore and upward, not an hour more or less;
And, to deal plainly,
I fear I am not in my perfect mind
WILLIAM SHAKESPEARE, 1564-1616, in *King Lear*, IV, 7

He that conceals his grief finds no remedy for it.

TURKISH PROVERB

Wine is only sweet to happy men.
JOHN KEATS, 1795-1821, in *To...(Fanny Brawne)*

It provokes desire, but it takes away the performance. Therefore much drink may be said to be an equivocator with lechery.
WILLIAM SHAKESPEARE, 1564-1616, in *Macbeth*, II:3

I smoke 10 to 15 cigars a day; at my age you have to hold on to something.
GEORGE BURNS, 1896-1996, U.S. comedian

As men draw near the common goal
Can anything be sadder
Than he who, master of his soul,
Is servant to his bladder

ANON, in *The Speculum, Melbourne*, 1938

The ultimate indignity is to be given a bedpan by a stranger who calls you by your first name.
MAGGIE KUHN, 1905-1995, activist and founder of the Grey Panthers

Old people, on the whole, have fewer complaints than the young, but those chronic diseases which do befall them never leave them.
HIPPOCRATES, c 460- c 357 BC, *in Aphorisms*

So we'll go no more a-roving
So late into the night,
Though the heart be still as loving,
And the moon be still as bright.

For the sword outwears its sheath,
And the soul wears out the breast,
And the heart must pause to breathe,
And Love itself have rest.

Though the night was made for loving,
And the day returns too soon,
Yet we'll go no more a-roving
By the light of the moon.
GEORGE GORDON, LORD BYRON 1788-1824,
"So We'll Go No More A-Roving"

15

Emergency Care

Teresita M. Hogan and Tonatiuh Rios-Alba

OBJECTIVES

Upon completion of this chapter, the reader will be able to:

- Understand the traditional emphases of emergency department (ED) care and the efforts in progress to address the ED needs of the elderly.

- Describe the differences between older adults' and younger adults' needs for emergency services, and how to address the more complex needs of the elderly.

- Identify specific geriatric emergencies, and discuss their management, focusing especially on whether to treat on site, to transfer to the ED (and if important, which ED), or directly hospitalize.

- Describe the optimal linkages between the primary care provider (PCP) and the ED or emergency physician (EP) in the transitioning of the care of specific geriatric emergencies.

- Navigate your **own** site-specific systems-based practice area (the places where you mainly do your clinical work and the EDs and hospitals available to you), and describe your criteria for choosing—in your own region—one ED or hospital relative to another for specific geriatric emergencies.

- Know your **own** region's arrangements for emergency transfer to the different levels of stroke and trauma care, especially your region's level 1 trauma center(s) and stroke center(s)] and the precise clinical criteria for their use in trauma and stroke emergencies.

- Detail the identification and initial management and the potential roles of the ED in the following geriatric emergencies, and apply the same principles of selective and often urgent use of the ED to the

---

Additional online-only material indicated by icon.

many other conditions in this book when emergencies occur: shortness of breath especially in chronic obstructive pulmonary disease (COPD); syncope with and without risk factors; trauma especially of the head; acute stroke; sepsis; hypo- and hyperthermia.

PRIMARY CARE AND THE EMERGENCY DEPARTMENT

Clinicians are most effective when working in the settings they use daily. Medical or surgical emergencies may be rare in some clinical settings, but every clinician (every "provider")—especially in the primary care environment—must master the appropriate use of their own emergency department (ED). This will prevent delay when minutes count. The urgent need is to decide which patients require the ED, and sometimes—if there are choices—which level of ED should be used, depending on the potential for definitive treatment. **The potential for local management without resort to the ED needs to be known**. The clinician "on the spot" needs to possess the ability to anticipate the immediate dangers and to be up to date about the potential for definitive treatment, to be able to initiate treatment and/or stabilize the patient if necessary, and to arrange the most direct transfer to optimal care. The decision as to when that does or does not require the ED depends on knowing the local circumstances as well as the patient's expressed preferences, if known. The clinician handling a potential emergency situation bears the grave responsibility of managing the efficient transition of care.

Know (or find out) what resources are available to YOU, the PCP, and what level the EDs and hospitals are in your region.

Identifying emergency conditions is especially demanding in older adults: atypical presentation makes early diagnosis of emergencies difficult; transitions of care to and from the ED require good communication of often complex medical, social, and personal information and knowledge of the medical care system—i.e., expertise in "systems-based practice". Mastery of these aspects will make a life and death difference to elderly patients.

Clinical situations requiring urgent, time-sensitive, definitive interventions include coronary revascularization, empiric antibiotic use, early goal-directed therapy, acute surgical intervention, fibrinolytic therapy, trauma resuscitation, advanced cardiac life support, and intubation. Identifying such situations, in which some often highly skilled technical procedure can be crucial and must occur rapidly in order to actually save lives of acutely ill or injured patients, is an essential skill for all clinicians—indeed health professionals of all types—and first responders. An informed public regarding the symptoms and illnesses in which urgent treatment is crucial is needed too!

Questions for readers of this chapter: Do YOU know how to rapidly identify the situations which may benefit from or require urgent, definitive treatment in a specialized setting, how to stabilize your patient, select the safest most rapid transport, communicate continuity of care with the emergency physician (EP), and ensure appropriate transition of care? Do you know what testing, treatment, consultation, and interventions are likely to be needed in such patients and how to assure expedited access to the service they need? Does your ED provide the service needed? If not where can you get it? Do you need to temporize and stabilize before ED transfer? Can you distinguish the patients in which definitive care can be provided by you, by a different location out of the ED, or only by the ED?

EDs Are Not Designed for Old People

The current model of emergency care, developed by the Committee on Trauma of the American College of Surgeons in 1962, was **intended to rapidly detect clear presentations of acute illness and injury requiring usually a single expedited intervention**. In the ED the best care of a previously unknown patient (triage, history, physical, medication reconciliation, stabilization, laboratory testing, imaging, acute consultation, initiation of definitive treatment, documentation of evaluation and actions, a preliminary diagnosis, and disposition to the appropriate level of care) optimally occurs in minutes to under 6 hours. This system is **not designed for the interwoven medical complexities, slowly evolving presentations, and convoluted social concerns that must simultaneously be addressed for optimal management of the old**.[1,2] The constant interruptions suffered by the EP (more than twice as many per hour as primary care physicians (PCPs) in one study) and the distraction of managing multiple patients simultaneously (more than three at a time, more than half of the time)[3] underscores the difference in the orientation of the ED and primary care settings: the ED is episodic, disease (and hospital) oriented, and urgent, whereas the primary care setting tries for continuity, complexity, care in the long term, and is dominantly subacute, and—ideally—interacts a lot with services out in the community.

A defining component of primary care,[4] continuity of care decreased markedly from 1996–2006 in the United States. This decrease was associated with a drop in patient satisfaction, an increase in medical errors, duplication of services, unwanted treatments, polypharmacy, and decreased autonomy, and undermined quality and outcomes.[5] The Institute of Medicine recommends that all participants in health care, including nursing and rehabilitation facilities, fully coordinate their activities and integrate communications; this would clearly improve elderly care.[6]

The PCP must ask before transfer: could the same care be provided in a non-ED setting? Sending a patient to the ED should not be a matter of convenience. The ED should not be used as the middle man: for example, a patient with a malfunctioning percutaneous endoscopic gastrostomy (PEG) tube could be sent directly to the gastrointestinal (GI) department or radiology (the same step the ED would have to take).

> **If you can refer directly to definitive care and avoid the ED you should.**

A study of PCPs' and emergency physicians' (EPs') ability to communicate and coordinate health care discovered haphazard communication and poor coordination, and that this situation undermines effective care and results in poor patient satisfaction and duplication of testing and treatment.[7] The use of hospitalists to care for admitted patients results in more direct and immediate communication at the start of the hospitalization. Efforts at coordination generally fall to the diligence and training of the professionals themselves. Such direct contact can make a life and death difference.

As PCP, your report to the EP provides critical information, often accumulated over time, which would otherwise take time and effort to discover. **Your direct report is the only guarantee this information will be known to the EP.** Your report helps counter the difficulties inherent in the hectic ED environment and the complexities presented by the old. When transferring a patient to the ED, convey your detailed knowledge of the patient including the baseline level of function, your evaluation and impression of the acute event, your specific goals of care for the ED, and the patient's overall goals of care as well.

EPIDEMIOLOGY

The aging of the United States population influences all segments of health care but especially the use of the ED.[8] Elders do have greater needs for emergency care than other age groups.[9] Currently, 20 million older Americans utilize EDs annually.[10] Studies overwhelmingly agree this high level of use by older adults

is appropriate.[11,12,13] The proportion of Emergency Medical Services (EMS) use in elders increases from 27% for age 65 to 84 to 48% among those 85 and older.[14,15,16] Elders require more ED staff time and resources, receive more medications, and have higher rates of admission to both the hospital and critical care units.[17,18] From 33% to 50% of elder ED visits result in hospitalization, which is up to 4.6 times higher than rates seen in younger adults.[19,20]

Older adults are likely to have a PCP. Most do consult their PCP prior to ED use and are referred to the ED by their PCP. The one exception to high ED use by older adults may be the rural setting, where there is a disproportionately lower rate of ED use by older adults.[19]

The strain placed by older adult utilization of already overcrowded EDs calls for a review of both the appropriateness and patterns of PCP ED referral as well as the model of ED systems of care.[20,21,22]

Comorbidities, polypharmacy, lack of access to care, lack of mobility, poor social support, and frailty all contribute to the vulnerability, with increased morbidity and mortality of our older patients. Fifty-one percent of "social admit" elderly patients were found to have an acute medical problem: infections in 24%; cardiovascular issues in 14%; a neurologic event in 9%; gastrointestinal problems in 7%; pulmonary problems were noted in 5%; and another 5% with fracture, anemia, acute renal failure, or uncontrolled pain.[22,23] **Patients sent to the ED for lack of social support suffered a 1-year mortality of up to 34%.**[24]

In the first 3 months after an index ED visit, 5% of discharged elder ED patients will die, 20% will require hospital admission, 20% require another ED evaluation, and from 10% to 48% suffer decline in functional abilities.[25,23,26] This high incidence of poor outcomes despite PCP follow-up suggests a complexity of need that far out spans the episodic ED visit.[27,28] **These outcomes suggest the underlying issue is not the acute event for which the ED was designed, but a quietly ongoing process.** Thus a substantial proportion of elders would likely be better served in non-ED settings and with active follow up, coordinated by their PCP,[29,30] who ideally should be vigilant for continued deterioration of older patients who attended the ED.

SYSTEMS-BASED PRACTICE (SBP)

This is one of six core competencies required in all physicians before they are certified to graduate by any residency program. SBP is defined by the Accreditation Council of Graduate Medical Education (ACGME) as: **an awareness of and responsiveness to the larger context and system of health care and the ability to effectively call on system resources to provide care that is of optimal value.**[31,32]

As a PCP, your distance from an ED, the specific services it provides, and the ease of transportation to and access of those services are critical components of SBP in your practice setting.

Access to the ED

Seventy-one percent of the U.S. population can access a general comprehensive ED within 30 minutes, and 98% has access within 60 minutes. Access to a teaching hospital ED is more difficult, with 16% access in 30 minutes and 44% within 60 minutes.[33] Such aspects can compromise the success of therapies for acute myocardial infarction, stroke, and sepsis. At least one rural study of three communities confirms that the more limited access of rural elders can be addressed using preplanned transport methods for acute emergencies, and by being well prepared to provide emergency care on site. In fact, there were probable advantages for these communities relative to nonrural settings.[34]

The "Geriatric Emergency Department" (GED)

Many attempts to optimize ED care for the old have been made; chief among these are geriatric service lines and development of a geriatric ED (GED). In addition to incorporating the Affordable Care Act's (ACA) focus on maximizing resources in the Medicare population, a further goal is to appropriately triage those requiring inpatient care, and to identify—and effectively implement—services for those who can be discharged. [35,36,37]

GEDs have the following characteristics:
1. Enhanced ED staffing and administration: geriatrically trained registered nurses (RNs), pharmacists, social workers, specialist geriatricians, and care coordinators. Geriatrician ED consults have resulted in avoidance of admission for 85% of the older patients evaluated.[8] Moderate improvements in the provision of physical and occupational therapy are also noted.
2. Screening: GEDs utilize screening to shift to being proactive rather than reactive. Screenings identify high risk individuals, decrease never-events, and identify need for specific services. Linkages to care for the problems identified are crucial; these generally involve primary care and community services.[36]
3. Case management: This is reported to improve the health, social, and service utilization outcomes arising from ED visits. Core components were reviewed as to their influence on effectiveness of interventions.[37] More than eight of these key components produced a trend toward better

outcomes: a validated risk stratification tool in a full geriatric assessment, significant nursing involvement in clinical evaluation, leadership roles, initiation of care and disposition planning from the ED, and having post-discharge follow-up mechanisms in place.
4. Staff education: In view of their recognized lack of geriatric-specific training,[38] many training programs and curricula have been developed for EMS providers, ED nurses, and EPs.[39-43]

The eight core competencies of emergency medicine care for the elderly are atypical presentations, medication management, trauma (including falls), emergency intervention modifications, effect of comorbidity, cognitive and behavioral disorders, and transitions of care.

COMMON EMERGENCIES IN GERIATRICS

The **three most common complaints** in elder ED patients are: chest pain, shortness of breath, and abdominal pain.[44,45] The differential of each of these obviously includes life-threatening emergencies.

The **most frequent medical diagnoses** made in older ED patients are: ischemic heart disease, congestive heart failure, cardiac dysrhythmias, syncope, acute cerebrovascular accidents, pneumonia, abdominal disorders, dehydration, and urinary tract infections.[46] **Surgical emergencies** in ED elders are primarily due to **injuries sustained in a fall**. Injuries are the seventh leading cause of death in the elder population.[8] Falls are a critical event in this population (see separate chapter) with the cause being as significant as the damage, due to high recurrence rates.

Is It An Emergency?

Vital signs can be difficult or misleading to interpret. Occult hypotension is common in the old. So is bradycardia from medications, and it can be excessive. Fever is notoriously unreliable in elders and sepsis may be heralded by temperatures of <36° or >38°C (<96.8° or >100.4°F). But, in general, a primary survey will reveal the majority of life-threatening issues.

"The ABCs"

A is for **Airway** compromise, the inability to move air through the mouth, nose, and upper airway into the lungs, as seen in stridor, mucosal edema, unconsciousness, anaphylaxis, and foreign body.
B is for **Breathing** and includes evaluation of respiratory rate. Danger exists at the extremes of <10 breaths/min or 30 and over breaths/min, or if the O_2 saturation is <93% on room air.

C is for **Circulation** and includes signs of decreased organ perfusion such as diaphoresis, new altered mental status, and cyanosis. **Shock** can be heralded by pulse <50 beats/min or >120 beats/min, or by a systolic BP <90 mm Hg.

D has been added for **(neurologic) Disability** and is noted by new decreased mental status, Glasgow coma scale[47] <13, or stroke-like symptoms.

> The ABCs are life threatening aspects of emergencies in the old: Airway, Breathing, Circulation (and D, neurologic Disability); in general, abnormalities in any of these (within the defined ranges) are to be RUSHED to the ED!!!

In general, patients with abnormalities of the ABCs should be rapidly triaged to an emergency department. The likely length of time until arrival of EMS, arrival in the ED, and initiation of treatment will indicate if you—as initial provider—should deliver stabilizing treatment prior to ED transport. Since elders may not manifest abnormal vital signs early in the course of illness, any acute deterioration in mentation or function should be evaluated as a possible emergency. Therefore these patients may be missed unless a baseline state is clearly known.

More difficult triage decisions are noted in patients with common life-threatening chief complaints such as chest pain, dyspnea, altered mental status, and abdominal pain, all of which are discussed in detail in other chapters. The differentiation of emergencies within these chief complaints often requires advanced laboratory testing, ECG, monitoring, and imaging. Only you can determine if such evaluation can be safely provided in your setting or if it requires further care. Highlights of cases demonstrating several other emergency conditions are discussed below.

ACUTE SHORTNESS OF BREATH

The wide differential diagnosis of acute shortness of breath in elders in the ED includes myocardial ischemia/infarction, COPD, congestive heart failure (CHF), pneumonia, pulmonary embolism, bronchitis, and dysrhythmia. The differential in the community is wider, containing more benign causes of shortness of breath (SOB), as well as less severe exacerbations of disease than are usually seen in the ED. How then does the PCP know who to send to the ED? In general if you have not reasonably excluded a life-threatening cause of shortness of breath, or stabilized a severe exacerbation of disease, you should transfer to the ED.

> If you cannot <u>exclude</u> a life threatening cause of <u>dyspnea</u>, or you cannot stabilize an acute exacerbation of disease, your patient <u>needs</u> the ED!!!

CASE 1

Shortness of Breath

Mr. Edward Harris is a 69-year-old male with COPD, who presents to your office with a complaint of shortness of breath. He states his family members have been sick with a cold, and he is concerned he may be catching it as well. He has been coughing up green mucus for the past 4 days, and he has been wheezing more and more each day. He has an albuterol inhaler at home, and he has had to use it every hour throughout the day. He has been having "low-grade fevers" but denies chills, vomiting, chest pain, or leg swelling.

He has a past medical history of hypertension, diabetes, and coronary artery disease (CAD). He admits to smoking 1–2 packs per day for the last 25 years. He denies illicit drug or alcohol use. He does require oxygen at home and uses 2L of O_2 by nasal cannula.

His vital signs are HR 105, BP 158/95, RR 26, Sat 85% on room air, which corrects to 90% on 2L and up to 92% on 6L. On exam, he is obese, looks uncomfortable, is able to speak only in 3–4 word sentences due to SOB, has moderate subcostal retractions, and has diffuse wheezing throughout. His peak expiratory flow rate (PEFR) upon arrival is measured at 160 L/min. He states his normal is around 400 L/min.

1. **What could have triggered this?**

2. **What specific dangers do you anticipate in this case?** ▪

COPD Exacerbations

Exacerbations are most often triggered by a viral or bacterial infection[48] but can also be triggered by cold weather, narcotic use, CHF, or anemia, among other triggers. It is essential to be able to differentiate between a mild exacerbation, which could be treated in the office, and a more severe one that requires transfer to the closest ED. The most life-threatening components of an exacerbation are hypoxemia and hypercarbia.[49]

Hypoxia and hypercarbia can present similarly with symptoms such as headaches, agitation, confusion, lethargy, and in severe cases, can lead to seizures or coma. Impending respiratory collapse will be manifested by the signs above plus tachypnea, tachycardia, hypertension, accessory muscle use, pursed lips, and altered mental status. The retention of CO_2 heralds acute respiratory failure. The idea that oxygen can induce hypercarbia is largely a myth.[50] Oxygen should not be withheld from patients with hypoxemia. However, do not apply high flow oxygen (defined as 8–10 L/min);

rather titrate oxygen treatments, which reduces mortality, hypercapnia, and acidosis in acute exacerbations of COPD.[51,52] Unless you can apply positive pressure or intubate the patient, maintain SpO_2 between 88% and 92% as this was found to reduce mortality by 58%.[53] Spirometry—to identify airflow obstruction—should be obtained in COPD patients with altered respiratory symptoms.[54]

Investigation

- Oxygenation: Initial measurement of oxygen saturation and, if available, arterial blood gas can serve to give a quick assessment of severity of the exacerbation.
- Pulmonary function tests: If patient is able to comply, obtaining a FEV1 or PEFR can help determine severity of the exacerbation. FEV1 is preferred but is rarely readily available in an acute setting. PEFR of <100 L/min, FEV1 <1 L, along with worsening function on sequential testing despite treatment, are all indicative of a severe exacerbation.[49,53]
- Ancillary testing: A chest x-ray can help identify underlying triggers of the exacerbation such as pneumonia or CHF. An ECG can help rule out ischemia or arrhythmias, such as multiple atrial tachycardia (MAT). Complete blood counts, electrolyte panel, and D-dimer should be performed when clinically indicated but should not be used to assess severity of a particular exacerbation.

Treatment: Interventions That Can Be Performed in an Outpatient Setting

- Oxygenation: Administer O_2 by nasal cannula, face mask, or by the most appropriate method.
- Bronchodilators: Short-acting beta 2 agonists such as albuterol[55] and anticholinergic agents such as ipratropium are both equally effective in acute COPD exacerbations and have been shown to lead to shorter stays in the ED and improved outcomes when used concomitantly.[56] Long-acting beta 2 agonist or long-acting anticholinergic agents have no role in acute COPD exacerbations.
- Corticosteroids: Administration of either IV or PO steroids during an exacerbation can help prevent return of symptoms after an exacerbation but do not prevent hospitalization in an acute setting. This is likely due to the onset of action of up to 6 hours from administration.[57] It is prudent to give steroids to a patient who is going to be discharged from the office. There is no difference in outcome or onset of action in using IV versus PO steroids.
- Antibiotics: Most common pathogens are streptococcus pneumonia, hemophilus influenza, and moraxella catarrhalis. Antibiotics should be given if concomitant infection is suspected from symptoms such as increased sputum or fever.[48]

Treatment: Interventions That Require Transfer to the Closest ED

- Noninvasive positive pressure ventilation (NPPV): Indicated for moderate to severe exacerbations as determined by worsening tachypnea >25 breaths/min, dyspnea with accessory muscle use, moderate to severe acidosis (pH<7.35), or hypercapnia (PaCO2 > 45mm Hg).[57] If a patient is deemed to require NPPV, he/she should be transferred to the nearest ED as soon as possible. Patients in respiratory distress that undergo NPPV have better short-term mortality, decreased intubation rates, and decreased length of hospital stay.[58]
- Mechanical ventilation: if a patient continues to deteriorate despite all the above interventions, endotracheal intubation is the next required therapy. This should always be determined by and performed in an ED or ICU setting.

If there is no improvement in clinical status after treatment with oxygen and bronchodilators, transfer to the nearest hospital is warranted for further treatment. In a patient who is stable without severe respiratory distress, stable oxygenation, and no requirement of continuous nebulizations, yet has persistent wheezing or lack of improvement, direct admission to an inpatient setting may be appropriate. For a patient who is continuing to deteriorate or a patient who shows signs of impending respiratory collapse as outlined above, immediate transfer to the nearest ED should be arranged.

CASE 1

Shortness of Breath (continued)

You start Mr. Harris on a combination albuterol/ipratropium nebulization, and your plan is to give him prednisone and an antibiotic before going home. However, after three intermittent 15-minute nebulizer treatments, he fails to improve. He is now experiencing worse SOB, and on exam, he is breathing around 30 breaths per minute, he is pursing his lips with each breath, can only say 1–2 words at a time and has more visible retractions despite the nebulized treatment. He starts to appear more confused, requiring repeated questions for him to comprehend what you are asking. He is unable to perform the PEFR measurement.

What could be the cause(s) of this decline? What is your next step?

You determine he would benefit from NPPV and further treatment, so you expedite a transfer to the closest ED. You call EMS who arrive within 7 minutes. They give him an albuterol nebulization and place him on a portable continuous positive airway pressure (CPAP) machine and take him to the closest hospital.

You follow up and find out he required admission to the ICU for continuous NPPV and nebulizations. He was able to avoid intubation but was subsequently treated for pneumonia. He stayed in the ICU for 2 days, after which he was transferred to the floor to continue treatment and was discharged home in a few days with PO steroids and antibiotics.

What precisely indicated that he should be transferred to the ED from the office? ▣

SYNCOPE

Syncope

Mrs. Vera Smith is a 72-year-old female who is brought to your office by her husband hours after experiencing syncope. The patient states she was napping on the couch, then awoke and walked to the kitchen. While walking, she became very dizzy and felt like her vision was closing in on her. Her husband noted she turned pale very quickly and then passed out. He was able to hold her so she did not fall. He laid her down gently and within a few seconds she was awake. Currently, she denies any discomfort. None of these symptoms has recurred since the event. She states there has been a "stomach bug" going around in her family, and she has had five episodes of vomiting and diarrhea during the last 2 days along with poor appetite. She has otherwise been well and denies any recent fevers, chills, chest pain, trouble breathing, and does not recall any other similar episodes of fainting. She has a history of GERD and asthma but is otherwise healthy. She does not smoke, denies illicit drug use, and only uses alcohol with family during holidays. Her vital signs are HR 105, BP 132/88, RR 18, O_2 Sat 99% on room air. On physical exam, you note the patient does have moderately dry mucous membranes but otherwise appears comfortable. Your examination of her heart, lungs, and abdomen is normal.

Her urine specific gravity is >1.02, with positive ketones and without glucose or leukocytes; an ECG shows sinus tachycardia without any other abnormalities. Upon standing, her BP drops to 105/70 and her HR increases to 120 and she reports feeling dizzy.

1. **Under what conditions is it reasonable to treat an elder with syncope in the office and discharge home?**

2. **What features of the patient's PMH define a high risk patient who warrants hospitalization for syncope evaluation?**

3. **In what circumstances is it safe to bypass the ED and directly admit an elder with syncope?** ▣

Syncope (continued)

You assess her as having probable simple dehydration, take blood for a BMP and Hgb, and advise her to return home, to not be alone in the house for a day or two (her husband is "always" there), to drink a lot of extra fluids (excluding her favorite fluids of tea and coffee), to stand up slowly after being recumbent in bed or in a chair, and to return for orthostatics by your nurse in 2 days. ▣

Management of Syncope

The 2008 American College of Emergency Physicians Clinical Policy: Critical Issues in the Evaluation and Management of Patients Presenting With Syncope,[59] recognizes the extremely low yield of non-directed testing in syncope evaluation.[59] On admitted syncope patients, the most commonly performed ED studies are ECG (99%), cardiac markers (95%), and CT head (63%). Markers and CT head affected diagnosis or management in less than 5% of cases and were diagnostic in <2%.[60] Although orthostatic blood pressure readings are obtained in about a third of patients, these evaluations affected diagnosis in up to 26%, management in up to 30%, and determined etiology in from 15% to 21% of patients. Obtaining an ECG and a hematocrit is warranted for most cases of syncope, with further testing normally being low yield. For suspected cardiogenic syncope, a chest x-ray and cardiac enzyme panel may be warranted. However, unless there exists a strong suspicion of neurologic cause or if head trauma is involved, a head CT is rarely warranted.

Generally, purely vasovagal or orthostatic hypotension syncope (or drug induced orthostasis) with a correctable cause has no increased risk for future adverse events.[49,61]

Symptomatic treatment and adequate follow-up is therefore appropriate. For orthostatic hypotension, hydration and re-evaluation is prudent. If symptoms improve with therapy, discharge home is appropriate.

On the other hand, cardiogenic or neurologic syncope requires immediate hospitalization for further evaluation. Ideally, if direct inpatient hospitalization can be arranged from the clinic or office, the patient can be sent straight for admission. Otherwise, sending the patient to the ED should be the next step.

If a clear etiology of the syncope cannot be determined, the patient should be risk stratified as low risk for adverse events. You should determine who can be discharged home with follow-up, who will need admission to an inpatient setting for further workup, and who requires ED intervention. Several clinical criteria and clinical decision rules (CDRs) exist to aid with risk stratification; unfortunately, there is no particular set of criteria that has been shown to be superior, and most have been proven to be inadequate to estimate risk in certain clinical settings.[49,61]

The San Francisco Syncope Rule[62] has five predictors of adverse events: (1) history of CHF; (2) hematocrit <30; (3) ECG changes consisting of any morphologic changes not seen on prior ECG, any dysrhythmias, or nonsinus rhythm either on strip or on monitor; (4) shortness of breath by history; and (5) systolic BP < 90 mmHg. If ANY of these criteria is met, the patient is considered high risk and warrants further evaluation. These rules have shown a 96% sensitivity and 68% specificity for serious outcomes defined as death, MI, arrhythmia, PE, stroke, SAH, hemorrhage, or any condition requiring return to the ED at 7 and 30 days.[3] However, the sensitivity and specificity of these rules have been shown to decrease significantly in the elder population.[63]

A different CDR, the OESIL score (Osservatorio Epidemiologico sulla Sincope nel Lazio), takes into account age >65, known CV disease, abnormal ECG, and lack of a presyncopal prodrome as high risk predictors—the higher the score, the higher the predicted mortality at one year. This tool had a sensitivity of 95% and specificity of 31%.[64]

CASE 3

Syncope with Risk Factors

Mr. Arthur Jones is an 81-year-old male with known congestive heart failure who presents after passing out earlier this morning. The patient was sitting on a park bench resting midway through his morning walk because he developed shortness of breath and chest pain. He suddenly became unresponsive. A neighbor who witnessed the episode reports that he was unconscious for about a minute. Since then, he has remained asymptomatic other than feeling weak and having some shortness of breath.

In addition to CHF, Mr. Jones also has hypertension, diabetes, is a smoker, and has been told he may need surgery for one of his heart valves that is "not working properly." His vital signs in your office are HR 87, BP 88/65, RR 22, SO_2 Sats 92% on room air. He looks a bit uncomfortable; on exam, you notice he has bibasilar rales and a systolic ejection murmur heard best at the right sternal border with radiation up towards his carotid. His ECG shows sinus rhythm with LVH and Q waves in the anterior leads without any ST changes. QTc is normal.

1. **He has multiple risk factors. What can you do in your office setting?**

2. **Do you admit him directly to the cardiology service?**

3. **Should he go to the ED first?**

4. **What is the likely course of action in either hospital location?** ◘

CASE 3

Syncope with Risk Factors (continued)

By history alone, you can determine high risk for adverse events. Further, on physical exam, his systolic BP

is <90 mmHg. You call the local hospital and arrange for transport and admission ED evaluation as you are concerned about his current hypotension. However, you know he will require admission to the cardiology service for further workup of his syncope. ◘

Workup of Syncope Risk Factors

The initial inpatient workup of patients with syncope with risk factors includes a full cardiac workup, including cardiac monitoring, trending out of cardiac enzymes, cardiac ECHO, and then a stress test. Vascular studies, head CT, and EEG may be warranted to further assess for neurogenic causes. For recurrent vasovagal syncope, tilt-table testing may be diagnostic.

In summary, any patients with structural heart disease, heart failure, abnormal ECG, anemia, or symptoms not consistent with benign causes of syncope are at high risk for adverse effects and should be hospitalized.

Trauma

CASE 4

Trauma

Mrs. Avril Green is a 72-year-old female with h/o HTN and atrial fibrillation on verapamil and warfarin. She comes to see you because she is having several episodes of vomiting every day. This has been going on for about 4 days. She has no infectious symptoms, abdominal pain, or diarrhea. There is no blood or bile in the emesis, and vomiting is not related to eating. No one else at home is ill. She has no history of gallstones or fatty food intolerance. She denies headache, visual changes, vertigo, or any focal neurologic complaint. She does complain of pain to her right buttock since she slipped in the shower about a week ago, but that is much better and does not interfere with her walking.

On exam VS: BP 146/92, P 86, R 14, pulse ox 96% on RA. HEENT shows PERRLA, EOMI and a 2x3 cm tender bump is noted on her right posterior scalp. She now mentions it hurts to brush her hair there. Neurologic, CV, pulmonary and abdominal exam are all normal. You note a resolving hematoma over her right buttock; there is no bony tenderness in that area, and her hip moves normally and her gait is normal.

1. **Is this an emergency a whole week after her fall?**

2. **What is the most dangerous cause for her symptoms?**

3. **You have a local hospital nearby, and a tertiary care teaching hospital 20 minutes away—which would you choose and why?** ◘

Overview

The decreased functional reserve in key body systems is well recognized both as the cause of atypical presentations in the old (e.g. the apathetic thyrotoxicosis, pneumonia presenting as falling, hypoglycemia presenting as mood changes) and as a characteristic which also diminishes the tolerance to bodily injury (e.g. trauma, acute CVA, etc.). The reduced reserve also contributes to overall reduced ability to fully recover from traumatic injury, or at least it delays recovery.[65] Link this characteristic to increased fragility (e.g. of bone, skin, and other tissues), often diminished muscular strength and support, reduced speed of response or even of awareness, impaired judgment from cognitive impairments, poorer balance, and reduced warning from hearing and visual impairments, and it can be seen to be predictable that severe injury may occur from seemingly nonserious incidents such as a fall from standing. The fifth most frequent cause of death in old people is trauma; failure to realize this among PCPs and first responders leads to failure to take older trauma victims directly to trauma centers, (or transfer them from ordinary EDs), and this failure has been linked to major increased risk of death.[66]

> **Failure to get elderly trauma victims to the highest level trauma center available is a remediable factor in their high death rate.**

Head trauma is particularly challenging. Cerebral atrophy—even in the presence of apparently normal cognitive function—is commonly found in old people. The brain (which is close to liquid at normal temperatures) moves more in the event of a car crash or fall, increasing the chance of hemorrhage. But there is also free space, so that intracranial hemorrhage (ICH)—by failing to cause raised intracranial pressure—often produces little or none of the expected neurologic clinical picture,[67-69] and yet if it is ICH, the mortality rate is 30% to 80%, even when the accident was a fall from standing height.[67,70]

> **Even in minor head trauma, vomiting is associated with increased risk of ICH.[68] Anticoagulation dramatically increases morbidity, mortality and difficulty of treatment.[71-73]**

> **Expedient trauma evaluation of apparently stable elders improves survival.[65]**

CASE 4

Trauma (continued)

Because of the vomiting and increased risk of ICH from anticoagulation, you do not send her to the closest hospital ED but have her transported 20 minutes away to a level 1 trauma center.

The ED evaluation consists of INR, type and cross-match, CBC, and expedited CT scan of the brain. The scan shows a large right subdural hematoma with collapse of the ventricles on the affected side but no midline shift. Rapid pharmacologic reversal of anticoagulation is indicated for any evidence of ICH.

Stabilization of the patient is achieved with aggressive reversal of anticoagulation using PCC. The vomiting is thought to represent increased intracranial pressure. Once clotting is controlled, an intracranial pressure bolt is placed. Within 6 hours of arrival, she is taken to the OR for evacuation of the subdural hematoma. On the third postoperative day, she is ambulatory, walking in the ICU hallway and awaiting transfer to a general bed.

1. **What do you learn from this case?**

2. **Does this affect your inclination to anticoagulate preventively in a patient in atrial fibrillation (AF)?** ▣

Under-referral to Trauma Centers

More, rather than less, medical and other health professional assistance will be needed in an injured older patient. Yet severely injured elders are less likely than younger but otherwise comparably injured patients to be transferred initially to a level 1 trauma center, as is extensively documented.[74-77]

Occult hypotension refers to normal blood pressure—but a reduction in the individual elder's BP—and normal heart rate being associated with reduced end organ perfusion—that is, acting like shock. In the old person, mortality increases if the systolic BP is <110 mm. Normal "vitals," such as heart rate and BP, are not reliable as the basis of estimating the need for a level 1 trauma center referral of an older patient, or of that patient's chance of dying,[78,79] as they may actually represent shock in an older person. Occult hypotension has been found in over 40% of injured older adults.[79] Failure to recognize it is one factor in the under-referral of older persons to trauma centers.

> **In elderly trauma, severe organ damage can occur at normal blood pressures, and the death rate goes up if the systolic is less than 110.**

Ground level falls and other low impact injuries, such as "fender benders" in crawling traffic, do cause severe traumatic injuries and result in high death rates in elders[80,81] (and under-diversion to trauma centers).

The new **Guidelines for Field Triage of Injured Patients 2012**[82] have added a fourth step about older adults to these guidelines for prehospital providers (EMS, et al) to better identify the correct destination facility and thus reduce the failures to get those most in need to the level 1 trauma center care they may need.[76,77,83,84] All PCPs should be aware of this, as they will—from time to time—be involved or even in charge of such decisions.

This is the wording of the statement about which injured elders in ANY of these conditions transport to a trauma center is recommended[82]:

- risk of injury/death increases after age 55 years
- SBP <110 might represent shock after age 65 years
- low impact mechanism (e.g., ground level falls) might result in severe injury
- high risk of **rapid deterioration in anticoagulated patients with head injury**

As spinal immobilization is so frequently carried out after accidents, PCPs should be aware that, whereas the elderly spine should be immobilized promptly and for fewer reasons than in younger patients, padding is necessary to increase immobilization as well as to guard against the real dangers of fragile skin breaking down.[85] Immobilization should thus be applied and used with considerable judgment, as those same frail patients whose skin can break down after 90 minutes on a backboard can also be ambulatory after trauma and yet have sustained a fracture.

Acute Stroke Care

CASE 5

Acute Stroke

Mr. Jeremiah Jones is a 65-year-old African American gentleman who is brought to your office by his wife with concern for trouble speaking. Mr. and Mrs. Jones were driving back home from grocery shopping when she noticed that all of a sudden, he began having "slowed speech" and seemed to struggle in getting certain words out. She got very concerned and had him drive straight to your office. Mr. Jones feels like there is nothing wrong with him other than his arm having "fallen asleep" from the way he was holding the steering wheel. When it is pointed out to him, he admits his words are coming out "very sluggishly" but dismisses this as lack of sleep. His right arm and neck feel numb, and according to him, he had some trouble walking up the steps to your clinic because his right leg feels heavy. Symptoms began around 45 minutes ago. He denies recent fevers, vomiting, shortness of breath, chest pain, headaches, or trauma to his head.

Mr. Jones has a past medical history of high blood pressure, hyperlipidemia, diabetes, and coronary artery disease. He is a smoker of 30 years, but denies drug or alcohol use. He has never had a stroke in the past. His vital signs are HR 88, BP 158/96, RR 16, Sat 98% on room air, Temp 37.2°C (98.9°F). On exam, he looks comfortable without distress. He has a slight droop to the right side of his lip when you ask him to smile. On more detailed neurologic exam, his cranial nerves seem intact other than decreased sensation on the right side of the face and the right facial droop. He has noticeably decreased (3/5) strength of his right arm compared to his left, and 4/5 strength of his right leg compared to his left, along with mild paresthesia of both right sided extremities. His pulmonary, cardiac, abdominal, and skin exams are unremarkable. You are of course concerned that Mr. Jones is having a stroke.

1. **How long do you have to get him to the most effective treatment facility for such a recent stroke?**

2. *Your local hospital is an "acute stroke hospital." Will they be able to give him the most effective treatment for this acute stroke?* ◘

Urgency of Stroke Care

An acute stroke is a time critical process in which "time is brain." The 2012 American Heart Association/American Stroke Association (AHA/ASA) guidelines[86,87] for the management of acute stroke has increased the time for rtPA administration to 4.5 hours from symptom onset. **A door to needle time of <60 minutes is emerging** supported by the National Quality Forum. Interventions delivered early in the course of stroke can prevent or decrease damage to critical brain structures preserving function.

Systems of care are evolving and the capabilities of acute stroke care at given hospitals are commonly divided into four levels. First are **comprehensive stroke centers** that can be certified by the Joint Commission of Hospital Accreditation. These centers offer 24/7 specialized care for **all stroke types**, beginning with tPA and ranging to a complex series of surgical and radiologic interventions. The second level of care is found at **primary stroke centers** that have 24/7 care for **ischemic stroke, without the interventional capabilities**. Third, there are **acute stroke hospitals** capable of evaluation and treatment. Finally **community hospitals** offer stroke care.

> COMPREHENSIVE stroke centers are the TOP, and can do EVERYTHING that can be done; primary stroke centers are good but lack some possible interventions; acute stroke hospitals evaluate and treat; don't be misled!

Different communities have varying support mechanisms to assist providers in instantiating stroke care. **Acute stroke patients must be dispatched to the highest level of care in the shortest time possible.** Providers must quickly diagnose stroke[88] and activate the stroke chain of survival, which in some instances may include air transport and hospital bypass.[89] **Drip and ship** is the term used for **initiating rtPA standard-dose before transfer** for invasive procedures or neuro intensive care including rigid BP control and assessment for potential intracranial hemorrhage. All EMS regions should be encouraged to build stroke systems to maximize accessibility of acute stroke care and all PCPs (indeed ALL providers) treating high-risk patients should be familiar with initiating the stroke chain of survival.

> "Door to needle" of sixty minutes; or "drip and ship" (give a dose of rtPA before transfer)

Emergency Detection and Management of Acute Stroke

Detection of stroke is essential given its varied presentations and potentially devastating sequel. Its identification process begins through patient education and awareness in the community, which, if done properly, can ensure early presentation and early treatment. If caught early, the neurologic deficits of the stroke can be minimized, whereas inability to properly identify can leave a patient with life-long disabilities.[86]

Management: Primary Care

- The diagnosis of stroke relies mostly on obtaining an accurate history and on performing a focused yet detailed physical exam. Its presentation can vary from gross unilateral paralysis to subtle findings easily overlooked in the busy office or clinic setting, without appropriate evaluation.[88,89]
- Traditional symptoms of stroke include unilateral paralysis of face, arm, legs, sudden confusion, aphasia, memory deficits, severe headache, or dizziness.
- **Atypical symptoms may include loss of consciousness, pain, palpitations, altered mental status, and shortness of breath.**[90]
- When symptoms are not immediately clear of a stroke and evaluation time is limited, several **prehospital stroke scales**[91,92] exist that can help aid in the diagnosis. The two most popular scales used by EMS systems are: Cincinnati Prehospital Scale (CPS)[91] and the Los Angeles Prehospital Stroke Screen (LAPSS).[92] The CPS has a sensitivity of 66% and specificity of 87% for acute stroke detection, whereas the LAPSS has a sensitivity of 91% and specificity of 97%.
- It is essential to be able to differentiate an acute stroke from other stroke mimickers. The **most common mimics are: seizures, confusional states, syncope, toxins, neoplasms, subdural hematomas. Hypoglycemia** can also cause neurologic deficits and must always be excluded.[90]
- The history should focus on **time of onset** of symptoms. This is essential as the definitive treatment of ischemic stroke with tPA administration depends on the length of duration of symptoms.
- Time of onset, as far as thrombolytics are concerned, is considered **the time last seen normal.** For example, if a patient wakes up with the symptoms, time of onset will be measured from the time the patient went to sleep.
- The presentation of **hemorrhagic versus ischemic** stroke can be identical. The differentiation of one versus the other needs to be made at a stroke center and should **not be of concern in an outpatient setting.** The management of acute stroke in a prehospital setting is the same regardless of the type of stroke.
- It is prudent to check a **point of care glucose** right away to exclude hypoglycemia as the cause of the symptoms.
- Once the diagnosis of stroke or concern for stroke has been identified, it is **essential to begin transfer** to the closest stroke center.
- Supportive care such as **oxygen, obtaining IV access, or giving fluid** to hypotensive patients is appropriate **as long as it does not delay the transfer** process.

Stroke Center Management

- Most stroke centers have a protocol in place to prioritize evaluation of a suspected stroke beginning with ensuring ABCs, IV access, oxygenation, cardiac monitoring, glucose and hemoglobin measurement, noncontrast head CT within 20 minutes of arrival to exclude hemorrhagic stroke, and basic blood work and history in order to determine tPA candidacy.
- There are criteria set by the AHA/ASA to determine **who is a candidate for tPA.** Inclusion criteria are **measurable stroke symptoms of onset < 4.5 hours with exclusion of hemorrhagic stroke in patients older than 18** years. Important exclusion criteria exist, including **hemorrhage of any kind, coagulopathies, and uncontrolled hypertension,** among many others.[86]
- Given that the AHA/ASA guidelines[86] for management of stroke in an ER setting call for a 60-minute time frame from arrival to evaluation and decision of management in acute stroke, and given the 3–4.5 hour time window for tPA administration, there exists a very short time available from time of onset of symptoms to outpatient evaluation to transfer to a stroke center. Because of this, **if you suspect acute stroke in your clinic, it is essential to expedite evaluation and effect immediate transfer to a stroke center over a lesser equipped emergency department.**
- Patients with **resolving or resolved symptoms consistent with a temporary ischemia attack (TIA), should still be transferred as soon as possible to the closest stroke center** for evaluation given the high risk of stroke in the near future, **particularly in the few days following the TIA.**[93]

Acute Stroke (continued)

You quickly obtain a finger stick glucose measurement which is 157. You know the capacity for stroke care in your nearest ED. You therefore decide that he needs immediate transfer to the closest emergency department given that the time of onset of symptoms was about an hour ago. You call EMS, who arrives within 10 minutes and take him to the ED.

When you follow up the next day, you learn that Mr. Jones was found to have an ischemic left-sided middle cerebral artery (MCA) stroke and that he was deemed to be a candidate for tPA. Administration was begun 2.5 hours from symptom onset thanks in part to your quick diagnosis and expeditious transfer. Two months later, during an office visit you see that Mr. Jones is recovering well, his speech is clear, and he has virtually no right-sided weakness. There are no limitations in his daily activities. You take this opportunity to reinforce stroke symptoms with both the patient and the wife. You discuss the importance to **act quickly and not let fear or denial interfere with prompt evaluation** by a doctor.

1. **What level of stroke care can YOUR local hospitals provide?**
2. **What are the local arrangements to get someone with an acute stroke to the nearest comprehensive stroke center?** ▣

Sepsis

The exact epidemiology of sepsis and septic shock in the ED is difficult to quantify due to **inconsistency in the definition** of sepsis. One study found ED infection frequencies in ED elders as follows: pneumonia (25%); urinary tract infection (22%); and sepsis and bacteremia (18%).[94] Infection presentation is, of course, frequently atypical in this population.[94] Vital signs consistent with serious illness are: **T >39.4°C (102.9°F), RR > 30, P >120. All such patients should be considered for expedited ED care.** Clinical findings associated with serious illness were **WBC >11 or presence of an infiltrate.** The most concerning feature is that absence of the above abnormalities in 46% of patients meaning **normal vital signs and lab values did not rule out serious infections.**[95] **Shaking chills, DM, major comorbidities, AMS, abdominal pain, and vomiting** are all predictive of bacterial infection.[96,97,98]

The Surviving Sepsis Campaign defines sepsis as the presence (probable or documented) of **infection together with systemic manifestations** of infection.[99] Screening for sepsis is recommended to increase identification and initiation of early therapy.[100] When initiated in the first 6 hours of diagnosis **Early Goal Directed Therapy (EGDT)** can improve survival.[101] As soon as hypoperfusion is recognized, aggressive fluid resuscitation should begin with goals of central venous pressure (CVP) 8–12 mmHg, MAP >65 mmHg, and urine output >0.5mL kg h^{-1}. Oxygenation as measured in the superior vena cava should be 70%. Antibiotic therapy should be initiated within the first hour of recognition of septic shock.

Sepsis

Mrs. Juanita Rodriguez is a 67-year-old female who presents to your clinic with cough. Mrs. Rodriguez has had a cough for a few days, along with runny nose, body aches, mild shortness of breath, and one episode of vomiting. Two people in her family have had similar symptoms. She has a history of diabetes and hypertension but is otherwise healthy. On exam, she appears well hydrated and nontoxic. Her vitals are HR 89, BP 138/72, RR 14, T 38.5 (101.3°F), Sat 97% on room air. Her HEENT, cardiac, pulmonary, and abdominal exam are benign. You diagnose her with the flu and send her home with supportive care.

One week later, Mrs. Rodriguez is brought into your clinic by her daughter. Her daughter tells you after you saw her she showed improvement for a few days but gradually experienced worsening shortness of breath, chills, and multiple episodes of vomiting. As a result, she has had very little fluid or solid food intake. For the past 2 days, she has been confused and not acting like herself. On exam, Mrs. Rodriguez looks pale, is oriented to person and place, has dry mucous membranes, is tachycardic, and has coarse crackles over the entire right lung base with decreased air movement on that side. Her vitals are HR 115, BP 105/55, RR 25, T 39.2 (102.6°F), Sat 93% on RA.

1. **Was the initial management appropriate?**
2. **What were her risk factors for this decline?**
3. **Can she still be managed at home?** ▣

Assessment

Elderly people are more prone to infection compared to younger people due to alterations in the immune response that occur with aging ("immune senescence").[102] The immune system may be further impaired by comorbidities, making adults with chronic disease more prone to infections than those without them.[103]

It is essential to risk stratify elderly patients who present to your clinic with signs of infection in order to **identify those that can be safely treated in an outpatient setting** and those that will need inpatient management. One way to categorize patients is by utilizing the concept of **SIRS** (Systemic Inflammatory Response Syndrome), **sepsis, severe sepsis, and septic shock**, which can be thought of as a severity of disease spectrum.

- **Systemic Inflammatory Response Syndrome** (SIRS) is defined as having at least two out of the four following criteria:[104,105]
  - Heart rate >90
  - Respiratory rate >20 (or PaCO2< 32)

- Temperature <36°C or >38°C (<96.8°F or >100.4°F)
  - Leukocyte count (WBC) >12 or <4, or with >10% bands
- **Sepsis** is defined as having SIRS **along with a suspected source** of infection.
- **Severe Sepsis** is defined as **sepsis plus either cardiovascular** organ dysfunction or **acute respiratory distress** syndrome or **dysfunction of two or more other** organs.
- **Septic Shock** is sepsis along with **hypotension of systolic BP < 90** despite appropriate fluid resuscitation (at least 40cc/kg).

A prospective study showed a mortality of 3% in patients with 0–1 SIRS criteria, 6% in those with 2 out of 4 criteria, 10% in those with 3 out of 4 criteria, and 17% in those meeting all four.[106] Thus it can be extrapolated that the more SIRS criteria in a given patient, the higher the expected mortality. Mortality rate from bacteremia is also higher in older patients: 37% to 50% versus 5% to 35% in young adults.[106]

Although the definitions above apply to all adults, it is important to keep in mind that **fever or chills may be less likely** to be present in older adults.[107]

Management

- Begin with the basics: Assess ABCs and check vital signs.
- Assess for signs of SIRS as this will help you to **risk stratify** a patient based on the SIRS-sepsis spectrum.
- Physical exam: Attempt to identify the source of infection. Pay attention to signs of hypoperfusion such as **dry mucous membranes, hypoxia, poor capillary refill**, and other signs of **shock or organ failure**.
- Ancillary testing: A **chest x-ray and urine analysis** can help identify the source of infection. At an advanced care facility, complete blood counts, electrolyte panel, blood cultures, urine cultures, blood gas, lactate, and an ECG are routine testing in a septic patient.
- It has been suggested that CRP may be used as an early marker for infection in elderly adults; however, there is wide variation in the sensitivity and specificity of this assay, and thus it adds little to clinical judgment.[108,109]
- Administer oxygen, control temperature, and address analgesia as needed.
- Focal infection: In an outpatient setting, if the source of infection is identified and if the patient does not meet sepsis criteria and does not show any sign of concerning systemic infection, it is reasonable to treat as an outpatient with prompt follow-up.

- Antibiotics: Direct therapy for known source, or empiric therapy for unknown source. **Antibiotics should be initiated as soon as possible** in order to improve outcome.[109]
- Once a patient has been deemed to be **septic, immediate transport to the closest ED** is necessary for appropriate treatment.
- Sepsis management: One of the most widely used approaches to manage sepsis is outlined by the **Surviving Sepsis Campaign** international guidelines.[99] These incorporate what is referred to as **Early Goal Directed Therapy**,[110] and include aggressive fluid resuscitation, broad spectrum antibiotics, +/− endotracheal intubation, central venous pressure monitoring through placement of a central line, and close hemodynamic management. In cases of septic shock, both vasoactive and ionotropic agents, as well as blood transfusions, may be indicated. This management is normally **begun in the ED and continued in the ICU.**

Summary: Sepsis

If you have a patient with a localized infection without signs of SIRS with good follow-up, it is reasonable to discharge them with treatment for their presenting infection.

If you identify a patient with sepsis (at least 2 out of 4 SIRS criteria), with altered mental status, blood pressure instability, or any other signs of end organ damage, you should transfer them immediately to the closest ED for further evaluation and workup.

CASE 6

Sepsis (continued)

You are concerned Mrs. Rodriguez has a post-influenza bacterial pneumonia and that she has developed sepsis based on her fever, tachycardia, tachypnea (3 out of 4 SIRS criteria). In addition, she has a lower blood pressure with a wide pulse pressure. If you have parenteral antibiotics at your disposal you should immediately initiate antibiotic treatment even as you call for ambulance transport to the nearest ED. You give her one dose of ceftriaxone in your office, one gram of acetaminophen for the fever, and begin to administer a liter of normal saline IV as EMS arrives for direct transport to the closest ED.

After the patient leaves, you wonder if you did the right thing by discharging her one week earlier. Given the fact that at the time the only vital sign abnormality was her fever (1 out of 4 SIRS criteria), that she looked well, that she had no systemic symptoms, and that she had symptoms typical of the flu, you conclude that there had been no indication to refer to the ED at that point. It is likely they may have sent her home as well.

You follow up on her hospital course and find out that on arrival she did in fact have a large right-sided bacterial pneumonia, had a WBC of 32,000, and an anion-gap metabolic acidosis with a lactate of 5.3. She was given 5 L of fluid in the ED. Broad spectrum antibiotics were initiated. She had a central line placed for hemodynamic monitoring and was admitted to the ICU, where she remained for 3 days. Her blood cultures grew out streptococcus species. She is recovering well on the general medicine floor with normal vital signs and improving symptoms of pneumonia. ▣

HYPOTHERMIA AND HYPERTHERMIA

All Boy Scouts learn (but possibly do not retain!) knowledge of the early symptoms of these two important, potentially lethal, and often seasonal syndromes.[111,112]

Not always seasonal, however. An old person fallen on the floor at night—even an ill, old person in bed in a hospital—can (sometimes insidiously) develop hypothermia, a diagnosis which can easily be missed (a rectal thermometer is essential to confirming and staging the diagnosis). In addition, heat stroke (the worst level of hyperthermia) can occur in a heat wave through sitting alone indoors without air conditioning, and—again—this can kill.

This section will help you recognize these syndromes, stage them, and thus decide if you or the Boy Scouts could handle it, or whether the patient needs the ED and often the ICU as well.

CASE 7

Hypothermia

Eric Fink is an eccentric old man of 92 who lives alone and does not welcome strangers. You see him rarely, but he is "yours." One morning in winter, he is found lying outside his barn in the snow. From a distance he looks dead. Neighbors are amazed to find he's alive, though mumbling incoherently. He is very cold to the touch. He is not shivering. His muscles are stiff. One neighbor starts rubbing his hands and legs "to get the circulation going." Another goes for a warm cup of coffee for him. The third neighbor calls you as they plan to carry him into a nearby kitchen.

1. **What do you tell them to do?**
2. **What will you do?** ▣

Hypothermia

Many illnesses and some drugs predispose to this illness, but the main cause is usually cold exposure. It is defined as a core temperature of less than 35°C (95°F).

Risk factors are: age, health, body size, undernutrition, dehydration, cognitive impairment, exposure,

low outdoor temperature, wind speed, humidity, alcohol, and a number of medicines.[111]

The **pathologic changes** are bradycardia, reduced reflexes, respiratory depression, and coma. Blood vessels constrict—a protective mechanism. Rewarming the skin and periphery dilates the surface vessels and acidotic, cold blood streams in, and the body temperature then drops ("core temperature afterdrop"), so the core needs to be warmed first. During warming, myocardial irritability from the cold predisposes to dysrhythmias and even cardiac arrest from ventricular fibrillation (VF).[113]

Diagnosis

This requires a rectal, low-reading thermometer, and gentle handling of the patient is crucial. Severity is measured by the core body (rectal) temperature, giving three stages:

Mild hypothermia: Core temperature 34–35°C (93–95°F). Patient is shivering, has muscle pains, is alert, and follows commands. This can be treated on site (indoors though).

Moderate hypothermia: Core temperature is 31–33°C (88-92°F). Patient may be confused, drowsy or hallucinating. No shivering and stiff muscles. Respiratory depression. Needs the ED urgently, as it may progress to:

Severe hypothermia: NOW it's an emergency: Core temperature is less than 31°C (88°F). Often unconscious, waxy skin or cyanosed, very stiff muscles, very depressed respiration, may appear dead. Needs ED and probably ICU urgently.[111]

CASE 7

Hypothermia (continued)

You tell them to cover him very gently with a blanket. He is very fragile and ill. Warming may induce cardiac arrest as clinically he's moderate, bordering severe. Don't rub the skin!! Don't give warm drinks!!! Just get him to the ED. He survives, but never remembers why or when he went out. He is friendlier to his neighbors afterwards. ▣

Management

Rewarming is the treatment but with cardiac arrest as a risk it must be the core first and slowly. Raise the core temperature by 0.5–2°C (0.25–1°F) per hour.[114]

Mild: Core temperature 34–35°C (93-95°F). Mild exercise. Warm bath. Glucose containing drinks. NO massage, NO alcohol or coffee.

Moderate: Core temperature is 31–33°C. In the ED, warm humidified air to breathe, warm IV boluses with dextrose, wrap trunk in warm blankets, or use a heated vest, warm limbs AFTER warming trunk. NO exercise, NO alcohol, NO cold air, NO cold drinks; watch for IV overload.

Severe: Core temperature is less than 31°C (88°F). Very gentle, may need intubation, and this too may precipitate VF. Heated humid air, peritoneal lavage with warmed K-free fluids, cardiopulmonary bypass with warmed fluids and blood, nasogastric (NG) tube with lavage and suction of warmed fluids; these are all possible techniques. Hyperkalemia, hemoconcentration, myoglobinuria, acute tubular necrosis (ATN), and hypercoagulable states complicate this potentially lethal situation.[111,114]

Hyperthermia

Hyperthermia

Daisy Meek is an *81-year-old* alcoholic who lives alone, and there's a heat wave in this *midwestern* town. She stays indoors "all the time," has no air conditioning, is sleepy, and smells of alcohol. You see her in the urgent care clinic. She is cool, clammy to the touch, and has had muscle cramps. She is thirsty but nauseous, alert but disoriented (but she is often confused, according to the neighbor who brought her to see you). BP is 165/90, P 96, T 37.5°C (99.5°F)

1. **The neighbor is willing to take her home to his place, which has *air conditioning*. Would the neighbor's offer be enough?**

2. **Is this heat stroke?**

3. **Should she be taken to the ED and, if so, why?**

4. **Can the local hospital deal with this? ▣**

Risk Factors

Heat waves in the Midwest have given us much of the data about this hot weather phenomenon. Lack of access to air conditioning and living alone with an illness are the big risk factors.[112]

Heart failure (HF), medications for hypertension and dysrhythmias, aged skin, and alcohol (which causes heat gain in a hot environment) are other factors.

Diagnosis

Heat fatigue: Exposure to high outside temperatures or over-exertion in the heat. The patient is pale, sweaty, cool and moist to the touch, weak, exhausted, but because he/she can sweat, the core temperature stays normal.

Heat syncope is a syncope, or dizziness, after exercising in the heat, sweating has lost fluid and electrolytes, and the patient is pale and sweaty, pulse is weak, heart rate is up, body temperature still normal.

Heat cramps are muscle cramps, still sweating; this is from fluid and salt loss; the pulse and BP are up, patient is thirsty. May need the ED as IV saline is part of the management.

Heat exhaustion is next, and turns the corner into a life-threatening phenomenon. Thirsty still, but altered mental state (dizzy, confused, weak), cool and clammy, tachycardic and maybe nauseated. Core temperature may be up a little. Patient needs the ED, for the IV saline and because it may morph into heat stroke.

Heat stroke is fatal if neglected, with the body temperature rising quickly and out of control. The temperature is often over 40°C (104°F), and the patient is hot and DRY, confused, combative, delirious, then comatose—plus tachycardia, hypotension, and hyperventilation—and there is end organ damage: acute renal failure (ARF) and hypercoagulation states occur.[115]

Management

Heat fatigue and **heat syncope** patients need drinks of electrolyte replacement fluids, a cool environment, and rest.

Heat cramps and **heat exhaustion** patients need a cool environment, oral liquids and IV saline, and rest.

Heat stroke patients need the ED and may need the ICU, but anyone can make a start with fanning and tepid water sprays, aiming to cool slowly, but with the EMS on the way.[116]

Hyperthermia (continued)

She clinically has the features of heat exhaustion, and although thirsty and alert, will need IV fluids; she was on the verge of heat stroke and so could easily have declined to that potentially lethal condition. She is already nauseous and, in addition, she is a known alcoholic and thus in danger of a withdrawal syndrome. Fortunately, she accepts direct admission to the local hospital, and—although her medical care was straightforward—her alcohol-associated dementia justifies a skilled nursing facility (SNF) level of care, and she is discharged to the safety and security of a local nursing home and settles in there without incident. ▣

TRANSITIONS OF CARE

All PCPs of older patients must acquire mastery of transferring care—not only sending a patient to other health professionals or to another care site but also taking over the care of a patient from someone or somewhere else. Poor transitions of care lead to failures in quality of care and medical errors, and augment disparities between patient needs and resource utilization.[117] The transferring professional must ensure adequate information exchange. This process typically involves prior discussion with the accepting facility as to what information is required for optimal care. As with many things, planning avoids predictable pitfalls.

Almost **25% of all nursing home residents are transported to the ED annually**.[118] In 2006, the Office of the Inspector General reported that approximately 34,500 patients annually are discharged and readmitted to the ED on the same day, costing over $226 million.[119] Clinicians have estimated that as many as **67% of NH hospitalizations are potentially avoidable**.[120]

However, the fee-for-service system, lack of ready provider contact with NH residents, and medical litigation together provide powerful incentives for an easy phone call ordering ED evaluation or hospitalization of NH residents. The high cost of care in NH patients, frail elders, and those at the end of life have spurred many efforts to create **disincentives for hospitalization**. Providers must be aware of these approaches to best position themselves for the future.

> In your nursing home and similarly frail home care patients, ensure that you have on record the patient's wishes about hospitalization, intubation, and other scope of treatment issues; you will be able to reduce ED visits and hospitalizations!

One tactic is to reduce transfers to ED and hospitals when care could have been delivered in another setting. The ACP is implementing quality assurance and performance improvement programs to prevent avoidable transfers from the nursing home to the hospital. Financing models that have been made to reduce hospitalization in frail elders include the Program of All-Inclusive Care for the Elderly (PACE).[121] INTERACT is another effort that has shown positive effects.[122] Other resources exist to aid in improving transitions of care. The National Transitions of Care Coalition (NTOCC), NTOCC.org, has **tools for health care professionals and patients addressing improved communications;** standardization of medical records and medication reconciliation; establishing points of accountability with PCPs, NHs, EDs, hospitalists, and SNFs; increasing use of case management; implementation of payment systems to align incentives; and developing performance metrics to ensure quality improvement in transitions. Finally, ED utilization can be decreased by initiation of geriatric assessments and geriatric case management during the routine care of older adults, thereby avoiding acute decompensation.[123] However, the payment system truly discourages even experienced clinicians from taking the appropriate preventive, anticipatory approach that these frail individuals both need and would wish to have. Good care would decrease the need for ED utilization. For good transitions of care to occur, you must have the knowledge of when to refer to the ED and when to treat on site, and the skills (and patience) to effect optimal communication, stabilization, and transport to the most appropriate level of care. This will ensure the best chance of survival for your patients, and a better chance of recovery to baseline function after the acute situation is over.

KEY REFERENCES

2. Grueneir A, Silver MJ, Rochon PA. Review: Emergency department use by older adults: A literature review on trends, appropriateness, and consequences of unmet health care needs. Med Care Res Rev 2011;68:131.

7. Carrier E, Tracy Y, Holzwart R. Coordination between Emergency and Primary Care Physicians. National Institute for Health Care Reform Research Brief No. 3; February 2011.

54. Qaseem A, Wilt TJ, Weinberger SE, et al. Diagnosis and management of stable chronic obstructive pulmonary disease: A clinical practice guideline update from the American College of Physicians, American College of Chest Physicians, American Thoracic Society, and European Respiratory Society. Ann Intern Med 2011;155(3):179-91.

83. Chang DC, Bass RR, Cornwell EE, et al. Undertriage of elderly trauma patients to state-designated trauma centers. Arch Surg 2008;143:776-81.

86. Jauch EC, Saver JL, Adams HP Jr, et al. Guidelines for the early management of patients with acute ischemic stroke: A guideline for healthcare professionals from the American Heart Association/American Stroke Association. Stroke 2013, Jan 31. (Epub ahead of print)

99. Dellinger R, Levy M, Rhodes A, et al. Surviving Sepsis Campaign: International guidelines for management of severe sepsis and shock, 2012. Intensive Care Med 2013;39:165-228.

References available online at expertconsult.com.

16

Delirium

Babar A. Khan and Malaz A. Boustani

OBJECTIVES

Upon completion of this chapter, the reader will be able to:

- Discuss the definition, the burden, and the pathophysiology of delirium among hospitalized older adults.

- Understand the delirium vulnerability-trigger interaction model, use this model to characterize the vulnerability of hospitalized older adults for developing delirium, and identify the precipitant factors that trigger delirium among these vulnerable individuals.

- Recognize the importance of using primary prevention to decrease the burden of delirium in hospitalized older adults, and the value of implementing proactive screening to identify at-risk persons at the time of hospital admission.

- Discuss the management of delirium in general and delirium-induced agitation in particular.

- Describe a multicomponent hospital system to decrease the burden of delirium, and discuss the process of implementing such a program at the reader's local acute setting.

Additional online-only material indicated by icon.

CASE 1

Elaine Fischer (Part 1)

Elaine Fischer is an 83-year-old woman with mild Alzheimer's disease. She lives at home with her daughter. She is independent in all of her basic activities of daily living (ADLs), and dependent on her daughter for shopping, finance management, and transportation. Today, Ms. Fischer comes to your office with her daughter. She is having paranoid delusions and has stopped eating because she is convinced that her daughter is poisoning her. She has been losing weight and feels weak. She also complains of shortness of breath on exertion. The remainder of her physical examination is normal.

What is the differential diagnosis for Ms. Fischer's paranoid symptoms? ▪

DEFINITION AND PATHOGENESIS OF DELIRIUM

Delirium or acute confusional state is a syndrome characterized by disturbance in consciousness, with reduced ability to focus, sustain, or shift attention that occurs over a short period of time and tends to fluctuate over the course of the day.[1] This disturbance affects numerous domains of brain function; thus *acute brain failure* is an accurate descriptive term for delirium.

Delirium induces various neuropsychiatric symptoms such as lethargy, aggression, and hallucinations. These symptoms can be used to divide delirium into hypoactive, hyperactive, or mixed types.[2,3] Delirium's neuropsychiatric symptoms are shared across various brain disorders such as dementia, depression, and psychosis. However, the acute and fluctuating nature of symptoms is the main feature differentiating delirium from depression, dementia, and other brain conditions. Box 16-1 summarizes the various categories of delirium neuropsychiatric symptomatology.

BOX 16-1

DELIRIUM SYMPTOMS

Acute change in mental status
Fluctuating course
Attention disturbance
Memory disturbance
Orientation disturbance
Perceptual disturbance
Thought disturbance
Sleep disturbance
Consciousness disturbance
Speech disturbance
Psychomotor activity disturbance

Studies of patients with delirium suggest that prefrontal cortex, basal forebrain, anterior thalamus, and nondominant parietal and fusiform cortex are involved in inducing delirium symptoms.[4-6] At present, stress is considered to be the cornerstone of delirium pathogenesis, leading to metabolic changes that modify the cerebral neurotransmission.[7-11] Common stressors include drugs, infection, hypoxia, hypoperfusion, trauma, and surgery,[6,9,12] with the final pathway being cholinergic deficiency and dopaminergic excess.[9,12] Thus, delirium can be considered a brain maladaptive reaction to acute stress.[12]

TABLE 16-1	Prevalence of Delirium among Hospitalized Older Adults
Setting and Population	**Delirium Prevalence Range**
Older adults hospitalized for medical illness[14-21]	11% to 41%
Postoperative: Older adults undergoing surgical repair of hip fracture[22-25]	40% to 52%
Postoperative: Older adults undergoing elective major noncardiac surgery[26-31]	10% to 39%
Postoperative: Older adults undergoing cardiac surgery[32-39]	13% to 44%

CASE 2

Mary Johnson (Part 1)

Your patient, Mary Johnson, an 82-year-old woman, is in the emergency room after having fallen and broken her hip. She is very healthy except for a history of hypertension. She is a widow who has been living in her house in a rural area. She has children who live elsewhere and see her only once or twice per year, and they report she has no problems with her ADLs, but they cannot assess her instrumental ADLs. She is taking no routine medications. Her labs on hospital admission show evidence of dehydration with sodium of 152 mmol/L and a BUN/creatinine ratio of >20:1. The nurse has administered the Mini-Mental State Examination (MMSE) and the Geriatric Depression Scale (GDS). The patient scored 21/30 on the MMSE and 7/15 on the GDS. She had no evidence of attention deficit or fluctuating mental status.

What is Ms. Johnson's probability of developing postoperative delirium? ▣

PREVALENCE AND IMPACT OF DELIRIUM

The 2007 National Hospital Discharge Survey conducted by the U.S. National Center for Health Statistics estimated 34.4 million hospital discharges. Patients aged 65 and older comprised 37% of all of the hospital discharges and 43% of hospital days.[13] The prevalence of delirium among the hospitalized older adults varied from 10% to 52%,[14-39] depending on the reason for hospitalization (Table 16-1). The rate increases dramatically among hospitalized older adults with dementia, with delirium occurring in 32% to 86% of this vulnerable population.[40] Of patients with delirium, 65% have the hypoactive type, 25% the hyperactive type, and 10% a mixed type.[41]

With the aging of the U.S. population, there will be an expected increase in the prevalence of age-related diseases.[42] Therefore, we can project an increase in the incidence and prevalence of delirium in the coming years.[43] According to the U.S. Centers for Medicare and Medicaid Services, hospitalization costs will exceed $1.3 trillion annually by the year 2019 because of the aging population.[44] The health care system is currently spending between $38 and $152 billion annually in delirium-related costs,[45] and with the rise in aging-related diseases, this expenditure is likely to go up.[43]

Delirium in the elderly increases the risk of death.[46-48] According to one study, the risk odds ratio (OR) of mortality for hospitalized patients with delirium, compared with nondelirious controls, have a higher risk of death (38% versus 27%; odds ratio [OR] 1.95; confidence interval [CI]: 1.51-2.52).[46] Patients with delirium are also at an increased risk of institutionalization (33.4% versus 10.7%; OR 2.41; 95% CI: 1.77-3.29).[46] These associations are independent of age, gender, comorbidity, severity of illness, and preexisting dementia. Coexistence of delirium with dementia increases the risk of rehospitalization and admission to long-term care compared to patients with dementia or delirium alone.[40]

CASE 1

Elaine Fischer (Part 2)

In your office you obtain laboratory results for a urinalysis, metabolic profile, and chest x-ray study; they are normal. You prescribe haloperidol 0.5 mg per day and send Ms. Fischer home with her daughter after providing reassurance and family education. However, Ms. Fischer continues to complain of shortness of breath and the delusions persist. The next day she "runs away" from home, and the police find her wandering in the neighborhood. She is brought to the emergency room for assessment, and a computed tomography scan of her head and a chest radiograph are negative. Pulse oximetry shows mild hypoxia, which is corrected by oxygen. Her haloperidol dose is increased to 0.5 mg twice a day. She is also started on trazodone 50 mg daily by the emergency department physician, and she is given codeine for off-and-on cough complaints. She is sent home with her daughter for follow-up in your office.

If Ms. Fischer does not currently have delirium, what is her current risk for developing delirium in association with hospitalization for an acute illness? ▣

RISK FACTORS AND PRECIPITATING FACTORS

Delirium among hospitalized older adults is the result of a complex interaction between various degrees of insult severity and different levels of patient's vulnerability.[49] This vulnerability-trigger interaction is responsible for the wide range (10% to 86%) of delirium prevalence rates reported among hospitalized older adults.

Finding a single factor responsible for the onset of delirium is rare. By using the vulnerability-trigger interaction model, clinicians can categorize the contributing factors of delirium into two groups. First is the cluster of predisposing or vulnerability factors (Table 16-2). Second is the cluster of precipitating or trigger factors (Table 16-3). However, some factors can act as both precipitating and predisposing. A common example of such a dual factor is a drug with anticholinergic properties. The delirium vulnerability of an older female adult who is taking anticholinergic drugs such as oxybutinine for urine incontinence is already high. Prescribing a sleeping pill such as diphenhydramine with anticholinergic properties to manage her postoperative sleep problem might be the factor that tips her into delirium during her hospital admission for elective knee replacement.

Because of the important role that anticholinergic medications play in the development of delirium as predisposing and precipitating factors, we have summarized the most common anticholinergic medications that are used in older adults (Table 16-4). The concept of total anticholinergic burden has been used to reflect the cumulative anticholinergic activities of all medications taken by an individual patient.[50,51] Thus both a single drug with strong anticholinergic properties and a combination of multiple drugs with a relatively small anticholinergic effect might lead to the development of delirium in older adults.[52-55]

Various methods are used to determine the anticholinergic activity of a given drug, and thus the anticholinergic burden faced by a particular patient. They

TABLE 16-2	Predisposing Factors for Delirium among Older Adults Hospitalized for a Medical or a Surgical Illness	
Risk Factor	**Odds Ratio (OR) Range***	**The Delirium Vulnerability Scale**
Cognitive Impairment:	3.5-5	Choose one score only
• Chart diagnosis of dementia	2-4	3 points
• MMSE <24	4	2 points
• Prior history of delirium		1 point
Current history of depression	2-4	1 point
Current history of alcohol abuse	3-6.5	2 points
Current and untreated hearing loss	2	1 point
Current and untreated vision loss	2-3.5	1 point
Need assistance in 2 basic activities of daily living	2.5	1 point
Current use of anticholinergic	1.5-2.7	2 points
Dehydration defined by BUN/creatinine >21:1	1.8-2	1 point
Sodium abnormality (Na <130 or Na >150)	2-4	1 point
Vascular risk factors: History of	2.3	Choose a score of 1 point if at
• Hypertension	1.3-2.9	least one risk factor was
• Congestive heart failure	1.3	present (maximum score is
• Diabetes mellitus	2.2	also 1 point)
• Cerebrovascular accident	1.4	
• Atrial fibrillation		
Admitted for		
• Urgent surgical repair of hip fracture	3	2 points
• Elective aortic aneurysm repair	6	3 points
Total Points		_____ [range 0-17]
Interpretation:	**Risk category**	**Probability of developing delirium****
• 0-1 point	Low	< 5%
• 2-3 points	Mild	5% to 20%
• 4-7 points	Moderate	21% to 40%
• >7 points	Severe	>40%

MMSE, Mini-Mental State Examination.
*OR estimates were based on review of the literature.
**Delirium probability estimates for each risk category were based on a literature review[17,20,21,24,26,29,31,36-40,52,54,66,75-79] and the authors' clinical and research experiences. The delirium vulnerability scale has not been validated in a prospective cohort study.

TABLE 16-3	Precipitating Factors for the Development of Delirium during Hospitalization for Medical or Surgical Illness[36,49,58,78,79]
Precipitating Factor	**Odds Ratio (OR)**
Use of physical restraints	4.4
Malnutrition	4
Using more than three new medications during hospitalization	2.9
Use of bladder catheterization	2.4
Exposed to any iatrogenic event	1.9
Intraoperative hypotension (at least 31% drop in mean perioperative BP or a SBP ≤80 mmHg	1.4
Postoperative Hct <30%	1.7
Untreated postoperative pain	5.4-9
Use of anticholinergic drug	1.5-2.7

BP, Blood pressure; *Hct*, hematocrit; *SBP*, systolic blood pressure.

include the use of a drug's in-vitro affinity to the muscarinic receptor,[56] opinion of clinical experts regarding the drug's clinical anticholinergic adverse effects,[54,56] and measuring the serum anticholinergic activity (SAA) secondary to the intake of a single or multiple drugs.[57,58] Table 16-4 integrates the results of different studies to categorize the anticholinergic activities of medications into drugs with definite central anticholinergic activity, assigned a score of 2 or 3, and those with possible central anticholinergic property with a score of 1. Based on recent evidence, each definite anticholinergic drug increases the risk of cognitive impairment by 46% over 6 years.[59] In addition, with each one point increase in the anticholinergic burden score, there is a decline in MMSE of 0.33 points over 2 years, and a 26% increase in the risk of death.[60]

CASE 1

Elaine Fischer (Part 3)

A week later you receive a call from the patient's daughter who reports that her mother is now very lethargic. You instruct the daughter to take her mother back to the emergency room to be evaluated. She again is hypoxic and has a rapid pulse, and is found to be somnolent and obtunded. In consultation with the emergency room physician you obtain a ventilation perfusion (VQ) scan, which shows a large right-sided pulmonary embolism with several small chronic emboli in the left lung.

What is the most urgent next therapeutic intervention? ◼

TABLE 16-4	Medications with Central Anticholinergic Activity*	
Score = 3 **High Anticholinergic Activity**	**Score = 2** **Moderate Anticholinergic Activity**	**Score = 1** **Mild Anticholinergic Activity**
Amitriptyline	Amantadine	Alverine
Amoxapine	Belladonna	Alprazolam
Atropine	Carbamazepine	Atenolol
Benztropine	Cyclobenzaprine	Bupropion
Brompheniramine	Cyproheptadine	Captopril
Carbinoxamine	Loxapine	Chlorthalidone
Chlorpheniramine	Meperidine	Cimetidine
Chlorpromazine	Methotrimeprazine	Clorazepate
Clemastine	Molindone	Codeine
Clomipramine	Oxcarbazepine	Colchicine
Clozapine	Pimozide	Diazepam
Darifenacin		Digoxin
Desipramine		Dipyridamole
Dicyclomine		Disopyramide
Dimenhydrinate		Fentanyl
Diphenhydramine		Furosemide
Doxepin		Fluvoxamine
Flavoxate		Haloperidol
Hydroxyzine		Hydralazine
Hyoscyamine		Hydrocortisone
Imipramine		Isosorbide
Meclizine		Loperamide
Methocarbamol		Metoprolol
Nortriptyline		Morphine
Olanzapine		Nifedipine
Orphenadrine		Prednisone
Oxybutynin		Quinidine

TABLE 16-4	Medications with Central Anticholinergic Activity (Continued)	
Score = 3 High Anticholinergic Activity	Score = 2 Moderate Anticholinergic Activity	Score = 1 Mild Anticholinergic Activity
Paroxetine Perphenazine Promethazine Propantheline Quetiapine Scopolamine Thioridazine Tolterodine Trifluoperazine Trihexyphenidyl Trimipramine		Ranitidine Risperidone Theophylline Trazodone Triamterene

*Based on the following methods: (1) the drug's in-vitro affinity to the muscarinic receptor,[56] (2) the opinion of clinical experts regarding the drug's clinical anticholinergic adverse effects,[54,56] and (3) the patient's serum anticholinergic activity (SAA) secondary to the intake of a single or multiple drugs.[57,58]

DIAGNOSIS AND ASSESSMENT OF DELIRIUM

Diagnosing delirium is difficult. This is evident from the fact that between one third and two thirds of delirium remains undiagnosed.[61] In order to differentiate between dementia, delirium, and other psychiatric illnesses with similar neuropsychiatric symptom profiles, clinicians need to be familiar with the core diagnostic features of delirium and understand that having a diagnosis of dementia does not rule out delirium.

There are several bedside tools available for delirium assessment.[62,63] The Confusion Assessment Method (CAM)[1] has the most evidence supporting its use as a bedside assessment. In contrast, the Folstein MMSE[64] (score <24) has little value in identifying delirium (likelihood ratio [LR] 1.6; 95% CI: 1.2-2.0).[65] Table 16-5 provides the CAM diagnostic algorithm for identifying delirium. This diagnostic approach has a sensitivity of 94% to 100%, a specificity of 90% to 95%, a positive likelihood ratio of 9.6 (95% CI: 5.8-16.0), and a negative likelihood ratio of 0.16 (95% CI: 0.09-0.29).[1,65]

> Delirium is associated with increased mortality, poorer functional status, limited rehabilitation, increased hospital-acquired complications, prolonged length of hospital stay, increased risk of institutionalization, and higher health care expenditures.

TABLE 16-5	The Confusion Assessment Method (CAM) Diagnostic Instrument*
Diagnostic Features	Definitions and Characteristics
(1) Acute Onset and Fluctuating Course	Presence is indicated by a positive response to one or more of the following questions: • Is there evidence of an acute change in mental status from the patient's baseline? • Did the (abnormal) behavior fluctuate during the day, that is, tend to come and go, or increase and decrease in severity?
(2) Inattention	Presence is indicated by a positive response to the following question: • Did the patient have difficulty focusing attention (e.g., being easily distractible) or have difficulty keeping track of what was being said?
(3) Disorganized Thinking	Presence is indicated by a positive response to the following question: • Was the patient's thinking disorganized or incoherent, such as rambling or irrelevant conversation, unclear or illogical flow of ideas, or unpredictable switching from subject to subject?
(4) Altered Level of Consciousness	Presence is indicated by any answer other than "alert" to the following question: • Overall, how would you rate this patient's level of consciousness? (alert [normal]), vigilant [hyperalert], lethargic [drowsy, easily aroused], stupor [difficult to arouse], or coma [unarousable])

Adapted with permission from Inouye SK, vanDyck CH, Alessi CA, et al. Clarifying confusion: The Confusion Assessment Method. A new method for detection of delirium. Ann Intern Med 1990;113:941-8.[1] Confusion assessment method: Training manual and coding guide, Copyright 2003, Hospital Elder Life Program, LLC.
*Delirium is defined as present if the patient has (1) + (2) + [either (3) or (4)].

After diagnosing delirium, a clinician can use the vulnerability-trigger interaction model to identify the underlying modifiable and nonmodifiable triggers. In one study of delirium among hospitalized older adults with a medical illness, fluid and electrolyte abnormalities were the possible trigger in 40% of cases, infection in 40%, drug toxicity in 30%, metabolic disorders in 26%, sensory and environmental problems in 24%, and low perfusion in 14%.[17] Among hospitalized older adults undergoing surgical repair of a hip fracture, 62% of the delirium cases had several triggers, with the most frequent causes being environmental issues, infection, medications, and fluid-electrolyte disturbances.[66]

> **Delirium is diagnosed if a patient has an acute change in mental status with attention deficit accompanied by disorganized thinking or a change in alertness.**

Table 16-6 provides a simple approach for delirium assessment. This approach is based on the authors' clinical experiences and their review of the literature.[48,62] The suggested assessment for delirium requires a face-to-face interview with the patients to identify the presence of emergent situation such as hypoxia, hypotension, or sepsis; this is followed by a comprehensive history and chart review to identify possible reasons that led to delirium development such as dehydration, electrolyte abnormality, heart failure, infectious process, or a new sedative or anticholinergic drug. Note that there is no routine recommendation for brain imaging or more invasive diagnostic tests without the presence of findings during the physical examination or chart review that suggest a new focal central nervous system process.

> **Brain imaging or more invasive diagnostic tests for delirium assessment are not indicated without the presence of positive findings during the history, physical examination, or chart review.**

CASE 2

Mary Johnson (Part 2)

Ms. Johnson undergoes hip replacement surgery. On postoperative day 2, she is rambling and incoherent but able to recognize the individuals caring for her. She has an oxygen mask that she keeps trying to take off; she tries to pull out her Foley catheter, and she keeps trying to get out of bed. She is administered lorazepam 1 mg intravenously to control her symptoms.

What are the safest and most effective strategies to manage the patient's delirium-induced agitation? ◫

TABLE 16-6	Identifying and Managing the Causes and Contributing Factors of Delirium in a Hospitalized Patient[48,71]
Assessment	**Treatment**
- Vital signs (pulse, BP, T, RR, and pulse oximetry) - Physical examination to diagnose and treat infectious process or other acute medical conditions (pneumonia, pressure ulcers, MI, CVA, etc.) - Urinalysis - Cr, Na, K, Ca, glucose - CBC with differential - Review old and new anticholinergic medications - Review old and new sedating medications - Review the need for Foley catheter, IV lines, and other tethers	<u>General Measures:</u> • Encourage sleep, orientation, and activity • Personalize the environment • Treat medical conditions such as dehydration, electrolyte disturbances, and infection • Discontinue catheters, IV lines, and other tethers if benefit does not outweigh harm • Discontinue sedating and anticholinergic medications when possible and appropriate • Identify and treat acute pain • Prevent and/or treat constipation <u>Interventions for Agitation:</u> • Consider professional sitter. • Assess the impact of agitation on patient safety and disconnect Foley and other tethers if possible • If history of alcohol use, consider lorazepam 0.25-0.5 mg PO/IM/IV q 4-6 hours PRN • If safety an issue, and sitter ineffective, and being treated for a reversible medical condition, consider haloperidol 0.25 mg PO/IM/IV q 4 hours PRN (maximum dose <3 mg/day, reevaluating every 24 hours and discontinuing haloperidol prior to discharge. <u>Interventions for Lethargy:</u> • Protect skin; check regularly for skin breakdown • Decrease dose of hypnotics and of other sedative medications

BP, Blood pressure; *CBC*, complete blood count; *CVA*, cerebrovascular accident; *IV*, intravenous; *MI*, myocardial infarction; *RR*, respiratory rate; *T*, temperature.

MANAGEMENT OF DELIRIUM

A number of reviews and guidelines have been published regarding the management of delirium in hospitalized older adults.[62,67,68] These reviews indicate that prevention and interdisciplinary system-based interventions constitute an effective and promising program to reduce the burden of delirium. The main evidence behind preventive strategies came from the Yale Delirium Prevention Trial,[69] in which an intervention was targeted toward minimizing six risk factors in elderly patients admitted to a general medicine service. These patients did not have delirium at the time of admission but were at risk for delirium development. The interventions included orientation activities for the cognitively impaired, early mobilization, preventing sleep deprivation, minimizing the use of psychoactive drugs, use of eyeglasses and hearing aids, and treating volume depletion. The incidence of delirium was 9.9% with this intervention compared with 15% in the usual care group (OR 0.60; 95% CI: 0.39-0.92). A randomized trial in which hip fracture patients were assigned to either standard care or a geriatrics consultation perioperatively showed a similar decrease in delirium incidence (32% versus 50%; OR 0.48; 95% CI: 0.23-0.98).[70]

Preventive interventions can be categorized into nursing policy interventions and physician-ordered interventions (Table 16-7). These interventions concentrate on modifying specific vulnerability or trigger factors such as the management of cognitive impairment, sleep deprivation, anticholinergic burden, pain, constipation, and restraints. Using such a preventive interdisciplinary

TABLE 16-7	Interventions to Prevent Delirium[7,48,70]
Factor	**Nursing Policy Interventions**
Sleep	Maintain 4-6 hours of uninterrupted sleep each night. If the patient complains of insomnia consider the following: • decrease the environmental noise at night • provide a drink of hot milk • provide a back rubbing for 15 minutes If the above failed then consider using a hypnotic drug.
Orientation	Orient patient about the date, place, and reason for hospitalization. Keep a clock and calendar inside the patient's room. Keep light on from 7 a.m. (sunrise) to 7 p.m. (sundown).
Environment	Encourage patient's family to bring personal items. Encourage patient's family to bring hearing aid and glasses. Encourage low-stimulating family visits.
Activity	Evaluate the appropriateness of restrictive activity order.
Tethers	Evaluate the necessity of using Foley catheter, restraint, IV line, and monitors.
Pain	Identify and manage adequately.
Constipation	Identify and manage adequately.
	Physician-Ordered Interventions
Cognitive Impairment	Continue or start cholinesterase inhibitors if patient has possible or probable Alzheimer's disease. Avoid, discontinue, or substitute all anticholinergic medications.
Anticholinergics	Avoid, discontinue, or substitute all anticholinergic medications.
Benzodiazepines	Avoid or assess the need for these drugs then taper off.
Pain	Maintain pain level of ≤3/10. Scheduled acetaminophen then scheduled narcotic if necessary. Avoid mepridine or codeine.
Constipation	Scheduled sorbitol or stimulant (if narcotics are used for pain control).
Insomnia	Low dose trazodone.
Mobility	Eliminate Foley catheter and physical restraints and order early mobilization if appropriate.
High risk for alcohol withdrawal	Consider scheduled short-acting benzodiazepine.
Dehydration	Maintain BUN/Creatinine <20/1. Maintain normal level Na.

program reduces absolute risk by 5% to 31%, with the total number of patients needing to be treated in order to prevent one delirium case number needed to treat [NNT] ranging from 3 to 20.[71] A cost effectiveness analysis of the multicomponent interdisciplinary interventions to prevent delirium, evaluated in the National Institute for Health and Care Excellence (NICE) guidelines,[68] showed that such interventions are cost-effective when applied to older medical patients at intermediate or high risk of developing delirium.[72] Therefore, an interdisciplinary hospital-based program is best suited to lowering the incidence of delirium in vulnerable elderly patients.

> The clinician's primary objective should be the prevention of delirium because once delirium symptoms have developed, the older patient is at risk for a poor clinical outcome.

Once delirium develops, managing it effectively is a very difficult task. Successful management of delirium (Table 16-7) depends on the accurate delivery of two types of interactive therapies:

- Treatment of the underlying causes, such as dehydration, infection, and/or the exposure to one or more of the anticholinergic medications, and providing safe and appropriate pharmacologic and nonpharmacologic care.[68,73]
- Supportive care targets the two types of delirium: hyperactive (agitation) and hypoactive (lethargy). For agitated delirium, the cornerstone of treatment is to provide safe and supportive care that allows the management of the underlying causes of delirium. Such supportive care includes an access to a trained professional sitter, involvement of family and caregivers, and administration of low-dose haloperidol (<3 mg/day). For hypoactive delirium, treatment focuses on skin protection, mobilization, and minimizing sedative medication.[74]

CASE 1

Discussion

Ms. Fischer's presentation is a typical example of delirium being the only manifestation of a life-threatening emergency. She is eventually found to have a pulmonary embolism, and with treatment her delusions disappear and her psychotropic medications can be reduced and eventually stopped. ■

CASE 2

Discussion

Ms. Johnson appears to have preexisting, undetected, mild dementia, which places her at increased risk for a postoperative delirium. Evaluation of her delirium symptoms reveals that she has a urinary tract infection. After starting an antibiotic, you arrange for a professional sitter to stay with Ms. Johnson in her hospital room, and prescribe haloperidol 0.25 mg q 6 hours as needed to manage her agitation. ■

SUMMARY

Decreasing the burden of delirium in older adults requires the implementation of a specialized delirium program that includes three crucial components: (1) implementing an active screening to identify patients with a high vulnerability for the development of delirium (using the delirium vulnerability scale); (2) educating the nurses and physicians on recognizing and diagnosing delirium and identifying its triggers; (3) structuring a consultation service that provides in-depth recommendations to prevent and manage delirium. Members of the consultation service should include at least a physician (geriatrician, geriatric psychiatrist, or a specialized hospitalist), a nurse, and an administrator.

Web Resources

www.americandeliriumsociety.org. American Delirium Society.
www.icudelirium.org. ICU Delirium and Cognitive Impairment Group at Vanderbilt University Medical Center.
www.europeandeliriumassociation.com/ European Delirium Association.

KEY REFERENCES

14. Thomas C, Kreisel SH, Oster P, et al. Diagnosing delirium in older hospitalized adults with dementia: Adapting the confusion assessment method to international classification of disease, tenth revision, diagnostic criteria. J Am Geriatr Soc 2012; 60:1471-7.
15. Naughton BJ, Saltzman S, Ramadan F, et al. A multifactorial intervention to reduce prevalence of delirium and shorten hospital length of stay. J Am Geriatri Soc 2005;53:18-23.
51. Campbell N, Boustani M, Limbil T, et al. The cognitive impact of anticholinergics: A clinical review. Clinical Interventions in Aging 2009;4(1):225-33.
62. Inouye SK. Delirium in older persons. N Engl J Med 2006; 354:1157-65.

References available online at expertconsult.com.

17

Alzheimer's Disease and Other Dementias

Christine Khandelwal and Daniel I. Kaufer

OBJECTIVES

Upon completion of this chapter, the reader will be able to:

- Understand the signs, symptoms, and diagnostic approach to the following common cognitive disorders of older persons: Alzheimer's disease, vascular dementia, frontotemporal dementia (FTD), Lewy body dementia (LBD), and Parkinson's dementia.

- Be able to conduct and interpret a screening examination for cognitive impairment, using the Mini-Cog and the AD-8.

- Be able to conduct and interpret a diagnostic evaluation of a patient with cognitive impairment using cognitive testing, laboratory studies, and brain imaging.

- Understand and be able to implement basic principles of dementia management, including medication use, nonpharmacologic management of behavioral symptoms, and working with community resources.

PREVALENCE AND IMPACT

Dementia is a progressive, global deterioration of cognitive ability in multiple domains including memory and at least one of the following: orientation, learning, language comprehension, and judgment.[1] The deterioration is severe enough to interfere with daily life. Approximately 5 million persons in the United States have dementia.[2] Dementia increases dramatically with age, so that the frequency of dementia among persons age 65 to 70 is approximately 2%, whereas for persons older than 85 it is more than 30%, costing $172 billion annually.[2] Not all cognitive complaints reflect dementia, however; in fact, nearly twice as many persons with cognitive impairment have milder symptoms that do not meet criteria for dementia.[3] Patients usually first discuss symptoms with their primary care physician. Among those diagnosed with dementia, 70% have Alzheimer's disease (AD).[4]

As the aging population grows, so will the number of dementia cases and the burden to family and caregivers. Care provided by family and friends often makes the difference between remaining at home and being placed in a long-term care facility.

Assessing cognitive impairment and diagnosing and managing dementia will be an increasingly important component of primary care medicine. Clinicians must be adept at assessing and monitoring patients who have mild cognitive symptoms, and identify those who develop a progressive dementia. Particularly challenging is the fact that the onset of dementia is insidious and the transition from normal age-related cognitive lapses to diagnosable dementia is gradual and, therefore, difficult to detect. Consequently, every clinician needs to develop a systematic approach to dementia screening and evaluating patients with cognitive impairment, and have a working knowledge of the common dementias.

Additional online-only material indicated by icon.

PATHOPHYSIOLOGY AND DIFFERENTIAL DIAGNOSIS

AD typically affects the hippocampus and adjacent temporal lobe regions initially, resulting in the loss of the capacity to learn and retain new information.[2] In AD, evidence suggests that there are two well-recognized pathophysiologic proteins present—neurofibrillary tangles and amyloid plaques— which are interconnected and lead to progressive neuronal death.[4]

Risk Factors for Alzheimer's Disease

Investigators have searched for decades for modifiable risk factors for AD. In general this research has been frustrating because of initial enthusiasm that was not substantiated in subsequent studies. A key limitation of much of the research is the challenge of distinguishing between association and causality, especially when factors associated with Alzheimer's are associated with aging (e.g., hyperlipidemia or arcus senilis). Sadly, relatively few risk factors have been definitively linked to AD, and even fewer are modifiable.

- Nonmodifiable risk factors include age, family history, the APOE-4 gene, and Down's syndrome.
- Modifiable or potentially preventable risk factors include prior head trauma, hypertension, diabetes mellitus, smoking, and depression.

> Modifiable or potentially preventable risk factors for AD include head trauma, hypertension, diabetes mellitus, smoking, and depression.

Age is the strongest known and best-studied risk factor.[2,5] The overall prevalence of dementia doubles for every 5-year increase in age after age 65. After age 85, the risk reaches nearly 50%.[5] A family history of AD is another strong risk factor; individuals with both parents having AD have a 54% cumulative risk of developing AD by age 80. First-degree relatives of patients with AD appear to have a cumulative lifetime risk of AD of 39%, twice the risk for the general population.[6]

Several genetic mutations have been associated with increased risk of AD. The risk gene with the strongest influence is apolipoprotein E-e4 (APOE-e4). Scientists estimate that APOE-e4 may be a factor in 20% to 25% of Alzheimer's cases.[7] Those who inherit APOE-e4 from one or both parents have a higher risk of AD, with homozygotes having a higher risk than heterozygotes. In addition to increasing risk, APOE-e4 is associated with an earlier onset of AD.[1] Scientists have also discovered genetic variations that directly cause rare, early-onset familial AD with onset of disease occurring prior to age 65. These mutations are found on the genes coding for three proteins: amyloid precursor protein (APP), presenilin-1 (PS-1), and presenilin-2 (PS-2).[8-10]

Down's syndrome is also a risk factor for AD, with 75% of people with Down's syndrome age 60 and older having AD.[11] Head trauma and traumatic brain injury are also risk factors for all dementias; the odds ratio is from 1.3 to 1.9.[5]

Clinicians should consider anxiety and depression to be premorbid risk factors of dementia. A case-control study suggested that a diagnosis of anxiety was strongly associated with a dementia diagnosis after adjustment for other risk factors (odds ratio 2.76; 95% confidence interval: 2.11-3.62).[12] What is unclear is whether these disorders represent a link in the causal chain or (as appears more likely) awareness of early cognitive loss.

Differential Diagnosis

Cognitive impairment results from altered brain function that affects one or more intellectual abilities. Isolated short-term memory deficits that go beyond mild forgetfulness but do not otherwise interfere with functional abilities are referred to as *mild cognitive impairment* (MCI). *Dementia* is defined as cognitive impairment that involves multiple domains and is associated with a decline in the ability to carry out everyday activities.

The most common cause of dementia in the elderly is AD, and many affected individuals exhibit isolated memory problems before developing full-blown AD. AD's course tends to be insidious in onset and slowly progressive, eventually leading to impairment of basic bodily functions, and finally—if no other illness intervenes—to death. In 2011 new criteria and guidelines for the diagnosis of AD were published by the Alzheimer's Association and the National Institute on Aging (NIA). The new guidelines focus on three stages of AD: (1) preclinical (presymptomatic) Alzheimer's dementia, (2) mild cognitive impairment (MCI) resulting from Alzheimer's, and (3) dementia resulting from Alzheimer's. Further recommendations by this group describe the use of biomarkers in Alzheimer's dementia and MCI caused by Alzheimer's as not intended for application in clinical settings at this time.[13]

> New guidelines for diagnosing AD focus on a three-stage model based on brain pathology in relation to the presence and degree of clinical signs.

- In a "preclinical" disease stage, the disease has not yet caused any noticeable "clinical" symptoms, because brain changes caused by the disease begin years before symptoms such as memory loss and confusion occur. The recommendations in the article on preclinical AD are intended for research purposes only. They have no clinical utility at this time.

- Mild cognitive impairment (MCI) caused by AD encompasses changes in memory and thinking abilities that are noticeable to the person and to family members and friends and that can be measured, but that do not affect one's ability to carry out everyday activities. Many, but not all, people with MCI go on to develop dementia caused by AD.[13]
- As AD pathology progresses, multiple cognitive domains become affected, leading to clinically significant functional impairment.[2,13] Behavioral problems frequently develop such as depression, apathy, anxiety, agitation, psychosis, and wandering.[2] Pathologically, these clinical manifestations are associated with the presence of extracellular amyloid plaques and intracellular neurofibrillary tangles, resulting in neuronal dysfunction and cell death.

Figure 17-1 graphically illustrates this new model of the time course of AD.

DIAGNOSTIC APPROACH
Screening for Cognitive Impairment

The suspicion that a person has cognitive impairment usually arises either because the clinician senses something abnormal during history-taking for an unrelated complaint, or because a family member brings up concerns about memory or thinking problems. When a suspicion arises or when the patient is at high risk for dementia (e.g., older than 75, family history), cognitive screening should be undertaken. The goal of cognitive screening is to identify persons who merit a more detailed diagnostic evaluation. When a person screens positive, care should be exercised to assure that a positive screen does not necessarily indicate a diagnosis of dementia, but rather, that further evaluation is indicated.

> The primary care physician has a key role in recognizing early signs and symptoms of dementia, and should use validated instruments for screening and diagnostic assessment.

Current recommendations by the American College of Physicians, the U.S. Preventive Services Task Force, and the Alzheimer's Association discourage routine screening for dementia on all older patients at a certain age. Screening is only recommended if a patient sees a doctor about some type of problem that could be resulting from dementia. However, a study that contradicted these current guidelines concluded that routine screening at primary care clinics led to a twofold to threefold increase in diagnoses of cognitive impairment.[14]

Diagnosing dementia in earlier stages will ultimately lead to preventative treatments, but current pharmacologic interventions address symptoms, not the underlying disease process. Behavioral interventions also have an important role in early disease management. One example is interventions to prevent financial loss caused by victimization from scams. In addition, early detection allows patients and families to plan, establishing goals of care, and

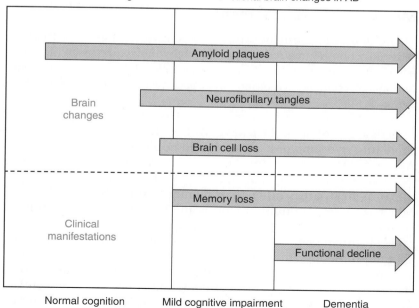

Figure 17-1 Schematic diagram for sequence of brain pathological changes beginning with asymptomatic (AD Stage 1) amyloid plaque deposition, followed by neurofibrillary tangle formation and associated neuronal dysfunction and destruction, resulting in initial memory disturbance (AD Stage 2), which progresses over time into clinically significant cognitive and functional changes, i.e., dementia (AD Stage 3).

Relative timing of structural and functional brain changes in AD

Brain changes
- Amyloid plaques
- Neurofibrillary tangles
- Brain cell loss

Clinical manifestations
- Memory loss
- Functional decline

Normal cognition   Mild cognitive impairment   Dementia (if desired) to participate in experimental treatment protocols.

The Mini-Cog provides a brief, valid, reliable, and uncomplicated measure for use in primary care as a routine screen for cognitive impairment.[15,16] The test consists of a 2-step assessment: a 3-item memory task (registration and later recall), with an intervening clock-drawing task serving as a distractor. The Mini-Cog is scored as a binary outcome (demented/not demented) based on the recall score alone (0/3 = demented, 3/3 = not demented) or in conjunction with the clock-drawing task, if recall performance is equivocal (1-2/3). The Mini-Cog is both highly sensitive and highly specific for dementia when used in a community-based elderly population.[15,16]

> Using the Mini-Cog and the AD8 provides the primary care physician with a rapid method of screening for cognitive impairment that is valid, reliable, and efficient.

The Mini-Cog can be supplemented by asking the patient's spouse or other family members to complete the AD-8. The AD8 is a brief, validated tool in which a family informant answers eight questions about the presence or absence of memory and other cognitive impairments.[17] The AD-8 is both sensitive (sensitivity >84%) and specific (specificity >80%). It has a positive predictive value of >85% and a negative predictive value >70% in detecting early cognitive changes associated with many common dementia-causing illnesses, including AD, vascular dementia, Lewy body dementia (LBD), and frontotemporal dementia (FTD).[2,18]

Mild Cognitive Impairment

Mild cognitive impairment (MCI) is present when cognitive function is impaired more than one would expect based on the individual's age and education level, but is not severe enough to interfere with activities of daily living.

It is estimated that as many as 10% to 20% of people age 65 and older have MCI.[19] MCI is classified into two subtypes: amnestic and nonamnestic. Amnestic MCI is present when the person has isolated memory loss; nonamnestic MCI involves impairment in areas other than memory. Amnestic MCI has a more ominous prognosis and is associated with a high risk of progression to AD.[20] The annual rate of progression to dementia among healthy community-living adults aged 55 and older is about 1% to 2% per year; in contrast, the annual conversion rate from amnestic MCI to dementia is 6% to 22% per year, with about 50% having dementia within 5 years.[19,20]

Diagnostic Evaluation of the Person with a Positive Screen for Cognitive Impairment

The differential diagnosis of cognitive impairment includes normal aging changes, mild cognitive impairment, delirium, and numerous dementia diagnoses. Table 17-1 summarizes these conditions.

The *Diagnostic and Statistical Manual of Mental Disorders, Fifth Edition* (DSM-V) replaces the term "dementia" with "neurocognitive disorder", broadly divided into a minor category (i.e., MCI), and a major category, commensurate with the syndromic definition of dementia.[13] These criteria accurately identify AD on clinical grounds, whereas diagnostic criteria for other dementias (e.g., vascular dementia, LBD, FTD) are not as robust.[21] Compared to AD, other dementias tend to have more variable clinical presentations, which makes defining diagnostic criteria more difficult.

Dementia, as defined in DSM-V, stands in contrast with delirium, which is distinguished by a primary alteration in attentional processing. Although dementia syndromes tend to be chronic, progressive, and irreversible, and delirium states tend to be acute to subacute, fluctuating, and reversible, these distinctions are more relative than absolute. Toxic, metabolic, and infectious disturbances associated with delirium are more likely to be potentially reversible than degenerative disorders. Brain dysfunction associated with dementia may render the patient more vulnerable to delirium-producing factors, highlighting the clinical challenge posed by the combination of dementia and superimposed delirium. Careful evaluation of persons referred for dementia can identify treatable or reversible disorders in up to 20% of cases, though treatment of the reversible component will rarely eliminate all deficits.[22]

Distinguishing cognitive impairment associated with an underlying brain disorder from potentially reversible cognitive symptoms (e.g., associated with depression) often demands ongoing evaluation, including appropriate diagnostic tests and perhaps therapeutic challenge with an antidepressant drug. Abrupt onset of thinking changes in temporal relation to a psychological stressor, poor effort on cognitive testing (particularly with demanding tasks), and prominent neurovegetative signs such as insomnia and anorexia are characteristic of depression-associated cognitive impairment. Drug-induced cognitive impairment occurring as a result of anticholinergic agents, sedative-hypnotic drugs (e.g., benzodiazepines), or opiate analgesics is common in the elderly and may variably cause or contribute to symptoms of dementia or MCI. A temporal association of cognitive symptom onset with the initiation or increase in dosing of such drugs should prompt withdrawal of any

TABLE 17-1		Common Diagnoses among Older Persons with Cognitive Complaints			
Diagnosis	Anatomic Location	History	Examination Findings	Brain Imaging/ Lab Findings	Comment
Normal aging changes	Diffuse	Forget names, occasional memory lapses	None	Mild generalized cortical atrophy and ventricular enlargement	White matter ischemic changes seen with HTN, DM
Delirium	Diffuse or multifocal	Identifiable toxic/ metabolic/ infectious etiology	Fluctuating attention, fidgety, agitated, tremulous, or apathetic/ obtunded	Diffuse EEG slowing, evidence of drug or metabolic toxicity, infection	Reversibility depends on etiology
Mild cognitive impairment	Medial temporal lobe	Impaired episodic short-term memory	None	Variable medial temporal atrophy (nonspecific)	50% or more risk of progressing to AD
Alzheimer's disease (AD)	Cortical (temporal and parietal)	Progressive memory and other cognitive deficits	Essentially normal (may have apraxia)	Medial temporal and parietal lobe atrophy	+ Amyloid brain PET scan
Vascular dementia (VaD)	Cortical and/or subcortical	Multiple stroke-like events and/ or vascular risk factors	Variable; sensory-motor, gait, cognitive dysfunction	Cortical/ subcortical infarcts, white matter lesions	Mixed AD /VaD commonly seen
Frontotemporal dementia (FTD)	Cortical (frontal and temporal)	Behavioral, personality, language changes	Variable, gait apraxia, frontal release signs	Marked atrophy in frontal and/ or temporal lobes	Speech/ swallowing problems late
Lewy body dementia (LBD)	Cortical and subcortical	Fluctuating attention, visual hallucinations, gait/motor/sleep disturbance	Limb rigidity, bradykinesia, may see intention tremor and gait disturbance	MRI imaging nondiagnostic	May have + Amyloid brain PET scan
Parkinson's dementia	Subcortical	Parkinson's disease with later onset cognitive dysfunction	Limb rigidity, bradykinesia, resting tremor, gait disturbance	MRI imaging nondiagnostic	+ Dopamine transporter PET scan

DM, diabetes mellitus; *EEG*, Electroencephalogram; *HTN*, hypertension; *PET*, positron emission tomography.

potentially offending agent. Accurately diagnosing dementia usually requires a systematic, longitudinal approach and, in many cases, targeted therapeutic additions or deletions. Multiple etiological factors are common, and the search for potentially reversible or modifiable conditions should be pursued vigorously (Table 17-2).

Making a Specific Diagnosis in Persons with Dementia

The earliest symptoms in AD are difficulty with higher cognitive functions such as memory, language, problem-solving, and reasoning. Memory loss is usually prominent early in the disease, and typically progresses over time. Also, patients with early AD often are disproportionately impaired in category fluency

(e.g., naming as many animals as they can in a minute) compared with letter fluency (e.g., naming words that begin with F).

> Looking carefully at patient performance of category fluency and letter fluency can help separate AD from other dementias.

Findings seen both in AD and in other disorders with more focal cortical involvement caused by strokes or degeneration include the following:
- Agnosia (inability to recognize and identify objects or persons despite having knowledge of the characteristics of those objects or persons)
- Aphasia (either a partial or total loss of the ability to communicate verbally or using written words)

TABLE 17-2	Potentially Treatable and/or Reversible Causes of Cognitive Impairment	
Cause	**Findings Raising Clinical Suspicion**	**Method of Diagnosing or Ruling Out**
Medication adverse effects	Patient is on anticholinergic drugs (e.g., diphenhydramine), sedative medication (e.g., benzodiazepines), or narcotic analgesics	Medication review Withdrawal challenge
Hypothyroidism	Fatigue, cold intolerance, constipation, weight gain, bradycardia (but typical signs may be absent in elderly)	History and physical TSH
Vitamin B$_{12}$ deficiency	Very poor diet/strict vegetarianism; paresthesias, ataxia, peripheral neuropathy	Vitamin B$_{12}$ level
Neurosyphilis	Grandiosity, confabulation, emotional lability, Argyll Robertson pupils	Serum FTA Spinal fluid FTA
Brain tumor	Headache, nausea/vomiting, seizures, focal neurologic signs	MRI or CT of the head with contrast
Normal pressure hydrocephalus	Wide-based gait, urinary incontinence early in course of cognitive impairment	MRI or noncontrast CT scan of the head Lumbar puncture
Subdural hematoma	History of trauma (often minor), fluctuating level of consciousness, headache, focal neurologic signs	Noncontrast CT scan of the head

CT, computed tomography; *FTA,* Fluorescent treponemal antigen; *MRI,* magnetic resonance imaging; *TSH,* thyroid stimulating hormone.

- Apraxia (total or partial loss of the ability to perform coordinated movements or manipulate objects in the absence of motor or sensory impairment)[23]

A general approach to dementia differential diagnosis can be outlined using short-term memory deficits (primary or secondary) and associated clinical signs and symptoms, obtained during a thorough history and physical examination with a detailed neurologic examination. Family and caregivers may provide more information regarding problems with daily life activities by filling out the AD8 questionnaire. A basic algorithm (Figure 17-2) can help guide a standardized approach to diagnosing dementia.

Using standardized instruments such as the SLUMS (Saint Louis University Mental Status),[17] the MOCA (Montreal Cognitive Assessment),[24] or the more common MMSE (Mini-Mental State Examination)[25] may help a provider distinguish an Alzheimer's dementia from a non-Alzheimer's dementia process. Furthermore, the SLUMS and MOCA are possibly better at detecting mild disorders compared to the MMSE.

AD is characterized by early, severe short-term memory difficulties that become worse over time. On testing, individuals with Alzheimer's typically do poorly on memory recall tests, and they are not usually helped when given recognition cues (e.g., "fruit" for apple).

Next to AD, the two most common dementias are vascular dementia and LBD (including individuals with Parkinson's disease–related dementia).

These "subcortical" dementias typically show less severe memory dysfunction, particularly early in the disease course, and tend to have greater deficits in attention, visuospatial skills, and executive function (initiation, planning, behavioral apathy).[2] Although poor spontaneous retrieval memory is common to both Alzheimer's and other dementias, preserved recognition is characteristic of non-Alzheimer's dementias. To capture this on testing, provide cues on testing (e.g., "fruit" to see if they then remember "apple" during recall testing). Selective deficits on verbal fluency testing may also help distinguish fronto-subcortical disorders from AD, as the former tend to exhibit greater difficulty with phonemic (letter) fluency tasks, which is relatively preserved in AD.[26]

Other features that may help distinguish non-Alzheimer's dementia are the presence of focal neurologic or motor signs, prominent psychiatric features, and a history of one or more strokes. Individuals with vascular dementia, LBD, or FTD tend to have sleep or behavior disturbances. Often caregivers and family will express more concern regarding sleep problems, behavioral changes such as apathy or anxiety.

Evaluating for Delirium and Depression

Delirium and depression are common comorbidities of dementia that deserve special attention as treatable problems (Table 17-3). Although prior emphasis has been on distinguishing depression and dementia as mutually exclusive and distinct entities, recent data suggest that depression may be an early sign of, or risk factor for, dementia.[27] The exact mechanisms linking depression and dementia are not well understood. An empiric trial of an antidepressant agent may be indicated when one is faced with a clinical presentation of conjoint cognitive and mood symptoms. Improved mood state without concomitant improvement in cognitive symptoms is suggestive of an underlying dementia. Table 17-3 compares delirium and depression and how they present differently with patients and on testing.

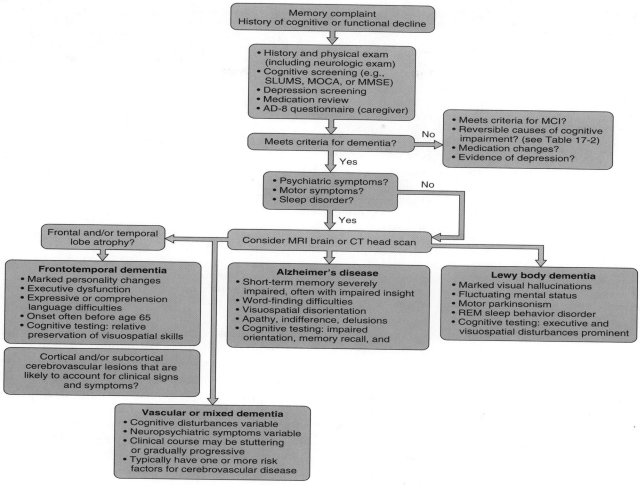

Figure 17-2 Algorithmic guide to diagnosing dementia.

TABLE 17-3	Distinguishing between Delirium and Depression	
Characteristics	**Delirium**	**Depression**
Presentation	Altered mental status/encephalopathy—fluctuating consciousness, impaired cognitive testing	"Pseudodementia"—appears demented but performs well on cognitive testing
Signs and Symptoms	Acute/subacute onset, fluctuating, sleep-wake disruption, often reversible	Gives up easily on cognitive tests, "I don't know," poor eye-contact, flat affect, cries easily
Time Course	More likely to occur in a person with dementia	May come on abruptly, often with major stressor (e.g., death of spouse, living relocation)
Prognosis	May "predict" dementia (e.g., postop delirium)	Independent risk factor for dementia

PREVENTION

Persons with a strong family history of dementia, including many family caregivers, are concerned about what they can do to prevent the disease. Most of the strategies that are supported by current research involve healthy life style and prevention of cardiovascular disease. These strategies (Table 17-4) have been divided into three areas: treatment of vascular risk factors, diet, and increasing neuronal reserves.

Treatment of Vascular Risk Factors

High blood pressure in midlife is a risk factor for cognitive impairment and dementia in late life, but research results are inconsistent for the effects of late-life blood

TABLE 17-4	Strategies for Prevention of Dementia	
General Strategy	Specific Actions and Goals	Level of Evidence Supporting Recommendations*
Treatment of vascular risk factors	• Treat hypertension to ≤140/90	A
	• Treat hypercholesterolemia to LDL ≤100	C
	• Treat diabetes to HbA_{1c} ≤7	C
	• Prescribe aspirin in persons with established cardiovascular disease	C
	• Manage heart failure optimally	C
	• Smoking cessation	C
Neuroprotection	• Folate and vitamin B_{12}	C
	• Mediterranean diet	B
	• Moderate alcohol consumption	B
Building up neuronal reserves	• Cognitive activity	B
	• Physical activity	B
	• Social and leisure activity	B

Adapted from Sloane PD, Khandelwal C, Kaufer DI. Cognitive impairment. In: Sloane PD, Slatt L, Ebell M, et al, editors. Essentials of family medicine. 6th ed. Baltimore, MD: Lippincott, Williams & Wilkins; 2011, p. 269-82. Reproduced with permission.
*A = consistent, good-quality patient-oriented evidence; B = inconsistent or limited-quality patient-oriented evidence; C = consensus, disease-oriented evidence, usual practice, expert opinion. For information about the SORT evidence rating system, see www.aafp.org/afpsort.xml.

pressure.[28] Several longitudinal observational studies showed significant reductions in the incidence of dementia in treated versus nontreated hypertensive patients; the Systolic Hypertension in Europe (Syst-Eur) trial concluded that long-term antihypertensive treatment decreased the incidence of AD and vascular or mixed dementia by 55%.[28,29] Similarly, primary and secondary prevention of stroke reduces dementia related to cerebrovascular disease either directly or as a comorbid factor in AD.[30] The relationship between cholesterol and dementia risk is less clear; study results have been inconsistent.[31]

Diet

Fish consumption is related to lower cognitive decline and a decreased risk of dementia.[32,33] Studies also suggest that the Mediterranean diet is associated with a trend for reduced risk both of developing MCI and of MCI conversion to AD.[34,35] Nutritional supplements such as vitamin E, omega-3 fatty acids, and other antioxidant nutrients generally do not have demonstrable benefits; however, vitamin B_{12} and folate supplementation in middle to late life may have a beneficial effect on dementia incidence or cognitive decline.[36] One to two daily alcoholic beverages may lower the risk of dementia due to salutary vascular effects, although chronic, excessive alcohol consumption may impair cognitive functioning due to direct toxic effects or through associated thiamine deficiency (i.e., Wernicke-Korsakoff syndrome).[37,38]

Increasing Neuronal Reserves

Social, cognitive, and physical activities are linked in small interventional and longitudinal studies with reduced risk of cognitive decline and improvement in cognitive function.[39] Whether these represent cause-and-effect or an association with other factors (e.g., socioeconomic status or education) is unclear. However, though the evidence is modest, a mentally, physically, and socially active lifestyle is recommended in late life, because even if the cognitive benefits are not yet entirely clear, this lifestyle should bring about improved quality of life and overall health.

TREATMENT

Management of Mild Cognitive Impairment

Current recommendations for management of MCI are similar to those presented above for prevention: healthy lifestyle and vascular risk factor reduction. In addition, careful medication review to minimize or eliminate drugs with sedative and anticholinergic properties is indicated.

However, once a patient has been diagnosed with MCI, the patient and his or her family often ask if any treatment can be provided to prevent the further progression of MCI to dementia. Unfortunately, numerous clinical studies testing the acetylcholinesterase inhibitors have been undertaken and none has been demonstrated to prevent progression from MCI to AD.[40] Consequently, no drug treatments are approved for MCI.

Management of Dementia

Management of cognitive disorders involves careful attention to cognitive status, general health, behavioral and family issues, and connection with community resources.

Management of dementia and related cognitive disorders involves careful attention to cognitive status, general health, behavioral and family issues, and connection with community resources. The approach must be individualized, because the needs and capabilities of the individual vary widely according to the stage of the disease and the background, interests, and living situation of the person with the disease and those who are providing care.

The primary goal of dementia management is to preserve function and independence, minimize risk factors, and help maintain quality of life for as long as possible. Pharmacologic interventions may be effective for improving cognitive function for certain dementias and useful in treating depression. Nonpharmacologic interventions, including measures to manage behavioral symptoms and ensure safety at home, are critically important, as is family support. Attention to long-term decisions regarding finances, nursing home placement, and caregiver stress is also important in the management of dementia. Table 17-5 summarizes the key available treatment strategies for dementia.

TABLE 17-5	Pharmacological Treatment of Persons with Dementia		
Target Conditions and/or Symptoms	**Intervention**	**Level of Evidence of Effectiveness***	**Comments**
Mild cognitive impairment	Cognitive enhancers (e.g., donepezil, memantine)	B	No consistent evidence of effect; most studies fail to show benefit.
Dementia: cognitive symptoms	Cholinesterase inhibitors (donepezil, rivastigmine, galantamine, memantine	A	Effective for mild, moderate, and severe dementia. Effect size equivalent to slowing cognitive decline by 6 months.
	Cognitive training	B	Improved ability specific to the abilities trained.
	Physical activity	B	Improved physical health and reduced depression.
Caregiver stress, burden, and depression	Caregiver support group programs and educational programs; use of respite services	A	Caregiver support groups and counseling can reduce psychological morbidity and delay nursing home placement. More intense and longer programs have greater effect.
Depression in persons with dementia	Selective serotonin reuptake inhibitors (SSRIs) (sertraline, citralopram)	A	Mild to moderate effects in reducing depressed mood; no effect on neuropsychiatric symptoms.
	Physical activity/exercise	B	A combination of exercise and caregiver education improved depression.
Agitation, aggression, and delusions in persons with dementia	Caregiver training in dementia management skills	A	Customized programs for caregivers focusing on nonpharmacologic interventions to decrease agitation.
	Antipsychotic drugs	A	Statistically significant effects in a minority of recipients, but unclear if benefits outweigh adverse effects.
	Benzodiazepine medications	C	Little evidence to support use in light of risk of worsening memory loss, confusion, and falls.
	Anticonvulsants	B	Carbamazepine has been found to reduce agitation, anxiety, and restlessness but the efficacy with long-term use is unknown; ataxia and hematologic toxicity occur. Valproic acid does not appear to be effective for neuropsychiatric symptoms.
	Cognitive enhancers (e.g., donepezil, memantine)	A	Donepezil and galantamine have been demonstrated to significantly improve agitation; effects are modest.
	Environmental modification	B	Music reduces agitation, aggression, and mood disturbance during eating and bathing.
	Physical activity	A	Physical activity and exercise programs significantly reduce agitation and aggressive events.

Adapted from Sloane PD, Khandelwal C, Kaufer DI. Cognitive impairment. In: Sloane PD, Slatt L, Ebell M, et al, editors. Essentials of family medicine. 6th ed. Baltimore, MD: Lippincott, Williams & Wilkins; 2011, p. 269-82. Reproduced with permission.

*A = consistent, good-quality patient-oriented evidence; B = inconsistent or limited-quality patient-oriented evidence; C = consensus, disease-oriented evidence, usual practice, expert opinion. For information about the SORT evidence rating system, see www.aafp.org/afpsort.xml.

Medication for Cognitive Symptoms

Although there is no treatment to slow or stop AD, the U.S. Food and Drug Administration has approved drugs that temporarily improve symptoms. Based on several randomized controlled trials and recent Cochrane reviews, cholinesterase inhibitors (donepezil, rivastigmine, galantamine) modestly improve cognition and global function in patients with mild and moderate AD; thus cholinesterase inhibitors are currently labeled for the treatment of mild to moderate AD.[41]

Memantine, an N-methyl-D-aspartic acid glutamate (NMDA) receptor antagonist, has been shown to delay clinical worsening of functional, behavioral, and cognitive components of AD-related decline.[42] Furthermore, studies using combination therapy with acetylcholinesterase inhibitors appear to demonstrate increased cognitive benefits compared to monotherapy.[43]

Several treatments originally thought to be promising have been demonstrated in randomized trials to not be effective. Dementia is associated with inflammation; however, studies of nonsteroidal antiinflammatory drugs (NSAIDs) have not clearly identified benefits,[44] and safety concerns have been raised regarding widespread NSAID use. Similarly, Ginkgo biloba appears to have no effect on cognitive decline.[45]

The drugs bapineuzumab and solanezumab were designed to treat AD by scavenging plaque-forming amyloid proteins; however, they have failed to demonstrate clinical benefit in patients with mild to moderate disease.[46]

Management of Behavioral Symptoms

AD and the related dementias are primarily behavioral disorders. It is the behavioral symptoms that cause the most challenges for families and professional caregivers, and whose management is the key to effectively maintaining someone with dementia living in the community. Unfortunately, although there are numerous medications available to treat behavioral symptoms (see next section), none is very effective and all have significant toxicity. Therefore, nonpharmacologic approaches are the mainstay of management and can often make a huge difference in terms of quality of life for persons with dementia and those who surround them.

Persons with dementia will often express themselves using agitation, aggression, or resistance to care. These behaviors should be understood as a form of communication, because they tend to result from a mismatch between environmental demands and the individual's ability to understand or cope with what is happening. Therefore, the first step in approaching these symptoms is to look for provoking factors, such as pain, infection, anxiety, or caregiver behaviors that are perceived as threatening. A good strategy in approaching such problems is to evaluate what may have precipitated the behavior and the initial reaction or response by care providers, as these factors are usually more easily remedied.

Behavioral interventions for dementia fall into several categories:

- *Creating a facilitative physical environment.* Here the goal is to structure the environment so the person with dementia is safe, has easily interpretable cues to know where he or she is, can make correct choices, and is not bombarded with unpleasant stimuli. Interventions in this category include such things as eliminating hazards, making the toilet visible from the bed, having lighting that reduces glare, and eliminating confusing noises. The implementation of an individualized, nonpharmacologic intervention appears to decrease agitation.[47] Small studies have shown that music seemed to reduce agitation, aggression, and mood disturbance during eating and bathing.[48,49] Furthermore, bright light appears to reduce aggression and agitation in residents with dementia.[50]
- *Stimulating cognitive function without overchallenging the individual.* Cognition-focused interventions, such as engagement in a range of group activities and discussions, are of great interest to persons with early-stage disease and can improve quality of life.
- *Facilitating success.* Depending on the stage of the disease, a variety of strategies can facilitate success. Examples include laying clothes out in the order they need to be put on, providing written reminders (for those who can read), and providing finger foods (for persons with apraxia who want to feed themselves).
- *Providing activities that promote feelings of pleasure.* Examples of such interventions include gardens, bird feeders, picture albums, and familiar books; and activities that enhance overall physical and cognitive health (e.g., dancing, going for a walk outside, preparing and eating a snack, reminiscence). To be successful, activities need to be suited to the cognitive level of the individual.
- *Providing care in a manner that is quiet, gentle, nonforceful, and respectful.* Care provision is a skill that requires both sensitivity to the individual and a toolkit of strategies to help avoid or abort agitated behaviors and resistance to care.

> Nonpharmacologic approaches are the mainstay of management of behavioral symptoms in dementia and can often make a huge difference in terms of quality of life for persons with dementia and those who surround them.

When nonpharmacologic methods are insufficient, physicians are often asked to provide a prescription to aid in management of behavioral symptoms. No drug is effective in even as many as 50% of cases and many of the medications used have adverse side effects. However, the following agents have some evidence supporting their use in select cases:

- Cholinesterase inhibitors appear to provide some improvement in behavior, especially in confusion-related symptoms, and these effects may persist even into advanced AD.[51-54]

- Selective serotonin reuptake inhibitors (SSRIs) as a class have shown efficacy in the treatment of depression but not in the treatment of behavioral symptoms.[55,56] However, citalopram has demonstrated efficacy in treating behavioral symptoms.[57]

- Antipsychotic medications are sedating, but their effectiveness in treating behavioral symptoms in dementia is modest. The atypical antipsychotics (clozapine, olanzapine, risperidone, quetiapine, ziprasidone, aripiprazole) are generally useful for short-term targeted therapy for agitation and psychosis. However, their use should be tempered by their increased risk of stroke and death relative to placebo, as well as possible cardiac conduction (Q-T interval prolongation) and adverse metabolic effects.[55,58] Typical antipsychotics (haloperidol, chlorpromazine, thioridazine, thiothixene, trifluoperazine, acetophenazine), on the other hand, have no clear evidence of benefit in treating neuropsychiatric symptoms. Although haloperidol may be an exception, it is unclear if this benefit outweighs adverse effects such as sedation and extrapyramidal motor dysfunction.[55,56] AD patients whose psychosis, agitation, or aggression has responded to the antipsychotic drug risperidone face a high risk of relapse if the drug is discontinued. This suggests that, though federal nursing home regulations mandate ongoing efforts to discontinue antipsychotics, this may at times be unwise.[59]

- So-called mood stabilizers such as carbamazepine and valproic acid, which are generally used to treat seizures, have been associated with modest reductions in agitation, anxiety, and restlessness, but their long-term effectiveness is unknown and the risk of ataxia and hematologic toxicity is a concern.[55,56]

- There is little evidence to support the use of benzodiazepines for behavior management, especially since they have been linked to worsening memory loss, confusion, and falls.

Management of Depression in Dementia

Recommendations for treatment of depression are based on limited, conflicting evidence and expert opinion.[60]

If a patient with dementia has depression, the first step should be to rule out causes of discomfort such as pain and medication side effects. For mild to moderate depression, nonpharmacologic approaches are recommended; several small studies have indicated that exercise, education, light therapy, and caregiver education may be helpful.

Pharmacologic therapies are reserved for moderate to severe depression, because the more severe the baseline depression the more robust the response to drugs.[61,62] SSRIs appear to be most effective for the treatment of depression in dementia patients.[63-65] In particular, sertraline and citalopram appear to have the most favorable effectiveness-to-toxicity profiles. Evidence suggests that treatment with SSRIs can improve emotional bluntness, confusion, irritability, confusion, anxiety, fear, restlessness, and depressed mood.[55,56,66]

There is little evidence that trazodone is effective in depression in dementia, though it may be used for sleep disturbances.[67] Agents with substantial anticholinergic effects, such as amitriptyline and imipramine, should be avoided because of their adverse cognitive effects.[68]

Working with Families and Community Resources

Providing support for the caregivers is an important aspect of the care for patients with dementia, because it is families, not institutions, that provide the majority of care to persons with AD and related dementias. Community support services play a critical role in the lives of many caregivers. Research has shown, for example, that counseling and support groups, in combination with respite and other services, can assist caregivers in remaining in their caregiving role longer, with less stress and greater satisfaction.[69] Extended involvement in counseling and support for caregivers of persons with mild to moderate dementia can improve caregiver mood and coping skills and may delay nursing home placement by as much as 12 to 24 months.[70,71] Short-term programs have little to no effect on patient outcomes; however, they improve caregiver knowledge and coping ability.[72]

For the primary care physician, an important element of dementia care is helping family caregivers gain access to home- and community-based services such as counseling, support groups, transportation, meals, home care, and respite. Table 17-6 provides specific suggestions for resources that are available in most communities. The Alzheimer's Association, with chapters nationwide, is a great resource for families and patients to obtain information and references for dementia care, education, and caregiver information.

Programs such as Project C.A.R.E. use a family consultant model to provide consumer-directed respite

TABLE 17-6	Partnering with Community Resources to Manage Common Problems in Persons with Dementia	
Management Problem	**What the Primary Care Provider Can Do**	**Resources**

Caregiver support needed	• Refer to community caregiver support groups; refer to local county Department on Aging or Alzheimer's Association for education and support groups.
	• For families who can afford to pay for services, especially if they live some distance away from the person with dementia, an option is to hire a geriatric care manager.
		Alzheimer's Association.
		  Phone: 800-272-3900
		  Website: www.alz.org
		National Center on Caregiving
		  Phone: 800-445-8106
		  Website: info@caregiver.org
		National Association of Professional Geriatric Care Managers
		  Website: www.caremanager.org

Driving concerns	• Write a prescription for a driving evaluation. • Write a letter to local or state department of motor vehicles expressing driving concerns and recommending an evaluation.	*At the Crossroads: A Guide to Alzheimer's Disease, Dementia, and Driving.* Available at www.thehartford.com/alzheimers.
Need for in-home help	• Refer to physical therapy/occupational therapy for an in-home safety evaluation. • Refer to a family caregiver specialist, local social service agency, or geriatric care manager.	Check with your local Area Agency on Aging.
Competency & legal issues	• Encourage assignment of health care and financial power of attorney early in the disease (before diagnosis is ideal). • Locate an elder attorney for documentation for advance directives, conservatorship issues/guardianship, financial and health power of attorney.	Follow your state guidelines for documenting advance directives. Web resource: www.caringinfo.org

Concern about safety at home	• Make a home visit.
	• Refer to an occupational therapist for an in-home safety evaluation.
		Centers for Disease Control and Prevention National Center for Injury Prevention and Control (NCIPC)
		  Phone: 800-232-4636
		  Website: cdcinfo@cdc.gov

Need for palliative, end-of-life care	• Plan ahead and document discussions about end-of-life wishes. Know criteria for hospice referral of persons with dementia and how to care for patients in residential care settings at end of life.	*End-of-life Care for People with Dementia in Residential Care Settings.* Available at www.alz.org/national/documents/endoflifelitreview.pdf.

care and comprehensive support to caregivers. The goal of that program is to increase quality, access, choice, and use of respite and support services to low-income rural and minority families caring for a person with dementia at home. Family caregivers can ask the physician about a variety of concerns that can often be addressed by community resources; the family physician should be able to direct caregivers to the appropriate assistance. The Tailored Activity Program, a customized program tailored for patients and their families to reduce behavioral symptoms, was effective in educating families to manage behavioral symptoms.[73] In another study, community consultants implemented a behavioral intervention with family caregivers, resulting in improvement in depression, burden, and reactivity to behavioral problems, and a reduction in the frequency and severity of care recipient behavior problems.[74]

SUMMARY

The primary care physician is often the first physician involved in making the diagnosis of dementia and is the primary link between the patient, the family, and supportive services. For the primary care physician, an important element of dementia care is helping family and caregivers be a part of the process for future planning to establish goals of care.

ACKNOWLEDGMENT

Portions of this chapter were previously published in Sloane PD, Slatt LM, Ebell MH, et al, editors. Essentials of family medicine. 6th ed. Baltimore, MD: Lippincott, Williams & Wilkins; 2011.

KEY REFERENCES

1. Daviglus ML, Bell CC, Berrettini W, et al. National Institutes of Health State-of-the-Science Conference Statement: Preventing Alzheimer's disease and cognitive decline. NIH Consens State Sci Statements 2010;27(4):1-30.

2. Galvin JE, Sadowski CH. Practical guidelines for the recognition and diagnosis of dementia. J Am Board Fam Med 2012;25:367-82.

13. Jack CR Jr., Albert MS, Knopman DS, et al. Introduction to the recommendations from the National Institute on Aging—Alzheimer's Association workgroups on diagnostic guidelines for Alzheimer's disease. Alzheimers Dement 2011;7(3):257-62.

14. McCarten JR, Anderson P, Kuskowski MA, et al. Finding dementia in primary care: The results of a clinical demonstration project. J Am Geriatr Soc 2012;60(2):210-7.

References available online at expertconsult.com.

18

Depression

Omair Abbasi and William J. Burke

OBJECTIVES

Upon completion of this chapter, the reader will be able to:

- Understand the impact of depression on a patient's general medical condition and quality of life.
- Identify risk factors for depression and suicide, and interventions for each.
- Describe the differences in presentation between late-life depression and early-onset depression.

- Assess for various types of depression including major depression, subsyndromal or minor depression, dysthymia, and depression secondary to substance use or a general medical condition
- List common screening tools and lab tests to be performed when considering a diagnosis of depression.
- Discuss treatment options for depression including medications, psychotherapy, electroconvulsive therapy (ECT), and rapid transcranial magnetic stimulation (rTMS).
- Identify cases that need referral to a psychiatrist or emergent psychiatric intervention.

PREVALENCE AND IMPACT

People age 65 and older currently make up 13% of the total U.S. population; that percentage is expected to rise to about 20% by the year 2030.[1] There are approximately 39 million elderly individuals in the United States and about 7 million of them are affected by depression.[2] Depression comprises the largest category of psychiatric disorder in the elderly and is currently the fourth leading cause of disability as estimated by disability-adjusted life years.[3] By 2020, depression will be second only to heart disease as a cause of disability in the global population.[4] In contrast, there will be approximately 2,640 geriatric psychiatrists in the United States by the year 2030, or 1 per 5,682 older adults with a psychiatric disorder.[5] It is therefore imperative that primary care providers are able to detect and treat depression in the elderly.

There is a common misconception that depression occurring in late life is a normal part of the aging process, or a normal reaction to stressors such as retirement, the loss of loved ones, medical ailments, and loss of independence. In fact, an enduring finding in epidemiologic studies is that only a small number of elderly people living in the community admit being depressed.[6] A Centers for Disease Control and Prevention report in 2006 estimated that approximately 5% of community-dwelling adults age 65 and older reported being currently depressed.[7] Rates of depression are higher in older adults who require more care or are in institutional settings. Fourteen percent of patients receiving in-home care[8] and approximately 20% of nursing home residents[9] meet criteria for depression. However, only a small percentage of older patients with depression receive proper treatment for their symptoms; those most likely to receive inadequate or no treatment for their depression are male, African

American, Latino, and those with a preference for counseling over antidepressant treatment.[10]

Depression in the elderly is often associated with significant morbidity and mortality. Schulz et al. followed a group of more than 5000 individuals over 65 years and found that those with higher baseline depressive symptoms were one and half times more likely to die.[11] The mortality rate coincided with the level of depression even when controlling for other factors. Older patients who report depressive symptoms are also more likely to report a lower quality of life, higher level of chronic pain, and increased disability.[12] Medically ill patients with depression have increased total health care costs. One study found that depressed patients with heart failure and diabetes had almost double the health care costs of nondepressed patients ($20,046 vs. $11,956).[13] In addition, it is estimated that friends or family members who are serving as primary caretakers of these patients provide approximately $375 billion of unpaid work annually.[14]

> Depression is a significant ailment that affects level of functioning, quality of life, cost of care, and mortality. It is not a normal part of aging and is the fourth leading cause of disability in the United States.

RISK FACTORS AND PATHOPHYSIOLOGY

Late-life depression shares much in common with depression occurring earlier in life but has unique, distinguishing characteristics in presentation, etiology, and risk factors. In younger adults, the stress-diathesis model is one of the more popular explanations for why people develop depression. This theory suggests that both genetic vulnerability and psychosocial factors play important roles. In contrast, whereas psychosocial factors play a part in the development of late-life depression, there is less consistent evidence for genetic predisposition, with studies showing little correlation between family history and late-onset depression.[15] However, other biological factors are important. For example, compromises in brain neurocircuitry, particularly in frontolimbic pathways, have a strong association with many depressive disorders in late life. This may explain the high incidence of depression in patients with neurologic conditions affecting these pathways such as stroke, Parkinson's disease (PD), and Alzheimer's disease (AD).[16]

Although the biological processes of late-life depression may separate it from early-onset depression, the aforementioned stress diathesis model is still useful in emphasizing the importance of psychosocial risk factors[15] (Table 18-1). These risk factors in turn can be modified by other factors including a patient's coping skills and the presence of ongoing stress outside of

TABLE 18-1	Risk Factors for Depression
Chronic medical illness	
Loss of a loved one	
Relocation	
Disability	

the context of the psychosocial risk factor. It should also be recognized that a majority of individuals with a given risk factor will not meet depressive criteria. Rather, the risk factors should be considered when suspecting depression and in the formulation of treatment.

CASE 1

Ms. Smith (Part 1)

Ms. Smith is a 68-year-old white female who lost her husband to cancer 15 months ago. Ms. Smith's daughter accompanies her to the office and states that since the loss of her husband, Ms. Smith has become short-tempered with her family. She skips family dinners and when she does attend, she tearfully discusses the loss of her husband. The daughter also mentions that Ms. Smith has refused to pack her husband's personal belongings and that they remain in the closet. Ms. Smith admits that she has feelings of bitterness about losing her husband and cannot seem to stop thinking about him. She often feels that if she had done something differently, her husband may have lived. Ms. Smith's daughter feels that her mother has refused to heal and is concerned about depression.

1. **What is your current differential diagnosis for Ms. Smith?**
2. **What additional questions would you want to ask?** ■

DIAGNOSIS OF LATE LIFE DEPRESSION

Diagnosing depression in the elderly at times can be a challenge. Although the *Diagnostic and Statistical Manual of Mental Disorders, Fourth Edition-Text Revision* (DSM-IV-TR) diagnostic criteria for major depressive disorder (MDD) are the basic construct for depression in the older population, there are distinctions in how depression may present. Older depressed individuals have a higher tendency to have somatic complaints (primarily gastrointestinal), hypochondriasis, and agitation but are less likely to have low self-esteem or guilt compared to younger persons.[17] In addition, older depressed patients tend to have a higher rate of psychotic and severe (melancholic) depression with more weight loss and decreased appetite.[18] Occasionally, depression in the elderly may be masked in that the patient denies any emotional disturbance but instead reports a multitude of physical symptoms. Family members may report that the patient has lost interest in activities or has had a change in affect. In such circumstances, there is an obvious barrier to recognition of the depressive illness, though when investigated, somatic complaints are out of proportion to the medical illness. There may also be a chronologic correlation between new or worsening physical complaints and the onset of an identifiable stressor that alerts the provider to consider depression as a diagnosis.

Two other subtypes of depression of importance are dysthymic disorder and minor or subsyndromal depression. Dysthymic disorder is a more chronic form of affective disorder (duration longer than 2 years) characterized by two or more of the following symptoms: poor appetite or overeating, sleep disturbance, low energy or fatigue, difficulty with concentration, indecisiveness, feelings of hopelessness, and low self-esteem (DSM-IV-TR). Unlike MDD, dysthymic disorder is associated with a younger age of onset[19] and presenting symptoms are similar to younger cohorts. Although dysthymic disorder is unlikely to occur in late life, it may persist from midlife into late life.[20] Subsyndromal depression is also known as minor depression in the DSM-IV-TR and is diagnosed when the number of depressive symptoms is below the number needed to establish a diagnosis of MDD (i.e., between two and four symptoms). Subsyndromal depression is often present with comorbid chronic medical illness leading to functional decline. One study identified vision loss as the illness most readily associated with this form of depression.[21] Subsyndromal depression may lead to the same level of disability as MDD and is associated with increased mortality.[22] Several epidemiologic studies have shown subsyndromal depression to have a 2 to 3 times higher prevalence than MDD in the elderly, with a point prevalence of approximately 9.8% in community-dwelling seniors and as high as 35% of primary care geriatric patients.[23]

> Elderly depressed patients are more likely to have somatic complaints or hypochondriasis rather than guilt or low self-esteem.

> Older people may develop masked depression in which there is a lack of reported depressed mood. Assessing for anhedonia and corroborating history with family members is vital.

> There is a higher incidence of minor depression than major depressive disorder in the elderly.

DIFFERENTIAL DIAGNOSIS
Normal Grief and Bereavement

Diagnosing depression can be particularly difficult in the setting of bereavement where the overlap of symptoms typical of normal grieving and major depression can be extensive. However, multiple studies have shown that the two can be differentiated and that persons who develop late-life depression after loss of a loved one have distinctive outcomes. What differentiates any normative process from psychopathology is its effect on functioning. Typically, the bereaved individual does not become functionally impaired or is minimally impaired. Grief and bereavement also do not typically involve active suicidal thinking; rather, the bereaved may have passive thoughts about "joining" their loved one. Although it is not uncommon for grieving individuals to feel that they have seen their loved one in a crowd or hear the deceased calling their name, florid psychosis in the form of prolonged auditory or visual hallucinations and delusions should raise suspicion of another underlying psychiatric disorder. Cultural background plays a major role in the length of time an individual will grieve, but it is generally expected that a person will begin recovery within 1 year after his or her loss.

Complicated Grief

An evolving concept in the study of grief is complicated grief, a protracted, severe form of grieving in which a person experiences strong feelings of anger or bitterness about the loved one's death, feelings of emptiness, a persistent longing to be with the loved one, recurring intrusive thoughts about the loss, and reclusiveness from family and friends.[24] To be diagnosed as complicated grief, these symptoms must persist for 6 months or more. Complicated grief differs from clinical depression in that the former's presenting symptoms are more focused on the loss. Although both diagnoses carry some level of dysfunction, the distinction is important because persons experiencing complicated grief have inconsistent responses to antidepressants and psychotherapeutic treatments useful for MDD.[25] Shear and colleagues proposed complicated grief therapy (CGT), as specific therapy in this condition.[26] CGT combines features of cognitive behavioral and interpersonal therapy in which patients revisit the loss of their loved one under guidance of a therapist to bring resolution. The therapist also aids the individual to engage in situations and activities that were once avoided because of the loss. Preliminary studies show that CGT has better results than standard interpersonal therapy for treatment of complicated grief.[26]

Depression and Cognitive Impairment

A particular challenge occurs when depression overlaps with cognitive impairment. In one scenario, depression may arise with co-occurring cognitive dysfunction. This presentation has a variety of names including depressive pseudodementia and dementia syndrome of depression. The initial view was that patients developed cognitive deficits as one element of a severe neurovegetative state related to a depressive disorder and that, as the depression resolved, so did cognitive impairments. What seems clear now is that this clinical presentation includes a number of conditions that can be distinguished largely by their outcomes. The classic presentation referred to above does occur and is important to identify because these patients have one of the truly reversible causes of dementia. It is now known that even those who have an excellent response to treatment and clear cognitively have an increased risk of developing dementia in ensuing years.[27] Another scenario is for patients to develop a depressive disorder and, over time, gradually become cognitively impaired and eventually develop dementia, suggesting that late-onset depression can serve as a prodrome or a forme fruste of a dementing disorder.

An interesting study further explored the relationship between depression and dementia by examining if depression that first occurred in midlife carried a different prognosis than that developed for the first time in the senium. The risk of developing dementia was increased by 20% when midlife depressive symptoms were present, by 70% when only late-life symptoms were present, and by 80% when depressive symptoms were present at both times.[28] When these risks were evaluated by type of dementia, subjects with late-life depression had only a twofold increase in risk of AD. However, patients with depressive symptoms in both midlife and late life had a more than threefold increase in vascular dementia risk. The authors concluded that depression occurring either in midlife or in late life is associated with a higher risk of developing dementia and that the pattern is important. New depression in late life is more likely to be part of an AD prodrome, and recurrent depression is more strongly associated with vascular dementia.[28]

Another common pattern is the group of patients with minimal to mild cognitive impairment (MCI) or early AD who, after diagnosis, become depressed. At times this reflects the overlap in symptoms that dementia and depression share: decreased energy, problems with concentration, psychomotor changes, and loss of interest.[29] Although families often feel that this constellation represents depression, apathy is frequently one of the most common behavioral and psychological syndromes that affects those with early AD.

Current theory suggests late-life depression can be either a prodrome or a risk factor for AD. Depression commonly occurs in AD, and late-life depression itself can include cognitive deficits. There is evidence that amyloid deposition begins decades before clinical diagnosis of AD is made. A study exploring the deposition of amyloid and tau protein using positron emission tomography (PET) scans found a higher binding rate in patients with a diagnosis of MDD.[30] Moreover, these protein depositions were found in the posterior cingulate and lateral temporal areas of the brain known to be involved in AD.[30] Additionally, a study by Gerritsen et al. exploring depression and its correlation with changes in hippocampal and entorhinal volumes noted that patients experiencing a first episode of depression in late life exhibited volume loss in entorhinal *rather* than hippocampal structures, the latter being seen in early-onset depression.[31] Although this preliminary evidence for an underlying biological correlation between AD and depression is intriguing, further studies are needed before a definite connection can be established.

> Depression and dementia are frequently intertwined in older people, with high rates of depression in patients with dementia, and depression itself being a risk factor for dementia.

Depression Secondary to a General Medical Condition

A common caveat in the DSM-IV-TR regarding a psychiatric diagnosis is that "the symptoms are not due to the direct physiological effects of a substance or a general medical condition." Given that comorbid illness itself is a risk factor for depression, it is difficult to differentiate whether a physical illness is *causing* depression or indirectly *adding* to it as a risk factor.

This relationship has been extensively explored in the setting of stroke. Approximately 20% of stroke victims develop MDD and another 20% develop minor depression.[32] Conversely, depression itself is a risk factor for stroke.[33] Those that develop poststroke depression tend to have a greater decline in activities of daily living (ADLs),[34] less recovery of functioning,[35] greater impairment of cognition,[36] and increased mortality[37] compared to nondepressed stroke patients. Adequate treatment of poststroke depression improves outcomes in both ADLs and cognitive impairment.[38,39] Additionally, preventative treatment after stroke with antidepressants may reduce incidence of significant morbidity and mortality. A multicenter randomized controlled trial (RCT) compared escitalopram to placebo or problem-solving therapy (PST) for prevention of depression 1 year after acute stroke. Patients receiving placebo were 5 times more likely to develop poststroke depression compared to escitalopram and those receiving PST were 2 times more likely.[40] A follow-up study showed patients given escitalopram were more likely to develop depression 6 months after discontinuation of treatment whereas patients receiving PST or placebo were not.[41]

Vascular depression has been proposed as a distinct form of depression related to cerebrovascular disease but not to a discrete stroke. These patients are clinically identified based on symptoms that include substantial psychomotor retardation, apathy, and pronounced disability. They have vascular lesions on neuroimaging, a poor response to treatment, unstable remissions, and a higher risk of developing dementia.[42] Vascular depression is felt to result from small vascular insults to cerebral structures leading to dysfunction in brain neurocircuitry, primarily in the frontolimbic and frontostriatal systems. Also, white matter hyperintensities on magnetic resonance imaging (MRI) have been correlated with a decreased response to antidepressants, although this has been inconsistent and requires further exploration.[43] Likewise, preexisting vascular burden may be a determining factor in whether executive dysfunction improves in older depressives in response to treatment.[44,45] Additionally, inflammatory markers (C-reactive protein [CRP]), fasting glucose, and the metabolic syndrome, which all have effects on vascular functioning, have been independently associated with the onset of depressive symptoms in the elderly.[46]

Other chronic medical illnesses with high rates of depression are arthritis, heart disease, and cancer; in these, the level of functional disability is strongly associated with depression.[47] The most robust data available is in patients with heart disease. Cardiac conditions such as heart failure and acute myocardial infarction (MI) are strongly correlated with depression; approximately 20% to 40% of individuals with these conditions have MDD.[48] Patients who develop depression shortly after an MI have increased mortality.[49] In fact, patients with ischemic heart disease taking selective serotonin reuptake inhibitors (SSRIs) have a reduced rate of MI.[50] Although heart disease and the other aforementioned conditions correlate with depression, it is not clear if the mental or the physical ailment is the causative factor.

> Both stroke and heart disease have a strong correlation with depression.

> Treatment of comorbid depression with antidepressants can significantly improve morbidity and mortality.

Delirium is a condition that is misdiagnosed as depression up to 40% of the time.[51] Although hyperactive delirium may present with agitation and bizarre behavior, hypoactive delirium displays symptoms similar to depression including apathy, indecisiveness, and psychomotor retardation, accompanied by memory and functional impairment. The clinical setting for these misdiagnoses is most often the inpatient setting where a patient suddenly begins to refuse interventions or participation in care and the assumption is that the patient has "given up." Delirium should be suspected if both mood and cognitive symptoms occur with rapid onset (hours to days) and have a fluctuating course. Cognitive screening tests can be serially administered to document changes in cognition. The primary treatment for delirium is to find the underlying cause. Antidepressants have no role in this setting.

Substance-Induced Depression

According to a 2012 report from the Institute of Medicine approximately 5.6 to 8 million older adults had one or more mental health or substance use conditions. This number is expected to increase 80% by the year 2030.[52] Substance abuse, although not as common among the elderly, is an important problem in late life that can lead to significant morbidity and mortality. As a result, mood disorders related to substance use should always be included in the differential diagnosis. Alcohol is overwhelmingly the most common misused substance in late life, although with baby boomers aging, marijuana use may become common. According to the DSM-IV-TR criteria, when considering substance-induced depression secondary to drug abuse or dependence, it is important to have chronologic evidence of mood symptoms "developing during, or within a month of, substance intoxication or withdrawal." In some cases, a patient may be using a substance to "self-medicate" the underlying mood disorder. It is important to elicit a history to establish if the mood symptoms were present during extended periods of sobriety.

In addition to substance abuse, iatrogenic depression may also occur from commonly prescribed medications such as benzodiazepines, opiates, and steroids. Although beta-blockers have received much attention for possibly inducing depression, this association is inconsistent.[53] Regardless of type of medication, if depression begins within 1 month of starting a medication, especially if a patient has no history of prior depression, it can be presumed that it may be medication induced. If depression is possibly secondary to a newly prescribed drug, the medication should be discontinued or substituted and the patient monitored for mood improvement.

ASSESSMENT

As with diagnosing any illness, thorough history taking is crucial to a correct depression diagnosis. In evaluating an older patient, collateral sources such as the patient's spouse, family members, and/or caretakers can provide key information, especially in the context of cognitive impairment. This should not, however, be performed in lieu of speaking to the patient but rather to correlate the patient's concerns with others' observations. When taking a history, the clinician should pay close attention to the chronology of the patient's symptoms, especially in regard to changes in level of functioning associated with said symptoms. Although older depressed patients may be preoccupied with physical ailments, a connection may be found between symptoms and an acute or chronic stressful event. Significant areas of questioning should include the patient's socialization pattern, activities of daily living (ADL), and level of physical activity. Appetite and weight loss are of high importance because these can be severe in geriatric depression and may even cause failure to thrive. In addition, asking about psychotic symptoms (e.g., delusions and hallucinations) is also important because psychotic depression typically requires intensive pharmacotherapy with an antidepressant and antipsychotic or electroconvulsive therapy.

It is important to screen for bipolar disorders by asking about a history of mania (Table 18-2). Presentation of bipolar depression is virtually identical to unipolar depression and only properly inquiring about a previous manic episode will differentiate the two. It is also important to avoid antidepressant treatment in bipolar patients, where mood stabilizers such as lithium and lamotrigine would be first-line treatment.

CASE 1

Ms. Smith (Part 2)

You ask about Ms. Smith's medical history. Ms. Smith states that she feels she may have some form of cancer but is unsure. She reports that she "feels tired and sore all the time" and that "there must be something wrong with me." Her daughter reports that Ms. Smith has worried about having cancer since the loss of her husband. Ms. Smith has had a thorough medical workup regarding the possibility of cancer and was provided with the report; however, she continues to worry. Ms. Smith does take ibuprofen occasionally for muscle aches but otherwise is not taking any medications on a regular basis and has no other past medical history. She admits to being treated for depression in the past with nortriptyline after divorcing her first husband 35 years ago. She denies other past psychiatric history. Ms. Smith also drinks about 4 oz of wine with dinner twice a week. She denies any other substance use. When asked about suicidal thinking, Ms. Smith admits she occasionally longs to join her husband, but denies any thoughts about ending her life.

1. **What screening tests may you want to administer?**

2. **What lab tests would you want to order?** ◻

Outside of the presenting complaint, additional inquiries regarding the patient's substance use—past and present—are essential because substances play a role in mood regulation, have long-term effects on the brain, and can negate the effects of psychotropic

TABLE 18-2	**Abbreviated Criteria for Identifying a Manic Episode**

- A distinct period of time (at least 7 days) where a person's mood becomes persistently elevated, expansive, and/or irritable. During this time the patient also displays at least three of the following symptoms:

  a. Inflated self-esteem and grandiosity— *Patient may start challenging authority at the workplace. May become suspicious that others are talking about or plotting against him/her.*

  b. Decrease in need for sleep—*Patient may sleep for only 3 hours per night without experiencing any tiredness during the day. Make sure to ask about daytime naps to rule out underlying sleep disorder.*

  c. Increase in distractibility—*Patient may have difficulty focusing on one task at a time.*

  d. Increase in goal-directed activity—*Patient may take on multiple projects at once.*

  e. Impulsivity—*Patient may partake in risky behaviors without considering the consequences.*

  f. Rapid thinking or racing thoughts—*Patient may have multiple unrelated thoughts at the same time and find it difficult to express these thoughts to others.*

  g. Talkativity—*Patient finds him/herself speaking rapidly, often forcing others to interrupt.*

Considerations

- Emphasize to the patient that these symptoms have to be both persistent and present together as an episode. Many depressed patients experience some of these symptoms between episodes of depression or from a comorbid anxiety disorder.

- It is important to verify that the patient was not using illicit substances during these episodes.

- In questionable cases, a collateral source can help in establishing a diagnosis.

treatment. Medications should also be reviewed, including correlation between onset of symptoms and the start or change in a medication.

Depression rating scales can be useful in identifying depression in an older patient. A commonly used scale is the Geriatric Depression Scale (GDS),[54] most typically used in its short, 15-item format although it is now available from the authors as a smartphone app (iTunes, 2012). The GDS is unique in that it does not emphasize physical symptoms of depression (e.g., sleep and appetite changes) but rather focuses on psychological factors to suggest the presence of depression. A score of 5 or more suggests a need for further evaluation. The GDS can be administered in 5 to 10 minutes or can be given to the patient to fill out. Other commonly used depression scales include the 9-item Patient Health Questionnaire (PHQ-9)[55] and the Beck Depression Inventory (BDI). Both the PHQ-9 and the BDI have the option of being completed by the patient. The PHQ-9 more closely follows DSM-IV-TR diagnostic criteria for MDD. A score of 10 or above on the PHQ-9 indicates the possibility of

MDD. An even more rapid, simplified screening test is the 2-item PHQ-2 questionnaire, which asks simply about lack of interest and depressed mood yet has a sensitivity of 83% and specificity of 92% for detecting depressive disorders.[56]

It is very important to test cognitive functioning during any assessment for depression using standard rating scales. As mentioned above, the relationship between mood and cognition is complex. Although more commonly tested scales such as the Montreal Cognitive Assessment (MoCA)[57] and the Mini-Mental State Exam (MMSE) require some time to execute, a more rapid test such as the Mini-Cog screening test can be useful.[58] In this test, the patient is provided three words that he or she is asked to remember. The patient is then instructed to draw a clock depicting a given time. The administrator of the test monitors the patient's accuracy in drawing the numbers on the face of the clock, the structure of the clock itself, and the appropriate lengths of the minute and hour hands. After completing this task, the patient is asked to repeat the three words provided previously. This abbreviated form of cognitive testing has screening utility similar to the MMSE.[59]

In addition to the score a patient receives, the patient's behavior during testing can provide some clues as to whether depression may be present. Depressed patients often show little effort during examination, readily answer, "I don't know," and have inconsistent memory loss and performance within the examination. Additionally, they may respond well to semantic prompts during recall, and their recognition memory may be relatively intact.[61]

Suicide

Suicide is a difficult topic to broach with patients; however, it is an important aspect of any psychiatric evaluation (Boxes 18-1 and 18-2). If asked, a majority of elderly patients will reveal suicidal thinking if it is present, yet physicians have been shown not to address this topic with their most ill and most disabled

---

BOX 18-1

SUICIDE PREVENTION

The following strategies are recommended:
1. Screening for depression
2. Limiting access to means for suicide (e.g., asking about and removing firearms from the home)
3. Addressing issues concerning aging, psychosocial losses, and increasing dependence on others
4. Inquiring about community and family support
5. Close follow-up after initiating mental health treatment

Derived from Erlangsen A, Nordentoft M, Conwell Y, et al. Key considerations for preventing suicide in older adults: Consensus opinions of an expert panel. Crisis 2011;32(2):106-9.

BOX 18-2

APPROACHING A PATIENT ABOUT SUICIDE—MASTERING THE DIALOGUE

1. *Break the ice:* "When someone is feeling low or depressed, it is not uncommon to have thoughts that life isn't worth living or of no longer wanting to be around. Do you ever experience this type of thinking?"
2. *Identify the presence or absence of a plan:* "Occasionally, when people have this type of thinking, they might also have thoughts about wanting to end their life. Have you ever found yourself thinking this way?"
3. *Have the patient expand in detail:* "Have you ever thought of a way that you might take your life?" (Providing examples such as overdosing, etc., is not shown to be harmful and may actually help the patient in providing details.)
4. *Establish intent:* "Have you ever tried to harm yourself in the past?" "Do you have any thoughts about doing so now?"

---

patients.[61] Although the number of suicide attempts is highest in middle-aged adults and suicide rates in the elderly have been trending down over the last 8 years,[62] suicide nonetheless has special significance in the elderly. The most vulnerable population segment is white males; in this group, suicide rates peak at 45 out of 100,000 in the oldest age segment. The rate of suicide among the oldest white males is 4 times the national age-adjusted rate.[62]

In comparison to younger age groups, in which 1 in 200 suicide attempters die by their own hand, the ratio for completed suicides in the elderly is 1 in 4. This could be because younger adults are more likely to attempt suicide impulsively or as a communicative act, whereas elderly patients make more lethal attempts that they have planned over time.[62] Elderly patients are also often frail and live alone, allowing for little chance of rescue or survival after a suicide attempt has been made. These facts may seem rather daunting, but awareness of this issue allows for interventions, including preventative strategies. Although it is not possible to accurately predict who will attempt suicide, retrospective studies of elderly suicide attempts have identified several potential risk factors. Psychiatric illness is present in most elderly suicides (71% to 97%) with depression being the most common diagnosis.[62] Importantly, whereas 94% of elderly suicide attempters have been seen by a health professional in the past 12 months, only 4% are diagnosed with a mood disorder before the attempt; 51% were diagnosed after the attempt.[63] Older patients are more likely to turn to their primary care provider than to seek treatment from a mental health specialist, emphasizing the importance of screening for both mood disorders and suicidal ideation by these services. It has been shown that although antidepressants have been associated with increased suicidal ideation or gestures in young adults, they actually significantly decrease its likelihood in older depressed patients,[64] making early identification and treatment imperative.

In addition to depression, other identifiable factors may alert the providing physician to carefully screen for suicide. Important is the patient's current physical health, with studies showing a threefold to ninefold increase in risk for suicide depending on the number of co-occurring ailments. Chronic severe pain is particularly important in elderly males, showing a strong correlation with suicidal thinking. Social factors also play a role, particularly those that may be more common in late life such as increasing dependence, financial stress, grieving the loss of loved ones, and disruption of social support from family members. An identified protective factor in the elderly is "social connectedness." Maintaining social relationships has been shown to decrease mortality by half in elderly patients[65] and is on par with other healthy habits such as quitting smoking or losing weight in its health-protective effects.[62] When involvement and collaboration with the patient's family, friends, and caretakers (i.e., nursing home staff) is encouraged, this process may also be able to provide additional information regarding the patient's potential risk.[66]

With the time constraints faced by many primary care physicians, collaborative care models for mental health suggest that treatment management, including measures for suicide prevention, can be facilitated by use of designated care managers or other forms of mental health support workers collaborating closely with primary care providers and psychiatric consultants. Studies also show that telephone encounters may substitute for face-to-face interventions for mental health follow-up.[67] In addition to these preventative measures, it is recommended that patients with a history of chronic suicidal ideation or previous suicide attempts be referred to a psychiatric provider. In cases where there is significant concern about a patient's safety, prompt referral to the emergency department for further mental health evaluation and possible psychiatric hospitalization is necessary.

Laboratory Testing

Laboratory testing is an integral part of assessment for depression. It is not used to arrive at a primary psychiatric diagnosis, but rather to rule out other causes for a patient's mood symptoms. There are many medical conditions that affect mood and may mimic depression. These should be ruled out before initiating antidepressant treatment. Common ailments presenting as depression and their respective lab tests are listed in Table 18-3.

TABLE 18-3

Medical Condition	Lab Test
Hypo-/Hyperthyroidism	TSH/Free T4
Vitamin deficiency	Serum B_{12}, 25-OH Vitamin D, Folate
Anemia, infection	Complete blood count with differential
Urinary tract infection	Urinalysis

TSH, thyroid-stimulating hormone.

CASE 1

Ms. Smith (Part 3)

Ms. Smith scores a 12 on the 15 item GDS. You also administer a MMSE and Ms. Smith scores 27/30, losing points only for serial 7s. Ms. Smith's electrolytes and liver function tests are within normal limits. You note, however, that Ms. Smith has an elevated TSH of 24.4 and a low Free T4 of 0.4. Other lab tests including Vitamin B_{12}, folate, and complete blood count are all within normal limits.

1. **What are Ms. Smith's treatment options?**
2. **What are some good and bad prognostic factors for Ms. Smith?** ▫

MANAGEMENT

The National Institute of Mental Health–sponsored Sequenced Treatment Alternatives to Relieve Depression (STAR*D) study revealed that approximately 30% of depressed adults of all ages treated in medical and mental health settings developed a complete remission of all depressive symptoms when initially treated with the antidepressant citalopram. In addition, 45% to 50% of patients showed response (i.e., had a 50% improvement in symptoms) to that first treatment. In those that did not remit, switching to another antidepressant or augmenting citalopram with buspirone or buproprion increased the remission rate to more than 50%. A post-hoc analysis of STAR*D showed no significant difference in remission rates between older participants (those older than 55 years of age) and their younger counterparts[68] and no differences in depression outcomes by treatment setting (mental health vs. primary care clinic). This reinforces the effectiveness of detecting and treating geriatric depression in all settings.

Our knowledge, however, concerning the specific efficacy of psychopharmacologic treatment of depression in the elderly is limited. There have been few adequately powered RCTs specifically targeting the treatment of late-life depression. Depression trials at all ages depend on careful subject selection to ensure comparability of treatment groups. This is much more challenging in older patients where heterogeneity is inherent, not only psychiatrically, but also in terms of medical and psychosocial comorbidities. Another characteristic of placebo-controlled trials of antidepressants in the elderly has been high placebo response rates.[69] As in other antidepressant studies, drug–placebo differences are greatest in patients with more severe illness.[70] Meta-analyses of available studies show mixed evidence of antidepressant efficacy. A meta-analysis by Nelson et al. showed overall improved outcome with antidepressant treatment over placebo; however, the level of improvement varied and was modest.[71] A literature review by Salzman and colleagues made similar conclusions with respect to the efficacy of antidepressants in minor depression and dysthymia.[72]

Efforts have been made to explore factors that may influence treatment outcome. Some suggest that the age of onset of late-life depression (>55 vs. >65 years of age) plays an important role in outcome, with later onset of depression leading to a decreased likelihood of improvement.[73] Poor outcomes with pharmacotherapy have also been associated with high anxiety at the time of depression onset and age of first episode.[74]

Keeping the above issues in mind, when antidepressants are used judiciously and with realistic expectations, they can be effective, with numbers needed to treat of 13 for response and 20 for remission.[71]

What Agent to Choose?

Overall, there are no significant differences in treatment efficacy between available antidepressants. Drug selection therefore is better based on other factors, such as those noted in Box 18-3.

SSRIs

SSRIs are among the most commonly prescribed drugs in medicine. SSRIs are generally well tolerated though they have both common and less well-known side effects that are important to consider when prescribing for older adults (Box 18-4). With a majority of serotonin receptors being located in the gut, the most common initial side effects of SSRIs tend to be gastrointestinal (GI) and transient. A temporary decrease in initial

---

BOX 18-3

CHOOSING AN ANTIDEPRESSANT

Choice of antidepressant should be made based on the following factors:
- Safety
- Side-effect profile
- Ease of discontinuing treatment
- Ease of administration (once-daily versus twice-a-day dosing)
- Safety in medically fragile patients
- Few dosage adjustment steps
- Minimal drug interaction potential

BOX 18-4

SSRI SIDE EFFECTS IN THE ELDERLY

- Gastrointestinal upset
- Jitteriness
- Hyponatremia
- Drug–drug interactions (because of effects on CYP450 liver enzymes)
- Gastrointestinal bleeding
- Extrapyramidal side effects (tremors, parkinsonism, bruxism)

---

dosing minimizes GI side effects for most patients while serotonin receptors in the gut are downregulated. Later emerging GI side effects include constipation with paroxetine, and diarrhea with sertraline. The latter can be quite persistent with an onset that is delayed enough that it is often poorly recognized as a cause. In addition, SSRIs can have an activating effect when initially prescribed, which may result in insomnia or jitteriness. Changes in dose and time of administration are usually sufficient to address these issues.

SSRIs have known effects on a number of hepatic CYP450 enzymes, most importantly CYP2D6, which is involved in the metabolism of several commonly used medications. Paroxetine and fluoxetine have the highest inhibitory effects on CYP2D6, whereas escitalopram, citalopram, and sertraline have little practical impact on the P450 system. For this reason, one of the latter drugs is often chosen as initial therapy for older adults, who are often taking other medications.

A particularly important side effect of the SSRIs (and the serotonin norepinephrine reuptake inhibitors [SNRIs]) in older patients is hyponatremia, caused by the syndrome of inappropriate secretion of antidiuretic hormone (SIADH). Case control and retrospective studies have suggested an incidence of between 10% and 40%.[75] Risk factors include old age, female sex, low weight, diuretic use, and lower baseline sodium levels.[76,77] In a majority of instances, onset of SIADH is within 2 weeks of starting treatment with an SSRI.[77,78] It is important to realize that most hyponatremic patients have very nonspecific symptoms such as fatigue, anorexia, and confusion. Only a minority will have persistent, severe hyponatremia that can result in seizures, coma, and death. Checking serum sodium after 2 weeks can be considered in patients starting an SSRI who have additional risk factors or who are taking other medications associated with antidiuretic hormone secretion (e.g., thiazides, nonsteroidal antiinflammatory drugs [NSAIDs]).[77]

SSRIs are also associated with an increased risk of upper GI bleeding, particularly in patients taking concomitant NSAIDs or aspirin. Estimates of the risk of these events have varied widely, but most recent estimates have suggested the risk is fairly low with a number needed to harm over a year of treatment being 411 for SSRIs alone and 106 for SSRIs used with NSAIDS.[79] Although the mechanism for this bleeding risk has focused on the known effect of SSRIs on serotonin depletion in platelets, with subsequent impairment of platelet aggregation, a more important effect may be the ability of these drugs to directly increase gastric acidity.[80] This latter effect may explain why the risk of GI bleeds occurs in the upper GI tract as well as the fact that proton pump inhibitors can reduce the bleeding risks.[80] Bleeding events can occur within the first month of treatment[81] but may occur over a much greater time frame (e.g., median time to bleeding in 101 spontaneous reports was 25 weeks). In instances where SSRIs and SNRIs are given with an NSAID, the time to a potential bleeding episode may reflect the time necessary for the peptic ulceration to occur.[80] If a patient is on a blood thinner such as warfarin, it is recommended that the patient's international normalized ratio be checked more frequently during the start of treatment and at dose changes.

Use of SSRIs can occasionally result in the induction or exacerbation of neurologic symptoms including parkinsonism, dyskinesias, akathisia, and bruxism.[82] Nevertheless, SSRIs and SNRIs can be useful to treat depression in PD and are well tolerated.[83] When SSRIs are used in patients with PD, studies show there is an approximately 3% chance of developing an exacerbation of extrapyramidal symptoms, primarily tremors.[84] Treatment options include dose reduction, discontinuation, or the addition of a benzodiazepine or beta-blocker.

SSRIs have generally been considered to have a safe cardiovascular profile. However, the Food and Drug Administration (FDA) has released recommendations regarding the dosing of citalopram based on its potential for dose-dependent prolongation of the QT interval.[85] The new FDA dosing guidelines call for a maximum dose of 40 mg per day in individuals up to age 65 and a per-day minimum of 20 mg in those older than age 65. The FDA also suggests more frequent electrocardiogram (ECG) monitoring in patients with heart failure or bradyarrhythmias, or who are on concomitant medications that prolong the QT interval. The latter recommendations may be relevant for patients taking acetylcholinesterase inhibitors for dementia, many of whom develop bradycardia with treatment. Note that as of this time, the FDA directives do not extend to the s-enantiomer of citalopram, escitalopram, though a conservative approach might be to keep doses of that medication to a maximum of 10 mg in older adults.

SNRIs

SNRIs (duloxetine, venlafaxine, desvenlafaxine) inhibit the synaptic reuptake of both norepinephrine and serotonin. Although there is no conclusive evidence that the SNRIs are any more efficacious than SSRIs in treating depression in the elderly,[86] this class does offer distinct benefits for chronic pain conditions with or without comorbid depression.[87] Venlafaxine predominantly affects serotonin uptake at doses less than 150 mg daily and accordingly at those doses its side effects are typical of SSRIs.[88] Duloxetine has a more balanced effect on both serotonin and norepinephrine at clinically relevant doses and is indicated for a number of pain indications including fibromyalgia, neuropathic pain associated with diabetic peripheral neuropathy, and chronic musculoskeletal pain.

Other Antidepressants

Other options for treatment of depression in the elderly include bupropion, which is mechanistically unique among antidepressants and the only agent with an additional indication for smoking cessation.[89] Bupropion has the additional benefits of having no sexual side effects, minimal weight gain potential, and negligible GI bleeding risk. On the other hand, it can be too activating for some patients, does not appear to be as effective for anxiety disorders, and has a moderate inhibitory effect on CYP2D6. Mirtazapine, also devoid of sexual side effects, is an alpha-2 antagonist and indirectly increases serotonin and norepinephrine transmission. It is also a potent inhibitor of histamine (H1) receptors, with subsequent effects on sleep and appetite. Sedation is greatest at lower doses (<15 mg daily) and is offset at higher doses by increased noradrenergic activity. Unlike the antidepressant effect, the impact on sleep is immediate, and, if not excessive, can provide for improved patient adherence. In one RCT, mirtazapine showed more pronounced improvement in depression when compared to paroxetine in the first few weeks of treatment, likely because of its effects on sleep, which is a major component of depression rating scales.[90] With both mirtazapine and bupropion, there is little information on long-term use and further study is needed.

TCAs. Tricyclic antidepressants (TCAs) have been extensively studied and there are numerous trials showing efficacy. However, TCAs have many safety issues and have a higher incidence of side effects, the most prominent of which are various anticholinergic effects and cardiac effects including increased heart rate, slowing of cardiac conduction, and orthostatic hypotension. ECGs should be monitored before and during TCA use and careful measurement of orthostatic blood pressure is mandatory. The two TCAs with the best safety profile for older patients are the secondary amines nortriptyline and desipramine. Both of these drugs can be measured in the blood stream and nortriptyline has a therapeutic window that can guide dosing.

Although TCAs are safe to use in the elderly, it is important to monitor pulse, orthostatic blood pressure, cardiac conduction, and anticholinergic side effects.

Psychostimulants. When the above treatments fail, psychostimulants are sometimes considered for monotherapy or adjunctive therapy in depressed elderly patients. One benefit with psychostimulants is that response to treatment is seen relatively quickly (i.e., within days). This may be helpful in cases where time to response is critical, such as with patients in rehabilitation programs or in end-of-life care. Trials, however, have been relatively short in total treatment time and number of patients treated.[91] Subsequently, long-term efficacy with this class of medications is unknown. There are several studies showing psychostimulants improving particular symptoms that may be seen with older depressed patients, such as apathy, fatigue, impaired executive functioning, and even gait dysfunction with a decreased incidence of falls.[91] However, these improvements do not necessarily correlate with overall improvement in depression and trials primarily included patients with comorbid medical conditions and hypoactive delirium. Precautionary measures when using psychostimulants include taking a thorough cardiac history because there is limited data about safe use of stimulants in the elderly; however, recent reports of use in younger adults have been largely reassuring. Blood pressure and heart rate should be monitored regularly because both can be increased by psychostimulant use.

Other Treatment Considerations

Box 18-5 suggests tips about how to educate patients and their families about the treatment of depression. Regardless of which medication is chosen as part of treatment, frequent monitoring and dose titration are vital.

When initiating treatment it is important to note that although geriatric patients can tolerate standard dosing of many antidepressants, they are more susceptible to side effects. As mentioned previously, SSRIs have a number of side effects that are transient in nature, such as jitteriness and nausea. Although these are not life threatening, they can certainly be uncomfortable for the patient and may lead to poor adherence or premature discontinuation of the medication. The general rule is to begin treatment at a low dose (e.g., start with 50% of the target dose) and titrate after 4 to 7 days to minimize initial side effects. Although the target dose for many older patients is lower than for younger adults, it is crucial to monitor the patient for both medication intolerance and improvement of depressive symptoms. If the patient reports no side

> **BOX 18-5**
>
> **CLINICAL TIPS FOR EDUCATING PATIENT/FAMILY ABOUT DEPRESSION AND ITS TREATMENT**
>
> 1. Explain that major depressive disorder is a medical illness (like diabetes or hypertension) and review specific signs and symptoms and treatment with patient and family. Reinforce that the patient is not simply being treated for "sadness."
> 2. When reviewing history with the patient, the provider may want to use phrases such as "How long have you been fighting/struggling with depression?" rather than "How long have you been depressed?" This should allow the patient to take a more proactive stance against the ailment.
> 3. Educate the patient that antidepressants should not be taken on an as-needed basis. They should not be doubled-up on "bad days" nor skipped on "good days."
> 4. Clarify to the patient that antidepressants do not solve problems. Review and prioritize acute and chronic psychosocial stressors with family and patient to create an appropriate treatment plan (e.g., social work referral, psychotherapy).
> 5. Preemptively educate the patient and family about common initial side effects such as jitteriness and GI upset, stressing the transient nature of these symptoms and dosing strategies to avoid them.

effects with the initial dose, yet does not show any improvement of depression, then it is prudent to continue increasing the antidepressant until a trial of the maximum tolerable dose of the medication is achieved. Although susceptibility to side effects is a concern on initiation of an antidepressant, once elderly patients have been established on a tolerable dose of the medication, they have a rate of discontinuation with continued treatment similar to that of the general adult population.[92]

A patient who has responded to antidepressant treatment should be continued on treatment for approximately 1 year for a first depressive episode. After a second or third episode, however, it has been recommended to extend treatment after reaching remission, with some patients requiring lifelong treatment.[93] For example, one study comparing treatment with paroxetine versus placebo in combination with psychotherapy 2 years after a depressive episode showed a relative risk of reoccurrence 2.4 times higher with placebo than with paroxetine.[94] It is therefore vital to continue antidepressants after remission of a depressive episode, especially for patients with a history of relapse.

For those patients who do not respond to an initial adequate trial of pharmacotherapy, choices include switching antidepressants or augmentation. For most patients who have taken an SSRI as a first agent, a simple choice is to switch to an alternative SSRI or different class of medication, such as an SNRI, or bupropion. These switching options had equivalent outcomes in the STAR*D trial. Alternatively, for a patient who has had a partial but incomplete response, augmentation with either buspirone or bupropion can be considered or a trial of cognitive behavioral therapy (CBT; see following section). In STAR*D, augmentation with these strategies appeared to be slightly more effective than switching to a new drug.

Psychosocial Interventions

Although antidepressants are a useful modality for treating late-life depression, they are not the sole option. Psychosocial interventions are often very effective and may be particularly useful in patients with less severe major depression, minor depression, or dysthymia, where the evidence for use of antidepressants is less robust. However, just as with pharmacotherapy, data on efficacy is limited using these interventions. Interventions that have been explored in an elderly population and have evidence of efficacy include problem-solving therapy (PST), which focuses on teaching patients strategies to solve everyday problems and deal with crisis; CBT, which focuses on behavioral activation and identifying and correcting automatic negative thought processes; and treatment initiation and participation (TIP) therapy, which focuses on education about health and medication.[95] Of these, PST has been shown to be useful in patients with cognitive impairment who would be less amenable to explorative types of therapy. CBT has also shown utility, with or without the concomitant use of desipramine, for even severe forms of depression.

Because of the heterogeneity of the elderly population, many individuals may have particular needs or additional psychosocial factors contributing to their depression. Case management is a valuable tool to aid with these concerns. Over the last decade, an initiative known as the Improving Mood, Promoting Access to Collaborative Treatment (IMPACT) care model[96] has proven quite beneficial and is being implemented in many settings. In this model, a care manager (most often a nurse) is present in the clinic and is assigned to patients diagnosed with depression. The care manager educates the patient about depression, monitors for improvement and adherence, and provides regular follow-up and counseling. The care manager typically consults with a psychiatrist on a regular basis. This model of care has been extensively studied and shown to decrease overall cost of care and significantly improve patient treatment response over what would be considered standard care.

Other Somatic Treatments

Electroconvulsive therapy (ECT) is often overlooked as a possible intervention in treatment of late-life depression (Box 18-6). ECT is highly effective and can be particularly beneficial for patients with active suicidal ideation and psychotic depression. It has the lowest incidence of mortality among all procedures performed

---

> **BOX 18-6**
>
> **ELECTROCONVULSIVE THERAPY (ECT)**
>
> 1. Useful when more rapid antidepressant effect is desired (failure to thrive, severe/psychotic depression, active suicidal ideation)
> 2. No absolute contraindications
> 3. Useful for frail elderly patients who may not be able to tolerate medications

---

under general anesthesia. There are no absolute contraindications to the use of ECT. It has been shown to be more efficacious in late-life depression than in the general adult population. It results in more immediate response in symptoms and may be effective for those patients experiencing significant disability from their depressive symptoms. ECT is also a useful alternative for frail elderly patients who may have multiple comorbid conditions and who are unable to tolerate antidepressant treatment. However, it should be noted that even after acute treatment and symptom improvement, there is an 85% chance of relapse in the first 6 months if the patient is not provided with adjunctive maintenance pharmacotherapy. Therefore, ECT is best seen as an acute intervention to hasten response. Primary side effects experienced by the older population are short-term memory loss and a possible increase in incidence of falls, particularly in nursing home patients.[97]

A newer form of somatic treatment, rapid transcranial magnetic stimulation (rTMS), has been FDA-approved since 2008. This treatment does not require anesthesia and can be performed on an outpatient basis. The patient is seated while magnetic pulses are used to stimulate the brain to induce change in mood. The procedure typically is prescribed as a total course of pulses delivered in 30- to 40-minute sessions daily over a period of 4 to 6 weeks. The patient is not sedated and can converse during treatments. Efficacy in the elderly is still being evaluated.[98,99] Given that the strength of the magnetic field falls off rapidly with distance and that many older adults have significant brain atrophy, this treatment modality may require higher doses in elderly patients than those used in younger adults for efficacy.

CASE 1

Ms. Smith (Part 4)

You begin Ms. Smith on thyroid replacement therapy while simultaneously starting her on nortriptyline, 25 mg by mouth at bedtime. You also perform a baseline ECG. You explain to Ms. Smith and her daughter about the signs and symptoms of major depression and the use of antidepressants including possible side effects and length of treatment. You also refer Ms. Smith for psychotherapy and educate her about its potential benefits when combined with antidepressants.

Ms. Smith returns to the clinic in 2 weeks and states that she has noticed some improvement in sleep, but she has not had much improvement in her other symptoms. She denies any side effects from the nortriptyline. You increase the dose from 25 to 50 mg and have her return in 4 weeks. At her next visit, you obtain a TSH level, which has returned to normal. Ms. Smith reports that she has been attending therapy once a week and has felt some resolution regarding the loss of her husband. She has started attending more family dinners and has been baby-sitting her grandchildren, which she enjoys. Under the direction of her therapist, she has made a scrapbook of her travels with her husband and has started sorting through some of his belongings, gifting a portion of them to her children. Her energy level has improved and she has been going on walks with her daughter as well. On repeat administration, Ms. Smith scores a 3 on her GDS and a 29/30 on her MMSE.

Discussion

Ms. Smith originally presented with what seemed to be complicated grief. However, when exploring Ms. Smith's symptoms further and using standardized scales, it was noted that Ms. Smith was suffering from depression. It was also discovered that the patient was hypothyroid; however, because Ms. Smith meets criteria for depression and has a history of depressive disorder, it would be optimal to treat both her hypothyroidism and depression simultaneously. Nortriptyline was selected as the treatment here given her prior good response and her willingness to accept treatment with that agent. Remember that use of tricyclic antidepressants necessitates baseline ECG and monitoring of orthostatic blood pressures. ■

SUMMARY

Depression continues to be recognized as a major contributing factor to both morbidity and mortality in the elderly. Simultaneously, there is a shortage of psychiatrists nationwide. Thus it is crucial that primary care physicians acquire the capabilities to both detect and treat depression. This is especially pertinent to depression in the elderly, which has unique presentations, prognoses, and higher likelihood of multiple medical comorbidities requiring a heightened sense of awareness. However, depression is a treatable condition; if medication and psychosocial interventions are optimized, it can be defeated. The patient's overall health and quality of life depend on appropriate treatment.

Web Resources

www.iom.edu/Reports/2012/The-Mental-Health-and-Substance-Use-Workforce-for-Older-Adults.aspx. The Institute of Medicine report on mental health care for older adults.
http://impact-uw.org. The IMPACT study and its protocols.
www.nimh.nih.gov/health/publications/depression/complete-index.shtml. National Institute of Mental Health pamphlet on depression in the elderly.
www.nrepp.samhsa.gov. Searchable database of evidence-based interventions for mental health.

KEY REFERENCES

32. Robinson RG, Spalletta G. Poststroke depression: A review. Can J Psychiat 2010;55(6):341-9.
63. Conwell Y, Van Orden K, Caine ED. Suicide in older adults. Psychiatr Clin North Am 2011;34(2):451-68, ix.
72. Nelson JC, Delucchi K, Schneider LS. Efficacy of second generation antidepressants in late-life depression: A meta-analysis of the evidence. Am J Geriatr Psychiatry 2008;16(7):558-67.
75. Andreescu C, Reynolds CF 3rd. Late-life depression: Evidence-based treatment and promising new directions for research and clinical practice. Psychiatr Clin North Am 2011;34(2):335-55, vii-iii. Review.
96. Kiosses DN, Leon AC, Areán PA. Psychosocial interventions for late-life major depression: Evidence-based treatments, predictors of treatment outcomes, and moderators of treatment effects. Psychiatr Clin North Am 2011;34(2):377-401, viii.

References available online at expertconsult.com.

Balance, Gait, and Mobility

Neil B. Alexander

OBJECTIVES

Upon completion of this chapter, the reader will be able to:

- Discuss the prevalence of gait/mobility deficits in older adults.
- List some of the deleterious impacts of gait disorders on the health of older adults.
- Discuss three risk factors for gait/mobility deficits in older adults.
- Describe common diagnoses and impairments contributing to gait disorders in older adults.
- Formulate a differential diagnosis to determine the cause of a gait disorder in the older adult.
- Describe and discuss some of the low-tech performance-based measures used to evaluate gait and mobility in the older adult.

- Describe and discuss some of the management options, including treatment outcomes, for gait and mobility deficits in the older adult.

CASE 1

Mrs. Henderson (Part 1)

Mrs. Henderson is a 78-year-old patient in your practice. She has had depression, backache, and neck pain for years, has a 1-year history of left hip pain on ambulation, and reports a recent onset of intermittent confusion. You have managed her depression and arthritic pain with a selective serotonin reuptake inhibitor antidepressant and antiinflammatory medications. At your suggestion she has been ambulating with a quad cane for the past year as needed. Six months ago you referred her to an orthopedic surgeon, who concurred with your diagnosis of moderately severe osteoarthritis of the hip and recommended a trial of physical therapy. She attended outpatient physical therapy three times a week for a month and had some relief with range of motion and strengthening exercises, although some residual pain remained. She now reports that the pain has become severe over the past 3 months, and that the exacerbation coincided with a fall at home 3 months ago. She went to the emergency room after the fall, but radiographs revealed no fractures. She reports no loss of consciousness after the fall. She is currently on multiple medications for pain, including acetaminophen with codeine and an as-needed muscle relaxant. Her chief complaints today are pain in the hip during ambulation, and headache and neck pain.

Your examination reveals a score of 22 on the Mini-Mental State Examination, with decreased attention and disorientation, suggestive of delirium. Her score on the Geriatric Depression Scale is 8, suggesting mild residual depression. Range of motion of the left hip is decreased when compared to the right hip, and all hip motions elicit pain. She is tender on palpation of the neck musculature, with reduced range of motion and pain on neck flexion and rotation. You order radiographs of the neck, which show signs of degenerative joint disease.

1. **What diagnoses would you place on her problem list?**

2. **What would you do next?** ▣

PREVALENCE AND IMPACT

The term *mobility* may encompass a variety of functional activities, such as transfers to and from a bed and chair, walking, stair climbing, getting in and out of vehicles, and others.[1] Difficulty ambulating and

---

Additional online-only material indicated by icon.

problems with general mobility are frequent complaints of older adults. Each year about 1 in every 100 older adults develops new severe mobility disability, defined as the inability to walk across a small room or the need for help from another person to do so.[2] Approximately 20% of noninstitutionalized older adults admit to having trouble walking or require assistance from another person or equipment to ambulate,[3] and the prevalence of walking limitations in noninstitutionalized adults 85 years and older can exceed 54%.[3] Finally, clinically abnormal gait, particularly with a neurologic etiology (identified later in this chapter), is associated with falls.[4]

The impact of gait and mobility deficits can be devastating for the older adult. Impairments in gait and mobility are associated with depressive symptoms,[5] falls,[6] functional dependence,[7,8] institutionalization,[9] and death strength of evidence (SOE) = B).[1,7]

> Having a problem with walking, particularly walking habitually slowly, is a strong predictor of adverse outcomes, including falls, functional dependence, and death.

TABLE 19-1	Diagnoses Contributing to Gait Abnormalities in Primary Care Geriatrics
Primary Diagnosis Contributing to Gait Disorder	**Percentage of Cases**
Osteoarthritis or an inflammatory arthritis	43
Sensory imbalances (e.g., peripheral neuropathy)	9
Parkinsonism	9
Orthostatic hypertension	9
Intermittent claudication	6
Postcerebrovascular accident	6
Congenital deformity	6
Postorthopedic surgery	3
Vertebrobasilar insufficiency	3
Heart disease	3
Idiopathic gait disorder: fear of falling	3
TOTAL	**100**

Adapted from Hough JC, McHenry MP, Kammer LM. Gait disorders in the elderly. Am Fam Physician 1987;35(6):191-6.

RISK FACTORS AND PATHOPHYSIOLOGY

Many adults maintain normal or near normal gait and mobility well into old age. Thus gait and mobility dysfunctions are not an inevitable consequence of aging, as is often thought, but in many cases are a reflection of chronic diseases[10] or of recent or remote trauma. Age-related declines in gait speed are well documented, and are a result of decreases in stride length, rather than decreases in cadence (steps per minute).[11] Shorter, broader strides, longer stance, and shorter swing durations are some of the gait characteristics apparent after age 75 or 80.[12,13]

Often the cause of a gait disorder is multifactorial. In one community-based sample, the prevalence of abnormal gait was 35%, split approximately evenly between neurologic and nonneurologic etiologies.[9] A number of diseases and impairments (Table 19-1) may contribute to decreases in gait speed, including cardiopulmonary or musculoskeletal disease, reduced leg strength, poor vision, diminished aerobic function, balance problems, physical inactivity, joint impairment, previous falls, and fear of falling.[15-21] Other less common factors contributing to gait disorders include metabolic disorders related to renal or hepatic disease, tumors of the central nervous system, subdural hematoma, depression, and psychotropic medications. Hypothyroidism and hyperthyroidism and B_{12} and folate deficiency may also be associated with reversible gait disorders.[11] Coimpairments, such as when leg weakness is found in the patient with balance deficits, may have a greater effect on deficits in mobility than the sum of the single impairments.[15]

DIFFERENTIAL DIAGNOSIS AND ASSESSMENT

One way of organizing a differential diagnosis for a gait disorder is to consider three levels of sensorimotor function—peripheral, subcortical, and cortical. Table 19-2 outlines for each of the three sensorimotor levels the most common conditions and gait characteristics associated with each condition.[22] To this must be added consideration of diseases of other organ systems that commonly affect gait. Finally, one must consider whether medication-related effects are contributing.

Peripheral sensorimotor deficits are divided into sensory and motor dysfunction, and include musculoskeletal (arthritic) and myopathic/neuropathic disorders (i.e., disorders distal to the central nervous system). With peripheral sensory impairment, unsteady and tentative gait is common; causes include vestibular disorders, peripheral neuropathy, posterior column (proprioceptive) deficits, and visual impairment.

With peripheral motor impairment, a number of classic gait patterns emerge, including obvious compensatory strategies. Examples of these strategies include the following:

- Trendelenburg gait (hip abductor weakness causing weight shift over the weak hip)
- Antalgic gait (avoidance of excessive weight bearing and shortening of stance on one side because of pain)

TABLE 19-2	Classification of Gait Disorders by Sensorimotor Level		
Sensorimotor Level	**Within-Level Classification**	**Condition (Pathology, Symptoms, Signs)**	**Typical Gait Characteristics**
Peripheral	Peripheral sensory	Sensory ataxia (posterior column, peripheral nerves)	Unsteady, uncoordinated, especially without visual input.
		Vestibular ataxia	Unsteady, weaving ("drunken").
		Visual ataxia	Tentative, uncertain.
	Peripheral motor	Arthritic (antalgic, joint deformity)	Avoids weight bearing on affected side, shortens stance phase. Painful hip may produce Trendelenburg gait (trunk shift over affected side). Painful knee is flexed. Painful spine produces short, slow steps and decreased lumbar lordosis. Other nonantalgic features: contractures, deformity-limited motion, buckling with weight bearing. Kyphosis and ankylosing spondylosis produce stooped posture. Unequal leg length can produce trunk and pelvic motion abnormalities (including Trendelenburg).
		Myopathic and neuropathic (weakness)	Pelvic girdle weakness produces exaggerated lumbar lordosis and lateral trunk flexion (Trendelenburg and waddling gait). Proximal motor neuropathy produces waddling and foot slap. Distal motor neuropathy produces distal weakness (especially ankle dorsiflexion, foot drop), which may lead to exaggerated hip flexion, knee extension and foot lifting (steppage gait), and foot slap.
Subcortical	Spasticity	Hemiplegia/paresis	Leg swings outward and in semicircle from hip (circumduction). Knee may hyperextend (genu recurvatum), and ankle may excessively plantar flex and invert (equinovarus). With less paresis, some may only lose arm swing and only drag or scrape the foot.
		Paraplegia/paresis	Both legs circumduct, steps are short shuffling and scraping, and when severe, hip adducts so that knees cross in front of each other (scissoring).
	Parkinsonism		Small shuffling steps, hesitation, acceleration (festination), falling forward (propulsion), falling backward (retropulsion), moving the whole body while turning (turning en bloc), absent arm swing.
	Cerebellar ataxia		Wide-based with increased trunk sway, irregular stepping, staggering, especially on turns.
Cortical	Cautious gait		Fear of falling with appropriate postural responses, normal to widened base, shortened stride, decreased velocity, and en bloc turns.
	Frontal-related gait disorders; other white matter lesions	Cerebrovascular; normal pressure hydrocephalus	Frontal gait disorder: difficulty initiating gait and short shuffling gait similar to Parkinson's but wider base, upright posture, preservation of arm swing, leg apraxia, may freeze with diversion of attention or turning. May also have cognitive, pyramidal, and urinary disturbances.

Adapted from Alexander NB. Differential diagnosis of gait disorders in older adults. Clin Geriatr Med 1996;12(4):689-703.

- Steppage gait (excessive hip flexion facilitating foot clearance of the ground in patients with foot drop caused by ankle dorsiflexor weakness)

These conditions involve extremity (both body segment and joint) deformities, painful weight bearing, and focal myopathic and neuropathic weakness. Note that if the gait disorder is limited to this low sensorimotor level (i.e., the central nervous system is intact), the person can adapt well to the gait disorder, compensating with an assistive device or learning to negotiate the environment safely.

Subcortical sensorimotor deficits result from lesions of the midbrain, brainstem, cerebellum, and spinal cord. At the middle level, the execution of centrally selected postural and locomotor responses is faulty, and the sensory and motor modulation of gait is disrupted. Gait may be initiated normally but stepping patterns are abnormal. Examples include the following:

- Diseases causing spasticity (such as those related to myelopathy, B_{12} deficiency, and stroke)
- Parkinsonism (idiopathic as well as drug-induced)
- Cerebellar disease (such as alcohol induced)

Classic gait patterns appear when the spasticity is sufficient to cause leg circumduction and fixed deformities (such as equinovarus), when parkinsonism produces shuffling steps and reduced arm swing, and when cerebellar ataxia increases trunk sway sufficiently to require a broad base of gait support. Recent attention has focused on the pathophysiology, diagnosis, and therapy for freezing of gait (FOG), found commonly in parkinsonian syndromes.[23]

Cortical sensorimotor deficits often involve cognitive dysfunction and slowed cognitive processing. Gait characteristics tend to be nonspecific. Behavioral factors such as fear of falling are also important, particularly in cautious gait. The presence of dementia and depression are often major contributors.

Frontal-related gait disorders tend to have a cerebrovascular component but may also result from dementia, normal pressure hydrocephalus, or a frontal mass. The severity of the frontal-related disorders run a spectrum from gait ignition failure (i.e., difficulty with initiation) to frontal dysequilibrium, where unsupported stance is not possible.

Cerebrovascular insults to the cortex and/or basal ganglia and their interconnections may relate to gait ignition failure and apraxia.[24,25] Cognitive, pyramidal, and urinary disturbances may also accompany the gait disorder. Gait disorders that might fall in this category have been given a number of overlapping descriptions, including gait apraxia, marche à petits pas, and arteriosclerotic (vascular) parkinsonism.

A vascular etiology has been proposed linking not only slowed gait and impaired cognitive (executive) function, but depressive symptoms as well.[26]

A number of studies have found age- and disease-associated deficits in gait speed, often using a measure of gait variability, particularly while performing a simultaneous cognitive task (dual tasking such as talking while walking). These deficits are linked to increased fall risk. Even mild cognitive impairment (either amnestic or executive) is associated with changes in gait, such as in variability.[27] Note that whereas declines in cognitive function, and executive function in particular, are associated with declines in gait speed, declines in gait speed can also predict declines in cognition.[28]

Approach to Patient Assessment

Patients consider pain, stiffness, dizziness, numbness, weakness, and sensations of abnormal movement to be the most common impairments contributing to walking difficulty.[14] In many cases, the older adult presents with a gait disorder as a manifestation of acute or chronic disease (or in some cases, multiple diseases). Thus the aim of the primary care practitioner should be to diagnose the underlying disease state to determine whether the gait disorder is cardiovascular, musculoskeletal, or neurologic in etiology, or a result of some other pathology. Components of the clinical assessment can include the traditional history and physical examination, performance-based assessments, and laboratory and imaging tests. All of these will assist the primary care practitioner in formulating a clinical and/or impairment-based diagnosis as it relates to the gait dysfunction.

History and Physical Examination

The evaluation should begin with a careful medical history. Enquire as to past medical history including history of injuries, accidents, and falls, because these may predispose the older adult to a mobility disorder. Determine if the patient uses an assistive device and if his or her level of physical activity is as expected in comparison to age-matched individuals. Enquire if they are fearful of falling, because this may cause older adults to limit their level of activity. Review medications, including adherence to the prescribed regimen.

A systems review is conducted to elucidate the multiple factors potentially contributing to the gait disorder. Systemic evaluation should include evaluation for acute cardiopulmonary disorders such as myocardial infarction, and other acute illness such as sepsis, because an acute gait disorder may be the presenting feature of acute illness in the older adult. Subacute and chronic cardiopulmonary disorders with dyspnea on exertion may also be present. Review auditory and visual systems, enquiring as to hearing and visual impairments, including Meniere's disease, vertigo, cataracts, and glaucoma. For the neurologic and musculoskeletal systems, inquire as to the following: lower extremity sensory changes including numbness and tingling, joint and muscle pain, stiffness, joint instability or muscle weakness limiting the patient's mobility during performance of daily activities such as ambulation, and poor balance and unsteadiness including dizziness during upright posture and gait. Evidence of subacute metabolic disease (such as thyroid disorders) also warrants evaluation.

The physical examination should entail a thorough evaluation of the patient's gait pattern, and should begin when the patient enters the room.[29] The examiner should first get an overall impression of the gait; does it seem abnormal? In this initial impression, one should consider global gait problems such as difficulty with initiation, unsteadiness, short or shuffling steps, asymmetric weight distribution, and poor toe clearance. Then a closer inspection is probably warranted, so observe the patient's gait pattern from the front, behind, and the sides, noting in each instance the motion from proximal to distal, that is, from the pelvis and lumbar spine down to the ankle and foot.[30] Observation from the front and behind enables the examiner to observe sideways swaying of the trunk, bowing of the femur or tibia, medial or lateral hip rotations, abduction or circumduction actions of the lower extremity during swing phase, width of the base of support, and foot position (toe and heel in or out). The classic Trendelenburg gait, in which there is weakness of the hip abductors (gluteus medius muscle) and which is characterized by trunk shift over the affected hip, is best visualized from behind or in front of the patient.[29,30] Observation of the patient's gait from the side enables the examiner to detect motions of the trunk and lower extremity in the sagittal plane, including the extensor or gluteus maximus lurch in which the patient thrusts the trunk posteriorly to compensate for weak hip extensors (gluteus maximus muscle).[29,30] Observation from the side also enables detection of ankle dorsiflexor weakness and foot drop leading to inability of the foot to clear the ground, which is compensated for by excessive lower extremity flexion to facilitate foot clearance of the ground (steppage gait).[29,30] Walking for a more extended period may exacerbate these deficits and also elicit dyspnea and oxygen desaturation, particularly in patients with active cardiopulmonary disease.

The examination should also include an attempt to identify motion-related factors, such as by provoking both vestibular and orthostatic responses. Visual screening should be performed. Musculoskeletal examination should include evaluation of the neck, spine, extremities, and feet for pain, deformities, and limitations in active and passive range of motion, particularly regarding subtle hip and/or knee contractures. Leg length discrepancies may occur following hip prosthesis surgery,[31] and can be measured with the patient in supine as the distance from the anterior superior iliac spine to the medial malleolus. The neurologic assessment should include assessment of strength, tone, reflexes, sensation (including proprioception), coordination (including cerebellar function), balance, and station and gait. Balance assessment should include determination of unipedal stance time; a time of less than 5 seconds is an indicator of increased risk for an injurious fall.[32] The Romberg test screens for simple postural control and whether the proprioceptive and vestibular systems are functional when the eyes are closed. Screening for mental status is also indicated.

Performance-Based Assessments

Timed or scored functional gait and mobility tests are often used in clinical settings to detect deficits in gait and mobility. These low-tech measures, quick to administer and requiring at most a stopwatch for timing, are used for screening and to track progress in response to interventions. Selection of the measure will depend on level of participant ambulation impairment (e.g., community ambulator versus homebound) and the need for simple (e.g., busy clinic or hospital setting) versus more time-consuming but informative multiple task assessments (e.g., rehabilitation setting). Underlying most of these tests is gait speed, which is consistently the most valid and reliable measure.

> Even without using formal timing, use the opportunity to watch patients rise from a seated position and walk to get a sense of their problems with transfers, balance, and gait.

Some experts advocate moving away from reliance on performance-based measures; for example, recent consensus conference guidelines for falls screening suggest that self-reported difficulty and/or unsteadiness with gait, rather than timed performance, is a key determinant of the need for subsequent fall risk assessment and intervention.[33]

Usual and Maximal Gait Speed

Usual gait speed performed from a standing start over a distance of 4 meters is a consistent risk factor for disability, cognitive impairment, institutionalization, falls, and mortality.[34] A recent pooled analysis of nine cohort studies of community-dwelling older adults found that usual gait speed predicted 5- and 10-year survival as accurately as a number of other important clinical variables such as age and chronic conditions. The likelihood of poor health and function increases at usual walking speed cutoffs of 0.8 or 1.0 m/s and particularly below 0.6 m/s; speeds above 1.0 m/s and perhaps 1.2 m/s are associated with better functional outcomes and increased life expectancy.[35] Note that fall risk may increase not just with slow gait but also with very rapid gait (>1.3 m/s), with slow walkers more likely to fall indoors and fast walkers more likely to fall outdoors.[36]

> If the gait pattern in an older adult seems abnormal, or at least slow, there are likely to be a number of contributors that can be determined from a history and physical assessment.

Changes in gait speed are increasingly used to evaluate intervention outcomes. Recent studies have estimated the extent to which a change in gait-related performance, such as gait speed, is clinically meaningful. For example, in cohorts that include mobility-impaired individuals, estimates range from 0.05 m/s to 0.10 m/s for small and substantial change respectively.[37] Using even a 0.10 m/s cutoff, however, may not coincide with perceived change in mobility in certain patient populations, such as patient's post–hip fracture.[38]

Timed Up and Go (TUG)

An indicator of functional mobility, the Timed Up and Go (TUG) test (also known as the Get Up and Go [GUG]) test, measures the time taken to stand up from a chair with armrests, walk 3 meters, turn, walk back to the chair, and sit down.[39] A cutoff score of 14 seconds or greater was originally proposed as predictive for falls.[40] However, a recent review suggests that in some studies, TUG may not predict falls, because of differences in study methodology, and the range of TUG cutoff times separating nonfallers and fallers can be wide, from 10.0 to 32.6 seconds.[41] Moreover, TUG may add little predictive value to relevant geriatric outcomes when gait speed is also measured.[42] A qualitative analysis (i.e., visual inspection by the clinician of aspects of the GUG), such as what might be done as part of a standard clinic visit, may be as predictive of falls as the timed test.[43]

Other Tests

The following are some other proposed mobility batteries that also include gait evaluation:
- The Performance-Oriented Mobility Assessment (POMA)—also known as the Tinetti Balance and Gait Scale. This is often used in clinical settings; however, in community-dwelling populations there is concern about ceiling effects and low sensitivity to change.[44] Moreover, although there may be a ceiling effect associated with the POMA, such as in moderately disabled Parkinson's patients, gait speed will continue to differentiate subtle changes in functional ability.[45]

- The Short Physical Performance Battery.[46] This is increasingly used in research but is not elaborated upon here because it includes tests of multiple rises from a chair and standing balance.
- The 6-minute walk test, a test of walking endurance, is the foundation of functional cardiopulmonary assessment,[47] whereas the 400-meter walk test has been increasingly used in research settings.[48]

Laboratory and Imaging Tests

Laboratory and radiologic testing may be warranted as part of the diagnosis and assessment of a gait or mobility issue, depending on the findings of the history and physical examination. Complete blood count, blood chemistries, and other metabolic studies may be useful when systemic disease is suspected.

If neurologic symptoms or signs were identified in the history and physical examination, head and spine radiographs, computed tomography, or magnetic resonance imaging (MRI) may be needed, and additional tests such as electromyography and nerve conduction studies considered. Ventricular enlargement, white matter hyperintensities, and subcortical and basal ganglia infarcts on MRI are associated with gait abnormalities.[49-51] Age-specific guidelines, sensitivity, specificity, and cost-effectiveness of these workups remain to be determined.

> Do not forget the brain and cognition as an important influence on walking.

MANAGEMENT

Treatable medical problems, such as medication side effects, B_{12} deficiency, folate deficiency, hypothyroidism, hyperthyroidism, knee osteoarthritis, Parkinson's disease, and inflammatory polyneuropathy, show improvement as a result of medical therapy.[11] However, many conditions predisposing the older adult to a gait disorder are only partially treatable, and the patient is often left with some degree of disability. In these patients, functional outcomes, such as reduction in weight-bearing pain, improvement in walking distance, or reductions in overall walking limitation, are the most relevant outcomes to seek (and evaluate) in treating patients with gait disorders.

Exercise and Gait Training

A variety of modes of physical therapy for diseases such as knee osteoarthritis and stroke result in modest improvement. Randomized controlled trials of exercise for osteoarthritis focus primarily on the knee, and may involve strengthening, walking, and aerobic training; these exercises all have shown positive impact on physical function, including walking (SOE = A).[52] The focus of exercise programs is on strengthening the extensor groups (especially knee and hip extensors) and stretching commonly shortened muscles such as the hip flexors.[53]

> Although the initial focus might be on physical therapy to reduce gait impairment, the practitioner must consider the contributions of other active comorbidities which, if treated, might also lead to gait improvement.

In Parkinson's disease, a range of physical therapy interventions, including treadmill training, are thought to improve gait in the short term (<3 months)[54] (Level B), but the results may not translate to improvements in daily function. For stroke patients, randomized controlled trials show small effects on gait speed from conventional overground physical therapy[55] and with electromechanical and robotic-assist devices[56] but little effect when using treadmill training or body support.[57]

Many investigators have also begun to test different exercise and cognitive-based interventions to improve dual task performance, including music-based multitask training.[28,58]

Participation in exercise groups can provide motivation for patients. A number of studies have demonstrated improvements in gait parameters such as gait speed, with the most consistent effects occurring when varied types of exercise are provided in the same program.[59-61] A 12-week combined program of leg resistance, standing balance, and flexibility exercises increased usual gait speed 8% in minimally impaired life care community residents.[59] A similar varied 16-week format with more intensive individual support and prompting in select older adults with dementia (mean MMSE 15) resulted in a 23% improvement in gait speed.[60]

Behavioral and Environmental Modifications

Improved lighting (particularly for those with vestibular or sensory impairment) and avoidance of pathway hazards (such as clutter, wires and slippery floors) are some behavioral and environmental modifications that can be used to make the environment safer for the older adult with a mobility disorder. Light touch of any firm surface like walls or furniture provides proprioceptive feedback that can often enhance balance.[62,63]

Shoes, Orthoses, and Assistive Devices

In general, to maximize balance and improve gait, well-fitting walking shoes with low heels, relatively thin firm soles, and if feasible, high, fixed heel collar support are recommended.[64] Assistive devices such as canes and walkers reduce load on a painful joint and improve stability.[65]

Use of orthoses and assistive devices may help ameliorate the effects of many gait disorders. Although there are few data supporting their use, lifts (either internal or external) to correct for limb length inequality may be helpful; they should be provided in a conservative, gradually progressive manner.[66] Ankle braces, shoe inserts, shoe body and sole modifications, and their subsequent adjustments are part of standard care for foot and ankle weakness, deformities, and pain.[67]

Surgical Management

The role of surgery in management of gait disorders is unclear. Improvement with some residual disability is commonly reported after surgical treatment for compressive cervical myelopathy, lumbar stenosis, and normal-pressure hydrocephalus (NPH). However, few controlled prospective studies and virtually no randomized studies address the outcome of surgical versus nonsurgical treatment for these disorders. Many of the concurrent cerebrovascular cardiovascular and musculoskeletal comorbidities (especially NPH) remain postoperatively and affect ultimate outcomes.

Outcomes for hip and knee replacement surgery for osteoarthritis are better although some of the same study methodology problems exist. In addition to pain relief, sizable gains in gait speed and joint motion can occur, although residual walking disability continues for a number of reasons, including residual pathology on the operated side and symptoms on the nonoperated side. For total knee replacements, despite rehabilitation postoperatively, some residual weakness, stiffness, and slowed/altered gait may remain.[68,69] Simple function may be maintained following a knee replacement, such as maintaining the ability to safely clear an obstacle, but usually at the expense of additional compensation by the ipsilateral hip and foot.[70] In terms of global functional measures not limited solely to walking, multidisciplinary rehabilitation post–knee replacement shows positive outcomes (SOE = B). One recent study found improvements in self-reported walking-related function (including Nagi items) in total hip replacement for osteoarthritis among Medicare beneficiaries,[71] but few other controlled studies exist. Based on a recent meta-analysis, the effect of therapy prior to elective knee or hip replacement for osteoarthritis is modest, and primarily improves pain and activity, rather than gait.[72]

CASE 1

Discussion

Your initial diagnoses are depression, delirium (possibly medication-induced), difficulty walking because of pain from hip osteoarthritis, and chronic headache, possibly associated with cervical spine arthritis. Your initial management is as follows: referral to the orthopedic surgeon for left hip arthroplasty; antidepressant medication; reassessment and removal of some pain medications (especially the codeine and the muscle relaxant). To reduce the likelihood of gastrointestinal side effects, you reserve antiinflammatory medications for exacerbations of neck symptoms, and prescribe around-the-clock acetaminophen for routine pain. Also, you document in your notes that, if these do not provide relief, you plan on referring her to a physical therapist specializing in manual therapy for further management of her neck/headache symptoms.

Your patient undergoes a left hip arthroplasty and, after discharge from the acute care hospital, 12 days of inpatient rehabilitation. She is educated in the precautions necessary to avoid hip dislocation, and engages in ambulation as tolerated with a walker, isometric and range-of-motion exercises, and transfer training. After discharge from inpatient rehabilitation, she receives 6 weeks of outpatient physical therapy for gait and lower extremity training.

She progresses satisfactorily in outpatient physical therapy, showing significant improvements in lower extremity strength, range of motion, and ambulation on level ground and up and down stairs. Her pain level has decreased significantly, but she elects to continue ambulation with the quad cane for safety. At the surgeon's instructions, she adheres to the hip dislocation precautions for at least 12 weeks. Six weeks postsurgery she sees you for follow-up. At that visit she displays no confusion and reports minimal headache/neck pain. She reports no loss of balance since the fall nearly 6 months ago. ■

SUMMARY

Problems with gait, and slowed gait in particular, are common in older adults and are a predictor of functional decline and death. The cause of the gait impairment in older adults is usually multifactorial; therefore, a full assessment must include consideration of a number of different causes, as determined from a detailed history and physical examination. A number of interventions, ranging from medical to surgical to exercise, can reduce the degree of impairment, although some residual impairment is often present.

KEY REFERENCES

23. Nutt JG, Horak FB, Bloem BR. Milestones in gait, balance and falling. Movement Disord 2011;26:1166-74.
28. Montero-Odasso M, Verghese J, Beauchet O, Hausdorff JM. Gait and cognition: A complementary approach to understanding brain function and the risk of falling. J Am Geriatr Soc 2012;60(11):2127-36.
35. Studenski SA, Perera S, Patel K, et al. Gait speed and survival in older adults. JAMA 2011;305:50-8.
37. Perera S, Mody SH, Woodman RC, Studenski SA. Meaningful change and responsiveness in common physical performance measures in older adults. J Am Geriatr Soc 2006;54:743-9.
41. Beauchet O, Fantino B, Allali G, et al. Timed up and go test and risk of falls in older adults: A systematic review. J Nutr Health Aging 2011;15:933-8.

References available online at expertconsult.com.

20

Falls

Laurence Z. Rubenstein and Della Dillard

OBJECTIVES

Upon completion of this chapter, the reader will be able to:

• Describe the incidence of falls among older adults.

• List the major risk factors for falls.

• Assess an older adult who has fallen.

• Identify effective evidence-based fall prevention interventions.

• Describe the American Geriatrics Society's clinical practice guideline for fall prevention.

• Develop an individualized plan for preventing future falls.

CASE 1

Opal Smith (Part 1)

Opal Smith, an 80-year-old woman, comes to your office as a new patient. She has hypertension, type 2 diabetes (diet-controlled), osteoarthritis, and mild hearing loss. Mrs. Smith's main reported symptoms are bilateral mild

knee pain and some sense of unsteadiness on walking. She denies dizziness, postural symptoms, or falls in the past year. She takes lisinopril 10 mg daily, a multivitamin, calcium with vitamin D, acetaminophen as needed for pain, and diphenhydramine as needed for occasional insomnia. She has lived alone since her husband died 3 years ago. She still drives and has several friends with whom she visits. One of her friends suffered a fall several months ago and fractured a hip, from which she is still recovering. Mrs. Smith is somewhat worried about her own unsteadiness and risk for falls.

On exam, her blood pressure is 136/78 mmHg, pulse 72, weight 150 lbs (68 kg), and height 5 ft 5 in. She is mildly hard of hearing but communicates well. She has some mild crepitus on motion of her knees; her gait is slowed with short steps and is somewhat wide based. The rest of her examination is unremarkable, as are all routine laboratory tests. At the end of her examination, Mrs. Smith asks you for fall prevention recommendations.

1. **What are Mrs. Smith's major risk factors for falls?**

2. **What would you recommend to minimize her risk?** ▣

PREVALENCE AND IMPACT

Falls rank high among serious clinical problems facing older adults. They cause substantial morbidity and mortality and contribute to immobility and premature nursing home placement. Unintentional injuries are a leading cause of death in older adults, and falls comprise two thirds of these deaths. In the United States, about three fourths of deaths resulting from falls occur in the 13% of the population that is aged 65 years and older, making injurious falls a true geriatric syndrome. At least a third of older persons living at home will fall at least once in a year, and about 1 in 40 will be hospitalized. Of those hospitalized after a fall, nearly half will die within a year. Repeated falls and instability are common precipitators of nursing home admission. Within long-term care institutions, fall rates are even higher, averaging almost two falls per patient year. Moreover, falls in institutions more commonly have serious complications—10% to 25% are associated with a fracture or laceration.[1]

The way a person falls often determines the type of injury sustained. Wrist fractures usually result from falls onto an outstretched hand; hip fractures typically result from falls to the side; and backward falls onto the buttocks have a much lower fracture rate.[2] Wrist fractures are more common than hip fractures in people between ages 65 and 75, whereas hip fractures predominate after age 75, probably because of slowed reflexes and loss of ability to protect the hip by "breaking the fall" with one's hands after age 75.

Remember when treating an elderly patient for a fall-related hip fracture to obtain a thorough history. The patient may have been pushed by his or her spouse with dementia as they argued over car keys, for example. The family may have to treat both parents or institutionalize one to protect them both.

The problem of falls in older persons clearly involves more than simply their high incidence, because young children and athletes fall more frequently than all but the frailest elderly groups. Rather it is a combination of a high incidence together with a high susceptibility to injury, resulting from a high prevalence of clinical diseases (e.g., osteoporosis) and age-related physiologic changes (e.g., slowed protective reflexes) that make even a relatively mild fall particularly dangerous in an older person. In addition, recovery from fall injury is often delayed in older persons, further increasing risk for subsequent falls through deconditioning. Another complication is the postfall anxiety syndrome, in which an individual downregulates activity in a perhaps overcautious fear of falling; this in turn further contributes to deconditioning, weakness, abnormal gait, and in the long run can further increase risk of falls.

The fear of falling not only socially isolates the patient; it may also overwhelm the family with increased responsibility physically, economically and emotionally. Family members may have to make major life transitions to care for an elderly parent. Encourage caregivers to seek support groups and respite as needed.

According to the U.S. Centers for Disease Control and Prevention, one in three adults aged 65 and older falls each year. Of these, 20% to 30% suffer moderate to severe injuries that reduce their functional capacity and increase their mortality risk, and 662,000 are hospitalized annually. The costs of falls are immense: in 2001 Medicare costs per fall averaged between $9,113 and $13,507, and by 2020 the annual direct and indirect cost of fall injuries is expected to reach $54.9 billion (in 2007 dollars).[3] The U.S. Public Health Service has estimated that two thirds of deaths resulting from falls are potentially preventable, based on a retrospective analysis of causes and circumstances of serious falls. Identifying and eliminating environmental risks in homes or institutions could prevent many falls caused primarily by environmental factors, and adequate medical evaluation and treatment for underlying medical risk factors, such as unstable gait and disabling medical conditions, could prevent many medically related falls.

Identifying and eliminating environmental risks in homes or institutions could prevent many falls caused by environmental factors.

PRECIPITATING CAUSES AND RISK FACTORS FOR FALLS

There are many precipitating causes of falls in older persons, as shown in Table 20-1, which summarizes data from 12 of the largest retrospective studies. Drawing conclusions across studies is limited by several factors, including differences in classification methods, patient recall, and the multifactorial nature of most falls. Although accidents or environmental hazards are the most frequently cited causes of falls, this is misleading because most falls attributed to accidents really stem from an interaction between environmental hazards and increased individual susceptibility to hazards from accumulated effects of age and disease. Older people tend to have less coordinated gaits than do younger people. Posture control, body-orienting reflexes, muscle strength and tone, and step height all decline with aging and impair ability to avoid a fall after an unexpected trip or slip. Age-associated changes such as impairment of vision, hearing, and memory also tend to increase the number of trips and stumbles. Because most elderly individuals have multiple identifiable risk factors predisposing to falls, the exact cause can often be difficult to determine.

In addition to looking retrospectively for causes, investigators have sought to identify specific risk factors that place individuals at increased likelihood of falling. In many ways, knowing about risk factors that can be identified before a fall is much more useful than identifying precipitating causes retrospectively, because prefall identification can allow preventive strategies to be devised and instituted. Table 20-1 also lists the major fall risk factors, displaying their relative importance in terms of mean odds ratio or relative risk, pooled from a large number of such studies.[1] The most important of these risk factors are muscle weakness, fall history, problems with gait and balance, visual deficits, arthritis, functional impairment, depression, and cognitive impairments. It should be noted that some of these risk factors are directly involved in causing falls (e.g., weakness, gait and balance disorders), whereas others are markers of other underlying causes (e.g., prior falls, assistive device, age >80). More recent analyses have confirmed these risk factors as well as the additional importance of taking psychoactive medications and polypharmacy, which are associated with odds ratios of between 1.5 and 1.8.[4] Figure 20-1 provides a visual schematic of the complex relationship among and between selected risk factors, precipitating causes, and falls. Such multifactorial causality is typical of geriatric syndromes generally, which explains why

TABLE 20-1	Factors Associated with Falls in Elderly Adults			
	Causes Identified in Retrospective Studies*		Risk Factors Identified in Prospective Studies**	
Cause	Mean%[†]	Range[‡]	Mean RR-OR[‡]	Range
Accident-/environment-related	31%	1-53%		
Gait/balance disorder or weakness	17%	4-39%		
Balance disorder			2.9	1.6-5.4
Weakness			4.4	1.5-10.2
Gait deficit			2.9	1.3-5.6
Uses assistive device for walking			2.6	1.2-4.6
Dizziness/vertigo	13%	0-30%		
Drop attack	9%	0-52%		
Confusion/cognitive impairment	5%	0-14%	1.8	1.0-2.3
Postural hypotension	3%	0-24%		
Visual disorder	2%	0-5%	2.5	1.6-3.5
Syncope	0.3%	0-3%		
Other specified causes[§]	15%	2-39%		
Arthritis				1.9-2.9
Depression			2.2	1.7-2.3
ADL deficit			2.3	1.6-3.5
Prior fall			3.0	1.7-7.0
Age >80			1.7	1.1-2.5
Psychoactive medication use***			1.7	1.6-1.9
Polypharmacy			1.7	1.5-2.0

*Summary of 12 studies that carefully evaluated elderly persons after a fall and specified a "most likely" cause. Adapted from Rubenstein LZ, Josephson KR. The epidemiology of falls and syncope. Clin Geriatr Med 2002;18:141-58.

**Summary of 16 controlled studies. Adapted from Rubenstein LZ, Josephson KR. The epidemiology of falls and syncope. Clin Geriatr Med 2002;18:141-58.

***Data from Bloch F, Thibaud M, Tournoux-Facon C, et al. Estimation of the risk factors for falls in the elderly: Can meta-analysis provide a valid answer? Geriatr Gerontol Int 2013;13(2)250-63.

§This category includes arthritis, acute illness, drugs, alcohol, pain, epilepsy, and falling from bed.

†Mean percent calculated from the 3628 reported falls.

‡Ranges indicate the percentages reported in each of the 12 studies.

ADL, Activities of daily living; *OR,* odds ratio (calculated from retrospective studies); *RR,* relative risk ratio (calculated from prospective studies).

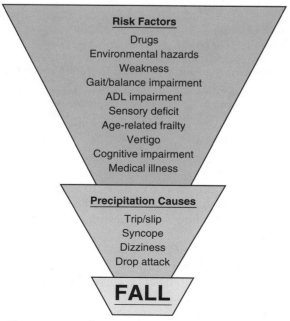

Risk Factors

Drugs
Environmental hazards
Weakness
Gait/balance impairment
ADL impairment
Sensory deficit
Age-related frailty
Vertigo
Cognitive impairment
Medical illness

Precipitation Causes

Trip/slip
Syncope
Dizziness
Drop attack

FALL

Figure 20-1 The multifactorial etiologies of falls.

fall prevention necessitates a systematic, multidimensional evaluation.

Leg weakness, one of the most important risk factors, is an extremely common finding among the aged population. Weakness often arises from deconditioning resulting from limited physical activity or prolonged bed rest, together with chronic debilitating medical conditions such as heart failure, stroke, or pulmonary disease, plus some age-related loss of muscle units. As a whole, healthy older people score 20% to 40% lower on strength tests than young adults,[5] and the reported prevalence of leg weakness was 57% among residents of an assisted living facility,[6] and more than 80% in a skilled nursing facility.[7] Gait and balance disorders are also extremely common among older adults, affecting between 20% and 50% of people older than age 65 years,[8] and are associated with a threefold increase in fall risk.[4] A simple screening test of gait and balance function, such as the Timed Up and Go or Tinetti's gait and balance test, is often useful in identifying risk and documenting need for treatment.[6]

A history of falls is also an important risk factor. Individuals who have already fallen have 3 times the risk of falling than that of persons who did not fall in the past year. Recurrent falls are frequently a result of the same underlying cause (e.g., gait disorder or orthostatic hypotension), but they can also be an indication of disease progression (e.g., parkinsonism, dementia) or a new acute problem (e.g., infection, dehydration).

Possibly even more important than identifying risk factors for falling per se is identifying risk factors for injurious falls, because most falls do not result in injury. Risk factors associated with injurious falls are the same as for falls in general, with the addition of female sex and low body mass, which are both related to osteoporosis.[2]

Most of the factors listed in Table 20-1 are amenable to improvement, suggesting ways that many falls can be prevented; moreover, the effectiveness of preventive strategies has been documented in a number of studies.

CASE 1

Opal Smith (Part 2)

Two years later, Mrs. Smith developed shortness of breath with fever. She was taken to the emergency department where radiography showed pneumonia with a loculated pleural effusion. After admission, she underwent chest tube placement to drain the empyema, and she was started on regular morphine for pain control to treat the discomfort associated with the chest tube. Two days after admission, Mrs. Smith requested a sleeping pill to overcome her insomnia, and she was treated with a benzodiazepine. Later that night, she got up from her bed alone to go to the bathroom and fell to the floor. Fortunately, no injuries were reported from her fall.

1. **What postfall assessment should be done?**

2. **What might the hospital have done differently to prevent this fall?** ▣

ASSESSMENT

Assessing the Patient Who Has Fallen

> Ask patients about near falls, slips, or catches. (Patients are more likely to admit to these incidents.) These may be early warning signs to help you implement appropriate adaptations to prevent or lessen severity of future falls.

When confronted with a patient after a fall, the physician's first job is to assess the acute situation. This process is summarized in Box 20-1. Once assured that the fall patient is out of immediate danger, it is crucial to obtain a full report of the circumstances and symptoms surrounding the fall. Reports from witnesses are important because the patient may have poor recollection of

---

BOX 20-1

POSTFALL ASSESSMENT

Immediate
- Call for help
- Basic life support: Danger, Responsiveness, Airway, Breathing, CPR, Defibrillate if indicated (DR ABCD)

Rapid Assessment
- Pain: grimacing, bracing, restlessness
- Bleeding: skin bruising, edema
- Injury: deformity of leg, inability to move
- Immobilize cervical spine if suspect any head injury before moving

Secondary Assessment
- Vital signs (VS): blood pressure (sitting and standing), pulse, respirations, pulse oximetry, temperature, pain scale
- Check blood glucose
- Neurologic checks (hourly × 4, then q4h × 24h)

History
- Can patient communicate effectively? Obtain patient's description of fall events
- Obtain witnesses' reports of events
- Description of area where patient was found after fall
- Was patient using/not using assistive device or help of another person on falling?
- Any medication or over-the-counter meds used in past 24 hours or recent illnesses
- Is the patient on anticoagulant, NSAID, aspirin, antiplatelet therapy, or known coagulopathy*
- Any acute change in behaviors, increasing confusion, lethargy, vomiting, or headache*

Notification/Verification
- Notify health care proxy if patient desires or does not have decision-making capacity
- Does the patient have an advance directive?
- Yes—Determine appropriate action consistent with expressed wishes
- No—To emergency room, clinic or observe per provider recommendation

Documentation
- Complete fall report
- Review incident with clinical leadership
- Implement changes as indicated for future prevention

Adapted from Clinical Excellence Commission. http://www.cec.health.nsw.gov.au/__documents/programs/falls-prevention/draft_revised_post_fall_algorithm_21_oct_2011.pdf.
*Computed tomography scan recommended.
NSAID, Nonsteroidal antiinflammatory drug.

---

the event. Fall circumstances that can suggest a specific etiology or help to narrow down the differential diagnosis include the following (suggested cause is noted in parentheses):

- Sudden rise from a lying or sitting position (orthostatic hypotension)
- Trip or slip (gait, balance, or vision disturbance or an environmental hazard)
- Antecedent cough or urination (reflex hypotension)

- A recent meal (postprandial hypotension)
- Drop attack (vertebrobasilar insufficiency or weakness)
- Looking up or sideways (arterial or carotid sinus compression)
- Loss of consciousness (syncope or seizure)

Symptoms, including the following, experienced near the time of falling may also point to a potential cause:

- Dizziness or giddiness (orthostatic hypotension, vestibular problem, hypoglycemia, arrhythmia, drug side effect)
- Palpitations (arrhythmia)
- Incontinence or tongue biting (seizure)
- Asymmetric weakness (cerebrovascular disease)
- Chest pain (myocardial infarction or coronary insufficiency)
- Loss of consciousness (any cause of syncope)

Medications, especially those with hypotensive or psychoactive effects, and existence of concomitant medical problems may be important contributing factors.

Elements of a Focused Fall-Related Physical Examination

On the postfall physical examination, it is especially pertinent to look for particular findings that may have directly contributed to the fall, as well as to note other fall risk factors. Important to look for are the following: orthostatic changes in pulse and blood pressure, visual acuity, presence of arrhythmias, carotid bruits, nystagmus, focal neurologic signs, manual muscle testing of the lower extremities, gait disturbances, and neurologic function. A quantitative mental screening evaluation, such as the Mini-Mental State Examination, is important to rule out cognitive impairment. It is often useful to attempt to reproduce (under careful monitoring) the circumstances that might have precipitated the fall (e.g., positional changes, head turning, or carotid pressure). Gait and stability should be assessed by close observation of how the patient rises from a chair (which is also a test of lower extremity strength), stands with eyes open and closed, walks, turns, and sits down. One should take particular note of gait velocity and rhythm, stride length, double support time (the time spent with both feet on the floor), height of stepping, use of assistive devices, and degree of trunk sway. Simple scored screening scales for detecting and quantifying gait and balance problems have been developed. Useful examples include the Performance Oriented Mobility Assessment[6] and the Timed Up and Go test,[9] both of which have been well validated for quantifying gait and balance impairment and assisting with diagnosis. The quantitative nature of these scales is useful for gauging severity of the problem and following progress over time. More detailed gait evaluation (see Chapter 19) can be useful among persons who fail the screen.

Assessing a Person for Future Fall Risk

The clinical practice guidelines on fall prevention and treatment of the American and British Geriatrics Societies recommend that a fall-risk assessment should be an integral part of primary health care for older persons, and that the intensity of the assessment should vary with the target population:[10]

- Low-risk community-dwelling older persons should be asked at least once a year about fall occurrence and circumstances.
- Older persons who report a single fall should be evaluated for mobility impairment and unsteadiness using a simple observational test, with those who demonstrate mobility problems or unsteadiness being referred for further assessment.
- High-risk populations (e.g., older persons who report multiple falls in the past year, have abnormalities of gait and/or balance, seek medical attention because of a fall, or reside in a nursing home) should undergo a more comprehensive and detailed assessment.

Figure 20-2 summarizes these recommendations.

The goals of the fall evaluation are twofold: (1) to diagnose and treat patients after a fall and (2) to identify risk factors for future falls and implement appropriate interventions. Most risk factors can be easily assessed in the physician's office using basic examination techniques or principles of comprehensive geriatric assessment; namely, a multidimensional assessment to quantify medical, psychosocial, and functional capabilities and problems in order to develop a comprehensive plan for therapy.

The core of the fall-risk assessment should be a directed history and physical examination aimed at uncovering any immediate precipitating cause as well as associated risk factors, as was discussed earlier in this section of the chapter.

In addition to identifying gait and balance deviations and other risk factors, it is important to assess functional mobility and physical activity. By determining the type of activities that a patient actually engages in, the clinician can make a more accurate appraisal of fall risk. Studies have suggested that patients with fall risk factors who are physically active are at somewhat greater risk of falling than similar patients who are more careful in restricting their activity.

CASE 1

Discussion

After a 10-day hospital stay Mrs. Smith was discharged home with physical and occupational therapy home visits, and her daughter agreed to stay with her until she recovered more fully. Two weeks after discharge she arrives at your office in a wheelchair along with her daughter for a follow-up visit. Her daughter reports that she had been

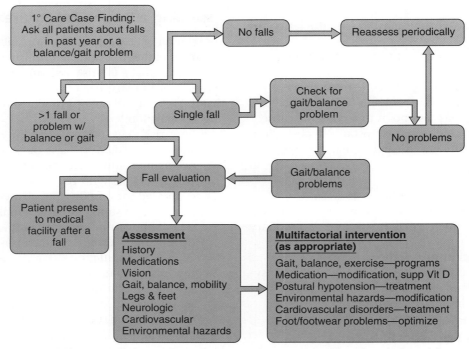

Figure 20-2   The American Geriatrics Society's fall assessment and prevention algorithm. (Adapted from Kenny RA, Rubenstein LZ, Tinetti ME, et al. AGS/BGS clinical practice guideline: Prevention of falls in older persons. J Am Geriatr Soc 2011;59:148-57.

improving during the immediate posthospital period. However, yesterday, while getting out of the bathtub, her legs caught in the edge of the bath mat, and she fell. She has no obvious bruises, no head trauma, and no loss of consciousness, but she is experiencing pain directly over her left hip and is unable to walk without assistance.

Mrs. Smith has now had two falls within a several-week period. This most recent fall is concerning for hip fracture, given her inability to walk. On examination, her legs are approximately of equal length and not rotated asymmetrically, there is no groin pain on hip flexion, and there is a 5-cm bruise visible over the left lateral hip. You send Mrs. Smith for an imaging study and it shows no evidence of a fracture. You prescribe pain medication, and in the next few days her ambulation improves.

> **Besides removing the bath mat and making sure the home physical therapy and occupational therapy recommendations (e.g., grab bars) are implemented, what else might you do for Mrs. Smith given that you have already completed a multifactorial fall assessment?** ◘

MANAGEMENT AND PREVENTION

Management of the Acute Faller

Once the cause(s) and/or risk factor(s) of falling are determined, specific therapy can be instituted.[11] For example, cardiac dysrhythmias clearly related to a fall should be treated with antiarrhythmic agents, a pacemaker, or both. Hypovolemia resulting from

hemorrhage or dehydration calls for treatment directed toward restoring hemodynamic stability. Parkinsonism usually responds to specific therapy; however, in advanced cases safe ambulation can require extensive assistance. Stopping drugs that cause postural hypotension, dizziness, confusion, or undue sedation is important whenever possible. For patients with gait and balance disturbances, specific assistive devices (e.g., walkers, canes, shoe modifications) are often helpful, as is a program of gait training under supervision of a rehabilitation therapist, individualized to deal with the underlying cause(s) (e.g., weakness, imbalance, arthritis).

> Recurrent falls are frequently a result of the same underlying cause but they can also be an indication of disease progression (e.g., parkinsonism, dementia, heart failure) or a new acute problem (e.g., infection, dehydration).

Several techniques may benefit patients with persistent orthostatic hypotension caused by autonomic dysfunction. These include sleeping in a bed with the head raised to minimize sudden drop in blood pressure on rising, wearing elastic stockings to minimize venous pooling in the legs, rising slowly or sitting on the side of the bed for several minutes before standing, and avoiding heavy meals and vigorous activity in hot weather. If conservative mechanical measures are ineffective, blood volume can be increased by liberalizing dietary salt. If this is ineffective, mineralocorticoid therapy (fludrocortisone increasing gradually from 0.1 mg per day) or an alpha-1 agonist such as midodrine (beginning at 2.5 mg three times a day) can help to maintain blood pressure, as long as associated medical conditions do not preclude these agents and that due care is taken to avoid side effects such as supine hypertension and fluid accumulation.

More difficult is managing and preventing recurrent falls among patients for whom a specific cause cannot be identified or who have multiple or irreversible causes. A careful search for and correction of other risk factors that predispose to falling (such as visual and hearing deficits) is essential. For disabilities that do not properly resolve with treatment of underlying medical disorders, a trial of short-term rehabilitation may improve safety and diminish long-term disability. Referral to physical therapy for gait training or an exercise regimen can often be very helpful in reducing risk factors and improving mobility. When irreversible problems exist, residual limitations should be explained and coping methods developed (e.g., slow rising from bed or use of assistive devices).

Physicians should advise patients to eliminate home hazards such as loose or frayed rugs, trailing electrical cords, and unstable furniture. Patients and their families should be educated on the importance of specific environmental improvements; adequate lighting, bathroom grab rails and raised toilet seat, secure stairway banisters, raised or lowered bed height, and an easily accessible alarm system are possibilities. A visiting nurse or other experienced person can perform a home evaluation to suggest modifications. Self-administered checklists to aid in this process are also available for use directly by the patient or caregiver.

Prevention of Future Falls

Fall prevention has been an area of active research since the mid-1980s. A number of programs (e.g., assessment, risk factor reduction, exercise, environmental modification, education) have been tested, and meta-analyses have documented the effectiveness of several approaches.[11-13] Effective approaches (Table 20-2) include multidimensional risk factor assessment tied to targeted interventions, exercise programs (including balance, strength, and endurance training), and environmental assessment and modification. Programs combining all of these approaches seem to have had the strongest effects. Clinical practice guidelines from the American Geriatrics Society and British Geriatrics Society (AGS/BGS) panel and other organizations have strongly advocated preventive approaches using these three components.[10] (See Figure 20-2 for a summary of these guidelines.)

Postfall assessments, as outlined above, can reveal many otherwise undetected treatable conditions and risk factors and can significantly prevent falls and reduce hospitalizations.[10,11,14,15] Exercise programs can clearly improve strength, endurance, and body mechanics, and several controlled trials have shown significant reduction in falls.[1,2,10-12,16] Table 20-2 summarizes effectiveness data from the 2012 iteration of the Cochrane Collaboration meta-analysis of community-based fall prevention interventions. In addition to the studies summarized in the Cochrane paper, there have been a number of other approaches to fall and injury prevention studied in single trials that were not combinable in the meta-analysis presented in the table. Several European trials of hip protector garments, conducted mainly in nursing home settings, have reported dramatic reductions in hip fractures.[17-19a] However, compliance has been an issue, especially in community settings, and some marketed hip protectors have been shown to have design flaws, necessitating caution in their recommendation.[20] Several studies indicate small but significant benefits from vitamin D on balance and fall reduction.[21] One study has shown the effectiveness of cataract surgery in reducing fall rates among patients with bilateral cataracts significantly impairing vision.[22] Another study showed that substituting single vision glasses for bifocals when outside has a small but significant effect on reducing falls.[23] A small study from an icy climate showed significant fall reduction through use of anti-skid shoe treads.[24] A large-scale public health fall-prevention trial in Connecticut showed significant reductions in fall-related injuries and use of fall-related medical services over a 5-year period in areas receiving a multicomponent senior and provider education program.[25]

TABLE 20-2	Preventive Interventions to Reduce Falls Risk*	
Preventive Intervention (N=number of studies in analysis)	**Fall Rate vs. Control (mean & 95% CI)****
Multifactorial fall-risk assessment and management program (N=19)	.76 [.68 - .86]
Multi-component exercise program (N=16)	.71 [.63 - .82]
Group tai chi program (N=6)	.72 [.52 - 1.0]
Group gait/balance training (N=3)	.73 [.54 - .98]
Individualized home exercise program (N=7)	.68 [.58 - .80]
Home safety intervention programs (N=6)	.81 [.68 - .96]

*Data from meta-analysis of intervention trials.
**Data from Gillespie et al, 2012.
CI, Confidence interval.

SUMMARY

Falls are common and often devastating to the elderly population, and systematic attention to fall prevention is a vital part of comprehensive care of the older adult. A number of important risk factors (e.g., weakness, gait/balance impairment, functional and cognitive deficits, psychotropic medications, and polypharmacy) will identify persons who are most likely to fall and therefore who most need prevention interventions. Substantial research has confirmed the clear effectiveness of fall-prevention measures, including fall-risk assessments tied to interventions, exercise programs, environmental inspection and modification, and combined interventions. The future looks bright in this area, as in so many areas of geriatrics.

Web Resources

http://www.adsa.dshs.wa.gov/pubinfo/falls/. Aging & Disability Services Administration, Clinical Excellence Commission. Provides resources for community fall prevention.

http://americangeriatrics.org/health_care_professionals/clinical_practice/clinical_guidelines_recommendations/2010. American Geriatrics Society. Contains updated clinical practice guidelines for fall prevention, based on work of an international interdisciplinary expert panel.

http://familydoctor.org. American Association of Family Physicians. A good resource for patient education for preventing falls, including a video on how to prevent falls.

http://www.cdc.gov/HomeandRecreationalSafety/Falls/index.html. Centers for Disease Control and Prevention. Provides current statistics on adult falls (e.g., nonlethal, bathroom falls, falls related to pets, etc.).

www.stopfalls.org/index.shtml. Fall Prevention Center of Excellence. Site contains a multitude of resources focused on senior fall prevention.

http://nihseniorhealth.gov/falls/toc.html. National Institute on Aging. Information on senior health and falls.

www.patientsafety.gov/SafetyTopics/fallstoolkit/notebook/05_fallspolicy.pdf. Veterans Affairs National Center for Patient Safety. Fall prevention advice and guidelines for hospitals and nursing facilities.

KEY REFERENCES

4. Bloch F, Thibaud M, Tournoux-Facon C, et al. Estimation of the risk factors for falls in the elderly: Can meta-analysis provide a valid answer? Geriatr Gerontol Int. 2012 Nov 27. doi: 10.1111/j.1447-0594.2012.00965.x., PMID 23185998.

10. Kenny RA, Rubenstein LZ, Tinetti ME, et al. AGS/BGS Clinical Practice Guideline: Prevention of Falls in Older Persons. J Am Geriatr Soc 59(1):148-57, 2011.

12. Gillespie LD, Robertson MC, Gillespie WJ, et al. Interventions for preventing falls in older people living in the community. Cochrane Database Syst Rev 2012 Sep 12;9:CD007146. doi: 10.1002/14651858.CD007146.pub3.

21. Cameron ID, Gillespie LD, Robertson MC, et al. Interventions for preventing falls in older people in care facilities and hospitals. Cochrane Database Syst Rev. 2012 Dec 12;12:CD005465. doi: 10.1002/14651858.CD005465.pub3.

25. Tinetti ME, Baker DJ, King M, et al. Effect of dissemination of evidence in reducing injuries from falls. N Eng J Med 2008; 359:252-61.

References available online at expertconsult.com.

21

Dizziness

Nadia Mujahid and Aman Nanda

CASE 1

Thelma Franklin (Part 1)

Thelma Franklin, age 82 years, complains of dizziness on and off for the last 4 to 5 months. She also gives a history of falling three times in the last 6 months while walking in the house. The falls were witnessed by her daughter who lives with her. The falls did not result in any head trauma or other serious injury and she denies any associated nausea or vomiting. The daughter reports some memory decline in her mother for the past 8 to 10 months. Medical history is notable for bilateral cataracts, coronary artery disease, hypertension, chronic backache, and diabetes mellitus. Ms. Franklin has been using a cane for the past 6 months. Medications include metformin 500 mg twice a day, a baby aspirin, metoprolol 12.5 mg twice a day, nifedipine extended release 60 mg once daily, ranitidine 150 mg twice a day, acetaminophen as needed, and a multivitamin.

1. **What anatomic structures may give rise to the type of dizziness reported by Ms. Franklin?**

2. **What are the risk factors in Ms. Franklin's medical history that can contribute to her dizziness?**

3. **What questions should you ask to identify the type of dizziness?**

4. **What is your differential diagnosis based on the clinical history thus far?** ▣

PREVALENCE AND IMPACT

Dizziness is one of the most common presenting complaints in older adults. Like other classic geriatric syndromes, dizziness is both a diagnostic and a management challenge. The complaint of "dizziness" is subjective, cannot be measured, and can be produced by several different mechanisms. In older adults multiple contributing factors are often involved.

Dizziness is reported more commonly by women than men; the overall prevalence ranges from 4% to 30%.[1-3] The likelihood of reporting dizziness increases by 10% for every 5 years of increasing age. Dizziness is associated with increased fear and increased risk of falling, orthostatic hypotension, syncope, strokes,

---

Additional online-only material indicated by icon.

worsening of depressive symptoms, disability, and of more unfavorable self-rated health.[4] In one study, after 2 years of follow-up, dizzy older persons were more likely to become disabled than those who were not. Another study showed that elderly people with dizziness had a higher prevalence of significant disability requiring assistance.[5]

Chronic dizziness has a negative effect on quality of life among older persons, and it has been associated with increased risk for falls, orthostatic hypotension, syncope, stroke, and disability.[6]

RISK FACTORS AND PATHOPHYSIOLOGY

Dizziness refers to a variety of abnormal or disturbing sensations related to the body's position, movement, or stability. Multiple body systems are normally involved in the maintenance of postural stability; disturbance of any of them can lead to dizziness. These postural control systems (Figure 21-1) include the cerebral cortex, brainstem, cerebellum, eyes and visual pathways, labyrinth and the vestibular pathways, and the proprioceptive fibers in peripheral joints and their associated pathways.

Because so many different body systems can give rise to dizziness, it is not surprising that the differential diagnosis is immense and that more than one body system is often involved. However, it can be narrowed by systematic history taking as described in the next sections.

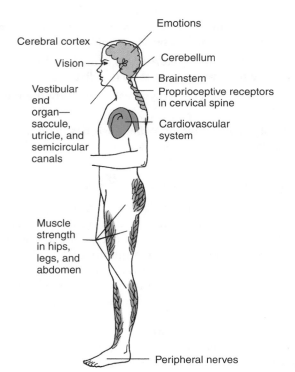

Figure 21-1   Components of the balance system.

It is important to keep in mind the most common conditions, and look for treatable causes (Table 21-1) and screen for potentially life-threatening conditions.

CHRONIC DIZZINESS AS A GERIATRIC SYNDROME

> Chronic dizziness is best considered as a geriatric syndrome, that is, a combination of symptoms and signs that often reflects impairment or disease in multiple systems.

In the past, clinicians assumed that dizziness arose from one or two specific diseases. However, chronic dizziness in the elderly arises from multiple conditions. In fact, dizziness will be present in 51% of persons who have four or more of the following common problems: depressive symptoms, cataracts, abnormal gait, postural hypotension, diabetes, past myocardial infarction, and use of three or more medications.[7,8]

CASE 2

Catherine Arnold (Part 1)

Catherine Arnold, an 84-year-old woman, presents to your office with several episodes of severe dizziness during the last 3 to 4 days. She reports that when she woke up one morning everything began to spin around her. She was nauseated and was unable to stand because of the dizziness. The symptoms subsided after 10 to 15 seconds. She reports feeling light-headed when she got up and had to sit on the bed for a while until symptoms subsided. She had another episode yesterday while cooking. When she felt that the room was spinning, she sat on a chair and symptoms subsided, but she still felt a little light-headed. She reports similar episodes when she turns her head or changes her position suddenly. Ms. Arnold had the same kind of experience 3 years ago lasting for a week. She denies head trauma, severe exertion, coughing, sneezing, loud noises, flulike symptoms, new medications, twisting or turning activities, or emotional stress.

1. **What other questions would you ask Ms. Arnold?**

2. **What is the likely diagnosis?**

3. **What will you do next?** ▣

DIFFERENTIAL DIAGNOSIS AND ASSESSMENT

Clinical History

Diagnosis of the cause of dizziness is often difficult at first. Some diseases require observation of a pattern

TABLE 21-1	Key Points in Taking a Dizziness History

1. Try to Classify the Dizziness Sensation

Sensation	Description	Mechanism
Vertigo	Spinning, sense of rotation	Impairment of vestibular system
Presyncopal light-headedness	Feeling one is about to pass out	Cerebral ischemia
Imbalance (disequilibrium)	Loss of balance	Multiple mechanisms; abnormal proprioception, cerebellar, motor or vestibulospinal function
		Anxiety, depression, or other psychosomatic disorders

Caution: About half of dizziness in older persons cannot be clearly assigned to one type. (Many have imbalance plus some other sensation.)

2. Determine If the Dizziness Is Episodic or Continuous

Temporal Nature	Common Causes
Episodic	Recurrent vestibulopathy, BPPV, TIA, Meniere's disease
Continuous	Medications, psychological

3. Ask What Other Symptoms Accompany the Dizziness

Symptom	Possible Diagnosis
Ear fullness	Meniere's disease, otitis media
Unilateral hearing loss	Labyrinthitis, Meniere's disease, acoustic neuroma
Weakness or diplopia, dysarthria	Vertebrobasilar insufficiency, TIA
Stiff, sore neck	Cervical osteoarthritis
Tinnitus	Meniere's disease, acoustic neuroma

4. Search for Factors that Bring on or Worsen the Dizziness

Factor	Suggested Cause
Nervousness, worry, or emotional stress	Psychological dizziness
Looking up (e.g., to a high shelf)	Cervical osteoarthritis
Rolling over in bed, bending over	BPPV, vestibulopathy
After meals	Postprandial hypotension
Standing from supine position	Postural hypotension, postural dizziness

BPPV, Benign paroxysmal positional vertigo; *TIA*, transient ischemic attack.

over time to make the diagnosis. Nevertheless, the initial evaluation should create a differential diagnosis from which a plan for further evaluation, treatment, or observation can be developed.[9]

Often, especially in chronic dizziness, the goal of assessment should be to identify factors that can be modified, some of which may not be the most immediate cause of dizziness. Associated symptoms should be sought (see Table 21-1). Certain factors about the onset, duration, and course of dizziness will, during the initial evaluation, help differentiate between the potential causes of dizziness (Tables 21-2 and 21-3). Physical deconditioning, visual problems, lack of use of proprioceptive aids (e.g., handrails or a cane), medications, and psychological problems are among the most common treatable factors contributing to dizziness.

In taking a clinical history and developing a differential diagnosis, the first steps involve reviewing the medications, identifying the dizziness subtype, establishing the duration of the symptoms (acute or chronic), and determining whether or not the dizziness occurs in episodes. Taking time to learn about these key characteristics will markedly narrow the differential diagnosis and will guide the remainder of the evaluation.

Medications

Medications should be reviewed early on, because dizziness is a known adverse reaction to many medications.[6,10,11] Common classes of medications contributing to or exacerbating dizziness are aminoglycosides, anxiolytics, antihistaminics, antidepressants, antipsychotics, antihypertensives, antiepileptics, chemotherapeutic agents, and nonsteroidal antiinflammatory drugs

TABLE 21-2	Common and/or Curable Causes of Dizziness in Older Patients					
Diagnosis	**Types of Dizziness**	**Episodic vs. Continuous**	**Frequency in Primary Care**	**Life Threatening?**	**Response to Treatment**
Anemia and/or hypovolemia	Presyncopal light-headedness	Continuous	M	Y	H
Anxiety (including panic disorder)	Light-headedness, often vague	Continuous	H	N	M
Benign paroxysmal positional vertigo	Vertigo	Episodes of <1 minute	H	N	M
Cardiac dysrhythmia	Presyncopal light-headedness	Episodic	M	Y	H
Cerebellar atrophy	Disequilibrium	Continuous	L	N	L
Cerumen against tympanic membrane	Variable, usually vertigo	Variable	M	N	H
Cervical vertigo	Vertigo, often with occipital headache	Episodic	M	N	H
Depression	Light-headedness, often vague	Continuous	M	Y	M
Drug adverse effect	Variable, often postural light-headedness	Variable	H	Y	H
Infection, systemic (viral or bacterial)	Presyncopal light-headedness	Continuous	H	Y	H
Meniere's disease	Vertigo (with hearing loss)	Episodes of 2-12 hours	M	N	M
Middle ear disease (e.g., serous otitis)	Vertigo or light-headedness	Continuous	M	N	H
Migraine	Vertigo	Episodic	L	N	H
Multiple neurosensory impairments	Disequilibrium	Continuous	H	N	L
Myocardial infarction (acute)	Presyncopal light-headedness	Continuous	L	Y	M
Neurolabyrinthitis	Vertigo; later disequilibrium	Continuous, abrupt onset	H	N	M
Neurosyphilis	Vertigo (with hearing loss)	Episodic	L	Y	H
Ocular	Light-headedness and/or imbalance	Continuous	L	N	M
Perilymphatic fistula	Vertigo	Episodes associated with Valsalva	L	N	H
Recurrent vestibulopathy	Vertigo	Episodes of hours to days	M	N	L
Transient vertebrobasilar ischemia	Vertigo	Episodes of 5-120 minutes	H	Y	L
Stroke, vertebrobasilar system	Vertigo, later disequilibrium	Continuous	L	Y	L
Tumor, acoustic nerve sheath	Unilateral hearing loss, occasionally with light-headedness or vertigo	Continuous	L	N	M
Vasovagal	Presyncopal light-headedness	Brief episodes	H	N	M

*Estimated frequency as a cause of dizziness in primary care.
H, High; *L*, low; *M*, moderate; *N*, no; *Y*, yes, at times.

TABLE 21-3	Evaluation and Management of Common Causes/Contributors of Dizziness		
Possible causes/contributors	History	Examination/Laboratory Tests	Therapy
Vestibular system			
Benign paroxysmal positional vertigo.	Sudden episodes of intense vertigo often associated with nausea or vomiting; provoked by changes in head positions (e.g., looking upward; rolling over in bed into lateral position; bending forward); episodes are recurrent and often last days to months.	Rotational nystagmus; definitive diagnosis by Dix-Hallpike maneuver.	Epley's maneuver or Brandt and Daroff's exercises is helpful in treatment. Sometimes a short course of vestibular suppressants is helpful.
Vestibular neuronitis / labyrinthitis / recurrent vestibulopathy (mostly viral or idiopathic).	Usually associated with upper respiratory infection; sudden onset of severe vertigo with nausea or vomiting; hearing is normal in vestibular neuronitis while impaired in labyrinthitis.	Spontaneous nystagmus with absence of auditory or neurologic signs; head thrust test; Fukuda stepping test. Unilateral reduced or absent caloric response.	Spontaneous recovery in few days; may need a short course of vestibular suppressants; vestibular rehabilitation.
Meniere's disease.	Episodic vertigo lasts for few hours; associated with tinnitus, fluctuating hearing loss, and sensation of fullness in ears.	Head thrust test and Fukuda stepping test is abnormal on the ipsilateral side. Tests: An audiogram will reveal a sensorineural hearing loss (low more than high frequencies).	During acute attacks vestibular suppressants may be helpful; salt restriction and diuretics are the mainstay. In severe cases may need surgical interventions, including intratympanic gentamicin ablation or transmastoid labyrinthectomy.
Vision			
Cataract; glaucoma; macular degeneration; presbyopia.	Abnormality in near or distant vision; use of bifocals.	Tests: Vision screening (Rosenbaum card); referral to ophthalmologist.	Appropriate refraction; avoid bifocals; cataract surgery; medical or surgical management for glaucoma.
Hearing			
Presbyacusis; otosclerosis; cerumen.	Difficulty in hearing on phone, in social situations; unilateral or bilateral deafness.	Otoscopy-cerumen; abnormal findings with whisper test, Rinne's test, Weber's test. Tests: Audioscopic examination; audiometry.	Ear wax drops; wax removal/irrigation of ears; hearing aids.
Hypotension			
Orthostatic-volume/salt depletion; medications; vasovagal episodes; autonomic dysfunction—Parkinson's disease, diabetes mellitus; Shy-Drager syndrome.	Near fainting/presyncope—most commonly when getting up from supine position, walking, exercising; medications history; complaints consistent with predisposing diseases.	Orthostatic changes in blood pressure and heart rate; signs of predisposing diseases. Tests: Investigations relevant to predisposing diseases	Proper hydration; dosage adjustment or removal of the offending drugs; treatment of relevant diseases; slow rising; graduated stocking; reconditioning exercises; drug therapy—fludrocortisone, etc. if needed.
Postprandial.	Light-headedness or dizziness within 1 hour of eating.	Postprandial orthostatic blood pressure changes.	Small frequent meals (5-6 times a day); have caffeine with meals; slow rising after meals.

Continued on following page

TABLE 21-3	Evaluation and Management of Common Causes/Contributors of Dizziness (Continued)		
Possible causes/ contributors	History	Examination/Laboratory Tests	Therapy
Peripheral Nerves			
Vitamin B_{12}, folate deficiency; diabetes mellitus; idiopathic.	Wooziness, disequilibrium; worse in dark or on uneven surfaces.	Abnormal vibration or position sense; gait and balance examination. Tests: Serum glucose; B_{12}, complete blood count folate levels.	Good lighting; appropriate walking aids; gait and balance training and exercises. Avoid high heels in footwear; treatment of specific disease.
Cervical spine			
Cervical spondylosis, degenerative or inflammatory arthritis.	Pain in neck on movement, episode of dizziness secondary to change in position of the neck; history of arthritis.	Limitation of range of motions of neck; abnormal vibratory or joint position sense; signs of radiculopathy or mylopathy. Tests: Cervical spine series.	Cervical collar; cervical or balance exercises.
Central Nervous System			
Vertebrobasilar insufficiency; transient ischemic attacks.	Transient episodes of dizziness; usually associated with diplopia, dysarthria, visual disturbances, etc.	Detailed neurologic examination can be normal or findings can be transient. Tests: Doppler ultrasound, arteriography are diagnostic for transient ischemic attack.	Depends upon the cause and site of lesion; low-dose aspirin and/or clopidogrel may be indicated.
Brain stem (vertebrobasilar insufficiency) and or cerebellar infarcts/hemorrhage.	History of dizziness (e.g., vertigo, near fainting) usually associated with slurred speech; visual changes; ipsilateral hemiparesis and/or gait ataxia	Neurologic examination to localize the lesion. Tests: Computed tomography or magnetic resonance imaging. Magnetic resonance imaging is preferred.	Low-dose aspirin and/or clopidogrel; rehabilitation therapy.
Cerebellopontine angle tumor; acoustic neuroma.	History of vertigo or imbalance or disequilibrium; unilateral hearing loss; tinnitus; may complain of parasthesias in trigeminal nerve distribution.	Detailed neurologic examination. Tests: Audiometery reveals sensorineural hearing loss (more with higher frequencies) in case of acoustic neuroma; brainstem auditory evoked potentials: magnetic resonance imaging.	Surgical excision.
Psychiatric disorders			
Anxiety, depression.	Usually continuous nonspecific dizziness; poor appetite; fatigue: sleep problems; somatic complaints.	Positive results on anxiety or depression screening (e.g., anxiety rating scales, Geriatric Depression Scale).	Psychotherapy; antidepressant therapy after considering risks and benefits.

(NSAIDs). Different classes of medications can provoke dizziness through different mechanisms. Aminoglycosides, loop diuretics, and NSAIDs can cause ototoxicity when used in higher dosages or for longer durations, especially when renal function is impaired. Antihistamines, tricyclic antidepressants, some cold remedies, and antihypertensives typically cause dizziness by contributing to orthostatic hypotension. Studies have also reported an independent association between the use of multiple medications and dizziness.[4,5]

Specifying the Cause of Dizziness

> Classically, dizziness is divided into four categories: vertigo, presyncopal light-headedness, disequilibrium, and "other." A fifth type, which is common in the elderly, is "mixed dizziness."

Vertigo

Vertigo is an illusion of movement, usually of rotation. It arises from the disturbance of the vestibular system or its connecting pathways. Patients usually talk about the environment spinning around; sometimes they can describe spinning inside their head or body, but this can also be a sign of psychogenic dizziness rather than true vertigo. The most common causes in older adults include acute neurolabyrinthitis, recurrent vestibular syndromes, benign paroxysmal positional vertigo (BPPV), and posterior circulation transient ischemic attacks.

Acute Neurolabyrinthitis. Caused by viral or vascular injury of all or part of one vestibular labyrinth, neurolabyrinthitis is characterized by rapid onset of vertigo accompanied by nausea, vomiting, sweating, and horizontal nystagmus. In young persons, the vertigo resolves within a week but in older adults it resolves more slowly and often leaves a residual disequilibrium. If the auditory portion of the labyrinth is also affected, hearing loss and tinnitus may be reported.

Treatment is supportive. Meclizine or promethazine may help during the acute phase; low-dose benzodiazepines may provide some relief of the more protracted disequilibrium and light-headedness, but must be used with caution because of sedation effects.

Recurrent Vestibular Syndromes. Recurrent attacks of vertigo, generally lasting hours to days, are common. When accompanied by hearing loss and tinnitus, they are referred to as Meniere's disease; when consisting purely of dizziness the syndrome is called recurrent vestibulopathy. Meniere's disease leads to progressive low-frequency hearing loss over time; recurrent vestibulopathy generally resolves over time. Meniere's generally responds to salt restriction and diuretics, but recalcitrant cases may require specialist care. Recurrent vestibulopathy tends to be milder and respond to symptomatic treatment using antihistamines such as meclizine. A common cause of recurrent vestibulopathy is migraine related. Migraine should be treated with control of triggers and possibly prophylactic medications. Consider sudden hearing loss with vertigo in the differential of vertigo and hearing loss. This is important because prompt treatment of sudden hearing loss with prednisone is associated with improved hearing outcomes.

Benign Paroxysmal Positional Vertigo (BPPV). An extremely common cause of dizziness among elderly patients, benign paroxysmal positional vertigo (BPPV) presents as bouts of vertigo lasting less than a minute, brought on by position change, such as by rolling over in bed or by bending over and straightening up. Attacks tend to come in flurries, lasting a week or two, separated by months to years without symptoms. Unilateral hearing loss, tinnitus, and cranial nerve deficits are generally absent. Most BPPV is caused by small, dense calcific particles (otoliths) from the saccule or utricle of the inner ear that break loose and migrate into the posterior semicircular canal, where they amplify rotational movements in the plane of the canal. With time, particles are absorbed, scarred down, or otherwise dealt with so that symptoms abate. A definitive diagnosis of BPPV can be made by Dix-Hallpike test (discussed later).

Posterior Circulation Disorders. In evaluating the older patient with acute or episodic vertigo, the possibility of a transient ischemic attack (TIA) or stroke in the posterior circulation must be kept in mind. These are discussed later in this chapter, because their dizziness is not always described as vertigo.

Presyncope

Presyncope is the sensation that one is about to pass out. It is described as a feeling of severe light-headedness and may be associated with unsteadiness or falling. The sensation arises because of temporarily decreased blood flow to the cerebral cortex leading to hypoxia. Most adults experience transient presyncope after rapid change in position (e.g., sudden standing from the lying or sitting position). Some aggravating factors include certain medications, excess alcohol intake, or even lying in hot sun. Common causes include orthostatic hypotension (OH), vasovagal episodes, carotid sinus syndrome (CSS), described below, as well as medications,[12] anemia, viral infections, and cardiac arrhythmias. See Chapter 22 for a detailed discussion of syncope and its differential diagnosis.[13]

Orthostatic Hypotension (OH). Orthostatic hypotension (OH) is a physical finding defined by the American Autonomic Society and the American Academy of Neurology as a systolic blood pressure decrease of at least 20 mmHg or a diastolic blood pressure decrease of at least 10 mmHg within 3 minutes of standing.

Some elderly patients may have dizziness because of impaired cerebral blood flow when standing even though they do not meet the above-mentioned criteria. Some take longer than 3 minutes to drop their blood pressure, and in others cerebral blood flow is impaired in spite of minimal reduction in peripheral blood pressure. The first step in treating these problems is elimination of medications that impair venous tone, including many cardiovascular medications (e.g., doxazosin [Cardura], clonidine [Catapres]).[14,15]

The next step is use of elastic compression stockings. If these measures fail then treatment with beta-blockers, disopyramide, transdermal scopolamine, and fludrocortisone can be considered.

Vasovagal Disorders. Vasovagal disorders result from either excessive vagal tone or impaired reflex control of the peripheral circulation. Episodes are characterized by a sudden hypotension, bradycardia, nausea, pallor, and diaphoresis. Most common precipitating factors are severe pain, emotional stress, extreme fatigue, or the process of micturition or defecation. The prognosis is usually favorable because vasovagal episodes are not caused by or indicative of cardiac disease. Excessive sympathetic activity causes cardiac hyperactivity and excessive stimulation of cardiac mechanoreceptors (afferent vagal C-fibers) leading to a sympathetic withdrawal and activation of parasympathetic activity resulting in hypotension and bradycardia. Low-dose beta-blocker treatment is often effective.

Postprandial Hypotension. Postprandial hypotension, defined as a decrease in systolic blood pressure of 20 mmHg or more in a sitting or standing posture within 1 to 2 hours of eating a meal, may also cause dizziness.[16] One study has shown that the effects of postprandial hypotension and orthostatic hypotension are additive but not synergistic, suggesting that the two entities may have different pathophysiologic mechanisms.[17]

Carotid Sinus Syndrome (CSS). Carotid sinus syndrome (CSS) is a controversial diagnosis, but one that probably causes considerable presyncope in older persons. There are two types—cardioinhibitory (caused by bradycardia or temporary asystole) and vasodepressor (caused by a marked reduction in systolic blood pressure). Studies indicate that between 36% and 48% of dizzy patients have CSS,[18,19] but the extent to which their CSS is incidental, contributory, or causal is uncertain.[20] Probably the most reasonable clinical conclusion to draw from this controversy is that older persons in general are more susceptible to vasovagal and other stimuli that reduce cerebral blood flow and that certain patients (i.e., those with demonstrable CSS) appear particularly susceptible.

Disequilibrium

Disequilibrium is a sense of imbalance. Patients with this type of dizziness can usually recognize that they are experiencing a body sensation rather than a head sensation. Disequilibrium is a multisensory disorder, which can arise from combinations of disorders of the musculoskeletal system interfering with gait, such as

arthritis, proprioceptive system abnormalities, diabetic peripheral neuropathy, cervical spondylosis, or cerebellar disorders. Vision problems or hearing disorders or neurodegenerative disorders such as Parkinson's disease are other important causes or contributing factors. Peripheral vestibulopathy is a common contributing factor to chronic unsteadiness.

Cervical Causes. Cervical vertigo arises from irritation of proprioceptive receptors in the facet joints of the cervical spine. Osteoarthritis or muscle spasm is usually responsible. Clinically, vertigo or a more vague lightheadedness is reported, accompanied by an occipital headache and neck stiffness or pain. Management involves treating the underlying arthritis or acute neck problem.

Two mechanisms have been proposed to explain cervical dizziness: proprioceptive deficits and vascular abnormalities.[15] Proprioceptive deficits in the cervical spine can cause dizziness secondary to stimulation of proprioceptive receptors in the facet joints of the cervical spine. In older persons, cervical osteoarthritis most likely causes dizziness via this mechanism. The patient usually complains of pain in the neck upon movement, along with a worsening of dizziness. There is often a history of arthritis or whiplash injury. Further examination may reveal a decreased range of motion of the neck or signs of radiculopathy or mylopathy and/or spastic gait.

A vascular cause of cervical dizziness is thought to result from impingement of the vertebral arteries. One theory is that when there is extensive blockage of one vertebral artery, rotation of the head can cause sufficient obstruction of the other vertebral artery to cause brainstem ischemia. Another theory is that when a person turns his or her head or neck, an osteoarthritic spur may press on the nearby vertebral artery, causing a transient disruption of the blood flow.

Vision Problems

The visual system plays an important role in spatial orientation and maintenance of equilibrium, especially when the vestibular and/or proprioceptive systems are not working optimally or when the individual is in a challenging situation (such as on a boat). Therefore, impaired vision can cause or contribute to dizziness and/or imbalance. Common ocular diseases that can cause dizziness include cataracts, macular degeneration, and glaucoma. Age-related visual changes that may contribute to dizziness include a decrease in visual acuity, dark adaptation, contrast sensitivity, and accommodation.

Causes of Dizziness That Often Do Not Fit Neatly into a Subtype

The "other" category of dizziness includes vague, difficult-to-categorize dizziness. Patients may describe feelings of dissociation, floating, swimming, or giddiness. In such situations the physician should not exclude vertigo, presyncopal light-headedness, or disequilibrium merely because the patient was not able to articulate the problem adequately. On the other hand, dizziness that is difficult to describe often accompanies a psychological condition such as anxiety and depression.

A feature of dizziness in the elderly, in contrast to younger adults, is greater difficulty in assigning patients to one dizziness subtype. Between 42% and 56% of older patients are unable to identify their dizziness as exclusively vertigo, presyncope, disequilibrium, or other; instead, they describe multiple dizziness sensations.[4] Persons with these multiple sensations can be categorized as having mixed dizziness.

Peripheral vestibulopathy is a common contributing factor in patients with nonspecific dizziness symptoms and anxiety. This is particularly true for patients with a history of panic disorder and/or migraine.

Anxiety and Depression. Psychological diagnoses have been reported to occur in as many as a third of persons with dizziness. The most common conditions in older persons are depression and anxiety. Patients with these conditions typically report a vague light-headed or floating sensation or continuous dizziness. Accompanying signs and symptoms may include headache, fatigue, neck soreness, and abdominal pain.

In older patients, psychological symptoms though common are usually secondary to the dizziness rather than a cause of it. Still, treating the psychological disorder may often reduce the disability when the dizziness itself cannot be cured.

Finally, there are several diagnoses whose symptoms do not fit neatly into one classical dizziness subtype. These include cerebrovascular disease and acoustic neuroma. Each is described briefly below.

Cerebrovascular Disease. Acute posterior circulation disease resulting from a TIA or stroke may present with main symptoms of vertigo; however, lacunar infarcts and small strokes in the same area often have the main symptom of a sudden or insidious imbalance. In severe acute disease, associated neurologic symptoms—such as diplopia, ataxia, dysarthria, unilateral weakness, or numbness of one side of the body—and perioral numbness occur frequently. However, their absence does not rule out a cerebrovascular event—up to a quarter of posterior circulation strokes begin as vertigo.

Dizziness caused by cerebrovascular disease is almost always a posterior circulation problem; TIAs involving the anterior circulation rarely produce vertigo. In fact, patients with vertigo who have carotid endarterectomies frequently fail to improve because the carotid disease is incidental.

The course of TIAs is variable. Less than half progress to a completed stroke, and symptoms frequently resolve completely. Therefore, although therapy is largely limited to antiplatelet agents and control of risk factors, the prognosis is by no means hopeless.

One circulatory disorder that is accompanied by severe vertigo (often including vomiting) is acute cerebellar hemorrhage or infarction. This diagnosis requires vigilance, because its initial presentation can look like vestibular vertigo. Look for gaze-evoked nystagmus, cerebellar coordination signs, or ataxia. If present, imaging test must be conducted immediately.

Acoustic Neuroma. A benign tumor of the eighth cranial nerve, acoustic neuroma typically has the symptom of progressive unilateral high frequency sensorineural hearing loss, and occasionally includes mild vertigo or disequilibrium.

Differences between Acute and Chronic Symptoms

Dizziness can be divided into acute or chronic, depending on its duration. Acute dizziness is defined by having been present for less than 2 months; chronic dizziness is defined by having been present for more than 2 months.

Acute dizziness usually results from a disorder of one system (e.g., acute labyrinthitis), and in older patients the approach to management is similar to that used in younger patients. Chronic dizziness in older persons, on the other hand, is most often secondary to the combined effects of disorders or impairments in the multiple systems responsible for maintaining equilibrium. The management approach is to intervene at multiple levels.

Importance of Determining the Episodic or Continuous Nature of Dizziness

If the patient has vertigo, it should be determined whether the dizziness is episodic or continuous. If dizziness is episodic, the duration and frequency of the episodes should be identified, along with any associated symptoms such as hearing loss, tinnitus, ear fullness, diplopia, dysarthria, and syncopal episodes.

- Episodes of vertigo lasting less than 1 minute suggest BPPV.
- Episodes of vertigo lasting between 15 minutes and several hours suggest TIA or migraine.
- Episodes of vertigo lasting between several hours and a couple of days suggest recurrent vestibulopathy or, if accompanied by tinnitus and hearing loss, Meniere's disease.

Continuous dizziness has a broad differential diagnosis. If dizziness begins abruptly and improves or remains the same, common causes include stroke, neurolabyrinthitis, cerebellar degeneration, peripheral neuropathy, physical deconditioning, drugs, anxiety, and depression. If onset is insidious, then psychological causes are particularly common, but other causes such as cerebellar degeneration from alcoholism or chronic effects of medications such as benzodiazepines should be considered, and acoustic neuroma should be ruled out.

Provocative or Precipitating Factors

Determining whether rolling over in bed or changing the position of the head or neck brings on the dizziness is useful; such patients usually have cervical or vestibular etiology. Dizziness on standing from the supine position is seen in postural hypotension. One should ask whether dizziness occurs after eating meals, as this would suggest postprandial hypotension. Dizziness developing after a change in medication needs careful review of side effects of that medication. Depressive disorders should be sought using a standardized instrument, such as the Geriatric Depression Scale (GDS). Dizziness on standing from the supine position suggests postural hypotension.

CASE 1

Thelma Franklin (Part 2)

On further questioning Ms. Franklin complains of head spinning or light-headedness. The episodes usually occur when she stands up from a sitting or lying position or with head and neck position changes. She denies nausea, vomiting, or a sensation of fullness in her ears, which is seen in Meniere's disease. Her daughter denies any loss of consciousness during the previous falls.

Case Discussion

One of the challenges a clinician faces in managing dizziness in the elderly is that they often are unable to specify one type of dizziness. Take Ms. Franklin for instance. If she had complained only of experiencing a spinning sensation, a vestibular lesion could be implicated. Sudden onset can suggest a vascular or traumatic process. Head stuffiness reported several weeks beforehand could indicate a viral process (neurolabyrinthitis) or the first episode of Meniere's disease. Other important points from her history include use of nifedipine, a calcium channel blocker (raising suspicion for postural hypotension), her living situation (potential stress), and bilateral cataracts (raising concern about the adequacy of compensation for a vestibular problem). Based on the initial history, Ms. Franklin's physician could construct the following list of most likely diagnoses: postural hypotension, cervical arthritis, vestibular causes, anxiety, and depression. ▪

CASE 2

Catherine Arnold (Part 2)

The remainder of Ms. Arnold's history is noncontributory. She is an 84-year-old grandmother who shares her home with another elderly woman for whom she serves as a part-time caregiver. She is generally healthy, does her own shopping, needs some help with housework, and has hypertension and left hip arthritis. She takes enalapril 10 mg by mouth once daily and acetaminophen as needed.

Based on her initial history the differential diagnosis includes BPPV, acute neurolabyrinthitis, TIAs or brainstem infarction, or cervical vertigo.

1. **What should be kept in mind during physical examination?**
2. **What are the bedside tests that can provoke dizziness?**
3. **What laboratory tests are helpful in the diagnosis?** ▪

PHYSICAL EXAMINATION

The physical examination has to be individualized. However, most patients with dizziness should have the following evaluations: testing for postural hypotension by measuring postural blood pressures; pathologic nystagmus; fundoscopy; hearing screening; bilateral otoscopic evaluation; testing for restricted cervical spine motion and tenderness; screening for a peripheral neuropathy; examination of the cranial nerves, peripheral arteries (especially the carotid arteries), and heart; gait and balance examination; Romberg's test (which if positive suggests vestibular or proprioceptive etiology); and a standardized instrument to evaluate for depressive symptoms.

Some bedside tests and maneuvers can provoke dizziness, and are useful if indicted by the clinical history. These include forced hyperventilation, head thrust test, marching in place with the eyes closed (Fukuda stepping test), and Dix-Hallpike maneuver.

- Forced hyperventilation is useful when anxiety is a possible diagnosis. Anxiety and, in some cases, depression can cause a light-headedness that probably arises from hyperventilation. Having such patients hyperventilate in the examining room may elicit the same dizziness they are concerned about, thus enabling the diagnosis. Deep breathing at a rate of 20 to 30 breaths per minute for 2 or 3 minutes usually provokes dizziness, often accompanied by finger and perioral numbness. Once dizziness develops, the patient should be asked if his or her dizziness symptoms are similar. In interpreting this maneuver, be aware that it may aggravate symptoms in certain vestibular disorders, and therefore is not specific for anxiety; therefore, other historical and examination data should be considered in interpreting the result of forced hyperventilation.
- The head thrust test helps to determine if the vestibuloocular reflex (VOR) is intact. The VOR helps to maintain visual stability during head

movement. It is impaired in patients with reduced peripheral vestibular function and some central nervous system diseases (e.g., stroke). This reflex depends on information relayed by the vestibular nucleus to the sixth cranial nerve nucleus in the pons and, via the median longitudinal fasciculus, to the third and fourth cranial nerve nuclei in the midbrain. In this test, the patient is asked to fix his or her eyes on the examiner's nose, and the head is rapidly rotated 10 degrees by the examiner to either the left or right side. Normally, the eyes will remain fixed on the target, but in a patient with a vestibular deficit the eyes move away from the target along with the head, followed by a corrective saccade back to the target. For example, in a patient with a left-sided vestibular lesion, head thrusts to the left will produce a movement of the pupils from the target to the left, along with the head, followed by a corrective movement back to the target, whereas head thrusts to the right will produce the normal response of continued fixation on the target.[21]

- The Fukuda stepping test (marching in place with the eyes closed) is a sensitive test for unilateral vestibular hypofunction (e.g., from a prior neurolabyrinthitis or from Meniere's disease). To conduct the test, the patient is asked to march in place for 30 seconds with his or her eyes closed and arms extended in front. Care must be taken not to orient the patient with sound, such as the examiner's voice, a radio, or a ticking clock. Patients with absent or reduced vestibular function rotate more than 30 degrees toward the lesion.

- The Dix-Hallpike maneuver is used to diagnose BPPV by provoking rotation in the posterior semicircular canals. In this maneuver, the patient is seated on the examining table so that he or she can be comfortably and rapidly eased backward to a recumbent position. Standing to the patient's right, the physician cradles the patient's head and neck in both hands, turning the head about 30 degrees to the right and advising the patient to hold the physician's upper arm for stability. At the count of three, the patient relaxes and the physician quickly lays the patient backward, maintaining the head position. This places the patient's right posterior semicircular canal in the vertical plane, causing that single canal to experience a rotatory stimulus-angular acceleration. The examiner maintains the patient in this head-hanging-right position for at least 10 to 20 seconds or until vertigo subsides. Then the patient is returned to the initial position, again holding the position for at least 10 seconds. Next, the procedure is repeated with the physician on the patient's left side to test the left posterior semicircular canal. A classic positive response to Dix-Hallpike maneuver includes four components: dizziness (vertigo), rotatory (torsional) nystagmus, latency (i.e., the dizziness and nystagmus do not begin immediately, but rather after a few seconds), and, fatigue such that repeating the same maneuver should result in reduced symptoms (i.e., if three or four repetitions are made, no more symptoms should be noted). A positive response to the Dix-Hallpike maneuver is diagnostic of BPPV. Because BPPV is generally unilateral, response is usually either limited to one side or unequal in intensity between sides. Negative Hallpike testing in BPPV is most common when an episode is mild or when the patient is already recovering. A recent population-based study in a U.S. emergency department reported that examination for BPPV is seldom conducted as part of the diagnosis when the patient's chief complaint is dizziness, vertigo, or gait imbalance, and when BPPV examination does occur, the Dix-Hallpike maneuver is underused in these patients. The author reports provider comfort as a major confounder.[22]

LABORATORY TESTING

> No laboratory test should be considered routine or mandatory in primary care patients with dizziness.

Test selection is guided by the presentation, duration, and severity of the problem and by the clinician's concern about possible progressive or life-threatening conditions. Among the laboratory tests useful in certain patients are the following:

- Hematologic and biochemical studies may be ordered to screen for systemic and metabolic causes of dizziness, such as anemia, hyperthyroidism, and syphilis.

- Audiometry with speech discrimination is the best screening test for acoustic neuroma, with a unilateral hearing loss suggesting the need for further evaluation. Hearing loss (unilateral or bilateral) that is especially prominent in the low frequencies in a patient with recurrent vertigo would help diagnose Meniere's disease.

- Electrocardiography (ECG) identifies rhythm disturbances such as atrial fibrillation, ventricular tachycardia, or complete heart block. In episodic dizziness, prolonged ambulatory cardiac monitoring may be necessary; however, the vast majority of cardiac monitoring for dizziness fails to identify a cardiac etiology.

- Brainstem auditory evoked potentials can isolate the anatomic site of a vestibular or auditory nerve deficit; they are useful in evaluation of unilateral hearing loss (to rule out eighth nerve tumor).

- Doppler examination of the cranial blood vessels and cerebral angiography can be used to diagnose vertebrobasilar disease. The usefulness of such information when the clinical picture already suggests posterior circulation TIA is questionable, however, because treatment is nonspecific. The greatest use of these tests is in differentiating migraine from vertebrobasilar insufficiency and in identifying subclavian steal, a surgically treatable cause of vertebrobasilar TIAs.
- Brain imaging is used to rule out a mass lesion, such as an acoustic neuroma, and to identify stroke. Magnetic resonance imaging (MRI) is preferred to computed tomography (CT) because clinically significant lesions (e.g., tumor or infarction) may be small and missed on CT scans. Demonstration of increased periventricular white matter signal in MRI presents a diagnostic challenge; how much is normal in older people and how much indicates lacunar infarct disease is unclear.
- Electronystagmography (ENG) is used to evaluate vestibular function by measuring the effect of selected stimuli on eye movements, using recordings from electrodes placed over the eye muscles. The test is based on the VOR, which, in many pathologic states, generates subtle oculomotor abnormalities that can be appreciated only with the eyes closed. The routine ENG can often differentiate between central and peripheral causes of vertigo; however, abnormal responses are so common in older persons that the test is highly nonspecific in this population.

> **Consultants can be helpful but tend to miss diagnoses outside their field.**

Consultation with an appropriate specialist can be fruitful particularly in patients with chronic dizziness and especially if the physician suspects a diagnosis within the province of a specific medical subspecialty, such as neurology, otolaryngology, or cardiology. Therefore, the importance of the generalist's role in integrating consultant opinions with the entire clinical picture cannot be overemphasized.

CASE 1
Thelma Franklin (Part 3)

On examination, Ms. Franklin's pulse is 82 beats per minute, supine blood pressure is 120/70 (standing 100/64), and temperature is 98.4° F. She complains of dizziness on standing. Cardiac and respiratory system are unremarkable.

Neurologic examination reveals difficulty in getting up from chair without using arms of the chair. Romberg's sign is negative, but she is not able to do a one-leg stand secondary to pain in the back. There is no nystagmus at rest or on head thrust test; Dix-Hallpike test is negative. She scores 27/30 on Mini-Mental State Examination (MMSE). She scores 3/15 on the GDS.

Case Discussion

The most likely cause of Ms. Franklin's dizziness is postural hypotension. Her gait abnormality secondary to backache and bilateral cataracts may be contributing factors. Her postural hypotension is most likely secondary to nifedipine extended release. Her blood pressure measured in the office suggests she may not need nifedipine at all; it should be discontinued. Her blood pressure should be monitored and, if needed, the dose of metoprolol can be increased. In addition, her backache should be adequately controlled with scheduled dosage of acetaminophen instead of using it as needed. She should also have her vision tested. ▪

MANAGEMENT

Treatment of dizziness depends on making the correct diagnosis. Many causes of dizziness are curable; examples include adverse drug effects, cerumen impaction, anemia, cardiac dysrhythmias, depression, and perilymphatic fistula. Other causes of dizziness, such as BPPV and many vasovagal phenomena, are benign and self-limited. When dizziness cannot be cured, treatment should strive to reduce disability and minimize symptoms. Box 21-1 identifies a general approach to treatment of the patient with dizziness.

Vision is the key adaptive mechanism for vestibular and proprioceptive deficits; cataract surgery and use of a night-light are two examples of ways vision can be enhanced. If loss of proprioception in the ankles and feet contributes to dizziness, the patient can get additional sensory input by touching the wall or another person, or by using a cane.

The extent to which anxiety and depression contribute to dizziness should not be overlooked. Dizziness is a common symptom of panic disorder, and vertigo is not an unusual description of the symptom. Admittedly, dizziness of purely psychiatric origin is relatively rare among older patients compared to younger adults; in fact, physicians often hesitate to make a psychiatric diagnosis without a long history of similar symptoms. However, secondary psychiatric problems such as anxiety and depression are common in older persons who are dizzy. One study of 56 elderly patients with chronic dizziness identified a psychological diagnosis meeting DSM-III criteria in more than one third of patients. In most cases, the diagnosis was a contributing factor to rather than the primary cause of the dizziness; anxiety disorders, depression, and adjustment reactions predominated.[23]

Pharmacologic Treatment

Antihistamines and sedatives are overused in the treatment of dizziness among elderly patients. Sedation, imbalance, and orthostatic hypotension are common side effects and can be more dangerous than the dizziness itself. Small doses of medication can, however, help in certain circumstances. Meclizine, dimenhydrinate, and other antihistamines provide relief for acute peripheral vestibular problems, such as labyrinthitis or attacks of Meniere's disease. Benzodiazepines reduce central sensitivity to some dizziness symptoms, but should be used with extreme caution because they cause sedation and increase the risk of falls; oxazepam and temazepam have short half-lives and are preferable to longer-acting agents. Antiemetics or antinausea medications are also sometimes useful.

Vestibular Rehabilitation

A growing body of literature indicates that physical therapy can result in significant functional gains in older persons with dizziness and imbalance.[24,25] Vestibular rehabilitation includes combinations of exercises involving head, neck, and eye movements designed to provoke dizziness and imbalance. Initially these exercises may worsen dizziness, but over a period of weeks to months dizziness improves, most likely because of central adaptation or desensitization.

Desensitization exercises seek to reduce the brain's responsiveness to the stimuli from the affected labyrinth, making use of a normal compensatory mechanism by provoking vertigo spells in a safe environment.

Specific dynamic balance exercises can help strengthen muscle groups that stabilize the patient, thereby reducing falls and fear of falling.

A randomized trial of vestibular rehabilitation (a specific group of exercises consisting of eye, head, and body movements designed to stimulate the vestibular system) resulted in a significant improvement in patients with chronic dizziness.[26] Another randomized trial found that physiotherapy aimed at reducing neck discomfort resulted in both improved symptoms and better postural performance among patients with suspected cervical dizziness.[27]

The modified Epley's canalith repositioning maneuver represents a specific treatment for BPPV[28] (Box 21-2). The purpose of this maneuver is to move free-floating debris by the effect of gravity from the posterior semicircular canal into the utriculus, where it will no longer affect the dynamics of the semicircular canals. There is a device called DizzyFIX that has been approved by the U.S. Food and Drug Administration that can be used by patients for home treatment. This device provides visual feedback and guides the patient in performing particle repositioning maneuver.[29] If the modified Epley's maneuver is not helpful, the patient can do Brandt and Daroff's exercises (Box 21-3). These exercises involve sitting on the bed and falling or rolling, in a controlled manner, toward the side of the injury, precipitating the dizziness, and doing this three or four times in a row. Typically this causes relief of symptoms, although relief may last only a few hours. The exercises likely work either by habituation or by dislodging debris from the posterior semicircular canals. There are other techniques, such as Semont's maneuver and Li's maneuver, that can be used for repositioning.[30,31] In Li's maneuver, the researchers developed a new series of movements to manage the BPPV of each semicircular canal individualized by the patient's report of vertigo on provocative head positioning.[31]

Surgical Therapy

Surgery is almost never indicated for dizziness. It is reserved for (1) persons with cerebellopontine angle tumors and (2) patients with severe Meniere's disease or refractory BPPV whose dizziness is so severe and chronic that an ablative (e.g., intratympanic gentamicin ablation, a common ablative procedure used in the geriatric population, or transmastoid labyrinthectomy) or nonablative (e.g., endolymphatic sac decompression and posterior canal occlusion) procedure is considered.[32,33]

Patient Education

Fearing a dizziness attack or a dizziness-related fall causes many older persons to give up activities crucial to their independence and self-image, such as going to church, shopping, visiting friends, and driving. For these reasons, the effective management of dizziness requires counseling the patient and family about these issues. Patients should be given basic education regarding the pathophysiology of dizziness and its provocation to help the patient understand and therefore be more realistic and less anxious about dizziness.

At times, modifying activities is indicated; for example, in case of postural dizziness, patients should be instructed to rise slowly from the sitting or supine position. Deconditioning plays an important role in the persistence of symptoms; accordingly, activities are to be encouraged. Finally, dizzy patients should avoid over-the-counter sleeping pills or cold medicines, and their prescription medications should be carefully reviewed.

CASE 2

Discussion

Ms. Arnold's vital signs are within normal limits, and no orthostatic hypotension is noted. Respiratory, cardiovascular, and neurologic examination findings are normal. Rapid positional testing using Hallpike maneuver reproduces her dizziness in the right head-hanging position. On further questioning, she admits to having greater difficulty rolling over to the right than to the left when in bed.

She is given instructions for positional exercises. These consist of reproducing her vertigo by rolling over rapidly to the right. After doing so, she is instructed to wait for her dizziness to resolve and then to roll over rapidly again in the same direction. She is instructed that, within five repetitions, the dizziness response should be fatigued temporarily and she can go about her day. As instructed, she performs the exercises every 3 hours while awake. Within 2 weeks she reports no more dizziness. ◪

SUMMARY

Chronic dizziness is one of the common problems in older persons. The majority of older persons are unable to identify their dizziness to a particular subtype. Chronic dizziness in older persons differs, in that impairments in multiple systems or multiple diseases usually contribute to the complaint and that is why it is considered a geriatric syndrome. Management of dizziness is aimed at trying to identify and treat or modify as many of the contributing impairments or diseases as possible to decrease the disability associated with dizziness.

Web Resources

www.youtube.com/watch?v=2o5qn9vb09k&feature=youtube_ gdata. Video demonstration of Dix Hallpike test.
www.youtube.com/watch?v=ZqokxZRbJfw&feature=youtube_gdata and www.youtube.com/watch?v=pa6t-Bpg494&feature=youtube_ gdata. Video demonstrations of Epley's maneuver.
www.youtube.com/watch?v=y0N-m8m_7Gw&feature=youtube_ gdata. Discussion about DizzyFIX, a home treatment for vertigo caused by BPPV.
www.youtube.com/watch?v=voZXtTUdQ00. Video demonstration of Brandt-Daroff habituation exercise.

KEY REFERENCES

1. Colledge NR, Wilson JA, Macintyre CCA, MacLennan WJ. The prevalence and characteristics of dizziness in an elderly community. Age Aging 1994:23;117-20.
3. Neuhauser HK, Radtke A, Brevern MV, et al. Burden of dizziness and vertigo in the community. Arch Intern Med 2008;168(19): 2118-24.
7. Tinetti ME, Williams CS, Gill TM. Dizziness among older adults: A possible geriatric syndrome. Ann Intern Med 2000;132:337-44.
8. Kao AC, Nanda A, Williams CS, Tinetti ME. Validation of dizziness as a possible geriatric syndrome. J Am Geriatr Soc 2001;49:72-5.
11. Gupta V, Lipsitz LA. Orthostatic hypotension in the elderly: Diagnosis and treatment. Am J Med 2007;120(10):841-7.
17. Maurer MS, Karmally W, Rivadeneira H, et al. Upright posture and postprandial hypotension in elderly persons. Ann Intern Med 2000;133:533.

References available online at expertconsult.com.

22

Syncope

Lorraine S. Sease

OBJECTIVES

Upon completion of this chapter, the reader will be able to:

• Describe the physiologic mechanisms that give rise to a complaint of syncope.
• Use key history and physical examination data to create a differential diagnosis for the patient experiencing syncope.
• Identify and describe the presentation, prognosis, and treatment of the common causes of syncope in the elderly.

Additional online-only material indicated by icon.

PREVALENCE AND IMPACT

Syncope is defined as the sudden loss of consciousness and postural tone with spontaneous recovery. It is distinct from dizziness, vertigo, seizures, prolonged decreased mental status, drop attacks without loss of consciousness, and cardiac arrest. During a 10-year period, approximately 6% of all adults have syncope. The prevalence rises steeply with age.[1] Older patients are more likely to present to their primary care provider or the emergency department for evaluation of their syncope, and they more often have life-threatening causes.[2] Syncope is not a disease, but it is a dangerous symptom whose underlying cause can be challenging to diagnose. In frail older adults it is more likely to lead to falls with injury and prolonged disability. Identification of the cause of syncope is important to allow treatment of the underlying disorder and prevent repeat events.

CASE 1

Lucia (Part 1)

Lucia is a 67-year-old woman who visits your walk-in clinic after having passed out at her granddaughter's wedding reception. Upon questioning, she tells you that the reception was held outdoors, in 85° heat. After standing for a long time in the sun, she felt flushed and a little nauseous. The next thing she knew she was lying on the ground.

Lucia's past medical history is significant for obesity and hypothyroidism. Her only medication is levothyroxine, at a stable dose for several years. Three months ago she was hospitalized overnight after an episode of chest pain. During that hospitalization she had a normal electrocardiogram (ECG) and a negative cardiac stress echocardiogram.

1. **Based on this history alone, what are the most likely type of syncope and the possible causes or contributing factors?**

2. **Is Lucia at high risk for cardiac syncope?** ▣

CASE 2

George (Part 1)

George is a 70-year-old man who reports that he passed out while eating lunch with a friend. His friend is with him at the appointment. He was talking normally and feeling well when, according to his friend, George suddenly slumped over onto the table into his food. His friend called for help and estimates that within 10 seconds George had awakened and lifted his head, looking very pale. His speech and actions were sluggish for another minute or two, but soon he was feeling back to normal. George adamantly rejected calling an ambulance, so his friend agreed to bring him to your office for a same-day appointment.

You have been George's physician for the past 15 years and know that he is an active retiree with longstanding hypertension, hyperlipidemia, and well-controlled diabetes. His medications include lisinopril, hydrochlorothiazide, lovastatin, aspirin, metformin, and glipizide. His last ECG was 5 years ago and was normal. This is his first episode of syncope.

1. **Which aspects of George's history put him at increased risk of syncope?**

2. **Based on the brief description of the syncopal event, what type of syncope do you suspect?**

3. **Could any of George's medications have contributed to the event?** ▣

RISK FACTORS AND PATHOPHYSIOLOGY

The underlying pathophysiology leading to syncope is inadequate oxygenation of the cerebral cortex and reticular activating system, resulting in loss of consciousness. A variety of mechanisms lead to this outcome, but the final common pathway involves reduced blood flow or reduced oxygen-carrying capacity. Figure 22-1 is a graphic identifying the main physiologic factors that can lead to inadequate brain oxygenation. The differential diagnosis is extensive; many diseases and conditions can lead to this outcome. They fall into these general categories: neurally mediated (reflex) causes, orthostatic hypotension, cardiac causes, central nervous system diseases, and psychiatric disorders.[3]

In a study of 655 cases of syncope among community elderly, a history of stroke or transient ischemic attack (TIA) was by far the greatest potential risk factor for syncope (odds ratio [OR] = 2.96). Use of cardiac medication (OR = 1.70) and a diagnosis of high blood pressure (OR = 1.50) were also significant predictors of a syncopal event.[4] The cause of these associations is probably multifactorial, with side effects from medications and autonomic insufficiency as possible contributing factors.

In addition to having more underlying chronic conditions and being on more medications than younger adults, older persons tend to have several age-related physiologic changes that increase their syncope risk. These include the following[5]:

• Atherosclerosis (impairing dilation of cerebral blood vessels in the face of reduced blood flow)
• Increased endothelin production (increasing vasoconstriction of cerebral arterioles)
• Left ventricular dysfunction, caused by longstanding hypertension and/or heart disease (resulting in decreased cardiac output)
• Cardiac valvular disease (increasing the likelihood of arrhythmias and heart block)
• Blunting of autonomic responses (predisposing the person to orthostatic hypotension

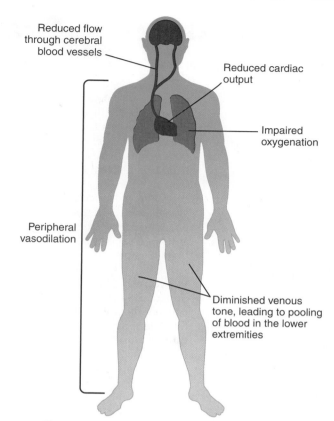

Figure 22-1 Mechanisms that lead to syncope.

DIFFERENTIAL DIAGNOSIS AND ASSESSMENT

Causes of syncope can be categorized as neurally mediated, orthostatic, cardiac, cerebrovascular, psychogenic, or multifactorial (Table 22-1). Some studies include drug-induced as a cause, though one could argue that drugs may cause increased susceptibility to all forms of syncope. Many etiologies of syncope go undiagnosed. Older patients are more likely to have multiple etiologies.

> Older patients are more likely to have multiple etiologies of syncope.

Neurally Mediated Syncope

Neurally mediated syncope is considered the most common form in all ages, including the geriatric population.[6,3] This usually involves the initiation of reflexes that lower blood pressure through venous pooling in the legs, or slow the heart rate through stimulation of the vagus nerve. A variety of physiologic stimuli can trigger this reflex: urination, defecation, cough, gastrointestinal stimulation (especially pain), stimulation of the carotid sinus (e.g., by a tight collar), and intense emotions. Neurally mediated syncope is often considered a benign

TABLE 22-1	Differential Diagnosis of Syncope		
Type of Syncope	Common Causes	Prevalence in Persons ≥65	Additional Notes
Neurally mediated	• Vasovagal • Situational—defecation, urination, coughing, eating • Carotid sinus syncope	44%	• Most common cause in older adults. • Precipitating factors and prodromal symptoms are clues.
Orthostatic hypotension	• Autonomic failure from underlying disease—Parkinson's, spinal cord injury • Drug-induced—alcohol, vasodilators, diuretics, phenothiazines, antidepressants • Volume depletion	23%	• More likely to occur in the morning. • More common in older ages.
Cardiac	• Arrhythmias—bradycardia, tachycardia • Structural heart disease—valvular disease, acute infarction, hypertrophic cardiomyopathy, cardiac mass, tamponade	15%	• Presence of chest pain or dyspnea is strong clue. • Less likely to describe nausea, sweating, blurred vision, awareness of impending syncope.
Drug-induced	• Alcohol, vasodilators, diuretics, phenothiazines, antiarrhythmics, QT-prolonging drugs	5%	• Drugs can affect susceptibility to all forms of syncope.
Multifactorial		4%	• Generally thought to be more common, especially in older adults, but most studies attempt to identify one primary cause.
Unexplained		10%	
Cerebral vascular disease	• Stroke • TIA • Seizure	None in this cohort	• Reported in 3% to 32% of cases in other studies including all adults.[15]
Psychogenic	• Pseudosyncope	None in this cohort	• Reported in 1% - 7% of cases in other studies including all adults.[15]

Source: Ungar A, Mussi C, Del Rosso A, et al. for the Italian Group for the Study of Syncope in the Elderly. Diagnosis and characteristics of syncope in older patients referred to geriatric departments. J Am Geriatr Soc 2006;54(10):1531-6.
TIA, transient ischemic attack.

etiology, but given its high prevalence it can be responsible for a large burden of morbidity and mortality. Multiple contributing factors may lead to this form of syncope.

The most common type of neutrally mediated syncope is vasovagal or neurocardiogenic syncope. This typically involves prolonged standing, emotional distress, or exertion in warm environments causing the peripheral venous pooling and a drop in blood return to the heart. As the heart recognizes a sudden decrease in preload, it tries to compensate by contracting harder. The quick increase in contraction activates mechanoreceptors in the ventricles that start a reflex mechanism causing the central nervous system to stimulate vasodilation and bradycardia. As the drop in cardiac output becomes more profound, syncope may occur.[7] When suspecting a neurally mediated syncope,

look for associated symptoms of nausea and/or vomiting, and a history that includes prolonged standing, hot environments, and/or unpleasant situations. You should be cautious to not assume this diagnosis in patients with known heart disease or repetitive episodes of syncope.

Neurally mediated syncope can usually be diagnosed by history and the initial evaluation alone.

Carotid sinus syndrome is often listed as a cause of syncope.[8] This is because manual stimulation of the carotid sinus can, in susceptible individuals, stimulate neurally mediated syncope. A few individuals (e.g., wearing tight collars) have true carotid sinus syncope; however, in most cases the provocation of syncope with carotid sinus massage indicates a susceptibility to neurally mediated syncope rather than a diagnosis.

Orthostatic Hypotension

Orthostatic hypotension is a drop in arterial pressure that occurs when an individual moves to an upright position. Typically, the autonomic nervous system rapidly compensates for this by increasing the venous tone in the legs; when this system fails, syncope may occur. When the circulating blood volume is depleted, as in dehydration, orthostatic hypotension and syncope may occur even with appropriate autonomic compensation.[9] This diagnosis should be considered in individuals who are on medications that can predispose to orthostasis, who have reason because of illness or blood loss to be dehydrated, or who have autonomic insufficiency from a neurologic disorder such as parkinsonism. A typical case occurs soon after standing up or after prolonged standing in a hot, crowded environment.

The traditional definition of orthostatic hypotension is a drop in systolic blood pressure of ≥ 20 mmHg, or a drop in the diastolic pressure of ≥ 10 mmHg, 3 minutes after assuming the upright position. While this definition remains in use, numerous studies have demonstrated that syncope resulting from orthostatic cerebral hypoperfusion can occur when the standard criteria for orthostasis are not met. Three general mechanisms can lead to this orthostatic syncope (or near-syncope) that does not meet the definition of orthostatic hypotension: early orthostasis, late orthostasis, and impaired cerebral perfusion with only mild decreases in systemic blood pressure.[10] Atherosclerotic narrowing of the carotid and/or vertebral arteries may increase the susceptibility to syncope from these mechanisms.

Cardiac Syncope

Cardiac syncope occurs when cardiac function is reduced by arrhythmia, myocardial death, or outflow obstruction, leading to decreased blood flow to the brain. Several studies have shown an increase in overall mortality and sudden death among patients with cardiac syncope compared to patients with syncope from other causes.[1,11] A cardiac cause should be considered when syncope is preceded by palpitations or chest pain, or when it occurs during exertion. Patients with known severe structural heart disease should be considered to have cardiac syncope until proven otherwise.

Cerebrovascular Disease

Cerebrovascular disease is a rare but plausible cause of syncope. Most TIAs or strokes do not cause loss of consciousness, but occasionally this can occur. There is a low yield in the use of neurologic testing in the evaluation of individuals with syncope unless it is directed at those with neurologic findings on initial evaluation.[3,12]

Psychogenic Syncope

Psychiatric causes should be considered in patients with repetitive syncope of unknown origin after cardiac causes have been effectively ruled out.[13] They are more common in younger patients. Prodromal symptoms, such as dizziness, are common. Several hypotheses exist regarding the connection between psychiatric disorders and syncope. Hyperventilation can increase susceptibility to neurally mediated syncope. There is also a term called pseudosyncope, which has been used to describe patients with syncope of unknown but presumed psychiatric origin, who have no pathologic findings on examination and documented syncope without any change in blood pressure or pulse.[14]

Drug-Induced Syncope

Drugs should always be considered as a cause or contributing factor in syncope. The older population is particularly sensitive to drug effects and is more likely to take more of them. Drugs such as alcohol, vasodilators, diuretics, phenothiazines, and antidepressants may lead to orthostatic hypotension as a cause of syncope. Antiarrhythmic drugs can lead to bradycardia, and QT-prolonging drugs may lead to torsades de pointes. There are many categories of drugs that can lead to a prolonged QT interval including antiarrhythmics, vasodilators, psychotropics, antimicrobials, nonsedating antihistamines, and methadone.[3]

CASE 1

Lucia (Part 2)

Lucia is lying on the examination table and appears comfortable, but tired. She is sipping water. She tells you that she "just got too emotional." Her initial vital signs were a pulse of 105 and a blood pressure of 122/76 with no significant difference between the supine and upright positions. The other vital signs were normal. Your nurse has already placed an intravenous line and administered 1 liter of normal saline at your request. You recheck Lucia's pulse and notice that it is down to the 80s and regular.

You find no abnormalities on Lucia's exam, including a comprehensive cardiac and neurologic exam. She is alert and well oriented. There are no signs of trauma from her fall. Her ECG shows normal sinus rhythm at 90 beats per minute, no conduction delays, and no signs of ischemia.

1. **Based on the history, physical examination, and ECG, what other testing is warranted?**

2. **Are there any new findings that make you think Lucia is at high risk for cardiac syncope?**

3. **Can you diagnose the cause of Lucia's syncope?**

4. **Will you hospitalize Lucia?** ▣

CASE 2

George (Part 2)

Upon entering the examination room, you find George sitting in his chair chatting with his friend and looking comfortable. He is fully alert and oriented. His vital signs are normal, including blood pressure in the supine and upright positions. There are no signs of trauma and his head, neck, and pulmonary examinations are normal. The cardiovascular examination is reassuring, with normal heart sounds, no murmur, and a regular rhythm. Carotid arteries are without bruits, and a comprehensive neurologic exam is negative.

The ECG reveals a heart rate of 72 beats per minute with a regular rhythm. Changes from his previous ECG include signs of left ventricular hypertrophy and a new left bundle branch block.

1. **What is the differential diagnosis for the etiology of George's syncope?**

2. **Based on the history and examination, what further testing is warranted?**

3. **What findings indicate that George is at increased risk of syncope caused by cardiac arrhythmia?**

4. **Does George need any additional neurologic workup, such as computed tomography (CT) or magnetic resonance imaging (MRI) of the brain, or electroencephalography?**

5. **Will you hospitalize George?** ▣

EVALUATION

The evaluation of the patient with syncope involves the parallel process of seeking a specific diagnosis and ruling out cardiac causes that are associated with a higher risk of sudden death. This can be done by taking a careful history, conducting a focused examination, and obtaining an ECG. However, patients without a diagnosis but who are at high risk of having cardiac disease should have additional studies (Table 22-2).

> All syncope evaluations should begin with a detailed history, examination, and ECG.

TABLE 22-2	Diagnostic Evaluation of Syncope		
Diagnostic	**Evidence Classification***	**Notes**	
History, physical exam, and electrocardiogram as initial evaluation on all patients	B	Electrocardiogram can be diagnostic; also used to risk-stratify for cardiac disease.	
Evaluation for orthostatic hypotension when suspected	B	Blood pressure measured supine and during active standing for 3 minutes.	
Carotid sinus massage	B	Recommended by European Guidelines for patients older than 40 after an initial negative evaluation.	
Tilt-table testing	B	To evaluate unexplained syncope in high-risk settings (occupational) or for recurrent syncope after cardiac causes ruled out.	
Electrocardiographic monitoring	B	When initial evaluation is suggestive but not diagnostic of arrhythmia as the etiology. Setting of monitoring chosen based on risk.	
Electrophysiologic study	B	For patients with known ischemic heart disease when arrhythmia is suspected. Not indicated if there is already an indication for a defibrillator.	
Echocardiography	B	To evaluate suspected structural heart disease or risk-stratify.	
Exercise testing	C	When syncope occurs during or soon after exercise.	
Psychiatric evaluation	C	When psychogenic cause is suspected.	
Neurological evaluation	B	Not recommended for routine evaluation of true syncopal event. Use only if history and exam suggests neurologic cause such as stroke or seizure.	

Source: Moya A, Sutton R, Ammirati F, et al. Task Force for the Diagnosis and Management of Syncope. Guidelines for the diagnosis and management of syncope (version 2009). Eur Heart J 2009;30(21):2631-71.

*Evidence classification: A = Consistent, good-quality patient-oriented evidence; B = Inconsistent or limited-quality patient-oriented evidence; C = Consensus, disease-oriented evidence, usual practice, expert opinion, or case series.

Historically diagnostic testing for syncopal events has been applied inconsistently and up to 34% of evaluations did not result in an etiology.[15] Through the use of guidelines and algorithms, the amount of undiagnosed syncope may drop to closer to 10% of cases.[6]

History and Physical Examination

A meticulous history and physical examination are inarguably the foundation of any syncope evaluation. Questions should help the clinician gain an understanding of the circumstances and symptoms that were present before, during, and after the attack, including association with position, particular situations, or activity. Witnesses of the syncopal event should also be questioned. The history alone can often diagnose syncope that is neurally mediated (vasovagal), caused by orthostasis, or drug-induced. Important aspects of the past medical history include a history of cardiac disease, neurologic disease, of metabolic disorder, a medication history, and an inquiry into recent ingestion of alcohol and nonprescription drugs. A comprehensive physical examination may provide clues to the presence of cardiac disease, underlying neurologic disorder, or vascular disease.

Assessing for Orthostatic Hypotension

To test for orthostatic hypotension, have the patient lie supine for 3 minutes, after which the blood pressure and pulse are checked. Then have the patient stand for 3 minutes, during which the pulse and blood pressure are monitored. Orthostatic hypotension is said to be present if the patient experiences a drop of at least 20 mmHg in systolic blood pressure or at least 10 mmHg in diastolic blood pressure within 3 minutes after standing from the recumbent position. This can also be demonstrated using the tilt table in the head-up position at a minimum 60-degree angle.

Multiple variables can affect the blood pressure readings, including the time of day, ambient temperature, postural deconditioning, and medications. Some patients may not show the diagnostic drop in blood pressure until they have been standing for at least 10 minutes. For these reasons it is important to repeatedly check for a significant orthostatic blood pressure reduction while keeping in mind when medications are taken, time of meals, and any other factors that may have contributed to the syncopal episode. Many patients who demonstrate a significant drop in blood pressure after standing will also have an increase in pulse rate, but it is not necessary for the diagnosis of orthostasis.

> **Always consider medications as a possible contributing factor.**

Ruling Out Cardiac Causes

Structural heart disease, defined as coronary heart disease, congestive heart failure, valvular disease, or

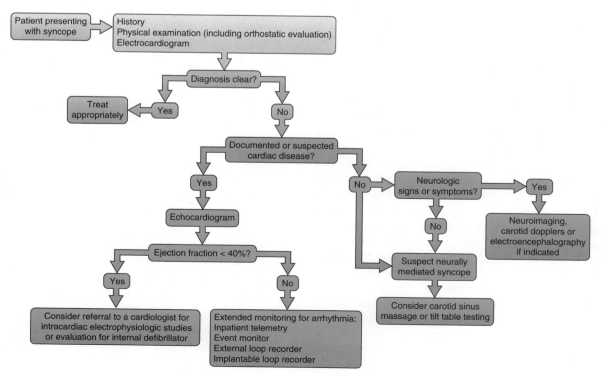

Figure 22-2 Syncope evaluation algorithm.

congenital heart disease, is the only independent risk factor for a cardiac cause of syncope. ECGs and echocardiograms may not be diagnostic in many cases, but they can stratify patients' risk by identifying who has structural heart disease. The intensity of the cardiac rule-out evaluation depends on the patient's risk status and the history of the event.

The ECG is an inexpensive and noninvasive test that can diagnose some cases of syncope and guide further testing in others. In a review of six inpatient and outpatient studies involving 1110 people with syncope, electrocardiography diagnosed only 5% of the cases, mostly arrythmias.[15] More important, the ECG is excellent at identifying who has structural heart disease. Abnormal findings include signs of previous myocardial infarction (i.e., Q waves or inverted T waves), bundle branch block, evidence of ventricular hypertrophy, atrioventricular blocks, bradycardias or tachycardias, premature ventricular contractions, pacemaker spikes, or significant ST abnormalities.[5,11,16] Patients with syncope and any of these ECG abnormalities should receive cardiac testing, whereas there is poor diagnostic yield from further cardiac testing of patients with a normal ECG and no cardiac history.

Patients with a cardiac history or abnormal ECG should have an echocardiogram if the etiology of syncope is still unknown after the initial history and physical examination. Similar to the ECG, echocardiography will diagnose a few rare causes of syncope such as critical aortic stenosis, myxoma, or tamponade. Additionally, the systolic function (i.e., ejection fraction) can be used as a marker of risk for arrhythmia. An ejection fraction of 40% or less places a patient at significantly higher risk of arrhythmia.[16]

The continued search for arrhythmia in patients with undiagnosed syncope may include in-hospital telemetry monitoring, 24- or 48-hour Holter monitoring, external loop recorders, and implantable loop recorders. These should be reserved for the select group of patients with unexplained syncope who are at increased risk for arrhythmia based on history and initial workup. The generalized use of these studies is inefficient and expensive. The finding of arrhythmia correlating with syncope or syncopal events without arrhythmia is both prognostically important and should be considered a successful test. The implantable loop recorder deserves special mention because it can be used for up to 36 months after implantation, increasing the likelihood of identifying another syncopal event. It can store data for 20 minutes prior to activation, allowing patients or their companions a longer time window to activate the device.[17]

Cardiac stress testing is rarely diagnostic in the evaluation of syncope. It should be considered in patients who have syncope during or after exercise or who experience chest pain associated with syncope.[3] These select patients may show cardiac ischemia or arrhythmias associated with exercise.

Intracardiac electrophysiologic studies are invasive and very expensive. They should be reserved for patients with known structural heart disease who have very high risk for arrhythmias because of depressed ventricular function. This will most likely include patients with previous myocardial infarction. In this procedure catheters are inserted from the femoral vein into the heart near the electrical conduction system. Atrial and ventricular pacing along with electrical stimulation are used to assess sinus node recovery time, sinoatrial conduction time, and atrioventricular node function. This allows detection of conduction abnormalities that can predispose to arrhythmia.[3,5,18]

CASE 2

George (Part 3)

Concerned that a cardiac arrhythmia may have caused George's syncope, you hospitalize him for cardiac monitoring and further risk stratification. The LVH and bundle branch block on the ECG, combined with his history of multiple cardiac risk factors, place him at high risk of having coronary heart disease and therefore of arrhythmia. His medication list is also worrisome because it contains drugs that could contribute to hypotension, electrolyte imbalances, and dizziness. A reflex-mediated situational syncope from swallowing is unlikely because George had no prodromal symptoms. The reassuring neurologic examination and lack of postictal symptoms eliminate the need for further neurologic testing at this time.

An echocardiogram shows an ejection fraction of approximately 40% with mild hypokinesis of the left ventricle and trace mitral valve regurgitation. You have George do a stress treadmill test along with the echocardiogram to make sure there is no reversible ischemia. George is able to exercise to about 80% of his maximum heart rate, but has to stop before goal because of fatigue. However, there are no signs of ischemia on the ECG or echocardiogram. George's serum sodium, potassium, chloride, blood urea nitrogen, creatinine, and magnesium are all within normal limits. His cardiac enzymes are also normal.

By this time George has been in the hospital for almost 24 hours on telemetry without event. You explain to George that you think he probably had a myocardial infarction at some point in the past couple years, and you are worried that he passed out from a cardiac arrhythmia. You decide to discharge him home with a 30-day event monitor and arrange for an appointment with a cardiologist. He is not to drive in the interim.

1. **What evidence do you have to make you more concerned about a cardiac arrhythmia?**

2. **What are your options to further investigate for a cardiac arrhythmia?**

3. **How do you defend your decision to hospitalize George? Could all of this have been done as an outpatient?** ▣

Evaluation for Neurally Mediated Syncope

Many cases of neurally mediated syncope will be diagnosed by the initial evaluation alone, based on a classic history. When the etiology of syncope is unknown and the syncopal events have become repetitive or dangerous, tilt table testing and carotid massage can be useful as confirmatory tests. It is important that cardiac syncope be effectively ruled out by prolonged cardiac monitoring if there is known or suspected cardiac disease.

Tilt table testing evaluates whether a patient is susceptible to neurally mediated syncope.[3,5] There are multiple protocols for tilt table testing, some including the use of drugs such as isoproterenol or nitroglycerin to increase susceptibility to syncope and improve the sensitivity of the test. The procedure involves baseline measurement of blood pressure and heart rate while supine, then quickly bringing the patient to an upright position by tilting to approximately 60 degrees. A foot board is in place for support. The patient is then kept in the tilted position for 45 minutes to observe for syncope or presyncopal symptoms while continuing to monitor heart rate and blood pressure. Some protocols include giving isoproterenol or nitroglycerin after the patient has been asymptomatic in the tilted position for 10 to 15 minutes, followed by further monitoring. If syncope symptoms occur during testing and correlate with a quick drop in blood pressure or pulse rate, it is considered a positive test. Likewise, if syncope occurs without a change in vital signs, a neurally mediated syncope is less likely and other etiologies should be considered. Arguments against the use of tilt table testing include variable sensitivity of the procedure, questionable diagnostic yield, and reproducibility of the test.[18]

Standardized carotid sinus massage (CSM) in the supine and upright positions can help differentiate carotid sinus syndrome, or carotid sinus hypersensitivity, another risk factor for neurally mediated syncope. The carotid sinus is located in the common carotid artery at the branching point of the internal and external branches. There are baroreceptors in the carotid sinuses that respond to changes in pressure. These, via nerve centers in the brain stem, stimulate the vagus nerve, causing inhibition of the sinus node of the heart or a reduction in blood pressure.[19] A positive cardioinhibitory result is present if a cardiac pause (asystole) of 3 seconds or longer occurs during or immediately after CSM; a positive vasopressor result is present if the systolic blood pressure drops 50 mmHg or more and is accompanied by symptoms.[20] This procedure requires continuous heart rate monitoring, frequent blood pressure monitoring, intravenous access, and the availability of atropine and transcutaneous pacing.

The presence of carotid bruits or known atherosclerotic disease of the carotids is a contraindication to the procedure.

Neurologic Evaluation

Neuroimaging and electroencephalography (EEG) have been used frequently in the routine workup of patients with unexplained syncope. Retrospective reviews have shown them to have a poor yield and high cost when used on unselected patients. In a review of 649 cases of syncope, 253 patients received EEG testing, and only six had abnormal results that explained the cause of syncope (i.e., a yield of 2%). All six of those patients had a history and physical examination that was consistent with seizure. In the same group, 283 patients had brain CT scanning, also with a yield of 2%; all had a history and examination consistent with acute stroke. Carotid Dopplers were done in 185 patients, with a 0% yield.[21] As a result, published recommendations for syncope evaluation limit neuroimaging and EEG testing to patients with symptoms or signs of acute stroke or seizure.[3]

Psychiatric Evaluation

Clues to a psychiatric origin include a history of anxiety or depression, repetitive syncope of unknown origin, a repeatedly negative cardiac workup, and multiple episodes of syncope without injury. In patients with suspected psychiatric disease, consulting with a psychiatrist is important both to identify or rule out a psychiatric diagnosis and to review the potential psychotropic effects of medications. Tilt table testing can also be helpful, because, if syncope is provoked, the physician can readily differentiate psychogenic (i.e., with no blood pressure or pulse changes) from neurally mediated syncope.[11,22]

CASE 1

Lucia (Part 3)

The history of Lucia's syncopal event is confirmed by her husband and daughter. They explain that Lucia had been standing in the sun for over an hour even though they had encouraged her to take a rest in the shade. It had been a long day, full of excitement and emotion, in the hot sun, and possibly with a glass or two of champagne. The bride and groom were just getting ready to leave the reception when Lucia passed out. This confirms your theory that Lucia most likely experienced a situational neurally mediated syncope. You have her get up and walk around, making sure that she feels steady on her feet. Then you send her home with her family with instructions to drink plenty of fluids and follow up with her primary physician within a week. ■

George (Part 3)

Two days later, George's wife calls you after he passed out again briefly while working in the yard. You are able to get the report from the event monitor and it shows that George had 30 seconds of ventricular tachycardia. You have George readmitted to the hospital immediately where an implantable cardiac defibrillator is inserted the following day. ◼

MANAGEMENT

Management of syncope involves first deciding on the appropriate setting for evaluation when not clear from your initial evaluation. The initial evaluation helps to estimate the patient's short-term risk of a severe event, including death. Patients without an established diagnosis of their syncopal event and with known or suspected cardiac disease are at high risk of death or a serious event and should be hospitalized for immediate evaluation. Others must be triaged based on risk factors. Numerous studies have looked at decision rules using age, history, symptoms, vital signs, laboratory results, and ECG results, among others, to help decide when patients should be hospitalized after presenting for evaluation of a syncopal event. The criteria most commonly cited are an abnormal ECG, shortness of breath, heart failure, abnormal vital signs, and older age.[23] Table 22-3 lists the symptoms or signs of heart disease that should prompt hospitalization.

> Consider hospitalization to evaluate patients with a high likelihood of cardiac syncope.

First-time syncope in patients without known or suspected heart disease usually warrants the reduction of risk factors for further syncope. This includes reducing polypharmacy and medication misuse, treating underlying illness, and education regarding avoidance of triggers. Further treatment for patients with recurrent

TABLE 22-3	Criteria That Suggest Cardiac Etiology of Syncope That Should Prompt Hospitalization[3,23,28]
Syncope while supine	
Syncope during exertion	
Palpitations prior to syncope	
Family history of sudden cardiac death	
History of previous myocardial infarction	
Low ejection fraction	
Signs of heart failure	
Abnormal ECG	
Systolic blood pressure <90 mmHg	

syncope or syncope in high-risk settings requires knowledge of the underlying mechanism of the syncopal event (i.e., type and cause of syncope).[24]

Treatment of Neurally Mediated Syncope

Lifestyle measures are the basis for treatment of reflex syncope. Awareness of the cause of the event and prodromal symptoms allow avoidance of triggers and possible prevention by abortive maneuvers. Education should also include information on drugs, including alcohol, that may increase susceptibility to syncope events. Physical counterpressure maneuvers can help increase blood pressure when prodromal symptoms occur; these include squatting, leg crossing, and hand gripping with arm tensing.[25] These isometric exercises can be taught easily to willing and functional patients to help them avoid or delay syncope. The exercises will be less useful in frail older adults.

Treatment of Orthostatic Hypotension

Treatment should begin with discontinuation of drugs that may be leading to orthostatic changes. Education about lifestyle changes can also make a significant difference in raising the standing blood pressure and preventing syncope. Increased intake of salt and fluids—including 2 to 3 liters of fluid and 10 grams of sodium per day—can help when cardiac disease or hypertension is not a contraindication.[26] The physical counterpressure maneuvers described in the previous section can also be used if prodromal symptoms occur. Abdominal binders and compression stockings can be worn regularly to decrease venous pooling in the legs and help prevent drops in standing blood pressure. Sleeping with the head elevated more than 10 degrees can help reduce nighttime polyuria, therefore increasing fluid volume.[3]

Two drugs, fludrocortisone and midodrine, have been show to be helpful in patients when lifestyle changes alone have not helped. They both work by increasing blood pressure and have been shown to prevent syncope from orthostatic hypotension. Midodrine works as an α-agonist to increase blood pressure. Fludrocortisone is a mineralocorticoid that expands fluid volume through its effect on the kidneys.

Treatment of Cardiac Syncope

Patients with syncope related to structural cardiac disease should have disease-specific interventions. Underlying disease such as acute myocardial infarction, pericardial tamponade, or aortic stenosis should receive appropriate therapy. Treatment of arrhythmias should be targeted to the cause. As in all types of syncope, drugs that may contribute should be discontinued when possible.

Cardiac defibrillators, catheter ablation, cardiac pacing, and antiarrhythmic drug therapy are additional treatment options.

Implantation of a cardiac defibrillator is indicated when syncope is caused by ventricular tachycardia or fibrillation and structural heart disease is present.[27] Severely depressed left ventricular ejection fraction alone, even without documented ventricular tachycardia, is also an indication for defibrillator placement. Unfortunately, patients are still at risk for recurrent syncope after defibrillator placement, but their risk of sudden cardiac death diminishes.

Catheter ablation should be considered in patients with syncope related to superventricular tachycardia or ventricular tachycardia when there is no structural heart disease. Some cases of rapid atrial fibrillation may also be treated with catheter ablation. Antiarrhythmic drugs include rate-controlling and rhythm-controlling drugs; they are used when catheter ablation fails and as first-line treatment in many cases of atrial fibrillation.

Cardiac pacemaker placement is indicated in the presence of syncope that has been correlated with bradycardia caused by sinus node disease. It should also be considered in patients with syncope who are found on monitoring to have asymptomatic pauses of ≥3 seconds, second-degree Mobitz II block, or complete atrioventricular block. Patients with bundle branch block who have abnormal electrophysiologic testing may also benefit from pacemaker placement.

Treating Other Causes of Syncope

As noted previously, cerebrovascular disease is an uncommon cause of true syncope. When it does occur, treatment should be directed to the underlying disease, such as stroke. Psychogenic causes of syncope necessitate psychiatric evaluation and help with treatment. Explanation of the psychological cause and acknowledgment that the syncopal acts are involuntary can help the patient accept the possibility of the diagnosis. This is important to make referral for treatment successful.[3]

CASE 1

Discussion

Lucia's case was fairly straightforward because of the circumstance of her event and her uncomplicated past medical history. After her initial medical history, examination, and ECG, you do not think the syncope is related to medications and you are fairly certain that she is at low risk for cardiac syncope. You believe that she was probably dehydrated from standing in the sun, and that a glass or two of champagne may have impaired her venous tone. As she became overheated and overcome by emotion, she was at risk for neurally mediated syncope.

The nausea she experienced prior to passing out is consistent with this explanation.

The lack of cardiac or neurologic findings on examination was reassuring. She had no signs or symptoms of trauma that would necessitate radiographic evaluation. Her slower pulse rate after receiving some fluids again suggest she was dehydrated. The normal ECG along with no history of heart disease and a recently normal echocardiogram convince you that she does not have structural heart disease that would put her at increased risk for cardiac syncope. Therefore, you feel confident diagnosing Lucia with situational syncope and sending her home with her family.

If similar syncopal events become a reoccurring problem for Lucia, you could consider tilt table testing to confirm your suspicion of her susceptibility to neurally mediated syncope. Educating her on prodromal symptoms and situations associated with neurally mediated syncope may help avoid injury. ◘

CASE 2

Discussion

George's case presents an example of syncope that cannot be diagnosed by history, examination, and electrocardiography alone. You should be concerned about cardiac syncope from the beginning after hearing about the sudden nature of his syncope and the lack of prodromal symptoms. Other red flags from George's history include his medical history that puts him at high risk of cardiac disease, and his medications. The abnormal ECG provides additional evidence that cardiac causes should be considered. The echocardiogram helps to risk-stratify George because his low ejection fraction is an additional risk factor for arrhythmia.

In this case, cardiac stress testing is not done as part of the syncope workup but to further investigate the new diagnosis of cardiac disease. If you already knew about George's cardiac disease and abnormal ECG, then the echocardiogram and cardiac monitoring would have been sufficient.

Hospitalization was warranted for George because of the high suspicion of cardiac syncope and the need to further evaluate his cardiac disease. On discharge, George had a support system in place and would always have someone around who could call for help and activate the event monitor if he became symptomatic again. Finally, do not forget to think of safety issues such as driving, flying, operating heavy machinery, and risk of injury from falls. ◘

SUMMARY

The multifactorial nature of syncope in older individuals makes it a challenging problem to diagnose and treat. For many patients, the etiology of syncope will never be clear. A directed approach to evaluating syncope after an initial history, physical examination, and ECG is well described. The future may bring increased use of algorithms and dedicated syncope units that will more efficiently risk-stratify patients with syncope and guide appropriate testing. This could reduce excessive use of resources, prevent hospitalizations, and help to more quickly diagnose a frustrating problem.

KEY REFERENCES

3. Moya A, Sutton R, Ammirati F, et al. Task Force for the Diagnosis and Management of Syncope. Guidelines for the diagnosis and management of syncope (version 2009). Eur Heart J 2009;30(21):2631-71.
6. Ungar A, Mussi C, Del Rosso A, et al. for the Italian Group for the Study of Syncope in the Elderly. Diagnosis and characteristics of syncope in older patients referred to geriatric departments. J Am Geriatr Soc 2006;54(10):1531-6.
12. Strickberger SA, Benson DW, Biaggioni I, et al. AHA/ACCF scientific statement on the evaluation of syncope: from the American Heart Association Councils on Clinical Cardiology, Cardiovascular Nursing, Cardiovascular Disease in the Young, and Stroke, and the Quality of Care and Outcomes Research Interdisciplinary Working Group; and the American College of Cardiology Foundation in Collaboration with the Heart Rhythm Society. J Am Coll Cardiol 2006;47(2):473-84.
15. Linzer M, Yang EH, Estes NA 3rd, et al. Diagnosing syncope. Part 1: Value of history, physical examination, and electrocardiography. Clinical Efficacy Assessment Project of the American College of Physicians. Ann Intern Med 1997;126(12):989-96.
23. Kessler C, Tristano JM, De Lorenzo R. The emergency department approach to syncope: Evidence-based guidelines and prediction rules. Emerg Med Clin North Am 2010;28(3):487-500.

References available online at expertconsult.com.

23

Urinary Incontinence

Catherine E. DuBeau

OBJECTIVES

Upon completion of this chapter, the reader will be able to:

- Discuss the prevalence and impact of urinary incontinence (UI) in older persons.
- Describe the impact of medical conditions and medications on continence.
- Perform an initial evaluation of incontinence in an older person.
- Develop and implement an initial patient-centered treatment plan for incontinence addressing multifactorial causes and tailored to the older person's goals of care.

Urinary incontinence (UI), the complaint of involuntary leakage of urine,[1] is one of the major geriatric syndromes. UI may be accompanied by other lower urinary tract symptoms (Table 23-1).

Additional online-only material indicated by icon.

PREVALENCE AND IMPACT

UI becomes more common with advanced age in both men and women, but is not a normal part of aging. Among women, the prevalence of UI is 15% to 30% in the community,[2] 50% among the homebound, and 70% in nursing home residents.[3]

In men, the prevalence is about one third that of women until age 85, when the ratio becomes 1:1. The prevalence of moderate to severe UI (at least weekly or monthly leakage of more than just drops) is 23% among women aged 60 to 79 years and 32% in those 80 and older.[3] Among nursing home residents, prevalence rates range from 43% to 77% (median 58%).[3] UI severity (i.e., frequency and volume of leakage) also increases with age.[4] In a significant number of affected individuals, UI severity will increase if not treated. One third of middle-aged and younger-old women (aged 54 to 79 years) with baseline UI once monthly progressed to leaking at least once a week over 2 years.[5] Little is known specifically about the incidence and severity of UI over time in older men. The most common type of UI in older persons is urgency UI[6]; however, the prevalence of stress UI in men is rising with increased surgical treatment of prostate cancer. The evidence is inconsistent whether race and ethnicity are associated with UI prevalence in older women,[7,8] and there are no data on their impact in older men.

> UI becomes more common with advanced age in both men and women, but is not a normal part of aging.

UI decreases health-related quality of life, with a negative impact on self-esteem, self-perception of aging, activities, and sexuality.[9] In older persons, the impact appears greatest in the area of coping with embarrassment with subsequent activity interference, rather than directly precluding activities.[10] Among frail nursing home residents, UI adversely impacts social interactions, an important aspect of quality of life in this setting.[11]

Persons with UI are at risk for urinary tract infections, skin breakdown, falls, and fractures. Associated caregiver burden can lead to depression and is associated with nursing home placement. Approximately 6% to 10% of nursing home admissions in the United States are attributable to UI.[12] Economic costs are significant for the individual and the health care system (nearly $20 billion in 2000),[13] and have nearly doubled for older persons in the last decade.[14] Unfortunately, the majority of the expenses (56%)

TABLE 23-1	Lower Urinary Tract Symptoms (LUTS)
Symptom	Description
Urinary incontinence	Involuntary leakage of urine.
Urgency	Compelling, often sudden need to void that is difficult to defer.
Urgency incontinence	Leakage preceded by/associated with urgency. Common precipitants include running water, hand washing, going out in the cold, even the sight of the garage or trying to unlock the door when returning home. The need to "rush to the toilet" and length of time one can forestall an urgency episode are less useful symptoms because they reflect cognition, mobility, toilet availability, and sphincter control as well as bladder function.
Stress incontinence	Leakage with effort, exertion, sneezing, or coughing. Leakage may be provoked by minimal or no activity when there is severe sphincter damage. Leakage coincident with cough, laugh, sneeze, or physical activity suggests failure of sphincter mechanisms. Leakage that occurs seconds after the activity, especially if difficult to stop, suggests a cough-induced uninhibited detrusor contraction.
Mixed incontinence	Presence of both urgency and stress UI symptoms. Patients vary in the predominance, severity, and/or bother of urge versus stress leakage.
Overactive bladder	Symptom syndrome (not a specific pathologic condition) consisting of urgency, frequency, and nocturia, with or without urge incontinence.
Frequency	Complaint of needing to void too often during the day, as defined by the patient.
Nocturia	Complaint of waking at night one or more times to void. If these voids are associated with UI, the term *nocturnal enuresis* may be used.
Slow (weak) stream	Perception of reduced urine flow, usually compared to previous performance.
Hesitancy	Difficulty in initiating voiding, resulting in a delay in the onset of voiding after the individual feels ready to pass urine.
Straining	Muscular effort either to initiate, maintain, or improve the urinary stream.
Intermittent stream	Sensation that the bladder is not empty after voiding.
Postvoid dribbling	Small amounts/drops of urine after voiding has stopped. More common in men.

UI, urinary incontinence.

are consequence costs (e.g., from nursing home admissions and loss of productivity). Treatment and diagnosis account for approximately one third of costs. Out-of-pocket expenses, predominantly for protective undergarments, have been estimated to run from $750 to $900 yearly, or almost 1% of the median annual household income.[15,16]

Optimal management of UI is hampered by the fact that at least half of persons with UI never mention it to their care providers, and in turn physicians often do not ask patients about it or fail to offer specific treatment.

CASE 1

Anna Roberts (Part 1)

Anna Roberts, a 78-year-old woman, returns to see you for follow-up of congestive heart failure. She has gained 4 lbs, has increased pedal edema, and complains of being fatigued and is not sleeping well. You review the status of her hypertension, hyperlipidemia, diabetes, and recent laboratory work. Her medications include lisinopril, amlodipine, furosemide, aspirin, atorvastatin, metformin, glipizide, and calcium with vitamin D. When asked about the weight gain, the patient admits to occasionally skipping

doses of furosemide when she is going out for the day for fear of wetting herself.

1. **What factors increase the risk for incontinence in Ms. Roberts?**
2. **What other information is needed to evaluate her symptoms?** ▪

> UI in older persons is multifactorial, resulting from interactions between lower urinary tract abnormalities, neurologic control of voiding, multimorbidity, and functional impairment.

RISK FACTORS AND PATHOPHYSIOLOGY

Risk factors for UI in older persons reflect the multifactorial nature of the problem. UI shares common risk factors with other geriatric syndromes (e.g., falls and functional dependence), including lower and upper extremity weakness, sensory and affective impairment,[17] and radiologic evidence of white matter signal abnormalities suggesting common etiologic pathways.[18] Along with age and functional impairment, the main risk factors for UI are female gender, obesity (women) diabetes, stroke, depression, fecal incontinence, and hysterectomy.[19-23] Nursing home residents with UI are more likely than continent residents to have impaired mobility, dementia, delirium, and receive psychoactive medications.[9] Parity increases the risk of UI in younger women but the impact attenuates with age. Although there is some evidence for a familial predisposition to UI,[24] this may not be a significant risk factor in older persons.

UI is common in persons with cognitive impairment, which is associated with a 1.5- to 3.5-fold increase in UI risk,[25] especially for bothersome UI.[26] At the same time, UI is not inevitable even in frail cognitively impaired persons, because the association between cognitive impairment and UI is at least in part mediated by functional impairment and disability.[27]

The pathophysiology of UI in older persons is multifactorial, resulting from interactions between lower urinary tract abnormalities, neurologic control of voiding, multimorbidity, and functional impairment. The lower urinary tract has two main functions, storage of urine and effective voiding. Key components of the bladder for continence are its detrusor smooth muscle and epithelial layer (the urothelium). Continence is mediated through the actions of the central and autonomic nervous systems (Figure 23-1).[28] Storage occurs through sympathetic stimulation of alpha-adrenergic receptors in the smooth muscle sphincter causing contraction, and beta-adrenergic receptors in the detrusor causing relaxation. Voiding occurs with parasympathetic stimulation of muscarinic receptors in the detrusor. The urothelium has rich and varied receptor signaling systems that conduct information about bladder filling and sensation through the sacral spinal cord to pontine and subcortical areas.[29] The prefrontal cortex is an important center for suppressing urgency and forestalling voiding.[30] The micturition center in the pons coordinates the cortical inhibitory inputs with the afferent signaling from the detrusor to allow storage of a large volume of urine at a low pressure, and adequate bladder emptying through detrusor contraction and sphincter relaxation.[28] Maintenance of urethral closure during storage is augmented by support by fascia and the levator ani.[31]

Very importantly, UI in older persons can be precipitated or worsened by factors outside of the lower urinary tract, including the following[19]:
- Mobility
- Environment (access to toilets)
- Medical conditions (Table 23-2)
- Medications (Table 23-3)
- Mentation
- Manual dexterity
- Motivation

There are three main types of UI:
- Urgency—leakage associated with a compelling, often sudden, need to void
- Stress—leakage associated with coughing, laughing, activity
- Mixed—both urgency and stress leakage

UI associated with impaired bladder emptying ("overflow" incontinence) is uncommon even among frail older persons and men with benign prostate disease.[19] Overactive bladder (OAB) is a syndrome defined by the symptom of urgency, usually with frequency and nocturia, with or without urgency incontinence.[1] Detrusor hyperactivity with impaired contractility (DHIC) is a type of urgency UI seen in frail patients, in which there is a concomitant elevated postvoiding residual volume (PVR).[32]

CASE 1

Anna Roberts (Part 2)

On further questioning, Ms. Roberts says that when she takes her "water pill" she "can't make it to the bathroom on time." She is wearing adult diapers, which she changes at least once during the day. She reports having to go to the bathroom at least three times during the night, which is affecting her sleep. She has no leakage when she coughs, denies dysuria, but reports more constipation lately. Her diabetic control has been good.

1. **What type of incontinence does this patient have?**

2. **What additional evaluation and testing are needed before recommending therapy?** ◘

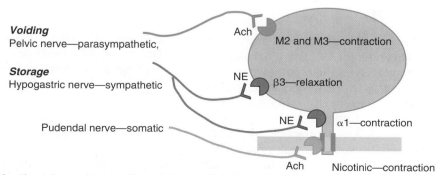

Figure 23-1 Physiology of micturition. Ach, acetylcholine; M, muscarinic; NE, norepinephrine.

TABLE 23-2	Medical Conditions Associated with Urinary Incontinence
Condition	**Effect on Continence**
Cardiovascular disease	
• Arteriovascular disease	Detrusor underactivity or areflexia from ischemic myopathy or neuropathy
• Heart failure	Nocturnal polyuria
Gastrointestinal disease	Impaired emptying/urinary from constipation; fecal and urinary incontinence commonly coexist
Metabolic diseases	
• Diabetes mellitus	Uninhibited bladder contractions (DO) with UUI; detrusor underactivity caused by neuropathy osmotic diuresis; altered mental status from hyper- or hypoglycemia; retention and overflow from constipation
• Hypercalcemia	Diuresis; altered mental status
• Vitamin B_{12} deficiency	Impaired bladder sensation and detrusor underactivity from peripheral neuropathy
Musculoskeletal disease	Mobility impairment; DO with UUI from cervical myelopathy in rheumatoid arthritis and osteoarthritis
Neurologic conditions	
• Cerebrovascular disease, stroke	DO with UUI from damage to upper motor neurons; impaired sensation to void from interruption of subcortical pathways; impaired function and cognition
• Delirium	Impaired function and cognition
• Dementia	DO with UUI from damage to upper motor neurons; impaired function and cognition
• Multiple sclerosis	DO, UUI, areflexia, or sphincter dyssynergia (concomitant sphincter and detrusor contraction), depending on level of spinal cord/CNS involvement
• Normal-pressure hydrocephalus	DO with UUI from compression of frontal inhibitory centers; impaired function and cognition
• Parkinson's disease	DO with UUI from loss of inhibitory inputs to pontine micturition center; impaired function and cognition; retention from constipation
• Spinal cord injury	DO with UUI, areflexia, or sphincter dyssynergia (depending on level of injury)
• Spinal stenosis	DO with UUI from damage to detrusor upper motor neurons (cervical stenosis); DO or areflexia (lumbar stenosis)
Obstructive sleep apnea	Nocturnal polyuria
Peripheral venous insufficiency	Nocturnal polyuria
Pulmonary disease	Conditions with chronic cough can worsen stress UI
Psychiatric disease	
• Affective and anxiety disorders	Decreased motivation
• Alcoholism	Functional and cognitive impairment; rapid diuresis and retention in acute intoxication
• Psychosis	Functional and cognitive impairment; decreased motivation

Adapted from DuBeau CE. Urinary incontinence. In:Durso SC, Sullivan GM, eds. Geriatrics Review Syllabus: A Core Curriculum in Geriatric Medicine, 8th ed. New York, NY: American Geriatrics Society; 2013, p 246.
CNS, central nervous system; *DO*, detrusor overactivity; *UI*, Urinary incontinence; *UUI*, urgency urinary incontinence.

DIFFERENTIAL DIAGNOSIS AND ASSESSMENT

Figure 23-2 provides an outline of diagnosis and assessment of UI. Active screening for UI in all older women is strongly recommended, given the high prevalence of UI and known quality gaps in treatment; screening for UI has been incorporated into health care quality process measures such as those from the Assessing Care of the Vulnerable Elderly (ACOVE) project.[33] Suggested screening questions are: "Do you ever leak urine/water when you don't want to? Do you ever leak urine on the way to the bathroom? Do you ever use pads, tissue, or cloth in your underwear to catch urine?"[34,35] Screening can be done by clinical staff and patient questionnaires.

> Acute onset of UI and the presence of suprapubic, lower abdominal, and/or pelvic pain are red flags for underlying neurologic or neoplastic disease, and should prompt quick referral.

Once a patient acknowledges UI, the next step is to characterize and determine the type of UI symptoms (see Table 23-1), including the frequency and volume of leakage. A proxy for the latter can be the

TABLE 23-3	Medications Associated with Urinary Incontinence
Medication	**Effect on Continence**
Alcohol	Frequency, urgency, sedation, delirium, immobility
α-Adrenergic agonists	Outlet obstruction (men)
α-Adrenergic blockers	Stress leakage (women)
ACE inhibitors	Associated cough worsens stress and possibly urgency leakage in older adults with impaired sphincter function
Anticholinergics	Impaired emptying, retention, delirium, sedation, constipation, fecal impaction
Antipsychotics	Anticholinergic effects plus rigidity and immobility
Calcium channel blockers	Impaired detrusor contractility and retention; dihydropyridine agents can cause pedal edema, leading to nocturnal polyuria
Cholinesterase inhibitors	Urinary incontinence; potential interactions with antimuscarinics
Estrogen	Worsens stress and mixed leakage in women
Gabapentin, pregabalin	Pedal edema causing nocturia and nighttime incontinence
Loop diuretics	Polyuria, frequency, urgency
Narcotic analgesics	Urinary retention, fecal impaction, sedation, delirium
NSAIDs	Pedal edema causing nocturnal polyuria
Sedative hypnotics	Sedation, delirium, immobility
Thiazolidinediones	Pedal edema causing nocturnal polyuria
Tricyclic antidepressants	Anticholinergic effects, sedation

ACE, angiotensin-converting enzyme; *NSAIDs*, nonsteroidal antiinflammatory drugs; *UI*, Urinary incontinence.
Adapted from DuBeau CE. Urinary incontinence. In: Durso SC, Sullivan GM, eds. Geriatrics Review Syllabus: A Core Curriculum in Geriatric Medicine, 8th ed. New York, NY: American Geriatrics Society; 2013. p 245.

frequency of pad changes. Most UI is relatively slow in onset and should not be associated with pelvic pain. Acute onset of UI and the presence of suprapubic, lower abdominal, and/or pelvic pain are red flags for significant underlying neurologic or neoplastic disease, and should prompt quick referral to neurology or urology/gynecology specialists.

Simple questions can differentiate urgency from stress and mixed incontinence with sufficient sensitivity and specificity for clinical practice.[36] The patient should be asked, "Do you leak urine. . . ."

- When you had the urge or feeling that you needed to empty your bladder but couldn't get there fast enough? [urgency UI]
- When you were performing some physical activity such as coughing, sneezing, lifting, or exercise? [stress UI]
- About as equally with a sense of urgency and physical activity? [mixed UI]
- Without either a sense of urgency or physical activity? [other]

There should be an assessment of the bother and quality of life impact of UI for the patient as well as the caretaker. This can be done informally, or through specific questions and questionnaires. Some patients, especially women, may report little bother because they "manage fine with pads." It is important to ask such persons about their concerns about treatment, the invasiveness and impact of which they may overestimate.

Nocturia is a bothersome symptom that can be caused by either lower urinary tract dysfunction (detrusor overactivity, bladder outlet obstruction), disproportionate nocturnal urine excretion (nocturnal polyuria), a primary sleep disturbance (e.g., pain, depression, disruptive bed partner) or a combination.[37,38] Nocturnal polyuria is a common driver of nocturia in older persons, and is defined as greater than one third of total 24-hour urine production occurring during hours of sleep.[37] Nocturnal polyuria can be assessed using a voiding diary (Table 23-4). The differential causes of nocturnal polyuria include excess fluid intake (especially beverages with caffeine or alcohol), pedal edema (often associated with medications—see Table 23-3), congestive heart failure, and—importantly—sleep apnea.[39] Sleep apnea should be considered in all patients with unexplained nocturnal polyuria, as this condition has significant morbidity and treatment with continuous positive airway pressure decreases nocturia.[40]

Other lower urinary tract symptoms, particularly slow stream, hesitancy, insufficient emptying, and postvoid dribbling, are less specific, but may be bothersome to the patient, and can be important to assess before treatment.

The evaluation should include a review of past medical history and medications for factors that may contribute to UI and/or its severity.[19] For some conditions (e.g., stroke) it is important to assess its relationship to the onset of UI, to determine whether the condition is related to UI. All patients with UI should be screened for depression and functional status.[19] Cognitive screening should be considered for the purpose of planning treatment.[19]

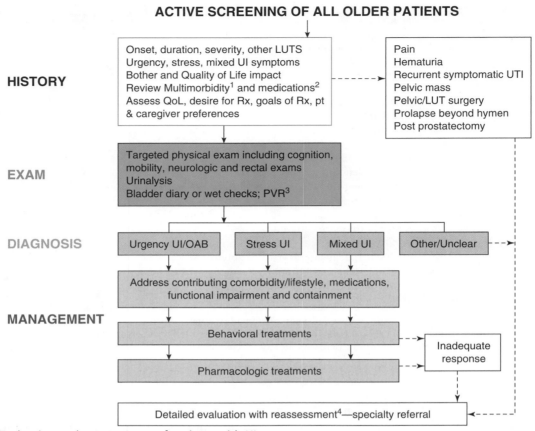

ACTIVE SCREENING OF ALL OLDER PATIENTS

Figure 23-2 Evaluation and management of patients with UI.
[1]See Table 23-2.
[2]See Table 23-3.
[3]Postvoid residual (PVR) test is optional; considered for women with marked pelvic floor prolapse, longstanding diabetes, history of urinary retention or high PVR, recurrent UTIs, medications that impair bladder emptying, chronic constipation, persistent or worsening UI on treatment with bladder antimuscarinics, or prior urodynamic study demonstrating detrusor underactivity and/or bladder outlet obstruction (Grade C). If PVR is elevated (e.g., 200 mL), consider trial of alpha-blocker (men), treat constipation, decrease or eliminate anticholinergic medications and calcium channel blockers, and consider catheter drainage followed by voiding trial if PVR 300 mL.
[4]Detailed evaluation with reassessment could include the following: bladder diary and PVR, if not previously done; revisiting/testing for comorbidity (e.g., sleep apnea if nocturia with nocturnal polyuria is present); trial of alternative medication for urgency incontinence (another antimuscarinic or switch to beta-3 agonist, if not contraindicated); or addition of biofeedback for pelvic muscle exercise training. (Adapted from DuBeau CE, Kuchel GA, Johnson T, et al. Incontinence in the frail elderly. In: Abrams P, Cardozo L, Khoury S, Wein A, editors. Incontinence. 4th ed. Paris: Health Publications; 2009, p. 961-1025.
LUT, lower urinary tract; LUTS, lower urinary tract symptoms; OAB, overactive bladder; PVR, postvoiding residual; Rx, treatment; UI, urinary incontinence.

The physical examination of older persons with UI focuses on (1) potential urogenital abnormalities and (2) detection and assessment of comorbid conditions that may be contributing to UI. All women with UI should have a pelvic examination.[19] The pelvic examination should include inspection of the vaginal mucosa for atrophy (thinning, pallor, loss of rugae) and inflammation (erythema, petechiae, telangiectasia, friability). A bimanual examination should evaluate for masses or tenderness. Pelvic organ prolapse can be assessed by a split-speculum examination, removing the top blade of the speculum and holding the bottom blade firmly against the posterior vaginal wall for support. Ask the woman to cough, looking for whether the urethra remains firmly fixed or swings quickly forward (urethral hypermobility) and

for bulging of the anterior vaginal wall either to or through the level of the hymenal ring (anterior wall support defect, or cystocoele). Check for a posterior wall support defect (rectocele) by turning the single blade of the speculum to support the anterior vaginal wall and having the patient cough again. Men should have a genital examination. A digital rectal exam can detect prostate nodules, rectal masses, and stool impaction, but does not provide reliable assessment of prostate size. It should be noted that an abdominal examination is not reliable for detecting bladder distension.

A detailed neurologic examination is not necessary in the initial evaluation of UI, but should be considered for patients with sudden onset of UI (especially urge), concomitant fecal incontinence, known neurologic

TABLE 23-4	**Using a Bladder Diary to Evaluate Nocturia**

Bladder diary of an older woman with complaints of urgency, occasional urgency UI (less than daily), and 4-5 episodes of nocturia. The diary demonstrates nocturnal polyuria (nocturnal excretion of >30% of total 24-hour urine output). Her nocturnal urine output (shaded areas, including all voids from bedtime up to and including first morning void) is 630-660 mL, or just over 50% of her 24-hour urine output on 10/2 (630 ÷ [630 + 570]). With a functional bladder capacity of 240 mL (largest voided volume on the diary), this amount of nocturnal polyuria necessitates that she void at least twice (630 ÷ 240) during the night. Thus, despite the presence of daytime urgency and rare urgency UI, the cause of her nocturia is nocturnal polyuria. Evaluation and treatment should focus on causes of the polyuria.

Date	Time	Measured Amount of Urine (mL)	Approximate Amount of Leakage (mL)	Comments	
10/1	3:50 PM	90			Total 450 mL
	6:05 PM	90			
	8:15 PM	120			
	10:20 PM	150			
10/2	12:00 AM	30			Total 630 mL
	2:15 AM	150			
	3:40 AM	120			
	5:00 AM	120			
	6:05 AM	240	Maybe a drop	Almost had accident	
	8:40 AM	120		Coffee	Total 570 mL
	12:50 PM	120			
	6:00 PM	120			
	9:20 PM	210		Dribbled on way	
	11:40 PM	120			Total 660 mL
	2:00 AM	150			
	4:50 AM	180			
	6:20 AM	180			

Adapted from DuBeau CE. Urinary incontinence. In: Durso SC, Sullivan GM, eds. Geriatrics Review Syllabus: A Core Curriculum in Geriatric Medicine, 8th ed. New York, NY: American Geriatrics Society; 2013 page 248.

disease (other than dementia), or new onset of neurologic symptoms.[19] Testing should include an evaluation of sacral root integrity, including perineal sensation, resting and volitional tone of the anal sphincter, anal wink (visual or palpated anal contraction in response to a light scratch of the perineal skin lateral to the anus), and the bulbocavernosus reflex (anal contraction in response to a light squeeze of the clitoris or glans penis).

All patients should have a urinalysis, with reflex urine culture if the patient has other symptoms of urinary tract infection (e.g., dysuria, fever) or if the UI is of new onset or new worsening. The primary purpose of this testing is to look for hematuria (and in diabetic patients, glycosuria, which can cause frequency).

Assessment of PVR is not necessary in the initial evaluation of persons with UI, including men, because of the low prevalence (prior probability) of a significantly elevated PVR (Level of Evidence D).[41] Furthermore, there is no agreed-upon definition of an "abnormal" or "clinically significant" PVR. Patients for whom a PVR should be considered are those with complex neurologic disease, long-standing diabetes mellitus (especially if poorly controlled), women with marked pelvic organ prolapse, and patients with a high burden of anticholinergic medications (Level of Evidence D).[19] PVR can be measured by bladder scan or catheterization, and should be done as soon after voiding as possible.

MANAGEMENT

Treatment of UI in older persons is a stepwise process, proceeding from addressing contributing comorbidity and medications, to lifestyle interventions, then behavioral treatment, pharmacologic treatment, and, if necessary, minimally invasive and surgical treatments. Management should be focused on the most bothersome aspects of UI for an individual patient, and patient (and/or caregiver)-defined goals of care.[42] Cure (complete persistent continence without continuing intervention) is, unfortunately, uncommon, and largely limited to surgical therapies or situations where a specific contributing factor (e.g., sleep apnea) is successfully treated or managed. However, many patients can experience continence with sustained interventions (behavioral, pharmacologic). For some patients, the goal may be (improved) contained incontinence, managed with protective garments.

> Optimal management of UI is hampered by the fact that at least half of persons with UI never mention it to their care providers.

Lifestyle Interventions

The only evidence-based lifestyle intervention is weight loss, which significantly reduces stress UI in obese, younger-old women (Level of Evidence A).[43] Other lifestyle interventions that may be helpful in individual patients, but for which strong supporting evidence is lacking, include the following: avoiding excessive or inadequate fluid intake (the latter can lead to concentrated urine, which may be irritating), caffeinated beverages, and alcohol; minimizing evening fluid intake for nocturia; and quitting smoking for patients with stress UI. Afternoon administration of loop diuretics may decrease the volume of nocturnal polyuria and perhaps nocturia episodes (Level of Evidence C), although it is not clear which patients are most likely to benefit.[37]

> Behavioral therapy should be the first-line therapy for most older patients with UI.

Behavioral Therapies

Bladder training (BT) and pelvic muscle exercises (PMEs) are effective for urge, mixed, and stress UI (Level of Evidence B),[44-46] including postprostatectomy UI (Level of Evidence B).[47,48] Behavioral therapy therefore should be the first-line therapy for most older patients with UI.[19] BT and PME are often used in combination (Table 23-5), with pelvic floor contraction used for urgency suppression and forestalling voiding.

Bladder training uses two principles: frequent voluntary voiding to keep bladder volume low, and urgency suppression using central nervous system and pelvic mechanisms. The initial toileting frequency can be every 2 hours or based on the smallest voiding interval on bladder diary. When urgency occurs, patients should stand still or sit down, do several pelvic muscle contractions, and concentrate on making the urgency decrease by taking a deep breath and letting it out slowly, or visualizing the urgency as a wave

that peaks and then falls. Once patients feel more in control, they should walk to a bathroom and void. After 2 days without leakage, the time between scheduled voids can be increased by 30 to 60 minutes, until the person is dry when voiding every 4 hours. Successful bladder training usually takes several weeks, and patients need reassurance to proceed despite any initial failure.

PMEs strengthen the muscular components of urethral support. They require patient instruction and motivation, although simple instruction booklets alone have had moderate benefit.

To do PMEs,[49] the patient (1) performs an isolated pelvic muscle contraction, without contracting buttocks, abdomen, or thighs (this can be checked during a bimanual examination in women), and holds it for 6 to 8 seconds (initially, only shorter durations may be possible); (2) repeats the contraction 8 to 12 times (one set), relaxing the pelvis between each contraction; (3) completes three sets of contractions starting 3 to 4 times a week, and continuing for at least 15 to 20 weeks. As patients progress, they should try to increase the intensity and duration of the contraction, perform PMEs in various positions (sitting, standing, walking), and alternate fast and slower contractions. Many experts believe biofeedback can improve bladder retraining and PME teaching and outcomes, but marginal benefit is unproven. Medicare covers biofeedback for patients who do not improve after 4 weeks of conventional instruction.

The only behavioral treatment with proven efficacy in cognitively impaired patients is prompted voiding.[50] A caregiver monitors the patient and encourages him or her to report any need to void, prompts the patient to toilet on a regular schedule during the day (usually every 2 to 3 hours) and leads the patient to the bathroom, and gives the patient positive feedback when he or she toilets. Patients most likely to improve void ≤4 times during the day (12 hours) and are able to accept and follow the prompt to toilet at least 75% of the time in an initial 3-day trial.[51] Toileting routines without prompting, such as habit training (based on a patient's usual voiding schedule) and scheduled voiding (using a set schedule) are not effective.

Pharmacologic Therapy

Pharmacotherapy is an important part of urgency UI management. There are currently no Food and Drug Administration–approved medications for stress UI; duloxetine is effective in reducing stress UI (Level of Evidence A)[44] but is not approved for this indication in the United States. Oral estrogen, alone or in combination with progestins, increases stress UI in women (Level of Evidence A).[52] Vaginal topical estrogen (cream, vaginal tablet, or slow-release ring) (Level of Evidence B)[53] is helpful for uncomfortable vaginal

TABLE 23-5	**Behavioral Treatments for Incontinence**		
Indication(s)	**Treatment**	**Level of Evidence for Effectiveness***	**Comments**
Cognitively intact; urge incontinence or urge-predominant mixed incontinence	Bladder training	A	For urge incontinence, ≥50% decrease in episodes; patient perception of cure at 6 mo, RR 1.69 [95% CI 1.21, 2.34]; for stress incontinence, ≥50% decrease in 75% of patients; all UI, ARR 0.51 [0.36, 0.66]
Urge incontinence or urge-predominant mixed incontinence; cognitively impaired	Prompted voiding	B	Average reduction 0.8-1.8 episodes/day, cure rare
Urge, stress, or mixed incontinence	Pelvic muscle exercises with bladder training	B	AHRQ: Meta-analysis difficult, "potential decreases" in UI episodes up to 1.9/day. For urge incontinence, up to 80% decrease; for stress incontinence, 56%-95% decrease; all UI, mean weighted effect size, −0.54 episodes/day [−0.71, −0.37], ARR 13% [7%, 20%]
Urge, stress, or mixed incontinence	Pelvic muscle exercises with bladder training and biofeedback	B	All UI, 50%-87% improvement, ARR 24% [8%, 39%], RR for continued UI 0.74 [0.6, 0.93]; compared with PME and biofeedback alone, better perception of improvement, RR 1.18 (1.01, 1.39)
Men: stress incontinence after prostatectomy		A	Continence achieved in 57% at 1-2 mo (relative benefit 1.54 [1.01, 2.34])

*A = supported by one or more high-quality randomized trials (RCTs); B = supported by one or more high-quality nonrandomized cohort studies or low-quality RCTs; C = supported by one or more case series and/or poor-quality cohort and/or case-control studies; D = supported by expert opinion and/or extrapolation from studies in other populations or settings; X = evidence supports the treatment being ineffective or harmful.

AHRQ, Agency for Healthcare Research and Quality; *ARR*, absolute risk reduction; *CI*, confidence interval; *PME*, pelvic muscle exercises; *RR*, relative risk; . *UI*, urinary incontinence.

atrophy and may decrease recurrent urinary tract infections.

Antimuscarinic agents are moderately effective for urgency UI, OAB, urgency-predominant mixed UI, and urgency associated with benign prostatic hyperplasia (BPH) (Table 23-6).[46,54] Their main mechanism of action is increasing bladder capacity by decreasing the basal excretion of acetylcholine from the urothelium; they do not decrease or ablate uninhibited bladder contractions.[55] There are conflicting data from randomized controlled trials whether combined antimuscarinic and behavioral therapy is better than either alone for reducing UI. The strongest evidence comes from well-conducted studies in older women comparing a BT/PME regimen and immediate-release oxybutynin, alone and in combination. In middle aged/young-old women combination was significantly better for improving quality-of-life outcomes (Level of Evidence B).

Antimuscarinics are contraindicated for patients with narrow-angle glaucoma (not open-angle), impaired gastric emptying, and known urinary retention. It is not necessary to routinely monitor PVR with antimuscarinic treatment (Level of Evidence D),[19] and

it is unclear at what volume it is safe to administer antimuscarinics (Level of Evidence D).[19] However, trials of antimuscarinics in men with BPH-associated lower urinary tract symptoms (LUTS) show no increased risk of retention with baseline PVR <200 mL. Patients complaining of worsening UI while taking antimuscarinics should have a PVR checked, because an elevated PVR decreases functional bladder capacity thereby increasing frequency and UI.

> The decision to use one antimuscarinic over another depends on avoidance of adverse drug effects (ADEs), drug–drug and drug–disease interactions, dosing frequency, titration range, and cost.

Antimuscarinics

Antimuscarinics with established efficacy are oxybutynin, tolterodine, fesoterodine, trospium, darifenacin, and solifenacin (see Table 23-6). Based on systematic reviews, these six antimuscarinic agents have generally similar efficacy in reducing urge UI frequency, but

TABLE 23-6	Pharmacologic Treatment for Urgency Urinary Incontinence

Antimuscarinic Agents

Indication(s)	Agent	Level of Evidence for Effectiveness*	Comments
Urgency UI OAB Urgency predominant– stress UI	All agents	A**	With baseline average UI episodes/day of 1.6 to 5.3, mean reduction in episodes/day with placebo 1.08 (95% CI 0.86-1.30); vs IR formulations 1.46 (1.28, 1.64), and ER formulations 1.78 (1.61, 1.94). Head-to-head comparison trials of agents of limited quality
	Antimuscarinics **Oxybutynin** Immediate release 2.5-5 mg three to four times daily Extended release (Ditropan XL) 5-20 mg once daily Topical patch (Oxytrol) 3.9-mg patch applied twice weekly Topical gel (Gelnique) 3% (84 mg, pump) and 10% (100 mg, sachet) once daily	A	Highest rate of dry mouth with immediate release, lowest with topical forms Application site rash in ∼ 15% with patch
	Tolterodine Immediate release (Detrol) 1-2 mg one tab twice daily Extended release (Detrol LA) 2-4 mg once daily	A	
	Fesoterodine (Toviaz) 4-8 mg once daily	A	Prodrug of tolterodine
	Darifenacin (Enablex) 7.5-15 mg once daily	A	Constipation
	Solifenacin (VESIcare) 5-10 mg once daily	A	
	Trospium Immediate release (Sanctura) 20 mg once to twice daily Extended release (Sanctura XR) 60 mg daily	A	Must be given on empty stomach
	Beta-3 Agonist		
Urgency UI OAB	Mirabegron (Myrbetriq) 25-50 mg once daily	A	ADEs include hypertension; should be used with caution in patients with known hypertension. Use with caution with metoprolol and digoxin.
BPH-associated urgency	**Tolterodine**	A	

ADE, adverse drug effect; *BPH*, benign prostatic hypertrophy; *CI*, confidence interval; *ER*, extended release; *IR*, immediate release; *OAB*, overactive bladder; *UI*, Urinary incontinence.

*A = supported by one or more high-quality randomized controlled trials (RCTs); B = supported by one or more high-quality nonrandomized cohort studies or low-quality RCTs; C = supported by one or more case series and/or poor-quality cohort and/or case-control studies; D = supported by expert opinion and/or extrapolation from studies in other populations or settings; X = evidence supports the treatment being ineffective or harmful.

**Although data comes from randomized controlled trials, a recent Agency for Healthcare Research and Quality systematic review rated the evidence as only moderate based on study quality.

Data from randomized controlled trials, a recent Agency for Healthcare Research and Quality differ in adverse events, metabolism, drug interactions, and dosing requirements.[46,54] Head-to-head trials are limited and all industry-supported.[54] Although older patients have been included in antimuscarinic trials, no study has included vulnerable or frail elderly. Anticholinergic adverse events impact both tolerability and safety.

Although anticholinergics as a class are associated with cognitive impairment, the risk, prevalence, type, and magnitude of cognitive changes from specific antimuscarinic UI medications in an individual patient are unknown.[56] Although one randomized study showed that extended-release oxybutynin 10-20 mg impaired memory while darifenacin 7.5-15 mg was not different than placebo (Level of Evidence B),[57] another found no increase in delirium in frail nursing home patients treated with extended-release oxybutynin 5 mg daily (Level of Evidence B).[58] No antimuscarinic is "safer" for all patients or those with dementia, nor has it been shown that the cognitive risk outweighs the potential treatment benefit (Level of Evidence D). Antimuscarinics should not be combined with cholinesterase inhibitors because of lack of efficacy and risk of increased functional impairment (Level of Evidence B).[59]

Chronic antimuscarinic use increases the risk of caries and tooth loss, and patients should have regular dental care.

All antimuscarinics except trospium are metabolized by cytochrome P-450 pathways, and can interact with drugs that induce CYP2D6 (e.g., fluoxetine) or are metabolized by CYP3A4 (e.g., erythromycin, ketoconazole). Fesoterodine is a prodrug that is metabolized to tolterodine by nonspecific peripheral esterases. Trospium is renally cleared and should be given once daily in patients with renal insufficiency; it should be taken on an empty stomach.

Given that overall the six antimuscarinic agents have similar efficacy in reducing UI, the decision to use one antimuscarinic over another depends on avoidance of ADEs for which a patient may be most at risk along with other geriatric prescribing factors including possible drug–drug and drug–disease interactions, dosing frequency, titration range, and cost. A lack of response to one agent does not preclude response to another.

Beta-3 Agonists

In 2012 a new class of medication, beta-3 agonists, became available in the United States for treatment of urgency UI and OAB. Stimulation of beta-3 receptors in the detrusor mediates bladder relaxation. Mirabegron (Myrbetriq 25-50 mg once daily) reduces UI (Level of Evidence B).[60] According to the package insert,[61] an important ADE with mirabegron is increased blood pressure. Hypertensive patients placed on mirabegron should have periodic blood pressure determinations, and mirabegron should not be used in patients with severe uncontrolled hypertension. Only the lowest dose should be used in patients with severe renal or moderate hepatic insufficiency. Mirabegron should be used with caution in patients on antimuscarinic medications and in men with bladder outlet obstruction from BPH because of risk of urinary retention. Mirabegron is a CYP2D6 inhibitor and if used with drugs metabolized by CYP2D6 (especially those with narrow therapeutic window, e.g., metoprolol), close monitoring is needed and dose reduction of these drugs may be necessary. Mirabegron can raise serum digoxin levels, which should be monitored.

Vasopressin (DDAVP)

Antidiuretic hormone is used to treat younger patients with bothersome nocturia associated with nocturnal polyuria. However, DDAVP should not be used to treat nocturia in older, especially frailer, patients because of the risk of hyponatremia (Level of Evidence A).[19]

Miscellaneous Agents

There is insufficient evidence for the efficacy of propantheline, dicyclomine, imipramine, hyoscyamine, calcium channel blockers, nonsteroidal antiinflammatory drugs, and flavoxate (Level of Evidence C).[19] Furthermore, several of these agents are highly anticholinergic and are potentially inappropriate medications for older persons.[62]

Minimally Invasive Procedures

There are several treatment options for patients with urgency UI refractory to behavioral and pharmacologic therapy. Intravesical injection of botulinum toxin can reduce UI with a slightly higher cure compared with antimuscarinics, although with a greater risk of urinary retention (Level of Evidence B).[63,64] Optimal dosing for specific patient groups such as the elderly is uncertain, and patients must be willing to do self-catheterization because of the risk of urinary retention.

Sacral nerve neuromodulation is used, paradoxically, for both refractory urgency UI and idiopathic and neurogenic urinary retention.[65] The mechanism of action is unknown. The procedure involves percutaneous implantation of a trial electrode at the S3 sacral root, which is connected to an external stimulator. Patients responding to the trial have a permanent lead with a pacemaker-like energy source implanted. Very small trials suggest a potential role for percutaneous tibial nerve stimulation for refractory urge incontinence.[66]

Surgery

Surgery has its largest role in the treatment of stress UI in women, for which it provides the highest cure rates. The most commonly used procedures are colposuspension (Burch operation) and slings (synthetic mesh, or autologous or cadaveric fascia, placed at the proximal or mid-urethra. Older woman can have comparable outcomes to younger women and age alone should not be a contraindication to surgery.[67] Periurethral injection of collagen is a short-term (≤1 yr) alternative and usually requires a series of injections.

CASE 1

Discussion

Ms. Roberts describes urgency (of note, she has no impaired mobility contributing to UI), with daily urgency-associated UI and nocturia. She denied leakage with coughing and activity; thus she does not have stress UI. UI is having a major impact on her, leading to worsening of her heart failure because of skipping diuretic doses. She also has the out-of-pocket expense of adult diapers.

Several comorbid conditions can contribute to her urge UI. The most common urologic dysfunction in persons with diabetes is urge UI. Her diabetes is well controlled, and therefore it is unlikely that osmotic diuresis contributes to daytime and nighttime frequency. Heart failure and associated peripheral edema may be a cause of nocturia. Amlodipine could be contributing to peripheral edema as well. Another potential cause of nocturnal polyuria to consider is sleep apnea.

Ms. Roberts's examination is normal except for an exacerbation of heart failure.

In terms of management of her UI, you explain to Ms. Roberts the association between heart failure and nocturia, and the importance of taking her diuretic, and prescribe compression stockings to reduce the edema. You also explain bladder training and give the patient a handout to follow.

When the patient returns to see you, her weight is down, and her pretibial edema is only a trace. She reports that she is getting up only twice a night now, but is still tired, and she is still leaking about once a day. She is willing to try an antimuscarinic, so you check her formulary, and select a preferred agent, which you start at low dose. You ask her to return in another month to review her progress, tolerance of the new medication, and adherence to the behavioral measures. ▪

SUMMARY

UI is common but never normal in older patients, and all older persons should routinely be directly asked about lower urinary tract symptoms. Evaluation should search for functional, comorbid, medication, and fluid balance factors that can precipitate and exacerbate incontinence. Behavioral therapies are effective for a variety of patients, especially when targeted to patients' functional and cognitive status. A combination of behavioral and drug therapy is more efficacious than either alone. Surgical treatment remains an effective option for older women with stress UI.

Web Resources

General: Each of these sites provides evidence-based guidelines and resources for providers to use in guiding patients.
- www.ics.org. International Continence Society; includes links to other continence organizations and resources.
- www.auanet.org. American Urological Association.
- www.augs.org. American Urogynecologic Association.
- www.amda.com. American Medical Directors Association; information about UI treatment in long-term care patients.

Patient advocacy
- www.nafc.org. National Association for Continence.
- www.simonfoundation.org. Simon Foundation for Continence.

KEY REFERENCES

21. Landefeld CS, Bowers BJ, Feld AD, et al. National Institutes of Health state-of-the-science conference statement: Prevention of fecal and urinary incontinence in adults. Ann Intern Med 2008;148:449-58.
34. Holroyd-Leduc JM, Tannenbaum C, Thorpe KE, Straus SE. What type of urinary incontinence does this woman have? JAMA 2008;299:1446-56.
38. Gulur DM, Mevcha AM, Drake MJ. Nocturia as a manifestation of systemic disease. BJU Int 2011;107(5):702-13.
42. Fonda D, Abrams P. Cure sometimes, help always—a "continence paradigm" for all ages and conditions. Neurourol Urodyn 2006;25(3):290-2.
44. Shamliyan T, Wyman J, Kane RL. Benefits and harms of pharmacologic treatment for urinary incontinence in women: A systematic review. Ann Intern Med 2012;156(12):861-74.

References available online at expertconsult.com.

24

Constipation and Fecal Incontinence

Alayne D. Markland

OBJECTIVES

Upon completion of this chapter, the reader will be able to:

- Define the various types of constipation and fecal incontinence (FI), along with associated bowel symptoms.

- Recognize subtypes and common conditions that may be associated with constipation and FI.

- Describe the clinical evaluation for older adults with constipation and FI, understanding when referral for further evaluation may be needed.

- Identify evidence-based nonpharmacologic and pharmacologic treatments for constipation and FI among older adults.

PREVALENCE, IMPACT, AND DEFINITIONS

Constipation and fecal incontinence (FI) can be classified as functional bowel disorders.[1] Functional bowel disorders are usually chronic (more than 3 to 6 months in duration at the time of presentation) and are attributable to the middle and lower gastrointestinal system. Constipation and FI are symptom-based diagnoses that may have multiple etiologies. Often, symptoms of constipation and FI occur simultaneously. Management will be discussed separately for constipation and FI, with a section on fecal impaction that can include symptoms of constipation and FI.

> Constipation and fecal incontinence are common, underrecognized, and underreported conditions.

Chronic constipation disproportionately affects the elderly, with an estimated 40% of people older than the age of 65 experiencing the condition.[2,3] Women have 2 to 3 times more constipation than men. African Americans also exhibit increased risk. Many community-dwelling older adults use over-the-counter preparations, such as stimulant and bulking laxatives. Nearly 85% of physician visits for constipation result in a prescription for laxatives and more than $820 million are spent per year on over-the-counter agents. Few resources are available to health care providers to guide them in an evidence-based approach to this common problem.

FI occurs in up to 15% of older women and men.[4,5] FI is distressing, socially isolating, and associated with a possible increased risk of dependency in activities of daily living, morbidity, and mortality. Many older individuals with FI do not volunteer the problem to their health care provider, and providers do not routinely enquire about the symptoms. The condition can affect care providers of home-dwelling patients, with FI being cited as a reason for requesting nursing home placement. Because frail, older adults frequently have coexisting urinary symptoms (most often urinary incontinence) and other bowel symptoms (constipation), evaluation and management of other urinary symptoms and FI should be done simultaneously (see Chapter 23).[4,6] Even when noted by health care professionals, FI is often managed with absorptive or containment products, especially in the long-term care setting where it is most prevalent.

FI can result from constipation with stool impaction and may be more common in certain frail, older populations.[7] In a recent study, 81% of residents in long-term care settings had symptoms of constipation and FI.[8] However, the true prevalence of impaction and FI in nursing home residents and home-care settings has not been clearly identified. Because constipation with FI is difficult to diagnose, treatments should target constipation.

CASE 1

Angela McDonald

Angela McDonald is a 76-year-old woman with a 15-year history of constipation symptoms who visits your office with new bowel complaints. She consistently has had one to two bowel movements a week for the last several years and often feels as though she has incomplete evacuation. Most of her stools are very hard and are rarely smooth in contour. She has never noticed any blood in her stool, has no pain with defecation, and has not had a change in the caliber of her stools. Her weight and appetite have been stable.

Over the last 6 to 8 months, she admits to having weekly FI episodes where she notes leakage of mushy stool consistency without any prior warning. She takes a stool softener on most days and occasionally uses milk of magnesia when she has not had a bowel movement in 6 to 7 days. She notices that the milk of magnesia is no longer providing as much relief for her symptoms. She has not started any new medications and has had no dietary changes. Her medical history includes hypertension, gastroesophageal reflux disease, and mild urinary incontinence. She is very bothered because her episodes of FI have caused her to start wearing adult diapers on most days (she previously wore mini-pads for her urinary incontinence).

1. **What is the most likely cause of Ms. McDonald's bowel symptoms?**

2. **Do her current symptoms warrant further evaluation with a colonoscopy or other bowel imaging?**

3. **What additional tests are needed (if any) for her bowel symptoms?**

4. **Given her current bowel symptoms, what is the best initial treatment for Ms. McDonald's symptoms?** ◨

Symptoms and Definitions

Constipation is often associated with other abdominal complaints (pain, bloating, and gas), as well as decreased overall well-being. It may involve infrequent defecation, difficulty in passing stool, or incomplete evacuation of stool. Physicians often define constipation as infrequent passage of stool; however, patients often define it as straining to defecate or sensation of incomplete evacuation. In order for chronic constipation (CC) to be diagnosed, symptoms should be present for at least 12 weeks.

The Rome III criteria, published in 2006, define CC as symptoms that have persisted for the last 3 months with an onset at least 6 months prior to diagnosis, with the following three criteria being met:

> **The most common subtype of constipation is normal transit constipation.**

1. Must include two or more of the following:
   - Hard or lumpy stool in ≥25% of defecations
   - Straining during ≥25% of defecations
   - Sensation of incomplete evacuation for at least 25% of defecations
   - Sensation of anorectal obstruction or blockage for ≥25% of defecations
   - Manual maneuvers to facilitate ≥25% of defecations (e.g., digital evacuation, support of the pelvic floor)
   - Fewer than three defecations per week
2. Loose stools are rarely present without use of laxatives
3. Insufficient criteria for irritable bowel syndrome (IBS)

Differentiating symptoms of chronic constipation from irritable bowel syndrome with constipation (IBS-C) and diarrhea (IBS-D) may not be as important in older adults, because age ≥50 years is associated with lower rates of IBS.[5] However, management can differ between the two diagnoses. IBS-C is defined by recurrent abdominal pain or discomfort for at least 3 days per month in the previous 3 months (onset ≥6 months prior to the diagnosis) that is associated with at least two of the following:

1. Improvement of pain or discomfort upon defecation
2. Onset associated with change in frequency of stool
3. Onset associated with a change in form or appearance of stool

The International Continence Society provides a definition of FI that is the "involuntary loss of liquid or solid stool that is a social or hygienic problem."[9] Flatal incontinence may also be a bothersome symptom but is usually excluded from the definition for FI. Other bowel symptoms that may present with FI include rectal urgency, seepage of stool after bowel movements, incomplete evacuation, and loss of stool without any sensory awareness.

PRIMARY AND SECONDARY CAUSES OF CONSTIPATION AND FECAL INCONTINENCE

Constipation and FI can be subgrouped as primary (subtypes of constipation or FI) or secondary (e.g., caused by a diagnosed medical condition or use of medications). Primary types of constipation are more clearly defined and are associated with specific diagnosis codes. The primary types of FI are more open to interpretation and are not associated with specific diagnosis codes. The primary types for constipation and FI are listed in Table 24-1 with secondary causes listed in Box 24-1.

Less is known about specific subtypes of FI.

Many prescription and nonprescription drugs impact stool consistency and cause hard or liquid/loose stools. Medications can slow transit time and contribute to a hard stool consistency (e.g., narcotics, anabolic steroids, anticonvulsants, anticholinergic agents, antihypertensive agents, tricyclic antidepressants). Nonprescription agents implicated in increased transit time and hard stools include antihistamines, calcium and iron supplements, antidiarrheals, nonsteroidal antiinflammatory drugs (NSAIDs), and some antacids.

Diarrhea-inducing medications include those that decrease transit time and cause loose stool consistency. Medications that induce diarrhea may be time-limited (i.e., a side effect that improves with time or with limited use of the medication); they may change intestinal bacterial flora, or the resulting diarrhea may be the result of a higher than normal serum concentration of the medication. Medications with associated time-limited diarrhea include metformin, high doses of proton pump inhibitors, acetylcholinesterase inhibitors, selective serotonin reuptake inhibitors, colchicine, and chemotherapeutic agents. Antibiotics may also cause loose stools and diarrhea by changing intestinal bacterial flora. Toxic levels of some drugs, such as digoxin, can cause loose stools. Nonprescription

---

BOX 24-1

SECONDARY CAUSES OF CHRONIC CONSTIPATION AND FECAL INCONTINENCE IN OLDER ADULTS

- Malignancy (including the treatments for malignancy—surgical bowel resection and radiation)
- Medications/polypharmacy (prescription and nonprescription drugs—including opioids)
- Endocrine/metabolic (diabetes mellitus, hyperthyroidism or hypothyroidism, hypercalcemia, hypokalemia)
- Neurologic disorders (Parkinson's disease, diabetic autonomic neuropathy, spinal cord injury, dementia, stroke)
- Nutritional (malabsorbtion syndromes, food sensitivities, fluid and dietary intake)
- Rheumatologic disorders (systemic sclerosis and other connective tissue disorders)
- Psychological disorders (depression, eating disorders, alcohol or substance abuse)
- Anatomic dysfunction (strictures, postsurgical abnormalities, anal fissures, megacolon, hemorrhoids, fistulas, rectal prolapse, occult obstetrical sphincter tears)
- Decreased mobility/sedentary lifestyle

TABLE 24-1	Primary Pathophysiologic Types of Chronic Constipation and Fecal Incontinence
Type of Chronic Constipation	**Characteristics**
1. Normal transit	• Most common subtype • Transit and stool frequency are within normal ranges but patients complain of constipation, bloating, and pain*
2. Slow transit	• Increased intestinal transit time • Reduced colonic motility • Multiple etiologies—gut, cellular, and protein-level responses
3. Defecatory dysfunction	• More common in older adults and women • Structural problems seen on anorectal manometry and defecography • Pelvic floor dyssynergia (failure to relax or inappropriate contraction of puborectalis muscle and external anal sphincter during defecation) • Pathogenesis not well understood
Fecal Incontinence Type	**Characteristics**
1. Urgency FI	• Often occurs with a strong urgency sensation to have a bowel movement • Liquid stool or diarrhea often associated with the inability to hold stool in the rectal vault*
2. Passive FI	• Bowel leakage without the sensation of the need to defecate • May not be able to differentiate passing gas from having a bowel movement • May also involve seepage after a bowel movement
3. Overflow FI	• More common in older adults with impaired mobility and functional impairments (i.e., long-term care residents) • May also involve seepage or smaller amounts of stool loss around an impaction • Associated with symptoms of constipation • May need to treat constipation symptoms to improve FI

*Presence of pain increases the likelihood of a diagnosis of irritable bowel syndrome with constipation (IBS-C) or diarrhea (IBS-D).

medications that cause loose stools include laxatives and some NSAIDS. Tube feedings may also be associated with loose stool.

History and Physical Examination

In most cases, patients with constipation and FI do not warrant extensive diagnostic evaluation. Older patients with a change in bowel symptoms who meet criteria for the warning or alarm symptoms should consider the benefits and risks of evaluation with colonoscopy or other invasive testing.

The clinical evaluation should consist of a thorough history for other potential causes and an appropriate physical examination and laboratory testing. Health care providers should inquire about constipation and FI, because many older patients do not seek treatment for their symptoms. Using appropriate patient-oriented terminology, such as the term "accidental bowel leakage," when asking about bowel habits is important. A focused history on stool frequency and consistency, and other bowel symptoms, helps exclude primary and secondary causes. Bowel symptoms should include excessive straining, incomplete evacuation, or self-disimpaction. Dietary intake may identify contributing factors (e.g., poor dietary intake of fiber or lactose intolerance). Symptoms such as persistent nausea, vomiting, and abdominal pain should broaden the differential and evaluation, especially for an intestinal obstruction.

> Specialized bowel evaluation testing can help differentiate causes of constipation and FI.

Constipation and FI symptoms that are new complaints and have occurred for less than 6 months should always prompt further evaluation for warning signs. Warning signs or red flag symptoms include hematochezia, a family history of colon cancer or inflammatory bowel disease, anemia, positive fecal occult blood test, unexplained weight loss ≥10 lbs, constipation that is refractory to treatment, and new-onset constipation/diarrhea without evidence of potential primary cause. These alarm symptoms may necessitate evaluation with more invasive testing. This should prompt shared decision making for evaluation with invasive testing in older adults with other chronic comorbid conditions.

Physical examination should include a rectal exam; palpating for hard stool; and assessing for masses, anal fissures, sphincter tone, prostatic hypertrophy in men, hemorrhoids, push effort during attempted defecation, and posterior vaginal masses in women. Laboratory testing should include a complete blood count, serum calcium, thyroid function tests, and fecal occult blood testing. Evaluation for causes of loose stool should look

for infection (including *Clostridium difficile* evaluation, fat malabsorption, and the presence of leukocytes). Other testing could involve serum tests to evaluate for celiac disease.

Abdominal radiographs may indicate significant stool retention in the colon and suggest the diagnosis of megacolon, a volvulus, or a mass lesion. Abdominal ultrasound could be ordered if acute or chronic cholecystitis symptoms are suspected as a potential cause for the change in bowel symptoms.

Referral for specialized testing for constipation and FI is rarely indicated. If indicated, colonoscopy may be needed to evaluate for colonic lesions, mass or obstruction, volvulus, megacolon, strictures, or for mucosal biopsy. Evaluation may be needed to identify anatomic abnormalities or factors such as sphincter tears/scarring, rectal sphincter muscle weakness, or dyssynergia.

The following four types of specialized testing may help with the diagnosis and etiology of constipation and FI symptoms. Although findings may suggest treatments, few have been evaluated for cost-effectiveness.

1. Marker studies or colonic transit studies in patients with constipation can help differentiate pelvic floor dyssynergia as a contributing cause for constipation. A marker study involves ingesting radiopaque markers with subsequent abdominal radiograph to detect the markers in the right, left, or rectosigmoid colon. Transit time evaluation with radioactive tracers and wireless motility capsule technologies (that record data after ingestion) are also available.
2. Anorectal manometry measures internal and external anal sphincter pressure at rest and during contraction. Sensation and rectal capacity can also be evaluated with a rectal balloon. Balloon expulsion tests can be used with anorectal manometry to evaluate pelvic floor dyssynergia and other defecation disorders.
3. Two- or three-dimensional endoanal ultrasound evaluates structural defects in the external or internal anal sphincters. Often, scarring or thinning of the muscle layers can also be detected. Endoanal ultrasound is done to evaluate patients with FI.
4. Defecography evaluates the defecatory process after a barium paste is inserted rectally and the patient defecates under fluoroscopy. Defecography can assess rectal emptying or structural abnormalities in the pelvic floor, such as obstruction or the presence of a rectocele.

TREATMENT OF CONSTIPATION

Once secondary causes of constipation have been evaluated and addressed, management of CC varies by type.[10] Treatment and prevention of slow transit constipation includes patient education about bowel habits, dietary changes, and drug therapies. Management of dyssynergic defecation involves biofeedback, relaxation exercises, and suppository programs. Patients with slow transit and dyssynergic defecation should receive treatment for the dyssynergia first before other measures.

> Nonpharmacologic treatments for constipation and FI should be the initial treatment option; these include bowel habit recognition, dietary considerations, and pelvic floor muscle control.

Nonpharmacologic treatment options or lifestyle modifications involve diet, exercise, bowel habit training, and biofeedback for dyssynergic defecation. Little clinical trial dietary modifications and physical exercise to prevent or treat constipation, especially in older adults.[11]

Dietary options include increasing fluid and fiber. In a study of 883 people older than 70 years, there was no association between estimated fluid intake and constipation; however, in 21,000 nursing home residents a weak association was found between decreased fluid intake and constipation. Adequate fluid may be an important general health recommendation and may impact treatment of constipation, especially with fiber supplementation. Recommended fiber intake is 20 to 35 g per day, but most Americans consume 5 to 10 g per day. Increasing dietary fiber is recommended. Information should be given on the fiber contained in common foods. Patients should increase fiber intake slowly—5 g per day at 1-week intervals until the recommended intake is attained. Patients should know that an immediate response is not expected, and that flatus and bloating may occur but are usually temporary. Increasing fiber intake gradually may reduce these unwanted side effects. Some providers suggest a mixture of dietary fiber and use of the natural cathartic effect of prune or pear juice. "Constipation recipes" mixing high fiber cereal (bran) and prune or pear juice (1 to 2 tablespoons of the mixture daily) with a warm beverage or oatmeal can be beneficial.

Probiotics have also been tested for the treatment of constipation. *Lactobacillus* and *Bifidobacterium* are symbiotic flora in the large intestine that may promote colonic mucosal health. Low levels of both have been reported in individuals with chronic constipation. Although properly controlled trials are lacking, some prospective evidence reports efficacy of probiotics (*Lactobacillus*) on constipation in nursing home residents. Survival and viability of probiotic bacteria in a commercial form have not been standardized for these treatments to have high levels of evidence.

Increased physical activity is associated with lower rates of constipation in older adults. Physical inactivity may also be associated with increased colonic transit time (harder stool consistency). Exercise should be encouraged in older adults, when appropriate.

Bowel habits and the use of bowel retraining are important initial steps, in addition to diet and exercise. Establishing and recognizing a regular bowel pattern is an important component for treatment. Older adults may need to be retaught how to recognize the postprandial gastrocolic reflex or urgency sensation because they may have ignored or no longer experience this sensation. Often, encouraging defecation shortly after the same daily meal and maintaining a schedule can be beneficial. Use of a glycerin suppository in the morning prior to the first meal may also help with bowel retraining and may improve bowel habits.

Caregivers and care providers in long-term care setting could be taught to use these bowel retraining techniques. A recent multicenter clinical trial, for improving FI and constipation in cognitively impaired nursing home residents (mean age 86 ± 10 years) compared a multicomponent intervention (toileting assistance, exercise, and food/fluid snacks every 2 hours for 8 hours/day for 3 months) to a usual-care group. The intervention group compared to the usual-care control group had improvements in bowel movement frequency and the percentage of bowel movements in the toilet, but not the frequency of FI episodes.

Biofeedback is an effective treatment for dyssynergic defecation, which is characterized by paradoxical contraction or failure to relax the pelvic floor muscles during defecation. In patients with dyssynergic defecation, biofeedback using coordinated therapy was consistently found to be more effective than continuous use of polyethylene glycol (PEG), standard therapy (other types of stool softeners and laxatives), sham therapy (aimed at overall body relaxation), or the use of diazepam in four randomized controlled trials. However, trials are needed to determine the efficacy of biofeedback in older adults.

Many people will have already tried fluids, fiber, and fitness, but often not in a sustained manner. Most Americans do not consume enough dietary fiber and increasing the intake of fiber and fluids may be enough to help prevent constipation in healthy older adults. Consideration may also involve nutritional expertise, physical therapy (when appropriate), and family/caregivers in making dietary and exercise changes for the treatment of constipation. Preventing and treating constipation with nonpharmacologic and pharmacologic treatments may be needed in specific situations (e.g., in the postoperative period, during hospitalization or other environments when decreased mobility is anticipated, and when using opioid medications).

Pharmacologic Treatments (Including Over-the-Counter Preparations)

The main categories of medications (including over-the-counter preparations) for prevention of constipation are bulking agents, stool softeners/emollients, and osmotic agents. The main categories for the treatment of constipation are bulking agents, stool softeners/emollients, osmotic agents, stimulants, chloride change activators, 5-HT$_4$ receptor agonists, and guanylate cyclase-C receptor agonists. Box 24-2 lists the pharmacologic treatments for constipation based on existing evidence from the American College of Gastroenterology Chronic Constipation Task Force.[12]

Bulking agents expand with water to increase the bulk of the stool and result in softer stools. Patients may need to try different types of fiber to achieve the desired outcome with minimum side effects. Some patients may better tolerate soluble and synthetic bulking agents than insoluable agents. Adequate hydration may be necessary for the desired outcome. Patients taking fiber need to increase fluid intake to 30 mL/kg of body weight daily to avoid worsening of constipation or impaction. Fiber may also inhibit the absorption of other drugs and should be taken 1 hour before or 2 hours after other medications. Bulking agents should be increased over weekly periods to avoid side effects, similar to increasing dietary fiber. Bulking agents are considered to be first-line agents for constipation. However, many older adults may not be good candidates for using a bulking agent. Some examples of when bulking agents may not be the first-line agent for older adults with constipation include the following: when taking high doses of narcotic medications, difficulty with swallowing or dysphagia (because of the consistency of certain types of fiber when mixed with water), anyone with surgical resection of the majority of the colon, patients who have a suspected rectal mass or possible bowel obstruction, and older adults who do not consume adequate amounts of fluid.

Stool softeners and emollients act by a detergent effect on stool consistency. This class of medications is well tolerated and does not interfere with other medications. No placebo-controlled trials exist and in a study of 170 patients, psyllium husk was as effective for softening stools and had similar overall efficacy as docusate. Mineral oil is also an emollient and may help lubricate the stool through the colon; however, aspiration and lipoid pneumonia are known risks to older adults. Stool softeners are often used when bulking agents do not work or are not preferred. Because of their mechanism of action as a detergent, stool softeners can also be used in combination with bulking agents. Like bulking agents, stool softeners alone are not good treatments for older adults on narcotic medications who have constipation.

Osmotic laxatives promote secretion of water into the intestinal lumen by osmotic activity and the hyperosmolar nature of these medications. PEG has the best evidence of use and is now available over the counter as a treatment for occasional constipation. It improves stool frequency and consistency in patients with constipation. Studies suggest that PEG can be dose adjusted or used every other day with efficacy. In an open-label study with 117 participants, people 65 years of age or older who used PEG over 12 months reported few side effects and no serious adverse events. A recent evidenced-based review concluded that PEG may be better for constipation symptoms than lactulose. In patients with congestive heart failure or chronic renal disease, PEG or magnesium hydroxide–containing preparations (milk of magnesia) should be used with extreme caution because these substances can cause electrolyte imbalances such as hypokalemia and diarrhea, further worsening

---

BOX 24-2

EVIDENCE-BASED PHARMACOLOGIC MANAGEMENT OPTIONS FOR CHRONIC CONSTIPATION

Therapy	Recommendations
Bulking agents	
Psyllium	Grade A
Calcium polycarbophil	Grade B
Methylcellulose	Grade B
Stool softeners/emollients	
Docusate calcium/sodium	Grade B
Mineral oil (linked with aspiration in older adults)	Grade C
Osmotic laxatives	
Lactulose	Grade A
Sorbitol	Grade B
PEG (polyethylene glycol)	Grade A
Magnesium hydroxide	Grade C
Stimulants	
Senna	Grade A
Bisacodyl	Grade A
5-HT$_4$ (serotonin) agonists	
Tegaserod maleate	Grade -*
Prucalopride (not available in U.S.)	Grade A
Chloride channel activator	
Lubiprostone	Grade A**
Guanylate cyclase-C receptor agonist	
Linaclotide	Grade A

*Tegaserod was approved for the treatment of irritable bowel syndrome with constipation (IBS-C) in women younger than 65. The Food and Drug Administration removed it from the market in 2007 because of increased risk of cardiovascular events.

**Data exist for adults older than 65 years of age without significant comorbid disorders.

fluid/electrolyte balances. Osmotic agents are useful when first-line bulking agents and/or stool softeners are not effective.

Stimulants, such as senna- and bisacodyl-containing compounds, increase intestinal motility by increasing peristaltic contractions. Stimulants also decrease water absorption from the lumen. Patients usually report more unfavorable side effects, including abdominal discomfort and cramping. Evidence exists for using bisacodyl given placebo-controlled studies. Evidence also exists for senna, although fewer clinical trials exist comparing senna to placebo than comparing bisacodyl to placebo. There is no evidence to support that long-term use of stimulant laxatives damages the enteric nervous system.[8] Stimulant laxatives have been associated with melanosis coli (seen on colonoscopy); this is a marker of chronic laxative use and may not indicate any other clinical consequences.

5-Hydroxytryptamine receptor subtype 4 (**5-HT₄ [serotonin]**) receptors are found in the colon and mediate the release of other neurotransmitters that enhance motility by increasing intestinal contractions. These drugs are no longer marketed in the United States and little data exist in older adults. Other prokinetic agents such as metoclopramide and erythromycin have not been formally evaluated for treatment of constipation. Because of side effects in older adults, metoclopramide should not be used for constipation.

Colonic Secretagogues

Chloride Channel Activators. Lubiprostone is a chloride channel activator that improves intestinal motility by increasing intestinal fluid secretion without altering serum electrolyte concentrations. Retrospective data from three pooled clinical trials of lubiprostone in elderly patients (n = 57) without significant comorbidities showed improvement in stool frequency and consistency, and decreased straining compared to placebo. Side effects include nausea, diarrhea, headache, abdominal distension, and abdominal pain but are generally well tolerated.

Guanylate Cyclase-C Receptor Antagonists. Linaclotide (another colonic secretagogue) stimulates intestinal fluid secretion and transit. Two large phase 3 trials in patients with constipation showed the treated groups had significantly higher rates of three or more complete spontaneous bowel movements per week and an increase in one or more complete spontaneous bowel movements from baseline during 9 out of 12 weeks compared with the placebo group. The most common adverse event was diarrhea, which led to discontinuation in 4% of patients. The long-term risks and benefits of linaclotide in constipation are unknown.

Opioid Antagonists. Alvimopan and methylnaltrexone are peripherally acting μ-opioid receptor antagonists that may have some role in treatment of opiate-induced constipation and paralytic ileus. Data are lacking in older adults. These medications do not cross the blood–brain barrier; thus they do not affect the analgesic properties of opioids.

TREATMENT OF FECAL IMPACTION

Constipation is an important factor in the development of fecal impaction in older adults, especially those who have limited mobility. Fecal impaction results from an individual's lack of ability to sense and respond to stool in the rectum.

To diagnose fecal impaction, a digital rectal examination is important, but this may not be the only evaluation necessary. Impacted stool may not have a hard consistency, and the key finding is a large amount of stool in the rectum. Fecal impaction can also occur in the proximal rectum or sigmoid colon, which would not be detected on digital rectal examination. If fecal impaction is suspected, obtaining an abdominal radiograph may help identify the area of impaction.

The management of fecal impaction involves disimpaction and colon evacuation, followed by a maintenance bowel regimen. Digital disimpaction can be used to fragment a large amount of feces in the rectum. Following digital disimpaction, a warm-water enema with mineral oil may be used to soften the impaction and assist with evacuating the impacted area. Very little evidence exists in guiding treatment of fecal impaction. However, if digital disimpaction and enemas fail, local anesthesia to relax the anal canal along with abdominal massage may be useful. In rare cases, colonoscopy with a snare to fragment fecal material in the distal colon may be needed. Abdominal tenderness or bleeding may indicate bowel perforation or ischemia, and surgery may be necessary.

TREATMENT OF FECAL INCONTINENCE (FI)

Given the multiple causes and contributors to FI, the treatments often include combinations of the following: dietary changes, behavioral interventions, biofeedback, pharmacologic treatments, perianal injectable bulking agents, and sacral neuromodulation (surgical and nonsurgical).[12] Special consideration is also given to managing skin problems such as incontinence-associated dermatitis.

Dietary and Behavioral Interventions for FI

Initial treatments for FI include conservative measures[12] (such as dietary modifications, bowel habit training, and pelvic floor muscle training with or without biofeedback and electrical stimulation) and pharmacologic treatments (such as constipating and/or stool-bulking agents). Conservative therapies are often combined and improve mild FI by 50% to 95% depending on the modality used.[13] Dietary modifications should focus on avoiding triggers for loose stool, such as lactose-containing products. Increasing dietary or supplementary fiber may improve loose stool and decrease diarrhea by bulking the stool. Solid stool may be easier to retain in the rectum. A small study comparing psyllium or gum arabic to placebo showed improved rates of FI in individuals with diarrhea-predominant FI. Bowel habit training and scheduled toileting with or without laxatives to empty the rectum may help those with cognitive or mobility problems.

Biofeedback

Biofeedback involves a trained provider who uses an instrument that gives a patient visual or auditory feedback on the proper control of voluntary muscle contraction and relaxation of the external anal sphincter and recognition of anal sphincter sensation.[13] Strength training, sensory training, and coordinated training (strength and sensory) occur in most biofeedback protocols for FI. The goal is improved external anal sphincter muscle contraction in response to rectal sensation or distension. Most centers use electromyographic or manometric biofeedback equipment. For success, patients who undergo biofeedback treatment need to have awareness of their defecation symptoms and be able to actively participate during the office-based treatments and adhere to a home exercise program. Older adults with cognitive problems and adults with spinal cord injury may not be good candidates for biofeedback.

Biofeedback has been compared to anal exercises and pelvic floor muscle exercises along with other conservative treatments.[13] A randomized controlled trial for FI management compared dietary and bowel habit advice alone, advice with exercises, and biofeedback, and showed that pelvic floor muscle exercises and biofeedback were no better than advice alone in improving FI frequency. However, 53% of all patients in this study had decreased FI frequency, better quality of life, and improved anorectal manometry pressures. In another trial of biofeedback compared with pelvic floor muscle exercises alone in 108 women who were not adequately treated with medication, education and behavioral strategies showed significantly greater reductions in FI severity, fewer days with FI, and more patients reporting adequate relief (76% vs. 41%) in the biofeedback group compared to exercises alone. A few studies show no improvement in FI with a home electrical stimulation unit over a sham unit or office-based treatment.

Pharmacologic Treatment

The most commonly used pharmacologic treatments involve antidiarrheal drugs for diarrhea-associated FI. Only three randomized crossover trials with adequate methodology have evaluated pharmacologic treatment of diarrhea-predominant FI in adults.[14] Trials compared drug versus placebo (one used diphenoxylate [n = 15], one used loperamide [n = 26], and one compared loperamide with codeine to diphenoxylate plus atropine [n = 30]). All had decreased frequency of FI episodes and volume, and improved stool consistency. More people treated with the drugs reported adverse events including constipation, abdominal pain, diarrhea, headache, and nausea. Given the anticholinergic properties of diphenoxylate plus atropine, this treatment should be avoided in older adults. Treatment of constipation-associated FI with laxatives can be very effective, especially in long-term care settings, when used with other behavioral interventions (see earlier section on the treatment of constipation).

Occasionally, when antidiarrhea drugs are not effective for improving diarrhea-associated FI, a trial with cholestyramine is warranted. Cholestyramine is a bile salt–binding medication used to lower cholesterol and can reduce diarrhea associated with the production of excess bile acid salts. Limited data exist on the use of this medication specifically for FI.

CASE 1

Discussion

Ms. McDonald has a long-standing history of chronic constipation symptoms, and fairly new onset (6 to 8 months) of worsening symptoms that are not responding to over-the-counter laxative therapy with milk of magnesia. The most likely explanation for her bowel symptoms may be overflow FI with fecal impaction. Her current symptoms do not warrant evaluation with a colonoscopy or other bowel imaging because she does not describe having any red flag symptoms. Even though you may not need further evaluation with endoscopy, you may consider doing further evaluation for worsening constipation and possible fecal impaction with an abdominal radiograph. Often fecal impaction is not identified on a digital rectal examination. In terms of additional testing you might consider thyroid function tests, serum calcium, and electrolytes. Ms. McDonald does not say she has diarrhea or loose stool so stool studies may not be indicated.

At the first visit you decide to treat her constipation symptoms. She may benefit from higher doses and more consistent laxative treatment with PEG (e.g., Miralax), which can be titrated to effect. She may also benefit from an enema or a stimulant suppository to help with her fecal impaction while treating her slow-transit problems with oral laxatives. She will also need to improve her overall bowel habits once her impaction has improved. Hopefully, with the treatment of the fecal impaction, she will no longer have the FI symptoms.

After using twice daily doses of PEG and rectal suppositories for 2 weeks after her initial visit, she had three to four bowel movements per week with a softer stool consistency and less complaints of incomplete emptying after a bowel movement. She also started drinking at least 40 to 50 oz of water daily. Although she was pleased with her current treatment, she still had some accidental bowel leakage that occurred after having a bowel movement. She noticed her leakage was not preceded by any fecal urgency symptoms. This passive leakage of stool occurred two to three times per month. Although she was only wearing the adult diapers when outside the house, she still wore sanitary pads daily.

Today she wants to know what else she could do to help with her symptoms. You know that long-standing constipation can increase compliance of the rectal wall and decrease the ability to have the same urgency sensation prior to bowel evacuation. However, she is having more leakage after having a bowel movement. This could indicate a rectal emptying problem. Problems with rectal emptying could occur from having a vaginal posterior compartment defect (vaginal rectocele), problems with loose or unformed stool consistency, or weakened rectal sphincter muscles.

In addition to educating Ms. McDonald about the importance of focusing on bowel habits including recognizing and responding to fecal urge, you decrease the dose of PEG to once every day or every other day. If the problem resulted from a posterior vaginal compartment defect or problems with stool consistency, you might consider increasing her total fiber content. Dietary fiber and supplementary fiber could be used, along with the PEG, to improve stool consistency in a motivated patient who is also drinking plenty of fluids. Biofeedback and a home rectal sphincter muscle exercise program would be indicated to increase rectal sphincter tone and to improve rectal sensation. ■

Injectable Agents

For use when conservative measures for FI have failed, a minimally invasive injectable agent has been approved. An office-based procedure involves the perianal injection of dextranomer microspheres and hyaluronic acid. Initial data are promising for reduced FI episodes, but more long-term data are needed. Studies involving other injectable agents into the perianal area have not shown significant improvements in FI episodes.[15]

Sacral Neuromodulation

Percutaneous tibial nerve stimulation (PTNS) and a surgically implanted device, Interstim, are used to treat FI by stimulating the nerves that help control defecation.[16] PTNS involves an office-based procedure to indirectly stimulate the sacral nerves through the posterior tibial nerve. A small, acupuncture-sized needle is inserted into the medial aspect of the lower extremity and attached to a stimulation device. Often, 12 weeks of treatment are needed to see improvement in FI symptoms. The eight small prospective studies (largest study, n = 32), involving a combined sample size of 129 participants, had significant variation in the study population, methodology, and outcome measures, as well as a large mean age range (38 to 60 years). Data collection from adequately powered randomized controlled trials for PTNS treatment for FI is ongoing and will add significantly to the evidence.

Interstim, a neuromodulation device that is surgically implanted, has been approved for use in Europe since 1994 and was recently approved in the United States for treatment of refractory FI.[17] This device stimulates the sacral nerves (at S3) and has shown improvement in symptoms compared to conservative measures.

> Surgical treatment for FI can be considered after more conservative treatment options fail.

Other Surgical Approaches

Other surgical therapies for FI include anal sphincter repairs, artificial bowel sphincter, and colostomy. Overlapping sphincteroplasty can be used to repair a torn anal sphincter, which most commonly results from an obstetrical injury and can be an occult finding in older women. Although short-term benefits may exist, longer term data on outcome are needed. Use of artificial bowel sphincter has significant associated morbidity. Colostomy is essentially used as a salvage procedure.

TREATMENT OF INCONTINENCE-ASSOCIATED DERMATITIS

Contact of fecal material with skin on the perineum can cause contact dermatitis, fungal infection, and pressure ulcers. Treatment of skin problems is dependent on correct classification and recognition. Incontinence-associated dermatitis in the perineal area can also occur from wetness and moisture exposure, which often results from the use of pads and other forms of containment. Use of skin barrier cream is recommended to help prevent and occasionally treat erythema and maceration that can occur with FI. Several moisture-barrier, skin-protectant creams and pastes are available for over-the-counter use; these often include zinc oxide and dimethicone.[18]

SUMMARY

Constipation and FI are common bowel symptoms that older patients experience. Older adults often resort to self-treatment and the impact of the symptoms is underrecognized by health care providers. Evaluation of potential causes and contributing factors is important. Evaluation with colonoscopy or other endoscopic procedures is often not warranted, unless alarm symptoms are present. Treatments often depend on the underlying cause of the constipation or FI. Conservative therapies are considered the initial treatment prior to using more invasive therapies, including medicine and surgery.

Web Resources

http://romecriteria.org. The Rome Foundation.
www.digestive.niddk.nih.gov/ddiseases/pubs/constipation. The National Digestive Diseases Information Clearinghouse, sponsored by the National Institute of Diabetes and Digestive and Kidney Diseases (NIDDK), National Institutes of Health.
www.digestive.niddk.nih.gov/ddiseases/pubs/fecalincontinence. The National Digestive Diseases Information Clearinghouse, sponsored by the National Institute of Diabetes and Digestive and Kidney Diseases (NIDDK), National Institutes of Health.

www.nia.nih.gov/health/publication/concerned-about-constipation. National Institutes of Health patient information website.
www.nafc.org/index.php?page=fecal-incontinence. National Association for Continence.
www.iffgd.org. International Foundation for Functional Gastrointestinal Disorders.

KEY REFERENCES

2. Lembo A, Camilleri M. Chronic constipation. N Engl J Med 2003;349(14):1360-8.
5. Whitehead WE, Borrud L, Goode PS, et al. Fecal incontinence in US adults: Epidemiology and risk factors. Gastroenterology 2009;137(2):512.
10. Gallegos-Orozco JF, Foxx-Orenstein AE, Sterler SM, Stoa JM. Chronic constipation in the elderly. Am J Gastroenterol 2012;107:18-25.
11. Wald A. Constipation in the primary care setting: Current concepts and misconceptions. Am J Med 2006;119(9):736.
12. Norton C, Thomas L, Hill J, Guideline Development Group. Management of faecal incontinence in adults: Summary of NICE guidance. BMJ 2007;334(7608):1370-1.

References available online at expertconsult.com.

25

Hearing Impairment

Timothy J. Lewis

Additional online-only material indicated by icon.

OBJECTIVES

Upon completion of this chapter, the reader will be able to:

- Identify effects of aging on the auditory system.
- Describe the psychosocial and functional consequences of hearing loss.
- Interpret common tests used to evaluate hearing impairment and disability.
- Distinguish presbycusis from other forms of hearing loss.
- Discuss the differential diagnosis for adult hearing impairment.
- List appropriate indications for audiology and otolaryngology referrals.
- Summarize effective hearing loss treatments.

PREVALENCE AND IMPACT

Hearing loss is common in older adults and has serious psychosocial and functional consequences. It affects one third of individuals 65 years or older and ranks as the third most common chronic disease in that age category. Hearing impairment rises geometrically with age from 16% at age 60, 32% at age 70, and 64% at age 80. The prevalence of hearing disability also rises with age (Figure 25-1). Functional deficits associated with hearing loss include diminished ability to recognize speech amid background noise and to locate and identify sounds that may have an important warning or alarm significance. The communication difficulties experienced by the hearing impaired also affect other people in their environment such as family members and coworkers. Hearing loss is associated with depression, social isolation, and poor self-esteem, as well as cognitive decline.

Despite the importance of hearing function in everyday life, hearing loss is often a poorly recognized and undertreated problem. The insidious onset and progression of age-related hearing loss (ARHL) likely contributes to its under-recognition. Although 26.7 million U.S. adults aged 50 years or older have clinically significant hearing loss, fewer than 15% use hearing aids.[1] In the United States, only about 40% of people with moderate to severe ARHL own hearing aids; that percentage drops to 10% among persons with mild ARHL.[2]

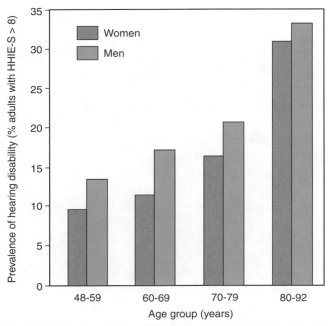

Figure 25-1 Prevalence of hearing disability (Hearing Handicap Inventory for the Elderly–Screening Version [HHIE-S] score >8) by age and gender. (Modified from Wiley T, et al. Self-reported hearing handicap and audiometric measures in older adults. J Am Acad Audiol 2000;11:67-75.)

BARRIERS TO THE EVALUATION AND TREATMENT OF HEARING LOSS

The subtle presentation of ARHL is rarely a call to action for either the afflicted person or his or her doctor. In the mild to moderate stages, ARHL is often characterized by the inability to understand words rather than the inability to hear, and the common refrain of "My hearing is fine. You're just mumbling." The functional consequences of hearing disability, however, should not be underestimated. When affected individuals do become aware of their hearing loss, initially they may try to compensate and conceal it, but symptoms eventually give their secret away. Persons wait on average 7 to 10 years between signs of hearing loss and audiologic consultation.[3] Affected persons may not be aware of the functional deficits or know what they are missing. Older persons who have ARHL but do not pursue hearing aids demonstrate less problem awareness on questionnaires of self-perceived hearing disability and have a greater tendency to deny communication problems. The high cost of hearing aids is an additional barrier to treatment for many older Americans.

Primary care providers can help with recognition and treatment of adults with hearing disability by routinely asking about hearing problems and watching for signs or symptoms of hearing disability, such as communication difficulties, social withdrawal, or

depressed mood. When the history and examination suggest ARHL, timely referral to an audiologist can help improve the outlook for persons with hearing disability.

> Timely primary care referral to an audiologist for formal hearing testing and evaluation of aural rehabilitation needs can help improve the outlook for older adults with hearing disability.

AGING CHANGES

Usual aging changes in the auditory system contribute to diminished hearing performance among older adults (Box 25-1). Prior noise exposure, middle ear disease, and vascular disease affect the progression of ARHL. Longitudinal studies demonstrate that hearing declines gradually in 97% of the population as evidenced by diminished pure-tone threshold sensitivities with age. Individuals under 55 years of age typically lose hearing at a rate of 3 dB per decade, and those over 55 years at a rate of 9 dB per decade.[4] The ability to understand speech in a backdrop of competing conversations begins to deteriorate slowly in the fourth decade of life, and accelerates after the seventh decade. As adults age, it also becomes increasingly difficult for them to understand speech that is rapid, poorly transmitted, or mispronounced.

CASE 1

Harry Jackson (Part 1)

Harry Jackson, a 70-year-old man, comes to your office accompanied by his wife of 45 years for evaluation of gradually worsening hearing loss. She has noticed that he has difficulty understanding speech, especially at a distance or in noisy social gatherings. He has been scaling back his work hours as a self-employed plumber in preparation for retirement. In his spare time he is an avid softball fan. He also enjoys the company of his grandchildren immensely but he has increasing difficulty understanding them. His wife is particularly concerned about Mr. Jackson's reluctance to participate in social activities. She has been encouraging him to have his hearing tested and thinks he needs a hearing aid. He denies ear pain, tinnitus, vertigo, or asymmetric hearing loss. His past medical history includes osteoarthritis, hypertension, and chronic stable angina. His only medications are 81 mg aspirin daily for heart attack prevention, metoprolol for hypertension, and Tylenol as needed for arthritis pain.

1. **What factors may be contributing to hearing problems in Mr. Jackson?**

2. **What assessments are needed to investigate this patient's hearing difficulty?** ▣

RISK FACTORS AND PATHOPHYSIOLOGY

The two major forms of hearing loss are sensorineural and conductive disorders; each has its own risk factors and causes. Disorders of the inner ear cause sensorineural hearing loss by damaging the cochlea, eighth cranial nerve, or internal auditory canal. Presbycusis is a distinct age-related sensorineural hearing loss that is the most common cause of ARHL. The hallmark of presbycusis is bilateral, symmetric, high-frequency sensorineural hearing loss. Advancing age is the predominant risk factor. The cochlea appears to be the primary site of pathogenesis, although the precise cause of presbycusis remains uncertain.

Noise-induced hearing loss (NIHL) is the second most common cause of sensorineural hearing loss among older adults. The pathogenesis of NIHL involves direct mechanical injury to the sensory hair cells of the cochlea. Continuous noise exposure poses greater risk than intermittent exposure.

Disorders of the external ear or the middle ear can cause conductive hearing loss by interfering with the mechanical transmission of sound in the inner ear. Conductive disorders typically have a mechanical cause. And occlusion of the external ear canal by cerumen is the most common cause of conductive loss. Other risk factors for conductive loss include perforated ear drum, fluid in the middle ear, and disarticulation of the ossicular chain. Specific disease entities causing conductive hearing loss are described in the following section.

DIFFERENTIAL DIAGNOSIS AND ASSESSMENT

Hearing loss can result from diseases of the auricle, external auditory canal, middle ear, inner ear, or central auditory pathways. Diseases of the inner ear or eighth nerve cause sensorineural hearing loss, whereas diseases of the auricle, external auditory canal, or middle ear generally cause conductive hearing loss.

BOX 25-2

DIFFERENTIAL DIAGNOSIS OF HEARING LOSS

Conductive Hearing Loss
Outer Ear Causes
Otitis externa
Trauma
Cerumen
Osteoma
Exostosis
Squamous cell carcinoma

Middle Ear Causes
Otitis media
Tympanic membrane
   perforation
Cholesteatoma
Otosclerosis
Glomus tumors
Temporal bone trauma
Paget's disease

Sensorineural Hearing Loss
Inner Ear Causes
Presbycusis
Noise exposure
Meniere's disease
Ototoxic drugs
Meningitis
Viral cochleitis
Barotrauma
Acoustic neuroma
Meningioma
Multiple sclerosis
Vascular disease

Mixed loss refers to a combination of conductive and sensorineural loss. Central auditory processing dysfunction is a major factor affecting speech perception in the seventh decade and beyond. Attention should be paid to memory function also because memory impairment affects central auditory ability.[5] Box 25-2 lists the differential diagnosis.

Conductive Hearing Loss

Conductive hearing loss results from obstruction of the external auditory canal (EAC) by cerumen, debris, or foreign bodies. Otitis externa causes conductive hearing loss when inflammation leads to canal edema that blocks the EAC. Tumors of the EAC such as squamous cell carcinoma can be mistaken for otitis externa. Conductive loss arises when such tumors occlude the canal. Diagnosis is by biopsy. Other causes of conductive hearing loss include perforations of the tympanic membrane; disruption of the ossicular chain from trauma or infection, fluid, scarring, or tumors in the middle ear; and otosclerosis.

Cholesteatoma is stratified squamous epithelium in the middle ear or mastoid. This nonmalignant, slowly growing lesion causes conductive hearing loss when erosion disrupts the ossicular chain. Cholesteatoma should be suspected when a chronically draining ear fails to respond to antibiotic therapy. Management is surgical.

Conductive hearing loss with a normal ear canal and intact tympanic membrane should raise concern for ossicular chain disease. Otosclerosis, a bony overgrowth involving the footplate of the stapes, leads to stapes fixation and low-frequency conductive hearing loss. Bone diseases such as Paget's disease and immunologic diseases such as rheumatoid arthritis can also lead to conductive hearing loss by causing ossicular pathology.

Tympanic membrane perforation causes conductive loss arising from trauma, and acute or chronic otitis media. Size and location of the perforation determine the degree of hearing loss. An audiogram determines the effect on hearing function. Small perforations tend to heal, whereas large perforations often require surgical repair. Otoscopy usually diagnoses tympanic membrane perforation, middle ear infection, and cerumen impaction.

Sensorineural Hearing Loss

The most common pattern of sensorineural hearing loss in adults is presbycusis. In the early stages the audiogram usually shows bilateral gentle or sharply sloping high-frequency hearing loss. Adults with presbycusis often complain of difficulty understanding speech, especially in noisy environments.

Sensorineural hearing loss also develops from damage to the hair cells of the organ of Corti from intense noise, ototoxic drugs, viral infections, meningitis, temporal bone fracture, or Meniere's disease. Noise is the second most common cause of sensorineural hearing loss after presbycusis; noise-induced sensorineural hearing loss is permanent but largely preventable. It begins at the higher frequencies (3000 to 6000 Hz) and develops gradually from cumulative exposure equal to an average decibel level of 85 dB or higher for an 8-hour period.

Older adults are at risk for ototoxicity from certain medications such as aminoglycosides. Tobramycin and amikacin are more cochleotoxic, whereas gentamycin and streptomycin are more vestibulotoxic. Additional medications with known ototoxicity are listed in Box 25-3.

Meniere's disease causes sensorineural hearing loss that classically affects low frequencies and is episodic with periods of vertigo, tinnitus, and aural fullness. The associated hearing loss may become permanent over time and involve other frequencies.

BOX 25-3

OTOTOXIC MEDICATIONS

- Antibiotics: aminoglycosides, erythromycin, tetracycline, vancomycin
- Antimalarials: chloroquinine,* quinine*
- Antineoplastics: cisplatin, bleomycin, 5-fluorouracil, nitrogen mustard
- Salicylates: aspirin*
- Diuretics: loop diuretics*

*Hearing loss and tinnitus are reversible when caused by these agents.

Tumors of the inner ear are usually benign. Acoustic neuroma is the most common benign tumor in the inner ear and originates from the eighth cranial nerve. Acoustic neuromas are commonly either asymptomatic or cause unilateral sensorineural hearing loss, but may also be associated with other symptoms such as unilateral tinnitus, dizziness, or headaches.

Sensorineural hearing loss may also be caused by meningiomas or other neoplasms, demyelinating or degenerative disease, or infections such as HIV. Endocrine or other metabolic disorders can also cause hearing loss. For example, diabetes can cause small vessel disease, which can induce cochlear ischemia.

CASE 1

Harry Jackson (Part 2)

To assess the self-perceived emotional and social impact imposed by Mr. Jackson's hearing impairment, you administer the Hearing Handicap Inventory for the Elderly–Screening Version (HHIE-S). Mr. Jackson obtains a total score of 10. Routine otoscopic examination reveals findings of bilateral cerumen impaction. Using a curette, you gently remove bilateral moderate cerumen plugs from the external auditory canal under direct vision of an otoscope. His tympanic membranes have normal landmarks. You proceed to perform screening audiometry using an otoscope with a built-in audiometer. He fails to hear the 2000-Hz pure-tone stimulus at a screening level of 40 dB in both ears on two trials. After discussing your findings with Mr. Jackson, he agrees to have a hearing assessment at a local audiology center. You make his referral.

1. **What is the significance of Mr. Jackson's score on the HHIE-S?**

2. **What is the traditional definition of an abnormal result on a screening audiometry test?** ▣

DETECTION AND EVALUATION OF HEARING LOSS

Screening

Although there is relatively sparse evidence that screening older adults for hearing loss changes outcomes, screening for ARHL appears advisable on epidemiologic grounds. Hearing impairment prevalence is high, as is the associated disease burden. Accurate and inexpensive screening tests for hearing impairment exist. Effective treatments for hearing impairment are also available. Furthermore, screening programs can likely reach the patients who could benefit, and appear feasible within the U.S. health care system despite significant barriers such as lack of medical insurance coverage for hearing evaluations and expensive treatments.[6]

Several professional organizations have advocated for greater use of audiologic screening among older adults. The American Speech-Language-Hearing Association 1997 guidelines recommend that adults older than 50 years have audiometric screening every 3 years.[7] The Canadian Task Force on Preventive Health Care also recommended screening older adults for hearing impairment. In 1996 the U.S. Preventive Services Task Force (USPSTF) recommended periodic screening of older adults for hearing loss. In 2012 the USPSTF issued a new recommendation stating "current evidence is insufficient to assess the balance of benefits and harms of screening for hearing loss in asymptomatic adults aged 50 years or older".[8,9]

An appropriate goal of a hearing screening program among older adults is to identify persons who need diagnostic hearing assessment to investigate possible untreated medical disease and/or hearing disability. There are two general screening strategies: audiometry and hearing disability self-report measures.

Screening Audiometry

Screening audiometry is a reliable and accurate physiologic test for identifying persons with hearing impairment. The Audioscope (Welch-Allyn) is a well-validated screening tool. This handheld otoscope with a built-in audiometer allows quick and accurate detection of hearing impairment when referenced against a conventional audiogram as the criterion standard. Adult subjects are considered to have failed screening testing if they do not hear a 40-dB tone at 2000 Hz in either ear. This criterion maximizes test accuracy, with excellent sensitivity (0.94) and good specificity (0.69 to 0.80). Screening with the Audioscope for >40 dB hearing loss is associated with a median positive likelihood ratio (LR) of 3.4 and a median negative LR of 0.05. [10,11]

The relationship between hearing impairment and hearing disability is imperfect. Some individuals experience disability and/or handicap even with a mild 25-dB-level hearing loss. Others with the same pure-tone threshold or worse may deny subjective hearing disability and lack motivation to try hearing aids. Auditory tests do not reflect the impact of hearing impairment on an older person's daily life. Validated questionnaires have been developed to help clinicians assess the handicap imposed by hearing impairment. Unlike pure-tone audiometry, these questionnaires focus on the functional and social implications of hearing impairment.

Hearing Disability Self-Report Measures

The Hearing Handicap Inventory for the Elderly–Screening Version (HHIE-S) is an accepted screening tool for hearing disability (Box 25-4). The 10-question HHIE-S can be administered in less than 2 minutes. Possible scores range from 0 (no handicap) to 40 (maximum handicap). A score of 10 or more suggests significant self-perceived hearing handicap, and should

---

BOX 25-4

HEARING HANDICAP INVENTORY FOR THE ELDERLY–SCREENING VERSION

- Does a hearing problem cause you to feel embarrassed when you meet new people?
- Does a hearing problem cause you to feel frustrated when talking to a member of your family?
- Do you have difficulty hearing when someone speaks in a whisper?
- Do you feel handicapped by a hearing problem?
- Does a hearing problem cause you difficulty when visiting friends, relatives, or neighbors?
- Does a hearing problem cause you to attend religious services less often than you would like?
- Does a hearing problem cause you to have arguments with family members?
- Does a hearing problem cause you difficulty when listening to television or radio?
- Do you feel that any difficulty with your hearing limits/hampers your personal or social life?
- Does a hearing problem cause you difficulty when in a restaurant with relatives or friends?

Note: Answers scored as yes (4), sometimes (2), and no (0). Total point range, zero to 40; zero to 8 = no self-perceived handicap; 10 to 22 = mild to moderate handicap; 24 to 40 = significant handicap.
Adapted from Ventry IM, Weinstein BE. Identification of elderly people with hearing problems. Am Speech Language Hearing Assoc 1983; 25:37-42.

---

prompt referral to an audiologist. Using the 10-or-more cutoff, the HHIE-S performs with a sensitivity ranging from 63% to 80% and a specificity ranging from 67% to 77%.[12]

Another screening option is to ask the patient a single question (SQ) about hearing loss. The performance of a positive HHIE-S (score >8) has been compared to a yes response to the question "Do you feel you have hearing loss?" using pure-tone average (PTA) hearing threshold as the gold standard in older people living independently in the community. In identifying a greater than 25-dB hearing impairment, the SQ had a higher sensitivity compared to the HHIE-S (54% vs. 44%). However, when using a PTA of greater than 40 dB as the gold standard, there were no significant differences in screening sensitivity between the HHIE-S and SQ (82% vs. 88%) and, furthermore, the HHIE-S >8 had significantly higher specificity than a positive SQ response (78% vs. 69%). In addition, the HHIE-S shows greater reliability than the single-question method. Based on these characteristics, it is preferable to use the HHIE-S rather than a single question about hearing loss as a screening tool for detecting hearing impairment in community-dwelling older adults.[13]

> The Hearing Handicap Inventory for the Elderly–Screening Version (HHIE-S) outperforms a single question about hearing loss in detecting hearing impairment (pure-tone average >40 dB) among community-dwelling older adults.

Screening Effectiveness

There is relatively sparse clinical outcomes research on effectiveness of hearing loss screening programs among older adults. The only randomized controlled trial of screening for hearing loss was in an outpatient veteran population. Screening led to significantly more audiology visits, confirmed cases of hearing loss, hearing aid fits, and hearing aid use 1 year later. Benefits of screening were especially strong in veterans 65 and older. In that subgroup, there were higher rates of 1-year hearing aid use compared to unscreened controls; the 1-year hearing aid use rates among participants in the otoscope, questionnaire, and dual screening trial arms were 11.7%, 7.1% , and 16.7% respectively, compared to 3.8% in controls (p <0.001). In the entire study population, despite fewer positive screening tests and fewer visits to audiologists, patients in the tone-emitting otoscope arm more frequently used hearing aids 1 year later (6.3%) than patients in the questionnaire-only arm (4.1%). Patients screened with both tests had the highest rate of 1-year hearing aid use (7.4%); the corresponding rate among the control patients was 3.3%. Screening using a tone-emitting otoscope was thus found to be more efficient in terms of the clinical outcome of hearing aid use after 1 year, possibly because of a higher false positive rate of the HHIE-S. In subgroup analysis, participants without self-perceived hearing loss at study entry, regardless of screening method, had low hearing aid use (only 1.6% at 1 year). Further research is needed to define the benefits and costs of screening asymptomatic adults for hearing loss compared with testing only those seeking treatment of perceived hearing impairment.[14]

Primary Care Evaluation and Referral

There are three steps in assessment of hearing function in the primary care office: history taking, physical examination, and screening for hearing impairment and disability. In the history, ask about difficulty understanding speech, especially in noisy environments, or during telephone use or soft conversation. Collateral history from a spouse or individuals familiar with the patient's hearing performance may be useful. Ask about confusion in social situations, excessive volume of television/radio/computer, or social withdrawal.

An otoscopic examination is essential. Otologic examination identifies reversible causes of conductive hearing loss including otitis externa, cerumen impaction, foreign objects obstructing the external auditory canal, and osteoma. Assessment of the integrity and mobility of the tympanic membrane is also indicated. Tuning fork tests such as the Rinne and the Weber allow differentiation of conductive and sensorineural hearing loss. Simple tests for hearing loss, such as the whispered voice test and the finger rub test, are quick to perform but difficult to standardize. In the whispered voice test, the examiner stands behind the patient at arm's length from the ear, covers the untested ear, fully exhales, and whispers a combination of three numbers and letters and then asks the patient to repeat the set. If the patient fails to repeat all three, the examiner whispers a second set; inability to repeat at least three of six test stimuli indicates impairment. There unfortunately is no reliable way to control the loudness of the whisper or finger rub, and strong data on interobserver variability and test-retest reliability are lacking. Identification of hearing impairment with pure-tone-emitting otoscope is a quick, reliable, and accurate alternative to the whisper test and the finger rub test. Patients with suspected or definite hearing loss should be referred for diagnostic audiometry and objective measurement of hearing function.

MANAGEMENT OF HEARING IMPAIRMENT

Cerumen Impaction

Earwax in normal amounts serves as a cleaning agent with protective, lubricating, and antibacterial properties. Earwax is formed in the outer third of the ear canal. When a patient has wax blockage deeper in the ear canal, this is often because the patient has probed the ear with a cotton-tipped applicator or another object that only pushed the wax deeper into the ear canal. Patients should be discouraged from probing ears with cotton-tipped applicators or other objects.

Cerumen impaction can usually be managed in the office. A small curette is used to remove cerumen if the clinician is familiar with the technique. Alternately, gentle irrigation with tepid water may loosen and remove cerumen if the tympanic membrane is visible and intact. Cerumen-dissolving drops such as 10% sodium bicarbonate can also ease cerumen removal. When severe cerumen impaction is identified, referral to an otolaryngologist may be advisable.

Counseling Older Adults about Hearing Health Services

A critical aspect of managing ARHL is promoting health-seeking behaviors. To be effective, clinicians must understand barriers to recognition of hearing loss, and help older adults become aware of hearing loss, its consequences, and available rehabilitative services. Patients should be counseled on benefits of hearing health services and their attitudes toward treatment such as hearing aids should be discussed. This is an opportunity to dispel pessimistic views about the benefits of hearing aids. The evidence supporting hearing aid effectiveness is strong, a fact that should be communicated to patients with suspected hearing impairment. Hearing aid use can reduce the adverse impact of hearing loss on quality of life among older adults.[15] Hearing aid recipients demonstrate significant improvements in social, emotional, and communication function, as well as depression.

Enhancing Communication with the Hearing Impaired

Communication with hearing-impaired older adults can be enhanced by optimizing speaking distance, sound environment, signal clarity, and visual cues. The speaker's face should be in full view of the listener and within 2 to 3 feet. Avoid backlighting as occurs when the speaker stands with his or her back to a bright window. Where possible, reduce background noise. Pause between sentences. Avoid shouting and speak clearly at a slightly louder than normal intensity. When repetition is necessary, paraphrase the message or write key words. Speaking directly into the good ear is not advisable because the speaker's face and lips are then no longer in view.

Myths about Hearing Aids

The common misconception that hearing aids draw attention to the individual and their hearing impairment merits discussion. To address this misconception, clinicians should advise prospective hearing aid candidates that not hearing when spoken to and not answering correctly are more conspicuous than wearing a hearing aid.

> If used appropriately, hearing aids can reduce hearing disability and thereby diminish the outward signs of hearing loss.

CASE 1

Harry Jackson (Part 3)

At his hearing aid evaluation, Mr. Jackson reported to the audiologist that he is hearing somewhat better since the wax removal. His wife was amused by her husband's recent comment that "we have to get these darn floors fixed." Since the wax removal, her husband became aware of the longstanding squeak of the floor boards in their century-old home. Audiometry revealed bilaterally symmetrical, mild to moderate, sloping high-frequency sensorineural hearing loss. On speech discrimination testing, Mr. Jackson recognized 87% of a monosyllabic word list in his right ear and 90% in his left ear with 40-dB amplification above his pure-tone thresholds. At normal conversational level, his word recognition score dropped to 70%. Mr. Jackson was then scheduled for a hearing aid evaluation.

At his hearing aid evaluation the audiologist recommended a behind-the-ear (BTE) hearing aid with a skeleton mold to fit the left ear. The patient preferred monoaural fitting and was left-handed. He experienced improved word recognition with use of the hearing aid. At a subsequent visit, the audiologist reviewed the care, use, and placement of the BTE unit and provided instruction on the benefits and limitations of amplification. Mr. Jackson and his wife elected to participate in an audiologic rehabilitation course to learn communication strategies to aid his engagement in social activities. He had a return appointment within the 30-day trial period for follow-up consultation.

1. **What are appropriate indications for audiology and otolaryngology referral?**

2. **What treatment options are there for hearing loss and are they effective?** ▣

MANAGEMENT OF HEARING LOSS

Patients with suspected hearing loss should see an audiologist, or an otolaryngologist for evaluation and treatment. Treatment options depend on the type and severity of hearing loss and may include assistive devices, environmental adaptations, training of communication partners, amplification via hearing aids, middle ear implants, electric acoustic stimulation, or a cochlear implant.[16]

Hearing Aid Use and Effectiveness

Hearing aids are the main treatment for ARHL. The goal of amplification is to improve communicative ability and quality of life. Hearing aids have been shown to improve speech perception, understanding, and social, emotional, and affective functioning related to hearing ability. For auditory rehabilitation to be a success, the amount of hearing loss is less critical than patient awareness and acceptance of hearing loss and communication difficulties, and motivation to try amplification. After completing an assessment, the audiologist will help select a hearing aid or aids based on the patient's hearing needs and goals and provide training in the use of amplification and other selected rehabilitative approaches. After fitting a hearing aid, the audiologist provides supportive follow-up during the trial period and after the purchase.

Types of Hearing Aids

Hearing aids come in a variety of styles with a range of features. The circuitry is either analog or digital. Most new models are digital. Digital hearing aids have performance advantages, including better sound quality, programs for different listening environments, better background noise reduction, less acoustic feedback, and the capacity for smaller size. Hearing aids come in several basic types, each with advantages and disadvantages. All aids are designed to increase the intensity of sound and deliver it to the ear with maximal fidelity. Behind-the-ear (BTE) hearing aids have a case containing the microphone and receiver (speaker), which conducts sound through a thin plastic tube to a molded ear piece. BTE aids have either an open or a closed ear canal fit. BTE aids offer more features compared to other styles including directional microphones, telecoils for use with phones, and direct audio input.

The receiver-in-the-canal type (RIC) aid is similar to an open-fit BTE type that has a thin wire connecting an amplifier resting behind the ear to the receiver that is housed separately in a bud inserted in the ear canal. Advantages include increased comfort with the open fit of the ear mold and higher signal amplification without as much feedback compared to aids that house the receiver and microphone closer together. Modern feedback cancellation systems have made the open ear fitting in RIC aids possible. Also, RIC aids have the advantage that the receiver can be changed if the person's hearing declines.

In-the-ear (ITE) aids are self-contained with all components in a single earpiece that covers the concha. ITE aids are convenient and easy for patients with limited dexterity. In-the-canal (ITC) aids are self-contained in an earpiece that partially covers the concha. They are smaller than the ITE models. They provide sound amplification similar to most BTE and ITE hearing aids, but pose a disadvantage for patients with dexterity problems because of their tiny size. Completely-in-the-canal (CIC) hearing aids are some of the smallest and most expensive aids and fit entirely within the ear canal. Only a small handle is visible for daily removal. They are suitable for patients with mild to moderate hearing impairment, good manual dexterity, and a healthy ear canal. Invisible-in-canal aids are a tiny molded unit placed deep inside the ear canal, typically by an audiologist, and replaced every 4 months.

> Cosmetic concerns have driven creation of smaller, less visible hearing aids, but smaller is not always better when it comes to performance and ease of use.

Hearing aid companies have introduced a number of new features, albeit at higher prices. The utility of new features for improved hearing often has not been well studied, and may depend on the specific needs of the individual. A qualified and reputable audiologist can help older adults identify a hearing aid that meets their needs and budget. Hearing aids that are labeled "entry level, basic, or mid-level" are sophisticated electronic instruments and often feature technologies that were considered "premium" only a few years ago.

Most hearing aid users will gain adequate hearing improvement with a basic to mid-level hearing aid at a considerable cost savings.[17] Unless a top-of-the-line hearing aid offers some feature that demonstrably benefits the person, a more basic hearing aid is likely a better value. Current high-end hearing aids come with features such as directional microphones that deemphasize sounds originating from the sides and back of a listener relative to those originating from the front. Some aids automatically switch from omnidirectional to directional mode depending on the location of sounds. "Binaural wireless connectivity" is a high-end feature where the user's hearing aids "talk" to one another wirelessly and work in concert. Hearing aids can also have programs that transpose high frequencies to lower frequencies where hearing may be better. Some hearing aids and features are more appropriate for persons with a given pattern or degree of severity of hearing loss. For symmetric hearing loss, most audiologists recommend binaural hearing aids, although the cost of two aids may be prohibitive.

> With so many hearing aid styles and features to choose from, it is important to refer patients to a qualified audiologist to assist them with selection to meet their unique hearing needs.

Insurance Coverage for Hearing Aids

In the United States, purchase of hearing aids is an out-of-pocket expense for most older adults. Medicare and most private health insurances do not cover hearing aids. Veterans Affairs insurance provides coverage if hearing loss is service connected. Medicaid covers hearing aids in 31 states but coverage is typically limited to one monoaural fitting.[18]

Managing Feedback in Hearing Aids

Acoustic feedback and its management are critical to hearing aid use and user satisfaction. Feedback causes hearing aids to whistle and can be a source of annoyance, frustration, and embarrassment and in extreme cases can lead to cessation of hearing aid use. Feedback occurs when amplified sound from the receiver leaks out of the ear canal, is picked up by the microphone, and amplified again. Common causes include an improperly inserted hearing aid, loss of proper hearing aid fit because of changes in ear canal shape, or earwax buildup causing sound to reflect back to the hearing aid. In hearing aid systems, feedback is a challenge because the microphone and speaker are close together. The BTE and RIC designs help control feedback by offering more separation between the microphone and speaker. A tight-fitting ear mold, as featured in a closed-fit hearing aid, is another strategy to prevent feedback. A closed-fit design occludes the external ear canal and helps direct sound away from the hearing aid microphone. Closed-fit hearing aids, however, are not as comfortable for some users as those with an open fit that allows sound to pass in and out of the ear. Open-fit aids feature an ear mold with tiny holes or vents.

The Occlusion Effect

Persons using closed-fit hearing aids sometimes complain of an auditory phenomenon known as the occlusion effect, which adds a "booming" or echo quality to their voices. Experts theorize that bone-conducted sound vibrations of one's own voice reflect off the unvented ear mold back toward the eardrum, in effect amplifying the loudness of the voice.[19] Open-fit or vented ear molds are less prone to the occlusion effect, but are more susceptible to feedback because they permit more amplified sounds to escape from the ear canal. Fortunately, feedback control circuits make a tight-fitting ear mold less critical, and allow control of feedback with open-fit aids. Hearing aids equipped with adaptive phase cancellation systems identify and suppress the offending signal responsible for feedback. They do so by generating an internal cancelling out-of-phase signal, suppressing feedback with minimum degradation of external sounds. Control of feedback for persons with severe hearing loss (thresholds in the 70 to 90 dB range), however, requires a well-fit mold that occludes the ear.[20]

Promoting Hearing Aid Use

Primary care providers can help set appropriate expectations about hearing aids to promote their successful use. Hearing aids will not correct hearing like glasses correct vision. Hearing aids do not restore normal hearing. However, even partial improvement can make a big real-life difference. Learning to use hearing aids requires patience and daily work and commitment to practice using them. Advise prospective hearing aid recipients to be patient and allow themselves to get used to the aids and the "new" sounds they will hear. New hearing aid users have to become acclimated to sounds that previously they were missing or had heard differently for years. They need to again become familiar with the high-frequency sounds of speech and the environment. There is a learning curve that takes from 6 weeks to 6 months. With practice, they should expect to be able to hear and understand others better. New hearing aid users may benefit from participation in group audiologic visits, which can improve adherence. Including a significant other in the fitting process can also improve the likelihood of use.

Assistive Listening Devices

A variety of assistive listening devices (ALDs) are available. Pocket-sized personal amplifiers contain a microphone that transmits amplified sound through headphones. These devices are a small fraction of the cost of a hearing aid and greatly facilitate communication with individuals with severe hearing impairment who cannot tolerate, afford, or properly manage hearing aids and should be standard equipment at primary care offices and other clinical sites caring for older patients. Other ALDs are useful adjuncts to hearing aids. They usually consist of a microphone placed close to the desired sound, and a means by which sound is transmitted directly to the listener. Examples of ALDs that improve signal-to-noise ratio via direct sound transmission include infrared, FM radio, and induction loop listening systems for televisions, stereos, concerts, public libraries, and church sermons. Hearing loop induction systems, a technology widely adopted in Northern Europe and increasingly available in public spaces in the United States, consist of a copper wire that is installed around the periphery of a room or other venue to transmit electromagnetic signals that are picked up by a telecoil receiver that is built into most hearing aids and cochlear implants. When the receiver is turned on, the hearing aid receives only the sounds coming from the microphone, not the background noise or reverberations. Other ALDs include hearing-aid compatible amplified phones, phone amplifiers, text telephones, systems that make lamps flash on and off when a phone or doorbell rings, vibrating alarm clocks, televisions with closed captioning, and flashing smoke detectors.

> Hearing aids do not completely restore normal hearing. Fortunately, however, even a partial improvement in hearing can make a big real-life difference.

Audiologic Rehabilitation Courses

Audiology centers may offer rehabilitation courses that focus on developing strategies to improve communication in everyday life situations. Such courses represent an important educational opportunity for hearing-impaired individuals and their families. Individuals should be encouraged to attend the course along with their communication partners because their participation helps reduce hearing handicaps for the referred individual and increases use of communication strategies. Findings from a randomized trial of Internet-based aural rehabilitative versus online discussion groups for hearing aid users suggest the Internet can be a useful tool to improve communication among the hearing impaired and help them make the most of their hearing aids.[21]

Indications for Otolaryngology Referral

Box 25-5 lists findings on the history or physical examination that should prompt referral for evaluation by an otolaryngologist. Referral is generally appropriate for patients whose hearing loss deviates from that characteristic of presbycusis (bilateral, symmetric, high-frequency hearing loss). Also, when ear inspection shows cerumen or a foreign body totally occluding the external canal, evaluation by an otolaryngologist may be beneficial.

Medical-Surgical Treatments for Hearing Loss

Cochlear implants are the standard of care for hearing rehabilitation in people with advanced sensorineural hearing loss who are unable to gain effective speech recognition with hearing aids. In appropriately selected patients, cochlear implants improve communication and lead to psychological and social benefits; furthermore, the surgery is safe and well tolerated in older patients. As of 2011, nearly 200,000 patients had received cochlear implants worldwide.[22] The surgery is now commonly done bilaterally to restore directional hearing that requires signals from two ears.

A healthy cochlea contains about 3000 hair cells that transmit data along 30,000 auditory neurons. Cochlear implants use 12 to 22 electrodes to stimulate a reduced number of spiral ganglion cells. The pattern of nerve activity produced by cochlear implants is crude compared to the complex resolution of the natural ear, yet recipients often achieve highly functional hearing allowing them to understand speech and talk on the phone. Even though speech is badly distorted by an auditory prosthesis, the pattern recognition of the brain overcomes the lack of fidelity and reconstructs the message. Cochlear implants restore speech understanding to a high level, but are poor at restoring perception of harmonic pitch in music, or voice quality, speaker identity, or the emotional content of speech.[23]

BOX 25-5
HISTORY OR EXAM FINDINGS THAT SHOULD PROMPT OTOLARYNGOLOGY REFERRAL
• Unexplained unilateral hearing loss • Hearing loss associated with ear pain, tinnitus, or drainage • Hearing loss associated with findings of middle ear disease such as cholesteatoma or tympanic membrane perforation • History of fluid-filled ears or painful draining ears within the past 3 months • History of sudden onset or rapidly progressive hearing loss within the past 3 months

---

CASE 1

Discussion

Mr. Jackson's increasing difficulty understanding his grandchildren's high-pitched voices is more likely a sign of presbycusis rather than his cerumen impaction, given that presbycusis predominantly affects perception of high pitches and the latter condition mostly affects low pitches. Although Mr. Jackson takes aspirin, a known cause of reversible hearing loss and tinnitus, hearing loss usually occurs only at doses such as 650 mg four times a day or more. This case also illustrates how cerumen impaction can worsen the hearing disability imposed by other diseases such as presbycusis. ■

SUMMARY

Accurate and reliable hearing screening tools exist to identify persons for whom hearing specialist referral is warranted. Clinicians can improve the outlook for hearing-impaired persons by recognizing the serious consequences of hearing loss, assessing routinely for hearing loss, and counseling patients about the benefits of hearing health services. Hearing aids significantly improve the quality of life of patients with sensorineural hearing loss.

Web Resources

www.nidcd.nih.gov. National Institute on Deafness and Other Communication Disorders, U.S. National Institutes of Health. Provides information on hearing disorders. Useful to laypersons and professionals. Includes links to more than 140 hearing-related organizations.

www.fda.gov/MedicalDevices/ProductsandMedicalProcedures/HomeHealthandConsumer/ConsumerProducts/HearingAids/default.htm. U.S. Food and Drug Administration—Protecting and Promoting Your Health: Medical Devices (Hearing Aids). Provides information for laypersons on types, benefits, and safety of hearing aids: how to get a hearing aid, hearing aids and cell phones, other products and procedures to improve hearing, and a checklist of steps to take before purchasing hearing aids.

KEY REFERENCES

3. Meyer C, Hickson L. What factors influence help-seeking for hearing impairment and hearing aid adoption in older adults? Int J Audiol 2012;51:66-74.
6. Pacala JT, Yueh B. Hearing deficits in the older patient. "I didn't Notice Anything." JAMA 2012;307:1185-94.
14. Yueh B, Collins MP, Souza PE, et al. Long-term effectiveness of screening for hearing loss: The Screening for Auditory Impairment—Which Hearing Assessment-Test (SAI-WHAT) randomized trial. J Am Geriatr Soc 2010;58:427-34.
16. Sprinzl GM, Riechelmann H. Current trends in treating hearing loss in elderly people: A review of the technology and treatment options—a mini-review. Gerontology 2010;56:351-8.
22. Carlson ML, Driscoll CL, Gifford RH. Cochlear implantation: Current and future device options. Otolaryngol Clin N Am 2012;45:221-48.

References available online at expertconsult.com.

26

Visual Impairment and Eye Problems

Karin Johnson and Stephen W. Record

OBJECTIVES

Upon completion of this chapter, the reader will be able to:

- Know changes to the eye, vision, and visual function that accompany aging.
- Understand the impact of contrast sensitivity, illumination, and glare on visual acuity and visual function.
- Be familiar with the three most common age-associated ocular diseases, their diagnostic features, and treatment.
- Understand optical and non-optical methods to enhance visual function.

VISUAL IMPAIRMENT WITH AGE

The eye is the window to the soul—and so much more. It is key to maximum functionality. With age, vision and functionality related to vision decline.[1,2] This has a major impact on quality of life and independence. Loss of vision is associated with depression, difficulties with activities of daily living and safe driving, as well as increased risk of injury, falls, and medication errors. Surprisingly, visual acuity is not a good predictor of visual ability.[2-4] Visual acuity is tested under high-contrast, ideal conditions that rarely exist outside of a doctor's office. Better predictors are contrast sensitivity, glare sensitivity, and performance under reduced illumination. Performance in these areas declines not only for older adults with visual impairment (visual acuity worse than 20/40) but also for older adults without visual impairment. Deficits worsen when low contrast, reduced illumination, and glare coexist. Treating refractive error and ocular disease is helpful but is not enough. Minimizing functional deficits related to the environmental conditions listed above will maximize function and independence. Success requires a team approach among the patient, family, primary care provider, eye care provider, and an occupational therapist trained in vision rehabilitation. The goal of this chapter is to provide the reader with the tools to easily deliver and coordinate such comprehensive care.

CASE 1

Wayne Knapp (Part 1)

Wayne Knapp is a 73-year-old white male who visits your office for a routine follow-up for hypertension, hyperlipidemia, and coronary artery disease. He has been free of chest pain but is occasionally short of breath. He continues to smoke cigarettes, but says he has decided to cut down because his first grandchild has been born and he does not want to expose her to the smoke. He notes that his vision is "not as good as it used to be" and that he has "to get right under the light to see anything." He reads the paper every morning and reports that some of the words look distorted, especially with his left eye. Furthermore, he notes that he has stopped driving at night

Additional online-only material indicated by icon.

because it is even harder to see, especially with headlights coming toward him.

You have him read a distance and near Snellen chart and realize you must examine his eyes with your ophthalmoscope.

1. **What is/are the most likely cause(s) of Mr. Knapp's visual complaints?**

2. **Which risk factors contribute to this/these conditions?** ▣

Prevalence and Impact

The Smith-Kettlewell Institute (SKI) Study evaluated vision and visual function in older adults aged 58 to 85 and older.[4] *Visual impairment* was defined as binocular acuity of 20/40 or worse. Among people age 40 and older, more than 3.6 million are visually impaired. After age 60, 89% of the SKI study patients had no visual acuity impairment. Unfortunately, this percentage declined steadily with increasing age as shown in Table 26-1. Thus, 40% of patients 85 and older had some form of visual impairment. The statistics are even worse for the nursing home population where it is estimated that the degree of legal blindness (visual acuity worse than 20/200) is 15% in those older than age 60 and up to 29% in those older than age 90. This is an increase of 15 times over community-dwelling older adults.[1] Such statistics highlight vision loss as the third leading cause of activity of daily living (ADL) impairment.[5] More than one half of the conditions that cause visual impairment or blindness in older individuals are surgically treatable or potentially preventable.[6] Additionally, one third of older adults with visual impairment improve vision with refraction alone. Thus simply increasing access to eye care would significantly improve vision and function in older Americans.

Risk Factors and Pathophysiology

Vision loss and decreased vision function in older adults are related to ocular disease and age-related physiologic changes.[1-5,7] Even older patients with good visual acuity (20/40 or better) and no significant ocular disease showed deficits in visual function.[4] Visual acuity is tested under maximum contrast (i.e., black target on white background) and illumination with minimal glare. Rarely in life do people operate under these ideal conditions. Real-life vision occurs more commonly under decreased contrast, decreased and changing illumination, and increased glare. Contrast sensitivity is the ability to distinguish an object from its background. A visual acuity chart and most street signs provide high contrast sensitivity whereas camouflage demonstrates low contrast.

Measurement of visual function (rather than visual acuity) correlates highly with success in performing many common and essential daily activities.[3,8]

> Even older patients with good visual acuity (20/40 or better) and no significant ocular disease show deficits in visual function.

Differential Diagnosis and Assessment

Standard visual acuity can be measured with a distance and near Snellen chart. Testing the effects of decreased contrast sensitivity, decreased illumination, and increased glare is not practical for the primary care provider, because the equipment necessary for such testing is specialized and is not widely available to primary care providers.[3,4] Rather, questioning older patients about their performance under these circumstances is easier. For contrast sensitivity, ask if a patient has much difficulty driving in the rain or seeing on a hazy day. For low illumination, ask if the patient has significantly greater difficulty seeing at dusk and at night. For glare, ask how debilitated the patient is by oncoming headlights, by walking from outside to inside on a sunny day, or by entering a tunnel from daylight.

Management

Enhancing visual function requires a team approach among the primary care provider, the eye care provider, and an occupational therapist trained in visual rehabilitation. Eye examination by an optometrist or ophthalmologist is key to providing best-corrected vision with refraction and treatment of visual deficits caused by ocular disease. Despite these efforts, some patients may not be correctable to 20/20. Performance can be enhanced for patients with low vision (worse than 20/70 visual acuity) and for patients with better acuity who have difficulty in certain circumstances or settings. An ideal approach would be to have a home evaluation by a vision rehabilitation specialist. Because this is not readily available for many older adults, a more practical approach educates the primary

TABLE 26-1	Visual Decline with Aging
Age (Years)	**Percent without Visual Acuity Impairment**
58-69	99
70-74	97
75-79	91
80-84	88
≥85	60

care provider, the patient, and the patient's family about simple measures to maximize visual acuity and function.

SPECIFIC OCULAR DISEASES ASSOCIATED WITH AGING

Age-Related Macular Degeneration

Prevalence and Impact

Age-related macular degeneration (ARMD) is the leading cause of severe vision loss in patients 75 years of age and older.[7,9] It is the most common cause of new visual impairment in patients older than age 65. More than 2 million Americans age 50 and older have advanced ARMD that can lead to severe vision impairment. More than 5% of older adults beyond age 65 have some form of visual impairment resulting from ARMD. The National Advisory Eye Council estimates that more older adults will become blind from ARMD than from glaucoma and diabetic retinopathy combined. ARMD targets the macula, and in particular the fovea, resulting in a loss of central vision first unilaterally and later bilaterally. This loss of central visual acuity is associated with impaired ability to perform ADLs, impaired mobility, increased risk of falls and fractures, increased medication errors, depression, and lower quality-of-life scores.[9] Also, visual function is adversely affected by distortion (metamorphopsia) and impaired ability to adapt to changing light levels.[4,9-10] Nonneovascular (dry) ARMD accounts for 90% of the cases and neovascular (wet) ARMD accounts for the remaining 10%.

> The National Advisory Eye Council estimates that more older adults will become blind from ARMD than from glaucoma and diabetic retinopathy combined.

Risk Factors and Pathophysiology

There is no gender predilection for the development of ARMD, but once present, nonvascular disease is more prevalent in women.[9] Additionally, there is a racial predilection for disease development, with older white Americans being affected twice as often as older blacks.[6,9] In general, risk factors for coronary artery disease and ARMD are similar. Patients with a history of hypertension, smoking, and atherosclerosis are more prone to acquire macular degeneration.[9] A supposition that oxidative damage to arterioles is causative played a role in studies examining the use of antioxidants in macular degeneration prevention and mitigation. Research also implicates phototoxicity, inflammation, and diet as other possible risk factors. A genetic link for ARMD is suspected in 50% of new cases.

Differential Diagnosis and Assessment

Ideally, the best way to diagnose ARMD is with a dilated fundus examination and the use of a slit lamp biomicroscope and special magnifying lenses. Optical coherence tomography (OCT) has become the standard for monitoring ARMD status and progression fluorescein angiography is also helpful.[9,10] Given the specialized equipment necessary for the diagnosis, a patient with suspected ARMD is best referred to an eye care specialist for establishment of the diagnosis.

CASE 1

Wayne Knapp (Part 2)

Mr. Knapp's acuity is 20/50 in the right eye and 20/40 in the left eye. With your ophthalmoscope, you find the red reflex, and in the retroillumination, you note that there appears to be a central density in both eyes. You adjust your ophthalmoscope to focus on the retina but note that the view in both eyes remains a little hazy despite your best efforts. You are able to detect yellowish, ground glass–like deposits in the macula as well as patchy white and black areas indicating disruption of the retinal pigment epithelium. You suspect Mr. Knapp has nuclear sclerosis cataracts and early dry macular degeneration. You refer him to a local eye care provider who confirms your diagnosis.

1. **After consultation with Mr. Knapp's eye care practitioner, what treatments do you advise?**

2. **What is the prognosis for his nuclear sclerosis cataracts and dry macular degeneration?** ▪

Management

Unfortunately, the treatment of dry ARMD is limited and the prognosis is poor. There is no medical management for dry ARMD. The Age-Related Eye Disease Study (AREDS) research group did show a reduction in the development of advanced dry ARMD in some patients with existing ARMD meeting certain specifications.[10] These patients were given an antioxidant mixture (vitamin C, vitamin E, and beta-carotene) with zinc. Pharmaceuticals to inhibit vascular endothelial growth factor (VEGF) are currently used to treat wet ARMD.[9] Over the past few years, anti-VEGF therapy for neovascular ARMD has become the standard treatment for wet ARMD.[11]

Cataracts

Prevalence and Impact

A cataract is any opacity in the lens that causes the lens to lose transparency or scatter light.[12] Cataracts affect nearly 22 million Americans age 40 and older. Prevalence is well known to be age related, occurring in one in six patients older than age 40 and 50% of patients age 80 and older. The Framingham Eye Study estimated the prevalence of cataracts causing acuity of 20/30 or worse to be 5% for ages 55 to 64, 18% for ages 65 to 74, and 46% for ages 75 to 80. Three main varieties of cataracts exist—nuclear sclerosis, posterior subcapsular, and cortical spoking. Cataracts reduce illumination, reduce contrast sensitivity, increase glare, and degrade blue-yellow color vision.[4,13] Any loss of visual acuity and visual function will impair ADL performance, driving ability, and mobility; increase fall risk and medication errors; and reduce quality of life. Additionally, cataracts are costly. Among Medicare beneficiaries, cataracts are the most common reason for eye examinations, and cataract surgery is the most frequently performed surgery. More than 43% of visits by older Americans to optometrists and ophthalmologists are for cataracts. Nearly $3.5 billion each year is spent on 1.35 million cataract surgeries.[13] http://www.cdc.gov/visionhealth/pdf/improving_nations_vision_health.pdf

Risk Factors and Pathophysiology

A number of risk factors exist for cataract development. They include more hours of sunlight exposure, smoking, heavy alcohol consumption, and a low educational level. Diabetics have a higher prevalence of cortical opacities, as do women and African Americans.[6,12] Diet and vitamin use appear not to play a role in cataract development. The AREDS research group showed no link between supplementation with a combination of antioxidants (vitamin C, vitamin E, and beta-carotene) and the development or progression of age-related lens opacities.[14] Pathophysiology is varied. Nuclear sclerosis results from the accumulation of high-molecular-weight protein. Subcapsular cataracts result from degenerative changes in the capsule epithelium. Cortical cataracts develop because of damage to the lens fibers caused by an increased accumulation of intracellular and extracellular water.

> A number of risk factors exist for cataract development. They include more hours of sunlight exposure, smoking, heavy alcohol consumption, and a low educational level.

Differential Diagnosis and Assessment

Cataracts are best diagnosed with a slit lamp biomicroscope through a dilated pupil. With retroillumination off of the retina, one or more types can be detected with an ophthalmoscope but this is clearly inferior to slit lamp examination. A nuclear sclerotic cataract appears as a yellowish-brown opacity in the lens center. It is football-shaped or circular depending on your view with the slit lamp or ophthalmoscope. A posterior subcapsular cataract looks like a smudge on the back of the lens. Cortical spiking appears as

whitish, triangular, or flecklike opacities around the lens perimeter.[12-16]

Management

The treatment of cataracts remains surgical. Extracapsular cataract extraction with posterior chamber intraocular lens implantation continues to be the standard. No medications are known to prevent or abolish cataracts. The criterion for surgery is functional visual impairment and not a specific visual acuity. In general, visual acuity of 20/50 or worse with glare testing is considered to be a surgical level of dysfunction.

Glaucoma

Prevalence and Impact

Primary open-angle glaucoma (POAG) affects approximately 6% of patients older than age 65.[7] Glaucoma affects almost 2.3 million Americans age 40 and older. It is the second most common cause of legal blindness in the United States and the leading cause of blindness among African Americans.[17] Unlike macular degeneration, which starts with a loss of central acuity, glaucoma destroys peripheral vision first and central vision in the end stages. It limits an older adult's useful field of view, making mobility and safe driving more difficult and increasing fall risk.

> Primary open-angle glaucoma affects approximately 6% of patients older than age 65; it is the second most common cause of legal blindness in the United States and the leading cause of blindness among African Americans.

Risk Factors and Pathophysiology

Open-angle glaucoma is characterized by progressive and initially asymptomatic optic neuropathy resulting in visual field loss in the presence of an open anterior chamber. Despite the open anterior chamber, there is resistance to aqueous outflow.[17] Intraocular pressure increases, resulting in damage to optic nerve fibers. Many risk factors exist.[18] The most well known is increased intraocular pressure (IOP). However, it is crucial to remember that the increase is relative. Some patients have low-pressure glaucoma and demonstrate optic nerve damage at pressures less than 21 mmHg, and others demonstrate ocular hypertension and have no damage at pressures greater than 21 mmHg. In general, patients with IOPs between 15 and 20 mmHg are at low risk, and patients with IOPs greater than 25 mmHg are at higher risk. Other contributory factors in addition to IOP and age are enlarged optic nerve cup (0.5 cup-to-disk ratio or larger), race (greater prevalence in African Americans), family history, and diseases affecting the vasculature such as hypertension and diabetes.

Differential Diagnosis and Assessment

Intraocular pressure measurement is essential for the diagnosis of open-angle glaucoma. However, measurement of IOP with a tonometer is not practical in the primary care setting. Neither is optic nerve head evaluation through a dilated pupil with a slit lamp biomicroscope and a special magnifying lens or visual field analysis with a computer. Use of a direct ophthalmoscope to view the optic nerve head is feasible but not ideal. Glaucomatous optic atrophy results in pallor and thinning of the neural retinal rim (the doughnut) with secondary widening and deepening of the cup (the doughnut hole). The rim should be thickest inferiorly, then superiorly, nasally, and lastly temporally (ISN'T). Deviation from this, as well as a cup-to-disc ratio of greater than or equal to 0.5, should raise suspicion of glaucoma. Differential diagnosis includes ocular hypertension, a congenitally large optic nerve cup, and a myriad of other types of optic atrophy.[16,17]

Management

Glaucoma is amenable to medical, surgical, and laser therapy. Beta-blockers are first-line medical therapy followed by prostaglandin analogs. Second-line agents include topical carbonic anhydrase inhibitors and alpha-2 agonists. Medications that were the standard 10 years ago, such as epinephrine, pilocarpine (a cholinergic agent), and oral carbonic anhydrase inhibitors, are now infrequently used.[18] All topical ocular medications have the potential for systemic absorption and side effects. Many of these side effects have been eliminated with the less frequent use of epinephrine and pilocarpine. Selective and nonselective beta-blockers may cause the same cardiovascular and pulmonary side effects as their oral counterparts. Additionally, the alpha-2 agonists may cause hypertension. When medical management is not sufficient, other treatment options include laser trabeculoplasty and filtration surgery.[18]

CASE 1

Discussion

Mr. Knapp's age and smoking are risk factors for both his cataract and his macular degeneration. His cardiovascular disease is a further risk factor for his macular degeneration. His difficulties in low light levels and with glare are consistent with cataract symptoms. The distortion he notes is typical of macular degeneration. It is not surprising that his visual acuity is reduced. When examining a patient's eyes, if the doctor has trouble seeing through the ocular media, then the patient will surely have trouble seeing out through it. If Mr. Knapp's vision is not improved with refraction, cataract surgery is a reasonable option. Unfortunately, no treatment exists for his dry macular degeneration. Mr. Knapp's best chance at mitigating progression is to quit smoking and get optimal treatment for his cardiovascular disease. In the future, he may need some of the optical and nonoptical aids discussed in the chapter. ■

SUMMARY

A basic principle of geriatric care is to identify functional impairment and maximize residual function. Vision care for the elderly is no exception. A difference exists between standard visual acuity and visual functional ability. Many older adults with good standard acuity will experience severe degradation resulting from everyday environmental factors. Thus it is important to know how the patient functions in his or her natural setting, and not just rely on office performance. Identifying and treating refractive errors and age-related ocular disease such as macular degeneration, cataracts, and glaucoma can go a long way toward improving function and quality of life. However, this is not enough. The vision of many older patients cannot be corrected to 20/40 or better despite treatment in these areas, and they need to be advised of other optical and nonoptical ways to enhance visual function. This requires a team approach among the patient, the family, the primary care and eye care providers and, where available, a vision rehabilitation specialist.

Web Resource

www.lighthouse.org. Lighthouse International.

KEY REFERENCES

2. Kamel HK, Guro-Razuman S, Shareeff M. The Activities of Daily Vision Scale: A useful tool to assess fall risk in older adults with vision impairment. J Am Geriatr Soc 2000;48(11):1474-77.

4. Schneck ME, Haegerstrom-Portnoy G. Practical assessment of vision in the elderly. Ophthalmol Clin North Am 2003;16(2): 269-87.

5. Crews JE, Campbell VA. Health conditions, activity limitations and participation restrictions among older people reporting visual impairment. J Vis Impair Blind 2001; 95: 453-467

6. Munoz G, West SK, Schein OD. Causes of blindness and visual impairment in a population of older Americans: The Salisbury Eye Study. Arch Ophthalmol 2000;118:819-25.

References available online at expertconsult.com.

27

Persistent Pain

Jerome J. Epplin, Masaya Higuchi, Nisha Gajendra, and Soumya Nadella

OBJECTIVES

Upon completion of this chapter, the reader will be able to:

- Define persistent pain and discuss its impact on older adults.
- Discuss the pathophysiology of persistent pain.
- Describe age-related changes that influence the presentation and treatment of persistent pain.
- Take an accurate pain history and use assessment tools to quantitate and monitor pain syndromes.
- Choose appropriate pharmacologic treatments to manage persistent pain.
- Apply nonpharmacologic approaches to the treatment of pain.

PREVALENCE AND IMPACT

Although pain is a ubiquitous experience, it remains a very complex and poorly understood phenomenon. The perception of pain is altered by many circumstances, such as the patient's prior experience with pain, cultural background, emotional status, possibility of secondary gain, and personality. Pain may be acute, usually precipitated by an acute illness or injury. This type of pain is often associated with autonomic responses such as tachycardia, elevated blood pressure, or diaphoresis. The management of such pain is often straightforward and usually the pain is alleviated once the precipitating factor is treated.

However, especially among the elderly, pain is often ongoing without a single incident that causes the pain. Previously this was referred to as chronic pain. However, because the term *chronic* is frequently associated with a negative connotation the preferred term to describe such pain is *persistent pain*. Contrary to common misconceptions, persistent pain has a distinct pathologic basis, causing changes in the nervous system that often worsen over time.[1]

Persistent pain is commonly encountered in a geriatric practice. It is estimated that 25% to 50% of the elderly may have persistent pain.[2] Sixty-five percent of nursing home residents report having inadequately treated pain.[1] However, a recent study[3] looked at the long-term persistence of musculoskeletal pain in community-dwelling older adults. Over a 6-year period, approximately 20% of the study participants had no musculoskeletal pain, one third had persistent pain, one third had intermittent pain, and one sixth had pain in each of the 6 years. However, half of those with pain during one of the years had no pain during any of the other 5 years. This could imply that pain, while common, may be a more dynamic symptom than previously thought.

Persistent pain has a significant negative impact on patients' lives (Box 27-1). Sleep disturbances, feelings of loneliness, depression, and social isolation are all more common in those with persistent pain. Patients with persistent pain have a reduced ability to carry out their social roles in their family or place of work. In addition, persistent pain often results in limited physical activity in patients, thereby worsening their physical conditioning.

Additional online-only material indicated by icon.

BOX 27-1

IMPACT OF PERSISTENT PAIN

Depression
Sleep disturbance
Worsening physical conditioning
Loneliness
Loss of productivity
Financial loss
Loss of social support
Potential of drug abuse/misuse

It is estimated that the total cost of pain in the United States is between $560 and $635 billion in 2010 dollars. The cost to Medicare is believed to be approximately $65.3 billion, which is 14% of the Medicare budget. These figures do not include lost productivity or lost tax revenue. Disability from all causes costs the United States $300 billion annually, with the persistent pain–related causes of arthritis and back/spine pain being the top two causes of disability.[4]

> Fourteen percent of the Medicare budget is consumed by pain treatment.

PATHOPHYSIOLOGY

It is sometimes helpful from a clinical standpoint to classify persistent pain in pathophysiologic terms.[2] *Nociceptive pain* comes about from stimulation of peripheral pain receptors and may be from tissue or joint inflammation or degeneration, continuing injury, or skin or internal organ noxious stimulation. Inflammatory or degenerative arthritis, myofascial pain syndromes, or ischemia are examples of such pain. Pain with this etiology responds to usual analgesic medications and nonpharmacologic strategies. *Neuropathic pain* results from abnormal nerve stimulation that involves peripheral or cranial nerves. Examples include diabetic or idiopathic peripheral neuropathy, trigeminal neuralgia, or phantom pain. Pain of this etiology is often more difficult to treat and may not respond completely to any treatment. Medications used include certain antidepressants or anticonvulsants. Another category is pain of mixed or uncertain etiology. Examples include recurrent headaches, vasculitis, somatization, or conversion reactions. Treatment of this category is difficult and should be individualized for each patient.

There is a difference in pain perception and tolerance when comparing the elderly with younger people. Myelinated and unmyelinated nerve fibers are decreased in density in the elderly with prolonged latencies noted in peripheral sensory nerves. This slows transduction and transmission of the pain signals.[5]

There is a lower density of descending pain inhibiting nerve fibers in the elderly. In addition there is a slower recovery from hyperalgesic states[6]; once pain is established these changes may make it more likely that persistent pain develops after a noxious insult.

Most studies indicate that there is an increase in pain threshold with aging.[2] There is also an age-related decrease in the willingness to endure strong pain. From a clinical standpoint, such changes may be evident in the different pain presentations that the elderly have with either an acute myocardial infarction or a ruptured appendix.

> Neuropathic pain refers to pain originating from abnormal peripheral or cranial nerve stimulation. Nociceptive pain refers to pain originating from stimulation of peripheral pain receptors.

CASE 1

Renee Peters (Part 1)

Renee Peters is a 78-year-old who comes to your office with increasingly severe low back pain. She has had low back pain for at least 5 years; the pain has intermittently interfered with her ability to do housework and leave her house. However, the pain worsened after she stepped down hard off a curb 1 week ago. There has been no radiation of pain to her buttocks or legs over the years.

1. **What is the pathophysiology of Mrs. Peters's pain?**
2. **How does the etiology of the pain influence therapy?**
3. **What do you expect to find on examination?** ◧

CASE 2

Bob Reid (Part 1)

Bob Reid is a 72-year-old who had an episode of shingles 4 months ago involving the right T7 dermatome. The rash cleared rapidly but severe pain persisted in the prior area of rash. He got only minimal relief with acetaminophen or ibuprofen. You had previously given him hydrocodone, which gave slightly more pain relief.

1. **What is the pathophysiology of Mr. Reid's pain?**
2. **How does the etiology of the pain influence therapy?**
3. **What do you expect to find on examination?** ◧

PAIN ASSESSMENT

Accurate assessment of pain is necessary to successfully treat it. This typically can include taking medical and pain histories, a physical examination with special attention to the painful areas, and using appropriate pain scales. Patients should routinely be evaluated for persistent pain (Level of Evidence B).

When taking a pain history, it is important that the clinician convey to the patient that his or her pain complaint is acknowledged and believed. It is also important that the patients know that pain is not a normal part of aging and they should not hesitate to discuss and describe their pain. Patients should be asked about a time line of the pain, acerbating and alleviating factors, and previous treatments. Descriptors of pain, such as sharp, burning, aching, radiating, or tightness should be sought (Level of Evidence D). Pain that awakens the patient from sleep may be particularly worrisome. How the pain affects the patient's everyday life should be assessed. The physical examination should pay particular attention to the painful areas and how function of those areas is affected (Level of Evidence D). Areas of inflammation or tenderness should be sought. Weakness or limitation of motion, numbness, paraesthesia, or change in reflexes is important. Simply observing the patient's gait can give information as to how the pain influences the patient's activities of daily living. The "get up and go" test can help quantify the patient's disability from the pain.

> **The patient must realize that his or her complaint of pain is taken seriously.**

CASE 1

Renee Peters (Part 2)

On physical examination Mrs. Peters ambulates slowly with obvious pain. She has diffuse tenderness and spasm throughout the lumbar spine. There is more pronounced tenderness over the L3 spinous process. Her sensation and muscle strength of her lower extremities are normal. Her deep tendon reflexes are also normal. You suspect that Mrs. Peters has a lumbar compression fracture superimposed on degenerative disc disease and osteoarthritis involving the lumbar spine. This would be considered to be nociceptive pain with no evidence of significant neuropathic involvement. The severity of her pain should be evaluated. Most likely she will require opioid therapy for her acute fracture. Once the acute pain has improved, her persistent, ongoing low back pain will need further evaluation.

1. **What further imaging or testing would you now recommend?**

2. **What other conditions relevant to Mrs. Peters should be addressed?** ◉

CASE 2

Bob Reid (Part 2)

On physical examination, Mr. Reid appears to be in pain and somewhat depressed. He has hyperalgesia involving the right T7 dermatome. There is no spine tenderness and his range of motion of the spine is normal. On further discussion with him, he admits that the constant nature of the pain has made him irritable and depressed.

1. **What further imaging or testing would you now recommend?**

2. **What other conditions relevant to Mr. Reid should be addressed?** ◉

PAIN QUANTITATION

There are many tools to assess pain in the elderly, both the cognitively intact and the cognitively impaired.[7] The most reliable way to evaluate the severity of pain of a cognitively intact patient is simply to ask the patient his or her estimate of the pain.[2] For those with mild to moderate dementia, reliable pain scales are available for use (Figure 27-1). Patients with advanced dementia are more difficult to evaluate, but clues from the patient's behavior or actions may be helpful.[8,9] Grimacing, grunting, or constant movement may be clues to uncontrolled pain. The mental status of the patient often deteriorates with persistent pain.

Because the pain intensity should be measured serially, keeping a pain log is useful. This should include the pain intensity, how activity affects the pain, results of medication or nonpharmacologic treatments, and how pain is affecting the patient's daily life. Also, with each office visit, the pain should be quantified and changes noted (Level of Evidence D).

CASE 1

Renee Peters (Part 3)

A plain film of Mrs. Peters's lumbar spine shows a moderate compression fracture of L3. Associated with this are facet arthritis and spurring of the lumbar vertebral bodies. Because she rates her pain prior to her fracture on most days 6 out of 10 and currently an 8 out of 10, you recommend hydrocodone therapy. Because she had a compression fracture without major trauma, a dual-energy x-ray absorptiometry (DEXA) scan was done, which revealed a T score of −2.9 over her lumbar spine. As part of further evaluation, a vitamin D level revealed a level of 20. Calcium, vitamin D, and bisphosphonates were recommended to prevent further fractures and pain. In order to address Mrs. Peters's ongoing back pain, physical therapy would be helpful after the acute pain of the fracture has improved.

What follow-up would you recommend? ◉

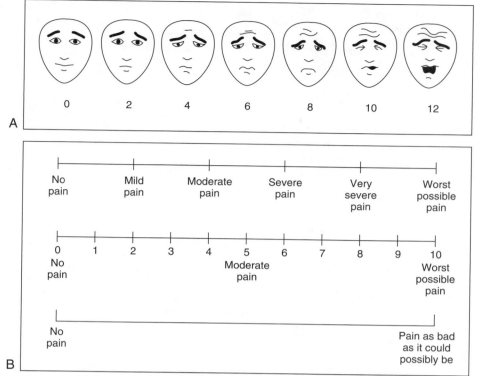

Figure 27-1 Pain intensity scales used in older patients. **A,** Faces scale. Ask the patient to "put an X by the face that best matches the severity of your pain right now." **B,** Visual analog scales. Ask the patient to "circle the number that best represents the intensity or severity of your pain right now." (**A** from the Pediatric Pain Sourcebook [copyright 2001], the International Association for the Study of Pain. **B** redrawn from Carr DB, et al. Acute pain management: Operative or medical procedures and trauma. Rockville, MD: Agency for Health Care Policy and Research; 1992 [AHCPR 92-0032], and Jacox A, et al. Management of cancer pain. Rockville, MD: Agency for Health Care Policy and Research; 1994 [AHCPR 94-0592].)

CASE 2

Bob Reid (Part 3)

By history, Mr. Reid has postherpetic neuralgia and further imaging is not indicated. However, because of a self-reported possible depression, a Geriatric Depression Scale was administered. This showed a score of 8 out of 15 (a score greater than 5 suggests depression). You discuss with Mr. Reid the possibility of using gabapentin for his neuralgia. He asks about using lidocaine patches rather than using an oral medication, and you prescribe the lidocaine patches. You also recommend discussing his depression with a counselor. He also agrees to try a selective serotonin reuptake inhibitor (SSRI) antidepressant. You had discussed with him the possibility of using the serotonin norepinephrine reuptake inhibitor (SNRI) duloxetine for both depression and possibly helping with the neuralgia, but the cost of the medication was prohibitive.

What follow-up would you recommend? ◙

PHARMACOLOGIC TREATMENT

Nearly all patients with persistent pain will require pharmacologic therapy, either constantly or intermittently. As with the treatment of any geriatric patient, the adage of starting low and slowly titrating upward on the dose applies. The drug that seems most effective and has the fewest side effects for the patient should be used, keeping in mind all the other comorbidities the patient may have. Also the type of pain the patient may have, either nociceptive or neuropathic, will dictate the type of medication used.

Nonsteroidal Antiinflammatory Drugs (NSAIDs)

Nonsteroidal antinflammatory drugs (NSAIDs) are a broad class of drugs (Table 27-1). Their main mechanism is to inhibit cyclooxygenase, which alters the transformation of arachidonic acid into prostaglandins, prostacyclins, and thromboxanes.

The primary use of NSAIDs is for inflammatory pain. They are more effective than acetaminophen for inflammatory pain such as that caused by rheumatoid arthritis[10] and are relatively effective in the short-term treatment of osteoarthritis and low back pain.[11-14]

NSAIDs are associated with gastrointestinal (GI), renal, and cardiovascular toxicity in the elderly, even more than in younger patients.[15] GI toxicity is less likely in nonacetylated NSAIDs such as salsalate when compared to aspirin, but the likelihood of GI toxicity is never zero.[16-18]

TABLE 27-1		Information on Commonly Used NSAIDs		
Drug	Route	Aging Effect	Precautions & Recommendations	Cost
Aspirin	PO, PR	GFR decreases, which results in decreased excretion	Evaluate risks and benefits Mostly used for cardiovascular protection	Generic
Ibuprofen	PO	Severity of GI toxicity increases with age and frequency	Treat acute or chronic inflammatory pain	Generic
Salsalate	PO	GI toxicity	GI toxicity lower than ASA	Generic
Naproxen	PO	COX-2 inhibitor, less GI toxicity; increases bleeding time	Moderate to severe inflammatory pain Low risk of cardiovascular events	Generic
Diclofenac	PO		Because of COX-2 selectivity has increased cardiovascular risk	Generic
Indomethacin	PO	More GI and central nervous system side effects	Not first-line drug for mild to moderate pain	Generic
Ketorolac	IM, PO	High GI toxicity and renal toxicity	Not recommended for long-term use	Generic
Nabumetone	PO	GI toxicity	Long half-life, low antiplatelet activity	750 mg 60 tabs $68.99
Celecoxib	PO	Selective COX-2 inhibitor	Fewer GI side effects	Generic

ASA, acetylsalicylic acid (aspirin); *GFR*, glomerular filtration rate; *GI*, gastrointestinal; *IM*, intramuscular; *PO*, by mouth; *PR*, per rectum.

Renal toxicity and hyperkalemia may be significant side effects of NSAIDs. This is more often seen in the elderly, those with congestive heart failure, hypertension, dehydration, preexisting mild renal dysfunction, and patients taking angiotensin-converting enzyme (ACE) inhibitors or diuretics. Fluid retention is also commonly seen in patients taking NSAIDs and may be severe enough to worsen congestive heart failure. If some of these clinical signs are noted in the absence of prescription NSAID use, the patient should be queried about the use of over-the-counter NSAID use. With the numerous potential side effects of NSAIDs, they should be used rarely and with caution for long-term use (Level of Evidence B).

A way to minimize the amount of GI side effects is to use COX-2 selective inhibitors such as celecoxib. Valdecoxib and rofecoxib have been removed from the market because of their increased adverse cardiovascular event rate.[19,20] Coadministration of NASIDs with gastroprotective agents such as proton pump inhibitors will help decrease their GI side effects.[21,22]

Acetaminophen

Acetaminophen is considered to be the initial drug of choice for management of mild to moderate persistent pain (Level of Evidence A). Although it is an effective, safe medication for musculoskeletal pain such as osteoarthritis and low back pain,[23,24] acetaminophen is not as effective for chronic inflammatory conditions such as rheumatoid arthritis.[25] It is not associated with significant GI bleeding, adverse renal effects, or cardiac toxicity. The maximum daily dose is 4 g but should not exceed 3 gm/day in those with significant renal or hepatic disease and in those with alcohol abuse. Side effects are minimal and may include transient elevation of alanine transferase, which does not translate into liver failure or dysfunction when maximum recommended dose is avoided. Chronic high-dose use for many years may rarely cause renal toxicity. A commonly prescribed combination is acetaminophen with codeine or hydrocodone. When given, it is important to monitor the total daily amount of acetaminophen the patient is taking.

Topical Agents

Topical agents may be useful for management of neuropathic pain or localized osteoarthritic pain (Table 27-2). They are generally well tolerated with few significant systemic side effects. Care should be taken to apply topical agents only to intact skin.

The 5% lidocaine patch is most useful for neuropathic pain, especially postherpetic neuropathy or diabetic neuropathy (Level of Evidence B). There are

TABLE 27-2[26-35]		Topical Agents			
Name	Route	Aging effect	Precaution	Comparison	Cost
Acetaminophen	Oral	Transient elevation of alanine amino-transferase	In hepatic insufficiency and alcohol abuse patient	No effects of GI bleeding, adverse renal effects, cardiac toxicity as of NSAIDs. Greater safety than NSAIDS so recommended as first-line therapy.[28] NSAIDs better for short-term pain—OA,[29,30] low back pain.[31,32] Acetaminophen less effective for chronic inflammatory pain than NSAIDs.[28]	OTC, 100 tablets for $17.99
Lidocaine 5% patch	Topical	Nontoxic with safe range of 4 patches in 24 hours	Skin irritation	Limited for neuropathic pain. Absence of toxicity, no drug interactions. Contraindicated in advanced liver disease.	Rx, $220.99 for a 30-patch box
Topical capsaicin cream	Topical		Burning sensation of skin	Some benefit in reduction of neuropathic and non-neuropathic pain.[33,34]	OTC
Topical NSAIDs	Topical	Reported toxicity is low when used in recommended doses.[35] Not fully understood.	Check renal and hepatic function periodically.	Effective and safe over short term (<4 weeks). Shown some efficacy in few studies of persistent pain management.[36,37]	Rx, 30 patches of 1.3% for $189.99

GI, gastrointestinal; NSAIDs, nonsteroidal antiinflammatory drugs; OA, osteoarthritis.

few controlled data for other types of pain. Up to three patches should be applied to the painful area for up to 12 hours daily. Capsaicin cream may be used for neuropathic or nonneuropathic pain (Level of Evidence B). Capsaicin is an inhibitor of substance P, which is a mediator of inflammation. Patients should be warned that they may notice a burning sensation at the site of application, which may take several weeks of use to dissipate. Topical NSAIDs (diclofenac and salicylate) are useful for localized nonneuropathic pain, particularly osteoarthritis. It is safe and effective, especially when used short term.[36,37] There is some systemic absorption so renal function should still be monitored.

Opioids

Opioids are the most effective analgesics with appropriate dosing and patient selection, especially for moderate and severe nociceptive pain[38] (Level of Evidence A). Because of the evidence that potential GI, renal, and cardiovascular adverse effects from NSAIDs and COX-2 inhibitors,[39] the role of opioid analgesics has been gaining acceptance even though data regarding long-term effectiveness for persistent noncancer pain is limited and controversial.

In addition to their potency, one other major advantage of opioids is the variety of routes available for delivery, including oral, subcutaneous, intravenous, transdermal, sublingual, intravenous, or rectal administration. This is valuable especially for the elderly with poor oral intake or dysphagia.

Long-term use of opioid analgesics often increases the risk of adverse events for the elderly. Central nervous system (CNS) side effects such as altered mental status, sedation, depression, delirium, and respiratory depression commonly occur, especially soon after initiation of the medication. GI side effects such as constipation and nausea are common. Constipation does not improve with continued use as CNS effects often will. It is worthwhile to anticipate this side effect and begin a bowel regimen consisting of physical activity, increased fluids, and osmotic or stimulant laxatives. Bulk-building agents are usually ineffective in these cases. Injections of methylnaltrexone, a selective peripheral μ-opioid antagonist, are available for severely ill patients with significant opioid-induced constipation.

After the patient's pain is stabilized, consideration could be given to the use of the longer acting opioids. These are available as a patch or in timed-release oral form. The dose should be titrated depending on both the amount of short-acting pain medication required by the patient for relief and the effectiveness of the long-acting medication.

Short-Acting Opioids

Commonly used and available short-acting opioids, along with precautions and changes expected in aging, are listed in table 27-3.

Long-Acting Opioids

Commonly used and available long-acting opioids, along with precautions and changes expected in aging, are listed in Table 27-4.

Drug Misuse and Addiction

Prescription opioid misuse and diversion have been a great burden for the primary care provider and health care system as a whole. Careful initial assessment for the risk of such behavior is critical and there have been tools, such as the Opioid Risk Tool (ORT),[40] to screen high-risk patients. Addiction is the behavior characterized as impaired control over drug use, compulsive use, continued use despite harm, and craving for higher doses of the medication.[41] It is worthwhile for the patient to sign a contract with the clinician promising he or she will not divert opioid medications. If there is any doubt, the patient could undergo periodic urine drug screens to ascertain if opioid metabolites are present.

Adjunctive Therapy

Adjunctive therapy should be strongly considered for specific types of pain, such as neuropathic pain or in order to alter and attenuate pain perception. Also, adjunctive therapy could be considered to decrease the use of analgesics that may have significant side effects. Therefore, this class of medication is primarily used in conjunction with other analgesic strategies.

In addition to topical agents (mentioned earlier in this chapter), various antidepressants and anticonvulsants are approved to use as adjunctive therapy.

Antidepressants

Tricyclic antidepressants (TCAs) have good evidence for efficacy in pain control,[42] but these drugs are associated with a significant risk of anticholinergic and cardiovascular adverse events. Because of these adverse events, TCAs should be used in geriatric patients with caution and only in those who do not tolerate other treatments. SNRI antidepressants, such as duloxetine or venlafaxin, may be useful for neuropathic pain and are better tolerated than TCAs. SSRIs have limited use in the management of persistent pain other than in the management of depression.

Anticonvulsants

The most commonly used anticonvulsants in the management of persistent neuropathic pain are gabapentin and pregabalin. Dosages should start low and titrate upward slowly as tolerated by the patient. Older anticonvulsants such as carbamazepine have more drug–drug interactions and bone marrow side

TABLE 27-3	Information on Commonly Used Short-Acting Opioids		
Drug	**Route Available**	**Aging Effect**	**Precautions and Recommendations**
Morphine	PO, SL, IV, SQ, PR	Active metabolite accumulation in renal insufficiency; more sensitive	Caution with low renal function; anticipate and treat constipation
Hydromorphone	PO, SL, IV, SQ, PR	Active metabolite accumulation in renal insufficiency; more sensitive	Caution with low renal function; anticipate and treat constipation
Oxycodone	PO, SL, PR	Active metabolite accumulation in renal insufficiency; more sensitive	Caution with low renal function; anticipate and treat constipation
Hydrocodone	PO		Usually comes in combination with other medication; caution
Fentanyl	PO, SL, intranasal, IV, SQ, PR	Can be twice as sensitive as other age group	Anticipate and treat constipation
Codeine	PO	Active metabolite accumulation in renal insufficiency	Monitor for nausea, anorexia; anticipate and treat constipation
Tramadol	PO	Active metabolite accumulation in renal insufficiency	Monitor for nausea, dizziness; use with caution in patients with history of seizure disorders

IV, intravenous; *PO*, by mouth; *PR*, per rectum; *SL*, sublingual; *SQ*, subcutaneous.

TABLE 27-4	**Information on Commonly Used Sustained Released Opioids**			
Drug	**Route Available**	**Aging Effect**	**Precautions and Recommendations**	
Sustained-release morphine	PO	Active metabolite accumulation in renal insufficiency	Escalate dose slowly because of possible drug accumulation; use immediate-release opioid for breakthrough pain	
Sustained-release oxycodone	PO	Active metabolite accumulation in renal insufficiency	Start at lower dose	
Hydromorphone extended release	PO		Use after stabilized dose with short-acting medication	
Fentanyl patch	Transdermal	Absorption may be variable, especially with thin subcutaneous fat	Start with lower-dose patch and supplement with short-acting medication after dose is stablized.	

PO, by mouth.

effects. However, carbamazepine may be especially helpful in the treatment of trigeminal neuralgia. Other anticonvulsants such as topiramate or lamotragine may have some utility in pain management if other medications fail. However, data are limited.

Other Medications

Corticosteroids may be useful as adjunctive therapy in some inflammatory conditions (Box 27-2). However, multiple side effects, such as osteoporosis, glucose intolerance, or cataracts, are associated with chronic use.

Baclofen is a centrally acting muscle relaxant that may be helpful in treating poststroke painful muscle spasms. Fatigue, weakness, and confusion may be side effects.

Other treatments that could be considered are intermittent joint injections or trigger point injections with local anesthetics, or corticosteroids may give relief for weeks or longer. The patient could be referred to pain management specialists for consideration of epidural steroid injections in cases of refractory back pain.

Methadone

Methadone has received more attention for use in the management of persistent pain. However, it has

unique pharmacodynamic and pharmacokinetic properties. It has a highly variable half-life with the potential for significant drug accumulation with resultant CNS depression. This drug should be used only in carefully selected patients educated in its use and prescribed only by clinicians experienced in dealing with its potential side effects.

> Clinicians must keep in mind the many side effects of long-term use of NSAIDs.

NONPHARMACOLOGIC STRATEGIES

Clinicians often think of pain relief only in terms of medications. However, excellent data support the use of ancillary treatments either alone or in combination with medications.[2] These treatments, which include physical and psychological therapies, require the patient to be actively involved. Patient education is an important part of any pain management program (Level of Evidence A). The patient can be informed about the nature of pain and the various modalities used for treatment. Appropriate expectations can be set for the patient.

Simple home therapies such as ice applied to affected areas after activity, or heat to the painful areas at other times, can give temporary relief. Stretching of the muscles around affected joints may help maintain mobility.

Cognitive behavioral therapy by a counselor can help the patient adjust to persistent pain. If patients have the attitude that the pain will never improve, their lives can be ruled by the pain. By helping patients cognitively take control of the pain, self-defeating attitudes such as helplessness, depression, anxiety, and low self-esteem may be improved by

BOX 27-2	
ADJUNCTIVE MEDICATIONS	

TCA antidepressants
SNRI antidepressants
Anticonvulsants
Corticosteroids
Muscle relaxants

SNRI, Serotonin norepinephrine reuptake inhibitors; *TCA*, tricyclic antidepressants.

actively altering behaviors. Relaxation and biofeedback are techniques that can be useful.

Physical or occupational therapists are invaluable in helping the patient manage persistent pain. Patients can learn energy-conserving techniques, stretching and exercises specific for their painful areas, and safe ways to work around their pain and manage activities of everyday living.

Participation in regular exercise programs can provide many benefits (Level of Evidence A). Physical deconditioning can contribute to generalized weakness and persistent pain. Better conditioning can also help improve the functional capabilities of those with persistent pain. In addition, participation in an exercise program can help with socialization, which is important for those with persistent pain.

Alternative therapies include homeopathy, acupuncture, chiropractic, naturopathy, and spiritual healing. Although these treatments are often used by patients, there are few controlled studies to support their efficacy. If patients use such therapies, it is important that clinicians not be disparaging if patients get relief. However, clinicians also must be diligent to make sure that patients are not harmed and do not abandon proven therapies (Level of Evidence D).

CASE 1

Discussion

When seen 3 weeks later, Mrs. Peters states her acute pain has improved to a level of 6 of 10. You recommend trying to decrease the use of hydrocodone and to start using acetaminophen on a regular basis up to 4 g daily. Physical therapy and regular exercise was recommended for her ongoing lumbar spine pain. In 2 years, you recommend repeating the DEXA scan for evaluation of her osteoporosis.

Mrs. Peters is an example of a patient with persistent pain who has an acute injury complicating her pain. Once the acute pain has improved, the persistent pain still needs to be dealt with. This can be done with a combination of modalities. Medications from different classes of pain medications, physical and/or occupational therapy, antidepressants, counseling, or various treatments from complementary and alternative medicine may be used solely or in combination. For nociceptive pain, exercise and muscle strengthening can be very helpful once acute pain or pain exacerbations have improved. ◘

CASE 2

Discussion

When seen 3 weeks later, Mr. Reid reports some relief of his neuropathic pain, but still rates it at a 6. He agrees to try gabapentin. When seen again 3 weeks later his pain is down to a 4 and he agrees to continue the gabapentin

and titrate the dose according to his pain level. In addition, talking with the counselor has helped him to better deal with his pain. He feels his mood has elevated with the use of the antidepressant.

Mr. Reid is an example of a patient with persistent pain resulting from neuropathic causes. Although opioids, NSAIDs, or acetaminophen may occasionally be helpful, other classes of medications such as anticonvulsants or antidepressants may be more beneficial. Also, because patients with neuropathic pain often do not get complete pain relief from medications, nonpharmacologic therapy such as counseling may be helpful. ◘

SUMMARY

Persistent pain is a common problem and sometimes challenging because of multiple complex issues related to aging changes and management options. However, persistent pain can be controlled; important factors include careful assessment of the etiology of the pain, selection of analgesics, their route of administration, and dose and frequency of medications. Drug effects and side effects should be carefully monitored. Reassessment for adjusting medication should be frequent enough to minimize the risk of potential side effects.

The clinician should understand that many aspects of the patient's life, such as interpersonal relationships, emotional health, and enjoyment of life, are affected. Nonpharmacologic therapies, such as physical and occupational therapy, counseling, and complementary and alternative treatments, can be used in certain patients. It should be emphasized that exercise is important for both general wellbeing and for strengthening of specific muscle groups that may be related to the painful area.

Optimized use of recommendations from the American Geriatrics Society (AGS) guidelines for persistent pain as well as various assessment and screening tools also are key to successful pain management and improving the quality of life of patients and their families and caregivers.

KEY REFERENCES

7. Hadjistavropoulos T, Herr K, Turk DC, et al. An interdisciplinary expert consensus statement on assessment of pain in older persons. Clin J Pain 2007;23(1):S1-43.
8. Herr K, Coyne P, McCaffery M, et al. Pain assessment in the patient unable to self-report: Position statement with clinical practice recommendations. Pain Manag Nurs 2011;12(4):230-50.
12. Towheed TE, Maxwell L, Judd MG, et al. Acetaminophen for osteoarthritis. Cochrane Database Syst Rev 2006;CD004257.
23. Chou R, Huffman LH. Medications for acute and chronic low back pain: A review of the evidence for an American Pain Society/American College of Physicians clinical practice guideline. Ann Intern Med 2007;147:505-14.
42. American Geriatrics Society Panel on Pharmacological Management of Persistent Pain in Older Persons. JAGS 2009;57:1331-46.

References available online at expertconsult.com.

28

Malnutrition and Feeding Problems

Migy K. Mathew and Matthew S. Jacobs

OBJECTIVES

Upon completion of this chapter, the reader will be able to:

- Understand the impact and prevalence of malnutrition and feeding problems in older adults.
- List the risk factors for poor nutritional status in older adults.
- Describe the pathophysiology of malnutrition and feeding problems in older adults.
- List the differential diagnosis for malnutrition and feeding problems in older adults.
- Identify assessment tools and management options to address malnutrition and feeding problems in older adults.

Additional online-only material indicated by icon.

Mr. Wells (Part 1)

Mr. Wells is an 88-year-old white male who lives at home with his wife. He has a history of prostate cancer, osteoarthritis, and iron deficiency anemia. He ambulates fairly well with a walker. He has lost 40 lbs over the last 2 to 3 months.

1. **Which factors place Mr. Wells at an increased nutritional risk?**

2. **How common is malnutrition in the ambulatory setting?**

PREVALENCE AND IMPACT

Malnutrition, more specifically undernutrition, appears to occur frequently in older adults, and has been associated with adverse health outcomes. The outcome of chronically poor nutritional status and unrecognized or untreated malnutrition is frequently considerable dysfunction and disability,[1] reduced quality of life, premature or increased morbidity and mortality,[2-5] and increased health care costs.[4-6]

When defined as a decrease in nutrient reserve, *malnutrition* is prevalent in 1% to 15% of ambulatory outpatients, in 25% to 60% of institutionalized patients, and in 35% to 65% of hospitalized patients.[7] Review of the current available incidence data suggests that unintended weight loss is a more frequent problem, especially in the older outpatient population, than previously thought. Malnutrition has been associated with increased mortality in numerous studies, with weight loss often remaining independently associated with mortality after adjustment for baseline health status, which suggests a potential causal role.[8-11]

Health outcomes other than mortality have also been associated with malnutrition in older adults. Data from National Health and Nutrition Examination Survey (NHANES) indicated that older women (baseline age 60 to 74, mean 66 years) who lost 5% or more of their body weight over a 10-year follow-up interval had a twofold increase in risk of disability compared to weight-stable women. This risk persisted after adjustment for age, education, smoking, and multiple health conditions.[12]

Sarcopenia has also been associated with malnutrition and diminished physical function, both of which are associated with geriatric functional decline and mortality. Sarcopenia is a syndrome defined as age-related muscle loss that contributes to functional decline and disability.[13]

RISK FACTORS AND PATHOPHYSIOLOGY

Many older adults undergo changes in their lives (e.g., physiologic, social, family, environmental, economic) that could affect their nutritional intake. Identifying risk factors for malnutrition helps direct further questioning. These risk factors, listed in Figure 28-1, are often multiple and synergistic; if left unchecked these risk factors could weaken nutrition status, increase medical complications, and result in loss of independence.[14]

CASE 1

Mr. Wells (Part 2)

During a routine visit Mr. Wells tells you that he has no appetite, has recently been depressed, and has not been eating much for the past 3 weeks. On physical examination you note mild to moderate temporal muscle wasting and moderate to severe clavicle muscle wasting as well as generalized loss of subcutaneous fat and lean muscle wasting. His recent laboratory work was significant for the following: albumin 2.8, prealbumin 14.3, and thyroid-stimulating hormone 5.68.

1. **What are the physiologic factors that may be influencing Mr. Wells's food intake?**

2. **What is the differential diagnosis for this patient regarding his malnutrition?** ▣

Normal Aging Changes

As one passes through the life span, changes often occur in body mass and percentage of body fat. Lean body mass declines at a rate of 0.3 kg per year beginning in the third decade. However, this decrease in lean body mass tends to be offset by an increase in body fat, which continues until at least age 65 to 70.[15,16] Body weight usually peaks at approximately the fifth to sixth decade of life and remains stable

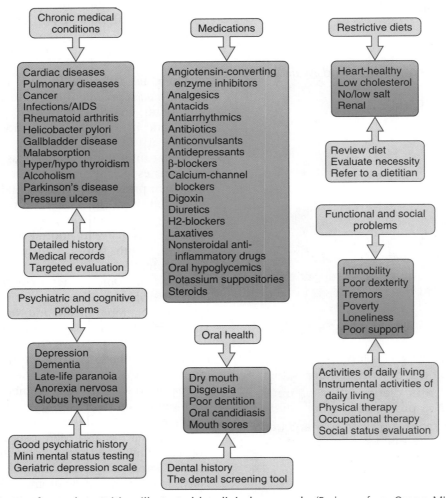

Figure 28-1   **Risk factors for undernutrition illustrated by clinical approach.** (Redrawn from Omran ML, Salem P. Diagnosing undernutrition. Clin Geriatr Med 2002;18:719-36.)

until 65 to 70, after which we see a slow decrease in body weight that continues for the remainder of life.[17]

Anorexia of Aging

Food intake is a motivated behavior between internal signals and environmental cues, and this occurs primarily through the senses of olfaction, taste, vision, and hearing. With aging we often see alterations in these hedonic qualities of food, specifically taste and smell.[15,17] The sense of smell declines dramatically with aging, with an increase in odor threshold and a decline in odor identification. Although changes in the sense of taste seem to be less important than changes in the sense of smell, many changes in taste do occur with aging. Among these changes are an increase in taste threshold, difficulty in recognizing taste mixtures, and an increased perception of irritating tastes. These chemosensory changes with aging lead to reduced appetite and subsequent weight loss.[18]

The regulation of appetite is a complex process involving feedback from a number of peripheral signals and the interactions of a variety of neurotransmitters within the central nervous system. Much of the anorexia of aging seems to be related to the changes in gastrointestinal activities that occur with aging,[18-20] with less antral distension, and thus earlier satiety.[18,21,22]

In addition, other factors, including depression and cognitive impairment, contribute to the phenomena of anorexia of aging. Older patients with decreased appetite, lessened food intake, and weight loss should be screened for depression.

Protein Energy Malnutrition

The physiologic anorexia of aging and its associated weight loss predisposes older persons to develop protein energy malnutrition (PEM). The prevalence rate for PEM is high and has been reported in 15% of community-dwelling older persons, 5% to 12% of homebound patients, 20% to 65% of hospitalized persons, and 5% to 85% of institutionalized older persons.[15] PEM has been defined as the presence of both clinical (physical signs such as wasting, low body mass index) and biochemical (albumin, cholesterol, or other protein changes) consistent with undernutrition.[23] It is a syndrome characterized by a person's having too little lean body mass, secondary to decreased energy or protein being supplied.

Within this PEM syndrome there are two clinical patterns that need to be distinguished: marasmus and kwashiorkor (hypoalbuminemic malnutrition). Marasmus is the PEM syndrome that develops gradually over months or years when energy intake is insufficient. Skeletal muscle, rather than plasma proteins or visceral protein, is metabolized, and thus there is generally a normal serum albumin level. Kwashiorkor is the more acute or subacute type of PEM and is frequently superimposed on marasmus, the precipitant being the stress of acute illness; it may develop over weeks but is often more acute. Because of elevated levels of hormones, monokines, and tumor necrosis factor, serum proteins are depleted, causing consequent edema and frequently no weight loss. Once developed, this PEM syndrome has a high mortality rate.

It must be emphasized that the symptoms and signs of PEM are nonspecific, and other conditions, such as underlying malignancy, malabsorption, hyperthyroidism, peptic ulcer, and liver disease, need to be ruled out.

> It must be emphasized that the symptoms and signs of protein energy malnutrition are nonspecific, and other conditions, such as underlying malignancy, malabsorption, hyperthyroidism, peptic ulcer, and liver disease, need to be ruled out.

DIFFERENTIAL DIAGNOSIS AND ASSESSMENT

Nutrition Screening and Assessment

Nutrition screening is the first step in identifying patients who are at risk for nutrition problems or who have undetected malnutrition. It allows for prevention of nutrition-related problems when risks are identified and early intervention when problems are confirmed.[24] Early detection and treatment are not only cost-effective but result in improved health and quality of life of the older patient.[24,25] An approach to the evaluation of weight loss in the elderly is illustrated in Figure 28-2.

Several screening and assessment tools specific to the older population are available. Regardless of the tool used, the screening process can be completed in any setting. Screening includes the collection of relevant information to determine risk factors and evaluates the need for a comprehensive nutrition assessment.[25]

Nutrition assessments are more comprehensive than nutrition screens and are generally completed by a registered dietitian. The mnemonic ABCD stands for anthropometric, biochemical, clinical, and dietary, the four primary components of a nutrition assessment.[26] Box 28-1 summarizes the most common data collected during a nutrition assessment of an older patient. Assessments vary in their detail and depth depending on the level of risk identified during the screening process, and the amount of information available at the time of the evaluation.

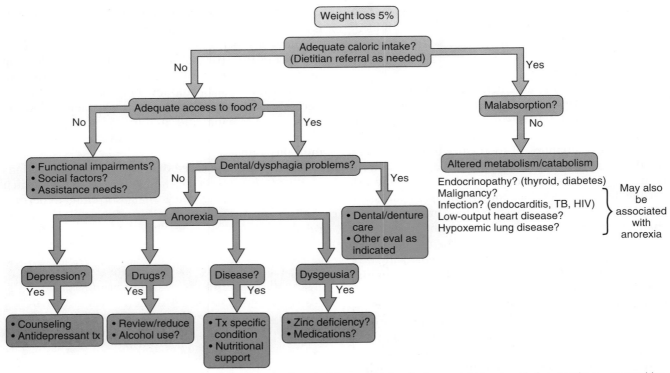

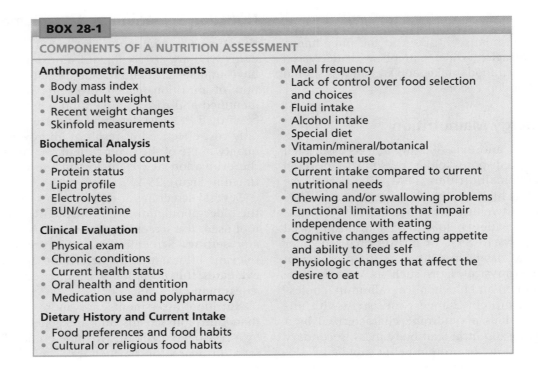

Figure 28-2 **Weight loss algorithm.** (Redrawn from Wallace JI, Schwartz RS. Involuntary weight loss in elderly outpatients—recognition, etiologies, and treatment. Clin Geriatr Med 1997;13:717-33.)

BOX 28-1

COMPONENTS OF A NUTRITION ASSESSMENT

Anthropometric Measurements
- Body mass index
- Usual adult weight
- Recent weight changes
- Skinfold measurements

Biochemical Analysis
- Complete blood count
- Protein status
- Lipid profile
- Electrolytes
- BUN/creatinine

Clinical Evaluation
- Physical exam
- Chronic conditions
- Current health status
- Oral health and dentition
- Medication use and polypharmacy

Dietary History and Current Intake
- Food preferences and food habits
- Cultural or religious food habits

- Meal frequency
- Lack of control over food selection and choices
- Fluid intake
- Alcohol intake
- Special diet
- Vitamin/mineral/botanical supplement use
- Current intake compared to current nutritional needs
- Chewing and/or swallowing problems
- Functional limitations that impair independence with eating
- Cognitive changes affecting appetite and ability to feed self
- Physiologic changes that affect the desire to eat

Once the nutrition assessment is complete, it is combined with data from other disciplines to be interpreted and evaluated for the purpose of developing a patient care plan to address identified risks and problems.[25]

Nutrition Evaluation Tools

The need for more than one nutrition evaluation tool exists because the older population can be divided into several subsets, such as the healthy community-dwelling group, those that live in the community but are frail, and those that are institutionalized.[26] Three popular tools developed for older Americans as part of the Nutrition Screening Initiative (NSI) are the Determine Your Nutritional Health Checklist (Table 28-1), and the Level I and Level II screens of the NSI. The NSI was a collaborative effort of the American Dietetic Association, the American Academy of Family Physicians, the National Council on Aging, and 35 other aging agencies. The checklist tool can be self-administered or used by any member of the health care team. For those patients identified to be at high nutritional risk, further information should be obtained by using a more in-depth assessment tool such as the Level I and Level II screens, or referring to a registered dietitian.[27]

A tool that is a combination of a quick screen and a detailed assessment is the Mini Nutritional Assessment questionnaire (MNA). It is an evaluation tool using 18 items to assess the malnutrition risk of an older patient.[28] It has also been shown to predict morbidity and mortality.[29] The MNA is only validated for patients over the age of 65.[30] Like the Determine

Checklist, the MNA provides a score on the screening section that determines the need for further assessment. Other tools include the Nutritional Risk Index, Nutritional Risk Score, Nutrition Risk Assessment Scale, Prognostic Nutritional Index, and Subjective Global Assessment. The tools vary in their length, type of data collected, and type of older patient being evaluated.

Feeding Problems

An important part of the nutrition assessment is determining barriers to eating a well-balanced diet. The loss of functional ability to eat caused by acute or chronic conditions of the oral cavity has an impact on diet and nutritional status.[31] Decayed or missing teeth, ill-fitting dentures, tooth erosion, periodontal disease, gingivitis, xerostomia, taste disorders, and oral infections are factors that can have a significant impact on a patient's willingness or ability to eat.[32] Certain prescription drugs have side effects such as dry mouth, disordered taste, anorexia, nausea, and drowsiness that can also impair the ability and desire to eat.[33] Edentulous patients are at a disadvantage when attempting to eat fresh fruits and vegetables and high-fiber foods. When a study compared the diets of denture wearers to fully dentate participants, the denture wearers had lower serum levels of beta-carotene, vitamin C, and folate as well as lower dietary fiber intakes.[34]

Other problems associated with feeding include general limitations in the ability to self-feed. Conditions that cause tremors or shaking, arthritis, loss of vision, loss of memory, sedation, changes in gastrointestinal tract motility, and generalized weakness can add to the challenges of feeding the older patient a well-balanced diet.[35]

TABLE 28-1	Determine Your Nutritional Health	
Questions		**Yes Points**
I have an illness or condition that made me change the kind and/or amount of food I eat.		2
I eat fewer than two meals a day.		3
I eat few fruits or vegetables or milk products.		2
I have three or more drinks of beer, liquor, or wine almost every day.		2
I have tooth or mouth problems that make it hard for me to eat.		2
I don't always have enough money to buy the food I need.		4
I eat alone most of the time.		1
I take three or more different prescribed or over-the-counter drugs a day.		1
Without wanting to, I have lost or gained 10 pounds in the last 6 months.		2
I am not always physically able to shop, cook, and/or feed myself.		2
Total score:		_____

Interpretation of scores:

0-2: Good. Recheck nutritional score in 6 months.

3-5: You are at moderate nutrition risk. Recheck in 3 months.

6 or more: You are at high nutritional risk. Review with a health care provider.

> An important part of the nutrition assessment is determining barriers to eating a well-balanced diet.

Swallowing Problems

The prevalence of swallowing disorders is 16% to 22% in adults over the age of 50 and up to 60% in nursing home residents.[36] Subtle changes in upper esophageal sphincter function and peristalsis can result in dysphagia.[37] Changes are associated with normal aging and with stroke, neuromuscular disorders, and central nervous system diseases.[37] Box 28-2 identifies the most common risks for swallowing problems, and Box 28-3 lists screening criteria used to evaluate swallowing problems.[38-40]

MANAGEMENT

Treatment of Common Feeding and Swallowing Problems

Once the assessment process is complete, the patient's plan of care with appropriate interventions is implemented.[25] Treatments may include environmental strategies, diet therapy, counseling, and the use of community services.

The environment in which meals are served can have an impact on intake. Eating the majority of meals alone is a risk factor for poor nutritional intake.[41] Encouraging companionship at mealtimes for those patients routinely eating alone is a primary strategy for improving nutrient intake. Congregate meal programs established by the Older Americans Act provide a nutritious meal 5 days each week and social interaction for the adult 60 years of age or older.[42] The program is available at no cost and also provides health screens and education. Home-delivered meals are available for those who qualify. Other agencies also provide mobile meals and in-home services. The local Area Agency on Aging can provide additional information.

Problems with the oral cavity, loss of taste and smell, and poor dentition are treated with a variety of food modification strategies. Foods may be mechanically altered by chopping, grinding, or pureeing to minimize or eliminate the need for chewing. Mechanical alteration affects the appeal of foods and may not be well accepted. Every attempt should be made to serve the food in an attractive way. Offering soft, nutritious foods such as fruit and vegetable juices, cooked fruits and vegetables, milk, yogurt, custard, tender moist meats, poultry, fish, and eggs will provide a palatable diet that is familiar to the patient. Food should be well seasoned to accommodate the loss of taste and smell. The patient with xerostomia should keep a water bottle close by and avoid dry and salty foods.[33] Special dishes, drinking cups, and eating utensils are available for patients who are physically impaired.

Feeding problems associated with dementia or Alzheimer's disease consist of problems with cognition and memory along with chewing and swallowing problems. The Alzheimer's Association website (www.alz.org) has a list of feeding strategies.[43] These include providing an environment that is not distracting (e.g., minimal noise, plain tablecloths or placemats) and offering one food choice at a time and one eating utensil. As the patient loses the ability to use eating utensils, finger foods are recommended. When the progression of the disease includes chewing and swallowing problems, the appropriate dietary modifications are made or aggressive nutrition support is introduced, if appropriate to the patient's condition and preferences.

The treatment of swallowing problems is an interdisciplinary approach involving the speech pathologist, the dietitian, the nurse, and the physician. Key strategies for successful eating include proper positioning and food consistency. The patient should be sitting up straight with the chin slightly down. Swallowing liquids of thin consistency requires the most coordination and control.[40] The registered dietitian should be involved in making recommendations for an appropriate diet, which may range in texture from pudding-like to nearly normal-texture solids, with liquids ranging from spoon thick, to honey-like, nectar-like, and thin. It is critical that food be thickened to the recommended consistency because aspirating food or liquid into the lungs may result in life-threatening aspiration pneumonia.[40] Commercial thickeners and thickened products are available.

> Key strategies for successful eating include proper positioning and appropriate food consistency.

CASE 1

Mr. Wells (Part 3)

Mr. Wells continues to have slow, involuntary weight loss. He has lost 45 lbs in 3 months. He states he does not have a desire to eat and food does not taste good. His current diet consists of canned soups, cold cereals, crackers, coffee, and ice cream.

1. **List strategies for improving Mr. Wells's dietary intake.**

2. **What suggestions can you offer to increase protein and calories in Mr. Wells's diet?** ▫

Nutrition Interventions

When malnutrition is identified and a course of action is planned, the first strategy to consider is a diet that is as liberal as possible without endangering the patient's life. Diet orders that restrict sodium, sugar, and fat can be liberalized to improve the palatability of the diet and thus improve intake.[44]

When patients are not eating enough to maintain weight and nutritional status, the introduction of nutrient-dense foods can be incorporated into the normal diet. Calories can be added without increasing the volume of food eaten. Strategies for increasing calories include adding fat in the form of butter or margarine to hot cereals, vegetables, and breads, using whole milk or half-and-half in cooking and for beverages, and using full-fat salad dressings and gravies. Carbohydrate calories can be added to beverages by using extra sugar, honey, corn syrup, or a commercial glucose polymer. Dry milk powder or commercial protein powder can be added to milk, creamed soups, hot cereals, and casseroles. Small nutrient-dense snacks can boost calories and protein without significantly diminishing intake at mealtime. Suggested snacks include eggnog, custard, pudding, peanut butter with bread or crackers, instant breakfast beverage, ice cream, and homemade milkshakes.

Adding calorie and protein boosters may still require some patients to eat and drink more volume than they desire or are capable of consuming. A variety of commercial supplements are available for these patients. Liquid supplements range from 1 to 2 calories per mL or approximately 250 to 500 calories per cup. Protein content ranges from 8 to 20 g per cup. Supplements that provide 1.5 to 2.0 calories per mL help the patient who is having a problem consuming much volume. Commercial supplements also provide micronutrients and the benefits that result from their intake.[16] Disease-specific commercial formulas are also available. Other supplemental dietary products include nutrition bars, fortified cookies, baked products, and even ice cream cups. A registered dietitian can help patients identify recipes and commercial products to meet their specific needs.

CASE 1

Mr. Wells (Part 4)

Mr. Wells is now in the hospital after his family found him in the bathroom after a fall. He is displaying confusion and is requiring assistance with meals. His nursing staff reports that he has been eating approximately 50% of his meals.

1. **How will you meet Mr. Wells's nutritional needs during his hospital stay?**

2. **What plans should be made regarding his continued nutrition support after discharge?** ▫

Nutrition Support

There comes a time for many patients when they are no longer able to meet their nutritional needs orally. At this point a decision must be made by the patient or caregiver regarding enteral or parenteral nutrition support. The position of the American Dietetic Association on ethical and legal issues in nutrition, hydration, and feeding is an excellent reference to guide the health care team when the wishes of the patient are not known.[45]

When the decision is aggressive nutritional support, enteral nutrition is the first option to consider for the patient who has a functioning gastrointestinal (GI) tract.[33] There are fewer infectious complications with enteral feedings compared to parenteral feedings (Level of Evidence A) and enteral feedings are more cost-effective (Level of Evidence B).[46] The patient's calorie, protein, fluid, vitamin, and mineral needs are all considered when selecting an enteral formula. Cost and product availability should also be considered.[4]

Parenteral nutrition support is indicated when the patient has an impaired GI tract that prevents enteral feedings.[33] Risks associated with parenteral nutrition in the older patient include impaired glucose tolerance, thin skin, and increased risk of infection.[47]

> The position of the American Dietetic Association on ethical and legal issues in nutrition, hydration, and feeding is an excellent reference to guide the health care team when the wishes of the patient are not known.

CASE 1

Discussion

Mr. Wells's case illustrates the classic presentation of an older community-dwelling person with multiple comorbidities (osteoarthritis, depression), along with physiologic changes in aging that may be contributing to his malnutrition. Also, as we often see in this age group, a catastrophic event can lead to a transition in living situations from independent to long-term care. Mr. Wells incurs an adverse event that leaves him debilitated and places him at an even greater risk for malnutrition, which will need to be addressed with supplementation and assistance with meals, either on a short- or long-term basis.

From this case, it is evident that an interdisciplinary team care approach will be necessary to provide optimal care for Mr. Wells. The realm of geriatric care extends well beyond the domain of the physician. The responsibility for preservation of health rests not only on the physician but also on other allied gerontologic professionals including registered dietitians, nurses, physical therapists, pharmacists, and social workers. ▣

SUMMARY

Age-related changes in physiology, metabolism, and function alter the older person's nutritional requirements. To evaluate the nutritional adequacy in older persons, clinicians must understand the general concepts of geriatric nutrition and the parameters of nutritional assessment for this age group. Nutritional care of the older person is indicated across the health care continuum and in all practice settings; therefore, clinicians need to work with other professionals from a variety of disciplines in addressing the nutritional health of older people.

Web Resources

www.aafp.org. American Academy of Family Physicians.
www.mna-elderly.com. Mini Nutritional Assessment.

KEY REFERENCES

14. American Dietetic Association. Nutrition, aging, and the continuum of care—position of American Dietetic Association. J Am Diet Assoc 2000;100:580-95.
15. Morley JE. Anorexia of aging: Physiologic and pathologic. Am J Clin Nutr 1997;66:760-73.
25. Council on Practice (COP) Quality Management Committee. Identifying patients at risk: ADA's definitions for nutrition screening and nutrition assessment. J Am Diet Assoc 1994;94:838-9. (Errata in J Am Diet Assoc 1994;94:1101.)
33. Niedert K, Dorner B, eds. Nutrition care of the older adult. 2nd ed. Chicago, IL: American Dietetic Association; 2004.

References available online at expertconsult.com.

29

Frailty

Jerry L. Old and Doug Woolley

OUTLINE

OBJECTIVES

Upon completion of this chapter, the reader will be able to:

- Describe the components of the two dominant theoretical concepts of geriatric frailty, and compare their approaches to defining or identifying frailty.

- Discuss the strengths and limitations of each of these two theoretical concepts for clinicians in identifying frail aged patients in their practices.

- Contrast the concepts of frailty and disability.

- Discuss whether and how the concept of frailty has usefulness in geriatric clinical care beyond a focus on specific diseases and disabilities.

- Describe examples of specific potentially treatable diseases that often silently amplify or even masquerade as generalized geriatric frailty.

- Discuss how patient-centered clinical decision making may be appropriately redirected when the patient, family, and physician agree that the patient is irreversibly quite frail.

- Give specific examples of recommendations to a patient and family when advanced and irreversible frailty is identified.

CASE 1

Frank Mills (Part 1)

Frank Mills is a 94-year-old widower who has been in your practice for many years. He is a retired army colonel, businessman, and college teacher with many awards and mementos on his walls in his continuing care retirement home. He requires daily support from the aides and nursing staff. He has cerebrovascular disease (CVD), hyperlipidemia, prostate cancer, glaucoma, and recurring deep venous thrombophlebitis (DVT). His diffuse degenerative lumbar arthritis with spinal stenosis has progressed and contributed to chronic back ache, leg weakness, gait instability with several recent falls, and bladder atony requiring an indwelling bladder catheter. His CVD is diffuse, with a history of transient ischemic attacks, scattered small deep lacunar infarcts, and white matter disease on magnetic resonance imaging. The CVD contributes to his gait slowness and instability. He receives bicalutamide (Casodex) and leuprolide (Lupron) treatments from an oncologist, and his prostate-specific antigen (PSA) has been low. He has not had a recurrence of his DVT or new transient ischemic attacks in the last couple years while on warfarin. His international normalized ratio is kept at around 2.0 and he has not suffered significant bleeds. For years his hyperlipidemia has been controlled with atorvastatin. His sight is declining significantly in spite of frequent ophthalmology consultations and adjustments of his glaucoma management. His mild chronic memory deficit has been more evident in recent months.

The nursing director notifies you that Mr. Mills is not eating as well as usual, and has lost about 5 lbs in 60 days. The fitness center director reports that he is not the usual enthusiastic exercise participant he had previously been.

1. **Would you consider Mr. Mills to be frail, and if so, why?**

2. **List significant possible contributors to Mr. Mills's functional and physiologic decline.**

3. **List key components of your multilevel plan of action to address this decline.** 🖥

Frailty is a general term that has been applied to certain elderly folks for quite some time. The term brings

---

to mind the image of a thin, stooped, slow-functioning 80- or 90-year-old. Although a precise and standardized definition of medical frailty is still a challenge, the simplest understanding is that frailty is a state of increased vulnerability to adverse outcomes.[1] The most widely used definition in clinical practice was suggested by Fried et al. in 2001. This definition identifies frailty as the presence of three or more of the following five criteria: weight loss, exhaustion, weak grip strength, slow walking speed, and low physical activity.[2] Some researchers and clinicians have suggested adding cognition, depressed mood, and pain to this list.[3-5]

> Clinically, frailty involves weight loss, exhaustion, weakness, slow walking speed, and low physical activity.

A basic tenet of geriatrics has been that age itself is not a good predictor of outcomes. Frailty is not synonymous with either *age* or *disease*. However, the prevalence of frailty seems to increase with chronologic age, and there comes a functional point at which frailty becomes likely for all individuals, making them vulnerable to adverse outcomes.[6] Even marathon runners who are in top physical shape tend to demonstrate an inevitable point at which physical reserves begin to deteriorate more rapidly.

It is estimated that in people older than 85 years of age, approximately 70% show signs of frailty; of that age group studied, 49% were living in the community, and 21% were living in nursing homes.[7,8]

These frail, older patients often pose a challenge to their health care provider, who may feel overwhelmed by the complex presentation of the patients' health status.[3] One of the major hurdles is that frailty does not fit the traditional medical model of single diagnosis or single organ system disease. There is almost never a chief complaint, and the manifestations of system failure within frailty occur in combination. Frailty refers to notable clinical losses in reserve in many systems that are interdependent for good health.[9-11]

> The medical problems of the frail patient often appear overwhelming because no single disease or organ system is involved.

Consensus does not yet exist regarding the medical components of frailty.[3,6,12] However, the term is increasingly recognized as progressively decreasing reserves in our aging population. The reserves of one system are no longer able to compensate for the decline in another system, as they do in the robust individual.

Although the recognition of frailty in a patient should not lead to decreasing care, it does generate a cascade of care needs, such as increased physician visits, hospital admissions, emergency room visits, prescription medications, and ancillary services.[1,8]

Primary care clinicians are well poised to identify frail patients in their practices. By identifying the frail patient, focused interventions (or avoidance of interventions), goal setting, and recommendations about medical management (Tables 29-1 and 29-2) can be made with discernment. There is good evidence that identifying frail patients will improve clinical outcomes and there is also increasing evidence that it is cost effective—in short, it is good medical care.[3,13,14]

ETIOLOGY OF FRAILTY

It has been proposed that aging is an accumulation of random damage to a complex system with overlapping parts. As defects accumulate with time, the organism loses its redundancy across multiple molecular, cellular, and physiologic systems.[15] Resilience is lost—systems no longer have the ability to compensate for one another. The individual then becomes frail as the decline in a majority of systems results in a negative energy balance, sarcopenia, and diminished strength and tolerance for exertion.[16] All systems are at or near the threshold of failure and homeostasis becomes difficult.

In healthy humans, the entire homeostatic network provides a flexible and timely response to any external threat. However, when frailty exists, the range of adaptive responses becomes much more limited. Frail adults have diminished capacity to withstand stress, which places them at risk for adverse health outcomes. This has been well known to astute clinicians throughout history.

> In the frail patient, reserves and redundancy of complex systems are lost, making homeostasis difficult to maintain—the body becomes less forgiving.

Recently, frailty has been viewed as a manifestation of an impaired energy pathway.[17] In other words, as persons become frail, more energy is needed to maintain homeostasis. Any pathology rapidly decreases the energy available in the system for healing, making the patient more vulnerable. In short, homeostasis becomes harder to maintain and the body becomes much less forgiving.

TABLE 29-1	Clinical Assessment and Management of Common Frailty Symptoms	
Symptom	**Assessment**	**Treatment**
Unintentional weight loss	Measure weight loss in the previous 6 months/year as a percentage of previous body weight (significant loss is >5%) Ask: "Have you lost more than 10 lbs in the past year—not on purpose?"	Inquire about food availability, preparation, and social aspects of eating Assess for dental problems Liberalized diet (encourage foods of choice) Recommend small frequent feedings Consider nutritional supplements
Exhaustion	Ask: "How often in the past week did you feel exhausted?" "How often would you say you just could not get going?"	Medication review to eliminate fatigue-causing medications Reordering tasks to conserve energy (e.g., eating first, resting, then bathing) Treat remediable conditions (COPD, CHF, anemia, insomnia) Modify daily procedures (e.g., sitting while showering rather than standing)
Weakness/low physical activity	Ask: "How often last week did you feel everything was an effort?" Measure grip strength (Jamar handheld dynamometer)	Increase physical activity (e.g., walking 20-30 min, 3-5 times per week) Strength training Modify environment to decrease energy expenditure (e.g., placement of phone, bedside commode) Adjust room temperature to patient's comfort
Slow walking speed	Timed walking at usual pace 15 feet: slow is >6 seconds for person of normal height (7 seconds for females under 62 inches and males under 68 inches)	Recommend referral for rehabilitation evaluation or physical therapy for strength training Recommend tai chi if available
Cognition	Mini-Cog screening MMSE, SLUM, or similar testing	Exclude reversible causes (medication toxicity, metabolic changes, depression, thyroid disease, subdural hematoma, etc.) Promote brain health by exercise, diet, stress reduction, etc. Nonpharmacologic interventions (behavior modifications, scheduled toileting, music, bathing in AM) Maximize and maintain functioning
Mood	Screen for depression (Geriatric Depression Scale, PHQ-9, etc.) Assess for helplessness, hopelessness, lack of pleasure, guilt, loss of self-esteem, social withdrawal, persistent dysphoria, and suicidal ideation	Prescribe SSRI alone or in combination with cognitive-behavioral therapy Schedule frequent encounters Listen to concerns Generally avoid TCAs in older adults Consider ECT if severe
Pain	Assess pain severity on scale of 1 to 10 Ask: "Describe how pain has interfered with your activities during the past 24 hours."	Educate on nonpharmacologic approaches to pain management (clean safe environment, decreased stimuli, back rub, therapeutic touch, etc.) If needed, prescribe oral analgesics for chronic and breakthrough pain in appropriate dosages—short-acting q3-4 hours; long-acting q8-12 hours (Initiate a stimulant laxative in all patients receiving opioids)

CHF, Congestive heart failure; *COPD*, chronic obstructive pulmonary disease; *ECT*, electroconvulsive therapy; *MMSE*, Mini-Mental State Examination; *PHQ-9*, Patient Health Questionnaire-9; *SLUMS*, St. Louis University Mental Status; *SSRI*, selective serotonin reuptake inhibitors; *TCAs*, tricyclic antidepressants.

MODELS OF FRAILTY

Within disciplines focusing on care and service to the aged individual, there has been a lively discussion for at least the past two decades about whether or not the term can be used to identify a subset of older people who deserve closer clinical monitoring and support.[18]

Various models of frailty have been proposed to predict the risk of poor clinical outcomes. The most well-known and widely used model, as discussed in the previous section, was proposed by Fried et al. in 2001 and describes frailty as a phenotype—a clinical syndrome or set of signs and symptoms that tend to

TABLE 29-2	Clinical Management of Frail Older Adults

- Identify frailty by screening all older adults for unintentional weight loss, weakness, exhaustion, slow walking speed, cognition, mood, and pain.
- Identify underlying treatable conditions that may be contributing to symptoms
- Treat symptoms until relief is obtained, or intolerable adverse effects of treatment occur
- Increase clinician availability:
  - More frequent or longer physician visits
  - Home/facility visits
  - Involve other health care professionals
    - Nurse contacts
    - Telephone contacts and tele-health devices
    - Community resources
    - Hospice agency
    - Other multidisciplines
      - Pharmacist
      - Rehabilitation
      - Mental health
      - Dentist
      - Podiatry
      - Wound care
      - Chaplain
      - Social worker
      - Medical aide
      - Dietary
      - Durable medical equipment
- Provide patient and family education
  - Self-management of symptoms
  - Long-term and short-term expectations
  - Warning signs that should prompt patients to contact a health care provider
  - Realistic hope
  - Harm reduction strategies
  - Advance directives

ful in research and policy planning, neither approach, to this point in time, has significantly benefited the primary care clinician. A simple, clinical, useful tool for frailty that will improve care and value patient-centered outcomes is still to be developed.[5,6]

CASE 1

Frank Mills (Part 2)

Mr. Mills requires careful broad-focused attention to his growing weakness, weight loss, and functional decline. His bladder catheter places him at risk for an occult bladder infection, which must be investigated. The status of his prostate cancer must be reviewed. Untoward effects of his medications on his appetite and well-being should be considered. The effectiveness of pain management, particularly the low back pain, must be reviewed. His ability to feed himself and swallow safely should be explored. His mood, never before a problem in his active life full of high achievements, should be assessed. With his declining gait and mental status, the possibility that a fall has led to an occult subdural bleed, particularly with his warfarin treatment, should be entertained. These issues are all addressed over the course of the following month, as is a thorough review of possible emerging new issues, but no new problems are unearthed. However, a mental status exam shows a significant decline from the previous year's score, consistent with his growing need for the supportive services.

1. **You are to meet with Mr. Mills and his daughter to summarize the findings of your investigation. What will be the major themes you will address?**

2. **What suggested care plan changes will you bring up?** ◘

occur together, thus characterizing a specific medical condition.[2] Components of the phenotype include the following five conditions: unintentional weight loss, exhaustion, weak grip strength, slow walking speed, and low physical activity. The presence of three or more of these factors equals frailty. In addition to assessing physical function, many clinicians believe that the definition of frailty should also include cognition, depressed mood, pain, and perhaps even advanced age.

Another popular model of frailty was proposed by Rockwood et al. in 2007.[9,19] In this model a frailty index (FI) is obtained—basically by adding all the multisystem biomarkers of decline together (disabilities and comorbidities) and coming up with a number. This concept views frailty as an accumulation of deficits—a quantitative approach using the number of health problems rather than the nature of health difficulties.

Each of these models, as well as other descriptions, has its own strengths and weaknesses. Although use-

IS RECOGNITION OF FRAILTY HELPFUL TO THE CLINICIAN?

Increasingly, the term *frailty* is being used to summarize health status and to provide useful clinical information.

Frailty has clinical consequences. It is widely accepted that recognizing frailty is important clinically, but recognizing physical frailty in clinical practice may not be as straightforward as first thought.[1,20] Many patients and families, as well as clinicians, may simply attribute declines in function to "old age" and not recognize frailty as an entity. Because of the often slow gradual decline, medical attention may not be sought. Other conditions, such as chronic disease, comorbidities, and disability, may overshadow the recognition of frailty. Also, there is often a general feeling that there is no treatment or intervention that is going to help with frailty anyway.[21]

However, recognizing frailty can be of tremendous benefit to the practicing physician. Because of frail patients' diminished capacity to withstand stress, they are at a high risk for adverse health outcomes. Not only are the decreased reserves of frailty important predictors of serious events such as falls, the presence of frailty also influences decision making about medication prescribing, and various interventions such as surgery, cancer treatments, coronary angiography, and others. As the body becomes less forgiving, the clinician must pay more attention to detail.

Timely recognition of frailty by the clinician may enable early identification of potentially treatable underlying conditions or open the possibilities of prevention and treatment. Primary care services for the oldest old are often reactive, and may not prove to have a significant impact on mortality or quality of life.[1] Identifying the frail patient may result in more proactive, preventive, or anticipatory clinical therapy decisions. Clinicians can potentially identify frail older adults by asking their older patients about declines in strength, endurance, nutrition, physical activity, fatigue or decreased energy, or slowed performance. Physical findings may include weight loss, slowed gait speed, and weakness.

> **Frailty is an important concept for the clinician to recognize—it is a more accurate predictor of adverse outcomes than age alone.**

Another important clinical area for early recognition of frailty involves the timely introduction of geriatric and palliative care approaches to care, if treatable options have been eliminated. Although not a substitute for a diagnostic workup, timely hospice and palliative care ensures that patients and families receive care that optimizes quality of life and relieves suffering.

CASE 1

Frank Mills (Part 3)

The discussion with Mr. Mills and his daughter centers around maximizing his current function and comfort and reassessing treatment goals for identified problems. In the latter discussion greater emphasis is now placed on reducing the risks of immediate harm from ongoing therapies rather than reducing the chance of later disease progression. Both the bicalutamide and leuprolide may be associated with weakness, anorexia, and weight loss. His PSA has remained low, and neither you nor his oncologist finds evidence of metastatic prostate disease. Thus you recommend that the bicalutamide and the leuprolide be stopped. Hyperlipidemia is now considered a low-priority problem, especially in the context of significant weight loss, so the

atorvastatin is stopped. Mr. Mills emphasizes the importance he places on continuing to walk with his walker and his daughter agrees, in spite of the risk of falls. The risk of major bleeds with a fall while on warfarin is now seen to be greater than that of DVT or transient ischemic attack if the warfarin is stopped. Considering Mr. Mills's cognitive decline, you, the care staff, and Mr. Mills's daughter agree that it is time to invoke his durable power of attorney for health care affairs. Mr. Mills agrees with this and the proposal that he move to the assisted living section of the home. In assisted living he will participate in a restorative program of daily exercises and nutritional support. He already has a do-not-resuscitate (DNR) order in place. You open a discussion with him and his daughter about considering a do-not-hospitalize (DNH) order (to be reviewed with any acute decline or injury that might provoke a hospital stay); they both agree to the DNH. ■

CASE 1

Discussion

Identifying Mr. Mills as frail and vulnerable has changed the course of his care substantially. He is no longer on the cancer drugs, disease-modifying drugs that are not likely to contribute to his immediate welfare but could be contributing to his decline. Warfarin, a high-risk drug that could lead to major immediate harm out of proportion to its short- and long-term benefit, has been stopped. He is receiving significantly more support with decisions and daily activities. He will now be less likely to end up in the hospital, a very high risk environment for frail, confused, and vulnerable aged patients. ■

TRANSITIONS TO FRAILTY

Clinically, frailty is a progressive dynamic process involving change over time, where individuals often transition from independence to focused assisted care, to more structured general care and finally into palliative care and hospice.[22]

Although many frail patients have chronic medical problems and may have disability when frailty is recognized, the Cardiovascular Health Study related that 63% of frail patients had no activities of daily living impairment and 32% had no or only one other common long-term disease.[5] The association of frailty with adverse outcomes seems to be independent of the presence of other medical conditions.

This has led to the concept of primary frailty, in which frailty occurs in the absence of significant overt disease, in contrast to secondary frailty, which is associated with known advanced disease. Individuals with secondary frailty may have a worse prognosis than those with primary frailty. This has been suggested by a study in which patients with diabetes, cancer, heart failure, and lung disease had worse 4-year survival independent of features such as low weight and decreased walking.[23]

> **Frailty is dynamic and changes over time, often leading to predictable outcomes.**

As individuals transition into frailty, the most common outcomes are institutionalization, debility, and death.[6] There is also increasing evidence linking frailty with falls, overprescribing of medications, and poor clinical outcomes of otherwise benign medical procedures.[24]

CASE 2

Lisa McDaniel (Part 1)

Lisa McDaniel is 89 years old, married, and was living with her husband at home until she suffered the latest of several recent falls. In that fall she suffered wrist and rib fractures, contusions, and skin tears. She has a several-year history of slow cognitive decline and a 1-year history of progressing stiffness, slowness, gait instability, and weight loss. Her 91-year-old husband, a retired college professor, has been her only caregiver. Her two children and grandchildren live on both coasts and do not often visit. Her family physician of many years retired last year and Mrs. McDaniel's husband is not fond of the young doctor who has replaced him. As a result, she has not visited the doctor for almost a year. Based on her long-standing dementia, her recent decline, and evident advanced frailty, the hospitalist and social worker brought up the suggestion to Professor McDaniel that Mrs. McDaniel be admitted to hospice, which he accepted.

You agree to care for Mrs. McDaniel in the nursing home after her four days of hospital care. The problem list you put together from the hospital records, Professor McDaniel's report, and her medication list includes:

- Dementia, diagnosed as Alzheimer's disease (treated with donepezil and memantine).
- Hyperlipidemia (treated with atorvastatin)
- Long-standing hypertension (treated with an angiotensin-converting-enzyme [ACE] inhibitor)
- Normocytic anemia (treated with iron)
- Osteoporosis (treated with calcium and vitamin D)
- Gait disorder and frequent falls, with four falls in the month before the hospital stay. Other falls have been associated with hip fractures and vertebral compression fractures. She used a walker intermittently before her recent fall.
- Malnutrition with a body mass index of 16 (treated with a multivitamin)

In the examination you find that her blood pressure is 110/60 mmHg and drops with standing. She is slow to respond to simple questions, but can do so given enough

time. She is very slow in eating, a process made more difficult by a large-amplitude tremor, noted at rest but particularly troubling when she tries to eat or drink. She has an expressionless face and diffusely increased muscle tone. Based on your examination the problem list now includes:

- Parkinson's disease
- Sarcopenia with major diffuse muscle loss
- Bilateral very dense cataracts
- High need for assistance in care for basic activities of daily living

1. **Does Mrs. McDaniel fit the picture of the "frail aged," and if so in what ways?**
2. **Considering your case review and exam, are you satisfied with the choice of hospice care for Mrs. McDaniel?**
3. **What other path of care might be productive for Mrs. McDaniel?** ■

TREATMENT OPTIONS FOR FRAILTY

Because frailty among older persons is a dynamic process, and is characterized by fluctuating losses of various reserves in multiple systems over time, there may be ample opportunity for prevention and remediation of frailty.[25] With timely recognition of prefrail and frail states, interventions and modifications may be made at many stages along this continuous process.[26,27]

As in Mr. Mills's case, the initial goal of treatment is optimal management of any underlying medical illnesses that may be contributing to frailty. The next goal is to intervene in areas that define frailty, including unintentional weight loss, exhaustion, weak grip strength, slow walking speed, low physical activity, cognition, mood, and pain. Nutritional education or supplements, exercise, and adequate therapy for depression and pain are all appropriate.

One of the most important goals is the prevention of muscle loss or sarcopenia, because it is a major cause of disability and frailty in older patients.[28] It is well accepted that exercise is beneficial along the entire spectrum of life, including the most aged and frail subsets.[29] A classic trial performed on nursing home patients with a mean average age of 87 years demonstrated that a high-intensity, progressive regimen of resistance exercise training improves muscle strength and size in frail people.[30] These changes were accompanied by improvement in mobility, strength, and physical activity. Even lower-level resistance training programs where older patients participated only two times per week demonstrated a lower progression of physical functional limitations.[31]

Early recognition and intervention are extremely beneficial if frailty is to be reversed.[32] The longer an individual is allowed to be in the frail state, the harder transition back out of frailty seems to be. Although transition to states of greater frailty seems to be more common in the already frail patient, transitions back out of frailty have been reported.[25]

Some interventions have been proven not to be beneficial. For example, increased caloric intake without any type of exercise program does not seem to improve function. Hormone replacement with testosterone and growth hormone has not shown significant benefits.[33]

The concept of frailty fits well into the philosophy of comprehensive, patient-centered, holistic medical care, integrating health and social care. Frailty provides a conceptual basis for not focusing exclusively on organ systems and disease, but on the complete patient. The concept of frailty aids in clinical decision making to assess risk factors and complication, to evaluate interventions for the individual unique patient, and to predict outcomes. It is a much better measure than chronologic age.[34]

> Close attention to detail in the older adult patient, can lead to interventions to delay, prevent, or possibly treat frailty.

Treatment and prevention of frailty will be enhanced by the development of a more formal, simple, clinical assessment tool. The concept of frailty in relationship to management of complex systems that are close to failure is growing in importance, and can be employed by the primary care practitioner to achieve better clinical care for frail older adults.

CASE 2

Lisa McDaniel (Part 2)

Mrs. McDaniel is very weak, easily fatigued, inactive, very slow, and emaciated. She also has a significant burden of impairing diseases. She would fit both Fried's and Rockwood's models of frailty. However, as her new physician, you have found a major unaddressed problem that could account for a significant portion of her progressing frailty: the Parkinson's disease. It is likely a major contributor to her gait problems and falls. Because of her slow eating and likely-to-progress swallowing problems, the Parkinson's is probably contributing to her weight loss. Because of her slow responses to questions, she may be considered more demented than she is. Moreover, in the last year, as her weight has dramatically declined, her blood pressure and lipid medications have not been reevaluated, and may be inappropriate now. Moreover, the donepezil and memantine should be reevaluated, especially because the former can be associated with anorexia. Mrs. McDaniel is taken off

hospice and placed on a Medicare A physical and occupational rehabilitation program. Her Parkinson's disease is treated with carbidopa/levodopa. She receives a swallow study. She receives assisted feeding, and food consistencies are adjusted based on the swallow study. Her medication list is dramatically reduced by eliminating the ACE inhibitor, the statin, the iron, and the dementia medications (the latter in a tapering fashion).

1. **What are your clinical expectations for Mrs. McDaniel?**
2. **When Mrs. McDaniel entered the nursing home, she had DNR and DNH status as part of hospice care. Should these be changed?**
3. **Does it make sense to address the dense bilateral cataracts?** ◉

After 2 months Mrs. McDaniel is feeding herself effectively. Her body mass index has moved up from 16 to 18. She is quicker to respond to others, and smiles during social interactions. She is able to engage in somewhat more complex discussions. She is back walking with a walker with assistance and has had no further falls. Her stiffness and tremor are much improved. Her interactions with her husband are much more rewarding for him. However, he and the care staff concur that the DNR and DNH will remain in place. An ophthalmology consult is scheduled to review the possibility of removing her cataracts, with the goal of possibly improving her quality of life and reducing her fall risk. Mrs. McDaniel remains frail, but she is not now on an accelerating course of decline. Identifying and addressing several reversible issues, particularly the high-impact Parkinson's disease, has served to reduce her frailty and vulnerability.

CASE 2

Discussion

Not all frailty is progressive and irreversible. When working with a frail aged patient, the clinician is responsible for identifying silent or undiagnosed diseases and deficiencies that may be playing a major reversible role in inducing or amplifying frailty. Moreover, the aged patient with progressive frailty may be on medications that are no longer, or never were, appropriate, and are contributing to the problem. Identifying a patient as frail does not mean "no further investigations or interventions."[35] ◉

FALLS AND FRAILTY

Walking upright in humans (bipedal ambulation) is of special importance because it requires higher order functions—a coordinated, integrated, and precise interaction among many components of a multifaceted system. Therefore, it is not surprising that there is increasing evidence linking frailty to falls when physical and cognitive deficits and loss of redundancy develop in this complex system.[25] The frailty concept explains why falls are not typically the result of a single cause, but rather the accumulation of many small deficiencies, each of which may be harmless on its own.

Falling in frail older people, then, should be recognized as an overall indicator of failure in the complex mobility system, rather than a specific disorder of a particular organ system. The same insult that can cause a fall in a frail patient will be compensated for in another system in the robust individual, where redundancy in the system has not been lost.

This understanding in the frail individual has great clinical significance when dealing with falls. Falls in the frail patient need to be seen as a complex system failure. Spending time and resources searching for the single cause of the fall is most likely futile, because a single cause does not exist.[8] Rather, if frailty is recognized as a failure of a multifaceted system, that concept provides a framework of understanding falls in the frail elderly (see Chapter 20).

THE ROLE OF PALLIATIVE CARE AND HOSPICE IN FRAILTY

Even though frailty may lend itself to a variety of medical interventions, the relationship between frailty and death has been well established.[36] Frailty has been found to be the most common condition leading to death in community-dwelling older people. Therefore it is important to recognize increasing frailty in clinical practice and the importance of advanced care planning, physician-patient communication about end-of-life issues, and appropriate and timely hospice referral.[37]

As frailty progresses and becomes severe, and potentially treatable underlying conditions have been reasonably eliminated, palliative care options become important. A multidisciplinary team-based approach to palliative care may enhance quality of life.

> With progressive frailty, death is a certain eventual outcome. Principles of palliative medicine and hospice should be applied early on before the patient is too sick to make appropriate end-of-life decisions.

Trajectories of decline and death at the end-of-life are variable, and the medical profession is not good at predicting life expectancy—even in the frail patient.[38,39] In the older frail population, death often follows a long progressive decline. Good end-of-life care must allow for the unpredictable timing of death. Goals change. The majority of older frail people have accepted death and are not afraid of it. However, they are fearful of pain and loss of dignity. Therefore, timely symptom-driven palliative care or hospice ensures that patients and families receive care that will optimize quality of life and relieve suffering.

When advanced frailty is recognized, frank communications with patients and their families may be as important as any other medical intervention. In addition to advance directives, it may be helpful to include topics such as limit setting or harm-reduction strategies in the discussions.[40,41] For example, statements such as these may be appropriate: "We want to help you live as long and as comfortably as possible, but in our opinion cardiopulmonary resuscitation would only harm you, and we recommend setting that as a limit."

The goal is not to take away a patient's hope, but to offer hope that is realistic. This allows the patient and family to plan realistically and to avoid the sudden "letdown" or "betrayal" from the medical profession that is sometimes felt when overly optimistic pictures are portrayed. "Hope but prepare" is always a good strategy (Figure 29-1): "Hope for the best; take care of the present; and prepare for the worst!"

CULTURAL CONSIDERATIONS

The baby-boomer generation that is just now beginning to impact geriatric medicine will usher in the most ethnically diverse population in the history of the United States. There is early evidence that frailty may occur at different rates in various ethnic groups.[42]

Cultural practices come to the forefront in certain seasons of life—births, weddings, and funerals. Frailty is viewed differently by different ethnic groups and the health care provider must remember that the patient and his or her family may not conceive of medical care in Western terms. For example, in some cultures the frail adult will be cared for at home by the

---

HOPE BUT PREPARE

- "Let's hope for the best"
  - Hope the medical options will work
  - Hope you get a miracle

- Attend to the present
  - Control pain and symptoms
  - Maximize 'quality of life'
  - Enroll in hospice

- And prepare for the worst!"
  - Advanced directive
  - Unfinished business

Figure 29-1 "Hope but prepare" is always a good strategy.

family—a nursing home is never a consideration. Preferences for disclosure of serious clinical findings may be different. Many cultures prefer that "bad news" discussions involve the children and not the elderly individual—the children are to do the worrying and decision making for the frail patient.

Western culture emphasizes direct communication— "Shall we leave your mother on the respirator, or pull the plug?" That would be extremely rude in most other cultures where indirect communication is preferred—"I had a patient with similar circumstances and this is what we did!"

Certainly practitioners cannot learn everything about all the various cultures and subcultures, but they can let the patient and family be their teachers. "I know different cultures have different ways of dealing with the problems of old age; please help me understand how you see things." Then listen.

> Health care providers cannot know everything about all cultures; however, they can ask the right questions and let the culturally diverse patients be their teachers.

It therefore behooves the wise practitioner to determine early on in the care of patients that are transitioning into frailty what their wishes will be. Be clear on such things as whether an interpreter will be needed, who the decision makers will be, and what the patient's or family's preferences in aggressive end-of-life care will be.

In many areas the term *AND* (allow natural death) is replacing *DNR*.[43] DNR has a negative connotation— "Do not do things!" AND, on the other hand, is more positive—"We should do all we can to make this person comfortable!"

PRESCRIBING FOR THE FRAIL PATIENT

Although frailty is not synonymous with either comorbidities or chronic disease, many frail older people have multiple chronic diseases and functional impairment and are prescribed long lists of medications.[8] However, older frail patients are routinely excluded from any drug trials.[44] Use of medications in frail patients is therefore generally based on evidence extrapolated from more robust patient groups with a lot fewer physiologic deficits and much stronger reserves.

Frailty is associated with altered pharmacokinetics that affects the bioavailability of medications. In frail patients there is an increase in body fat as compared to lean body mass, which affects the distribution of drugs. Low albumin levels in the frail patient reduce drug binding and the activity of enzymes responsible

for drug metabolism. It is not surprising that the risk of adverse drug reactions increases with increasing patient frailty. Studies have shown adverse drug reactions to be as high as 20% of older people living in the community,[45] up to 33% of hospitalized patients, and 50% of those in long-term care.[46] The frail patient tolerates adverse drug reactions less than a more robust individual with overlapping reserves.

The goal of prescribing should be kept well in mind when prescribing medications for the frail patient— the improvement in quality of life through symptom control.[47] However, the goal of secondary prevention may not apply to all frail patients, who statistically may not survive long enough to see any benefit. For example, the risk of adverse drug reactions in the frail patient may exceed the intended benefit from long-term goals; this is sometimes true in the case of statins or bisphosphonates.[48,49] The notion of "time until benefit" becomes very useful to the clinician in decision making for the frail elderly.[50]

> Medications are tested one at a time in healthy individuals—their effects in frail patients are only extrapolations. Stopping medications should always be a viable clinical consideration.

Stopping medications, even though that idea runs contrary to the expectations of physicians and patients, as in Mr. Mills, may be desirable. There is little research on the best clinical approach to stopping medications, but common geriatric wisdom supports a gradual dose taper rather than abrupt discontinuation.[51] It is reassuring, however, that available studies to this point have found very few adverse drug consequences from stopping medications in the frail elderly. Most medications are safe to withdraw, and withdrawing medications in the frail patient may make the patients better.[52]

COORDINATION OF CARE

Routine office visits, hospital stays, and even nursing home stays do not seem to fulfill the personal and practical needs of patients who are frail and experiencing multisystem failure. Extended measures such as provider home visits, home health services, and comprehensive care programs such as PACE (Program of All-Inclusive Care for the Elderly) are attempts to fill this void.[8]

In the frail patient, the coordination of services for management of cognitive, physical, and psychosocial conditions and functions is invaluable. There is evidence that the use of such services for ongoing care can actually reduce decline in physical function and decrease the necessity of nursing home placement for vulnerable older adults.[53]

Medications, which are more likely to have adverse reactions in the frail patient, are often inappropriately prescribed, misused, and inadequately monitored during transitions between care settings.[54] To avoid such problems, pharmacy and geriatric consultants may provide decision support to the primary care clinician. Electronic medical records databases may also help to eliminate some of these problems in the future.

Continuity of care is also important in the frail vulnerable patient to prevent the danger of iatrogenic harm. A personal knowledge of the patient can be invaluable in preventing unnecessary hospitalizations, unwanted diagnostic procedures, duplication of tests and procedures, and medication hazards. Knowing the patient's goals is important in advising about advance directives or AND orders. On the patient side, continuity allows the avoidance of unfamiliar clinicians and hospitals, which can be extremely agitating to someone with already diminished cognitive skills.

SUMMARY

Although there is not yet a clear consensus regarding the definition of frailty, the concept of frailty continues to grow in importance. There is good evidence that if we do not succumb to other pathologies first, frailty will eventually affect us all, making us medically vulnerable. Clinicians need a better understanding of the health and functional status of older persons in order to make better informed treatment and prognostic decisions. By recognizing frailty, health care providers can identify older persons at elevated risk for numerous adverse outcomes. In addition, perhaps some treatment, prevention, or at least delay in the onset of late life frailty and adverse consequences can be undertaken.

Currently, work is being done to develop an operational definition of frailty that is simple enough to be used clinically to guide prevention and care. In a health care system that is increasingly dependent on guidelines, screening tools, and evidence-based protocols, a precise, dependable clinical definition of frailty can only improve the clinical management of the older patient.

KEY REFERENCES

1. De Lepeleire J, Iliffe S, Mann E, et al. Frailty: An emerging concept for general practice. British J of General Practice 2009;59(562):177-81.
3. Lacas A, Rockwood K. Frailty in primary care: A review of its conceptualization and implications for practice. BMC Med 2012;10:4.
5. Fried LP, Ferrucci L, Darer J, et al. Untangling the concepts of disability, frailty, and comorbidity: Implications to improved targeting and care. J Gerontol A Biol Sci Med Sci 2004;59:255-63.
6. Sternberg SA, Schwartz AW, Karunananthan S, et al. The identification of frailty: A systematic literature review. J Am Geriatr Soc 2011;59:2129-38.
18. Bergman H, Ferrucci L, Guralnik J, et al. Frailty: An emerging research and clinical paradigm—issues and controversies. J Gerontol A Biol Sci Med Sci 2007;62(7):731-7.
26. Van Kan G, Rolland Y, Bergman H, et al. The JANA Task Force on frailty assessment of older people in clinical practice. J Nutr Health Aging 2008;12:29-37.

References available online at expertconsult.com.

30

Pressure Ulcers

Aimée D. Garcia and E. Foy White-Chu

OBJECTIVES

*Upon completion of this chapter, the reader
will be able to:*

- Define the stages of pressure ulcers.
- Identify the risk factors that place a patient
  at risk for pressure ulcer development.
- Recognize and implement appropriate
  pressure redistribution strategies for the
  prevention of pressure ulcers.
- Develop and implement a care plan for
  pressure ulcer management.

CASE 1

Kevin Maloney (Part 1)

Kevin Maloney, an 89-year-old man, comes to the emergency room with altered mental status. He lives alone in his own home and his children check on him daily. The daughter

---

Additional online-only material indicated by icon.

reports that he has become incontinent over the last few days and that she found many wet undergarments throughout the house. When she went to see him today, she found him confused and lying on the floor in his room. She saw no evidence of trauma, and the patient stated he "was tired and lay down on the floor." She is not sure how long he was there. On evaluation, the patient is oriented to name only. His vital signs are as follows: temperature 99.1° F, blood pressure 125/82, respiration rate 18, pulse 82.

On physical examination, Mr. Maloney is found to have skin breakdown on the left buttock. The wound measures 6 cm × 5 cm × 0.1 cm. The wound bed is in the dermis and is pink without necrotic tissue visible. It appears to have minimal serous drainage, and no odor.

1. **What stage would you document for Mr. Maloney's skin ulcer?**

2. **What treatment recommendations would you make, and why?** ▣

CASE 2

Meryl Curry (Part 1)

You are seeing Meryl Curry, a 75-year-old woman who resides in an assisted living facility, for an initial evaluation. She has diabetes, hypertension, chronic obstructive pulmonary disease (COPD), and a history of a stroke with left-sided hemiparesis. She is on 2 L per minute of home oxygen for the COPD. She is incontinent of bladder and wears protective undergarments. She is continent of bowel and is able to toilet herself. Mrs. Curry recently lost her husband and has been depressed. She does not like to leave her apartment and sits in an easy chair most of the day. Since the loss of her husband, her appetite has diminished. The patient has had two admissions in the past 6 months for COPD exacerbation. She is a thin, frail-appearing woman with a flat affect.

On physical examination, the patient has very pronounced bony prominences. She is found to have skin breakdown on the sacral/buttocks area measuring 8 cm × 9 cm which is covered with 100% necrotic tissue. There is erythema surrounding the site and foul-smelling drainage.

1. **What stage would you document for Mrs. Curry's skin ulcer?**

2. **What treatment recommendations would you make, and why?** ▣

EPIDEMIOLOGY AND DIFFERENTIAL DIAGNOSIS

With an aging population and a trend to provide more health care services in the home, primary care providers find themselves increasingly providing care for patients with pressure ulcers. Incidence rates of pressure ulcers vary widely. In previous studies, pressure ulcers were noted to occur most frequently in acute care settings, with incidence rates as high as 38% in older persons. Efforts have reduced these rates considerably—in the past 10 years hospital incidence rates among older persons have dropped to between 2.8% and 9%. Long-term care and home care settings, in comparison, have incidences that range from 3.6% to 59% and 4.5% to 6.3% respectively.[1]

The primary care provider, when taking care of a patient with a pressure ulcer, must be mindful of the litigious nature surrounding this geriatric syndrome. Often these ulcers are seen by family and patients as a sign of neglect. Careful assessment, documentation, and multidisciplinary care planning are therefore important both to educate patients and to optimize healing and prevent litigation.[2]

Pressure ulcers are devastating to the patient and the health care system. The Centers for Medicare and Medicaid Services estimate that the cost per stay for hospitalized beneficiaries with a secondary diagnosis of pressure ulcer is $40,381.[3] Annual costs as high as $129,000 have been estimated for the treatment of stage IV pressure ulcers.[4] In the Netherlands, where the proportion of elderly persons in the population equals that projected for the United States in 25 to 30 years, one report identified pressure ulcers as that country's most costly condition, surpassing cancer and cardiovascular disease.[5]

As of October 2008, the Centers for Medicare and Medicaid Services have stopped reimbursing acute care facilities for treatment of pressure ulcers that developed in-house. In 2011 the National Quality Forum considered recommending an expansion of this legislation to include post-acute and long-term care.[6] This legislation was based on the belief that pressure ulcers are largely preventable. Although these efforts to improve quality are to be applauded, it continues to be unclear how this decision will impact pressure ulcer prevention and treatment.

Pressure ulcers develop when pressure forces exceed capillary blood flow, causing ischemia, and subsequent tissue necrosis occurs. This most readily happens over bony prominences such as the coccyx, sacrum, heels, hips, and elbows. Depending on the overall health and mobility of the patient, and on the hardness of the surface on which the patient is sitting or lying, tissue ischemia and necrosis can occur in as little time as 2 hours. Pressure ulcers can also occur wherever skin is damaged by excessive friction or shear and moisture. Pressure ulcers are the only wound type that should be staged (i.e., venous leg ulcers and other wound types are not staged).

> **When an open ulcer is seen on a geriatric patient, the clinician needs to consider not just pressure ulcer but other potential sources of skin breakdown.**

When an open ulcer is seen on a geriatric patient, pressure ulcer should be at the top of the differential diagnosis. However, there are other causes of skin breakdown, including moisture-associated skin damage, an open abscess, comorbid illness, and malignancy. Table 30-1 reviews the differential diagnoses of ulcerations that are commonly misdiagnosed as pressure ulcers. Of these, several merit note:

- Moisture associated skin damage (MASD) and abrasions are the most common misdiagnosis. Although MASD and friction put the patient at risk of pressure ulcers, a discrete ulceration needs to form to delineate pressure ulcer from these conditions.[7]
- A diabetic foot or arterial foot ulcer can be difficult to distinguish from a pressure ulcer; however, it is important therapeutically to determine the primary underlying cause. In the case of a diabetic foot ulcer, this would be neuropathy. For an arterial foot ulcer, the cause would be poor arterial flow, with weak or absent pulses a corroborating sign.
- Skin changes at life's end—also known as skin failure—is another increasingly recognized syndrome.[8] Thus far it has been challenging to diagnose this condition as distinct from pressure ulcers.

The National Pressure Ulcer Advisory Panel states that some pressure ulcers are unavoidable. The panel also recognizes pressure ulcers as being separate from skin failure, but that the two diagnoses can coexist. For patients who have an illness that has caused poor tissue perfusion and thus low tissue tolerance to any pressure, the provider should consider documenting the pressure ulcer as "unavoidable" and that skin failure may be occurring.[9]

RISK FACTORS AND PREVENTION

> **Prevention efforts in every care setting should be used to limit the development of pressure ulcers.**

Aggressive, 24-hour-a-day prevention efforts in every care setting are critical to limit the development of pressure ulcers. The first step is to be aware of the factors that place patients at high risk. Risk factors are numerous and can be separated between intrinsic and extrinsic risk factors (Table 30-2).

- *Intrinsic factors* are those that alter skin integrity. They include limited mobility; medical comorbidities such as diabetes, chronic obstructive pulmonary disease, congestive heart failure or other medical conditions affecting

TABLE 30-1	Differential Diagnosis of Pressure Ulcers	
Diagnosis	**Typical Location**	**Characteristics**
Moisture-associated skin damage (also known as incontinence-associated dermatitis)	Perineum—sacrum, coccyx, gluteal folds, groin folds	Moisture must be present Indistinct edges No necrosis Typically diffuse superficial excoriation, possible fungal appearance
Old pilonidal cyst excision	Gluteal cleft—inferior to coccyx	There is a history of pilonidal cyst excision or a scar is visible
Diabetic foot ulcer	Heel, plantar surface, toes	Neuropathy must be present
Arterial insufficiency–related foot ulcer	Heel, toes	Nonpalpable pulses
Venous insufficiency–related ulcer	On the lower extremity below the knee	Superficial ulcerations with ragged edges Associated hemosiderin deposition noted on extremity
Edema/blisters	Anywhere on the body	Superficial ulcerations Tend to be clean Usually round
Abrasion/friction	Anywhere on body	Skin flap present or abraded/excoriated skin surface
Malignancy	Anywhere on body	Will not heal despite offloading and local wound care
Herpes simplex or zoster	Anywhere on body	Both simplex and zoster have punched out appearance Tend to start out as blister or painful lesions Zoster is dermatomal
Abscess	Anywhere on body	Starts as blister or localized swelling that will drain on its own

perfusion and oxygenation, malignancy, and renal dysfunction; poor nutrition; and aging skin changes.

- *Extrinsic factors* are those factors that affect tissue tolerance. They include pressure, friction, shear, and moisture.

Clinical Tools to Estimate Pressure Ulcer Risk

For pressure ulcers, there are two validated and widely used risk assessment tools: the Braden scale and the Norton scale.[10] Neither has undergone randomized trials to look at their impact on pressure ulcer incidence.[11] Risk assessment should be done on a regular basis and whenever the patient's condition changes, and the score provided by the tool should be considered supplemental to clinical judgment.

The Braden scale has six domains: sensory perception, moisture, activity, mobility, nutrition, and friction/shear. The first five domains are rated on a scale from 1 to 4, with 1 being worst and 4 being best; friction/shear is rated from 1 (problematic) to 3 (not a problem). The maximum score is 23. Typically, patients are considered at risk of pressure ulcer development if their Braden score is 18 or lower. Therefore, scores at or below 18 should trigger nursing and other support staff to put in place more aggressive preventive measures, such as frequent

turning, a specialized mattress, and perhaps a nutrition consult.

The other tool that is often used to assess pressure sore risk is the Norton scale. This uses a 1-to-4 scoring system in rating five domains: physical condition, mental condition, activity, mobility, and incontinence. A score of less than 14 usually indicates a high risk of pressure ulcer development. The Norton scale tends to identify more patients at high risk than the Braden scale.[12]

For both of these tools, individual item scores are important in planning care. For instance, a patient may score high in nutrition and have no sensory impairments but also be very immobile with poor activity and friction/shear forces at work. By looking at the items that engender risk, the provider can target interventions to the most important risk factors for that individual patient. However, when a patient "rules in," every risk factor identified by the Braden or Norton scale should have an action plan prepared and implemented.

Preventive Measures

Seventy percent of pressure ulcers occur from the waist down. The main areas to examine when considering a patient's potential for skin breakdown are the sacrum, the trochanters, and the heels. If the patient is often in a seated position, the coccyx and ischial tuberosities become a site for greater risk of breakdown.

TABLE 30-2	Risk Factors for Pressure Ulcers	
	Factor	**Examples**
Intrinsic Factors (factors within the body)	Limited immobility	Delirium Sepsis/critical illness End-stage dementia CVA with hemiplegia Para/Quadriplegia Severe osteoarthrosis Spinal stenosis
	Sensory loss that reduces signaling to brain to reposition oneself	Hemi/Para/Quadriplegia Diabetes mellitus with neuropathy
	Comorbid illness that reduces tissue oxygenation or immune response to injury	Diabetes mellitus Coronary artery disease Congestive heart failure Peripheral arterial disease Chronic obstructive pulmonary disease Chronic kidney disease stage IV/ESRD with dialysis Autoimmune disease Malignancy Urinary or fecal incontinence
	Body type	Underweight or obese Older age
Extrinsic Factors (factors in the immediate environment that affect the body)	Pressure	Standard mattress Wheelchair that is too small or too large Wheelchair seating
	Friction and shear forces	Rubbing heels in bed Drag with repositioning Aggressive hygiene cleansing Head of bed greater than 30 degrees (body slides down in bed) Reclining a wheelchair
	Moisture	Incontinence Diaphoresis caused by pyrexia, autonomic instability, or ambient temperature
Both Intrinsic and Extrinsic	Inadequate nutrition	Hypercatabolic state (malignancy, infection, critical illness) Low protein
	Supplemental nutrition	Patients on total parental nutrition (TPN) or gastrointestinal tube feeds

CVA, Cerebrovascular accident; *ESRD*, end-stage renal disease.

Once at-risk patients are identified, the health care provider can effectively put preventive interventions into practice. These include the following:

- *Maximizing treatment of the patient's medical conditions.* This is the first step. All medical conditions that could affect healing and skin integrity should be optimized. The provider and patient should make every effort to optimize diabetes control (for older adults a HbA1c of 7% is adequate), blood pressure, and respiratory status. A review of medications may find ones that cause easy bruising or skin tears, such as warfarin or prednisone. If so, the provider should inquire as to whether they can be stopped, in consultation with the patient and other providers, and in consideration of the goals of care.

- *Nutrition consultation.* This should be considered early in the course of prevention, especially if there is concern that the patient's nutritional level is compromised. A systematic review found that many randomized controlled trials were poorly designed when addressing nutritional supplementation as a preventive measure for pressure ulcers. The review concluded that a nutrition consultation is reasonable for patients at risk.[13]

- *Frequent repositioning.* If the individual is bedbound or chairbound, the patient and his or her caregivers should be educated about effective offloading strategies. While in the bed, the patient should be turned and repositioned every 2 to 4 hours. A patient who spends most of the day in a wheelchair, recliner, or gerichair needs to be repositioned every hour. This can be easily done by reclining the chair, tilting the legs, or simply having the patient stand for about 30 seconds and then sit back down again.[14] Despite the lack of high-quality randomized controlled trials to support frequent repositioning, it is still considered a standard of care. The exception would be a dying patient who has significant discomfort with frequent repositioning; that person should be kept comfortable even at the expense of skin integrity.

- *Management of incontinence.* Urinary, and especially fecal, incontinence alters the pH balance of the skin surface, thereby increasing the risk of breakdown and pressure ulcer formation. Incontinence is best managed through toileting programs and, if needed, containment systems.

Pressure Redistribution Systems

Pressure redistribution surfaces are a mainstay of prevention and treatment for pressure ulcers. Unfortunately, insurance plans will pay for these devices only when a pressure ulcer is present. Many hospitals and health care facilities have purchased pressure redistribution surfaces on their own as part of their prevention protocols, however, in spite of the lack of insurance coverage.

> Despite the use of a pressure redistribution system, patients will still need to be turned and repositioned if they cannot do so themselves.

There are numerous different surfaces, ranging from gel mattress and overlays to low-air-loss and air-fluidized mattress systems. Clinicians will need to become familiar with the types of mattresses and features available within their health care system or refer the patient to a wound care specialist to obtain the appropriate device. Only a few high-quality randomized controlled trials have been done, however, and the question remains unanswered as to whether powered versus nonpowered mattresses are best for prevention or treatment.[13,15]

The other element of pressure redistribution is seating cushions, because patients who spend many hours in a wheelchair, gerichair, Broda chair, or a regular chair at home are at risk for skin breakdown. The provider needs to take a thorough history and ask about decreasing mobility, especially in older patients with worsening musculoskeletal disorders, cardiac/pulmonary disorders, or dementia. The patient should have a cushion to prevent skin breakdown at the coccyx and ischial tuberosities. Again, there are many varieties of pressure redistribution cushions, and referral to a physical therapist or physiatrist for determination of the most appropriate type is warranted.

EVALUATION, STAGING, AND DOCUMENTATION OF PRESSURE ULCERS

Assessment and Documentation

There are a multitude of assessment frameworks available for wounds in general and pressure ulcers in particular. Prior to assessing the ulcer, the provider must thoroughly cleanse the wound of any excess drainage or wound care product. The key components to each assessment and documentation should include the following:

- Measurement—There are a variety of measurements techniques available. Budgetary constraints for the primary care provider may determine the choice. Regardless of the chosen device, there must be inter- and intra-rater reliability between the providers and nurses when measuring the progress of the ulcer.
- Appearance—Describe the wound location accurately. Location can be key to what is causing the pressure. For instance, sitting tends to cause ischial and coccyx pressure ulcers, whereas lying down causes heel and sacrum pressure ulcers. Pressure ulcers on the earlobes tend to be from oxygen tubing or glasses. The provider should describe the borders (surrounding erythema or maceration) and the edge (well demarcated, or erosive/evolving, undermining). Undermining may be evidence of shear/friction forces. Describe the wound bed and percentage of presence of necrotic slough (wet, stringy tissue), necrotic eschar (dry yellow/brown/black tissue), or granulation tissue. Does the wound bed bleed easily, meaning it is friable? Is there scant, moderate, or heavy drainage, as evidenced by the dressing? What color is the drainage? And is there odor—this is an important patient concern that should be addressed, because odor and drainage may be indication for patient isolation.
- Photo documentation—This is becoming increasingly popular, and family members may also document wounds with cellular or other portable devices. If you choose to photograph pressure ulcers in your clinic or facility, consultation with nursing and risk management representatives is important to develop a policy regarding written consent (if considered necessary), record-keeping, and storage.[16]

When documenting the incidence of a pressure ulcer, the physician must also document whether the patient is in the midst of severe illness or has significant comorbidities that would reduce the tissue tolerance to any pressure.[17] Determining the exact cause of the pressure ulcer is important in formulating a care plan. If the cause cannot be reversed, then the wound will not heal.

> Patients' medical status will impact their risk for development of a wound, as well as their ability to heal.

In addition, the clinician should estimate if the underlying causal process is reversible. This is done by carefully reviewing the care plan in collaboration with the family and direct care providers. For example, if a patient with end-stage Alzheimer's disease has progressed to where he or she is no longer eating or drinking, then despite all repositioning efforts the skin may still break down. These wounds may not have the potential to heal, and this should be clearly stated to the family and documented. The primary goal should be one of comfort and infection prevention, if possible.

Staging

The most widely used staging system for pressure ulcers is the one created by the National Pressure Ulcer Advisory Panel (NPUAP).[14] The stages are based on the degree of tissue damage (Figure 30-1).

- Stage I—*Intact skin with nonblanchable redness of a localized area usually over a bony prominence.* The key to this definition is that the skin is intact. If there is any break in the surface of the skin, it is no longer stage I. A physical exam of high-risk patients must include a tactile assessment of the skin, because the stage I pressure ulcer may be tender and indurated. Special attention must be paid to dark-skinned individuals. In darker pigmented patients, the presence of nonblanchable erythema may not be as prominent, but the patient may have skin areas that are warmer, cooler, tender, firm, or boggy, indicating an area of stage I damage.
- **Stage II**—*Partial thickness loss of dermis presenting as a shallow open ulcer with a red pink wound bed, without slough. May also present as an intact or open/ruptured serum-filled blister.* A stage II skin ulcer is superficial, and the wound bed is clean. There is no necrotic tissue within the wound bed. If a blister is present, it is filled with clear fluid. If the blister is filled with blood, it is not a stage II. A wound is also not identified as a stage II if the site is a skin tear, tape burn, moisture-associated skin damage, or excoriation.

- **Stage III**—*Full thickness tissue loss. Subcutaneous fat may be visible but bone, tendon, or muscle is not exposed. Slough may be present but does not obscure the depth of tissue loss. May include undermining and tunneling.* The depth of a stage III pressure ulcer will vary by the anatomical location. On the nose or ankle, where there is little subcutaneous tissue, a stage III may be very shallow. In an area such as the buttock, a stage III may be very deep but still be in the subcutaneous tissue.
- **Stage IV**—*Full thickness tissue loss with exposed bone, tendon, or muscle. Slough or eschar may be present on some parts of the wound bed. Often includes tunneling and undermining.*
- **Suspected deep tissue injury**—Purple or maroon localized area of discolored intact skin or blood-filled blister resulting from damage of underlying soft tissue from pressure and/or shear. The key to this stage is "suspected." Sometimes with offloading these lesions will disappear. However, the provider must be aware that in the event that deep tissue injury has occurred, the wound will progress in a matter of days to weeks to full thickness (i.e., stage III or higher) tissue loss. The provider should prepare family and support staff of this possibility, emphasizing that although the damage may have been done, efforts regarding offloading and care for the individual can be put into place.
- **Unstageable**—*Full thickness tissue loss in which the base of the ulcer is covered by slough (yellow, tan, gray, green, or brown) and/or eschar (tan, brown, or black) in the wound bed.* The depth is unknown. This appearance often occurs after suspected deep tissue injury has evolved or if an ulcer has progressed in the setting of continued pressure, friction/shear, and moisture forces. Until the necrotic tissue is removed to expose the base of the wound, the depth cannot be determined.

An important aspect of pressure ulcer staging is that once a pressure ulcer is staged at a higher level of skin damage, the wound cannot then be backstaged. For example, if a wound is found to be involving muscle and tendon, it is a stage IV. If a month later, with good treatment, the wound is covered in granulation tissue, it is still a healing stage IV. Once closed, it is a healed stage IV.

Appropriate staging of the pressure ulcer is important, not only for care of the patient, but because reimbursement for many support surfaces and modalities is dependent on the staging of the ulcer. There is also the issue of litigation. Appropriate documentation of wounds is an important piece in preventing and defending lawsuits associated with pressure ulcers. Depending on the severity of the wound and whether infection is present, the wound can be reassessed every 2 to 4 weeks.

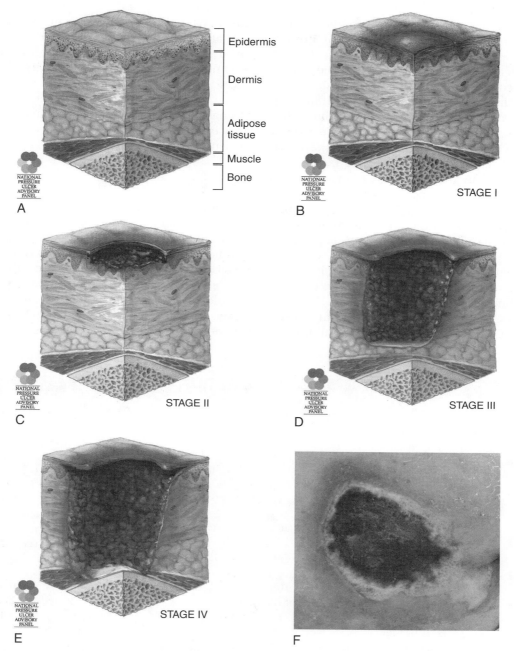

Figure 30-1 Staging of pressure ulcers. **A,** Normal skin, showing layers. **B,** Stage 1—redness without a break in the skin. **C,** Stage 2—superficial, confined to skin (can include dermis). **D,** Stage 3—penetrating into the subdermal tissues. **E,** Stage 4—down to the bone. **F,** Photograph of an unstageable ulcer—one whose base is covered by necrotic material. (Diagrams reproduced with permission of the National Pressure Ulcer Advisory Panel; photographs copyright Drs. Garcia and White-Chu.)

CASE 1

Discussion

In Mr. Maloney's case, the pressure ulcer would be a stage II ulcer. ▣

CASE 2

Discussion

In Mrs. Curry's case, the wound would be considered unstageable. ▣

TREATMENT STRATEGIES

For wounds where the underlying cause is reversible and thus healable, treatment strategies need to be put in place quickly and effectively that will promote healing and prevent further progress of skin damage. The cornerstones of pressure ulcer treatment are listed below. Note that what the physician does with the wound locally is not nearly as important as reversing underlying conditions that are causing or worsening the wound. These include, as has been noted previously, managing underlying medical conditions, optimizing nutrition, and controlling fecal and urinary incontinence.

As also noted previously, comorbid conditions such as uncontrolled diabetes mellitus, hypertension, congestive heart failure, malignancy, and inflammatory disorders will put greater demands on the body and affect the functioning of cell lines critical to wound healing. The clinician should therefore make every effort to optimize each condition. These factors also will have impact on the clinician's estimate of the wound's prognosis for healing.

Nutrition is critical. Many geriatric patients are nutritionally compromised for multiple reasons, including dentition, anorexia-inducing medications, depression, lack of access to tasty and nutritious food, or other underlying comorbidities. A nutrition consult, where available, should be done early in the course of treatment to maximize protein and fluid intake.

Management of incontinence is important to keep fecal and urinary contamination to a minimum. In an outpatient setting, a Foley catheter or fecal containment system is not optimal because of patient discomfort and risk of infection. However, if the health care team is unable to manage the incontinence and it is leading to skin breakdown, temporary use of these devices is sometimes needed. If the level of skin breakdown is advanced (stage III or higher), and the provider is unable to contain fecal contamination, consideration may need to be given to a diverting colostomy until the patient is healed.

Pressure Offloading

As previously stated, turning and repositioning of patients who cannot reposition themselves is essential for alleviating pressure. Small shifts in weight and use of positioning devices such as pillows can be very effective in offloading a bony prominence. The most appropriate pressure redistribution system(s) for the patient should be implemented promptly, taking into consideration comfort and cost (Table 30-3). It is important to note that despite the use of a pressure redistribution

TABLE 30-3	**Support Surface Recommendations for Pressure Ulcer Prevention and Treatment**			
Type	**Indications***	**How It Works**	**Cost**	**Level of Evidence****
Nonpowered specialized mattress or overlay (filled with gel, foam, or combination)	Prevention to stage II	Redistributes pressure at boney prominences	$-$$	Prevention—A (better than standard mattress) Treatment—Has not been studied against standard mattress
Low-air-loss mattress or overlay	Stage III or higher	Air sacs allow warmed air to pass through	$$$$	Prevention—B (no better than nonpowered specialized) Treatment—B (no better than nonpowered specialized overlay)
Alternating pressurized mattress	Stage III or higher	Alternates between high and low pressures, thus reducing time at high pressure	$$$$	Prevention—B (no better than nonpowered specialized) Treatment—A (no better than nonpowered specialized overlay)
Air-fluidized mattress	Stage III or higher	Silicone-coated beads liquefy when air passes through them	$$$$$	Prevention—B (no better than nonpowered specialized) Treatment—B (better when compared to alternating pressured mattress covered with foam)
Rotating bed	Critical illness	Bed rotates lateral for pulmonary toileting; not intended to replace turning and repositioning	$$$$$	Prevention—X (no better than standard hospital or ICU beds) Treatment—D (expert opinion)
Specialized wheelchair cushion (foam, gel, air, or combination)	Prevention to stage IV	Redistributes pressure at boney prominences	$-$$$	Prevention—A (if combination gel/foam) Treatment—D (expert opinion)

*The National Pressure Ulcer Advisory Panel guidelines and other guidelines do not recommend a particular support surface for a particular stage of pressure ulcer. The indications listed here are regarding typical use of these surfaces.
**A = supported by one or more high-quality randomized controlled trials (RCTs); B = supported by one or more high quality nonrandomized cohort studies or low-quality RCTs; C = supported by one or more case series and/or poor-quality cohort and/or case-control studies; D = supported by expert opinion and/or extrapolation from studies in other populations or settings; X = evidence supports the treatment being ineffective or harmful.

system, patients will still need to be turned and repositioned if they cannot do so themselves.

Debridement

Necrotic tissue in the wound must be debrided. This tissue contains a high bacterial load and can lead to further breakdown of the surrounding tissue. Debridement methods include mechanical debridement, sharp debridement, enzymatic debridement, biologic debridement, and autolytic debridement; Table 30-4 summarizes key aspects of each method. Conservative debridement, meaning debridement of only the necrotic tissue and not to the point of causing bleeding tissue, is indicated in almost every wound regardless of its potential to heal.

> Necrotic tissue in the wound must be debrided.

Depending on the clinical environment and the extent of tissue necrosis, referral to a surgeon may be necessary for debridement. Factors that may affect the need for surgical referral include the following: the physician's comfort level with debridement, the patient's pain level, the extent of necrosis, the underlying goals of care (i.e., cure vs. comfort care), the patient's ability to tolerate a surgical procedure, and use of anticoagulants.

Provision of Moist Wound Healing

Once the wound is cleared of necrotic tissue, the goal of therapy is to achieve moisture balance and moist wound healing. If the wound has a lot of drainage, a dressing should be chosen that absorbs drainage, such as an alginate or foam. If the wound bed is dry, a dressing such as a film, hydrocolloid, or hydrogel can be used. The choice of dressing is going to depend on the care setting and the wound characteristics. There are more than 1000 wound care products on the market. Collaborating with nursing staff can help the primary care provider to determine the best local wound care dressing.

Diagnosing and Managing Infection

Infection continues to be a challenge in the care of patients with open wounds. There are different levels of bacterial invasion into wounds, and the majority of wounds do not require the use of systemic antibiotics. The levels of bacteria in the wound can be classified as follows:

- *Colonization.* All wounds are colonized, because bacteria live on our skin and in the environment. Colonization describes a bacterial level that is not affecting wound healing. Topical antiseptics or antimicrobials can effectively decrease bacterial load in the wound bed. Systemic antibiotics are not indicated.
- *Superficial infection.* The bacteria are now at a concentration that is negatively impacting wound healing. The wound may appear clean but is not progressing toward healing. There may be increased drainage or odor. Aggressive local care (debridement and topical antimicrobials) is indicated. There are multiple dressings that can be used, including cadexomer iodine, Manuka honey, or ionized silver products. Dressings such

TABLE 30-4	Methods of Debridement for Geriatric Skin Ulcers		
Type of Debridement	**Examples**	**Advantages**	**Disadvantages**
Sharp debridement	• scalpel, scissor, curette	• Fast • Selective	• Requires expertise • Level of comfort of practitioner • Availability of equipment • Painful • Slower acting
Autolytic debridement	• Manuka honey • Hydrocolloid • Hydrogel • Film	• Painless • Does not require expertise	
Enzymatic debridement	• Collagenase	• Selective • Does not require expertise	• Slow acting • Availability • Cost
Mechanical debridement	• Wet-to-Dry • Pulsatile lavage • Whirlpool	• Easily accessible • Does not require expertise (except pulsatile lavage)	• Nonselective • Painful • Infection control problems can occur
Biologic debridement	• Maggot therapy	• Very selective	• "Ick" factor • Often unavailable

as Dakin's, clorpactin, or betadine can be used for a very short time to decrease bacterial load in the wound bed, but long-term use of these products can impair wound healing.

- *Cellulitis.* Bacteria have now invaded the soft tissue and are causing the classic signs and symptoms of soft tissue infection, which may include erythema, pain, increased drainage, odor, fever, or elevated white count. For these patients, systemic antibiotics plus aggressive topical treatment are indicated.

SUMMARY

Key points in pressure ulcer prevention and care include the following:

- Not every wound on an older adult is a pressure ulcer. Consider other diagnoses such as incontinence-associated dermatitis, friction/shear, or arterial ulcers.
- Seventy percent of pressure ulcers occur from the waist down. Always look at the sacrum, ischial tuberosities, hips, and heels.
- Sitting surfaces are often overlooked in pressure ulcer prevention. Patients who are up in a wheelchair or spend the majority of their day sitting are at risk for skin breakdown.
- Devices such as oxygen tubing and Foley catheters can lead to pressure ulcers over nonboney prominences.
- Nutrition is an important part of wound healing. Obtain a nutrition consult early in the treatment of a pressure ulcer to maximize the patient's ability to heal.
- Debridement of necrotic tissue is crucial for wound healing. Wet to dry dressings are a form of nonselective debridement, are painful, and

provide no antimicrobial balance; they are no longer the standard of care for pressure ulcer debridement or management.

- Remember that the "hole" is part of the "whole" patient, and that pressure ulcer prevention and treatment requires a comprehensive, interdisciplinary approach.

Web Resources

www.npuap.org. National Pressure Ulcer Advisory Panel website with photos, staging guide and pressure ulcer white papers, position statements, as well as a searchable database on pressure ulcer–related research.

http://aawconline.org/wp-content/uploads/2011/09/AAWCPU-Qwik-Ref-Final-23Sep11.pdf. Association for the Advancement of Wound Care's pressure ulcer prevention and treatment quick reference guide.

https://www.nursingquality.org/NDNQIPressureUlcerTraining/default.aspx. This National Database of Nursing Quality Indicators website has modules on pressure ulcer education. It was developed for nurses but is a great resource for all clinicians.

KEY REFERENCES

9. Black JM, Edsberg LE, Baharestani MM, et al. Pressure ulcers: Avoidable or unavoidable? Results of the National Pressure Ulcer Advisory Panel Consensus Conference. Ostomy Wound Manage 2011;52:24-37.

11. Moore ZE, Cowman S. Risk assessment tools for the prevention of pressure ulcers. Cochrane Database Syst Rev 2008;CD006471.

13. Reddy M, Gill S, Rochon P. Preventing pressure ulcers: A systematic review. JAMA 2006;974-84.

14. National Pressure Ulcer Advisory Panel and European Pressure Ulcer Advisory Panel. Prevention and treatment of pressure ulcers: Clinical practice guideline. Washington, DC: National Pressure Ulcer Advisory Panel; 2009.

15. McInnes E, Bell-Syer SEM, Dumville JC, et al. Support surfaces for pressure ulcer prevention. Cochrane Database Syst Rev 2008;4:CD001735. doi:10.1002/14651858.CD001735.pub3.

References available online at expertconsult.com.

31

Sleep Disorders

Jennifer L. Martin and Cathy A. Alessi

OBJECTIVES

Upon completion of this chapter, the reader will be able to:

- Recognize common causes of sleep problems in older people.
- Understand diagnostic testing and appropriate treatments for common sleep disorders in older people.
- Differentiate between sleep complaints that can be managed in primary care versus those requiring referral to a sleep specialist.

Additional online-only material indicated by icon.

Jonathan Chen (Part 1)

Jonathan Chen, a 72-year-old retired, Asian-American engineer, comes to your office for a routine visit. Near the end of his appointment, with prompting from his wife, he states that he is "up all night" and asks you for "something to help me sleep." He is clearly concerned about his inability to sleep. He reports having sleep problems since his retirement 3 years ago, and notes spending much of his daytime "resting" in order to "catch up on sleep," which limits the couple's social activities.

> **How common are sleep problems in older adults and to what extent do they affect the well-being of older people such as Mr. Chen?**

Charles Banker (Part 1)

Charles Banker, a 79-year-old African-American man, arrives 1 hour late for his first appointment in your office, and apologetically explains he fell asleep at home. He reports falling asleep during conversations and card games with friends. He is a retired security guard, and he was fired from a job several years ago for "falling asleep on the job." He sees a psychiatrist, who is treating him for depression. Mr. Banker wonders whether there is an "energy pill" that will help him stay awake during the day.

> **What are the potential causes of Mr. Banker's sleepiness?**

PREVALENCE AND IMPACT

Sleep is an essential biological process, and sleep deprivation leads to neurologic, autonomic, and biochemical changes. Older people generally report more nighttime awakenings and more daytime sleeping than younger people. The primary care provider needs to understand common underlying causes of sleep problems, appropriate treatments, and indications for referral to a sleep specialist.

The prevalence of sleep complaints among older adults may be 50% or more.[1] Also, across the life span, women report more problems with insomnia than men. Insomnia is the most common sleep disturbance in the older population, with up to 40% of persons older than age 60 complaining of difficulty falling asleep and/or maintaining sleep, and more than 20% reporting severe insomnia.[1,2] The prevalence of primary sleep disorders, such as sleep apnea and restless leg syndrome (RLS), also increases with age, and the magnitude of sleep problems is higher in long-term care facilities than in community settings.

Sleep disruption in old age is not benign. It can have a significant impact on overall quality of life. In correlational studies, sleep disturbance and sleep disorders have been associated with cognitive impairment, poor health status, low quality of life, and increased mortality.[3,4]

CASE 1

Jonathan Chen (Part 2)

Mr. Chen's physical examination reveals mild arthritis in his left knee, for which he takes ibuprofen as needed. He denies pain at night. He does not have hypertension or a history of heart disease. He denies a history of depression, anxiety, or other psychiatric problems. He states that his current mood is "great, except for this sleep thing," and that he is worried about his son's job and his grandchildren's education.

Are Mr. Chen's sleep complaints age-related? ▣

CASE 2

Charles Banker (Part 2)

Mr. Banker describes his mood as "tired." He is obese, with a history of hypertension, gastroesophageal reflux, high cholesterol, and diabetes. He takes glipizide, metformin, atenolol, omeprazole, aspirin, and atorvastatin. On physical examination, his blood pressure is 134/76 mmHg; he is 5 feet 8 inches tall and weighs 190 lbs. Heart and lung examination is unremarkable.

Are Mr. Banker's sleep complaints age-related? ▣

RISK FACTORS AND PATHOPHYSIOLOGY

Human adult sleep is composed of two separate states: rapid eye movement (REM, or stage R) sleep and non-REM (NREM, or stages N1 to N3) sleep. NREM sleep is further divided into three stages, which roughly parallel a "depth of sleep" continuum, including a "light" stage of sleep (stage N1), a stage of sleep where the majority of time asleep is spent (N2), and deep sleep (stage N3). REM sleep is normally characterized by electroencephalogram (EEG) activation, muscle atonia, and rapid eye movements. Normal adults generally progress from NREM stages N1 to N3, then return briefly to lighter sleep (typically stage N2) before entering REM sleep, in a cycle of approximately 90 minutes, which repeats throughout the night.

One of the most notable changes in sleep structure with aging is a decrease in deep (stage N3) sleep. Other common changes with age include taking longer to fall asleep, having decreased sleep efficiency (percentage of time asleep out of time spent in bed),

being awake more during the night, waking earlier than desired in the morning, and having more intentional and inadvertent daytime napping.[5] Age-related neuronal loss in the suprachiasmatic nucleus (SCN) of the hypothalamus and reduced melatonin production by the pineal gland weaken circadian (24-hour) rhythms, contributing to these changes. In addition, a host of other factors often cause or aggravate sleep difficulties.[6] Box 31-1 lists medical, pharmacologic, psychiatric, and psychosocial factors that commonly contribute to sleep problems in older people. Table 31-1 summarizes age-related changes in specific organ systems and the impact of these changes on sleep.

CASE 1

Jonathan Chen (Part 3)

On further questioning, Mr. Chen reports that he has not been sleeping well for several months. He drinks a glass of wine with dinner, and then later dozes in a chair while

---

BOX 31-1
FACTORS THAT INCREASE RISK OF SLEEP PROBLEMS AND SLEEP DISORDERS IN OLDER ADULTS

Medical Conditions
Chronic pain (e.g., from arthritis, other rheumatologic disorders, or neuropathy)
Dyspnea of cardiac or pulmonary origin
Gastroesophageal reflux
Obesity
Nocturia and/or incontinence
Neurodegenerative diseases such as Alzheimer's disease and Parkinson's disease

Psychiatric Disorders
Depression and other mood disorders
Anxiety disorders
Drug or alcohol abuse or dependency

Psychosocial, Psychological, and Lifestyle Factors
Retirement
Bereavement
Poor sleep habits/inadequate sleep hygiene
Daytime sleeping, extended napping
Inaccurate, maladaptive beliefs about sleep changes with advancing age

Medications and Nonprescription Agents
Benzodiazepines
Antihistamines
Tricyclics and other antidepressants
Analgesics
Clonidine
Theophylline
Methylphenidate
Anticonvulsants
Antiparkinsonian agents
Diuretics
Nicotine
Caffeine
Alcohol

TABLE 31-1	Impact of Specific Physiologic Changes in Older Adults and Possible Effects on Sleep	
System	**Changes**	**Consequences**
Circadian rhythms	Phase advance (shift earlier) is normal with aging	Problems maintaining sleep; early morning awakening
Upper airway physiology	More fatty tissue, reduced muscle tone	Obstructive sleep apnea (nighttime awakenings and daytime sleepiness)
Musculoskeletal	Arthritis, other conditions causing chronic pain	Problems with falling asleep and nighttime awakenings
Genitourinary	Increased nighttime urination (e.g., with benign prostatic hyperplasia)	Nighttime awakenings
Menopause	Hot flashes	Nighttime awakenings, night sweats

watching television. He goes to bed at 10:00 PM most nights, and lies awake thinking about his family as "the hours tick by" until he is able to sleep. He generally awakens at 4:00 AM to urinate, and often has trouble falling back to sleep after using the restroom. He and his wife get up at 6:00 AM, and he "rests" on the couch after breakfast. He generally exercises in the afternoon, and then rests on the couch while his wife prepares dinner. He does not drink coffee or consume other caffeine. He snores softly on some nights, but his wife has not witnessed loud snoring or periods when he stops breathing while asleep. He denies leg discomfort at night, and his wife has not noticed that he kicks his legs during sleep.

What is your differential diagnosis and what tests should be ordered for Mr. Chen? ◾

CASE 2

Charles Banker (Part 3)

Mr. Banker reports sleeping "off and on" throughout the day and night. He falls asleep in his recliner in the evenings, and then goes to bed around midnight. He falls asleep quickly, but awakens "too many times to count" during the night. He urinates several times during the night, but also awakens for other unknown reasons. He gets out of bed around 4:30 AM, and then falls back asleep in his recliner until about 9 AM. He reports being told in the past that he snores loudly, although he currently sleeps alone.

What is your differential diagnosis and what tests should be ordered for Mr. Banker? ◾

DIFFERENTIAL DIAGNOSIS AND ASSESSMENT

Sleep problems are common among older adults,[7] but older patients often do not spontaneously report problems with sleep to their primary care providers. Because of this, screening for sleep complaints is recommended. This should include asking about satisfaction with sleep, daytime fatigue and sleepiness,

and unusual behaviors during sleep (especially snoring, interrupted breathing, and/or leg movements).[8] Persistent sleep problems require a detailed sleep history from the patient and the bed partner or caregiver, if available. In addition, a "sleep diary," in which the patient tracks sleep-related behaviors for 1 to 2 weeks, can be informative.

> Older adults seldom spontaneously report problems with sleep to their primary care providers; therefore, screening for sleep complaints is recommended.

The initial evaluation of sleep should focus on medical conditions, substance abuse, mental health problems, and medications that may be contributing to sleep complaints (see Box 31-1). Patients should be queried about their usual sleep patterns and events during sleep such as limb movements, respiratory distress, panic attacks, pain, nocturia, shortness of breath, headache, or symptoms of gastroesophageal reflux. Recent stressors and symptoms of depression, anxiety, and other psychiatric disorders need to be identified, and psychosocial factors such as bereavement, loss of social supports, and lifestyle changes (e.g., retirement) should be considered. A mental status examination to identify cognitive impairment is also indicated. A full medication history, including the use of over-the-counter and herbal medications, is essential. The focused physical examination should be based on evidence from the history. For example, reports of nocturia disrupting sleep should lead to evaluation for cardiac, renal, or prostate disease. Prior treatments for sleep-related complaints should be reviewed.

Referral for an overnight sleep study (polysomnography [PSG]) is indicated when evidence suggests a primary sleep disorder, such as sleep-disordered breathing or periodic limb movement disorder (discussed later in the chapter).[9] PSG is the gold standard for the evaluation of sleep and generally involves spending a night in a sleep laboratory, where physiologic measures are recorded, including an EEG, electrocardiogram (ECG), electrooculogram (EOG), electromyogram (EMG), respiratory effort and airflow, and oxygen saturation. PSGs are performed and interpreted by sleep specialists. Many portable, home monitoring systems are available, particularly to test for sleep-disordered breathing (e.g., sleep apnea).

Insomnia

Insomnia is a complaint that can include one or more of the following:

- Difficulty falling asleep
- Difficulty staying sleep
- Waking up too early
- Sleep that is nonrestorative or poor in quality, that results in some form of daytime impairment, such as fatigue, irritability, impairment in attention or concentration, or daytime sleepiness[8]

In older adults, chronic insomnia commonly coexists with other medical or psychiatric problems, so it is often termed "comorbid insomnia." The diagnosis of insomnia is made based on a thorough sleep history, sometimes in conjunction with a sleep diary.

The American Academy of Sleep Medicine recommends PSG in the evaluation of insomnia only when a sleep-related breathing disorder or periodic limb movement disorder is suspected as an underlying cause, the initial diagnosis is uncertain, initial treatment has failed, or precipitous arousals occur with violent or injurious behavior.[9]

True primary insomnia is quite rare among older adults, accounting for only 5% to 20% of cases. Most insomnia complaints are comorbid with specific medical conditions, neurologic disorders, primary sleep disorders (described later in the chapter), substance abuse, prescription medications, or psychiatric conditions; multiple factors may coexist. In depression, early morning awakening is the most characteristic pattern, along with increased sleep latency (time to fall asleep) and more nighttime wakefulness. Chronic pain at night is a common medical cause of insomnia, particularly in older patients with rheumatologic disorders, neuropathy, or cancer.

> Most insomnia complaints in older adults are comorbid with specific medical conditions, neurologic disorders, primary sleep disorders, substance abuse, prescription medications, or psychiatric conditions; multiple factors may coexist.

Drug and alcohol use are thought to account for 10% to 15% of cases of insomnia. Chronic use of hypnotics can lead to fragmented sleep and rebound insomnia when stopped abruptly. Many over-the-counter medications produce side effects that are either sedating or stimulating. Older patients often take multiple medications, which may be prescribed by multiple providers, compounding the situation. Caffeine (an ingredient in many nonprescription analgesics and dietary supplements, teas, chocolate, and beverages) increases sleep latency and sleep fragmentation. Although older adults sometimes try alcohol as a sleep aid, it actually leads to fragmented sleep. The use of alcohol combined with hypnotics may further exacerbate sleep difficulties, and may worsen sleep-disordered breathing.

Sleep-Disordered Breathing (Sleep Apnea)

Sleep apnea is characterized by repeated episodes of either a cessation or marked decrease of airflow during sleep.[10] Apneas (complete airflow cessation for 10 seconds or more) and hypopneas (partial decrease in airflow for 10 seconds or more with a drop in oxygen saturation) during sleep can result from either upper airway obstruction (obstructive apnea) or a loss of ventilatory effort (central apnea).

Obstructive sleep apnea (OSA) is characterized by recurrent episodes of upper airway collapse and a reduction or cessation of airflow despite persistent ventilatory efforts. When the number of apneas/hypopneas per hour of sleep (the apnea-hypopnea index, AHI) is ≥15, or when the AHI is ≥5 and is associated with symptoms such as daytime somnolence, OSA can be diagnosed. An increased body mass index (BMI) and large neck circumference are both risk factors for OSA. However, in older adults OSA is not as tightly linked with BMI and neck circumference. OSA may be aggravated by alcohol (especially near bedtime), sedatives, sleep deprivation, nasal congestion, and supine sleeping posture (in some cases). Consequences of OSA include hypertension, cardiac arrhythmia, heart failure, memory impairment, and other problems. Excessive daytime sleepiness, ranging from subtle drowsiness to falling asleep in unsafe circumstances (e.g., while driving), is a common complaint of OSA patients, but older adults with OSA may also have insomnia resulting from fragmentation of sleep.

> Older patients with obstructive sleep apnea may not be obese or have a large neck circumference.

Loud snoring, nocturnal gasping, and witnessed apneas may be reported by bed partners or caregivers and serve as an additional important clue to OSA. Apneic episodes are usually terminated by gasps, chokes, snorts, and/or brief awakenings, which may lead to complaints of insomnia. Patients may also experience morning headaches; impaired attention, memory, or judgment; or personality changes, such as irritability, anxiety, or depression.

Clinical examination of a suspected OSA patient should include an evaluation of body habitus (height, weight, and neck circumference), and a careful upper airway examination to identify structures or abnormalities that potentially narrow the airway. Patients suspected of having sleep apnea should be referred to a sleep laboratory for PSG (Level of Evidence A) or should undergo home portable testing (Level of Evidence B), from which an AHI can be determined and used to inform treatment decisions.

Sleep-Related Movement Disorders

Among older patients, periodic limb movements during sleep (PLMS) are common.[11] PLMS involves episodes of repetitive, highly stereotyped movements (primarily of the legs) during sleep. Although PLMS may be asymptomatic, when PLMS is associated with a complaint of insomnia and/or excessive sleepiness with no other disorder to explain the symptoms, it is referred to as periodic limb movement disorder (PLMD). Restless legs syndrome (RLS) is characterized by an irresistible urge to move the legs while awake (often when in bed trying to sleep). The restless feeling in the legs is usually associated with uncomfortable paresthesias of the legs. The symptoms worsen at rest, and movement of the limbs relieves symptoms. For many patients, symptoms are worse later in the day, making it difficult to fall asleep. RLS runs in families and, in some cases, an underlying medical disorder, such as uremia, iron deficiency, or peripheral neuropathy, may predispose a person to RLS. The diagnosis of RLS is made based on history, whereas diagnosis of PLMD requires both history and overnight PSG. RLS and PLMD are distinct syndromes that frequently coexist. Approximately 80% of individuals with RLS have evidence of PLMD on PSG as well.

Circadian Rhythm Sleep Disorders

These disorders result from desynchronization between patients' endogenous circadian clock and the external environment. Circadian rhythms are entrained to the 24-hour day by time cues or *zeitgebers*, the most important of which is the light–dark cycle.[12] Older adults often have an advanced sleep phase, where they go to sleep early in the evening and wake up early in the morning. On nights when they do stay up late, their biological clock usually still causes them to awaken in the early morning hours, making them sleepy during the day. In contrast, people with a delayed sleep phase (which is thought to be less common in older people) fall asleep late and wake up late in the morning. Sleep diaries and wrist activity

monitoring (Level of Evidence A) can be used to detect these sleep patterns.

REM Sleep Behavior Disorder

The presenting symptoms of REM sleep behavior disorder are usually vigorous sleep behaviors associated with vivid dreams. This "dream enactment behavior" is associated with a lack of the normal muscle atonia that should occur with REM sleep. The vigorous nighttime behaviors may result in injury to the patient or bed partner, and there may be a family history of the disorder. Toxic-metabolic abnormalities, drug or alcohol withdrawal or intoxication, and certain medications (e.g., tricyclic antidepressants, monoamine oxidase inhibitors, cholinergic agents, and serotonin specific reuptake inhibitors) can cause acute REM sleep behavior disorder. The chronic form is usually idiopathic or associated with other neurologic disorders, such as Lewy body dementia, Parkinson's disease, and multiple system atrophy. PSG is indicated when this disorder is suspected; PSG is used to test for key features of this disorder, including the pathologic absence of the muscle atonia that should occur during REM sleep.

CASE 1

Jonathan Chen (Part 4)

Mr. Chen's sleep problems may have been precipitated by lifestyle changes after his retirement, which resulted in development of problematic changes in his sleep habits, in particular daytime napping, and worry about sleep. These factors likely perpetuate his sleep problems and have led to chronic insomnia.

What treatment strategies should be initiated for Mr. Chen? ◨

CASE 2

Charles Banker (Part 4)

Mr. Banker has classic symptoms of sleep-disordered breathing, including daytime sleepiness and snoring. PSG reveals an AHI of 45 events per hour of sleep, which indicates severe OSA.

What treatment strategies should be initiated for Mr. Banker? ◨

MANAGEMENT

Following careful assessment, primary care clinicians should be able to determine whether a sleep-related problem can be managed within the primary care setting, or whether a referral to a sleep specialist is indicated (Figure 31-1). The following discussion will

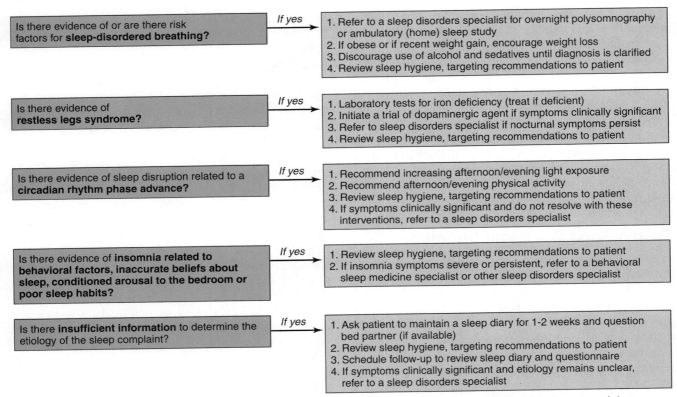

| Is there evidence of or are there risk factors for **sleep-disordered breathing**? | *If yes* → | 1. Refer to a sleep disorders specialist for overnight polysomnography or ambulatory (home) sleep study
2. If obese or if recent weight gain, encourage weight loss
3. Discourage use of alcohol and sedatives until diagnosis is clarified
4. Review sleep hygiene, targeting recommendations to patient |

| Is there evidence of **restless legs syndrome**? | *If yes* → | 1. Laboratory tests for iron deficiency (treat if deficient)
2. Initiate a trial of dopaminergic agent if symptoms clinically significant
3. Refer to sleep disorders specialist if nocturnal symptoms persist
4. Review sleep hygiene, targeting recommendations to patient |

| Is there evidence of sleep disruption related to a **circadian rhythm phase advance**? | *If yes* → | 1. Recommend increasing afternoon/evening light exposure
2. Recommend afternoon/evening physical activity
3. Review sleep hygiene, targeting recommendations to patient
4. If symptoms clinically significant and do not resolve with these interventions, refer to a sleep disorders specialist |

| Is there evidence of **insomnia related to behavioral factors, inaccurate beliefs about sleep, conditioned arousal to the bedroom or poor sleep habits**? | *If yes* → | 1. Review sleep hygiene, targeting recommendations to patient
2. If insomnia symptoms severe or persistent, refer to a behavioral sleep medicine specialist or other sleep disorders specialist |

| Is there **insufficient information** to determine the etiology of the sleep complaint? | *If yes* → | 1. Ask patient to maintain a sleep diary for 1-2 weeks and question bed partner (if available)
2. Review sleep hygiene, targeting recommendations to patient
3. Schedule follow-up to review sleep diary and questionnaire
4. If symptoms clinically significant and etiology remains unclear, refer to a sleep disorders specialist |

Figure 31-1 Suggestions for the evaluation and management of primary care patients with sleep complaints.

review the management of sleep problems within primary care and will provide some detail on situations in which referrals are needed.

Behavioral Treatment of Insomnia

Because insomnia is associated with a variety of medical, psychological, and psychiatric conditions, it is crucial to identify underlying conditions, which can lead to specific treatments, such as analgesics for nocturnal pain or treatment for depression. Treating insomnia with hypnotic medications without addressing comorbid conditions can result in treatment failure and even exacerbation of the problem. For chronic insomnia, after underlying problems have been addressed, the first-line approach should be nonpharmacologic, as described below. For short-term, stress-related transient insomnia, such as during acute hospitalization or other acute stressors, short-term use of sedative-hypnotic medications may be appropriate.

The focus of the primary care provider should be on identifying behaviors that directly contribute to sleep disruption, and providing education and instructions on healthy sleep practices in combination with a regular sleep schedule (Box 31-2).[13,14] Patients should be made more aware of health practices (e.g., lack of exercise, substance abuse) and environmental factors (e.g., light, noise, temperature, mattress) that impact sleep.

Evidence suggests that patients with severe, chronic insomnia are unlikely to respond to sleep hygiene education alone. Additional nonpharmacologic approaches address behavioral and cognitive factors that may underlie the chronic insomnia, and these approaches are well supported by multiple randomized controlled trials in both younger and older adults (Level of Evidence A).[15] Several are described in the following list.

- Cognitive behavioral therapy for insomnia (CBT-I) combines behavioral techniques with methods to identify and address inaccurate beliefs about

---

BOX 31-2

BASIC RECOMMENDATIONS TO IMPROVE SLEEP

Maintain a regular morning rising time.
Avoid daytime naps, or limit napping to the early afternoon for less than 1 hour.
Exercise or increase activity level during the day, but not in the evening or immediately prior to bedtime.
Increase exposure to bright light during the day or early evening.
Take a hot bath about 2 hours before bedtime.
Avoid caffeine, nicotine, and alcohol in the evening.
Avoid excessive food or fluid intake at night.
Practice a relaxing bedtime routine.
Minimize light and noise exposure in the bedroom at night.

sleep such as "staying in bed longer will help me sleep better." These treatments are typically provided by psychologists, sleep medicine specialists, or advance practice nurses with specialized training.

- Stimulus control therapy involves instructing the patient to reserve the bed and bedroom only for sleep and sexual activity with the goal of breaking the association between the bedroom environment and anxiety about sleep.
- Sleep restriction therapy involves curtailing the amount of time in bed to match the amount of time the patient actually sleeps. This approach addresses the common mistake patients make in increasing their time in bed in an effort to "catch up" on sleep.
- Relaxation techniques such as progressive muscle relaxation, yoga, and meditation can be useful for insomnia patients with high physiologic arousal at night, although these methods are not universally effective.

Implementation of these techniques requires motivation on the patient's part and close follow-up by the clinician; involvement of a specialist trained in behavioral sleep medicine is likely most effective.

> The management of chronic insomnia in older adults should address comorbid conditions, and the first-line therapy for chronic insomnia in older adults is behavioral/nonpharmacologic.

Bright Light Therapy

When sleep problems are characterized by early morning awakening and there is no evidence of another sleep disorder, evening bright light exposure may be considered,[16] although evidence for effectiveness is mixed. Light therapy targets the underlying circadian rhythm changes that result in an advanced sleep phase. Exposure to either outdoor or artificial light via commercially available bright light boxes can be effective. The light intensity (brightness) used in research studies is generally between 2500 and 10,000 lux,

which is comparable to daytime outdoor light levels. Potential side effects include transient headache and eye strain. Light exposure may be inappropriate for patients taking photosensitizing agents (e.g., amiodarone, hydrochlorothiazide), and a routine eye examination is recommended prior to treatment.

Pharmacologic Treatment

The decision to initiate drug therapy for insomnia should be based on the presence and severity of daytime symptoms and their impact on functioning and quality of life. Short-term hypnotic therapy may be appropriate in conjunction with improved sleep hygiene in cases of transient situational insomnia, such as during bereavement.[2,14,17] In older adults with chronic insomnia, sedative/hypnotic agents should be considered cautiously, because of the complications associated with long-term use in older people. Fall risk is increased by some commonly prescribed hypnotics, and confusion may result, especially in persons with underlying cognitive impairment. Altered metabolism of drugs, high rates of polypharmacy, and increased sensitivity to central nervous system depression all contribute to the high rate of adverse effects in older persons. When hypnotic agents are used, careful follow-up is essential, and a plan for discontinuation should be discussed when the initial prescription is provided.

Table 31-2 lists commonly used sedative-hypnotic medications. In general, medication factors associated with fewer adverse effects include receptor selectivity, a shorter half-life, and lack active metabolites. Benzodiazepines shorten the time to fall asleep and increase total sleep time; however, most change sleep architecture such that more time is spent in the lighter stages of sleep. Short-acting nonbenzodiazepines/benzodiazepine receptor agonists may be useful for treating difficulty falling asleep; they have fewer daytime effects and are less likely to be associated with falls and hip fractures than longer-acting agents. Intermediate-acting agents are recommended for problems with sleep maintenance; using the lowest effective dose and tapering the dosage prior to discontinuation of the drug can reduce the potential for rebound insomnia. Long-acting agents

TABLE 31-2	Some Medications Commonly Used for Insomnia in Older Adults		
Agent	**Chemical Class**	**Dose (Range), in mg**	**Half-Life or Range, in hours**
Temazepam	Benzodiazepine	7.5 (7.5-30)	3.5-18.4
Eszopiclone	Nonbenzodiazepine	1 (1-2)	6.0
Zolpidem	Nonbenzodiazepine/benzodiazepine receptor agonist	5 (5-10)	1.4-4.5
Zaleplon	Nonbenzodiazepine for eszopiclone, zolpidem and zaleplon	5 (5-10)	1.0
Ramelteon	Melatonin receptor agonist	8	1.5-2.6
Doxepin	Sedating antidepressant	3 (3-6)	15.3 (31 for metabolite)

(e.g., quazepam, flurazepam) should not be used in older people because these medications have active metabolites and a half-life of more than a day.

Newer nonbenzodiazepine hypnotics may have advantages in terms of safety and effectiveness over the older benzodiazepines. They also reduce the time to fall asleep, and some increase the duration of sleep and may be less likely to disturb sleep architecture. Zolpidem and zaleplon should only be taken immediately prior to bedtime or after the patient has gone to bed and has been unable to fall asleep. No evidence of tolerance has been observed with either medication; however, psychological dependence may develop with continued use. Eszopiclone can be helpful for maintaining sleep during the night and has been approved for long-term use.

Sedating antidepressants (e.g., trazodone, doxepin, and mirtazapine) are sometimes used off label to treat insomnia, and a low-dose formulation of doxepin has also been approved for the treatment of insomnia. These agents may be helpful as sleep aids in patients with depression who are taking another antidepressant (at a therapeutic dose for depression) during the daytime. Other than the newer formulation of doxepin, there is little evidence to support the use of sedating antidepressants in nondepressed individuals with insomnia.

Most over-the-counter sleep aids contain a sedating antihistamine such as diphenhydramine. They should not be used in older persons, because of their potential for causing adverse anticholinergic effects, daytime sedation, and confusion.

Melatonin is a popular over-the-counter nutritional supplement marketed as a sleep aid. It may be helpful for individuals suffering from circadian rhythm–related sleep disorders. Melatonin has had mixed results when used as a hypnotic agent for sleep problems unrelated to circadian rhythm changes, but there is recent evidence for effectiveness with a prolonged-release formulation.[18] A melatonin receptor agonist (ramelteon) is also available for the treatment of insomnia.

Obstructive Sleep Apnea

Positive airway pressure (PAP) is the treatment of choice for sleep apnea (Level of Evidence A).[2,6,10] Positive pressure is used as a "splint" for the airway, reducing airway collapse during sleep. PAP is extremely effective and should be recommended as a first-line treatment for OSA, regardless of the patient's age. Other general measures consist of weight loss (if overweight) and avoiding sedatives, hypnotics, and alcohol. Some patients will have positional OSA that improves by avoiding the supine sleeping position. Oral and dental appliances that reposition the jaw or tongue may be appropriate in mild cases or in patients who refuse PAP. In a few severe cases, surgical treatments such as uvulopalatopharyngoplasty may be considered; however,

successful resolution of OSA may occur in only about half of surgically treated patients.

> Positive airway pressure (PAP) is the established treatment of choice for sleep apnea.

PLMD and RLS

Dopaminergic agents are the initial agents of choice for both PLMD and RLS, when treatment is warranted. Potentially causative or contributory factors need to be addressed. Patients with RLS in association with low ferritin levels may respond to iron replacement therapy. A nighttime dose of carbidopa/levodopa can be used on an as-needed basis for infrequent RLS symptoms, but carbidopa/levodopa may increase the risk of RLS symptoms occurring during the daytime and may cause other side effects, so it is not currently recommended in most cases. First-line treatment for RLS (particularly in patients with clinically significant, chronic symptoms) are dopamine agonists, such as pramipexole or ropinirole (Level of Evidence A). Benzodiazepines (e.g., clonazepam) and opioids (e.g., oxycodone) may also be effective, but these may have higher risks in older people. There is also some evidence regarding the use of gabapentin in the treatment of RLS (Level of Evidence B).

Other Sleep Disorders

Patients with an advanced sleep phase may respond to evening bright light exposure. In patients with REM sleep behavior disorder, steps should be taken to keep their home sleeping environment safe, because vigorous movements may occur during sleep. Clonazepam is reported to be highly effective in the treatment of REM sleep behavior disorder, with little evidence of tolerance or abuse over long periods of treatment.[19] There is also evidence for the successful use of melatonin in older patients with REM sleep behavior disorder in conjunction with neurodegenerative disorders (Level of Evidence C), which may be a safer alternative than clonazepam.

CASE 1

Discussion

You recommend that Mr. Chen give up his evening alcohol and limit his daytime napping to 30 minutes in the early afternoon. You also recommend that he get up at the same time every morning. Two weeks later, Mr. Chen reports that, after "a few rough days and nights," he is generally sleeping better at night, and feeling better during the day. You let him know that referral to a behavioral sleep medicine specialist is also available if his insomnia symptoms return. ■

Discussion

Mr. Banker is prescribed a PAP machine, and receives close follow-up from the sleep clinic to help encourage his adherence. When you see him for follow-up, he reports marked improvement in his daytime sleepiness and fatigue, but some discomfort with the face mask for his PAP. You refer him back to the sleep clinic to consider changes in his PAP mask, which helps encourage his long-term adherence. ▣

CHANGES IN SLEEP WITH DEMENTIA AND IN THE NURSING HOME

Patients with dementia have frequent sleep disruption and arousals, lower sleep efficiency, more stage N1 sleep, and less N3 (deep sleep) compared to individuals without dementia.[5] Disturbances of the sleep–wake cycle are common, resulting in both fragmented nighttime sleep and frequent, brief episodes of daytime sleeping. This may be especially challenging for family caregivers and can precipitate nursing home placement. Some dementia patients may "sundown," or experience an exacerbation of confusion and agitation during the evening or nighttime hours, which can also be extremely difficult for caregivers.[20] Evaluation and treatment of sleep problems among patients with dementia should include input and participation from the caregiver, and should focus on improving quality of life for both. Initial evaluation should seek to identify medical causes, such as infection, polypharmacy, and fecal impaction. Once they are excluded, sleep disturbances should be managed similarly to individuals without dementia, and recent findings suggest that, with caregiver support, dementia patients can benefit from nonpharmacologic treatments, bright light therapy (if indicated), and even PAP treatment for sleep apnea.[21,22]

> Evaluation and treatment of sleep problems among patients with dementia should include input and participation from the caregiver and should focus on improving quality of life for both.

In nursing home residents, marked disruption in sleep patterns can be seen, perhaps even beyond what is found in dementia patients living at home.[23,24] In the nursing home, many of the same factors contribute to sleep problems; however, additional environmental and caregiving factors are also important to consider.[25,26] In many nursing homes the nighttime environment is noisy; lights are frequently left on (or turned on) in residents' rooms during the night; and caregiving activities frequently interrupt sleep. In addition, daytime inactivity, excessive in-bed time, and minimal time spent outdoors exposed to bright light contribute to the commonly seen pattern of continual dozing and waking over the day and night. There are, however, few data on the effectiveness of sleep medications and specific management of sleep disorders in the nursing home setting, and side effects of sedative-hypnotics can be significant in frail older people. Behavioral factors and environmental interventions should, therefore, be the treatments of choice, and sleep medications should be considered with caution.[2]

SUMMARY

Most sleep disturbances in older adults are comorbid with other conditions, which should be properly evaluated. Obtaining a good sleep history is essential. Referral should be made when appropriate. Accurate diagnosis and appropriate therapy of sleep disorders may substantially improve sleep and quality of life in older people.

Web Resources

www.aasmnet.org. American Academy of Sleep Medicine: Click on "Practice Guidelines" to access free evidence-based reviews of many common sleep disorders.

www.nhlbi.nih.gov/sleep. Free educational materials on a variety of sleep topics provided by the National Institutes of Health, National Center on Sleep Disorders Research, for providers (under the heading "Professional Education") and for patients (under the heading "Patient and Public Information").

www.sleepresearchsociety.org. Sleep Research Society: This organization of sleep researchers provides information on sleep research activities, and a variety of educational courses and products on various sleep-related topics.

KEY REFERENCES

2. Bloom HG, Ahmed I, Alessi CA, et al. Evidence-based recommendations for the assessment and management of sleep disorders in older persons. J Am Geriatr Soc 2009;57(5):761-89.
10. Epstein LJ, Kristo D, Strollo PJ Jr, et al; Adult Obstructive Sleep Apnea Task Force of the American Academy of Sleep Medicine. Clinical guideline for the evaluation, management and long-term care of obstructive sleep apnea in adults. J Clin Sleep Med 2009;5(3):263-76.
13. Morin CM, Bootzin RR, Buysse DJ, et al. Psychological and behavioral treatment of insomnia: Update of the recent evidence. Sleep 2006;29(11):1398-414.
14. Schutte-Rodin S, Broch L, Buysse D, et al. Clinical guideline for the evaluation and management of chronic insomnia in adults. J Clin Sleep Med 2008;4(5):487-504.
15. Morgenthaler T, Kramer M, Alessi C, et al; American Academy of Sleep Medicine. Practice parameters for the psychological and behavioral treatment of insomnia: An update. Sleep 2006;29(11):1415-9.

References available online at expertconsult.com.

32

Sexual Health

Thomas Mulligan and Michael P. Feloney

OBJECTIVES

Upon completion of this chapter, the reader will be able to:

- Be aware of the prevalence and pathophysiology of sexual dysfunction.
- Understand how to evaluate a patient with sexual dysfunction.
- Be knowledgeable of the treatment strategies for sexual dysfunction.

Our understanding of sexual function and dysfunction in older men has increased greatly in recent years. There is less available information on the sexuality of older women. Nevertheless, we now have a better understanding of the pathophysiology of age-associated sexual dysfunction and various effective treatments.

CASE 1

Clifford Johnson (Part 1)

Clifford Johnson is a 68-year-old man and a new patient in your practice. During his initial visit he mentions that he will soon be remarrying and is concerned that he will not be able to have sex with his new wife. His first wife died

of breast cancer 5 years ago. He has not engaged in sexual activity since her death, except for occasional masturbation. He reports strong interest in sex since meeting his fiancé about 9 months ago. However, he fears his erections are not adequate to complete intercourse. Medications include hydrochlorothiazide 25 mg daily for hypertension, atorvastatin 10 mg orally daily for hyperlipidemia, and amitripty 50 mg daily for prolonged bereavement.

How can you discern if Mr. Johnson is sexually functional and what is the most likely etiology if he is dysfunctional? ◻

MALE SEXUALITY: AGE-ASSOCIATED CHANGES

As men age, their sexual function changes. The frequency of intercourse and the prevalence of any sexual activity decrease. Young married men report intercourse 3 to 4 times per week, whereas only 7% of men aged 60 to 69 and 2% of those older than age 70 report this same frequency (Level of Evidence A).[1,2] However, sexual interest often persists despite decreased activity. Factors contributing to a man's decreased sexual activity include poor health, decreased partner availability, decreased libido, and erectile dysfunction (ED). Though aging is associated with changes in sexual behavior and response (e.g., refractory period between erections is longer),[3] erectile failure is not a part of healthy aging but rather is caused by age-associated disease (e.g., peripheral arterial disease) or treatment (e.g., radical prostatectomy for prostate cancer) (Level of Evidence B).[4]

> Normal age-associated changes lead to decreased sexual interest and ability; however, complete loss of sexual function is not a part of healthy aging.

ERECTILE PHYSIOLOGY AND DYSFUNCTION

In brief, testosterone, mental health, and an attractive partner stimulate libido. Fantasy as well as visual, tactile, or other erotic stimuli trigger neural impulses from the brain or spinal cord to the penis. Neural impulses cause release of neurotransmitters (e.g., nitric oxide, cGMP), which induce arterial vasodilation. Increasing arterial inflow dilates the corpora cavernosa, which impedes venous outflow. As the intrapenile (i.e., intracavernosal) pressure equilibrates to mean arterial pressure, the penis becomes rigid as blood is trapped in the penis.

Additional online-only material indicated by icon.

ED, the inability to maintain an erection adequate for sexual intercourse, is the most common sexual problem of older men. The prevalence of ED increases with age; by 70 years of age, 67% of men have ED.[5] The common causes of ED in older men are outlined in Table 32-1.

The most common cause (30% to 50%) of ED in older men is vascular disease (Level of Evidence A).[6] Risk of vascular ED increases with traditional vascular risk factors (e.g., diabetes mellitus,[7] hypertension, hyperlipidemia, and smoking).[8,9] Obstruction from atherosclerotic arterial disease impedes the intracavernosal blood flow and pressure needed to achieve a rigid erection. Venous leakage[10] leading to vascular ED can result from Peyronie's disease, arteriovenous fistula, or trauma-induced communication between the glans and the corpora. In anxious men who have excessive adrenergic-constrictor tone and in men with injured parasympathetic dilator nerves, ED can result from insufficient relaxation of trabecular smooth muscle.

> **Neurovascular problems are the most common causes of ED.**

The second most common cause of ED in older men is neurologic (17% to 37%).[10] Disorders that affect the parasympathetic sacral spinal cord or the peripheral efferent fibers to the penis impair penile smooth muscle relaxation and prevent the vasodilation necessary for erection. In patients with prostate cancer, all forms of (curative) treatment frequently cause neurogenic erectile failure (brachytherapy or external radiation, 50%; radical prostatectomy with nerve sparing, 45% to 80%) (Level of Evidence B).[4] Common health problems such as diabetes mellitus and stroke can cause autonomic dysfunction,[11] and surgical procedures such as prostatectomy, cystectomy, and proctocolectomy commonly disrupt the autonomic nerve supply to the penis, resulting in postoperative ED.

Many medications are associated with erectile dysfunction.[12] Medications with anticholinergic effects, such as antidepressants, antipsychotics, and antihistamines, can cause ED by blocking parasympathetic-mediated vasodilation and trabecular smooth muscle relaxation. Almost all antihypertensive agents have been associated with ED; of these, clonidine and thiazide diuretics have higher incidence rates,[13,14] whereas angiotensin-converting enzyme (ACE) inhibitors and angiotensin-receptor blockers have lower incidence rates (Level of Evidence B).[15,16] Numerous over-the-counter medications can cause ED. Cimetidine acts as an antiandrogen[17] and increases prolactin secretion; thus it has been associated with loss of libido and erectile failure. Ranitidine can also increase prolactin secretion, although less commonly than does cimetidine.

The prevalence of psychogenic ED correlates inversely with age. Common causes[18] of psychogenic ED include performance anxiety, fear of sexually transmitted diseases, and "widower's syndrome,"[19] in which the man involved in a new relationship feels

TABLE 32-1	Causes of Sexual Dysfunction in Older Men
Causes (in order of prevalence)	**Characteristics**
Vascular disease	Gradual onset
	Vascular risk factors: diabetes mellitus, hypertension, hyperlipidemia, tobacco use
Neurologic disease (e.g., radiation therapy, spinal cord injury, autonomic dysfunction, surgical procedures)	Gradual onset (unless postsurgical)
	Neurologic risk factors: diabetes mellitus; history of pelvic injury, surgery, or irradiation; spinal injury or surgery; Parkinson's disease; multiple sclerosis; alcoholism
	Loss of bulbocavernosus reflex
Medications (e.g., anticholinergics, antihypertensives, cimetidine, antidepressants)	Sudden onset
	Lack of sleep-associated erections or lack of erections with masturbation
	Temporal association with a new medication
Psychogenic (e.g., relationship conflicts, performance anxiety, childhood sexual abuse, fear of sexually transmitted diseases, "widower's syndrome")	Sudden onset
	Sleep-associated erections or erections with masturbation are preserved
Hypogonadism	Gradual onset
	Decreased libido more than erectile dysfunction
	Small testes, gynecomastia
	Low serum testosterone concentration
Endocrine (e.g., hypothyroidism, hyperthyroidism, hyperprolactinemia)	Rare, <5% of cases of erectile dysfunction

guilt as a defense against subconscious unfaithfulness to his deceased spouse. A patient suffering only from "widower's syndrome" should be able to achieve rigid erections with masturbation.

Hypogonadism, hypothyroidism, and hyperprolactinemia have been associated with ED. However, less than 5% of ED is caused by endocrine abnormalities.[20] Thus endocrine evaluation of men with ED but intact libido is of limited value (Level of Evidence B). Even men with castrate levels of testosterone can attain erections in response to direct penile stimulation. It may be that erection from direct penile stimulation is less androgen dependent, whereas erection from fantasy is more androgen dependent. Thus testosterone plays a large role in libido and a smaller role in ED.[21]

Therefore, if a man has complaints of low libido (more likely the man's spouse urged him to seek evaluation for this problem), assessment of serum testosterone is warranted. Ideally, blood should be obtained in the morning to account for circadian rhythm and the result carefully interpreted. For example, a serum total testosterone concentration less than 200 ng/dL in a symptomatic man strongly suggests hypogonadism that will likely respond to treatment. A serum total testosterone concentration less than 300 ng/dL in a symptomatic man likely also represents hypogonadism but response to treatment is less predictable.

EVALUATION OF ERECTILE DYSFUNCTION

Sexual history should clarify whether the problem consists of decreased libido, inadequate erections, or orgasmic failure. The onset and duration of ED, the presence or absence of sleep-associated erections, and the associated decline in libido are clues to the likely cause.

Sudden onset (in the absence of pelvic surgery) suggests psychogenic or drug-induced ED. A psychogenic cause is likely if there is a sudden onset but retention of sleep-associated erections or if erections with masturbation are intact (Level of Evidence A).[22] If sudden-onset erectile failure is accompanied by lack of sleep-associated erections and lack of erection with masturbation, temporal association with new medication should be investigated. A gradual onset of ED associated with loss of libido suggests hypogonadism. Gradual onset associated with intact libido (the most common presentation) suggests vascular, neurogenic, or other organic causes.

Medical history is directed at discerning those factors likely to be contributing to ED. Vascular risk factors include diabetes mellitus, hypertension, coronary artery disease, peripheral arterial disease, hyperlipidemia, and smoking. Neurogenic risk factors include diabetes mellitus; history of pelvic injury, surgery, or radiation; and spinal injury or surgery. A complete medication review, including over-the-counter medications, is essential. Finally, the history should assess the patient's relationship with the sexual partner, the partner's health and attitude toward sex, economic or social stresses, living situation, alcohol use, and affective disorders.

On physical examination, attention should be paid to signs of vascular, neurologic, or endocrine diseases. A femoral bruit and diminished (or absent) pedal pulses suggest an arterial etiology. Palpation of penile plaques (i.e., Peyronie's disease) suggests venous etiology. Orthostatic hypotension and loss of the bulbocavernosus reflex suggest neurologic etiology. Small testes and gynecomastia suggest hypogonadism or hyperprolactinemia.

CASE 1

Clifford Johnson (Part 2)

On further questioning of Mr. Johnson, you determine that his libido and orgasmic function are intact but he has lost sleep-associated erections and is not able to get a rigid erection with masturbation. On examination you note a unilateral femoral bruit with good pedal pulses. He assures you he has no claudication.

What diagnostic testing should you perform? ▣

Laboratory evaluations should target relevant comorbid conditions such as diabetes mellitus and vascular disease or disorders suggested by the physical examination. The measurement of serum testosterone should be considered in men with low libido.

An at-home therapeutic trial of a phosphodiesterase inhibitor (sildenafil or vardenafil) is considered first-line evaluation and treatment.[23] The initial dose should be low (sildenafil 25 to 50 mg or vardenafil 5 to 10 mg) in men suspected of having neurogenic ED. A poor response suggests vasculogenic ED. Further therapeutic trial with sildenafil at 100 mg or vardenafil at 20 mg may prove to be effective.

More extensive diagnostic testing is not commonly used. The penile-brachial pressure index[24] can be helpful in assessing arteriogenic ED. This index measures the loss of systolic pressure between the arm and the penis. When measured before and after exercise, it can be used to assess pelvic steal syndrome, which is the loss of erection associated with initiation of active pelvic thrusting, presumably because of the transfer of blood flow from the penis to the pelvic musculature. More invasive and expensive tests such as Doppler ultrasound to assess penile arterial function, dynamic infusion cavernosometry to assess venous leakage syndrome, and penile arteriography are generally reserved for research or penile vascular surgery candidates.

CASE 1

Clifford Johnson (Part 3)

Now that you know your patient's ED is likely caused by a combination of "widower's syndrome," medication adverse effects, and possible mild vascular disease, what treatments are likely to help him regain adequate erectile function? ▣

TREATMENT OF ERECTILE DYSFUNCTION

Multiple effective therapeutic options are available for the treatment of ED.[25] Treatment should be individualized and based on etiology, personal preference, partner issues, and cost (Table 32-2). Oral therapy for ED with sildenafil, vardenafil, tadalafil, or avanafil has revolutionized treatment of male sexual dysfunction. Sildenafil is a phosphodiesterase inhibitor that potentiates the penile response to sexual stimulation. It improves the rigidity and duration of erection. It is taken 1 hour before sexual activity and has little effect until sexual stimulation occurs. Vardenafil is a more potent and specific phosphodiesterase inhibitor. A lower effective dose and better adverse-event profile (no effect on color vision) make vardenafil a reasonable option. Tadalafil is a longer-acting phosphodiesterase inhibitor with an adverse-event profile similar to that of vardenafil but with the added potential problem of muscle pain. Avanafil is a more recently approved phosphodiesterase inhibitor; it is taken 30 minutes before sexual activity. All four of these agents are contraindicated for concomitant use with nitrate

TABLE 32-2	Treatment Options for Erectile Dysfunction					
Treatment	Route/ Administration	Applicable Conditions	Onset	Duration of Action	Dosage	Selected Adverse Events
Sildenafil	Oral	N, A?, V?	60 min	4 h	25-100 mg	Headache, flushing, rhinitis, dyspepsia, transient color blindness; contraindicated with nitrate use and α-blockers
Vardenafil	Oral	N, A?, V?	45 min	4 h	5-20 mg	Headache, flushing, rhinitis, dyspepsia; contraindicated with nitrate use and α-blockers
Tadalafil	Oral	N, A?, V?	45-60 min	24-36 h	5-20 mg	Headache, dyspepsia, flushing, rhinitis; contraindicated with nitrate use and α-blockers
Avanafil	Oral	N, A?, V?	30 min		100 mg	Headache, flushing, prolonged erection; contraindicated with nitrate use and α-blockers
Vacuum device	External	P, N, V, A?	<5 min	30 min	—	Petechiae, bruising, painful ejaculation
Papaverine	Intracavernosal	N, A?, V?	10 min	30-60 min	15-60 mg	Prolonged erection, fibrosis, ecchymosis
Alprostadil	Intracavernosal	N, A?, V?	10 min	40-60 min	5-20 mcg	Prolonged erection, pain, fibrosis
Phentolamine	Intracavernosal	N, A?, V?	10 min	30-60 min	0.5-1 mg	Prolonged erection, fibrosis, headache, facial flushing
Medicated urethral system for erection (MUSE)	Intraurethral	N, A?, V?	10-15 min	60-80 min	250-1000 mcg	Penile pain or burning, hypotension
Penile prosthesis	Surgical	N, A, V		Replacement in 5-10 years	—	Infection, erosion, mechanical failure
Sex therapy	Counseling	P	weeks	years	weekly	Anxiety

A, arteriogenic; *N,* neurogenic; *P,* psychogenic; *V,* venogenic.

medications, because the combination can produce fatal hypotension. In addition, combined use of α-blockers with phosphodiesterase inhibitors should be done with caution, starting with the lowest dose; hypotension may occur with higher doses. All phosphodiesterase inhibitors result in sufficient penile rigidity for an approximately 50% success rate. Because of the longer duration of action of tadalafil, men tend to select it when given the choice (Level of Evidence B).[25] Daily dosing regimens have gained Food and Drug Administration (FDA) approval for select phosphodiesterase inhibitors. The higher cost of daily dosing and the rapid onset of as-needed dosing suggest that as-needed dosing would be preferable for most patients.

Vacuum tumescence devices are another option. This consists of a plastic cylinder with an open end into which the penis is inserted. A vacuum device attached to the cylinder creates negative pressure causing blood to flow into the penis to produce penile rigidity. A penile constriction ring placed at the base of the penis then traps the blood in the corpora cavernosa to maintain an erection. The vacuum device is effective for psychogenic, neurogenic, and venogenic ED, but it requires a lot of manual dexterity. Local pain, swelling, bruising, and painful ejaculation are adverse events. It is important to remove the constriction ring after 30 minutes.

> **Type-5 phosphodiesterase inhibitors are now first-line therapy for ED. Combined use of α-blockers with phosphodiesterase inhibitors should be done with caution, starting with the lowest dose; hypotension may occur with higher doses.**

Intracavernous injection of drugs such as papaverine, phentolamine, and alprostadil are effective in producing erections (Level of Evidence A)[26] but are used much less frequently since oral therapy has become available. Alprostadil, the only agent approved by the FDA for intracavernosal injection, produces erections that last 40 to 60 minutes. Intracavernosal therapy should be reserved for patients in whom oral therapy with a phosphodiesterase inhibitor is not effective. Alprostadil can also be administered intra-urethrally using a medicated urethral system for erection (MUSE). This system contains a small pellet of alprostadil that is placed within the urethra and is rapidly absorbed through the urethral mucosa to produce an erection within 10 to 15 minutes. Possible adverse events are penile pain, urethral burning, and a throbbing sensation in the perineum.

Testosterone supplementation increases libido and can improve ED in men with hypogonadism (Level of Evidence B). It is available as an intramuscular injection (testosterone enanthate or cypionate) or transdermal patch and gel. Possible adverse events associated with testosterone include polycythemia, prostate enlargement, and fluid retention. It is important to obtain a baseline prostate-specific antigen level before beginning therapy. If prostate-specific antigen or hematocrit increases with testosterone therapy, it usually does so within the first 6 months. Therefore, these levels should be checked every 3 months during the first year of therapy.

Surgical implantation of a penile prosthesis is an option, but is rarely done since the introduction of alprostadil and, more recently, phosphodiesterase inhibitors. Nevertheless, long-term patient satisfaction with penile prosthesis is actually higher than with oral therapy (Level of Evidence B).[27] Penile revascularization surgery has limited success.

Men with psychogenic ED should be referred to a mental health or other professional specializing in treatment of sexual disorders for further evaluation and treatment.

CASE 1

Discussion

You refer Mr. Johnson to a counselor for his "widower's syndrome." You also stop amitriptyline (started after his wife's death) to decrease the anticholinergic burden, and change his antihypertensive from hydrochlorothiazide to lisinopril. The patient reports a return of erectile rigidity with masturbation. To provide additional assurance for his honeymoon, you offer a prescription for sildenafil 50 mg to be taken by mouth 1 hour before sexual activity if he finds that he needs it. ▫

FEMALE SEXUALITY: DEFINITION AND EPIDEMIOLOGY

As women age and go through menopause, there is decreased sexual interest, responsiveness, and intercourse frequency.[28,29] In addition, there is an increase in urogenital symptoms, such as difficulty with lubrication (44%), inability to climax (38%), lack of pleasure during sex (25%), and pain during intercourse (12%).[30]

CASE 2

Gloria Dean (Part 1)

Gloria Dean, a 70-year-old woman, is seen in your office for an annual examination. During your review of systems, she admits to a lack of sexual interest. For several years intercourse has been painful and she has been unable to achieve orgasm. Past medical history includes hypertension, hyperlipidemia, seasonal allergies, overactive bladder, and recurrent urinary tract infections. She takes lisinopril, simvastatin, cetirizine, and solifenacin. She is not on hormone replacement therapy. She had a hysterectomy with oophorectomy at age 39.

1. **Are there additional elements in the history that will be helpful in making a diagnosis?**

2. **What other steps will be essential in identifying the etiology of Mrs. Dean's problem?** ■

EVALUATION AND TREATMENT

> Many older women have sexual dysfunction but do not report it to their primary care provider unless asked.

Dyspareunia (pain with intercourse) can result from postmenopausal atrophic vaginitis as a consequence of estrogen deficiency. With each subsequent encounter the woman with this condition anticipates pain, causing inadequate arousal with decreased lubrication. Other causes of dyspareunia include vaginal infection, cystitis, Bartholin cyst, uterine or vaginal prolapse, endometriosis, dermatoses (lichen simplex chronicus, lichen sclerosus, lichen planus), excessive penile thrusting, and vaginismus (involuntary contraction of the perineal and paravaginal muscles).[31] Vulvar or pelvic tumors are less common causes of dyspareunia, but important problems in themselves, the treatment of which may produce sexual dysfunction.[32]

Systemic or local estrogen therapy can improve symptoms of vulvovaginal atrophy (dyspareunia),[33,34] but estrogen therapy has little effect on libido or sexual satisfaction (Level of Evidence B).[35] Libido is thought to depend on testosterone (even in women), rather than on estrogen.[36] The ovaries and adrenals are the main sources of androgens in women.

> Systemic or local estrogens are first-line therapy for vulvovaginal atrophy, but estrogen therapy has little effect on libido or sexual satisfaction.

Many common medical conditions seen in older women may affect sexuality. Women with diabetes mellitus report decreased libido and lubrication and longer time to reach orgasm.[37] Rheumatic diseases affect sexuality via functional disability. After mastectomy for breast cancer, 20% to 40% of women[38] experience sexual dysfunction, possibly because of disruption of body image, marital and family problems, spousal reaction, adjuvant therapy, or the psychological impact of a breast cancer diagnosis. Several drugs can adversely affect sexual function, including antidepressants, antipsychotics, antiestrogens, antiandrogens, and anticholinergic drugs.[39] Psychosocial factors also have an important role in sexual dysfunction. Women live longer than men. Consequently, older women spend the last years of their lives alone. Widowhood has a major influence on the frequency of sexual activity for women, but not for men.[1] Even when a partner is available, he might have erectile dysfunction (ED). Finally, lack of privacy can be a problem when an older couple lives with their children or in a nursing home.[40,41] Therefore, medications, relationship issues,[42] the partner's health, and mood disorders are all important in the evaluation of women with sexual dysfunction, as they are in men.

CASE 2

Gloria Dean (Part 2)

On further questioning Mrs. Dean describes pain on initial penetration. You perform a general examination, which is unremarkable. Pelvic examination shows no vulvar lesions, the vaginal mucosa thin and friable with visible veins, and a poorly distensible vaginal vault. Pressure at the introitus reproduces her pain.

What are your next steps in evaluation and treatment? ■

The history is the most important part of the evaluation. Clinicians should ask about dyspareunia, lack of vaginal lubrication, and previous negative experiences, such as rape, child abuse, or domestic violence. Asking if dyspareunia occurs with initial penetration or if it occurs with deep thrusting helps to locate the pain as superficial or deep. Medications should be carefully reviewed for those potentially interfering with sexual function (Table 32-3), including the commonly prescribed antidepressants (selective serotonin reuptake inhibitors).[43]

A woman with dyspareunia should undergo a pelvic examination that includes inspection of the external genitalia for atrophy and vulvar dermatoses. After providing a careful explanation, attempt to localize the source of pain. Apply gentle pressure against the inner thighs and then the external genitalia including the vulvar vestibule in a systematic fashion in an attempt to replicate the pain. Also examine pelvic floor muscles for tenderness; the uterus and cervix, ovaries, bladder, and rectum for pathology; and note the general elasticity of the vaginal tissue.

Therapy follows identified pathology. Vulvar dermatoses generally should be biopsied to distinguish malignant or premalignant lesions from benign conditions. Benign conditions (e.g., lichen sclerosis) respond to topical steroids. Tender pelvic floor muscles are a sign of high-tone pelvic floor dysfunction and patients should be referred to physical therapists specializing in pelvic floor muscle dysfunction.

TABLE 32-3	Drugs Associated with Sexual Dysfunction in Men and Women		
Therapeutic Class	**Agent**	**Effect**	**Notes**
Acid suppressants	Cimetidine, ranitidine, famotidine	ED Loss of libido	Gynecomastia, which is rarely reported with some proton pump inhibitors
Anticonvulsants	Carbamazepine, phenytoin, phenobarbital, primidone	ED Reduced libido	Increase metabolism of androgen
Anticholinergics		Vaginal dryness	
Antidepressants	SSRIs	Reduced libido Delayed orgasm	Sildenafil may reduce this side effect in both men and women
Antihistamines		Vaginal dryness	
	Lithium	ED	
Antihypertensives	Spironolactone, centrally acting sympatholytics (e.g., clonidine)	ED Reduced libido	Any antihypertensive can reduce genital blood flow
Antipsychotics		Orgasmic dysfunction	More common with 1st generation (e.g., haloperidol) than 2nd generation (e.g., quetiapine)
Aromatase inhibitors		Vaginal dryness Arousal issues	
Lipid-lowering agents	Fibrates Statins	ED Gynecomastia	
Opioids	All	Reduced libido Anorgasmia	Reduced testosterone
Other	Alcohol Digoxin Metoclopramide	Reduced libido Gynecomastia Hyperprolactinemia	At high doses

ED, erectile disfunction; *SSRIs,* selective serotonin reuptake inhibitors.

Decreased lubrication, vaginal discomfort, itching, and dyspareunia caused by atrophic vaginitis respond well to topical estrogen therapy (Level of Evidence A).[34] Improvement of symptoms can be expected within 2 to 4 weeks. The vaginal ring (replaced every 90 days) delivers low-dose estradiol locally with lower systemic absorption and risk of adverse events than conjugated estrogen cream. The estradiol ring may be preferred over topical estrogen creams because of ease of use. When creams are prescribed, they should be at a minimum dose to avoid systemic effects. Typically patients are instructed to apply a dime-size amount to the vaginal introitus daily for 2 weeks, then two to three times per week. Topical estrogens also reduce the risk of recurrent urinary tract infection.

If the patient is not a candidate for or does not want to use topical estrogen, water-soluble vaginal lubricants (e.g., Astroglide, K-Y Jelly, Replens) are beneficial. Vaginal lubricants are also first-line treatment for women with hormone-sensitive cancers. Importantly, local stimulation through regular intercourse helps maintain a healthy vaginal mucosa. Longer foreplay allows more time for vaginal lubrication.

Decreased libido without identifiable cause may respond to testosterone, but no androgen preparation is approved by the FDA for hypoactive sexual desire disorder in women. Several placebo-controlled, randomized trials showed that a low-dose testosterone patch delivering 300 mcg used twice weekly or daily improves sexual desire in women with natural or surgical menopause and on systemic estrogens (Level of Evidence A).[44,45] Androgenic adverse events such as acne and hirsutism were uncommon. Although the testosterone patch seems effective, there are only limited data on the long-term safety of the testosterone patch in women. Phosphodiesterase-5 inhibitors have no proven benefit in treatment of disorders of sexual arousal in women (Level of Evidence A),[46,47] although they are effective for women with antidepressant-associated sexual dysfunction (Level of Evidence A).[48] Finally, older women should receive education about male sexual aging in addition to female sexual aging. Otherwise, an older woman might mistakenly attribute her partner's diminished erection and need for more genital stimulation to her own inability to arouse her partner. Other psychological issues, including depression,[49] history of sexual abuse, and relationship problems, should be addressed and treated with antidepressants, psychotherapy, and marital therapy, as necessary (Level of Evidence C).[50-52]

CASE 2

Discussion

After the examination, you discuss with Mrs. Dean the potential benefits and safety of low-dose vaginal estrogen and the option of using water-soluble lubricants. For this patient, estrogens may provide the additional benefit of reduced risk for recurrent urinary tract infections. You also provide written information to educate her and her spouse about aging and sexuality. She agrees to begin topical estrogen and to return in 2 months to have you assess her progress. ◼

SUMMARY

Normal aging is associated with decreased sexual interest and ability; however, sexual dysfunction is not normal and often has treatable causes in both men and women. Knowledge of those causes combined with a careful history and focused examination often provides a diagnosis that directs treatment without additional testing.

Web Resources

www.mayoclinic.com/health/erectile-dysfunction/DS00162. The Mayo Clinic website provides good and detailed information. (Many websites are biased or inaccurate; the reader is advised to use a critical eye and look for websites from reputable sources.)

www.nia.nih.gov/health/publication/sexuality-later-life. The National Institute on Aging offers a patient handout to help patients understand the normal and common pathologic changes in sexual function with age.

KEY REFERENCES

4. Alemozaffar M, Regan MM, Cooperberg MR, et al. Prediction of erectile function following treatment for prostate cancer. JAMA 2011;306(11):1205-14.
10. Albersen M, Orabi H, Lue TF. Evaluation and treatment of erectile dysfunction in the aging male: A mini-review. Gerontology 2012;58(1):3-14.
23. Lee M. Focus on phosphodiesterase inhibitors for the treatment of erectile dysfunction in older men. Clin Ther 2011;33(11):1590-1608.
29. Walsh KE, Berman JR. Sexual dysfunction in the older woman: An overview of the current understanding and management. Drugs Aging 2004;21(10):655-75.
33. Johnston S, Farrell S. The detection and management of vaginal atrophy. J Obstet Gynaecol Can 2004;26:503-8.

References available online at expertconsult.com.

33

Mistreatment and Neglect

Sonia R. Sehgal and Laura Mosqueda

OUTLINE

OBJECTIVES

Upon completion of this chapter, the reader will be able to:

- Know the caregiver, care recipient, and social factors associated with elder mistreatment.
- Know the different types of abuse and neglect.
- Recognize components of the history and physical examination that raise concern for possible abuse.
- Explain and overcome barriers to the identification of abuse.
- Propose initial assessment and management strategies.

Abuse and neglect of older adults is a common yet underreported problem that will be growing in scope. Although the number of older adults is increasing, the number of available trained caregivers is decreasing. This demographic trend of more vulnerable adults and fewer people to care for them combined with a national trend of decreasing social services is a harbinger of a new epidemic.

Additional online-only material indicated by icon.

CASE 1

Doris Johnson (Part 1)

Doris Johnson is an 86-year-old woman who comes to your office for a routine visit. She has been living in her own home by herself since her husband died 12 years ago. Although she has Parkinson's disease, diabetes, and hypertension, she has remained independent. Over the past year, she has had some decline in her function and requires meals-on-wheels and other services to remain at home. Her daughter Betsy recently moved from another state to live with Ms. Johnson and provide assistance.

The physical examination reveals a pleasant woman who has a moderate amount of tremor at rest and who ambulates slowly with the aid of a walker. You notice that Ms. Johnson seems withdrawn during this visit, and she tells you that it has been difficult to adjust to having a new person in the house even though she knows she needs help to stay there. Ms. Johnson's next visit is an urgent appointment because she fell and has multiple large bruises on her upper arms and forehead. Betsy brings her to see you and reports, "I just found Mom on the floor this morning." Ms. Johnson nods in agreement but says little else. No medical treatment is needed and she goes home. Three weeks later another urgent appointment is made: Ms. Johnson has a dislocated shoulder and bruises on her upper chest wall. Again, her daughter reports that Ms. Johnson fell. In spite of Betsy's protests, you ask her to leave the exam room so that you may speak privately with Ms. Johnson. When you ask Ms. Johnson what happened, she breaks down in tears and reports that her daughter has been taking her money for years. You discover that Betsy moved in because she had no other place to live but promised that she would care for her mother in exchange for room and board. Once she was living there, Betsy asked her mother to sign over bank accounts. Initially, Betsy "just yelled at me and threatened to put me in a nursing home. But over the past month, Betsy became more aggressive and pushed me down several times. Last night she grabbed me and punched me because I would not sign the house over to her. I'm so ashamed.... I never thought my own daughter would do this to me."

1. **Did you notice anything at the first visit that may have led you to worry about the possibility of abuse?**

2. **Do you think Ms. Johnson would have told you what happened if Betsy had been in the room?**

Translating the definition of abuse (Box 33-1) to a diagnosis of abuse is not easy nor is it straightforward: It is often difficult to distinguish between injuries that

ELDER MISTREATMENT: DEFINITION

- Intentional actions that cause harm or create a serious risk of harm (whether or not harm is intended) to a vulnerable elder by a caregiver or other person who stands in a trust relationship to the elder.
- Failure by a caregiver to satisfy the elder's basic needs to protect the elder from harm.

From Bonnie R, Wallace R. Elder mistreatment: Abuse, neglect and exploitation in an aging America. Washington, DC: National Academy Press; 2003.

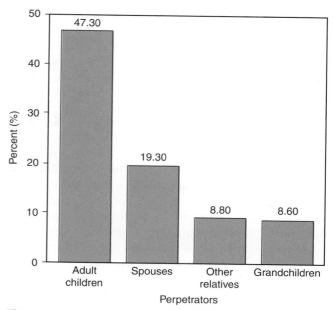

Figure 33-1 Breakdown of suspected perpetrators of elder abuse. Note: Only 16% of perpetrators are nonfamily members. (Adapted from National Center on Elder Abuse. National Elder Abuse Incidence Study: Final report. Washington, DC: Department of Health and Human Services Administration for Children and Families and Administration on Aging; September 1998.)

occur through innocent mechanisms (e.g., tripping and falling) and those that occur as a result of abuse (e.g., being punched). Although some acts of commission or omission are blatantly abusive, there is no simple method to tell when some acts, such as poor care, cross the line to become abuse. However, this does not excuse the need to make a diagnosis at the earliest possible time. Primary care providers are in a unique position to prevent, recognize, and respond to mistreatment. They are often the first to identify both victim and perpetrator and, therefore, must be mindful of the possibility of abuse as well as be able to respond to its occurrence. Physicians are among the least likely to report suspicion of abuse to Adult Protective Services (APS).[2]

> Clinicians in primary care are in a unique position to prevent, recognize, and respond to abuse. However, health care professionals, particularly physicians, are among the least likely to report suspected abuse to Adult Protective Services.

INCIDENCE AND IMPACT

Best estimates suggest that between 1 and 2 million Americans age 65 and older have been the victim of elder mistreatment or neglect by a caregiver.[1] Only 1 in 24 cases is reported to local authorities for intervention.[3] Several studies have evaluated the prevalence of specific forms of elder mistreatment in community-dwelling older adults. The National Elder Mistreatment Study published in 2010 projected the prevalence of emotional mistreatment at 4.6%, physical mistreatment at 1.6%, sexual mistreatment at 0.6%, and financial abuse at 5.2% per year.[4] Prevalence of verbal mistreatment has been found to be as high as 9%.[5] Contrary to popularly held perceptions, family members, particularly adult children and spouses, are the most common perpetrators of abusive acts (Figure 33-1).[2] Unfortunately, victims of abuse face increased mortality rates as compared to unabused

patients.[6] When all other risk factors are taken into account, elder abuse by itself imposes a threefold increase in the risk of death of community-dwelling older adults.[7] These patients have more psychiatric and physical disorders manifested by increased numbers of hospitalizations and emergency department visits. With increased life expectancy, it is projected that the older adult population will almost double in size to 20% of the U.S. population by 2030.[8] The pool of potential victims is growing at a rapid rate.

CASE 1

Discussion

As primary care provider for Ms. Johnson, you correctly evaluated her. You were observant, noting that the patient was withdrawn and that the bruises were in unusual locations for a fall; you had the daughter leave the room so that Ms. Johnson could tell her story; you were reassuring but direct in asking Ms. Johnson what happened. This case illustrates the common finding that victims of abuse are often subjected to multiple types of mistreatment over a prolonged period of time. As is quite common in elder mistreatment, Ms. Johnson experienced financial, psychological, and physical abuse for many years. ◙

> The primary care clinician is in an excellent position to prevent abuse if warning signs are recognized. Although caregiver stress may trigger abuse, it is not an excuse for abuse.

RISK FACTORS AND PATHOPHYSIOLOGY

Risk factor assessment is important to identify potential elder mistreatment victims and initiate treatment. Risk factors are found in the victim, perpetrator, and sociocultural environment in which they are embedded (Box 33-2). Dementia is a known risk factor for mistreatment. In a study published in 2010, 47% of patients with dementia were found to be mistreated by their caregiver. Associated factors thought to increase the risk of abuse in people with dementia include caregiver depression, anxiety, and perceived burden of care; and care recipients with physically aggressive behaviors. This study found that when asked, caregivers of patients with dementia will acknowledge abuse.[9] Alcohol and/or drug abuse among perpetrators of elder mistreatment is also common.[10] Furthermore, several studies have demonstrated that perpetrators are more likely to be dependent on the victim they are mistreating. Additional risk factors for elder mistreatment include advanced age (80 years and older), physical or mental disability, and depression.

> Simply having a dementing illness places a person at increased risk for mistreatment, particularly if the person with dementia displays disruptive behavior.

CASE 2

Alan Greenwood (Part 1)

Alan Greenwood, age 84, has been your patient for many years. You diagnosed him with Alzheimer's disease 3 years ago, and lately he has been quite agitated. He requires assistance with some activities of daily living but he gets upset when his daughter Camille tries to help. He also follows her around the house and asks her the same questions repeatedly.

Camille brings him in for his appointments, and it is clear that she is unhappy and resentful. You ask how she is doing with her dad; she tells you "My father was never around when I was growing up. Now that he needs help he has come back into my life and is ruining it! I can't spend the time I want to with my own kids, and my husband is getting annoyed because the house isn't as organized as I used to have it." You smell alcohol on her breath when she was telling this to you. Although you have seen no evidence of abuse, you recognize that the potential exists.

1. **What interventions might you implement to help calm this situation?**
2. **What issues might you discuss with Camille during this office visit?** ▣

BOX 33-2

RISK FACTORS FOR ELDER MISTREATMENT

Victim
- Advanced age
- Dependent for basic activities of daily living
- Dementia
- Combative behavior

Perpetrator
- Depression/mental illness
- Alcohol or drug dependence
- Financial dependence

DIFFERENTIAL DIAGNOSIS AND ASSESSMENT

Barriers to Diagnosis

Given the complexity of elder mistreatment cases and the short length of most outpatient visits, detecting, questioning, and confronting issues of abuse and neglect can be daunting. However, the primary care provider may be the only person with adequate contact to suspect and protect when abuse is present. Often the primary care provider is uncertain as to what constitutes abuse. Few training programs have dedicated instruction on the detection and management of elder mistreatment. Bruises and fractures can be clues to incidents of abuse, but these also commonly occur among frail older adults as a result of falls or injury to delicate tissues. Medical personnel may attribute the injury to "old age" rather than mistreatment.

Cognitive impairment may interfere with a person's ability to disclose abuse or understand that abuse has occurred. People with dementia or depression are often dependent on their abuser for essential daily activities and socially isolated from third-party observers who may detect mistreatment.

Alternatively, cognizant victims often hesitate disclosing details of the abuse sustained or abuser. Many feel ashamed and embarrassed that the abuse occurred or that it was inflicted by a trusted loved one. In addition, fear of nursing home placement may cause the older adult victim to hesitate reporting abuse inflicted by an in-home caregiver. Many elders would rather be abused than be taken out of their home. Many older adult victims are depressed and find it difficult to confront their abuser or voice concerns to a health care provider.

In children, retinal hemorrhages and long bone fractures make up a constellation of findings that would trigger an immediate suspicion of abuse. Unfortunately, such pathognomonic findings do not exist for abuse of an older adult. Awareness, suspicion, and a comprehensive assessment are required to detect elder mistreatment. If it is not on our differential, we will fail to make the diagnosis.

CASE 2

Discussion

Camille and her father historically have had a strained relationship. He is now ill, forgetful, and resistant to care. She feels overwhelmed, angry, may be abusing alcohol, and her family is pressuring her to spend more time with them. Because you have recognized these as red flags for possible abuse (see Box 33-2), you intervene to prevent this situation from escalating. You ask Camille if she has ever hurt her father, and she tells you that she has not but that she is worried she might hit him when she gets upset and feels out of control. After empathizing with her situation and thanking her for her honesty, you explain how you will help her: You give Camille information about adult day care programs close to her home, support groups through the Alzheimer's Association, books on Alzheimer's disease, an appointment with a counselor, and information on assisted living facilities specializing in caring for people who have dementia and providing respite care. You have them follow up with you in 1 week. As a result of your efforts, Mr. Greenwood starts attending the day care program 3 days a week, Camille understands more about the illness her father has, and she gets appropriate emotional support. When you see them again several months later, both Mr. Greenwood and his daughter are calmer and happier. ■

> Elder abuse should be included on the differential diagnosis list of many common conditions.

Assessment

Abuse can span many years or occur as a one-time, isolated incident. If a medical provider suspects abuse it is prudent to make a report to local authorities. Cases of abuse and neglect may be found during a routine visit at a primary care provider's office or a regular visit to a long-term care facility. A thorough evaluation is required for patients suspected to be victims of abuse. The patient should be examined alone, away from family members and/or other caregivers, because the victim may be embarrassed or may fear retaliation.[10] Direct questioning by the primary care provider in a caring, nonthreatening manner should be conducted. Home environment and safety issues should be evaluated. Information regarding inciting factors, frequency, and type of abuse should be elicited. Factors suggestive of abuse include a delay in seeking treatment, confusing or unlikely causes of injury, or a past history of suspicious incidents.[11] A history of "doctor shopping"

and caregiver avoidance of appointments should also raise suspicions of abuse.[12]

A complete physical examination should be performed on all patients suspected of being abused (Box 33-3). A full skin assessment is undertaken. Areas hidden from plain sight are examined, including soles of feet, inner thighs, axillae, and palms, with all areas of bruising, burns, tenderness, or abrasions documented. Weight loss, hygiene, and a history of fractures are noted. Sexual abuse cannot be overlooked and a gynecologic evaluation may be necessary. Assessment of patients suspected of being abused warrants not only a physical but also a cognitive evaluation. Cognitive impairment as well as visual or auditory deficits can make an already challenging evaluation that much more difficult.

Care providers should be asked about their level of stress and their ability to function in the role of caregiver. Financial difficulties, anger, and resentment toward the patient should also be assessed. Caregiver burnout should be suspected when primary caregivers begin to complain about the patient and blame the patient for situations that are out of the patient's control.[13]

Confirmatory laboratory testing can be done to corroborate unusual findings. A complete blood count, blood urea nitrogen, creatinine, total protein, and albumin levels can help establish whether dehydration or malnutrition is present. Radiographs depicting old and new fractures can help suggest patterns of long-term abuse.

Contextual factors are often as important as the injury itself. For example, if a person has a stage IV pressure ulcer of his coccyx, the health care provider may know that this person is in hospice care, and that all appropriate steps are being taken to prevent and treat skin breakdown. However, if a patient who had been ambulatory and in good health 2 months prior suddenly appears in the office with the same wound,

---

BOX 33-3

POSSIBLE ABUSE INDICATORS

- Weight loss
- Dehydration
- Poor hygiene/elongated toenails
- Depression
- Inappropriate attire (e.g., not dressed warmly in cold weather)
- Abrasions/lacerations
- Hematomas
- Traumatic alopecia
- Bruises in unusual locations (e.g., breasts/genital area)
- Welts
- Burns
- Pressure ulcers
- Rectal/vaginal bleeding
- Signs of sexually transmitted diseases

this is an unexpected finding that deserves careful questioning.

> Factors suggestive of abuse include a delay in seeking treatment, confusing or unlikely causes of injury, or a past history of suspicious incidents.

CARE

When elder mistreatment is suspected, the first step in evaluating abuse is an open conversation with the patient. It is important to establish a safe and private setting in which to conduct the interview. Patients cognizant of their circumstances can often take an active role in future care planning. For those patients who may be unable to fully understand or participate in decision making, a multidisciplinary team consisting of social workers, physicians, and legal counsel is available in many communities to assist with difficult management issues.

Health care workers are mandated reporters of elder mistreatment and neglect in almost all states. The definitions and elder mistreatment reporting requirements vary from region to region. It is important for medical providers to be familiar with the laws in their area. APS is the agency responsible for taking and investigating reports of abuse in community-dwelling older adults. In some states, APS also investigates abuse in licensed facilities; in other states this is done by the state ombudsman. Police should be contacted in addition to APS in emergent situations. It is not a violation of the Health Insurance Portability and Accountability Act to share medical information with police or APS when abuse is suspected.[14]

Careful documentation of physical findings, such as bruises or abrasions, is important. Photographs should be taken of unusual skin findings with a reference object in the visual field for an estimation of size. All lesions should have accurate documentation of their dimensions and locations. Diagrams are also helpful in charting locations of skin lesions. Areas of pain or tenderness should be noted. All facets of the history and physical examination can be entered as evidence if a case goes to trial, a rare but important event. For this reason, records should be legible and complete. Objective information should be recorded, including statements made by both the victim and perpetrator.

PREVENTION AND EARLY DETECTION

Most primary care providers and emergency room personnel do not routinely screen for elder abuse. In 1992 the American Medical Association encouraged physicians to "incorporate routine questions related to

elder abuse and neglect into daily practice."[15] Although current screening tools are limited—several of them require accurate responses from victims who may be cognitively or emotionally impaired, as well as from their caregivers—providers can ask: "Are you afraid of anyone? Has anyone threatened you or harmed you?"

Prevention strategies should be employed during routine medical visits. At each visit, both the caregiver and patient should be questioned regarding stress in the living environment and observed for signs of feeling overwhelmed or discouraged. Respite services should be readily offered. Senior centers, adult day health care services, and other community programs may offer the caregiver and patient much-needed time away from each other.

> Even under the best of circumstances (loving family, adequate resources), abuse can happen to anyone by anyone.

SUMMARY

Elder mistreatment is a national tragedy that has a serious impact on the health and happiness of elders and those who love them. Victims suffer from more illness and premature death as compared to unharmed patients. A reasonable suspicion, identification of risk factors, and a multidisciplinary team approach will help victims and abusers obtain the treatment they need.

Web Resources

www.ncea.aoa.gov. National Center on Elder Abuse.
www.preventelderabuse.org. National Committee for the Prevention of Elder Abuse.

KEY REFERENCES

1. Bonnie R, Wallace R. Elder mistreatment: Abuse, neglect and exploitation in an aging America. Washington, DC: National Academy Press; 2003.
4. Acierno R, Hernandez MA, Amstadter AB, et al. Prevalence and correlates of emotional, physical, sexual, and financial abuse and potential neglect in the United States: The National Elder Mistreatment Study. Am J Public Health 2010;100:292-7.
15. American Medical Association (AMA). American Medical Association diagnostic and treatment guidelines on elder abuse and neglect. Chicago: AMA; 1992.

References available online at expertconsult.com.

34

Alcoholism

James W. Campbell, Barbara Resnick, and Gregg A. Warshaw

OBJECTIVES

Upon completion of this chapter, the reader will be able to:

- Identify risk factors and diagnostic criteria for alcoholism in older persons.
- Discuss screening instruments and laboratory tests used in the diagnosis of alcoholism and the effects of aging on their clinical use.
- Describe the mechanisms of initiating treatment and the types of treatment available.
- Discuss the relationship of alcohol dependency to other common syndromes of old age: dementia, depression, suicide, polypharmacy, falls, and multiple medical illnesses.

Additional online-only material indicated by icon.

PREVALENCE AND IMPACT

The diagnosis of alcoholism is often missed in older patients. Many of the classic clues are mistaken for age-related changes or diseases. The psychosocial factors that are often pivotal in moving younger alcoholics into treatment (spouse, job, and legal pressures such as being charged with driving while intoxicated) are less likely to occur in older adults. Age-associated pharmacokinetic changes make the quantity of ethanol used a less reliable indicator of problems, falsely reassuring the health care professional. Moreover, diagnosis, prognosis, and treatment are complicated by comorbid conditions commonly found in older adults. Clinicians must be alert to the significance of features such as falling, incontinence, poor social support, cognitive decline, depression, noncompliance, and others.

Alcoholism is difficult to diagnose, and yet can be successfully treated in older adults. Treatment modalities may be different than those used with younger individuals.

CASE 1

James Beem (Part 1)

James Beem is a 79-year-old seat-belted driver involved in a car crash. He has suffered a femur fracture, unilateral rib fractures, and a laceration of the left arm. He has been stabilized in the trauma bay and is currently in the surgical intensive care unit for monitoring. You have been asked to consult on hospital day 2 regarding his mental status (Mini-Mental State Exam [MMSE] 17/30) and hypertension (blood pressure 202/106 mmHg, pulse 96). He has a past history of hypertension, glaucoma, cataracts, and hyperlipidemia.

1. **Which of the many completed laboratory investigations do you seek first?**

2. **A family member is waiting to see you. What questions will you ask first?** □

Definition

Alcohol dependency is a medical syndrome. This is most important. It determines the types of treatment and professional responsibility for care. Early in the twentieth century, alcoholism was defined in moralistic terms: treatment involved condemnation and punishment, and was in the scope of the religious and criminal justice systems. Although Benjamin Rush launched a health education campaign that warned the public about the hazards of alcoholic beverages in the early nineteenth century, it was not until the rise of Alcoholics Anonymous (AA) in the 1930s and the recognition of AA in 1956 by the American Medical Association that alcohol dependency became clearly categorized as a disease.[1] Alcoholism was thus moved from the legal system and placed in the purview of public health. The medical community then developed diagnostic criteria and prevalence and natural history data, and screening and treatment modalities were defined.

In 1975 the World Health Organization defined the drinking behaviors characteristic of alcohol-dependence syndrome: drink-seeking behaviors, increased tolerance of alcohol, repeated withdrawal symptoms, repeated relief or avoidance of withdrawal symptoms by further drinking, subjective awareness of a compulsion to drink, and reinstatement of the syndrome after abstinence.[2] In this chapter the terms *alcoholism*, *alcohol dependence*, and *alcohol addiction* are used synonymously. These terms imply development of tolerance, withdrawal reactions, loss of control of alcohol use, and psychosocial decline.[3]

A practical classification scheme for elderly alcoholics identifies four patterns: (1) chronic, (2) intermittent, (3) late onset, and (4) reactive.[4] Reactive alcoholism, implying impaired use after psychosocial stressors, has not been a clinically useful term. Many individuals categorized as "reactive" alcoholics, with further investigation, are found to have a prior significant history of alcohol use. Although some studies simply distinguished late from early onset in terms of the four-part classification, chronic and intermittent alcoholism are almost always early onset, and reactive may be either late or early onset because the drinking is in response to a biopsychosocial stress. Two thirds of older alcoholics fall in the chronic or intermittent class, and one third are true late onset.[5]

Current (past month) use of alcohol is defined as at least one drink in the past 30 days. Binge use is five or more drinks on the same occasion (i.e., at the same time or within a couple of hours of each other) on at least 1 day in the past 30 days. Recent studies have emphasized the negative effects of binge use.[6] Heavy use of alcohol refers to five or more drinks on the same occasion on each of 5 or more days in the past 30 days.[7]

> Only one third of elderly alcoholics can truly be categorized as "late onset."

Prevalence

Of the elderly, 5% to 10% are heavy alcohol users. It is estimated that there are a half million elderly alcoholics in the United States.[5] Alcoholism is the third most prevalent psychiatric disorder among elderly men (15%), surpassed only by dementia and anxiety disorders.[8] Elderly alcoholics often present to the health care system through associated diagnoses.[9] Older persons hospitalized for general medical and surgical procedures and institutionalized elderly demonstrate a prevalence of approximately 18% of

alcohol abuse.[3] One third of older alcoholics are estimated to have begun their alcohol abuse after age 65.[5] The binge drinking rate for older adults is still substantial despite being lower than it was in 2009, when it was 9.8%.[7] Being female, older, college educated, and African American were associated with a lower risk of being a heavy or binge drinker. Conversely, having depression, being a current smoker, and having an alcoholic parent were associated with increased risk of being a heavy or binge drinker.[10] Retirement is not consistently a contributor to heavy or binge drinking behavior.[11]

The older alcoholic is likely to drink only five to six times per week and only four to five drinks per occasion,[12] yet ethanol has greater pharmacologic impact as we age. Ethanol absorption does not change with increasing age. However, at an unchanged rate of ethanol intake, peak blood concentration is on average higher in the elderly. This is a result of the smaller volume of distribution. Ethanol is distributed in body water, which is decreased in elderly persons.[4]

The rate of illicit drug use continues to be quite low (1%) among older adults, and decreases with increasing age.[7] The alcohol-dependent elderly patient is unlikely to be cross-addicted to other illicit drugs; however, the possibility of misuse of prescription medications must be considered. Misuse of prescription medications is estimated to occur in more than 10% of elders.

Table 34-1 summarizes the factors contributing to the low reported rates of alcoholism and to the increased impact of drinking in old age. Many of these factors arise from society's unwillingness to label older persons as alcoholics because of the continued stigma. The mistaken thought that older alcoholics are untreatable is prevalent and therapeutic nihilism reduces detection. In addition, health care providers do not frequently consider alcohol as a possible comorbid condition in patients presenting to the clinic or acute care setting with a clinical problem (e.g., uncontrolled hypertension, increased confusion, nausea).

> The mistaken thought that older alcoholics are untreatable is prevalent and reduces detection.

Impact of Alcohol Use

Moderate alcohol use (one or more drinks per day) is associated with gastritis, stomach ulcers, and liver and pancreatic problems. Heavier drinking (two or more drinks per day) is associated with depression, gout, gastroesophageal reflux disease, breast cancer, insomnia, cognitive problems, and falling. Excessive drinking (three or more drinks per day) is associated with hypertension, hemorrhagic stroke, and several other cancers. In some epidemiologic studies, moderate alcohol use among older adults is associated with some

TABLE 34-1	Factors Affecting Reported Rate and Impact of Alcoholism		
Age-Related Factors	**Other Factors Causing Low Reported Rates**	**Other Factors Increasing Impact**	
Increased biologic sensitivity (lower body water ratio, less efficient liver)	Institutionalized people excluded from community surveys	Institutionalized people not being diagnosed or treated	
Underdiagnosis by health care providers	Less overall driving, so less driving while intoxicated	Coexisting conditions limit sensory input while driving	
Cohort values and underreporting	Cognitive impairment	Increased concomitant disease	
Less socialization and less awareness by peers of drinking behaviors	Spontaneous remission	Increased prescription and nonprescription drug use	
Less job or legal pressure to initiate treatment	Selective survival		
Family unwillingness to report	Ill health Financial constraints		

potential benefits including reduction in cardiovascular disease, diabetes, and dementia, as well as a reduction in all-cause mortality.[13-15]

RISK FACTORS AND PATHOPHYSIOLOGY

Etiology

Alcoholism is best understood as a medical condition. In the past, attempts to treat alcoholism in a moral mode or in a model of a personality disorder have been unsuccessful. The medical model removes patient blame and enables patients to be more participatory in recovery.

Evidence suggests that alcoholism is an inherited tendency: an increased number of direct relatives of alcoholic individuals have the disease. The genetic nature of the disease helps patients and families to understand and accept the diagnosis and allows them to be more active in their recovery. Ingestion of alcohol triggers the genetic tendency. There is increased endorphin production in response to alcohol intake; this is consistent with the model of the unified theory of addiction. The full illness manifests as the inability to practice controlled usage. Approximately 8% of the American population is unable to ingest alcohol in a controlled-use, "social" pattern. Genetic predisposition is estimated to account for 40% to 60% of patients with alcoholism.[16]

Changes in body fat to water ratio alter the pharmacokinetics of alcohol consumption in the elderly. Clearance is decreased as a result of decreased liver blood flow and the decrease in liver mass, which results in higher blood alcohol concentration with similar alcohol ingestion. The same quantity of ingested alcohol in an older person leads to a higher blood alcohol concentration than it does in a younger person, because alcohol is water soluble and body water is relatively reduced in the elderly. These changes explain the paradox that older people appear to be drinking the same amount and yet are experiencing more negative effects from the alcohol.

Specific late-life and life history factors can identify older adults at risk for future excessive alcohol consumption. In one study, middle-aged adults who had more friends who approved of drinking, used alcohol to relieve anxiety and tension, and were better off financially were more likely to engage in high-risk alcohol consumption. Also, drinking problems by age 50 were associated with late-life alcohol abuse. Middle-aged adults who had attempted to cut back on their alcohol use or had participated in Alcoholics Anonymous were at less risk of late-life alcohol problems.[17]

DIFFERENTIAL DIAGNOSIS AND ASSESSMENT

Screening and Detection

Screening questionnaires have been shown to differentiate people suffering from alcoholism from people who are not, although such screening tests are less sensitive in older persons. Such questionnaires cover the quantity consumed, alcohol-related social or legal difficulties, alcohol-related health problems, symptoms of drunkenness or dependence, and self-recognition.[18,19] Certain questions on the CAGE (the name is an acronym formed from its four items) questionnaire[14,20] and the Michigan Alcoholism Screening Test (MAST)[15,16] are significantly less likely to be answered in the affirmative if the subjects are elderly.

The shorter 24-item MAST-G (Geriatric MAST) test is age-appropriate and therefore widely used.[21] An even shorter version (S-MAST-G, Figure 34-1) has been developed for use in busy practices.[22] A systematic office assessment flow for alcoholism is summarized in Figure 34-2. The Alcohol Use Disorders

	Yes (1)	No (0)
1. When talking with others, do you ever underestimate how much you drink?		
2. After a few drinks, have you sometimes not eaten, or been able to skip a meal, because you didn't feel hungry?		
3. Does having a few drinks help decrease your shakiness or tremors?		
4. Does alcohol sometimes make it hard for you to remember parts of the day or night?		
5. Do you usually take a drink to relax or calm your nerves?		
6. Do you drink to take your mind off your problems?		
7. Have you ever increased your drinking after experiencing a loss in your life?		
8. Has a doctor or nurse ever said they were worried or concerned about your drinking?		
9. Have you ever made rules to manage your drinking?		
10. When you feel lonely, does having a drink help?		
TOTAL S-MAST-G SCORE (1–10)		
SCORING: 2 or more "YES" responses indicate an alcohol problem.		

Figure 34-1 Short Michigan Alcoholism Screening Test–Geriatric Version (S-MAST-G). (Redrawn from The Regents of the University of Michigan. Ann Arbor: University of Michigan Alcohol Research Center; 1991. Selzer ML, Vinokur A, Van Rooijen L, A self-administered short Michigan Alcoholism Screening Test (S-MAST), Journal of Studies on Alcohol, 1975 36: 117-126.)

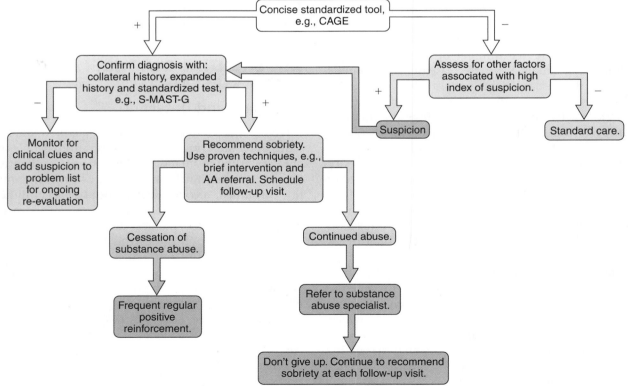

Figure 34-2 Flow diagram for alcoholism evaluation in context of new patient assessment or clinical suspicion. CAGE = Four screening questions (> = 2 Yes responses is positive screen): C (needed to **C**ut down on drinking); A (people **A**nnoyed you by criticizing drinking); G (felt **G**uilty about drinking); E (needed **E**ye-opener in morning). AA, Alcoholics Anonymous.

Identification Test (AUDIT) has also been developed with corrected scores to improve screening efficacy among older adults.[23]

A number of clinical clues to alcoholism that are often misinterpreted in elders are summarized in Box 34-1. The genetic component of alcoholism renders the family history especially significant. The most helpful clinical clue to the presence of alcoholism in an elderly person is often the presence of the disease in a child or grandchild. Families whose rituals and behaviors became distorted as a result of alcoholism are more likely to transmit the disease familially.[24]

Laboratory Testing

In contrast to self-report questionnaires, clinical laboratory procedures provide objective evidence of problem drinking. When alcohol-abuse problems are suspected in older adults, the most useful laboratory tests are gamma-glutamyl transferase (GGT) and the mean corpuscular volume (MCV). The serum GGT is elevated in patients who use alcohol excessively. MCV also has been used as a marker of heavy alcohol consumption, although it is less sensitive than is the GGT level and should not be used alone to indicate alcohol abuse. Carbohydrate deficient transferrin (CDT) serves a role in monitoring recovery compliance, or in conjunction with the GGT, as a screening tool.[25] Four to seven drinks per day for at least 1 week can significantly elevate CDT levels in patients with alcoholism.[26] CDT seems to be useful as a first-line biological marker to confirm or disprove suspected alcohol misuse. High CDT and GGT is indicative of alcohol dependence, whereas high CDT with a GGT below normal is evidence of alcohol abuse.[27] The accuracy of these markers is affected by various factors such as nonalcoholic liver damage, use of medications or drugs, and by metabolic disorders.[28] Blood alcohol levels, although more specific, lack adequate sensitivity as a screening tool.

> The most helpful clinical clue to the presence of alcoholism in an elderly person is often the presence of the disease in a child or grandchild.

Alcoholism and Other Illnesses

When assessing a patient with suspected alcohol-abuse problems, the medical problems associated with alcoholism must be specifically sought: diseases of the esophagus, stomach, pancreas, or liver, as well as cognitive impairment, blackouts, and cerebellar dysfunction. Alcoholism has a significant effect on health; problem drinkers have poor overall health and significant mental health problems.[29]

Alcoholism is distinctly related to dementia; it is estimated that 10% of the instances of dementia in older persons are alcohol related. Cognition usually improves after treatment, but at the very least, progression can be aborted.

Depression is commonly the medical illness that is comorbid with alcohol abuse; alcohol is an easily available, nonprescription psychotropic. Although alcohol has mood-elevating effects in moderate doses,[4] it is primarily a central nervous system depressant. Among clinically depressed people, 10% to 15% use alcohol for self-medication.[30] One study found that more than 50% of patients admitted for alcoholism treatment had symptoms of depression that persisted for at least 1 year after alcohol treatment.[31] Alcohol is also associated with suicide. Similarly, factors associated with a diagnosis of depression include alcohol or substance abuse.[32]

Alcoholism has a definite relationship to falling. Interestingly, there is a significant association of hip

---

BOX 34-1

ALCOHOLISM CLINICAL CLUES MISATTRIBUTED TO OTHER CAUSES

Clues Misattributed to Common Problems of Old Age

- Dementia
- Confusion
- Memory loss
- Disorientation
- Falls
- Bruises
- Fractures
- Incontinence
- Malnutrition
- Polypharmacy
- Use of sedatives and anxiolytics
- Use of analgesics

Clues Misattributed Because of Age-Biased Views

- Treatment ineffectiveness
- Resistance to treatment
- Self-neglect
- Functional decline
- Sleep impairment
- Anxiety
- Postoperative problems

Clues Misattributed to Coexisting Diseases Common in Older Persons

- Depression
- Hypertension
- Malnutrition
- Sleep disturbances
- Chronic fatigue
- Peripheral neuropathy
- Cerebellar degeneration
- Seizures
- Sexual dysfunction
- Repeated infections
- Cardiomyopathy

fracture with heavy alcohol consumption in younger persons; after age 65 the association is less strong.[33] Hip fracture occurs at a substantially younger age among older individuals with comorbid alcoholism diagnoses.[34]

> Laboratory procedures provide objective evidence of problem drinking. The most useful laboratory tests when alcohol-abuse problems are suspected in older adults are gamma-glutamyl transferase (GGT) and mean corpuscular volume (MCV). No laboratory test has adequate sensitivity and specificity to function as a stand-alone screening tool for alcohol abuse.

CASE 1

James Beem (Part 2)

Mr. Beem was initiated on a delirium tremens protocol including close observation and as-needed lorazepam and he has not experienced withdrawal symptoms. He has been transferred from surgical intensive care to a regular floor. His tachycardia and hypertension have both improved. He reports a history of drinking. His cognition has improved, and he is resistant to the possibility that his alcohol consumption may be causing negative consequences. He insists that he drinks the same amount now as he did when he was younger.

How can you help Mr. Beem and his family understand the increase of alcohol-related symptoms in the context of stable alcohol intake? ▣

MANAGEMENT

Three significant barriers to management of elderly alcoholics have been defined: (1) physicians are less likely to identify elderly alcoholics; (2) if identified, the elderly patient is less likely to be referred for treatment; and (3) the elderly are less likely to be accepted into treatment programs.[2] The first step in treatment is recognition. One study found that the diagnosis may be missed in three out of four elderly hospital patients with alcohol dependence.[3] Management of alcoholism involves effective treatment of individuals, controlled alcohol availability and advertising, control by price and tax, as well as health and safety warning labels.[35]

Overall Treatment

Older adults who do engage in treatment to abstain from alcohol have been noted to have substantially better outcomes and are more likely to complete treatment compared with younger adults.[35,36] In one study, a multifaceted intervention in a primary care setting

was able to reduce alcohol intake in older problem drinkers. The intervention consisted of education materials, drinking diary, advice directly from the primary care provider, and telephone counseling from a health educator.[37]

No known published studies have been completed to consider the impact of alcohol cessation programs with cognitively impaired older adults. For impaired individuals it is not certain that cognitive-behavioral interventions are effective. Structured interventions, however, that remove access to alcohol and provide alternative activities can be very effective in preventing ongoing high-risk alcohol intake in these individuals.[38] This requires a strong interdisciplinary team approach and must include support from family and friends.

CASE 1

James Beem (Part 3)

Mr. Beem is resistant to referral for more in-depth alcoholism assessment.

How will you help guide him into treatment?

The family is not only helpful in making the diagnosis but is the key element of the treatment plan. In fact, using the family is the most significant advance in treatment and rehabilitation of the alcoholic patient. The effective approach to the patient and family is to avoid being judgmental and to emphasize the disease model and the need for further evaluation. It is important to initiate the treatment plan on the same day that the patient is confronted with the diagnosis. The physician can facilitate this by maintaining relationships with existing AA members who can be called upon to help. AA is appropriate for older patients; one third of AA members are older than age 50. The treatment plan must include family and friends. Legal commitment is occasionally necessary; recovery rates for such patients approximate those for persons who seek help voluntarily.[39] Recent evidence demonstrates that older persons respond to brief interventions in the primary care office with positive net results for such patients.[40]

The essential principle of treatment is abstinence; controlled drinking is not recommended unless this is done in very rigidly controlled environments in which the alcohol is dosed as any other pharmaceutical intervention would be dosed. Many successful modalities redirect the dependency from the alcohol onto others: "Replace drinking with people." Group therapy is the choice in most situations, including settings involving the elderly. Therapy may require more time in elders. Late- and early-onset alcoholism do not appear to differ substantially in terms of treatment outcomes. ▣

Detoxification

Initial treatment may require hospitalization for control of drinking or detoxification.[41] Adverse functional and cognitive complications during alcohol withdrawal occur more frequently in elderly patients. Delirium tremens is a significant disease with a known mortality and may occur in older adults. Standard screening tools for withdrawal symptoms are available for use in hospital settings (see Chapter 10).

Self-Help

Self-help groups for family members (Al-Anon for spouses, Alateen for children, and ACOA for adult children of alcoholics) are important because a family-centered approach is universally recommended.

Medications

Pharmacologic treatments have not traditionally played a major role in the long-term treatment of older alcohol-dependent adults. Until recently disulfiram (Antabuse) was the only medication approved for the treatment of alcoholism, but it was seldom used in older patients because of concerns about cardiovascular adverse effects from acetaldehyde toxicity. In 1995 the opioid antagonist naltrexone (Revia) was approved by the U.S. Food and Drug Administration for the treatment of alcoholism and was found to be safe and effective in preventing relapse and reducing the craving for alcohol in older adults.[42-44] Acamprosate (Campral), which was approved for the treatment of alcohol abuse in 2004, has likewise been used effectively with older adults.

Treatment Efficacy

Evidence of effectiveness of alcohol treatment includes data from alcoholism treatment facilities that indicate that patients who seek or achieve reduced or moderate drinking tend to have consumed less alcohol, have fewer lifetime alcohol problems, and be more socially stable. Successful community-dwelling abstainers reported more drink-related problems and higher consumption than facility-based abstainers. They were also more likely to drink in order to reduce the negative effects of the alcoholism itself, whereas other drinkers drank for psychosocial reasons during evenings out and in family settings.[45] Thus, current debate focuses on the value of an elderly-specific treatment milieu. Advantages could include the management of associated medical problems.

It is often thought that older alcoholics are more resistant to treatment; however, using 6 months of sobriety as the definition of success, subjects older than age 60 do at least as well as 20- to 60-year-old subjects.[24] Improved treatment success rates among older alcoholics are likely in part attributable to the lower incidence of polysubstance abuse among older adults. Compliance in early- versus late-onset alcoholism treatment in elders is similar.[46]

CASE 1

Discussion

Mr. Beem accepts referral to AA. He attends one meeting daily for the first 3 months. After 3 months, his MMSE is 29/30, and his blood pressure is 138/82 mmHg; he is taking hydrochlorothiazide 12.5 mg by mouth daily. He has had no further trauma. ■

SUMMARY

Alcoholism is common and can cause significant cognitive and physical impairment in older adults. Unfortunately, it is underrecognized and undertreated by the health care system, despite the fact that older alcoholics are at least as treatable as (and probably more than) younger alcoholics. Essentials of effective treatment include recognition and screening, involving the family/caregivers, emphasizing that this is an inheritable medical illness, use of existing AA members, abstinence (controlled drinking is not recommended), group therapy, and "replacing drinking with people." Many common problems of older adults are worsened or often caused by alcoholism, and treatment can significantly improve the outcomes and quality of life of these individuals.

Web Resources

http://store.samhsa.gov/product/Older-Adults-and-Alcohol-Use-Pocket-Screening-Tools/SMA02-3621. Accessed August 8, 2013. Pocket screening guide for alcohol use among older adults.

www.niaaa.nih.gov/alcohol-health/special-populations-co-occurring-disorders/older-adults. Guidelines on alcohol use and abuse, including those specifically for older adults, from the National Institute on Alcohol Abuse and Alcoholism.

KEY REFERENCES

10. Sacco P, Bucholz KK, Spitznagel EL. Alcohol use among older adults in the national epidemiologic survey on alcohol and related conditions: A latent class analysis. J Stud Alcohol Drugs 2009;70:829-38.
11. Kuerbis A, Sacco P. The impact of retirement on the drinking patterns of older adults: A review. Addictive Behaviors 2012;37:587-95.
17. Moos RH, Schutte KK, Brennan PL, et al. Late-life and life history predictors of older adults of high alcohol consumption and drinking problems. Drug Alcohol Depend 2010;108:13-20.
37. Moore AA, Blow FC, Hoffing M, et al. Primary care-based intervention to reduce at-risk drinking in older adults: A randomized controlled trial. Addiction 2010;106:111-20.
38. Resnick B. Alcohol use in a continuing care retirement community. J Gerontol Nurs 2003;29:22-9.

References available online at expertconsult.com.

35

Driving

Alice K. Pomidor

OBJECTIVES

Upon completion of this chapter, the reader will be able to:

• Recognize important risk factors for driving disability in older adults.

• Describe a risk assessment strategy for fitness to drive.

• Identify strategies for risk reduction and counseling of older adult drivers and their caregivers.

• Discuss legal and ethical issues involved in reporting impaired drivers.

Driving has become an instrumental activity of daily living for all of us. Changes normally seen with age and the medical morbidities that occur commonly can make driving difficult, reducing human contact, social life, access to nutrition and health care, and impairing independence and the enjoyment of life. Primary prevention of loss of driving ability, secondary

Additional online-only material indicated by icon.

detection and treatment of impaired driving skills, and tertiary management of lost driving capacity are essential if driving capacity and safety are to be maintained; achievement of these goals can be challenging and time consuming in health care settings. Driving is a skill, and its loss is a social problem, which does not fit typical health care paradigms; it is obviously difficult to assess this skill in the office, especially when we all have significant time constraints. Legal and ethical questions also deter health care professionals from addressing driving. However, early intervention can prevent fatalities, injuries, unnecessary disability, and potentially the premature loss of driving skills and privileges, with their serious adverse effects on the quality of life.

CASE 1

Evelyn Harris (Part 1)

Evelyn Harris, age 74 years, comes in to your office for her annual health maintenance visit. The nurse screens her instrumental activities of daily living; Mrs. Harris reports that "It is getting very hard for me to drive at night. I don't think it's safe. What should I do?" She reports being blinded from oncoming headlights and having trouble clearly seeing familiar landmarks at night.

Are Mrs. Harris's safety concerns and actions regarding driving justified? ▣

PREVALENCE AND IMPACT

The number of people older than age 65 is projected to increase from 40 million in 2010 to 72 million by 2030 and 88 million by 2050, and more than 80% of this age group is licensed to drive.[1] Motor vehicle accidents are the leading cause of death from unintentional injury in those ages 65 to 74, and the second leading cause of death from unintentional injury in those older than age 75.[2] In 2010 almost 5500 people age 65 and older were killed (17% of all traffic fatalities) and 189,000 were injured in crashes.[3] Older drivers hospitalized after crashes have significantly higher mortality rates and longer hospital stays, and are less likely to be discharged directly home.[4] The crash risk of older adults is similar to that of those ages 24 and under, although this is mostly because of the higher risk, urban nature of their lower average number of miles traveled (referred to as low-mileage bias).[5,6] Adults over age 70 make an average of 3 trips per day, with average mileage 6400 a year; adults in their 40s take a mean 4.5 trips a day and average more than 15,000 miles a year.[7] Older women are at higher risk of crash-related injury and fatality compared to older men; such incidents most often occur during moving violations (missing signs and signals, crossing lines while passing, and making left-hand turns). Accidents of older drivers are usually lower speed and multive-hicular, reflecting city traffic.[8] However, a larger proportion of older compared to younger adults have safe driving habits, including seat-belt use, and avoiding night driving, rush hour, bad weather, and unfamiliar areas; they also tend not to drive while under the influence of alcohol or other intoxicants.[9]

CASE 1

Evelyn Harris (Part 2)

Mrs. Harris has had no changes in her basic activities of daily living. She does report more trouble reading recently and has begun wearing her drugstore reading glasses for other activities as well. She has no chronic illnesses other than osteoarthritic changes in her hands and neck, takes an aspirin and calcium with vitamin D daily, and uses acetaminophen as needed for her neck and hand pain.

What findings do you expect on vision testing? Does Mrs. Harris have other risk factors for future driving disability and injury? ▣

RISK FACTORS AND PATHOPHYSIOLOGY

The main medical factors affecting an older adult's ability to drive safely are age-related loss of physical and cognitive functions, increased prevalence of medical conditions, and the use of multiple medications. Behavioral and environmental factors influence safety, but are rarely assessed with regard to their effect on driving; these factors include choice of vehicle, how often and where to drive, road and weather conditions, and distractions in the vehicle (such as eating, the radio, passengers, and cell phones), and the driver's own values on safety versus risk.[10]

Physical Function

Impaired vision is the most clearly identified function placing older drivers at increased risk for crashes, particularly severe visual field loss and restricted useful field of view (UFOV).[11] Visual field loss may be present because of glaucoma, macular degeneration, or retinopathy in 18% to 30% of those 70 and older.[12] A UFOV test takes visual processing speed and cognitive skills (such as divided visual attention) into account, by measuring speed of response to two vehicles simultaneously displayed on a monitor. If UFOV is reduced by more than 40%, the risk of motor vehicle collision increases by about 1.5 to 2.5 times.[11] Static visual acuity does not predict crash involvement, although it is

the most commonly used measure of vision and generally the only one assessed by departments of motor vehicles. Diminished static visual acuity may decrease driving performance when lower than 20/40, particularly because of difficulty reading signage.[13] Glare and contrast sensitivity impairment from cataract disease, present in two thirds of adults in their 70s, strongly affects driving performance and is reversible with treatment.[14]

The National Highway Traffic Safety Administration (NHTSA) evaluated several aspects of physical functioning measured in the Assessment of Driving-Related Skills (ADReS) published by the American Medical Association (AMA)[15]: the Rapid Pace Walk, and testing of manual muscle strength and range of motion (ROM).[16] Motor strength testing was not found to correlate with behind-the-wheel testing. However, impaired ROM (especially the neck) and inability to walk 10 feet and back in less than 9 seconds did correlate with impaired driving skills. NHTSA guidelines summarize the available evidence for physical limitations and in particular note that any condition that affects the upper or lower limbs, the neck, and the back may have an effect on the patient's fitness to drive.[3] Arthritic conditions, common in older adults, have been associated with a twofold increase in risk for injurious crash,[1] although NHTSA notes that almost any condition may be compensated for with adaptive equipment.

> Impaired range of motion of the neck and inability to walk 10 feet and back in less than 9 seconds do correlate with impaired driving.

CASE 1

Discussion

On examination, Mrs. Harris's visual acuity has worsened from 20/70 last year to 20/100 at this visit and you see significant cataracts. She is unable to reach both hands behind her head, to touch her chin to her shoulders, or to fully close her hands. Her height has decreased by one half inch over the course of the past year. After your referral to physical therapy, her range of motion improves substantially. She also makes seat and mirror adjustments after attending a community CarFit event. Mrs. Harris's confidence in nighttime driving activity improves after her cataracts are removed, and she returns to evening social activities. ▣

Cognitive Function

Cognitive skill is universally acknowledged to be essential for safe driving. The primary issues are which cognitive abilities can be easily and reliably evaluated and how to know which disabilities predict on-the-road driving impairment and crash risk. For example, slower speed of processing may reduce driving safety, whereas greater caution may improve it.[10] Neuropsychological testing scores that reflect actual performance and are not adjusted for age or demographics better predict driving impairment and risk, because the hazards that are inherent in the road and traffic do not adjust to the driver.[17] Speed and precision of visuospatial processing and attention, such as measured by the UFOV and by copying complex drawings, are key cognitive functions. The Trails Making Test–B (Trails B) evaluates processing speed, visual and motor function integration, symbol recognition and sequencing, and the ability to focus on two thought processes at once.[18] Memory dysfunction appears to be an indicator of underlying neurologic illnesses impairing multiple cognitive domains, rather than an independent predictor of driving ability, because even patients with severe memory problems can perform most aspects of driving well.[19] This is consistent with the characteristically much later loss of procedural memory relative to the early loss of event memory in dementias of the Alzheimer's type. Executive decision-making is a critical function for planning and choosing what actions to perform, but this skill is not age dependent, and variability is high within age groups.[20]

The well-known Mini-Mental State Examination (MMSE)[21] is one of the most frequently administered cognitive screening tools to investigate impairment of the elderly (and of their ability to drive), but it was certainly not designed to assess driving skill. It focuses mainly on orientation, language, and memory, and omits the other domains of cognitive functioning important for driving competence. As such, the MMSE does not consistently predict future crashes or traffic violations.[22] The Porteus Maze, Snellgrove Maze Task, Clock Drawing, Trail-Making Test Parts A or B (TMT-A, B), UFOV, and Neuropsychological Assessment Battery tests do correlate significantly with on-road driving performance.[23,24] Of these, the Clock Drawing test and TMT-B as described in the AMA's ADReS are easily administered in the office or emergency room settings and are sensitive, identifying 92% of those who failed the behind-the-wheel test, although specificity was low at 50%.[16,18] The UFOV is commercially available. The Montreal Cognitive Assessment (MoCA) combines features of the MMSE, Clock Drawing, and Trails B, as well as testing abstract ability and verbal fluency (which tests retrieval speed), and is freely available in multiple languages. The MoCA has been found to have higher sensitivity than the MMSE for detection of early cognitive impairment, but it has not yet been studied specifically for prediction of on-the-road driving performance.[25-27] It is also important that any evaluation strategy for age-related cognitive function be applicable to measuring the functional impact on driving when one is following the course over

time of neurodegenerative diseases such as Alzheimer's and Parkinson's disease, for which the exact time of onset and speed of progression are unknown.[17]

CASE 2

Jerry Rucker (Part 1)

Jerry Rucker is an overweight 78-year-old man here for his quarterly checkup for his known 10-year history of hypertension, low back pain, atrial fibrillation, and mild depression. His daughter waits for you in the hall outside her father's room so she can talk to you without her father hearing the conversation. "You have to talk to Dad about his driving when you go in. He almost got himself hit the other day, and I feel like he shouldn't take the children out anymore." She tells you that he has become more absentminded over the past year, sometimes forgetting to take his daily medications.

Mr. Rucker attributes this to "dizzy" spells that started a couple of months ago and occur almost every week, but never yet while driving. Although willing to admit to being "a little slower on the brakes" than he used to be, he does not recall the incident described by his daughter until half way into the story. Mr. Rucker does then admit to turning left in front of an oncoming car while attempting to beat someone else to the parking spot he wanted at his grocery store. He is upset that his daughter is no longer willing to let him drive his grandchildren to activities and thinks she is "making a big deal out of nothing."

1. **What driving skills appear to be already impaired in Mr. Rucker, and what risk factors does he have for additional driving disability and injury?**

2. **What additional information would be most useful?** ◼

Medical Conditions and Medications

Many medical conditions that are more prevalent with increasing age are associated with an elevated risk of crash, and so is the use of multiple medications (Box 35-1).[28] The natural history, time course, severity, stage, and treatment of a medical disorder influence its

---

BOX 35-1
CLASSES OF MEDICATION THAT SHOULD BE AVOIDED OR MINIMIZED IN OLDER DRIVERS
Anticonvulsants Antihistamines Antipsychotics Tricyclic antidepressants Antispasmodics* Benzodiazepines Muscle relaxants Barbiturates
*Both urinary and gastrointestinal (i.e., ALL anticholinergics, including OTC).

effect on driving.[29] Interactions of medications and medical conditions with other (often multiple) comorbidities and medications are also significant.[30] Medical conditions that affect driving fall into three categories: those causing (1) acute loss of function (e.g., syncope, seizure, fracture with cast), (2) chronic functional limitations (e.g., neuropathy, dementia, sleep apnea, heart failure), and (3) the use of unsafe substances (medications, street drugs, alcohol).[3,30] Older adults taking any medication were 1.43 times more likely to be involved in a crash than those taking none, and those taking three or more potentially driving-impairing medications were 1.87 times at risk of a crash.[31] In a trauma population, those on two or more central nervous system–acting medications had 7.99 times the risk of crash.[32]

Several organizations have recently reviewed the available evidence about medical conditions and driving fitness. The Federal Motor Carriers Safety Administration (FMCSA) has an ongoing series of comprehensive reviews of the crash risk associated with a variety of disorders[33]; these focus on commercial drivers, whereas the NHTSA and AMA recommendations focus on drivers of private vehicles.[15] All three organizations have developed medical report forms that reflect the medical conditions of greatest concern with respect to driving (Box 35-2).

The FMCSA advises physicians to consider the following: (1) the nature and severity of the condition (e.g., loss of strength); (2) the degree of limitation caused (e.g., range of motion); (3) the likelihood of progression; and (4) the likelihood of sudden incapacitation occurring.[33,34]

CASE 2

Jerry Rucker (Part 2)

Mr. Rucker's medications include warfarin, digoxin, amiodarone, cyclobenzaprine, citalopram, and as-needed acetaminophen. He reports no shortness of breath with exertion or limitations in his ability to ambulate or perform his basic activities of daily living. His sense of lightheadedness is accompanied by palpitations and it tends to occur in the morning approximately 1 hour after taking his medications, when standing up. He has never passed out and denies any changes in his vision both during the episodes and since his vision was corrected by his ophthalmologist 4 months ago. On questioning, Mr. Rucker describes still feeling tired when he wakes up in the morning, before he "gets going for the day" with his back pain medication. He claims that this is why he is nodding off during the visit while you speak with his daughter. He reports no other traffic incidents and denies being pulled over or ticketed, but does volunteer that he has stopped driving on high-speed roads because he does not like the busy traffic, and prefers to only travel on well-known routes between his house and his daughter's home. He has stopped attending exercise classes at the senior center, which is now "too much bother." Your physical examination reveals orthostatic changes in heart rate and blood pressure that reproduce his sensation of dizziness and palpitations. Other routine physical examination findings are unchanged from his baseline. Clock drawing is normal, but the rest of the visuospatial section of the MoCA, as well as the attention and delayed recall sections, are impaired, with an overall score of 24 out of 30. He is able to walk 10 feet and back in 15 seconds.

What should be done to help reduce Mr. Rucker's driving disability and/or compensate for his decreased skills? Should he continue to drive? ◘

CASE 2

Discussion

Mr. Rucker has impairment of several driving skills, some of which may be improved with a combination of medical interventions and driving rehabilitation. His description of lightheadedness is of particular concern as a risk for syncope, which may be reversible with medication adjustment, but it could also reflect progression of his cardiovascular disease. Decreased alertness with daytime sleepiness and fatigue could be from sleep apnea, a side effect of central nervous system–acting medications, or from worsening depression. Slower reaction time braking, mild cognitive impairment, and poor judgment on a left-hand turn reflect cognitive/neurologic impairment; this impairment may be the first symptoms of neurologic illness such as dementia or Parkinson's disease, neuropathy related to his low back pain, or medication side effects. In view of his multiple risks, Mr. Rucker should be (1) counseled to not drive, (2) referred to a driving rehabilitation specialist if possible, and (3) assisted with finding alternative transportation until he is able to go through a workup and treatment targeted at these concerns. If he does not accept these recommendations, Mr. Rucker must be counseled regarding the safety risks of continued driving and about restrictions that might reduce his risk (Box 35-3). ◘

BOX 35-2

CONDITIONS WITH AN INCREASED RELATIVE CRASH RISK

Slight to moderate (odds ratio 1.2 to 2.0): cardiovascular disease, cerebrovascular disease, traumatic brain injury, depression, diabetes mellitus, musculoskeletal disorders, vision disorders
Moderately high (odds ratio 2 to 5 or higher): alcohol abuse and dependence, dementia, epilepsy, schizophrenia, obstructive sleep apnea

Data from Marshall SC. The role of reduced fitness to drive due to medical impairments in explaining crashes involving older drivers. Traffic Injury Prevention;2008;9(4):291-8; and U.S. Department of Transportation. How medical conditions impact driving (report). Available at www.fmcsa.dot.gov/rules-regulations/topics/mep/mep-reports.htm.

BOX 35-3

HOW THE CLINICIAN CAN REDUCE DRIVING RISK

1. Identify medical conditions producing driving disability.
2. Treat those conditions to maximally restore functional ability and prevent functional decline.
3. If a medication is probably producing impairment, reduce the dose if possible, substitute a different therapy, or discontinue the medication.
4. Counsel the patient about the risks to driving safety.
5. Recommend driving restrictions, alternative transportation, or driving cessation.
6. Refer to a driver rehabilitation specialist if available for driving evaluation and rehabilitation.

CASE 2

Jerry Rucker (Part 3)

Mr. Rucker works through several adjustments in his medical management over the next 6 months and also sees a driving rehabilitation specialist, resulting in improved driving performance as evaluated by on-the-road testing and resolution of most of his previous areas of concern. After an uneventful 18 months of routine care, he is brought in by his daughter to see you for follow-up after an emergency room visit for involvement in a crash, where witnesses report he drifted into a neighboring lane and was rear-ended at moderately high speed by a following vehicle. "My neck is so sore from that fender-bender. The emergency room said that I had to come in and see you if the pain didn't go away after a few days." Mr. Rucker denies all other complaints except mild right-sided chest pain with movement only. On inquiry, his daughter reports that she believes he is not taking his medication accurately by her observation of his half-full pill bottles at home, even though he should have completely run out a month ago. She states that he had another incident 2 months ago, which she only just found out about by finding on his mail table the traffic ticket for running a red light. Although he was not given any restriction by the emergency room, his daughter would not let him drive today, because she does not feel he is a safe driver. On physical exam he appears upset but generally cooperative. Physical findings are unremarkable except for blood pressure of 200/90, irregular heart rate (104), and right-sided chest wall tenderness. He is able to perform his 10-feet walk and return without difficulty but blames his slower time of 20 seconds on soreness from the accident. His score on the MoCA has declined to 20 out of 30. On repeat questioning at the end of the visit, he is uncertain about why he is here in your office today.

> **Why has Mr. Rucker's driving ability changed? Is it possible to restore and/or compensate for his driving disability? Should he continue to drive?** ◼

Dementia and Driving

Cognitive impairment that progresses to dementia is an especially challenging issue for driving disability evaluation and management. A diagnosis of early Alzheimer's disease (AD) does not necessarily preclude safe driving, but it is always a risk factor. Driving impairment in adults with AD has been correlated with neuroimaging changes in regional cortical function. Neuropsychological tests of visuospatial ability, executive function, and attention such as clock drawing and TMT-B that assess corresponding frontal and right hemisphere resources are more accurate predictors of driving competence than global measures of cognition. However, types of dementia other than AD, such as frontotemporal, Lewy body disorders, and vascular dementias, may create different patterns of cognitive deficits.[35]

Several professional societies and consensus groups (e.g., American Academy of Neurology, American Association for Geriatric Psychiatry, AMA, American Geriatrics Society, and the Alzheimer's Association) have published practice guidelines for clinicians regarding how to detect drivers with dementia and remove them from active driving for their own safety as well as that of other road users. However, although there is broad consensus that moderately severe dementia precludes safe driving, there is no consensus about managing those with questionable or mild dementia who are minimally or mildly dependent on others for assistance with their other daily living activities.[36] Pooled data from two longitudinal studies involving 134 drivers with dementia show that 88% of drivers with very mild dementia (Clinical Dementia Rating [CDR] scale score = 0.5) and 69% of drivers with mild dementia (CDR = 1.0) are still able to pass a formal road test. In one study, 77% of early driving terminations at 18 months (sooner than the mean of 2 years found in the study) were caused either by hazardous driving (55% were related to road test failure and 2% were related to motor vehicle accident) or family decisions based on the progression of dementia symptoms (20%). The median time to discontinuance of driving for those with very mild dementia was 2 years after dementia diagnosis, and for those with mild dementia the mean discontinuance was 1 year.[37] Even if the perceptual motor skills are unimpaired, such drivers often lack insight into their limitations or make poor judgments about their capacity to manage complex or challenging situations.[38] It is therefore both desirable and reasonable to follow such patients every 6 months to reassess their ability to drive safely.

DIAGNOSIS AND ASSESSMENT

Medical evaluation of fitness to drive must be thorough enough to detect undiagnosed conditions that could affect driving, yet also must screen for specific driving skills. Multiple assessment algorithms have been developed. Box 35-4 summarizes aspects of assessment commonly recommended.

The AMA's *Physician Guide for Assessing and Counseling Older Drivers* is the most accessible, comprehensive, and straightforward guidance available for medical

DRIVING RISK ASSESSMENT AREAS

- Questionnaire about driving habits and events plus traditional medical history
- Visual screen: acuity, fields, contrast sensitivity, processing speed
- Auditory screen: whisper test or audioscope
- Cognitive screen: MoCA (best) or MMSE plus visuospatial and executive function tests (e.g., clock draw, mazes, complex drawing, or TMT-A or B)
- Psychological screen: depression scale (e.g., GDS, others)
- Functional assessment: ADLs, IADLs, and AADLs
- Musculoskeletal screen: timed walk and range of motion of neck, shoulder, legs
- Sleep history: sleep habits, Epworth scale. (see Chapters 31 and 34)
- Alcohol and drug use: CAGE, urine testing, etc. (see Chapters 31 and 34)
- Medications (prescribed and OTC) that could impair

AADLs, Advanced activities of daily living; *ADLs*, Activities of daily living; *CAGE*, cut down, annoyed by criticism, guilty about drinking, eye-opener drinks (a test for alcoholism); *GDS*, Geriatric Depression Scale; *IADLs*, instrumental activities of daily living; *MMSE*, Mini-Mental State Examination; *MoCA*, Montreal Cognitive Assessment; *OTC*, over the counter; *TMT*, Trail-Making Test.

professionals; it is freely available online in its 2010 format and as an interactive video released June 2012.[39]

MANAGEMENT

A general approach to risk reduction and counseling is summarized in Box 35-5.

> Advise the caregiver: You may have to lie, such as "The car's being fixed" or "The insurance turned you down."

Jerry Rucker (Part 4)

Mr. Rucker contends that he still needs to drive to accomplish his daily activities, and is very reluctant to become a transportation burden to his daughter. However, he does concede that he has not fully recovered from his accident and agrees to not drive for 6 weeks while receiving therapy for his neck injury and while taking pain medication for his chest wall contusion. You support him in maintaining this decision by writing a prescription stating that he agrees not to drive for 6 weeks because of his acute injury, and both of you sign it. Your copy remains at the office, his daughter keeps a copy taped to the steering wheel, and Mr. Rucker has a copy taped to his kitchen table as a reminder. During his therapy, you review his medical conditions and treatment to ascertain whether there are any contributing factors that may have led to the accident, refer him at age 80 to an ophthalmologist for comprehensive vision testing, and arrange for consultation with the local Area on Aging office to investigate alternative transportation. At the end of the 6 weeks of therapy, Mr. Rucker informs you that he has decided to avoid the

RISK REDUCTION AND COUNSELING STRATEGIES FOR THE OLDER DRIVER

- Treat reversible deficits
- Eliminate potential problem medications when possible
- Proper safety belt use
- Avoid severe weather conditions
- Avoid driving if sleep-deprived or acutely ill
- No driving with alcohol or when impairing meds could still be present
- No radio or music
- One quiet adult passenger at most and no unrestrained children or uncaged animals
- No night driving and no cell phone
- Avoid freeways
- Avoid high mileage drives (or have a co-driver)
- Plan your route: avoid left turns and overtaking; avoid school bus times
- Encourage driving refresher courses
- Use alternative transportation; buses, trains, and planes are safer per mile for long trips
- Use occupational therapist or driving rehabilitation specialist for formal evaluation and for rehabilitation after an immobilizing illness of any kind
- Know your state's mandatory reporting laws and other legal requirements
- If all else fails, recruit caregivers to assist: confiscate or grind keys down, park car out of sight, discontinue insurance, disable or sell car, inform DMV (license withdrawal)

expenses of maintaining a vehicle in the face of his increased insurance rates post-crash, and that he is trading in his car to the local affiliate of ITN*America** for ride credits that will pay for transportation whenever he needs it.

> **What are the potential risks for Mr. Rucker when he stops driving? Would a co-driver have been a reasonable alternative solution? What would you have done if he had not agreed to stop driving?** ◉

LEGAL AND ETHICAL ISSUES

Older adult drivers in the United States have "driving life expectancies" of approximately 11 years at age 70, meaning that most will drive until their early 80s, but will continue to need alternative transportation for probably an additional 5 to 10 years of life. Latino older adults are an exception to this, with far fewer drivers overall in this age group and those who do drive stopping sooner with apparently worse health.[40] For many people, driving symbolizes freedom, independence, and having control. Educational, driving refresher, and training programs aimed at promoting the adoption of safe driving practices and strategies are popular ap-

---

*The Independent Transportation Network (ITN) is a nonprofit, membership-based organization committed to the independence and mobility of older adults and people with visual impairment. Dignified transportation is available 7 days a week, 24 hours a day, for any purpose.

proaches to the safe mobility of older drivers. Although their effectiveness on crash risk and driver performance is not well validated, they are regarded as an essential component of any strategy, particularly those that focus on improving driving awareness and behavior.[41] Overall, driving retirement is an expected but still highly stressful transition associated with depression, social isolation, and reduced access to services.[42,43]

Many physicians do not feel comfortable when having to confront a patient regarding his or her driving retirement and potentially reporting the patient for legal intervention by the state. In Canada, about 75% of physicians surveyed feel that reporting a patient as an unsafe driver places them in a conflict of interest and negatively impacts both the patient and the physician–patient relationship and 72.4% agreed that physicians should be legally responsible for reporting unsafe drivers.[44] In the United States, a survey of vision care providers in Michigan found that when a change in driving status is deemed necessary, more than half recommend their patients modify their driving rather than stop driving altogether. More than half of these vision care providers were concerned that reporting would negatively influence the health of the provider–patient relationship, and more than 40% considered that reporting unsafe drivers breached physician–patient confidentiality. Because the main victim (should injury or death occur) is the driver, and because the death of innocent bystanders is unacceptable in a civilized nation, it is a relief to know that most physicians believe the risks posed to the patient, his or her passengers, and the public by failing to report outweigh such negative consequences.[45]

Of course, older drivers may have symptoms incompatible with safe driving that could occur at any age, such as syncope or presyncope, vertigo, arthritic or irrecoverable injuries, narcolepsy or the sleep attacks of undiagnosed sleep apnea, seizures, or transient ischemic attacks. If the patient does not mention driving or forgets to ask, the clinician should take the initiative in patients with these symptoms and advise against driving. If the problem is persistent, patients will need to be advised to seek alternate transportation, including taxis, rides from family and friends, and medical transportation services. Hospitalized patients and patients treated in the emergency room should routinely be advised about driving (or not) prior to discharge, especially when they are taking newly prescribed sedative or narcotic medications. Even when a patient's symptom or treatment appears to clearly preclude driving, it should *not* be assumed that the patient is aware of that. The clinician should counsel the patient and discuss a future plan regarding when to resume driving or how to arrange driving rehabilitation. Mandated reporting varies from state to state; these requirements are available through the American Automobile Association (AAA),[46] at the Insurance Information Institute,[47] or may be found in the AMA's *Guide*. Only a handful of states have any type of required reporting of vision or dementia

changes.[48] However, Maryland and Florida are exceptions and are pursuing driving safety for their older residents, with the stated mission of the Florida Safe Mobility for Life Coalition being to "improve the safety, access and mobility of older adults and to reduce their crash, fatality and injury rates."[49]

SUMMARY

Primary prevention of loss of driving ability, secondary detection and treatment of impaired driving skills, and tertiary management of lost driving capacity are essential. The main medical factors affecting an older adult's ability to drive safely are age-related loss of physical and cognitive functions, and increased prevalence of medical conditions and use of multiple medications. Driving retirement is a highly stressful transition associated with depression, social isolation, and reduced access to services. Mandated reporting varies from state to state. Clinicians should (1) identify medical conditions producing driving disability; (2) treat those conditions to maximally restore functional ability and prevent functional decline; (3) reduce or discontinue impairing medications or substitute a different therapy; (4) counsel the patient about the risks to driving safety; (5) recommend driving restrictions, alternative transportation, or driving cessation; and (6) refer to a driver rehabilitation specialist if available for driving evaluation and rehabilitation.

Web Resources

www.ama-assn.org/ama/pub/physician-resources/public-health/promoting-healthy-lifestyles/geriatric-health/older-driver-safety.page. Older Driver Safety information presented by the American Medical Association.

www.nhtsa.gov/Driving+Safety/Older+Drivers. National Highway Traffic Safety Administration's Older Drivers page.

http://seniortransportation.easterseals.com/site/PageServer?pagename=NCST2_older_directory. National Center on Senior Transportation.

www.driver-ed.org. The Association for Driver Rehabilitation Specialists.

www.safeandmobileseniors.org/FloridaCoalition.htm. Safe Mobility for Life Coalition.

www.fmcsa.dot.gov/rules-regulations/topics/mep/mep-reports.htm. U.S. Department of Transportation: Federal Motor Carrier Safety Administration Medical Reports.

http://lpp.seniordrivers.org/lpp.htm. Accessed September 1, 2013. American Automobile Association Foundation for Traffic Safety: Driver Licensing Policies and Practices.

KEY REFERENCES

3. American Association of Motor Vehicle Administrators Driver Fitness Working Group. Driver Fitness Medical Guidelines. U.S. Department of Transportation. Washington, DC: National Highway Traffic Safety Administration; 2009.

15. Carr DB, Schwartzberg JG, Manning L, Sempek J. Physician's Guide to Assessing and Counseling Older Drivers, 2nd edition, Washington, D.C. NHTSA. 2010.

33. U.S. Department of Transportation. How medical conditions impact driving (report). http://www.fmcsa.dot.gov/rules-regulations/topics/mep/mep-reports.htm

References available online at expertconsult.com.

UNIT 3

Selected Clinical Problems of the Organ Systems

Whenever a man's friends begin to compliment him about looking young, you may be sure that they think he is growing old.
WASHINGTON IRVING, 1783-1859, U.S. writer, in *Bracebridge Hall*

I never accept lengthy film roles nowadays, because I am always so afraid I will die in the middle of shooting and cause such awful problems.
SIR JOHN GIELGUD, 1904-2000, in *The Independent, March 26,* **1994**

I think your whole life shows in your face and you should be proud of that.
LAUREN BACALL, b.1924, U.S. film actress, remark in 1988

Better is a poor and a wise child than an old and foolish king, who will no more be admonished.

The Bible, Ecclesiastes 4:13

To live effectively, with a real purpose and not merely to exist, you must be active, interested, involved – both physically and mentally.
LAWRENCE J. FRANKEL, 1904-2004, exercise in old age pioneer,
in *Be Alive as Long as you Live*

I was so much older then, I'm younger than that now.
BOB DYLAN, b 1941, in *My Back Pages*

I grow old… I grow old…I shall wear the bottoms of my trousers rolled.
T. S. ELIOT, 1888-1965, U.S.- born British poet, in
The Love song of J. Alfred Prufrock

The wise, for cure, on exercise depend.
God never made his work for man to mend!
JOHN DRYDEN, 1631-1700, English poet

To get back my youth I would do anything in the world, except take exercise, get up early or be respectable.
OSCAR WILDE 1854-1900, in *The Picture of Dorian Gray*

Last scene of all,
That ends this strange eventful history,
Is second childishness and mere oblivion;
Sans teeth, sans eyes, sans taste, sans everything.

WILLIAM SHAKESPEARE, 1564-1616, in *As You Like It, II, 7*

36

Hypertension

Margaret Helton

OBJECTIVES

Upon completion of this chapter, the reader will be able to:

- Define hypertension and its pathophysiologic impact on the cardiovascular system.
- Discuss the evidence that treating hypertension is beneficial to the elderly.
- Discuss the different types of hypertension.
- Discuss the treatment approach, including adjusting therapy in specific clinical conditions common in older people.

PREVALENCE AND IMPACT

Hypertension is one of the most common medical conditions in the geriatric population. The percentage of adults with hypertension rises steadily and progressively as people age (Figure 36-1).[1] Data on postmenopausal women in the Women's Health Initiative (WHI) study identified prevalence rates of 27% for women 50 to 59 years of age, 41% for women 60 to 69 years of age, and 53% for women 70 to 79 years of age.[2]

Compared with whites, blacks of all ages are more likely to have hypertension, a trend that continues as people age.[3] Mexican Americans generally have hypertension rates that are lower than those of both whites and blacks.[4] Asian Americans are a diverse group, but generally their rates of hypertension are about the same as those of whites, or a little lower, and their risk of death from cardiovascular disease is 50% lower than that of whites.[5] The main complication of hypertension in Asian Americans is stroke, whereas in white people it is coronary heart disease.[6] Black individuals have the highest rate of hypertension-related mortality.[7]

Adverse Outcomes

Population data consistently show that people with hypertension have a higher rate of all cardiovascular events including myocardial infarctions, stroke, peripheral arterial disease, and heart failure, and that risk of cardiovascular disease associated with hypertension increases markedly with age.[8] Among people 80 years of age or older, major cardiovascular events occur in 9.5% of those with normal blood pressure, 19.8% of those with prehypertension, 20.3% of those with stage 1 hypertension, and 24.7% of those with stage 2 hypertension. Hypertension is also linked to functional issues that affect quality of life such as impotence,[9] renal function,[10] and vascular dementia.[11]

Additional online-only material indicated by icon.

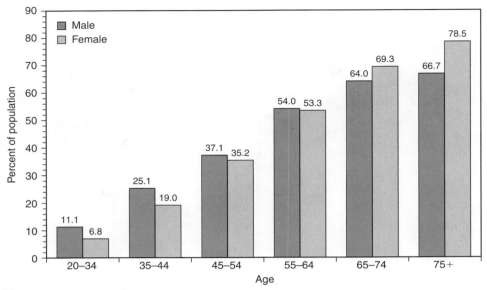

Figure 36-1 **Prevalence of high blood pressure in adults age 20 and older by age and sex.** (Source: Roger VL, Go AS, Lloyd-Jones DM, et al; on behalf of the American Heart Association Statistics Committee and Stroke Statistics Subcommittee. Heart disease and stroke statistics 2012 update: A report from the American Heart Association. Circulation 2012;125(1):188-97. doi:10.1161/CIR.0b013e31823ac046. Available at http://circ.ahajournals.org/content/125/1/e2.full.pdf+html.)

Whether hypertension increases the risk of Alzheimer's disease is not clear,[12] though cognitive impairment in late life is often a mixture of Alzheimer's disease and microvascular brain damage, the latter of which is worsened by hypertension.

These adverse outcomes lead to increased death rates. In 2008 hypertension was the primary or contributing cause of death for almost 350,000 Americans.[1] The death rate associated with hypertension increased 20.2% from 1998 to 2008, and the actual number of deaths rose 49.7%, reflecting increasing numbers of older Americans and their higher prevalence of hypertension.

> Hypertension is common in the elderly and associated with increased cardiovascular morbidity and mortality.

Low Rates of Successful Treatment

Despite the prevalence of hypertension and evidence of its serious impact on health and mortality, the rate of successful treatment remains low in all ages. Among persons older than 80, only 38% of men and 23% of women have blood pressures that meet targets set by the National High Blood Pressure Education Program's clinical guidelines.[8] Only 29% of older hypertensive women (70 to 79 years of age) in the WHI study had blood pressures within the goal range compared to 41% and 37% of those 50 to 59 and 60 to 69 years of age, respectively.[2] The good news is that the percentage of hypertensive adults of the three major race and

ethnic groups (non-Hispanic white, non-Hispanic black, and Mexican American) who achieved blood pressure control has steadily increased over recent years as has that of adults age 60 or older.[13]

Rationale for Treatment

The benefits of treating hypertension in older individuals were established in the 1990s when large trials showed that treatment significantly lowered the rate of strokes and cardiovascular disease by 30% to 40% (Table 36-1).[14-20] These trials firmly established the benefits for individuals in their 60s and 70s, but concern remained regarding treatment in individuals over age 80 until the Hypertension in the Very Elderly Trial (HYVET) was published in 2008.[21] In this older age group, treatment was associated with a 39% reduction in the rate of death by stroke, 23% reduction in rate of death from cardiovascular diseases, 64% reduction in rate of heart failure, and 21% reduction in the rate of death by any cause.

> Blood pressure treatment and control can lower the risk of cardiovascular events and mortality in all age groups, including the elderly.

CASE 1

Betty Johnson (Part 1)

Betty Johnson is an 82-year-old white woman who lives in an assisted living facility. She moved to the area 3 years ago to be near her adult daughter. She has macular

TABLE 36-1 Large Randomized, Blinded, Placebo-Controlled Trials of Pharmacologic Hypertension Treatment in the Elderly

	HYVET	SHEP	STOP HTN	MRC	Syst-Eur	Syst-China	STONE	EWPHE
No. of patients	3,845	4,736	1,627	4,396	4,695	2,394	1,632	840
Mean age (years)	84	72	76	70	70	66	66 (women) 67 (men)	72
Type of hypertension	Systolic	Systolic	Systolic and/or diastolic	Systolic and/or diastolic	Systolic	Systolic	Systolic and/or diastolic	Systolic and/or diastolic
Treatment regimen	Thiazide diuretic ± ACE inhibitor	Thiazide diuretic ± β-blocker, reserpine	Thiazide diuretic ± β-blocker	Thiazide diuretic ± ACE inhibitor	Calcium channel blocker ± ACE inhibitor, diuretic	Calcium channel blocker ± ACE inhibitor, diuretic	Calcium channel blocker	Diuretic ± methyldopa
Relative Risk Reduction of:								
Stroke	30%	36%[a]	47%[a]	25%[ab]	42%[a]	38%[a]	—	36%
Coronary artery disease	—	27%[a]	13%	19%[b]	30%	—	—	20%
Congestive heart failure	64%[a]	49%[a]	51%[a]	Not reported	29%	—	—	22%
Other significant reduction	Coronary artery disease mortality	Coronary artery disease mortality	Major cardiovascular events; total mortality		Vascular dementia	Cardiovascular mortality	Cardiovascular events	Fatal coronary events; cardiovascular mortality

Adapted from Harvey P. Woodward M. Management of hypertension in older people. Aust J Hosp Pharm 2011;31:212-9.

EWPHE, European Working Party on High Blood Pressure in the Elderly[20]; *HYVET*, Hypertension in the Very Elderly Trial[21]; *MRC*, Medical Research Council[16]; *SHEP*, Systolic Hypertension in the Elderly Program[14]; *STONE*, Shanghai Trial of Nifedipine in the Elderly[19]; *STOP-HTN*, Swedish Trial in Old Patients with Hypertension[15]; *Syst-China*, Systolic Hypertension in China Trial[18]; *Syst-Eur*, Systolic Hypertension in Europe Trial[17].

[a]Statistically significantly at p < 0.05.

[b]This reduction was noted only in the thiazide arm.

degeneration, breast cancer for which she underwent lumpectomy and radiation 10 years ago (and has remained disease-free), and arthritis in her knees, which requires her to use a rolling walker. Her only medication is a vitamin recommended by her eye doctor. Today her blood pressure is 165/85 mmHg. In reviewing your last three visits with her, you notice that those blood pressures were 142/82 mmHg, 146/82 mmHg, and 150/80 mmHg. She feels well and has no new complaints.

Does Ms. Johnson need medication? ◨

Charlie Williams (Part 1)

Charlie Williams is a 77-year-old African-American man with a long history of hypertension. He had a heart attack 4 years ago after which he received a stent in his left anterior descending artery and continues to be medically managed with metoprolol 25 mg twice daily, aspirin 81 mg daily, and clopidogrel 75 mg daily. He had a stroke last year that left him with mild left-hand weakness. He reports feeling more short of breath and tired over the past months. His blood pressure is 150/100 mmHg.

What other information would be helpful in Mr. Williams's history and examination? ◨

RISK FACTORS AND PATHOPHYSIOLOGY

Effective treatment of hypertension in older individuals requires an understanding of the pathophysiology that leads to increased blood pressure. Some of these changes occur with normal aging but most are heavily influenced by lifestyle factors.

Arterial blood pressure consists of a forward wave generated by the heart and reflective waves returning to the heart from peripheral sites. In young people, the artery is distensible so the pressure wave travels slowly and is reflected back in diastole. Aging is associated with a progressive increase in stiffness of the large vessels.[22] With this arterial stiffening, the waves move faster and reflect back to the proximal aorta during systole, augmenting the systolic pressure and lowering the diastolic pressure.

Whereas systolic hypertension is associated with an increase in large vessel resistance, diastolic hypertension is associated with an increase in resistance of small peripheral vessels, which hypertension further compounds because the resultant vascular hypertrophy can lead to high resistance and even closure of small vessels.[23] Before age 50, most people with hypertension have elevated diastolic hypertension, but as people age the systolic pressure continues to rise and diastolic pressure tends to fall, causing isolated systolic hypertension to be the predominant problem (Figure 36-2).[24] These changes lead to a widening pulse pressure (the difference between systolic and diastolic blood pressure) as people age. Framingham data indicate that with increasing age, pulse pressure becomes a better predictor of heart disease than either systolic or diastolic blood pressure.[25,26]

With age, blood vessels become less responsive to the vasodilatory effects of β-adrenergic stimulation,[27]

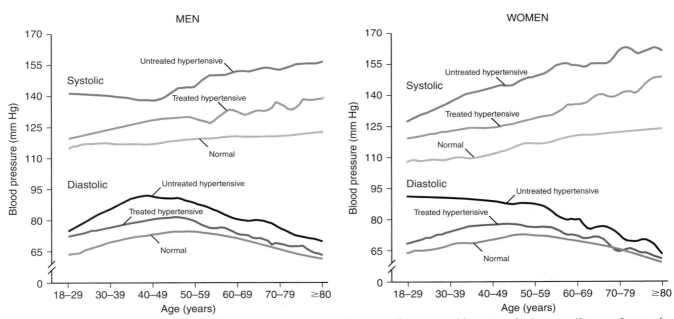

Figure 36-2   Mean systolic and diastolic pressure for men and women, by age and hypertension status. (Source: Centers for Disease Control and Prevention, National Center for Health Statistics, National Health and Nutrition Examination Survey, 2001-2008.)

changes that also contribute to hypertension. Plasma renin activity declines with age, probably because of age-associated nephrosclerosis, and plays less of a critical role in hypertension than the previously described vascular changes.[28,29] The decline in the aldosterone level leads to a greater risk of hyperkalemia in older individuals, especially when associated with the overall age-associated decline in renal function.

Lifestyle significantly influences blood pressure. Smoking, excessive alcohol intake, and obesity have a complex and deleterious interplay with hypertension, all synergistically negative in the impact on health.

DIAGNOSIS AND ASSESSMENT

Definitions and Criteria

Hypertension

Hypertension is defined as an average blood pressure of 140/90 mmHg or higher, based on at least three readings taken on three separate occasions. Table 36-2 describes blood pressure classifications per the Joint National Committee on the Prevention, Detection, Evaluation, and Treatment of High Blood Pressure (JNC).[30] The JNC is convened by the National Heart, Lung, and Blood Institute and issues the most widely accepted definitions, guidelines, and recommendations in the United States. The most recent report (JNC 7) was released in 2003 and the next report (JNC 8) is in development.

Isolated systolic hypertension, seen commonly in geriatric care, means the systolic blood pressure is elevated (>140 mmHg) with a normal (<90 mmHg) diastolic blood pressure.

Essential Hypertension

The vast majority of people with high blood pressure have essential hypertension, which is defined as a rise in blood pressure of unknown cause. It is likely the result of an interaction between environmental and genetic factors and tends to coexist with other cardiovascular risk factors such as aging, being overweight, insulin resistance, diabetes, and hyperlipidemia.[31] The term *essential* dates back to the time when it was thought that an increase in blood pressure was a necessary and appropriate response to guarantee adequate perfusion of organs.

Secondary Hypertension

Hypertension resulting from an identifiable secondary cause is uncommon in elderly individuals but can be considered if there is a sudden rise in blood pressure or a lack of response to three-drug therapy. Probably the most common cause of secondary hypertension in older people is renal disease, although it is often hard to tell if the renal disease is causing the hypertension or vice versa. Renal artery stenosis caused by atherosclerotic disease should be suspected if there is an acute decline in renal function (a rise in serum creatinine of greater than or equal to 0.5 to 1 mg/dL) after starting an angiotension-converting enzyme inhibitor (ACE-I) or angiotension receptor blocker (ARB).[30] The renal arteries can be evaluated with computer tomography angiography, magnetic resonance imaging, or ultrasound. However, medical management is as effective as revascularization with similar rates of blood pressure control and cardiovascular deaths and without the risks associated with surgery.[32] Thus, diagnosing renal artery stenosis may be of little value in most elderly patients.

Thyroid disease can cause hypertension and can occur in middle or older age. Thyroid-stimulating hormone (TSH) is a sensitive measurement for diagnosis. Parathyroid disease can also increase blood pressure and can be evaluated by measuring calcium and parathyroid hormone levels.

Hypertension owing to medications should be considered. Nonsteroidal antiinflammatory agents, steroids, and decongestants can increase blood pressure and are commonly used by elderly individuals.

Pseudohypertension

In rare cases, peripheral arteries may be so stiff and rigid that measuring blood pressure with the arm cuff may lead to an overestimate of the arterial pressure because of incomplete compression of the brachial artery.[33] This should be considered in patients whose hypertension does not respond to treatment or who have postural symptoms with treatment.

Markedly Elevated Blood Pressures

Patients with systolic blood pressure greater than 179 mmHg or a diastolic blood pressure greater than 109 mmHg are at especially high risk of cardiovascular

TABLE 36-2	Classification of Hypertension		
Hypertension Classification	Systolic Blood Pressure (mmHg)		Diastolic Blood Pressure (mmHg)
Normal	<120	*and*	<80
Prehypertension	120-139	*or*	80-89
Stage 1 hypertension	140-159	*or*	90-99
Stage 2 hypertension	≥160	*or*	≥100

Source: Chobanian A, Bakris G, Black H, et al. The seventh report of the Joint National Committee on prevention, detection, evaluation and treatment of high blood pressure. JAMA 2003;289:2560-72.

disease and therefore need rapid treatment. These situations are classified as hypertensive urgencies in the absence of acute end-organ damage and as hypertensive emergencies if there is evidence of end-organ damage, such as chest pain, shortness of breath, headache, visual changes, altered mental status, or acute renal failure.[30,34] The distinction guides therapy: patients with hypertensive urgency should have blood pressure reduced within 24 to 48 hours and can be treated with oral medications in the outpatient setting, whereas patients with a hypertensive emergency require parenteral drug treatment, usually in a hospital or emergency room setting.

Assessment

Blood Pressure Measurement

A diagnosis of hypertension should be based on at least three different blood pressure readings taken on at least three separate occasions. The principles of blood pressure measurement have changed little since Korotkoff introduced the procedure 100 years ago.[31] Mercury sphygmomanometers remain the gold standard but their use is being phased out in many countries because of environmental and health concerns. Aneroid and electronic devices do not use mercury but still report values in millimeters of mercury (mmHg) and are commonly used for safety and convenience. Aneroid sphygmomanometers use auscultation and a dial and require regular calibration to maintain accuracy. Electronic, or digital, devices are widely used and base readings on oscillometric measurements with the device placed at the upper arm or wrist. They do not require auscultation so can be used in noisy environments but may not be accurate in patients with arrhythmias. An up-to-date evidenced-based assessment of specific blood pressure measuring devices is available online at www.dableducational.org.

Proper technique starts with an appropriately sized cuff, with the length at least 80% of the upper arm circumference. Too small a cuff may produce an artificially elevated systolic blood pressure. The patient should be quietly seated for at least 5 minutes with the blood pressure cuff at heart level. The cuff should be inflated until the brachial artery is occluded and then slowly released. When blood starts to flow in the artery a pounding sound is heard (first Korotkoff sound) indicating the systolic blood pressure. With further release of the cuff pressure, eventually no sound is heard, indicating the diastolic blood pressure.

Inappropriately low systolic blood pressure readings in older individuals can occur because of an ausculatory gap, which is the interval of pressure where the Korotkoff sounds that indicate systolic pressure fade away and reappear at a lower pressure point. This gap is related to arterial stiffness and is associated with

an increased risk of cardiovascular disease, especially carotid atherosclerosis.[35] The true systolic pressure can be obtained by palpating the radial artery pulse, which is recommended whenever a manual blood pressure is taken and is usually around 10 mmHg lower than the pressure heard with auscultation; or, the gap can be avoided by making sure the blood pressure cuff is always inflated to about 30 mmHg higher than that needed to occlude the brachial artery.

Office measurement of blood pressure may not accurately reflect a patient's baseline blood pressure. The blood pressure in the office may be elevated because of patient anxiety ("white coat hypertension"), a phenomenon that is thought to be even more common in the elderly. Conversely, office blood pressure measurement may systematically fail to identify patients with blood pressures that are usually higher than that measured in the office because of a masking effect, which can only be detected with out-of-office readings.[36] For accurate diagnosis and monitoring, it is reasonable for nearly all patients to obtain out-of-office blood pressure measurements.[37] This can be done by 24-hour ambulatory blood pressure monitoring or intermittent blood pressure monitoring with a validated oscillatory device, the latter being easier and just as reliable.

CASE 1

Betty Johnson (Part 2)

On physical examination, Ms. Johnson weighs 116 lbs and is 5 feet two inches in height. You decide to start her on hydrochlorothiazide 25 mg daily.

What laboratory and other investigations are appropriate in Ms. Johnson's case? ▣

CASE 2

Charlie Williams (Part 2)

Further history reveals that Mr. Williams was a one-pack-a-day smoker for 50 years but successfully stopped after his heart attack. On physical examination, he has moderate arteriovenous nicking in the fundi. He has normal carotid upstrokes. On chest examination he has bibasilar rales and a soft systolic murmur over the aortic outflow area. He has mild pitting edema around his ankles and diminished pulses in his feet.

What laboratory and other investigations are appropriate in Mr. Williams's case? ▣

Past Medical History

The initial and ongoing evaluation of the patient with hypertension should assess for other cardiovascular risk factors and concomitant diseases affecting prognosis and treatment, identifiable causes of hypertension, and end-organ damage. The duration of hypertension and previous treatment history are also important.

Lifestyle Factors

Behaviors that affect blood pressure should be ascertained, including smoking, diet, and exercise. Level of education, income, and family support can influence treatment and should be reviewed.

Physical Examination

Physical examination should include assessment for possible end-organ damage. Cardiovascular assessment should include examination of optic fundi, palpation of apical impulse, abdominal pulsation, and peripheral pulses, and auscultation for heart murmurs and abdominal or carotid bruits. The thyroid gland should be palpated and the lungs auscultated. Neurologic examination should look for any deficit that might indicate previous stroke. Mental status testing is often indicated in the elderly individual if you, the family, or the individual have concerns regarding memory and cognition.

Clinical Tests

Laboratory studies can help in the assessment of target organ damage and should include creatinine, potassium, and urinalysis. Potential contributing cardiovascular risk factors can be identified with fasting glucose and lipid levels. An electrocardiogram (ECG) will identify left ventricular hypertrophy or signs of previous cardiac events. TSH and other endocrine testing can be obtained if a secondary cause of hypertension is suspected, but this is not common in the older patient.

MANAGEMENT

Goals of Treatment

Although JNC 7 recommends a blood pressure goal of 140/90 mmHg for all patients, in older patients these goals may need to be modified based on individual factors and comorbidities. Individuals older than 80 years of age are likely to benefit from treatment, but the data on patients older than 85 years of age are limited, particularly those who are frail or have multiple comorbidities. Based on available data, it is recommended that patients older than 80 years of age with a systolic blood pressure greater than 150 mmHg are candidates for antihypertensive drugs with a target systolic blood pressure of 140 to 145 mmHg.[38] For frail or medically compromised patients it may be reasonable to withhold treatment. There is little evidence that people greater than 90 years of age benefit from antihypertensive drugs.

An algorithm for treatment of hypertension in the elderly is presented in Figure 36-3.

> ### CASE 1
> #### Betty Johnson (Part 3)
>
> About 3 months after starting the hydrochlorothiazide, Ms. Johnson appears in the clinic with her daughter who expresses concerns that her mother seems more confused. Blood work reveals a sodium of 128 mmol/L with a creatinine of 0.66 mg/dL. Her medication is changed to metoprolol 12.5 mg twice daily. You see Ms. Johnson in follow-up and she complains about the new medicine, saying it is making her tired. Her blood pressure is 155/87 mmHg.
>
> **What are the next steps in managing Ms. Johnson's case?** ▣

> ### CASE 2
> #### Charlie Williams (Part 3)
>
> An ECG on Mr. Williams shows an old anteroseptal myocardial infarction, diffuse nonspecific ST and T wave changes, and left ventricular enlargement. You order a chest radiograph because of the crackles on his lung examination. It shows moderate cardiomegaly, fluid in the fissures, and small bilateral pleural effusions. His blood pressure is 152/88 mmHg.
>
> **What are the next steps in managing Mr. Williams's case?** ▣

Nonpharmacologic Treatment

Given the cost, poor adherence, and unwanted side effects of many medications, it is important to emphasize lifestyle changes that can effectively reduce blood pressure (Table 36-3). Research is ongoing to investigate the effects of these behaviors not only on lowering blood pressure but improving morbidity and mortality outcomes, but it seems likely that these lifestyle interventions can help with health problems and increase overall quality of life, though change is notoriously challenging for people.

Weight Loss

In the United States, the prevalence of obesity (body mass index [BMI] >30 kg/m^2) is 36% with rates increasing as people age, especially for women over 60, where the rate of obesity is 42%.[39] How this epidemic will interplay with the aging of the population is complex but it is certain that being overweight or obese complicates the aging process.

The evidence that being overweight increases blood pressure is overwhelming at all ages. The syndromes that go along with obesity such as metabolic syndrome and diabetes affect the heart, vascular system and the kidneys, worsening the risks already associated with hypertension.[40] Whether weight loss can blunt the age-related rise in blood pressure is

Target systolic blood pressure is ≤140 mmHg in patients aged 55 to 79

Target systolic blood pressure is ≤140 mmHg in patients aged 80+
but for some in this age group, 140 to 145 mmHg can be acceptable

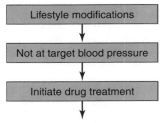

| Lifestyle modifications |
| Not at target blood pressure |
| Initiate drug treatment |

Without Compelling Indications	
Stage 1 Hypertension SBP 140 to 159 mmHg or DBP 90 to 99 mmHg	**Stage 2 Hypertension** SBP ≥160 mmHg or DBP ≥100 mmHg
Diuretic, CCB, ACEI or ARB, or combination	Most older patients require at least two medications if untreated BP is more than 20 mmHg above target.

With Compelling Indications	
Comorbidity	Initial therapy options
CAD or high CVD risk	THIAZ, BB, ACEI, CCB
Post myocardial infarction	BB, ACEI, ALDO ANT, ARB
Angina pectoris	BB, CCB
Heart failure	THIAZ, BB, ACEI, ARB, CCB, ALDO ANT
Aortic aneurysm	BB, ARB, ACEI, THIAZ, CCB
Diabetes	ACEI, ARB, CCB, THIAZ, BB
Recurrent stroke prevention or TIA	THIAZ, ACEI, ARB, CCB
Chronic kidney disease	ACEI, ARB
Benign prostatic hypertrophy	Alpha blocker

ACEI indicates angiotensin-converting enzyme inhibitor; ALDO ANT, aldosterone antagonist; ARB, aldosterone receptor blocker; BB, beta blocker; CAD, coronary artery disease; CCB, calcium channel blocker; CVD, cardiovascular disease; DBP, diastolic blood pressure; SBP, systolic blood pressure; and THIAZ, thiazide diuretic.

Figure 36-3 **Algorithm for treatment of hypertension in the elderly.** (Modified from Chobanian A, Bakris G, Black H, et al. The seventh report of the Joint National Committee on prevention, detection, evaluation and treatment of high blood pressure. JAMA 2003;289:2560-72.)

TABLE 36-3	**Effects of Lifestyle Modifications on Blood Pressure**	
Lifestyle Modification	**Specifics**	**Approximate Reduction in Systolic Blood Pressure**
Weight loss	Maintain BMI <25 kg/m²	5-20 mmHg per 10 kg weight loss
Physical activity	At least 30 minutes per day	4-9 mmHg
Reduce salt intake	Limit sodium to 2.4 g per day	2-8 mmHg
DASH eating plan	Low-fat diet with fruits and vegetables	8-14 mmHg
Stop smoking		1-6 mmHg
Moderation of alcohol consumption	Limit alcohol to ≤2 drinks/day for men and ≤1 drink/day for women	2-4 mmHg

Modified from Chobanian A, Bakris G, Black H, et al. The seventh report of the Joint National Committee on prevention, detection, evaluation and treatment of high blood pressure. JAMA 2003;289:2560-72.
BMI, body mass index; DASH, Dietary Approaches to Stop Hypertension.

unclear.[41] Still, although most weight loss studies involve middle-aged adults, several were conducted in older persons and demonstrated that older persons can successfully achieve and maintain weight control and reduce blood pressure.[42,43]

Physical Activity

Multiple trials have reported that blood pressure is reduced with physical exercise even when participants do not lose weight.[44] Though these trials were not limited to older adults, the benefits of exercise are legion and include reduction in lipids and insulin resistance, improvement in mental health, and lower risk of falls, with an overall improvement in quality of life that benefits elderly individuals, including those with chronic disease.

Reduced Salt Intake

The relationship between dietary salt (sodium chloride) intake and blood pressure is direct and progressive and it is recommended that salt intake be limited to 2.3 grams per day.[45] The effects of salt restriction on blood pressure reduction are most pronounced in blacks, older persons, and people with hypertension, diabetes, or chronic kidney disease. Reduction in salt consumption is challenging in our society because of the high consumption of processed foods, so individual efforts to reduce added salt will be limited without a strategy to reduce salt in processed foods from food manufacturers and restaurants.[30,46]

DASH Eating Plan

The Dietary Approaches to Stop Hypertension (DASH) eating plan has been shown to reduce blood pressure. It emphasizes fruits, vegetables, low-fat dairy products, whole grains, poultry, fish, and nuts with reduced intake of fats, red meat, sweets, and sugar-containing beverages.[47,48] The diet is rich in potassium, phosphorus, and protein, so it is not recommended for persons with stage 3 or 4 chronic kidney disease. Similarly, though multiple trials have documented an inverse relationship between potassium intake and blood pressure, leading to a recommendation that individuals have a potassium intake of at least 4.7 grams per day, this advice should be taken with caution in the elderly who are susceptible to hyperkalemia because they often have conditions or take medications that impair renal excretion of potassium.[45]

Smoking

Tobacco use is the most common, avoidable cause of death in society, yet 45 million adults in the United States smoke cigarettes, including 9.5% of adults over the age of 65.[49] Smoking works synergistically with hypertension to increase the risk of coronary artery disease and stroke another twofold to threefold above the twofold to threefold increased risk of hypertension alone.[50] Smoking cessation lowers blood pressure in the elderly and should be strongly encouraged.[51] Medicare covers tobacco cessation counseling and prescription medications for treating tobacco dependence, but smokers over age 65 are less likely to be prescribed smoking cessation medications.[52,53] This may be a result of the belief that older smokers have given up or that it is too late to have meaningful positive effect; however, this is a mistaken impression, because age does not seem to diminish the desire to quit or the benefits of quitting.[54,55]

Alcohol

Drinking alcohol, especially outside of meals, causes a dose-dependent increase in blood pressure in all age groups. Alcohol consumption should be limited to no more than 2 drinks per day for men and no more than 1 drink per day for women.[45]

Caffeine

Slight elevation in blood pressure because of coffee consumption has been reported in elderly individuals but it is not clear that this is of clinical significance.[56]

> Lifestyle interventions are important, but most older people with hypertension will require medications.

Pharmacologic Treatment

Overview of Medications

Reduction of end-organ disease from hypertension depends on successful reduction of blood pressure rather than on the choice of any specific medication. Table 36-4 lists the most commonly used antihypertension drugs and Table 36-5 provides an overview of head-to-head trials between different classes of drugs used for treatment in the elderly.

CASE 1

Betty Johnson (Part 4)

At the last visit you changed Ms. Johnson's medication from metoprolol to lisinopril, but she called the nurse 2 weeks later, explaining that the lisinopril was making her "feel hot." You instructed the nurse to have Ms. Johnson stop the lisinopril and begin amlodipine 2.5 mg daily. You see her in follow-up today and she reports that the amlodipine is making her legs swell and she wants to stop it. You change her to losartan but she calls the nurse again 2 weeks later and reports it is making her "swimmy headed." You have her come in to the office and her blood pressure is 139/82.

How will you address Ms. Johnson's concerns? ◉

CASE 2

Charlie Williams (Part 4)

Mr. Williams has coronary artery disease, a previous stroke, probable peripheral vascular disease, and now signs of congestive heart failure. You realize he is at high risk for further cardiovascular events if his blood pressure and other risk factors are not better controlled. You congratulate him on stopping smoking, and advise that he reduce salt consumption and review with him the principles of the DASH eating plan, though he admits it does not sound very appealing to him.

What medications will you add to Mr. Williams's regimen? ◉

TABLE 36-4	Antihypertensive Drugs		
Drug Class	Common Names	Mechanism of Action	Possible Adverse Effects
Diuretics			
Thiazide	Hydrochlorothiazide Chlorthalidone	Inhibit sodium and chloride reabsorption in the kidney, reducing intravascular volume and peripheral vascular resistance	Volume depletion hypotension, hyponatremia, hypokalemia, hypomagnesemia, hyperuricemia (gout), hyperglycemia, renal impairment
Nonthiazide	Indapamide		
Loop	Bumetanide Furosemide		
Potassium sparing	Triamterene Spironolactone		
Angiotensin-converting enzyme inhibitors (ACE inhibitors)	Benazepril Captopril Fosinopril Lisinopril Ramipril	Inhibit angiotensin-converting enzyme, interfering with conversion of angiotensin I to angiotensin II, reducing vasoconstriction	Hyperkalemia (with impaired renal function), cough, angioedema, rash, renal impairment, altered taste
Angiotensin II receptor blockers (ARBs)	Candesartan Irbesartan Losartan Valsartan	Antagonize angiotensin II AT1 receptors, reducing vasoconstriction	Hyperkalemia, renal impairment
Beta-Blockers			
Nonselective	Nadolol Propranolol	Antagonize β-1 and β-2 adrenergic receptors	Sinus bradycardia, heart block, fatigue, bronchospasm, hyperglycemia, confusion
Beta₁ selective	Atenolol Metoprolol	Selectively antagonize β-1 adrenergic receptors	
Dual acting	Carvedilol Labetalol	Antagonize α-1, β-1 and β-2 adrenergic receptors	
Calcium channel blockers Non-Dihydropyridines Dihydropyridines	Diltiazem Verapamil Amlodipine Felodipine Nicardipine Nifedipine	Inhibit calcium influx, relaxing vascular smooth muscle and decreasing peripheral resistance, dilating coronary arteries. Prolong AV node refractory period (non-dihydropyridines).	Sinus bradycardia, heart block, heart failure, rash, GERD, constipation, gingival hyperplasia
Alpha-adrenergic agonists, centrally acting	Methyldopa Clonidine	Stimulate α-2 adrenergic receptors centrally	Sedation, dry mouth, constipation
Alpha₁ selective adrenergic antagonists, peripherally acting	Doxazosin Prazosin Terazosin	Antagonize peripheral α-1 adrenergic receptors	Orthostatic hypotension

GERD, Gastroesophageal reflux disease.

Treatment in Specific Clinical Circumstances

Uncomplicated Hypertension. Diuretics are the cornerstone of hypertension treatment in the elderly and should be used when initiating therapy.[30] They are inexpensive, effective, well-studied, and generally well-tolerated, though electrolytes, especially potassium, should be monitored, especially after initiation of therapy and before a homeostatic balance is reached. Other potential side effects in the elderly are increased uric acid with possible symptomatic gout. Alternative first-line choices in the elderly are calcium channel blockers (CCBs), angiotensin-converting enzyme inhibitors (ACE inhibitors), or angiotensin-receptor blockers (ARB), though the latter two classes are potentially less effective in the elderly given that older people have a less active renin-angiotensin system than younger individuals.

Most elderly individuals with hypertension need two or more drugs to effectively lower their blood pressure.[30] A second drug can be chosen from among the other classes suggested for initial therapy.

Beta-blockers are not recommended as first-line therapy for uncomplicated hypertension in patients

TABLE 36-5	Head-to-Head Trials of Hypertension Treatment in the Elderly				
	ANBP-2	ALLHAT	STOP-2	LIFE	INVEST
No. of Patients	6,083	42,418	6,614	-	-
Mean Age (years)	76	67	76	70	66
Type of Hypertension Treatment Regimen	Systolic and/or diastolic ACE inhibitor vs. thiazide diuretic	Systolic and/or diastolic ACE inhibitor vs. thiazide diuretic vs. calcium channel blocker vs. alpha-1 blocker[a]	Systolic and/or diastolic ACE inhibitor vs. thiazide diuretic vs. calcium channel blocker ("new drugs") vs. thiazide diuretic or β-blocker	Systolic and/or diastolic Angiotensin receptor blocker vs. β-blocker ("old drugs")	Systolic and/or diastolic ACE inhibitor and calcium channel blocker vs. thiazide diuretic and β-blocker
Median Follow-up (years)	4	5	5	4	2
Reductions in Stroke	No difference	Thiazide > ACE	No difference	ARB > BB	—
Reductions in Cardiovascular Events	ACE > diuretic (for men only, and $p = 0.05$)	No difference	No difference between newer and older drugs, except ACE > CCB for MI	ARB > BB	No difference
Reductions in Congestive Heart Failure	No difference	Thiazide = best	No difference between newer and older drugs, accept ACE > CCB	-	-
Reductions in Total Mortality	ACE > diuretic (for men only, and $p = 0.05$)	No difference	No difference	No difference	No difference

Adapted from Dickerson L, Gibson M. Management of hypertension in older persons. Am Fam Phys 2005;71(3):469-76.
ALLHAT, Antihypertensive and Lipid-Lowering Treatment to Prevent Heart Attack Trial[61]; *ANBP-2,* Second Australian National Blood Pressure study[81]; *CCB,* calcium channel blocker; *INVEST,* International Verapamil-Trandolapril study[84;] *LIFE,* Losartan Intervention for Endpoint Reduction in Hypertension[83]; *STOP-2,* Swedish Trial in Old Patients with Hypertension-2.[82]
[a]Alpha-1-blocker arm stopped early because of significantly higher incidence of major cardiovascular events.

60 years of age or older. A meta-analysis of 13 randomized controlled trials reported an increased risk of stroke with beta-blockers compared with other antihypertensive agents in this older age group.[57] Their use is recommended in older patients with compelling indications owing to concomitant conditions such as certain arrhythmias, essential tremor, symptomatic coronary artery disease, recent myocardial infarction, or congestive heart failure.

> A thiazide diuretic should usually be part of treatment, with additional agents based on comorbidities.

Isolated Systolic Hypertension. Arterial stiffness associated with aging causes systolic blood pressure to rise and diastolic pressure to fall, and isolated systolic hypertension predominates. In the Systolic Hypertension in the Elderly Program (SHEP), treatment with the diuretic chlorthalidone in patients with systolic pressure of 160 mmHg or greater and diastolic pressure below 90 mmHg had impressive reductions in the incidence of stroke and heart disease.[14] Similarly positive results were demonstrated with a calcium channel blocker.[17,18]

Wide Pulse Pressure. Widened pulse pressure, whether pretreatment or treatment induced, is independently predictive of increased risk of stroke, heart failure, and other cardiovascular disease.[58,59] Data from large trials suggest that thiazide diuretics are more effective in reducing pulse pressure than ACE inhibitors or CCBs.[60,61]

Coronary Artery Disease. Recall that arterial stiffening with age causes the systolic pressure to increase and the diastolic pressure to decrease. Lowered diastolic pressure can impair coronary blood flow and predispose to myocardial ischemia which may be why the relationship between diastolic pressure and cardiovascular risk is bimodal in older individuals, with diastolic pressures of greater than 90 mmHg associated with similar increased risk as that associated with diastolic pressures lower than 70 mmHg.[62,63] Studies on hypertension have repeatedly found a paradoxical increase in cardiovascular events with lower blood pressure, known as the J-curve hypothesis. No J-curve effect was seen regarding the incidence of stroke, which may be because of the fact that the heart is perfused mostly during diastole and is therefore more susceptible to reduction in diastolic pressure.[64] In the INVEST study, the HOT study, the ACTION study, and the Syst-Eur trial, the risk of death and myocardial infarction but not stroke rose progressively with low diastolic pressure readings in patients with coronary artery disease and hypertension.[65-68]

With these precautions in mind, elderly patients with hypertension and stable angina and/or prior myocardial infarction should be treated with a beta-blocker followed by a long-acting dihydropyridine calcium channel blocker if hypertension or angina persists.[30] They should also be given an ACE inhibitor, especially if left ventricular function is compromised.

Congestive Heart Failure. In patients with systolic heart failure (impaired cardiac pumping), both preload and afterload should be reduced, and the preferred antihypertensive medications are diuretics, ACE inhibitors, and beta-blockers. In diastolic heart failure (limited diastolic filling because of ventricular stiffness) patients may benefit from rate reduction (which allows more time for filling and emptying the heart chambers) with a beta-blocker or calcium channel blocker. The role of ACE inhibitors, ARBs, and diuretics in diastolic heart failure is less clear, and they should be used with caution because a patient with diastolic dysfunction can develop hypotension with excessive preload or afterload reduction.

Previous Stroke or TIA. Elderly patients with hypertension and previous stroke or transient ischemic attack (TIA) can have their risk of ischemic stroke reduced by 37% and their risk of hemorrhagic stroke reduced by 54% with effective lowering of their blood pressure. Any medication works, though diuretics and ACE inhibitors are generally recommended.[30,69]

Diabetes. Because patients with diabetes are already at significantly increased risk of cardiovascular events, guidelines often suggest aggressive reduction in blood pressure to less than 130/60. However, the INVEST trial reported that tight control of systolic pressure was not associated with improved outcomes in older patients (mean age 62) with hypertension, diabetes, and coronary artery disease compared to usual control and could potentially be hazardous over the long term.[70]

Like other conditions, the reduction of vascular complications in elderly diabetics with hypertension depends more on reducing blood pressure rather than on the type of drug used, though ACE inhibitors and ARBs are usually recommended because they not only treat blood pressure but also slow the progression of renal disease.[30]

Chronic Renal Disease. Hypertension can worsen the decline in renal function that accompanies aging and both are independent risk factors for cardiovascular events and adverse outcomes. Blood pressure control itself is the most important goal in slowing progression of kidney failure and there are no specific data that outcomes are better with one type of medication over another in the elderly.

Expert consensus advises that ACE inhibitors or ARB therapy is most effective in slowing the progression of chronic kidney disease in patients with proteinuria.[30] However, the benefit of these medications in older adults is uncertain because most of these patients do not have proteinuria and most trials did not enroll patients over the age of 70.[71] If these agents are used, renal function should be monitored because ACE inhibitor or ARB therapy can cause a decline in the glomerular filtration rate (GFR), although the medication may be continued if the GFR decline over 4 months is less than 30% from baseline.[72] Alterations in potassium metabolism can occur with ACE inhibitors or diuretic treatment so potassium levels need to be monitored in all patients on these therapies but especially so in the older patient with renal disease. Hypokalemia is readily correctable with potassium supplementation. Hyperkalemia occurs less frequently but may require discontinuation of the medication. With careful management, the cardioprotective effects of treatment outweigh potential problems caused by the alteration of potassium metabolism.[73]

Dementia. The role of role of antihypertensive treatment in preventing dementia remains uncertain.[74] In some studies, a U-shaped curve was reported between blood pressure and risk for dementia, presumably caused by cerebral hypoperfusion with low blood pressure.[75,76] The HYVET study did not show a significant reduction in the onset of dementia in treated patients.[77] Other studies such as the Syst-Eur, PROGRESS, and SHEP showed a modest trend toward reduction in dementia with treatment.[14,78,79] These studies, along with a few other smaller studies, report that calcium channel blockers seem to be the most effective in delaying dementia, perhaps because of an effect independent of blood pressure such as reduction of excess intracellular free calcium in neurons, which may happen in patients with Alzheimer's disease.

Part of the challenge in generating hypotheses, clinical trials, and treatment guidelines is separating Alzheimer's disease, which results from neurodegeneration, from vascular dementia, which is caused in part by hypertension. It is not always possible to tell which form of dementia the patient has and many have both. The different pathophysiologic processes of the dementias cloud any hypotheses regarding treatment for hypertension. For now, the data are inconclusive but worthy of further investigation.

Frail Elderly. While the HYVET study provided clear evidence that blood pressure lowering with antihypertensive medication reduced the risk of stroke, congestive heart failure, and cardiovascular disease in the very elderly, subjects in this study were in relatively good physical health for their age and did not include frail and medically compromised patients. The use of medications in frail patients should be judicious with close follow-up.

Benign Prostatic Hypertrophy. Although they can be helpful in reducing urinary symptoms related to prostatic hypertrophy, the use of alpha-adrenergic blockers should be limited in the elderly. The ALLHAT study showed doxazosin was associated with 25% excess cardiovascular events compared with the diuretic chlorthalidone.[80]

> Deciding how aggressive to be in treating hypertension in the elderly requires considerable clinical judgment.

CASE 1

Discussion

After trying numerous medications over the past year, Ms. Johnson is now on hydrochlorothiazide 12.5 mg daily and enalapril 2.5 mg daily. She reluctantly agreed to take them after you gently encouraged her to do so, educating her on the risks of untreated hypertension. Although both drugs belong to medication classes that she did not tolerate in the past, she seems to be tolerating them presently and you are monitoring her electrolytes.

Ms. Johnson's case illustrates a common scenario in hypertensive management in older adults. Medication adherence is challenging and patients often stop medications because of real or perceived side effects. Time,

patience, and a willingness to listen and work with older individuals builds trust, which can help increase adherence and therefore successful treatment.

> Strategies to improve medication compliance include education on potential side effects, once-daily dosing, avoiding expensive medications, considering a combination pill if a two-agent regimen is established, and a plan for medication management such as a pillbox, calendars, and use monitoring by a nurse, pharmacist, or family member.

CASE 2

Discussion

Mr. Williams's symptoms of congestive heart failure along with his suboptimally controlled hypertension lead you to add furosemide 20 mg daily to his treatment, while continuing the metoprolol. You suggest adding an ACE inhibitor (benazepril), which will help with both his congestive heart failure and his hypertension. You advise him that his kidney function and fluid status will need close monitoring, so you arrange to check his electrolytes and creatinine in a week.

SUMMARY

Hypertension, especially systolic hypertension, is prevalent in elderly people and is associated with increased cardiovascular morbidity and mortality. These risks can be reduced with treatment. Lifestyle interventions are appropriate but most older people will require pharmacologic management. Considerable clinical judgment is required regarding treatment decisions because comorbidities and tolerance to medications must be considered.

Acknowledgment

Minor portions of the hypertension chapter from the fifth edition of this text were retained in this chapter. The fifth edition chapter was authored by Amrit Singh.

Web Resources

www.dableducational.org. Includes a list of validated blood pressure measuring devices.
www.nhlbi.nih.gov/about/nhbpep. U.S. Department of Health and Human Services, National Heart, Lung, and Blood Institute. National High Blood Pressure Education Program.

KEY REFERENCES

30. Chobanian A, Bakris G, Black H, et al. The seventh report of the Joint National Committee on prevention, detection, evaluation and treatment of high blood pressure. JAMA 2003;289: 2560-72.
38. Aronow WS, Fleg JL, Pepine CJ, et al. ACCF/AHA 2011 Expert Consensus Document on Hypertension in the Elderly. A Report of the American College of Cardiology Foundation Task Force on Clinical Expert Consensus Documents Developed in Collaboration with the American Academy of Neurology, American Geriatrics Society, American Society for Preventive Cardiology, American Society of Hypertension, American Society of Nephrology, Association of Black Cardiologists, and European Society of Hypertension. J Am Soc of Hypertension 2001;5(4): 259-352.
45. Appel LJ, Brands MW, Daniels SR, et al. Dietary approaches to prevent and treat hypertension: A Scientific Statement from the American Heart Association. Hypertension 2006;47:296-308.

References available online at expertconsult.com.

Coronary Artery Disease and Atrial Fibrillation

George E. Taffet

OBJECTIVES

*Upon completion of this chapter, the reader
will be able to:*

- Appreciate the potential for the altered
  presentation of coronary artery disease
  (CAD) in older patients.

- Know and understand the main risk factors
  for CAD in older patients, and current strategies for risk factor reduction.
- Be up-to-date regarding assessment and
  treatment of the various clinical manifestations of CAD.
- Understand the risk factors for development
  of atrial fibrillation (AF).
- Be able to assess the risk benefits for
  anticoagulation and stroke prevention
  in patients in AF.

CORONARY ARTERY DISEASE (CAD)

CASE 1

Corinne Watson (Part 1)

Corinne Watson is an 80-year-old African-American woman who lives alone and is completely independent in her activi-ties of daily living (ADLs) and her instrumental activities of daily living (IADLs). She always comes to your office accom-panied by her daughter. You see her now because of recent dyspnea and fatigue on walking to the bathroom of her home; this has occurred four times in the past week. The dyspnea is relieved by rest and is not accompanied by chest pain. Ms. Watson's medical history is positive for hyperten-sion, diet-controlled type 2 diabetes mellitus, and degenera-tive joint disease of the knees and hip that is treated with acetaminophen. Her average blood pressure in your office has been in the range of 146/85 mmHg. She has been fairly compliant with your treatment program of low-salt diet, triamterene-hydrochlorothiazide (37.5/25 mg) daily, and amlodipine 5 mg daily. Two months ago her blood count, urinalysis, electrolytes, electrocardiogram, and chest x-ray examination (CXR) were normal. Physical examination shows the following: weight 10 lbs over ideal weight; blood pressure 150/82, pulse regular (52 per minute), respiratory rate 16, no signs of congestive heart failure (CHF), an S_4 gallop, good distal pulses, and good nutrition of the skin of the feet.

1. **Is this an emergency?**
2. **Which facts suggest a cardiovascular cause for Ms. Watson's symptoms?**
3. **What social factors should influence your thinking?**
4. **What do you do (and say) next?** ▣

Prevalence and Impact

Coronary artery disease (CAD) is so prevalent in older persons that it should be considered as a primary,

---

Additional online-only material indicated by icon.

contributing, or potentially complicating factor in many clinical scenarios encountered by primary care clinicians in their care of older patients. The 6% of Americans older than 75 years of age account for 60% of the CAD-related deaths.[1,2]

Recent data suggest that clinically recognized myocardial infarctions constitute only one half of those with evidence of a scar on magnetic resonance imaging (MRI). In a group of Icelanders aged 67 to 93 without diabetes, 9% had a recognized infarct, 23% had infarcts by MRI.[3] A similar ratio was seen in those with diabetes. The impact of these "subclinical infarcts" remains to be determined but these findings are consistent with the high prevalence of CAD in this population.

A note about the evidence base in CAD: Caution should be exercised in interpreting the level of evidence for published articles regarding treatment, as well as guidelines published by various highly respected organizations. We and others recommend caution because very few (and sometimes no) older patients were included in the studies cited and guidelines often do not apply to older patients who have multiple interacting medical problems. We do not cite level of evidence for this reason. As always, the results of studies and guidelines offered should be noted, but their application to a specific older patient must be left to the clinician's judgment.[1,2]

> **Many respected studies and guidelines do not apply to the multiple-problem older patient!**

Risk Factors and Pathophysiology

Risk factors for CAD have been well defined although calculation of absolute risk in the elderly, especially older women, may not be as accurate as it is for middle-aged people[4,5] (Box 37-1). In older persons, the etiology of CAD is almost always atherosclerosis. Age is so important to the chance of developing CAD that a normotensive, normal lipid, nonsmoking 80-year-old man has a slightly higher risk than a 40-year-old hypertensive, hypercholesterolemic, inactive, diabetic male smoker. Other than for hypertension, the proportion of those older than age 75 who have the other risk factors decreases prominently.[1,2] Whether CAD produces angina pectoris, unstable angina pectoris, myocardial infarction (the last three combined are called acute coronary syndrome [ACS]), or sudden death depends on the extent of the coronary obstruction, which is determined by the following pathologic features: atherosclerosis, propensity of the atherosclerotic plaque to incite platelet aggregation and clotting, the degree to which the blood itself is prone to clot formation (hypercoagulable states), and the cardiac workload (demand).

BOX 37-1

RISK FACTORS FOR CORONARY ARTERY DISEASE

Age
Gender (male/female disparity narrows with age)
Hypertension
Diabetes mellitus
Left ventricular hypertrophy on ECG
Hyperlipidemia
Smoking
Elevated homocysteine[1]
Obesity
Metabolic syndrome[2] (central obesity, blood pressure ≥130/85, insulin resistance, dyslipidemia (increased triglycerides, decreased HDL)
Sedentary lifestyle
Lipoprotein abnormalities[3] with normal total cholesterol (small dense LDL, increased lipoprotein(a), increased postprandial VLDL and IDL)
Use http://hin.nhlbi.nih.gov/atpiii/calculator .asp?usertype=pub to calculate risk score, although this tool is less accurate in patients older than 80 years.

ECG, Electrocardiogram; *HDL*, high-density lipoprotein; *IDL*, intermediate-density lipoprotein; *LDL*, low-density lipoprotein; *VLDL*, very-low-density lipoprotein.

Age is such a dominant risk factor that it alone, in the absence of other risk factors, should make one consider CAD. Atypical symptoms of angina pectoris are more common with increasing age. In cognitively impaired patients, anxiety or poorly described distress may be the presenting symptom.

Differential Diagnosis and Assessment

Angina Pectoris

Angina pectoris, sometimes called silent ischemia, in CAD is well described, but the clinical diagnosis of CAD requires an index symptom or symptoms. The index symptom of angina pectoris—as classically described—is chest pain (CP). Less than 50% of older patients have the chest pain typical of angina pectoris.[5,6] Commonly, it is dyspnea, fatigue, diaphoresis, nausea, or syncope—without chest pain—that is the index symptom of CAD in older patients, especially elderly patients with diabetes (Table 37-1).

The broader differential diagnosis of angina pectoris is outlined in Box 37-2. Initial tests when the clinical diagnosis is angina pectoris are listed in Box 37-3 along with notes on the rationale for ordering them.

CASE 1

Corinne Watson

Discussion

Ms. Watson has important risk factors for CAD: age, hypertension, and diabetes mellitus. Your first consideration should

TABLE 37-1	Presenting Symptoms of Angina Pectoris in the Old	
	Classical	Atypical
Chest pain	Present	Absent
Pain radiating to jaw or arm	Often present	Absent
Sweating	Often present	Absent
Dyspnea	Often present	Often the only symptom
Fatigue	Often present	May be the only symptom
Syncope or presyncope	Atypical	May be the only symptom
Symptoms related to exertion and relieved by rest	Present	Present

BOX 37-2

CONSIDERATIONS IN THE DIFFERENTIAL DIAGNOSIS OF CHEST PAIN

- Ischemic cardiovascular disease
  - Acute MI, unstable angina, and stable angina pectoris
- Nonischemic cardiovascular disease
  - Dissecting or atherosclerotic aortic aneurysm, mitral valve prolapse, hypertrophic cardiomyopathy, pericarditis
- Gastrointestinal disorders
  - Esophageal spasm, reflux, cholecystitis, peptic ulcer disease
- Musculoskeletal disorders
  - Cervical disk disease, costochondritis, fibrositis
- Pulmonary diseases
  - Pleuritis, pulmonary embolus, neoplasm, pulmonary hypertension
- Psychiatric illnesses
  - Anxiety disorders and depression

MI, myocardial infarction.

BOX 37-3

STUDIES TO CONSIDER IN PATIENTS NEWLY DIAGNOSED WITH ANGINA PECTORIS

- To exclude associated acute myocardial infarction
  - Troponin I, total CK, MBCK, and ECG
- If dyspnea a prominent symptom, assess for CHF
  - BNP, echocardiogram
- If needed to exclude chest pain arising from GI tract
  - Ultrasound of gallbladder, esophagram, UGD
- If statins are being considered for therapy
  - LFTs, CK, aldolase
- To confirm diagnosis and quantify risks of adverse CAD events
  - CRP, pulse oximetry, CBC
  - Exercise or pharmacologic stress test
  - Echo (for wall motion abnormalities)
  - Coronary angiography

BNP, brain natriuretic peptide; *CBC*, complete blood count; *CHF*, congestive heart failure; *CK*, creatine kinase; *MBCK*, myocardium-based creatine kinase; *CRP*, C-reactive protein; *ECG*, electrocardiogram; *GI*, gastrointestinal; *LFTs*, liver function tests; *UGD*, upper gastro duodenal endoscopy.

Ms. Watson has stable vital signs and is in no distress now. She walks 100 feet in your office suite, which does not produce dyspnea or pain. There is no indication for hospitalization at this point.

1. **What is the cardiovascular working diagnosis at this point?**

2. **Are there still some potential noncardiovascular diagnostic possibilities?**

3. **What are your next steps?** ◘

Severe (or unrecognized) dementia may prevent the patient from giving an accurate history; it may also affect their ability to understand your questions.

CASE 1

Corinne Watson (Part 2)

Ms. Watson's diagnosis is now angina pectoris caused by CAD. Although the prognosis is relatively good at the moment, because patients with CAD may sustain unpredictable, sudden changes in the coronary circulation, leading to unstable angina, MI, or sudden death, you obtain permission from Ms. Watson to include her daughter in the discussion of diagnosis, prognosis, and treatment. You have previously determined that Ms. Watson has the capacity to make judgments for herself. You ask about treatment preferences. She wants to be resuscitated in case of a cardiac arrest but declines for the moment either stress testing or coronary angiography. In these circumstances, there is no immediate necessity for cardiac consultation.

be CAD. Given this history of risk factors coupled with recent onset of dyspnea on ordinary exertion, CAD must be considered as the most likely diagnosis. CHF is unlikely on the basis of physical examination, but you will order a CXR and a brain natriuretic peptide (BNP) test. Remember, "silent" myocardial infarctions (MIs) are common in older persons, especially those with diabetes. The patient's anginal equivalent (dyspnea) is not rapidly increasing nor severe and prolonged, excluding, on clinical grounds, ACS or unstable angina pectoris.

Underlying pulmonary disease as a cause of intermittent dyspnea is unlikely, and previous chest x-ray films are normal. Pulmonary emboli may deserve consideration but are not your first concern in the overall setting. Anemia as a cause of dyspnea is unlikely, but you will do another blood count just to be sure.

Regarding social factors, Ms. Watson lives alone and is a somewhat unwilling patient, but has a concerned daughter nearby.

Discussion

In addition to routine studies of blood and urine and a CXR, other tests are indicated. It is helpful to have the results back before the patient leaves your office. In patients where there is more uncertainty about the diagnosis, you may want the laboratory tests back in 1 to 2 hours or you may choose to send the patient to an emergency room. At this point, office or ambulatory care (and home care) could be safe and sufficient. ■

CASE 1

Corinne Watson (Part 3)

Ms. Watson's blood count, urinalysis, and CXR are normal. The ECG is unchanged from previous tracings, showing nonspecific ST and T wave changes in the lateral chest leads. Normal values for troponin I, creatine kinase (CK), C-reactive protein (CRP), liver function tests (LFTs), and BNP are returned in 2 hours. The homocysteine level will be sent to your office in the morning. You are now anticipating that Ms. Watson will not need hospitalization. You schedule a right upper quadrant (RUQ) ultrasound (US) even though cholecystitis is not high on the list of differential diagnoses. If the patient had not declined to have stress testing, you would have ordered it. Her average blood pressure is 146/85 mmHg.

1. **Which antihypertensive agent(s) would be the best choices(s) and why?**

2. **What approaches are indicated for Ms. Watson's diabetes and general health?**

3. **Are more cardiovascular medications indicated at this point? If so, which ones and why?**

Discussion

Raised BP

Because of the elevated blood pressure, a beta-blocker is a consideration, given the diagnosis of CAD, but the heart rate is 53 per minute. The amlodipine could be increased, but adding an angiotensin-converting enzyme (ACE) inhibitor or substituting it for the amlodipine is a better choice because ACE inhibitors offer beneficial effects for the diabetic kidney and the heart compromised by CAD, in addition to reducing blood pressure.[7] Because coronary perfusion is dependent on diastolic pressure, diastolic hypotension should be avoided.

Diabetes mellitus.

Weight loss and (eventually) exercise will be good first steps in treating a patient with CAD. If the HbA$_{1C}$ is not 6.0 or lower, an oral agent such as glipizide should be considered, remembering that the adverse effects of hypoglycemia may be greater in those with heart disease.

Nitrates.

A long-acting nitrate (isosorbide mononitrate 20 mg twice a day) and nitroglycerin 0.4 mg sublingually for dyspneic episodes should be prescribed, after instructing the patient to sit or lie when taking the first several doses of nitroglycerin. A visiting nurse should monitor the blood pressure and pulse, both sitting and standing, at home, to determine if this dose of isosorbide mononitrate causes postural or sustained hypotension.

Statins.

In the presence of diabetes, overweight, and age, it is unlikely that the lipids in Ms. Watson's case will be too low to start a statin now. Statins decrease low-density lipoprotein (LDL), raise high-density lipoprotein (HDL), stabilize atherosclerotic plaques, and may even cause them to regress.[8] In addition, statins have a beneficial effect on endothelial function, promoting coronary flow.

Aspirin.

A daily 325-mg aspirin (ASA) helps protect against untoward cardiovascular events such as heart attack and stroke. A smaller dose of ASA (100 mg/day) has been found to be effective in reducing risk of stroke, but not of cardiovascular events, in women.[9]

Ivarbradine.

Ivarbradine acts to slow the heart rate and has been used to decrease symptoms in patients over 80 with angina.[10] Drugs in this class can produce syncope or other manifestations of bradycardia in the elderly. Two other agents, nicorandil and ranolazine,[11] have good potential to assist in angina management in the elderly, but their roles need to be further clarified in studies of the elderly with CAD.

Exercise.

Ms. Watson should continue her usual activities to the extent that they do not produce dyspnea (or chest pain).

Diet.

An American Diabetes Association diet to slowly reduce overweight and get patients down to their ideal weight should be used. The diet should also meet American Heart Association recommendations for total fat and cholesterol intake, but should give enough for nutritional content for the patient's needs. Folic acid will reduce the concentration of homocysteine, but, unfortunately, does not alter the cardiovascular risk.[12] ■

CASE 1

Corinne Watson (Part 5)

You add ramipril (2.5 mg daily) and arrange for periodic checks on Ms. Watson's electrolytes, blood urea nitrogen (BUN), and creatinine. You refer Ms. Watson and her daughter to a dietitian. You instruct the patient on what to do and whom to call if the pain is not controlled, and you arrange for an appointment in 1 week.

You prescribe simvastatin (10 mg daily) with the intent of going higher if necessary and if side effects permit, plus isosorbide and nitroglycerin as needed. You arrange for the visiting nurse to check blood pressure. You prescribe aspirin (325 mg per day) to reduce Ms. Watson's risk for heart attack and stroke.

Ms. Watson returns in 1 week and reports only one mild episode of exertional dyspnea and that it was short-lived. She has no muscular aches or pain. She has been compliant with your suggestions with respect to diet and medications. Her blood pressure is 138/76 mmHg.

The results of the laboratory tests you ordered are as follows: BNP 200 pg/mL (5-100 pg/mL is normal range); RUQ US is negative; total cholesterol is 200, LDL 111, and HDL 50 mg/dL; triglycerides 109 mg/dL; homocysteine 18 μmol/L (5-15 μmol/L is normal range).

You follow her closely, with scheduled appointments. ▪

> Regular, scheduled appointments are needed for unwilling patients whose ongoing medical care is crucial to their health, and if they "no show" you contact them!

CASE 1

Corinne Watson (Part 5)

Over the next year, Ms. Watson does well. Exertional dyspnea occurs about once every 2 weeks, mostly with extended walking, but it is mild and short-lived. Blood pressure is 130/78 mmHg. She fails to sustain a 5-lb weight loss. Hemoglobin A_{1c} level is 5.8%. Electrolytes, BUN, creatinine phosphokinase (CPK), LFTs, and creatinine remain normal. Her lipid levels are total cholesterol 171, HDL 50, LDL 100 mg/dL, and triglycerides 72 mg/dL on simvastatin therapy. You consider further LDL reduction, but Ms. Watson does not tolerate higher doses of the statin.[13]

About a year after her first visit to your office, her daughter calls because her mother has noticed mild anterior chest discomfort while at rest and her daughter has noticed her mother to be anxious, dyspneic, and diaphoretic for about 15 minutes each episode, then recovering yet remaining fatigued.

1. **Is this an emergency?**

2. **Should you see Ms. Watson today?**

3. **Has Ms. Watson's likely cardiovascular diagnosis already changed a little and if so what is it at this point, before you see her?**

Part 5 Continued

You are suspicious that these symptoms are the result of progression of her CAD—specifically that they represent unstable angina pectoris or ACS, a medical emergency. You advise the daughter to call 911. She drives her mother to the emergency room (ER) where you will see her. You have ER privileges.

1. **What do you do first, before leaving your office?**

2. **If admitted will Ms. Watson need more than a telemetry bed?** ▪

Diagnosis and Assessment of Acute Coronary Syndrome

Acute coronary syndrome (ACS) includes unstable angina and acute MI. Unstable angina is a clinical diagnosis based on a significant change (instability) in the frequency or severity of the patient's angina. If the angina is new in onset, frequent, and precipitated by trivial exertion, one may also use this diagnosis. Unstable angina is a serious condition, frequently leading to death or MI if not promptly treated, and is almost always a reason to admit the patient to an intensive care unit (ICU).[2]

Changes in the pattern of angina may be caused by factors that increase the work of the heart (e.g., hyperthyroidism, anemia, or high blood pressure) and are independent of the progression of the CAD. More frequently, unstable angina is caused by a significant reduction in blood flow to the myocardium. Commonly, an existing atherosclerotic plaque will rupture, inducing thrombus formation in the artery, leading to a more critical obstruction of that artery.

The patient should be admitted to an ICU; cardiology consultation is advisable. Laboratory studies should include a complete blood count, basic metabolic panel, thyroid function studies, ECG, myocardial enzymes, and CXR. Treatment should include aspirin, nitrates (given intravenously or orally), and beta-blocking drugs. After stabilization, an ACE inhibitor should be given to patients with diabetes mellitus. Echocardiography and coronary arteriography are almost always indicated; if the left ventricular ejection fraction (LVEF) is decreased then an ACE should be started because ACE inhibitors decrease the frequency of heart failure and adverse remodeling. Exercise or chemical stress ("non-stress") testing is useful when the diagnosis of CAD is in doubt.

CASE 1

Corinne Watson (Part 6)

You call the ER and order the following: troponin I, CK, myocardium-based creatine kinase (MBCK), and an ECG, and ask for a cardiologist to see Ms. Watson with you. When Ms. Watson arrives in the ER her vital signs are blood pressure 140/84 mmHg, pulse 62, respiratory rate 20, and temperature 98.0° F. O_2 saturation is 99% on 2 liters nasal oxygen begun by the ER team. She is not symptomatic. Physical examination is unchanged as is the ECG. While waiting for the myocardial enzyme values to be returned, you order another 325-mg tablet of enteric-coated aspirin and an infusion of nitroglycerin 0.25 mg/kg per minute with instructions to reduce the infusion rate if the systolic blood pressure reaches 100 mmHg.

The cardiologist is delayed in responding to the consultation. You again ask for treatment preferences from Ms. Watson in the daughter's presence, having again established that Ms. Watson has the capacity to make medical decisions for herself. She still does not want a stress test or coronary angiography.

While the nitroglycerin drip is being started, Ms. Watson suddenly becomes pale, her heart rate increases from 62 to 96 while remaining regular, and her blood pressure is found to be 90/70. She is anxious, diaphoretic, and dyspneic. Inspiratory rales are now present at the bases of the lungs. The ECG now shows ST-segment elevation in leads I, AVL, and V2-6.

The cardiologist is late! The patient has suddenly declined.

1. **Did you mismanage anything?**
2. **What do you do next?**
3. **What do you say to your patient and her daughter?** ◙

Diagnosis and Assessment of Acute Myocardial Infarction

Because unstable angina and MI are so closely related, they are grouped into ACS. Admission to an ICU and cardiac consultation are essential in most cases. Sixty percent of MIs in those older than age 85 go unrecognized. This is one reason why many of the improved outcomes that have resulted from modern ACS care have been seen in patients younger than 65 and not the elderly.[1,2] Some patients may insist on home treatment of MI: home treatment of acute MI is not optimal. Diagnosis and assessment are carried out in large measure as for unstable angina. However, the clinician should exercise care in making the diagnosis of MI solely on the basis of a small and persistent elevation of troponin I (i.e., troponin leak).

> Almost *all* patients diagnosable with unstable angina and/or acute MI require ICU admission. (Some ERs may be preferable initially with the truly unstable patient. Know your ER!)

Management of Angina, Unstable Angina, and Myocardial Infarction

Treatment of angina pectoris includes the prescription of exercises to increase skeletal muscle efficiency in using oxygen; slowing, stopping, or reversing atherosclerosis; medications to restore the balance between myocardial oxygen demand and supply; and medications that reduce cardiovascular morbidity and mortality in selected patients.

Exercise

Cardiac oxygen demands should be reduced to the extent possible by treating elevated blood pressure and tachycardia, and by reducing the patient's level of stress. Exercise—usually but not necessarily walking—in a frequency and amount appropriate to the patient's cardiac and general health status is recommended.

Medications

Unless there is a contraindication, aspirin (to prevent plaque-related thrombosis) is prescribed. Angina may be controlled with short- or long-acting nitrates alone or in combination, and beta-blocking drugs.

LDL cholesterol should be reduced to below 100 mg/dL by diet alone or, more commonly, by diet and statins. In certain groups, even lower targets are recommended.

ACE inhibitors reduce cardiovascular morbidity and mortality in patients with CAD who have left ventricular dysfunction and those without left ventricular systolic dysfunction who have diabetes mellitus (confirmed in the HOPE trial).[13a,13b] There is accumulating evidence that patients without either diabetes or left ventricular systolic dysfunction will also show reduction in death, MI, and stroke on ACE inhibitors.

Emergencies

The treatment plan for angina pectoris provides the basis for longer-term treatment of the other two clinical manifestations of coronary artery atherosclerotic disease. However, the initial treatment of unstable angina and acute MI poses different challenges for both the cardiologist and the primary care physician. In both conditions, time is of the essence. In unstable angina prompt treatment is essential to prevent myocardial infarction and death; in acute MI prompt treatment is essential to prevent death as well as limit infarct size.

Primary Care Physician Roles

The PCP has several responsibilities in the prehospital phase of angina, unstable angina, and myocardial infarction, including the following: (1) to educate the patient and family in the initial symptoms of each of these conditions and to ensure that they know how to contact the physician or an emergency medical service without delay, and (2) to know the capabilities of the hospital(s) to which he or she may refer patients with unstable angina or MI. The primary care physician may have critical input in assessing the risk:benefit ratio of any emergent procedure for the patient.

Unstable Angina

The patient with unstable angina (UA) should be given an initial or an additional dose of aspirin and admitted to an ICU with cardiac consultation. Clopidogrel added to aspirin may have benefit but increases bleeding in patients who may require coronary artery bypass grafting (CABG). The decision to use clopidogrel (or glycoprotein IIb/IIIa antagonists) is best made after the patient's initial evaluation in the hospital.

For example, the PURSUIT study showed a 23% *increase* in mortality or MI with selective inhibitors of platelet glycoprotein (GP) IIb/IIIa receptors in addition to a 70% increase in bleeding for the elderly.[14] Overall the combination of the glycoprotein IIb/IIIa antagonists and fibrinolytic therapy has a prohibitively high bleeding rate (including hemorrhagic stroke) and should be avoided in those older than age 75.[15]

> Streptokinase within 12 hours of onset may benefit the AMI patient who cannot be brought to a hospital with angioplasty capability.

Acute Myocardial Infarction

Patients with acute myocardial infarction (AMI) at home should call an emergency medical service promptly (Box 37-4). The patient should be taken by the emergency medical service to a hospital with the capability of performing angioplasty. TACTICS-TIMI showed a marked cardiac advantage for invasive treatment for those older than 75 years of age with angioplasty, though this was also accompanied by a threefold increase in bleeding.[16] However, a community-based study did not confirm this benefit for those older than 75,[17] nor did a substantial review for reperfusion in general for those older than 75.[18] Thus caution should be used in extrapolation to decisions for the old; targeting the major therapies to those most likely to benefit may provide optimal results.[19,20] If the patient cannot be admitted directly to a hospital with the capability of performing angioplasty, then consideration of streptokinase is appropriate because it may be better than no treatment if it is administered within 12 hours of the onset of symptoms.[15]

Guidelines for in-hospital treatment of AMI, as well as contraindications to fibrinolysis, can be found at the website of the American College of Cardiology (www.acc.org).

CASE 1

Corinne Watson (Part 7)

Ms. Watson's diagnosis now is AMI with ST-segment elevation (STEMI). She is admitted to the cardiology care unit

BOX 37-4

IDEAL TIME GOALS FOR ACUTE MI MANAGEMENT

EMT on scene, 8 minutes
If fibrinolysis, EMT to needle time, 30 minutes
If angioplasty, EMT to balloon, 60 minutes

EMT, Emergency Medical Technician.

(CCU) under your care with the cardiologist as the primary consultant. She now will consider coronary angiography and whatever other therapy is indicated including thrombolytic therapy and percutaneous transluminal coronary angioplasty (PTCA), but she still hesitates about accepting coronary artery bypass grafting (CABG). Ms. Watson is stabilized in the CCU, undergoes coronary angiography, and is found to have triple-vessel CAD. The proximal left anterior descending coronary artery (LAD) has a critical stenosis, and a successful PTCA with stent placement is carried out. Ms. Watson leaves the hospital on a regimen of the following: 325 mg of enteric-coated aspirin, clopidogrel 75 mg/day, metoprolol 12.5 mg/day (heart rate 50), simvastatin 10 mg/day, ramipril 2.5 mg/day, a low-salt American Heart Association heart-healthy diet, and isosorbide mononitrate 30 mg/day.

1. **What input can and should you as the PCP have in the CCU and ICU where many or all of the medical decisions are made by others?**

2. **How could you improve Ms. Watson's understanding of the proposed procedures—especially the definitive CABG?** ▪

Role of the PCP in the Care of the Patient in ICU

The PCP (or equivalent) remains as the advocate for the patient and serves as an important information link between the care in the ICU and CCU and the patient and her family. This includes communication about prognosis. The in-hospital mortality of a STEMI is 20 times higher in an 85-year-old man than in a 55-year-old,[21] although this difference has narrowed over the past decades. Similar relationships are seen for women.

The primary care physician can help improve outcomes. The PCP's role when his or her patient is in the ICU/CCU includes the following functions: periodically assess the patient for capacity to make medical decisions; continue to supervise other aspects of care, that is, other than those directly related to the AMI; recognize the frequency with which CHF is caused in hospitalized elderly patients by vigorous IV fluid administration (i.e., monitor IV fluid orders of the cardiologist); keep an eye out for contrast-induced kidney damage; recognize and treat delirium; assure that the patient is adequately nourished; and, when appropriate, limit treatment or transfer the patient to a palliative care unit. Advocating in favor of treatment, when appropriate, can be critical because almost 50% of those eligible for certain treatments may have a relative contraindication; the most common relative contraindication is patient preference,[18] which may really mean inadequate education.

Corinne Watson (Part 8)

Ms. Watson is followed by you and the cardiologist and does well for the first 6 months. Her functional state gradually decreases, and you ask for a home health nurse to see her regularly. The home health visiting nurse is called by Ms. Watson's daughter because her mother wakes up one morning complaining of weakness, shortness of breath, and episodic sweating. The nurse advises that Ms. Watson should take a 325-mg aspirin and they should call 911 so that Ms. Watson can be taken immediately to the ER for evaluation and treatment. However, Ms. Watson, who still has the capacity to make decisions, refuses to go to the hospital. The visiting nurse alerts you to the situation. You speak to both the patient and her daughter and confirm that Ms. Watson wishes to stay at home, even after you clearly explain the diagnostic possibilities and the risks of not going to the hospital. The nurse finds Ms. Watson to have mild chest pain, but no dyspnea or other clinical signs of CHF. She is lucid and fatigued, but firm in her decision to not go to the hospital. Her blood pressure is 160/90 mmHg, heart rate 110, respiratory rate 22, and oxygen saturation 92%. Portable ECG shows ST elevation in leads II, III, and AVF.

What could be motivating Ms. Watson's refusal of hospitalization at this point?

Discussion

The clinical picture corresponds to an acute inferior MI. If Ms. Watson had not declined the possibility of going to the ER, she would have been a suitable candidate to receive immediate reperfusion therapy with percutaneous coronary intervention (i.e., PTCA) preferred to thrombolysis. ▣

Corinne Watson (Part 9)

You order oxygen 2 L by nasal cannula, and arrange for both formal and family caregivers to be with Ms. Watson 24 hours per day. Although you discuss the possibility of hospice care, Ms. Watson and her daughter wish to accept active treatment in the patient's home. You prescribe 1 to 2 mg morphine intramuscularly for pain control, and continue her beta-blocker, aspirin, statin, and ACE inhibitor. Forty-eight hours after her AMI, the charge nurse calls you to let you know that Ms. Watson's mental status has changed: she became transiently unresponsive and lost movement of her left arm and leg. Physical examination reveals an irregularly irregular heartbeat. Her daughter, to whom Ms. Watson had given durable power of attorney for health care decisions, now requests care for comfort only, and asks you to contact a hospice program.

1. **What are the benefits (and potential difficulties) of hospice services at this point in Ms. Watson's illness?**

2. **Should hospice have been involved earlier?**

Discussion

Clearly Ms. Watson has developed a stroke that may be ischemic or embolic secondary to atrial fibrillation. With hospice actively involved in Ms. Watson's care, you may elect to withdraw as the physician of record in favor of the hospice physician, or you may wish to maintain your role as physician of record and work collaboratively with the hospice physician and the hospice team. Ms. Watson is now no longer able to make decisions for herself. ▣

Strokes occur in more than 1%[22] of patients with AMI, despite anticoagulation and typically 2 to 7 days after the MI event. In the elderly, the most common complications are cardiac arrhythmias such as atrial fibrillation, CHF, stroke, and death.

Corinne Watson (Part 11)

Ms. Watson is enrolled in home hospice care and dies peacefully at home in the presence of her daughter. ▣

CORONARY ARTERY DISEASE SUMMARY

Significant CAD, often subclinical but nonetheless pathologic, is so common in the elderly that CAD must be considered a primary, contributing, or possibly complicating factor in most clinical situations. Risk factors are dominated by age, but important contributing risk factors are hypertension, diabetes, and hyperlipidemia, whereas other factors play important but lesser roles. The primary care clinician plays a vital role in the early diagnosis of CAD, and therefore must be aware of the frequently atypical presentation of this common disorder in older persons. The primary care clinician and a team including nurse, nurse practitioner, dietician, physical therapist, cardiologist, cardiac surgeon, and social worker play important roles throughout all phases of treatment (including the CCU and ICU, and palliative and hospice care when appropriate). To play these roles effectively, the primary care clinician must know the capacity of the patient to make decisions and needs to express the patient's wishes to the other clinicians. If the patient lacks capacity to make decisions, it is the primary care clinician who should be closely involved in defining (and communicating with) a surrogate or, if a surrogate cannot be found, assisting the clinical team with such decisions.

ATRIAL FIBRILLATION (AF)

Stanley Cooper (Part 1)

Stanley Cooper is an 86-year-old white male with CAD, benign prostatic hyperplasia, hypertension, and dementia who presents for the first time in your clinic with his wife of 63 years. His main complaints are his memory problems and knee pain; he also wears a diaper for his urinary incontinence. His medications include donepezil, finasteride, tamsulosin, aspirin, hydrochlorothiazide, isosorbide dinitrate, lisinopril, and simvastatin. He is pretty much independent in all his ADLs, except for his incontinence issue. He still drives with navigational help from his wife. He has difficulty remembering new events and names. He has a good appetite and no weight loss. His echocardiogram was a few years ago and showed a normal LVEF with an enlarged left atrium.

Blood pressure is 125/61 mmHg, heart rate 88, respiratory rate 18, temperature 95.6° F, and weight 240 lbs. Mr. Cooper was in no acute distress and has no signs of CHF, and no localizing or lateralizing neurologic signs. Montreal Cognitive Assessment (MOCA) is 17/30. (See Chapter 17 *Alzheimer's Disease and Other Dementias*.)

Fasting labs were BUN 21.0, creatinine 1.4, HgA$_{1C}$ 6.9, total cholesterol 124.0 with HDL 28.0 and LDL 59.6.

1. **What risk factors does Mr. Cooper have for atrial fibrillation?**

2. **Are there other risk factors you should look for?**

3. **Does he have dementia and if so how severe is it?**

Discussion

Mr. Cooper has many of these risk factors for AF (except no sleep apnea)—see discussion below. The enlarged left atrium five years ago adds to his already elevated risk of developing atrial fibrillation. ▣

Risk Factors for Atrial Fibrillation

Atrial fibrillation (AF) is an increasingly common dysrhythmia; its prevalence rises to above 10% in those older than age 80. The lifetime risk of developing AF is now 25% from age 40.[23] Increasing age is the strongest AF risk factor, but diabetes, hypertension, cigarette smoking, and alcohol consumption also increase the risk of developing AF.[24,25] Sleep apnea will increase AF risk fourfold,[26] and obesity increases AF risk in part through sleep apnea. More than half of the incidental AF was attributed to inadequate control of the modifiable risk factors in the longitudinal ARIC study.[26] Statins have antiinflammatory and antioxidant effects, and a meta-analysis investigating their use in primary and secondary AF prevention found an astounding 60% reduction in the incidence or recurrence of AF with statin use (Level of Evidence A). This has been confirmed in prospective fashion,[27] providing another reason to be on a statin. AF can also be a manifestation of hyperthyroidism, cardiac amyloid, or other primary processes.

Structural changes in the heart also increase the risk of developing AF. Atrial enlargement occurs with aging and in response to left ventricular or mitral valve changes. With each centimeter of increase in left atrium (LA) dimension or in LA volume, the risk of development of AF increased significantly. Those older patients in sinus rhythm with the highest LA volumes and the largest LA dimension had 20 times the risk of those with the smallest left atria.[28]

CASE 2

Stanley Cooper (Part 2)

Mr. Cooper returns to you 4 months later. An ER visit a few weeks ago was precipitated by shortness of breath only occurring at night when he returned to bed after urinating without any evidence of shortness of breath during the day. The ER physician started him on furosemide 20 mg with concerns for CHF and atenolol 12.5 mg by mouth daily for AF with rapid ventricular response. Since the ER visit he notes an increase in daytime sleepiness and a decrease in energy level, without shortness of breath. His mood and appetite have been good. He does not snore and wakes rested. The furosemide (instead of hydrochlorothiazide) and atenolol are the only changes in medications. He is now dependent on his family for his IADLs. He is now ambulating with a walker and has had no recent falls.

Blood pressure is 116/76 mmHg, pulse (radial) 62, respiratory rate 18, temperature 94.7° F, weight 242 lbs.

He has crackles at both bases; an irregularly irregular rhythm with apical rate over 90 and radial pulse of 62, no S3 appreciated, 2+ edema to the knees. His gait is unsteady without the walker. ▣

Rate Control for Atrial Fibrillation

AF may be classified as paroxysmal or chronic (persistent). Because the probability of stroke and overall management are similar, the differentiation for our purposes is not critical. Large studies have now shown that we overestimated the benefits of returning typical patients with AF back into sinus rhythm. The studies have also underscored the difficulty in maintaining sinus rhythm for those patients. Amiodarone is the most effective agent for maintaining sinus rhythm, but even in the trials where amiodarone was most successful, AF recurred in more than one third of cases.[29] Because the older heart relies more on atrial systole to maintain filling than the young heart, one might expect the benefits of maintaining sinus rhythm to be obvious in the elderly. Unfortunately these data are not available for the elderly, but hints of benefit are suggested by a reanalysis of the AFFIRM study wherein those who stayed in sinus rhythm were better and lived longer independent of which group they were randomized to (rate control or rhythm control).[30] Furthermore, the incredibly long half-life of amiodarone means that adverse effects (other than the frequently seen hypothyroidism) persist long after the drug is discontinued. The role of dromenadone instead of amiodarone for the elderly is yet to be clarified.

Therefore, control of **ventricular rate has become the dominant goal**. Targets are ventricular rates of 80 to 100 beats per minute at rest and 90 to 110 beats per minute during moderate exercise, based on the results of the Rate Control versus Electrical Cardioversion (RACE) trials (<100 beats/min at rest in the RACE-I study; in RACE-II the strict control strategy targeted heart rate <80 beats/min at rest and <110 beats/min during moderate exercise).[31] Drugs frequently used to accomplish this include digoxin, nonhydropyridine calcium channel antagonists (e.g., diltiazem), and beta-adrenergic antagonists. The pulse deficit (between the apical or ECG-derived heart rate and that perceived at the radial pulse or by the blood pressure cuff) remains a clinically useful measure. When the interval between contractions is too brief to allow adequate filling, there is functionally no blood ejected. Reducing the heart rate to obviate the pulse deficit is a reasonable goal.

Catheter ablation is emerging as an exciting alternative to rate control and the early data show select individuals older than 80 have had fairly good success (70% still in sinus at 18 months) without increased risk.[32] Those ablated may avoid anticoagulation but may still need antiarrhythmic therapy. Other investigators have been unwilling to stop anticoagulation for elderly ablated patients, removing one of the key advantages to the procedure.[33]

While **cerebrovascular accidents** (CVAs) are the most dreaded adverse effect of AF, the **precipitation of CHF** is also very frequent.[34] In the Framingham Heart Study about 40% of those with AF developed CHF and about the same percentage with CHF developed AF. The combination may be associated with worsened survival,[34] but trying to keep patients in sinus rhythm has not improved survival in patients with reduced LVEF.[35]

Anticoagulation and Atrial Fibrillation

AF is associated with cardiovascular morbidity and mortality and is a major risk factor for cardioembolic stroke.[36] The use of anticoagulants in patients with AF precipitates some challenging risk/benefits discussions with patients and families. Clearly CVAs are a dreaded outcome for patients with AF and anticoagulation reduces that risk. Using the CHADS2 (*C*ongestive heart failure; *H*ypertension; *A*ge ≥75 years; *D*iabetes mellitus; prior *S*troke or transient ischemic attack [*2* points]) score,[37] the likelihood of such an event and the yield of anticoagulation can be calculated and compared to the adverse events of major bleeding and fall-related bleeding. For older women the CHA₂DS₂-VASc may be more useful[38] (Table 37-2). Critically, a halfway approach is not supported by the evidence;

TABLE 37-2	CHAD Scores	
Score	CHA$_2$DS$_2$-VASc (%/y)	CHADS2 (%/y)
0	0	1.9
1	1.3	2.8
2	2.2	4
3	3.2	5.9
4	4	8.5
5	6.7	12.5
6	9.8	18.2
7	9.6	
8	6.7	
9	15.2	
C	Congestive Heart Failure	1
H	Hypertension	1
A	Age >75	1
D	Diabetes	1
S	Stroke	2
V	Vascular disease	1
A	Age 65-74	1
Sc	Sex category, female	1

titrating to a low international normalized ratio (INR) (less than 2.0) increases risk of embolic events without markedly decreasing the hemorrhagic events, especially hemorrhagic stroke.

Almost unique to the elderly is the concern about falls and traumatic hemorrhage. Gage and colleagues used a database to assess the risks. Patients that were at high fall risk on anticoagulants had a sixfold increase in hemorrhage (2.0 vs. 0.34 per 100 patient years), but those who were at high risk for falls had an extremely high risk of embolic stroke (13.7 per 100 patient years), the equivalent of having a CHADS2 score of five.[39] That is, in this retrospective study, being at high fall risk was an (additional) risk factor for embolic stroke.

Overall physicians are hesitant to start anticoagulation in the elderly, especially those with elevated fall risk. The evidence supporting their (and the patient's) trepidation is modest, especially if high fall risk is shown to increase stroke risk in prospective studies of the elderly.

CASE 2

Stanley Cooper (Part 3)

Mr. Cooper had the indication for anticoagulation to be started even considering his unsteady gait, and thus elevated fall risk, but after a discussion with Mr. Cooper he and his family chose to see how he would do continuing just on his aspirin.

1. **Was this the right decision?**

2. **How would you explain anticoagulation in order to encourage the family and the patient to agree to it?**

3. **What alternatives should be considered?** ■

The introduction of new antithrombotic agents has modified stroke prevention, and novel AADs, LA appendage occlusion devices, and upstream therapies could also enhance stroke prevention. Antithrombotic therapy is the only treatment for AF associated with reduced mortality. Unlike when using vitamin K antagonists, monitoring the INR has no role in assessing the therapeutic levels of the other drugs, but when the INR is above 2.5 in a patient on dabigatran, that means dabigatran levels above 500, and in our experience over-anticoagulation and elevated bleeding risk.[40] The ultimate roles of the newer agents will be refined in the coming years.

ATRIAL FIBRILLATION SUMMARY

AF is increasingly common. Prevalence is greater than 10% in those older than 80 years of age. The strongest risk factor is age, with diabetes mellitus, hypertension, cigarette smoking, and alcohol, as well as obesity and sleep apnea all increasing the risk (sleep apnea increases AF risk by a factor of four). The benefits for typical patients of returning to sinus rhythm have been overstated and ventricular rate control is now the major goal. With CVAs the most feared complication, families, patients, and physicians overestimate the danger of hemorrhage (2 per 100 patient years); a meta-analysis shows that patients at high risk of falling have an extremely high risk of stroke (13.7 per 100 patient years)! This emphasizes the much greater risk of stroke if the patient is not anticoagulated, compared to the small but increased risk (times 6) of hemorrhage associated with anticoagulation. CHF is a frequent complication of AF: 40% of AF patients developed CHF and 40% of CHF patients developed AF in the Framingham Heart Study.

Web Resources

www.acc.org/clinical/guidelines/stemi/Guideline1/index.htm#top. American College of Cardiology CardioSource. Includes guidelines for care of acute myocardial infarction.

www.americanheart.org. American Heart Association.

www.nhlbi.nih.gov/about/ncep. National Heart, Lung, and Blood Institute's National Cholesterol Education Program.

www.nhlbi.nih.gov/guidelines/hypertension. National Heart, Lung, and Blood Institute's Seventh Report of the Joint National Committee on Prevention, Detection, Evaluation, and Treatment of High Blood Pressure.

www.framinghamheartstudy.org. Framingham Heart Study, a project of the National Heart, Lung, and Blood Institute and Boston University.

KEY REFERENCES

CAD

1. Alexander KP, Newby LK, Armstrong PW, et al. Acute coronary care in the elderly, part II: ST-segment-elevation myocardial infarction: A scientific statement for healthcare professionals from the American Heart Association Council on Clinical Cardiology: In collaboration with the Society of Geriatric Cardiology. Circulation 2007;115(19):2570-89.
2. Alexander KP, Newby LK, Cannon CP, et al. Acute coronary care in the elderly, part I: Non-ST-segment-elevation acute coronary syndromes: A scientific statement for healthcare professionals from the American Heart Association Council on Clinical Cardiology: In collaboration with the Society of Geriatric Cardiology. Circulation 2007;115(19):2549-69.
6. Canto JG, Rogers WJ, Goldberg RJ, et al. Association of age and sex with myocardial infarction symptom presentation and in-hospital mortality. JAMA 2012;307(8):813-22.
15. Franken M, Nussbacher A, Liberman A, et al. ST elevation myocardial infarction in the elderly. J Geriatr Cardiol 2012;9(2):108-14.
16. Bach RG, Cannon CP, Weintraub WS, et al. The effect of routine, early invasive management on outcome for elderly patients with non-ST-segment elevation acute coronary syndromes. Ann Intern Med 2004;141(3):186-95.
18. Forman DE, Chen AY, Wiviott SD, et al. Comparison of outcomes in patients aged <75, 75 to 84, and ≥85 years with ST-elevation myocardial infarction (from the ACTION Registry-GWTG). Am J Cardiol 2010;106(10):1382-8.

AF

36. Fuster V, Rydén LE, Cannom DS, et al. 2011 ACCF/AHA/HRS focused updates incorporated into the ACC/AHA/ESC 2006 Guidelines for the management of patients with atrial fibrillation: A report of the American College of Cardiology Foundation/American Heart Association Task Force on Practice Guidelines developed in partnership with the European Society of Cardiology and in collaboration with the European Heart Rhythm Association and the Heart Rhythm Society. J Am Coll Cardiol 2011;57(11):e101-98.
37. Gage BF, Waterman AD, Shannon W, et al. Validation of clinical classification schemes for predicting stroke: Results from the National Registry of Atrial Fibrillation. JAMA 2001;285(22):2864-70.
38. Mason PK, Lake DE, DiMarco JP, et al. Impact of the CHA2DS2-VASc score on anticoagulation recommendations for atrial fibrillation. Am J Med 2012;125(6):603, e1-6.
39. Gage BF, Birman-Deych E, Kerzner R, et al. Incidence of intracranial hemorrhage in patients with atrial fibrillation who are prone to fall. Am J Med 2005;118(6):612-7.

References available online at expertconsult.com.

38

Congestive Heart Failure

Robert J. Luchi and George E. Taffet

OBJECTIVES

Upon completion of this chapter, the reader will be able to:

- Understand how the clinical features of congestive heart failure (CHF) are altered in the older patient and how brain natriuretic peptide (BNP) levels may aid in making the diagnosis of CHF.

- Appreciate that CHF may be caused by systolic dysfunction or diastolic dysfunction of the heart.

- Understand the important role of angiotensin-converting enzyme (ACE) inhibitors in the prevention and treatment of CHF associated with left ventricular systolic dysfunction.

- List and justify the important additional roles of angiotensin receptor blocker (ARBs) drugs, beta-receptor blocker drugs, spironolactone, nesiritide, and biventricular pacing in the treatment of CHF associated with left ventricular systolic dysfunction.

- Implement treatment strategies for treatment of CHF associated with normal left ventricular systolic function.

CASE 1

Betty Postle (Part 1)

Betty Postle is an 83-year-old white woman who is a new patient for you, brought in by an out-of-town daughter, who notes her mother's decreasing ability to take care of herself. Mrs. Postle is now dyspneic with minimal exertion. Her caregiver had a recent motor vehicle accident, and both Mrs. Postle and her daughter are unclear about Mrs. Postle's medication regimen. On examination, her heart rate is 100 and blood pressure is 89/43 mmHg. She has crackles bilaterally extending halfway up the lung fields, jugular venous distention (JVD), and pedal edema. A II/VI pansystolic murmur is appreciated over her entire precordium with both S_3 and S_4 gallop. Chest x-ray (CXR) cardiac enlargement, pulmonary venous vascular congestion (enlarged hila that appear indistinct because of perivascular edema), and increased prominence of the pulmonary veins draining the upper lobes (cephalization of flow). Hemoglobin is 13 g, white blood cell count is normal, and urinalysis shows 1+ protein without active sediment. Blood urea nitrogen (BUN) and creatinine are 30 mg/dL and 1.6 mg/dL, respectively. Serum albumin is 3.6 g/dL.

1. **What is the significance of the S_3 gallop? And the S_4?**

2. **What is the significance of the pedal edema?**

3. **How should treatment be initiated?**

4. **What further tests will guide optimal treatment? Why?**

5. **What factors precipitating congestive heart failure (CHF) should be ruled out?** ◻

PREVALENCE

CHF is the most common reason for hospitalization in Medicare patients. Prevalence is typically between 10% and 20% in elderly cohorts. The incidence increases tenfold from age 45 to age 85.[1] Five-year survival is less than 50% in both systolic and diastolic CHF.[2]

RISK FACTORS AND PATHOPHYSIOLOGY

Asymptomatic left ventricular systolic dysfunction (ALVSD) frequently progresses to congestive heart failure (CHF). This progression can be retarded by angiotensin-converting enzyme (ACE) inhibitors.[3]

Additional online-only material indicated by icon.

ALVSD is a function of age. In community-based studies, almost all the young people with left [ventricular] systolic dysfunction (left ventricular ejection fraction [LVEF] greater than 30) are asymptomatic; in men older than age 65, half were asymptomatic, and in older women, only 27% were asymptomatic.[4] This may be because the symptoms of CHF are manifestations of compensatory mechanisms used to maintain cardiac output. Data for patients older than age 75 are not available.

Left ventricular systolic dysfunction is the cause of CHF in the elderly patient in 50% to 60% of CHF cases. In the remainder, LVEF is normal but evidence of impaired ventricular filling is present.[5] If significant valvular or pericardial disease is absent, CHF is then attributed to diastolic dysfunction. Normal LVEF, determined by echocardiography or nuclear techniques, is generally 50% or more. Significant left ventricular systolic dysfunction is defined as an LVEF less than 40%. There is no simple measure of diastolic function. CHF resulting from diastolic dysfunction may be so common in the elderly because aging itself results in a stiff, poorly relaxing left ventricle. Disease processes add to these aging effects.

CHF, a more advanced stage of heart failure (strictly defined as impairment in heart function leading to symptoms such as fatigue and dyspnea because of inadequate cardiac output), is defined as the presence of evidence of fluid retention manifested clinically by edema and congestion of the veins of the pulmonary and systemic circuits.

DIFFERENTIAL DIAGNOSIS AND ASSESSMENT

Diagnosis

Classically, the diagnosis of CHF is based on history, physical examination, and chest x-ray (CXR) examination.[6] Brain natriuretic peptide (BNP) testing has altered this approach. Diagnosis of CHF in the elderly may be difficult because the history is often atypical (Box 38-1), or unobtainable, or because the symptoms are minimized by the patient or attributed to age. One of the most common atypical presentations of CHF is delirium, which is frequently superimposed on preexisting dementia.

Physical signs of CHF are often overlooked. Jugular venous distention (JVD) and hepatojugular reflux are excellent signs of "right-sided failure." S_3 gallop remains reliable but is often difficult to hear. In contrast, the S_4 is a common finding in otherwise healthy older patients. Crackles or rales on lung auscultation are nonspecific. Ankle edema often merely reflects inactivity or associated dependency of the legs.

BNP testing has revolutionized CHF diagnosis.

BOX 38-1

CLASSIC AND ATYPICAL MANIFESTATIONS OF CONGESTIVE HEART FAILURE IN THE ELDERLY

Classic (Noncerebral)	Atypical	Atypical (Cerebral)
Dyspnea	Chronic cough	No history
Orthopnea	Insomnia	Falls
Paroxysmal nocturnal	Weight loss	Anorexia, dyspnea
Peripheral edema	Nausea	Behavioral disturbances
Unexplained weight gain	Nocturia	Decreased functional status
Weakness	Syncope	
Poor exercise tolerance		
Abdominal pain		
Fatigue		

A good-quality CXR may be difficult to obtain, especially in frail, older patients. Persistence until an adequate film is obtained pays rich diagnostic dividends. Consider performing the CXR examination with the patient sitting upright in the wheelchair. Key findings are an enlarged heart, enlarged hila with indistinct margins (perivascular edema), and prominent veins draining the upper lobes (cephalization of flow).

The measurement of BNP has revolutionized the diagnosis of CHF. BNP is specific to the ventricles, reflects stretch or tension of the left ventricle, and correlates well with the severity of CHF. BNP is elevated in both systolic and diastolic CHF. Patients with dyspnea and normal BNP are unlikely to have CHF as the cause of their symptoms. BNP levels decrease as CHF patients improve so monitoring BNP may be helpful. Healthy women have higher levels than do men, and BNP increases with age; thresholds used to discriminate normal from CHF may need age and sex adjustment. In addition, BNP is cleared by the kidneys so renal function influences BNP. Various parts of the peptide have been assayed but all appear to provide similar information.[7] BNP has beneficial effects: natriuresis, diuresis, vasodilation, and antagonism of endothelin, aldosterone, and renin. Nesiritide (recombinant human BNP) produces these effects when infused in decompensated patients despite their preexisting BNP elevations. Nesiritide may be less arrhythmogenic than is dobutamine, but experience in elderly patients is limited. BNP, for diagnosis and monitoring, is valuable in the elderly, whereas the use of nesiritide is still being defined.[7]

Beta-blockers help function and survival in CHF.

Precipitating Factors

Conditions increasing cardiovascular demand or interfering with compensatory mechanisms can precipitate CHF in otherwise compensated patients (Box 38-2). Frequent precipitating factors form the mnemonic DAMN IT:

Drugs—including withdrawal of ACE inhibitors, digitalis, or beta-blockers, and the administration of steroids or nonsteroidal antiinflammatory drugs (NSAIDs)

Arrhythmias—bradyarrhythmias, including heart block and tachyarrhythmias, especially atrial fibrillation

Myocardial ischemia—often presenting atypically (consider stress testing if suspicion is high)

Noncompliance—such as with diet, fluid restriction, or medications

Intravenous fluid administration

Thyroid—hyperthyroidism (thyroid-stimulating hormone and free T_4 should be considered) (Box 38-3).

Pharmacologic stress testing can be used if exercise testing is not obtainable. Once precipitants are treated, the ongoing CHF regimen may need to be modified.

> CHF precipitants: Drugs, Arrhythmia, MI, Noncompliance, IV, Thyroid (DAMN IT!).

CASE 1

Betty Postle (Part 2)

You find that Mrs. Postle has a long history of CHF owing to coronary artery disease and hypertension. Current medications include an ACE inhibitor, furosemide, digoxin,

---

BOX 38-2

FACTORS THAT PRECIPITATE CONGESTIVE HEART FAILURE

Anemia
Arrhythmias
Exacerbation of chronic obstructive pulmonary disease
Digoxin withdrawal
Drugs: cardiac depressants (e.g., antiarrhythmics, antineoplastics)
Hypoxia
Hyperthyroidism
Intravenous fluid overload[a]
Infection
Myocardial infarction/ischemia
Dietary or medication noncompliance[b]
Pulmonary embolism
Renal insufficiency
Sepsis

[a]Most common precipitating cause in hospitalized patients.
[b]Most common precipitating cause outside hospital.

BOX 38-3

MNEMONIC OF FREQUENT PRECIPITATING FACTORS OF CONGESTIVE HEART FAILURE (DAMN IT)

Drugs
- withdrawal of ACE inhibitors, digoxin, or beta-blockers
- administration of steroids and NSAIDs

Arrhythmias
- bradyarrhythmias, including heart block
- tachyarrhythmias, especially atrial fibrillation

Myocardial ischemia
- often presents atypically; consider stress testing

Noncompliance
- with diet, fluid restriction, or medications

Intravenous fluids
Thyroid: hyperthyroidism
Once the precipitants are treated, review the ongoing CHF regimen; it may need modification.

---

spironolactone, low-dose beta-blocker, and nitrates. Her electrocardiogram (ECG) reveals sinus tachycardia and prolonged QRS duration. Her BNP is 3030 pg/mL. You control symptoms initially by prescribing a low-sodium diet and increasing her furosemide. As the edema clears, Mrs. Postle's "dry" weight is 105 lbs. The LVEF is 20%, confirming that CHF is caused by systolic dysfunction. You increase her ACE inhibitor, ramipril, to 2.5 mg twice a day.

1. **Why should ACE inhibitors be used in this case?**

2. **What other medications or considerations should be made at this time?** ◘

MANAGEMENT

General treatment measures for CHF include sodium restriction and appropriate exercise after acute symptoms have been controlled. Patient education and support groups help promote compliance. Prognosis should be discussed openly and completion of advanced directives regarding health care preferences encouraged.

Dietary sodium intake should be restricted to 3 g or less per day. The person preparing the patient's food should be instructed by a dietitian. Reduction in alcohol intake is recommended, and smoking is discouraged. Mild aerobic exercise, mainly walking or cycling, increases functional capacity and quality of life.

Repetition of the therapeutic program essentials is necessary for success. Information needs to be given concerning diet, drugs, prognosis, and safe level of activity.[2] This information is best given over several office visits.

There is little randomized clinical trial data directly relevant to very old patients. Extrapolation should be performed cautiously. Because each decision is a risk-benefit analysis, and the impact and likelihood of risks depend on the individual, it seems reasonable to take advantage of published data, but an actual evidence base upon which to make treatment decisions is not available.[8] The risk of medication use in the elderly is complicated by altered pharmacokinetics and by pharmacodynamics resulting from age- and disease-related changes in various organ systems.[6] The goals of treatment are increased quality of life and improved survival.

> **Diuretics in CHF: keep the first dose low and follow magnesium as well as potassium.**

Loop diuretics (furosemide, bumetanide, torsemide, indapamide, ethacrynic acid) are used most frequently because glomerular filtration rate (GFR) in the elderly is often less than 30 mL per minute, rendering thiazides ineffective. The goal is gentle diuresis, avoiding hypotension and its consequences. Equivalent doses of loop diuretics are furosemide 40 mg, bumetanide 1 mg, and ethacrynic acid 50 mg. Whether given orally or intravenously, the first dose should be small because of the danger of an exaggerated "first dose diuresis." Usual maintenance dose is 20 to 40 mg furosemide daily, but 160 mg per day is not unusual. Bumetanide has a shorter duration of action. Ethacrynic acid is rarely used because of ototoxicity, but it is of use in patients allergic to furosemide and bumetanide. Major toxic effects include hypotension, hypokalemia, hyponatremia, and hypomagnesemia. Hypotension can be avoided by orthostatic blood pressure and BUN/creatinine monitoring and reduction of the diuretic dose at the first sign of volume depletion. Removing the last trace of peripheral edema or pleural effusion may decrease preload to the point at which cardiac output decreases. Serum magnesium and potassium should be measured routinely and replaced as indicated. The treatment of hyponatremia depends on the cause: sodium depletion from excessive diuresis calls for reduction in diuretic dose and lessening of sodium restriction; hyponatremia secondary to relative retention of free water is treated by fluid restriction. Diuretic-related incontinence can be avoided by timing of diuretics or giving bumetanide. Other drugs with hypotensive effects can produce serious interactions. NSAIDs can completely inhibit the diuresis by their action on GFR. Potassium-sparing diuretics are useful, in combination with loop diuretics, to reduce potassium loss. Their major side effect is hyperkalemia, which can be additive to the hyperkalemia of ACE inhibitors (see the following paragraph). When the patient is resistant to loop diuretics, metolazone may be added. A 2.5-mg test dose of metolazone is recommended to avoid profound volume depletion. Subsequently, 5 mg is given by mouth 1 hour before the loop diuretic.

ACE inhibitors improve survival and quality of life in patients with CHF with reduced LVEF. Side effects include hypotension, often precipitated by concurrent use of diuretics. ACE inhibitors should not be given to patients with volume depletion. It may be best to begin the ACE inhibitors after the patient enters a stable state, after diuresis. Doses should be started low and progressively raised while the clinician monitors the patient closely. ACE inhibitors are frequently underprescribed, and reaping the benefits requires reaching target doses or at least the maximally tolerated dose.[9] Hyperkalemia and mild to severe angioedema occur, and cough is a symptom of mild airway edema. This may be a bradykinin effect because ACE inhibitors also inhibit kininase II, which breaks down bradykinin.[9] Other ACE inhibitor effects may also be bradykinin mediated.

> **ACE inhibitors: be careful not to underdose!**

CASE 1

Discussion

The calculated creatinine clearance for Mrs. Postle is below 40 mL per minute. Because ramipril and the active metabolite ramiprilat are excreted in urine, correction for renal function is necessary. Therefore, the starting dose should be 1.25 mg twice a day, gradually increasing over time. Her renal function does not contraindicate a trial of ACE inhibitors, but electrolytes, BUN, and creatinine should be monitored regularly.

Aldosterone antagonists are used because the end result of activation of the renin-angiotensin system is aldosterone production by the adrenals. Aldosterone is a potent sodium- and water-retaining steroid with additional actions that are deleterious to the heart and blood vessels. Spironolactone and eplerenone are aldosterone antagonists with utility in moderate or severe CHF[10]; in this study, spironolactone added to an ACE inhibitor improved functional status, reduced total death rate and death from cardiovascular causes, and reduced CHF hospitalizations. Although the mean age of study participants was only 65 and just one fourth were women, in older (age greater than 67) or female subgroups, spironolactone was still effective.

ACE inhibitors should eliminate aldosterone production but they do not. The dose of ACE inhibitor may be insufficient or aldosterone can escape regulation with sustained ACE inhibitor treatment, so aldosterone production takes place in the absence of angiotensin II. Spironolactone also allows loop diuretic doses and potassium to be decreased. In the Randomized Aldactone Evaluation Study (RALES), hyperkalemia in patients treated with spironolactone was infrequent; subsequently, in real world application, it frequently produced life-threatening hyperkalemia. In older patients, especially those with renal impairment or diabetes, aggressive monitoring of potassium and careful patient selection is advised.

Digoxin's role has changed from a first-line drug in CHF treatment when a regular sinus rhythm is present to a second-line drug. Digoxin may improve quality of life and reduce hospitalizations in patients taking diuretics and ACE inhibitors. The dose of digoxin must be reduced when renal function is impaired, and the dose should be further reduced if renal functional impairment increases. Only serum digoxin levels obtained 12 to 24 hours after the dose are useful to evaluate if the dose of digoxin is acceptable.

Beta-blockers have beneficial effects on survival for patients with a history of myocardial infarction that may be additive to the effects of ACE inhibitors. Beta-receptor blocking agents also improve function, improve survival, and reduce hospitalizations for systolic CHF patients. Metoprolol or atenolol are the drugs commonly used. Carvedilol, which blocks both α- and β-adrenergic receptors, reduces rates of hospitalization and improves survival for patients with mild to moderate heart failure secondary to ischemic heart disease.[11] Carvedilol is known to reach 50% higher concentrations in the elderly.[11] Nebivolol, a β-adrenergic antagonist with nitric oxide mediating effects, had modest efficacy in the Study of the Effects of Nebivolol Intervention on Outcomes and Rehospitalization in Seniors with Heart Failure (SENIORS), one of the few studies to feature typical elderly patients. Presently these investigators begin beta-receptor blocking therapy with metoprolol and reserve carvedilol (as a substitute for metoprolol) for those situations in which symptoms worsen in the face of maximal treatment. With all the beta-receptor antagonists, it may take 2 or 3 months of therapy before clinical benefit is noticeable.[9] ▣

CASE 1

Betty Postle (Part 3)

Mrs. Postle does well on a therapeutic program now including metoprolol 12.5 mg twice a day and digoxin 0.125 mg daily. Fourteen days after initiating this daily loading dose of digoxin, her serum digoxin level is 1.6 ng/mL and serum potassium is 3.7 mEq/L. She complains of a cough without sputum production. You discuss the possibility that cough may result from treatment with ACE inhibitors, but Mrs. Postle states that the cough is not that annoying and wishes to continue the ACE inhibitor. Two weeks later she calls to complain that the cough has become quite bothersome and asks if something can be done about it. Physical examination and CXR are negative.

1. **What can be done about the cough without significantly impairing the therapeutic program?**

2. **What additional measures are indicated now to complete the therapeutic program and patient instruction?** ▣

Angiotensin II receptor blocking drugs (ARBs) do not exhibit all of the actions of an ACE inhibitor (e.g., they do not inhibit kininase II), but they do improve the outcome in systolic CHF. In clinical trials, patients taking ARBs have much less cough; however, angioedema, although rare, may occur.[12] Those who develop angioedema on an ACE inhibitor are more likely (up to 10%) to develop angioedema with an ARB than is the general population.[13] ARBs share other side effects of ACE inhibitors, such as hyperkalemia, hypotension, and renal dysfunction, but in general ARBs are tolerated well. In African Americans the use of hydralazine and long-acting nitrates is clearly of benefit in study populations.[14]

CASE 1

Betty Postle (Part 4)

You discontinue Mrs. Postle's ramipril and substitute losartan 25 mg daily. She no longer has a cough. Her CHF remains controlled. You refer Mrs. Postle to a dietitian for counseling about a low-sodium diet. You add aspirin 81 mg and a statin for additional prophylaxis against ischemic cardiac or cerebral events. You prescribe a walking program of gradually increasing distance and time, with the exercise intensity not to produce dyspnea (patient unable to complete a sentence while exercising) or a heart rate greater than 100 beats per minute, and consider a referral to an invasive cardiologist and to a home health agency. ▣

Biventricular pacing or cardiac resynchronization therapy (CRT) is a relatively new intervention for patients with systolic CHF and heterogeneity in the timing of cardiac activation; such patients may have wide QRS on ECG, or dyssynchrony on echocardiography or nuclear study. Conceptually, one can imagine a large left ventricle, activated in an uncoordinated fashion so that blood just sloshes around the ventricle instead of being ejected by a well-timed, homogeneously activated ventricle. CRT electrodes are placed in the right ventricular apex and in the coronary sinus. The delay between impulses is manipulated to optimally activate the ventricle to contract in a more coordinated fashion.

Some patients derive significant benefit from CRT, whereas 25% do not respond. Criteria for choosing between those likely to benefit and the nonresponders are still being defined. In addition to short-term benefit, CRT may remodel and improve the heart in the long term. Older patients, especially women, are underrepresented in published studies so data for decision making are inadequate. Nevertheless, for patients with dilated ventricles and dyssynchrony, CRT may be discussed (if only to be discounted).

Automatic implantable cardiac defibrillators (AICDs) recognize arrhythmias and electrically terminate them.

Sudden death is a very common cause of mortality in patients with heart failure. Because the experience with antiarrhythmic drugs was so discouraging, the research focus turned toward AICDs. A 25% decrease in mortality for CHF patients can be realized with AICDs. This benefit was similar in the oldest subgroup (those older than age 70). Perhaps the optimum in the very select subgroup in whom one should consider these expensive options would be the combined CRT-AICD device if there is dyssynchrony or the AICD alone if there is not. AICDs and CRTs will provide end-of-life challenges; these should be addressed beforehand, rather than in crisis.

Home care–based multidisciplinary efforts are effective in keeping patients out of the hospital and improving their quality of life.[15] Nurses, therapists, and pharmacists contribute to a team effort, supporting the patient in his or her regimen. Adjustments of diuretics or other medications can be made on a daily basis according to protocols.

CASE 2

Gladys Alden (Part 1)

Gladys Alden, a 73-year-old white woman, has mild hypertension and diabetes mellitus controlled with oral hypoglycemic agents. She had a myocardial infarction 1 year ago. She has shortness of breath, nocturnal cough, and lower-extremity edema. Vital signs include blood pressure 150/80 mmHg; pulse 92 regular; resting respiratory rate 26; and temperature 97° F. She has peripheral edema, JVD, positive hepatojugular reflux, bilateral basilar rales, S$_4$ gallop, and a 2/6 systolic ejection murmur heard best at the base of the heart. ECG shows a regular sinus rhythm with evidence of an old anterior myocardial infarction.

You control Mrs. Alden's symptoms of heart failure initially by means of a low-sodium diet and furosemide 40 mg daily. Potassium chloride 25 mEq per day is added to counteract diuretic-related hypokalemia. As her edema clears, her "dry" weight is 110 pounds. You order an echocardiogram to determine if the CHF is related predominately to systolic dysfunction or diastolic dysfunction. The LVEF is 67% without evidence of pericardial or valvular disease, confirming that the CHF is primarily caused by diastolic dysfunction.

1. **What factors in the history and examination would allow you to discriminate between CHF caused by systolic dysfunction and CHF caused by diastolic dysfunction?**
2. **What is Mrs. Alden's prognosis compared to a similar patient with systolic heart failure?** ■

Diastolic Heart Failure

Diastolic heart failure is the more frequent type of heart failure in the elderly; in this type, cardiac contraction is maintained but filling is impaired. This may happen because of problems in active relaxation,

passive stiffness of the ventricle, dyssynchrony of relaxation, or possibly coupling between the arterial tree and the ventricle. Thus diastolic heart failure is probably just as heterogeneous as is systolic heart failure; some of the more promising interventions are directed outside the heart.[16]

The clinical signs and symptoms of diastolic heart failure are, for the most part, identical to those of systolic CHF, and no historical features are unique to one or the other. For example, in our experience with older male veterans, past myocardial infarctions were equally common in both groups.[17] BNP levels may be lower for patients with diastolic CHF, although still clearly elevated.[18]

> **Diastolic heart failure is as common as systolic heart failure in the elderly.**

The mortality of diastolic CHF in the elderly is very high, almost as high as that of systolic CHF, and these outcomes are converging as advances are made in the management of systolic CHF while little progress is made in diastolic heart failure management. Also, in many older patients with systolic CHF, there is a significant component of diastolic dysfunction; interventions focused at diastolic CHF may thus help most such patients.

Treatment

The first line of treatment for diastolic CHF is decreasing the pulmonary congestion and venous pressures with diuretics. Because of the dependence of cardiac output on filling pressure, aggressive diuresis is very likely to result in hypotension or prerenal azotemia. Obviously, if myocardial ischemia is present, this should be addressed promptly; if hypertension is present, reducing afterload may improve cardiac function.

Tachycardia will worsen or precipitate diastolic CHF because diastole (the time for ventricular filling) is disproportionately shortened. Reducing heart rate permits increased time for filling. If atrial fibrillation is present, then calcium channel blockers and beta-blockers may be used.

A few small, short-term studies of patients with diastolic CHF resulting from hypertension, ischemic disease, or both suggest calcium channel blockers, ACE inhibitors, or angiotensin receptor blockers can improve exercise capacity modestly,[17] but overall the published data to direct management are limited.

CASE 2

Discussion

You add an ACE inhibitor, ramipril, in a dose of 1.25 mg twice daily. No hypotension is noted at this dose. The dose of ramipril is then progressively increased to 2.5 mg twice a day. ACE inhibitors are also indicated in this diabetic patient because she has microalbuminuria. Mrs. Alden does well on a regimen including metoprolol 12.5 mg twice a day. Fourteen days later, her BUN is up to 62 and her serum potassium is 5.7 mEq/L. She complains of weakness and lightheadedness when standing up. On physical examination, she has no edema.

The tendency is to dry out patients with diastolic CHF, decreasing filling pressures and compromising cardiac output. It is likely that for Ms Alden to feel her best, she will need to have some pedal edema. ◼

SUMMARY

Left ventricular systolic dysfunction, during its asymptomatic phase (ALVSD), can be slowed in its development into CHF by treatment with ACE inhibitors. CHF in elders is the result of LVSD in more than one half of patients. LVEF is normally more than 50%: significant LVSD exists if the LVEF is less than 40%. Heart failure (i.e., when there are symptoms related to poor cardiac output) often progresses to CHF (i.e., heart failure with evidence of fluid retention). CHF is the most common reason for hospitalization of Medicare patients. In both systolic and diastolic CHF, 5-year survival is less than 50%. Diagnosis of CHF has been revolutionized by BNP measurement: it is elevated in both systolic and diastolic CHF. Diastolic dysfunction is as common as systolic dysfunction in elders. Precipitants of CHF are described by the mnemonic DAMN IT (*d*rugs, *a*rrhythmias, *m*yocardial ischemia, *n*oncompliance, *i*ntravenous fluid, *t*hyroid [hyperthyroidism]). Loop diuretics and ACE inhibitors are the main therapeutic agents for CHF, with aldosterone antagonists (e.g., spironolactone), digoxin, beta-blockers, and ARBs having significant roles. The place of pacing or CRT in therapy of older patients is not yet clarified.

KEY REFERENCES

7. de Denus S, Pharand C, Williamson D. Brain natriuretic peptide in the management of heart failure: The versatile neurohormone. Chest 2004;125:652-68.
9. Yan A, Yan P, Liu P. Narrative review: Pharmacotherapy for chronic heart failure: Evidence from recent clinical trials. Ann Intern Med 2005;142:132-45.
12. Brunner-La Rocca H, Vaddadi G, Esler M. Recent insight into therapy of congestive heart failure: Focus on ACE inhibition and angiotensin-II antagonism. J Am Coll Cardiol 1999;33:1163-73.
15. Rich MW, Beckham V, Wittenberg C, et al. A multidisciplinary intervention to prevent the readmission of elderly patients with congestive heart failure. N Engl J Med 1995;333:1190-5.
18. Aurigemma G, Gaasch W. Diastolic heart failure. N Engl J Med 2004;351:1097-105.

References available online at expertconsult.com.

39

Peripheral Vascular Disease

Jason M. Johanning

OBJECTIVES

Upon completion of this chapter, the reader will be able to:

- Describe the three most common types of peripheral vascular disease.
- Describe the current diagnostic strategy for workup of peripheral vascular disease.
- Describe the indications for treatment including minimally invasive and open surgical options.

PERIPHERAL VASCULAR DISEASE

CASE 1

Fred Jones (Part 1)

Fred Jones is a 73-year-old former maintenance worker who comes to your office with complaints of lower leg cramping with activity. He is obese with a long-standing history of type 2 diabetes mellitus treated with oral medications. He is also hypertensive with a reduced glomerular filtration rate.

What are the ideal diagnostic studies with which to confirm the presence of significant peripheral vascular disease? ◻

Peripheral vascular disease (PVD) is primarily a disease of the aged. The average age of patients seeking treatment is approximately 70 years of age. With the expected increase in our elderly population, the diagnosis and treatment of PVD will become a priority. A working knowledge of the most common sites of disease, the initial diagnostic tests, and options for treatment as well as their outcomes are necessary to provide optimal guidance for these patients.

Additional online-only material indicated by icon.

A basic framework for diagnosis of vascular disease relies heavily on the vascular laboratory. The majority of structures involved in vascular disease, including retroperitoneal vascular structures, can be imaged because of the increasing resolution of ultrasonography. Additionally, in the periphery and supraclavicular region, vessel proximity to the skin level and the dynamic image acquisition often allow diagnosis and treatment without need for advanced imaging modalities. In fact, the vascular laboratory should be able to document the presence and extent of carotid, aortic, and lower extremity disease for the vast majority of patients, with advanced imaging (computed tomography [CT] and magnetic resonance imaging [MRI]) reserved for those patients in whom diagnosis is in question or for pretreatment planning. With regard to CT and MRI, these techniques also have increased in accuracy and clarity. Thus noninvasive imaging has essentially replaced diagnostic angiography for the detection of vascular disease, with angiography primarily reserved for confirmation of disease during planned endovascular intervention.

> Noninvasive imaging has essentially replaced diagnostic angiography for the detection of vascular disease, with angiography primarily reserved for confirmation of disease during planned endovascular intervention.

Similar to the increasing role of noninvasive imaging, there has been an increasing shift in vascular disease treatment to less invasive interventions. Vascular interventions for all patients can follow four different paths. All patients with vascular disease benefit both at disease location and systemically from treatment with antiplatelet agents and from cholesterol-lowering agents, primarily in the form of statin agents. Increasingly, patients are being treated especially in the lower extremities with solely percutaneous interventions requiring arterial access via catheters and guidewires. Although decreasing in usage, open surgical revascularization still remains the gold standard against which all techniques are judged. Lastly, a combination of open and percutaneous endovascular interventions can be combined to create a hybrid operation chosen to address complex vascular disease where outcomes are best served by a unique approach. The important point to remember is the patient at any time can be served by any of these techniques and therefore clinical judgment and informed consent are paramount in choosing the appropriate intervention.

CORONARY ARTERY DISEASE
Indications for Diagnostic Study

CASE 1

Frank Johnson (Part 1)

Frank Johnson is a 70-year-old retired custodian who has transient monocular blindness that he describes as a window shade covering his eye intermittently. He smokes one pack per day despite having coronary artery bypass grafting 10 years previously.

You discuss with Mr. Johnson next steps regarding diagnostic testing.

What are the options specific to the expected outcome for surgical treatment of carotid stenosis? ▣

Carotid Stenosis

Proper diagnosis, management, and treatment of carotid stenosis are important for reducing risk of ischemic stroke in elderly patients. Stroke is the third leading cause of death in the United States and results in significant disability. Generally 80% of strokes are ischemic and 20% hemorrhagic. Of the 80% of ischemic strokes, 20% to 30% are attributed to atheroembolic disease resulting from stenosis of one carotid artery more than 50%. Focus has been placed on risk stratification for proper selection of appropriate treatment. Treatment will vary depending on degree of stenosis and presence of symptoms and comorbid conditions that could potentially increase operative risks.

> Of the 80% of ischemic strokes, 20% to 30% are attributed to atheroembolic disease resulting from stenosis of one carotid artery more than 50%.

History

A complete history is important to identify those patients at increased risk for carotid disease and stroke. It is important to determine if the patient is symptomatic or asymptomatic because this information in combination with imaging studies will dictate what types of treatment are appropriate for patients with varying degrees of stenosis. Patients with prior or current cardiovascular disease may be at increased risk for concurrent carotid disease; therefore, knowing a patient's cardiac history is critical. Neurologic symptoms such as unilateral weakness, numbness or parasthesias, aphasia or dysarthria, history of transient ischemic attack (TIA), prior stroke, or amaurosis fugax (transient unilateral loss of vision) are all significant historical findings. Patients with TIA, stroke, or amaurosis fugax in the past 3 months are at greater risk for stroke and this warrants further workup for carotid disease. Symptoms not usually associated with carotid disease are vertigo, ataxia, diplopia, nausea, vomiting, decreased consciousness, or generalized weakness.

Risk Factors

Risk factors for carotid disease are similar to those of atherosclerosis in other peripheral arteries and include smoking history, advanced age, male gender, and positive family history. Risk factors for stroke risk are multifactorial, but for patients with carotid disease, the most important are a history of neurologic symptoms, the degree of carotid stenosis, and plaque characteristics.

Physical Examination

Complete physical examination is important to determine the possibility of carotid disease as well as to assess the general health of patients who could potentially undergo a procedure. Focused physical examination includes auscultation of heart, palpation of distal pulses, cranial nerve examination, neurologic examination, musculoskeletal examination for overall strength and symmetry as well as examination of face for unilateral weakness or facial droop. Ocular examination can identify Hollenhorst plaques, but may not, and carotid auscultation for bruit is a classic finding, but its absence does not rule out potentially significant carotid disease.

Optimal Diagnostic Study

Multiple radiologic studies can be used to assess the carotid arteries including duplex ultrasonography (DUS), angiography with CT or MRI, and conventional digital angiography (DA). Each has utility in specific situations and these studies should not be used interchangeably. Imaging aids the clinician by providing information about the degree of stenosis and the plaque's morphology and location.

DUS

Ultrasound is an accurate, reliable, noninvasive imaging modality used to characterize carotid vascular disease. It is often the initial study to identify patients with disease. The degree of stenosis is determined by peak velocity through a narrowed lumen. DUS is also very useful for determining plaque morphology. It is operator dependent and can assess only the extracranial carotids.

CT

CT imaging alone is not sufficient to evaluate; contrasted angiography must be used for accurate imaging of the carotid arteries. This may preclude some patients with contrast allergy or preexisting renal disease from this imaging modality. When possible, it is a very effective imaging technique with high resolution and allows full examination of neck and cranial arteries. High calcium content in plaque can obscure contrast and thus occasionally makes identifying plaque morphology difficult. This modality, although noninvasive, does expose the patient to ionizing radiation and can be expensive.

MRI

MRI is a good alternative to CT because contrast is not required for evaluation of arteries, but is required for concurrent soft tissue evaluation. An MRI is noninvasive and allows for plaque morphology analysis as well as examination of intracranial arteries. Magnetic resonance angiography can tend to overestimate the degree of stenosis. It is limited by cost and availability, and because it cannot be used with any implanted ferrous devices. MRI should not be used for first-line imaging.

DA

Conventional peripheral catheter-based DA is considered the gold standard for carotid imaging. It provides excellent images that are easy to interpret. The degree of stenosis and location and morphology of plaque can all be assessed with this modality. It is most useful in patients with conflicting imaging prior to operation. Major limitations are cost, risk associated with a percutaneous intervention under mild sedation, and possibly poor vascular anatomy that could preclude a percutaneous study.

Current recommendations for screening of asymptomatic patients are in constant debate. It is generally agreed that population screening examinations for asymptomatic patients are not cost effective. Highly selected patient populations may benefit from screening. This includes patients older than 60 years with one or more risk factors such as hypertension, coronary artery disease, current smoker, a first-degree relative with history of stroke, or if they may be undergoing a planned coronary artery bypass grafting procedure. Screening is not recommended for patients based solely on presence of an abdominal aortic aneurysm, presence of a carotid bruit, or prior head and neck radiotherapy.

> Asymptomatic patients that may benefit from screening for coronary artery stenosis include those older than 60 years with one or more risk factors such as hypertension, coronary artery disease, current smoker, a first-degree relative with history of stroke, or if they may be undergoing a planned coronary artery bypass grafting procedure.

Surveillance recommendations include postoperative DUS within 30 days to assess status of the artery as well as contralateral imaging to monitor any disease progression when there is greater than 50% stenosis. Specific timing for surveillance DUS is not established; however, with little risk associated and minimal cost, there is little concern about timing as long as it is done.

Treatment

Once a diagnosis of carotid stenosis is made several factors are examined when considering optimal treatment. First is whether or not the patient's stenosis is symptomatic or asymptomatic. Second pertains to the degree of stenosis. Lastly, comorbidities, location of plaque, and patient preferences must be considered. Generally medical management is reserved for low-grade stenosis (less than 50%) in asymptomatic patients. Surgical correction of stenosis is performed for patients with symptomatic stenosis greater than 60% or in asymptomatic patients with stenosis of 70% to 90%.

Endovascular

Carotid artery stenting (CAS) via percutaneous approach has become an acceptable way to manage carotid stenosis. This approach allows for a less invasive technique for potentially poorer operative candidates. CAS also allows for angiography, angioplasty, and stent placement all with one procedure, but it does have limitations. Anatomic conditions of femoral vessels, the aorta, and the aortic arch must be appropriate. Furthermore, plaque characteristics such as long segment lesions may lead to multiple stents, and soft plaques can rupture, increasing perioperative stroke risk. CAS may be more beneficial in asymptomatic patients with greater than 60% stenosis and for symptomatic patients with greater than 50% stenosis with coronary artery disease or prior head or neck radiation. CAS can reduce the number of perioperative myocardial infarctions, but it does have a higher risk of periprocedural stroke.

Open Repair

Carotid endarterectomy (CEA) is the gold standard operative procedure for correction of carotid stenosis. It has been shown to reduce stroke risk to 7% over 2 years from 17% when compared with medical management alone. CEA is generally preferred for patients with carotid stenosis because of the improved outcomes with reduction in overall stroke risk and risk of periprocedural death. The procedure requires excision between the plane of the inner and outer medial layers, resulting in removal of intima, plaque, and part of the media. A patch is sewn in place to close the carotid artery. CEA is preferred in patients with longer segment disease, or with occlusions of greater than 70% stenosis. Patients are monitored overnight in the hospital and can be discharged the following day barring any complications or concerns.[1]

Medical

Medical management is important for all patients with carotid disease regardless of the degree of stenosis. Treatment is aimed at decreasing stroke risk and minimizing progression of stenosis. Treating underlying comorbid conditions is important. Hypertension, diabetes mellitus, and lipid abnormalities are all treatable conditions. Smoking nearly doubles stroke risk and cessation will markedly improve patients' risk. Universal anticoagulation recommendations have not been adopted because there is no evidence suggesting antiplatelet agents other than aspirin have improved benefit in asymptomatic carotid stenosis patients. Antiplatelet agents are recommended for patients with non-cardioembolic ischemic stroke or TIA associated with carotid atherosclerosis. Aspirin is the most commonly used antiplatelet therapy but should not be used in combination with clopidogrel for this indication because no benefit has been shown.

Outcomes

Complications associated with surgical repair include stroke, cranial nerve injury, hematoma, reocclusion, and complications with anesthesia. As noted earlier, risk of myocardial infarction is higher in CEA patients, and perioperative stroke rates are higher in CAS. Morbidity and mortality can range from 1% to 2% to as high as 10%. Accepted 30-day stroke and death risk is about 3% or lower for patients with greater than 60% stenosis and who are expected preoperatively to live more than 5 years.[2]

ABDOMINAL AORTIC ANEURYSM

CASE 1

Frank Roberts (Part 1)

Frank Roberts is a 75-year-old male who on workup for an unrelated disease was found to have a 6-cm asymptomatic abdominal aortic aneurysm. He was a previous smoker who quit 40 years ago. His past medical history includes hypertension and hypercholesterolemia.

Mr. Roberts is reluctant to think about surgery.

What information can you provide Mr. Roberts about the risk that his abdominal aortic aneurysm will rupture? ▣

Indications for Diagnostic Study

Abdominal aortic aneurysm (AAA) is a degenerative disease of the aorta in which progressive remodeling of the arterial wall leads to progressive dilatation and possibly rupture. AAA is defined by increase in vessel diameter by more than 50%, generally more than 3.0 cm. AAA is a progressive disease that can result in a long indolent period or unexpected rupture, which is associated with high morbidity. It is most commonly seen in men older than age 65. Common presenting symptoms are abdominal pain radiating to the back or a pulsatile abdominal mass.

History

A thorough history is helpful in determining a patient's risk for developing an AAA as well as his or her risks associated with complications; the history is also useful for identifying comorbidities that may affect surgical repair. Estimation of the patient's functional and cardiac status is critical in order to assess the patient's preoperative reserve and ability to tolerate surgical repair. The metabolic equivalent unit, or MET, is a standard criterion for assessing a patient's activity level and is frequently used to assess a patient's preoperative status. A complete cardiac history is important because coronary artery disease is the leading cause of mortality after AAA repair. Other comorbidities that contribute to morbidity and mortality are chronic obstructive pulmonary disease and diabetes mellitus.

Risk Factors

Identifying patients at risk for an AAA is part of a complete history. Development of an AAA is associated with smoking, advanced age, coronary artery disease, atherosclerosis, high cholesterol, hypertension, first-degree relative affected, and male gender. Risk factors for expansion include advanced age, severe cardiac disease, prior stroke, and tobacco use. Independent risk factors for rupture of AAA include female gender, large initial diameter, low forced expiratory volume (FEV_1), current smoking, and elevated mean blood pressure. Patients with family history for inherited disorders such as Marfan's syndrome, Ehlers–Danlos syndrome, and familial thoracic aortic aneurysm and dissection (TAAD) are also at increased risk for developing AAA at a younger age.

Physical Examination

Complete physical examination is critical to assess overall patient function. Abdominal exam may or may not reveal a pulsatile mass in the mid-abdomen. This is highly dependent on patient body habitus and size of the AAA if present. AAAs between 3.0 and 3.9 cm are detected only 29% of the time, whereas an AAA larger than 5.0 cm can be detected 76% of the time. In addition to abdominal examination, peripheral pulses, femoral pulses, and cardiac and pulmonary examinations should be performed at a minimum.[3]

Optimal Diagnostic Study

Multiple radiologic studies can be used to assess AAA including ultrasound (US), CT and MRI. Each has utility in specific situations and they should not be used interchangeably.

Ultrasound

US is an inexpensive, noninvasive, and accessible means to detect an AAA. Sensitivity and specificity for detection are close to 100%. Limitations include operator skill level, variability from examiner to examiner, and nonvisualization resulting from bowel gas or body habitus. US is ideal for screening, but it is not good for preoperative anatomic assessment or for determining exact AAA growth rate over time.

CT

CT is an excellent means of imaging AAA and is generally more reproducible than US with more consistent measurements between examinations. CT also allows for examination of the entire aorta, intraabdominal/pelvic structures, and allows for three-dimensional reconstruction of vessels. Use of intravenous contrast allows for greater detail and information about the aneurysm, arterial calcification, and presence of thrombus. CT also provides excellent imaging of related anatomy such as femoral, iliac, and renal vessels, which are important for preoperative planning when undergoing endovascular repair. CT has become more accessible yet still can be expensive and exposes the patient to radiation.

MRI

MRI can be used to evaluate AAA; however, because of expense, time, and limited access, MRI should not be first-line imaging for AAA.

Current recommendations for screening are ever changing because no screening protocol has been demonstrated to be more beneficial than another. Generally US exam should be done on men older than 65 who have a smoking history or men older than 55 with family history. Women should be screened with US at 65 if there is a family history or smoking history. Currently Medicare offers US screening as part of its Welcome to Medicare physical examination to men who have smoked at least 100 cigarettes or to any patient with a family history.

> Ultrasound AAA screening should be done on men older than 65 who have a smoking history or men older than 55 with family history. Women should be screened with US at 65 if there is a family history or smoking history. Currently Medicare offers US screening as part of its Welcome to Medicare physical examination to men who have smoked at least 100 cigarettes or to any patient with a family history.

No definitive recommendations have been established for surveillance if an AAA is detected. Current practice is to follow up at 12-month intervals for 3.5- to 4.4-cm AAAs and 6-month intervals for 4.5- to 5.4-cm AAAs. Three- to five-year follow-up is appropriate for 2.6- to 3.3-cm AAAs. All follow-up should include repeat imaging to accurately assess any change in AAA diameter. Should an AAA become symptomatic, imaging may be indicated sooner.

Treatment

Treatment for AAA is specifically aimed at reducing a patient's risk of rupture. Therefore general principles of treatment weigh the risk of rupture for a patient's AAA with the risk of morbidity and mortality associated with the surgical repair. Size is the major determining factor for risk of rupture, but rate of expansion can also be used. Larger AAAs have a higher yearly risk of rupture, with aneurysms smaller than 4.0 cm having a 0% to 0.5% yearly rupture risk, 5.0- to 6.0-cm AAAs having a 3% to 15% yearly rupture risk, and AAAs larger than 8 cm having up to a 50% yearly rupture risk. It is generally accepted that AAAs between 5.0 and 5.5 cm for men and 4.5 to 5.0 cm for women have a high enough yearly risk for rupture that surgical intervention is indicated on an elective basis. Any AAA that enlarges 0.05 to 0.07 cm in 6 months or 1 cm in 12 months, regardless of size, is also an indication for surgical repair.[4]

Endovascular Aneurysm Repair (EVAR)

First described in 1991, the endovascular aneurysm repair (EVAR) approach uses the femoral arteries as access points for catheters and wires, allowing for a graft to be placed intraluminally under fluoroscopy. This technique has numerous benefits over the traditional open approach. Benefits include no abdominal incision, less postoperative pain, shorter hospital stay, and lower 30-day mortality. These benefits allow for patients who could not tolerate an open procedure to have their AAA repaired, as well as quicker recovery for ideal surgical candidates. In spite of these perioperative benefits, numerous studies have not shown any improvement in quality of life or long-term morbidity and mortality. Endovascular repair is limited to patients with specific aneurysm characteristics and locations, and can also be limited by less favorable femoral and iliac artery anatomy. Control of ruptured AAAs can also be managed endovascularly with quick access and avoidance of a large incision that could possibly depressurize a rupture that has tamponaded in the retroperitoneum. Risks associated with EVAR include rupture, graft migration, endoleaks, perforation, infection, femoral artery aneurysm, hemorrhage, infection, and others.

Open Aneurysm Repair

Open repair of an AAA requires either a transperitoneal or retroperitoneal approach, with midline laparotomy common. Open approach is generally used for patients who do not meet anatomic specifications for EVAR, or for those who require more complex repairs. This approach may also be indicated for redo procedures on the aorta. Once the aorta has been dissected from the retroperitoneum it can be clamped to stop blood flow into the aneurysm. The AAA is then opened and a graft is sewn intraluminally proximally and distally with the aneurysm sac closed over the newly placed graft. Patients are monitored in the intensive care unit postoperatively and generally do well both short and long term, although there is a higher 30-day morbidity and mortality when compared with EVAR. Risks associated with open repair include iatrogenic injury, bowel ischemia, hemorrhage, infection, hernia and others.

Medical

Optimal medical management is indicated for all patients with AAA. This includes smoking cessation, hypertension control, lipid control, diabetes management, diet and exercise lifestyle modifications, and regular follow-up with the primary care provider. New evidence also suggests that small asymptomatic AAAs may be amenable to medical therapy. Matrix metalloproteinases (MMPs) have been found to play a critical role in development of AAA. These enzymes can be inhibited with doxycycline; this property is independent from the drug's antimicrobial properties. Research has shown decreased rate of growth and even reversal of AAA size in some cases. Currently no recommendation for use of doxycycline for management of small AAAs exists, but clinical trials are currently under way.[5]

Outcomes

With proper diagnosis, surveillance, and medical management, patients can go years without needing surgical repair for their AAA. For those who do qualify for elective repair, discussion with patient and surgeon to address the best approach is critical. EVAR has more short-term perioperative benefits. However, the cost for fewer short-term complications is more complications over the long term and secondary interventions associated with graft durability. The reintervention rate at 6 years for EVAR patients was 29.6%, versus 18.1% for those who had had open repair. In a recent prospective trial, 6-year survival for EVAR was 68.9%, versus 69.9% for open repair.[6]

LOWER EXTREMITY ARTERIAL DISEASE

Indications for Diagnostic Study

Lower extremity arterial disease is commonly referred to as peripheral arterial disease (PAD). It is clearly a disease of the elderly, with various studies documenting a 15% to 20% incidence in patients older than age 70. The presentation of PAD varies over a continuum. The most common presentation is that of claudication, or cramping of the lower extremity muscles. The cramping or aching occurs primarily in the calves and buttocks and is relieved within 10 minutes of cessation of activity. Although claudication secondary to arterial disease may seem significant and can cause the patient significant distress, the rate of progression of disease to rest pain (severe ischemic pain caused by insufficient arterial inflow), gangrene, and subsequent amputation is low and on the order of 10% even in the absence of any intervention.

History

A focused history of ambulation is able to confirm the diagnosis of claudication in the majority of patients. The patient with true vasculogenic claudication will complain of pain with ambulation that starts after a known distance (often at presentation this will be on the order of two to three blocks, a distance that commonly interferes with activities of daily living). Upon cessation of activity and with simple standing, the pain will subside and the patient will be able to ambulate again a similar distance. This cycle in vasculogenic claudication can be repeated indefinitely. In the elderly patient, coexistent disease is common and must be distinguished. The two most common conditions are neurogenic claudication secondary to spinal stenosis and osteoarthritis of the hip or knee. Osteoarthritis is more easily differentiated from claudication as the pain of osteoarthritis generally localizes to the joint, improves with pain medications, and has a varying course of improvement and worsens throughout the day. Neurogenic claudication is the most difficult to differentiate from vasculogenic disease because of the frequency of spinal stenosis in the elderly population. The most common presenting symptom of neurogenic claudication is pain in the calves and posterior thigh and buttocks. In contrast to vasculogenic disease, neurogenic claudication has a variable distance to onset, often takes 15 minutes to more than several hours to relieve the pain, and claudication distance can be significantly increased with the use of an assistive device such as a shopping cart on which the patient can lean and relieve the pressure on the nerves within the spinal canal. Unfortunately, often all three conditions in the elderly patient can coexist and then diagnosis of the primary limiting condition is of utmost concern to achieve an optimal outcome and maintain ambulatory independence.

Risk Factors

Risk factors for PAD are similar to those of atherosclerosis in other peripheral arteries and include smoking history, advanced age, male gender, and positive family history.

Physical Examination

Lower extremity examination and documentation includes inspection of the legs to assess for and document lesions consistent with arterial ischemia. Arterial lesions are primarily located on the toes or distal foot and tend to be painful because of loss of arterial flow. Loss of hair on the toes and distal ankles is also a common finding in patients with arterial compromise. Palpation of pulses in the femoral, popliteal, and tibial (dorsalis pedis and posterior tibial) allows a relatively quick determination of location of disease (loss of femoral pulses = aortoiliac disease, loss of popliteal pulses with preservation of femoral pulse = superficial femoral artery disease, loss of tibial pulses with preservation of popliteal pulse = tibial arterial disease of the lower leg).

Optimal Diagnostic Study

Multiple radiologic studies can be used to assess the lower extremity arteries including DUS, angiography with CT or MRI, and conventional DA. Each has utility in specific situations and should not be used interchangeably. Although these are noninvasive, simple Doppler analysis in the form of segmental arterial pressures and ankle brachial index (ABI) can be very useful in providing an adequate physiologic picture of the peripheral vasculature.

DUS

Ultrasound is an accurate, reliable, noninvasive imaging modality used to characterize carotid vascular disease. It is often the initial study to identify patients with disease. The degree of stenosis is determined by peak velocity through a narrowed lumen. DUS is also very useful for determining plaque morphology. It is operator dependent and can assess only the extracranial carotids.

CT

CT imaging alone is not sufficient to evaluate for lower extremity arterial disease; contrasted angiography must be used for accurate imaging of the carotid arteries. This may preclude some patients with contrast allergy or preexisting renal disease from this imaging modality. When possible, CT is a very effective imaging technique with high resolution and allows full examination of neck and cranial arteries. High calcium content in plaque can obscure contrast and thus occasionally makes identifying plaque morphology difficult. This modality, while noninvasive, does expose the patient to ionizing radiation and can be expensive.

MRI

MRI is a good alternative to CT because contrast is not required for evaluation of arteries (but contrast is required for concurrent soft tissue evaluation). MRI is noninvasive and allows for plaque morphology analysis as well as examination of intracranial arteries. Magnetic resonance angiography can tend to overestimate the degree of stenosis. MRI is limited by cost and availability, and cannot be used in patients with any implanted ferrous devices. MRI should not be used for first-line imaging.

DA

Conventional peripheral catheter-based DA is considered the gold standard for carotid imaging. It provides excellent images that are easy to interpret. The degree of stenosis and the location and morphology of plaque can all be assessed with this modality. DA is most useful in patients with conflicting imaging prior to operation. Major limitations are cost, risk associated with a percutaneous intervention under mild sedation, and possibly poor vascular anatomy that could preclude a percutaneous study.

Current recommendations for screening asymptomatic patients for lower extremity arterial disease are in constant debate. It is generally agreed upon that population screening examinations for asymptomatic patients are not cost effective. Highly selected patient populations may benefit from screening. This includes patients older than 60 with one or more risk factors such as hypertension, coronary artery disease, current smoker, a first-degree relative with history of stroke, or if they may be undergoing a planned coronary artery bypass grafting procedure. Screening is not recommended for patients based solely on presence of an abdominal aortic aneurysm, presence of a carotid bruit, or prior head and neck radiotherapy.

Surveillance recommendations include postoperative DUS within 30 days to assess status of the artery as well as contralateral imaging to monitor any disease progression when there is greater than 50% stenosis. Specific timing for surveillance DUS is not established; however, with little risk associated and minimal cost, there is little concern about timing as long as it is done.

Treatment

Once a diagnosis of PAD is made, initial treatment should consist of medical management of the patient's atherosclerotic disease and a thorough assessment of the patient's cardiac status should be conducted; 90% of patients with PAD will have documented coronary artery disease based on angiographic evaluation with absence of overt symptoms secondary to lack of activity.

Medical management should consist of an antiplatelet agent in conjunction with a statin agent. Secondly, a walking program in which the patient is encouraged to walk 30 minutes at a time, preferably three times a week, should be initiated. With a walking regimen that is followed, patients can double or triple their maximal walking distance. Additionally, exercise itself

has outcomes that are comparable to iliac angioplasty and stenting. Drugs such as cilostazol (Pletal) may be prescribed, taking into account side effects and contraindications. If tolerated, there is evidence that these agents do improve ambulation in patients with claudication; however, the maximal gain in walking distance is somewhat limited compared with exercise therapy. Interventions to restore blood flow are indicated (1) in patients with significant disease that limits ambulation thus resulting in subsequent lifestyle changes that are unacceptable, (2) in patients with pain at rest, or (3) in patients with gangrene and tissue loss.

> Exercise consisting of a 30-minute walk three times a week can double or triple maximal walking distance in patients with lower extremity arterial disease and can have outcomes that are comparable to iliac angioplasty and stenting.

Endovascular

PAD treatment via the percutaneous approach has become the preferred initial treatment modality for those patients with both lifestyle-limiting claudication and rest pain/tissue loss. The approach is usually from the femoral arteries for both iliac and femoral/tibial lesions. Short focal stenosis responds very well to angioplasty and stenting, whereas long segment stenosis and occlusions are more challenging to treat and have a reduced patency rate. Although generally believed to be less durable than open surgical approaches, the endovascular approach provides a lack of major complications compared with open surgery and can be repeated two to three times after the initial revascularization procedure while still maintaining the ability to perform open surgical bypass in the future.

Open Repair

Open surgical bypass of occluded or stenotic segments still remains the gold standard against which percutaneous interventions are gauged. Bypass of iliac stenosis using aorto-bifemoral bypass or bypass of the occluded superficial femoral artery or proximal tibial arteries is the most commonly performed procedure to provide pulsatile flow to the distal leg in the setting of lesions or gangrene. The downside to open surgical revascularization is the definite risk of mortality and morbidity that accompanies these procedures despite the much more reliable provision of blood flow.

Outcomes

Complications associated with percutaneous intervention include vessel thrombosis, embolization, dissection, and rupture. Although complications can be serious, they are worth tolerating because of the severity of PAD; acute complications of PAD can necessitate amputation and the patient should be made aware of the potential for limb loss. Outcomes for percutaneous intervention are improving, with patency rates of intervened segments approaching 80% at 2 years for iliac stents and 70% at 2 years for superficial femoral artery (SFA) stents. Aortoiliac revascularization using aorto-bifemoral bypass has a 90% 5-year patency. Femoral popliteal and femoral tibial bypass have 70% to 80% and 60% to 70% 5-year patency respectively. More important, limb salvage is greater than 90% in the majority of patients at 2 years and this is confirmed by large-scale data documenting a reduction in amputation rates in population-based studies.[7]

SUMMARY

Knowing how to diagnose and manage peripheral vascular disease is important for the geriatrician because there is a high incidence of the disease in the elderly population. A trend toward noninvasive diagnosis and minimally invasive approaches is noted. However, a treatment plan based on knowledge of current treatment paradigms with attention to provider- and patient-specific factors should be taken into consideration to achieve optimal treatment outcome.

KEY REFERENCES

2. Ricotta JJ, AbuRahma A, Ascher E, et al. Updated society for vascular surgery guidelines for management of extracranial carotid disease. J Vasc Surg 2011;54(3):e1-31.
3. Chaikof EL, Brewster DC, Dalman RL, et al. The care of patients with an abdominal aortic aneurysm: The society for vascular surgery practice guidelines. J Vasc Surg 2009;50(4 Suppl):S2-49.
7. Silva MB, Choi L, Cheng CC. Peripheral arterial occlusive disease. In: Townsend C, Beauchamp RD, Evers BM, Mattox KL, editors. Townsend: Sabiston textbook of surgery. 19th ed. Philadelphia, PA: Elsevier Saunders; 2012, p. 1725-84.

References available online at expertconsult.com.

40

Transient Ischemic Attacks and Stroke

Susana M. Bowling and Janice Weinhardt

OUTLINE

OBJECTIVES

Upon successful completion of this chapter, the reader will be able to:

- Use appropriate stroke terminology.
- Identify appropriate classification of strokes as a guide to selection of secondary stroke prevention measures.
- Define transient ischemic attack (TIA) in physiologic terms and discuss its appropriate management.
- Identify individualized risk factors for stroke and outline appropriate management of these factors.
- Describe a step-wise approach to hospitalized stroke care that maximizes recovery, minimizes complications, and uses principles of accountable care and transitions of care.

Additional online-only material indicated by icon.

PREVALENCE AND IMPACT

Stroke occurs when there is a rapid loss of neurologic function corresponding to a localized area of the brain caused by disturbance of its blood supply. This can be caused by either an interruption of blood flow (ischemic stroke) or an extravasation of blood outside of the vessel (hemorrhagic stroke). Hippocrates (circa 400 BC) wrote about "apoplexy" to refer to symptoms of what we now know as stroke. Four centuries ago, William Cole (1635-1716), first coined the term *stroke*, which continues to be the only appropriate term. Unfortunately, for a short period of time in the 1970s, a series of acronyms were introduced: SFR, RIND, PRIND, PRINS, TRINS, IRINS, CVA, as well as terms such as *stroke in evolution, completed stroke*, and *incomplete stroke* or *mini stroke*. These have been abandoned among experts, not only because of their lack of anatomic, physiologic, and prognostic implications, but most importantly because they were inconsistently defined and applied. This has led to chaotic communication among health professionals and confusion among patients. Despite its inadequacy, the outdated term *cerebrovascular accident (CVA)* continues to be used. There is nothing "accidental" about strokes.

Every year, AHA/ASA publishes epidemiologic updates revealing a progressive increase in stroke incidence. As of 2012, 795,000 people had experienced a new or recurrent stroke per year and approximately 76% of these are first attacks. This increase is most likely related to more aggressive evaluation and better imaging technology. Of the types of strokes, 87% are ischemic, 10% intracerebral hemorrhage (ICH), and 3% subarachnoid hemorrhage (SAH).[1]

Hospital admissions for ICH have increased by 18% in the past 10 years. This is attributable to increases in the number of elderly people (many of whom lack adequate blood pressure control) as well as to the increasing use of anticoagulant and antiplatelet therapies. Mexican Americans, Latin Americans, African Americans, Native Americans, Japanese, and Chinese continue to have higher incidences of ICH than do white Americans.[1]

> Despite the increase in stroke numbers over the last year, mortality has decreased and stroke is now the fourth leading cause of death in the United States. Stroke remains a leading cause of disability.

PATHOPHYSIOLOGY

Rudolf Virchow, Amédée Dechambre, and Miller Fisher are some of the contributors to the current understanding of the mechanisms of ischemic stroke: description of thrombosis, (Virchow's triad), characterization of lacunar infarction, and understanding of carotid occlusion and embolism, respectively. Their work led to the etiopathogenic classification of cerebrovascular diseases as landmarked by the World Health Organization in the 1980s and by the AHA/ASA Scientific Committee in 2010. Location of blood in hemorrhagic strokes determines the subclassification of either intracerebral, ICH (blood within the parenchyma), or subarachnoid (SAH, blood in the subarachnoid space).[2-4]

Atherothrombosis refers to the development of atherosclerotic plaque. This plaque can be located anywhere along the cerebrovascular tree, intracranial or extracranial, independent of the size of the vessel. Most commonly, however, plaque forms in areas of flow turbulence such as bifurcations because of injury to the endothelium. Plaque rupture—with or without artery-to-artery embolization, intraplaque hemorrhage, ulceration, or luminal thrombosis— heralds acute occlusions of a vessel.

Lacunar infarctions result from the long-term effect of high blood pressure and diabetes on small penetrating vessels leading to thickening of the medial layer of the blood vessel by means of lipohyalinosis and fibronecrosis. Ultimately the lumen of the vessel becomes compromised and affects flow and consequently causes tissue ischemia and stroke.

Cerebral embolism results from the obstruction of a cerebral vessel by particles moving upstream, most typically originating from a cardiac source. Approximately 20% of strokes are embolic. Of these, 80% will affect the anterior circulation and 20% the vertebrobasilar system. Debris can be made of platelet aggregates, thrombus, cholesterol, calcium, bacterial, neoplastic cells, or mixomatous material. Different conditions can be classified as medium to high risk for cardiac embolism.[4] The aortic arch can also be a source of debris particularly plaque and plaque-thrombus embolus. A transesophogeal echocardiogram (TEE) assists in the identification of aortic arch pathology as a potential cause of stroke. Paradoxical embolus refers to the origin of particle being venous rather than arterial. Emboli detour into the arterial system by means of a shunting mechanism, most typically through a patent foramen ovale (PFO), or pulmonary arteriovenous malformation. In such cases, characteristics of the embolus could be very diverse: air, fat, amniotic fluid.[4]

Approximately 5% of strokes are the result of other causes such as arteritis, vascular dissections, sickle cell anemia, cerebral venous thrombosis, vasospasm, and genetic vasculopathies. When the cause of a stroke is not identified, strokes are referred to as cryptogenic. Cryptogenic classifications may be given when the evaluation was considered incomplete, there is more

than one cause of stroke identified, or the cause remains in question after complete evaluation.[2-4] The etiopathogenesis of hemorrhagic stroke, ICH, and SAH are listed in Box 40-1. The most common cause of ICH is hypertension; the most common cause of SAH is aneurysmal rupture.[4]

> **A second stroke cannot be prevented without understanding the mechanism that led to the first stroke.**

CASE 1

Mrs. Hernandez (Part 1)

Mrs. Hernandez, an 83-year-old Hispanic woman, comes to your office with her daughter. She denies any active problems other than severe arthritis for which she takes over-the-counter medication. She has not seen a physician since relocating and moving in with her daughter 2 years ago following the death of her husband. The daughter reports that her mother is depressed, inactive, and forgetful, which is particularly worse in the morning. Her history includes laryngeal cancer that was treated with radiation 10 years ago. She has no other documented medical or surgical conditions. Her family history includes coronary artery disease and stroke in both parents. She complains of hypersomnolence and fatigue during the day.

Box 40-1

ETIOLOGY OF HEMORRHAGIC STROKES

Hypertension
Vascular malformation
Saccular aneurysm
Arteriovenous malformation
Venous angioma
Telangiectasias
Cavernomas
Bleeding disorders
  Genetically acquired
  Iatrogenic (anticoagulants, antiplatelets)
  Inflammatory, acute illness (DIC)
Autoimmune (TTP, ITP)
Liver failure/alcohol abuse
Dural venous fistulas
Arterial dissections
Cerebral venous thrombosis
Hemorrhagic infarctions
Hemorrhagic contusions
Neoplastic/metastatic
Infections (particularly viral)
Autoimmune (vasculitis)
Drugs (particularly cocaine, NSAIDs)
Amyloid angiopathy

DIC, Disseminated intravascular coagulation; ITP, idiopathic thrombocytopenic purpura; NSAIDs, nonsteroidal antiinflammatory drugs; TTP, thrombotic thrombocytopenic purpura.

The patient has been independent but uses a walker for long distances because of the fatigue and arthritis. She rarely drinks alcohol but is a two-pack-a-day smoker. Her only fluid intake is coffee and she eats a careless diet. Her physical exam is significant for being unengaged with conversation, cooperative but demonstrating some difficulties following complex commands. Her Mini-Mental State Examination is 29/30 based solely on word-finding problems. The rest of her exam includes: blood pressure 150/90 mmHg, body mass index above 30, significant arthritic changes, poor dental care, soft bruit on left, and II/IV systolic left parasternal ejection murmur that diminishes with squatting and increases upon standing. She has no clear focal findings other than mild apraxia of fine motor movements with the right hand, loss of reflexes S1 bilaterally, decreased vibratory, proprioception, and temperature sensation to the ankles, and mild unsteady gait with interrupted turns resulting in part from her arthritis.

1. **What are Mrs. Hernandez's risk factors for stroke?**
2. **What working diagnosis should you consider for further evaluation?**
3. **What elements of counseling and education should be discussed in the first visit?** ◘

DIFFERENTIAL DIAGNOSIS AND ASSESSMENT

Stroke symptoms appear abruptly, are focal in nature, and depend on the location and function of the damaged brain cells. The most common signs and symptoms include the following:
- Sudden weakness of arm, leg, and/or face, usually on one side of the body
- Sudden sensory loss, usually on one side of the body
- Sudden speech abnormalities
- Sudden and unusual headache
- Sudden dizziness or loss of balance
- Sudden loss of vision or double vision

Limb-shaking transient ischemic attacks (TIAs) may precede an anterior cerebral artery (ACA) occlusion and are caused by intermittent compromised flow through a critically narrowed vessel. Compromised flow to the vertebrobasilar system can result in drop attacks. Transient retinal ischemia caused by compromised flow to the ophthalmic artery results in amaurosis fugax, a transient loss of vision in one eye. Dizziness in a patient older than age 60 should raise the concern for vertebrobasilar insufficiency. Examination findings such as unidirectional nystagmus, test of skew (vertical strabismus), and head impulse testing can help discern peripheral from central causes of vertigo.[5]

Stroke mimics are common sources of diagnostic errors, suboptimal treatments, and readmissions. Tumors, metabolic disorders, and in particular, rapid changes in glucose values, hemiplegic migraine, infection, seizures/Todd's paralysis, and conversion disorders are among the most common alternative diagnoses. Seizures should be considered if the patient has an altered level of consciousness, involuntary movements, and positive symptoms such as tingling. Consider musculoskeletal disorders in the presence of pain.

> Stroke symptoms appear abruptly, are focal in nature, and depend on the location and function of the damaged brain cells.

Identification of the vascular territory responsible for the stroke is important in guiding decisions for treatment strategies and for counseling patients/families regarding therapeutic options, risks and expectations for complications, morbidity, and mortality. Distinction must be made regarding the vascular territory involved: large vessel versus small vessel injury, cortical versus subcortical, and anterior versus posterior circulation (Table 40-1, Boxes 40-2 to 40-5).

Table 40-1	Anterior Circulation
Anterior Circulation—LMCA	**Anterior Circulation—RMCA**
• Language dysfunction • Right hemiparesis/hemiplegia • Right sensory loss • Face and arm more than leg • Variably, contralateral homonymous hemianopsia • Impaired rightward gaze	• Left hemiparesis/hemiplegia • Left sensory loss • Dyspraxia • Neglect • Face and arm more than leg • Variably, contralateral homonymous hemianopsia • Impaired contralateral gaze

LMCA, Left middle cerebral artery; *RMCA*, right middle cerebral artery.

Box 40-2
CORTICAL SIGNS OF STROKE
• Aphasia (can the patient repeat)   • Neglect   • Extinction   • Spatial disorientation/acalculia   • Face and arm vs. face, arm, and leg   • Graphesthesia, two-point discrimination   • Horizontal gaze preference   • Hemianopsia

TRANSIENT ISCHEMIC ATTACKS (TIAs)

These "transient" episodes of focal neurologic deficits have been the subject of research, as well as discussions of origin, significance, accuracy of diagnosis, evaluation and treatment guidance. Sir William Osler and Miller Fisher were contributors to the evolution of the field of neurology. They emphasized the importance of temporary attacks as a warning that often precedes stroke and the association of these attacks with carotid artery occlusion and large strokes in 1951.

The term *TIA*, inadequately substituted for terms such as *mini stroke*, has been the subject of discussion for decades, beginning with the first Princeton Conference (biannual academic stroke conference sponsored by the National Institute of Neurological Disorders and Stroke) in 1954, to the final recognition of the term in 1965. That the mechanism of attack is a temporary reduction in blood flow to a local area of the brain was agreed upon in the 1960s. As part of the definition of TIA, the complete resolution of symptoms as a distinguishing factor from a stroke is clear. However, time from onset to resolution of symptoms remains under discussion. At a time when imaging for detection of tissue injury was unavailable, postmortem pathology was the only way to prove or disprove the presence of stroke. Initially symptom resolution times varied from 1 hour to 3 weeks. In 1964 John Marshall defended the definition of TIA to include symptoms that lasted up to 24 hours. This definition was finally agreed upon by the National Institutes of Health in 1975, despite existing data of tissue injury present in 60% of patients whose symptom duration had been less than 1 hour.

The arbitrary selection of 24 hours resulted in a lack of urgency to activate the emergency response system and the nihilistic attitude of health care professionals to urgently treat stroke symptoms. Although patients were being taught about the need to run for help in the setting of chest pain, they were less alert to stroke symptoms. Twenty years later this would become the major obstacle to providing acute stroke treatments.

The invention of computed tomography (CT) scanning in 1972 marked the beginning of the neuroimaging era. Explosion of research in this field has led to availability of techniques that allow detection of early ischemic injury as soon as 5 minutes after symptom onset. Better understanding of flow dynamics and cellular physiology in combination with functional imaging leads to the detection of tissue committed to injury before its death. It is not surprising in this setting that old terminology based on phenomenology would be considered obsolete and would be substituted by definition based on demonstrated pathology. The current AHA definition of TIA is tissue based as opposed to time based.

The American Heart Association/American Stroke Association defines a TIA as "an acute onset of focal neurological deficits from brain, cord, or retina of presumed vascular origin, which resolves with no evidence of acute ischemic changes in imaging evaluation."[6]

Everything a patient might refer to as a "spell" should *not* be considered a TIA. Before a diagnosis of TIA is made, several questions need to be answered. Are the patient's complaints considered to be a *focal neurologic deficit*? Can onset and resolution times be clearly determined? And most importantly, can it be presumed there is a vascular etiology of symptoms? If the answer to all of these questions is yes, then it is reasonable to suspect a TIA. In such cases, thorough evaluation of the cause of symptoms is crucial for appropriate treatment prevention.

Giving a wrong diagnosis of TIA can result in high readmission rates, increased costs, unnecessary testing, and morbidity. Patients who have no focal deficits but have an altered level of consciousness are commonly misdiagnosed as TIA. Other diagnoses to consider include radiculopathies, neuropathies, hyperglycemia or hypoglycemia, malignant hypertension, presyncope, gout, deep venous thrombosis, toxic metabolic encephalopathy, vestibular neuropathy, labyrinthitis, seizures/Todd's paralysis, conversion reactions, hemiplegic migraine, or malingering and recurrent symptoms of prior strokes in the setting of infection.

The estimated prevalence of self-reported, physician-diagnosed TIA was 2.3% (approximately 5 million people). The true prevalence is likely greater because many who experience focal deficits consistent with TIA fail to report these to their health care provider.[1,4,6]

Quantification of the risk of stroke after TIA has been the subject of multiple studies. On average, the risk of stroke is 3.5% to 9.9% in the first 24 hours, 8% to 13.4% in the first 30 days, and as high as 17% at 90 days. Those who survive the initial high-risk period have a 10-year stroke risk of roughly 19%. Seventeen percent of patients report having had TIA symptoms in the prior 24 hours, and as many as 43% report having had symptoms of TIA within the prior 7 days.[7,8]

It is also important to recognize TIA as a warning sign of cardiac pathology, with up to 2.6% cardiac event risk within 90 days. The combined 10-year stroke, myocardial infarction, or vascular death risk after TIA is 43% (4% per year). Within 1 year of TIA, approximately 12% of patients will die.[9,10]

Independent predictors of stroke after TIA have been identified from retrospective and prospective studies. These include age older than 60, diabetes, weakness, speech impairment, duration of symptoms longer than 10 minutes or less than 60 minutes, and systolic blood pressure higher than 140 mmHg or diastolic blood pressure higher than 90 mmHg at the time

of presentation. The Age, Blood Pressure, Clinical Features, Duration, Diabetes (ABCD2) scale has gained recent popularity in predicting stroke risk after TIA. Although this scale is intended to serve as a guide for urgency of evaluation, criticism has been raised about the true validity of the score (Table 40-2). General consensus remains that stroke risk is highest during the first few hours and days after TIA and therefore evaluation should not be delayed.[7,8,11]

> General consensus remains that stroke risk is highest during the first few hours and days after TIA and therefore evaluation should not be delayed.

STROKE RISK FACTORS
Nonmodifiable Risk Factors

Stroke risk factors can be subdivided into nonmodifiable and modifiable. Stroke risk doubles in each successive decade after age 55; however, strokes can occur at any age. An increased incidence of obesity and associated comorbidities such as hypertension and diabetes has led to an increase in the number of young stroke patients. Each year more women than men have a stroke. Women suffer stroke at an older age than men with resulting increase in morbidity and mortality, and loss of independence with subsequent need for placement.[1,12]

Modifiable Risks

Stroke shares many of the same risk factors as coronary artery disease. Control of these modifiable risk factors is

TABLE 40-2	ABCD2 TIA Risk Assessment			
		ABCD2 Score		
Risk Factor	*Points*	*ABCD2 Score*	*2-Day Stroke Risk*	
Age		0-3	Low	
≥60 years	1			
Blood Pressure		4-5	Moderate	
Systolic BP ≥140 mmHg *or*	1			
Diastolic BP ≥90 mmHg				
Clinical features of TIA *(choose one)*	2	6-7	High	
Unilateral weakness with *or* without speech impairment *or*	1			
Speech impairment without unilateral weakness				
Duration				
TIA duration ≥60 minutes	2			
TIA duration 10-59 minutes	1			
Total ABCD2 Score	0-7			

ABCD2, Age, Blood Pressure, Clinical Features, Duration, Diabetes; *TIA,* transient ischemic attack.

the basis of secondary prevention.[13] Traditionally, treatment strategies have focused on better control of blood pressure, diabetes, and dyslipidemia, as well as smoking cessation. Of equal concern is aggressive treatment of physical inactivity, obesity, alcohol consumption, depression, and obstructive sleep apnea (OSA). Sleep medicine research has associated OSA with an increased risk for stroke. [1] The role of inflammatory states in the etiopathogenesis of artherosclerosis is becoming clearer. An association exists among poor dental care, chronic inflammatory diseases, and chronic infections (particularly HIV and its treatments) as potential contributors of stroke.[14] Concerns exist regarding an increase in relative risk for stroke of up to 2.5-fold in the 3 months following infections such as urinary tract infection or pneumonia. Special attention should be given to patients considered high risk who suffer these conditions (Table 40-3).

Atrial fibrillation (AF) remains the number one cause of cardioembolic strokes. In the Framingham study, a 4.8-fold increase in stroke risk was reported across all ages in patients with nonvalvular AF and an annual rate of stroke as high as 11.7%. Paroxysmal atrial fibrillation (PAF) is present in 9.2% of patients older than age 55 with stroke or TIA. Presence of multiple old brain infarctions on magnetic resonance imaging (MRI) helps predict the presence of PAF in patients with cryptogenic stroke. Risk for continuous AF is equivalent to paroxysmal AF. Incidence of AF increases with age. Age older than 75 is identified as an independent risk factor for stroke in patients with AF. The risk for hemorrhagic complications related to treatment with systemic anticoagulation in these patients is also considered to be higher. However, prospective studies of anticoagulation in octogenarians still demonstrate benefit of anticoagulation. The calculated stroke risk per year can be as high as 18%. The combination of stroke risk assessment scores (e.g., CHADS2, CHA2DS2-VASC), along with bleeding risk assessment scores (e.g., HAS-BLED), should be used to assist in treatment decisions for these patients.[1,15-20]

> Good secondary prevention starts with the identification of the individual risk factors, and interventions aim for the control of each of them.

STROKE ASSESSMENT

An accepted validated and reliable tool for assessing stroke severity is the National Institutes of Health Stroke Scale (NIHSS). It is a nonlinear ordinal scale that has a score range from 0 to 42. The severity of stroke increases with a higher score (0 = no stroke symptoms; 1-4 = minor stroke; 5–15 = moderate stroke; 16-20 = moderate to severe stroke, 21–42 = severe stroke), although a score of 4 in a patient who is mute is a devastating disability. The tool measures five areas of neurologic function: level of consciousness, vision, motor, sensory, and language.

Using this assessment assists the practitioner in identifying deficits at baseline, improvements, and deterioration.[21,22]

MANAGEMENT

The urgency in evaluation and aggressiveness of secondary stroke prevention treatment of TIA is the same as for stroke. Current AHA/ASA guidelines for antithrombotic therapy should be followed.[6]

Hyperacute Management

Hyperacute management is defined as the time from symptom onset to emergency department (ED) arrival. This is the period of time where public education has the biggest impact. One minute of brain ischemia can kill 2 million nerve cells and 14 billion synapses! Time is brain. Recognition of stroke symptoms and rapid activation of the emergency response system is essential to survival and prevention of disability. Emergency

TABLE 40-3	Risk Factors for Stroke	
Nonmodifiable	**Modifiable**
Age 55 or older	High blood pressure
Family history	Diabetes
Female gender	Cigarette smoking
Genetics	Alcohol consumption
Prior stroke or TIA	Dyslipidemia
	Atrial fibrillation
	Cardiac disease
	Overweight/Obesity
	Physical inactivity
	Sleep apnea
	Contraception and HRT
	Socially isolated women
	Adult onset of asthma
	Depression
	Presence of migraine history, particularly migraine with aura
	Carotid bruit
	Illicit drug use
	Pregnancy
	HIV/Poor dental care
	Chronic inflammatory diseases
	Syphilis
	Urinary tract infection
	Pneumonia
	Sepsis
	Hypercoagulability

HIV, Human immunodeficiency virus; *HRT*, hormone replacement therapy; *TIA*, transient ischemic attack.

Medical Service (EMS) staff have expertise in the evaluation and treatment of stroke in the field. EMS alerts the receiving ED of the estimated time of arrival and the severity of the patient's symptoms using a prehospital stroke scale. Intravenous (IV) fluids are initiated, supplemental oxygen given, and the patient is placed in a neutral position. While in transport basic laboratory tests and ECG can be collected. EMS is able to provide a higher level of care if complications such as seizures, vomiting, rapid deterioration, or coma should occur.[23]

Acute Management

From ED arrival to definitive therapy, the goal of this phase is recanalization. Optimization of collateral flow to ischemic penumbra with fluid resuscitation using crystalloids or colloids is a priority in stroke resuscitation. Because 30% of acute stroke patients are dehydrated, fluids help to optimize renal function and prepare the patient for potential use of nephrotoxic contrast agents. Optimal hydration during hospitalization has been linked to better outcomes.[24] Actively decreasing blood pressure may result in loss of collateral flow and enlargement of the area of infarction with subsequent neurologic deterioration (Box 40-6).

Immediate imaging is obtained with the goal of answering the following questions. Is it a stroke? If so, is it hemorrhagic or ischemic? Is there already demonstration of tissue injury that would limit the chances for aggressive treatments? More sophisticated but time-consuming studies may be needed to determine the specific occluded vessel, cause of the occlusion, and identification of the core versus penumbra (salvageable) areas. Current treatment options are time limited. Modern imaging techniques assist in the selection of patients by means of physiologic windows, as opposed to time windows.[25-27]

IV infusion of tissue plasminogen activator (tPA) within the first 3 hours of symptom onset was approved in 1996 after the National Institute of Neurological Disorder and Stroke trial results were published. Considering that it takes an average of 60 minutes to complete the initial evaluation, patients would have had to arrive at the ED within 2 hours of symptoms to be candidates for treatment. Success rates of IV tPA depend on the size of occluded vessels. Middle cerebral artery (MCA) vessels may have a

recanalization rate as high as 17%. However, risk for hemorrhagic complications may vary from 3% for patients with an NIHSS score below 10, to 17% for those with a NIHSS score higher than 20. Risk for bleeding due to tPA must be weighed against a greater than 60% unfavorable outcome without treatment. The European Cooperative Acute Stroke Study III (ECASS III) trial in 2010 demonstrated safety and favorable outcomes for the use of tPA within the first 4.5 hours of symptom onset. This extended time-window is currently used with additional exclusion criteria in stroke centers.[28-31]

In posterior circulation infarcts, IV infusion of tPA, or endovascular recanalization, has been approved in the first 6 hours from symptom onset and up to 24 hours. Controversy remains regarding the true benefit of these procedures. Angiographic success is not always paired with clinical success. Careful selection of patients with the aid of imaging protocols is crucial for optimization of outcomes.[32-35]

If tPA or endovascular recanalizations are not indicated, then what? When patients do not meet the criteria for acute intervention with medications or mechanical intervention, treatment with antiplatelet therapy is essential. The Chinese Acute Stroke Trial (CAST) and International Stroke Trial (IST) both demonstrated the benefit of a simple aspirin (ASA) in reduction of mortality and disability. ASA should be given to patients with the same acuity as tPA when the former is no longer an option.[29,36-38]

Subacute Management

From intervention to discharge, the goal during this phase is the management and prevention of complications and comorbidities, as well as determination of stroke cause and risks. Aspiration pneumonia, urinary tract infections, venous thromboembolisms (VTEs), depression, deconditioning, malnourishment, dysphagia, and fever are common comorbidities. Nutrition support and rehabilitation therapies (physical, speech, and occupational therapy) should be initiated as soon as possible (see Chapter 13). VTE prevention and screening need to be applied to all patients in accordance with their level of disabilities. Overlooking depression treatment may lead to decreased patient participation in therapy and worsening outcomes.

Stroke risk assessment refers to the search for identification of individual stroke risks and potential causes of stroke. Hematologic studies should include a lipid profile, HgA$_{1c}$, complete blood count and differential, prothrombin time (PT), partial thromboplastin time (PTT), international normalized ratio (INR), and basic metabolic panel (BMP). Hypercoagulability studies are costly and should not be part of an initial evaluation. All patients should be admitted to a stroke unit equipped with telemetry. Echocardiography should be

---

Box 40-6
BLOOD PRESSURE GOALS IN STROKE
Acute Ischemic Stroke
If not a candidate for thrombolysis = 220/120
If candidate for thrombolysis = 185/110
After thrombolysis = 180/105
After revascularization = 140/80

done if no data are available in the prior 6 months, or if changes are suspected. For determination of the area of infarction MRI studies should be performed. When MRI is not possible, a repeated CT may help. Carotid ultrasonography provides minimal anatomic information and is inappropriate as an isolated tool for evaluation of cerebral vasculature. When ultrasounds are used, more information than just the flow velocities and estimation of stenosis is needed. Plaque characteristics and the presence or absence of intimal thickening is of value but seldom reported. Vessel anatomy is best obtained with either magnetic resonance angiography (MRA) or computed tomography angiography (CTA) technology. When using MRA, contrast aids improve the positive predictive value of the test. In both cases angiographic data should be collected from the aortic arch to the second and third divisions of intracranial circulation. As of 2012, cerebral angiography remains the gold standard, although not so frequently used.[25,27,29,39]

What represents a complete evaluation of stroke? In some centers, all patients with stroke undergo TEE. The cost benefit of including this invasive study in all stroke patients is questionable. Some would argue that it should only be performed when routine mechanisms of stroke as causative agents have not been identified. Almost 30% of cryptogenic strokes are characterized as cardioembolic after prolonged cardiac monitoring and findings of PAF. Because of cost, genetic testing for stroke risk is reserved for patients with a high level of suspicion. Cerebral vasoconstriction syndromes, vasculitis, or arteriopathies may require arteriography and biopsy studies. No tests can substitute for a thorough history and physical examination.

Late Subacute and Chronic Care

Forty percent of stroke patients are left with moderate functional impairments and 15% to 30% with severe disability. Effective rehabilitation interventions initiated early after stroke can enhance the recovery process and minimize functional disability. Improved functional outcomes for patients also contribute to patient satisfaction and reduce potentially costly long-term care expenditures.[40] Although most of the recovery occurs in the first 6 months after a stroke, improvement processes can take years (see Chapter 13).

> One minute of brain ischemia can kill 2 million nerve cells and 14 billion synapses! Time is brain.

CASE 1

Discussion

Mrs. Hernandez's MRI demonstrates an old cortical infarct in the territory of the left anterior branch of the middle cerebral artery. Her MRA demonstrates less than 50% stenosis of the left internal carotid artery. Her ECG, however, showed atrial fibrillation and a depolarization defect; the echocardiogram demonstrates a left atrium size of 4.3 and left ventricular hypertrophy with an ejection fraction of 50%. Laboratory studies are significant for the presence of anemia with hemoglobin 9 g/dL, hematocrit 35, a mean corpuscular volume of 103, vitamin B_{12} level of 202 pg/mL, and HgA_{1c} of 8%. Her renal function clearance is less than 55 mL per minute. Her sleep study is positive for obstructive sleep apnea.

1. **What can be done to optimize compliance and prevent complications of systemic anticoagulation in Mrs. Hernandez?**

2. **Which subspecialties should be involved in her interdisciplinary care?**

3. **In addition to anticoagulation, what treatments should be included in the plan of care?** ■

Quality Improvement/Accountable Care

In an accountable care environment, the Centers for Medicare and Medicaid Services (CMS) has established core performance measures to award outcomes of care that are based on evidenced-based practice. The Joint Commission (TJC) also uses these measures to award hospitals advanced stroke certification.[41]

SUMMARY

Cerebrovascular disease is the leading cause of disability with high cost to individuals, families, and society in the form of mortality, morbidities, loss of independence, and diminished quality of life. Risk factor identification and aggressive management of these are imperative for primary and secondary prevention. Understanding the etiology of each individual stroke leads to appropriate secondary prevention. Education of patients on signs, symptoms, and emergent activation of the emergency medical system is the first step to optimize outcomes. Care of stroke patients is best provided in stroke-certified centers by stroke-trained physicians and personnel with a multidisciplinary approach to care.

KEY REFERENCES

6. Albers GW, Easton JD, Saver JL, et al. Definition and evaluation of transient ischemic attack. Stroke 2009;40:2276-93.
13. Adams RJ, Albers GW, Kasner SE, et al. Guidelines for the prevention of stroke in patients with stroke or transient ischemic attack. Stroke 2011;42:227-76.
23. Acker JE III, Crocco TJ, Pancioli AM, et al. Implementation strategies for emergency medical services within stroke systems of care: A policy statement from the American Heart Association/ American Stroke. Stroke 2007;38:3097-115.
29. Adams HP Jr, Alberts MJ, del Zoppo G, et al. Guidelines for the early management of adults with ischemic stroke. Stroke 2007;38:1655-1711.
40. Duncan PW, Zorowitz R, Bates B, et al. Management of adult stroke rehabilitation care: A clinical practice guideline. Stroke 2005;36:e100-43.

References available online at expertconsult.com.

41

Diabetes Mellitus

Imaad Razzaque, John E. Morley,
Konrad C. Nau, and Heather B. Congdon

Additional online-only material indicated by icon.

OBJECTIVES

Upon completion of this chapter, the reader will be able to:

- Understand the changing epidemiology of adult diabetes mellitus (DM) and the impact it has on the elderly.
- Identify the risk factors for DM in older persons.
- Understand the continuum of the disease process in diabetes and how this affects the diagnostic criteria for DM.
- Be able to assess the elderly diabetic in a multisystem and multidisciplinary fashion, including the common geriatric syndromes.
- Describe the roles and contraindications for pharmacologic and nonpharmacologic treatments of DM.

CASE 1

Maria Sweetly (Part 1)

Maria Sweetly is a 72-year-old Hispanic woman who comes to your office for hypertension follow-up and remarks that for 2 months she has had bilateral burning and numbness of her feet and that she has fallen recently at home, without injury. Medications include hydrochlorothiazide 25 mg daily and metoprolol 50 mg twice a day. Her blood pressure is 160/88 mmHg, pulse 60 beats per minute, weight 173 lbs, and body mass index 30; monofilament and light touch sensation is diminished in a stocking distribution, Achilles reflexes are +1 dorsalis pedis pulses are +1 and the remainder of the examination is unremarkable. Fasting serum glucose is 130 mg/dL, blood urea nitrogen 19 mg/dL, and creatinine 1.2 mg/dL, and electrolytes are normal.

1. **Can you name at least four of Mrs. Sweetly's risk factors for diabetes?**
2. **Can you make the diagnosis of diabetes at this time?**
3. **What additional laboratory tests would you order?** ▣

PREVALENCE AND IMPACT

The prevalence of diabetes continues to increase steadily in the general population with a peak occurring between 60 to 74 years of age (Figure 41-1). Between 1995 and 2007 diabetes mellitus in the nursing home increased from 16.9% to 32.8% of residents.[1] Males tend to have a higher prevalence than females, and Hispanics and African Americans have a higher prevalence than whites.

This increase in diabetes prevalence largely parallels the U.S. obesity epidemic.

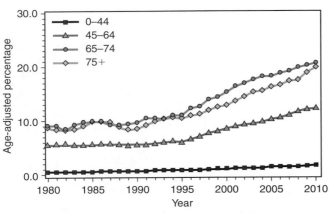

Figure 41-1 Increasing prevalence of diabetes.

Elderly persons diagnosed with diabetes have a similar spectrum of macrovascular and microvascular complications as is seen in their younger counterparts; however, the risk of cardiovascular disease is substantially higher. Older persons with diabetes are more likely to have an excess of functional disability, mobility impairment, depression, falls, incontinence, cognitive impairment, and cataracts.

More than half of direct medical expenditures on diabetes are for those persons over 65. One dollar in every $10 spent on health care in the United States in 2002 was for diabetes. Nineteen percent of personal health care expenditures in the United States are for diabetes mellitus (DM), although only 4.2% of the U.S. population is known to have diabetes. Adjusting for age, sex, and race/ethnicity, people with diabetes had medical expenditures 2.4 times higher than those without diabetes.[2]

The life expectancy at birth of people with diabetes was 64.7 and 70.7 years for men and women, respectively, compared with 77.5 and 81.4 years in those without diabetes in a 2004 Ontario study.[2] A British study of persons older than age 85 found that only 32% of the remaining life of persons with diabetes was active, whereas it was 42% for those without diabetes.[3]

PATHOPHYSIOLOGY

There is a progressive continuum from the asymptomatic prediabetic state, with insulin resistance, through mild postprandial hyperglycemia and/or mild fasting hyperglycemia, to diagnosable type 2 diabetes.

Both an increased resistance to insulin-mediated glucose disposal and a decrease in non–insulin-mediated glucose uptake play a role in the development of diabetes mellitus in older persons.[4,5] Both aging and obesity play a role in producing these effects. The resistance to insulin-mediated glucose disposal is, in part, caused by triglyceride infiltration into muscle and mitochondrial defects in the muscle. However, older persons with diabetes mellitus are much less likely to be obese than middle-aged people with the disease. In older persons a reduction in glucose-induced insulin release from the pancreas is a larger component of the pathophysiology than is seen in middle-aged persons with type 2 diabetes mellitus. Older persons have fewer abnormalities in fasting hepatic glucose output compared to middle-aged persons. The differences in how diabetes mellitus manifests in older persons compared to how it appears in "classical" manifestations are highlighted in Table 41-1.

Adiponectin, a hormone produced from adipocytes, reduces insulin resistance. Recently, fetuin-A (a hepatic alpha-fetoprotein) has been shown to produce insulin resistance, decrease adiponectin production, and increase inflammatory cytokine production from adipocytes. These findings suggest a number of factors are involved in the insulin resistance of aging.

DIFFERENTIAL DIAGNOSIS AND ASSESSMENT

Presenting Symptoms

Atypical or asymptomatic elders account for 30% of undiagnosed elders with diabetes. They do *not* have the "3 P's" (polyphagia, polydipsia, polyuria).

The renal threshold for glucose increases with age because older persons often have a higher thirst threshold; thus glycosuria may not occur.[5] Polydipsia can be absent; presentation in the elderly may be dehydration with altered thirst perception and delayed fluid supplementation. Polyuria can present as incontinence. More often, changes such as dry eyes, dry mouth, confusion, incontinence, or diabetic complications are the presenting symptoms.[6]

TABLE 41-1	Diabetes in Old Age Compared to "Classical" Types 1 and 2		
Age	**Young**	**Old**	**Middle Aged**
Body habitus	thin	thin or mild visceral obesity	obese
Coma	ketoacidotic	mixed/lactic acidosis	hyperosmolar
Glucose induced insulin release	very low	low	incr. but insufficient to overcome insulin resistance
Insulin mediated glucose disposal	normal	mild or decreased	markedly decreased
Fasting hepatic glucose output	increased	normal	increased

Elderly patients may occasionally have the presenting symptoms of weight loss or hyperosmolar nonketotic coma (HONKC). The common age-associated syndromes of persistent pain, urinary incontinence, cognitive impairment, depression, injurious falls, and polypharmacy are all increased in persons with diabetes; thus they are often the presenting problem.

Conversely, all elderly diabetics should be screened for these common syndromes within 3 to 6 months of diagnosis.[7]

Screening for and Confirming the Diagnosis

The laboratory diagnosis, similar to the pathophysiology, involves a continuum from prediabetes to the diabetic threshold (Boxes 41-1 and 41-2). The fasting blood glucose (FBS) of 126 mg/dL or greater is still the preferred test to screen for prediabetes and diabetes.[8] It is easily available, and has a 95% confidence interval ($\pm18\%$) when performed on fasting venous plasma glucose samples (FPG).[9]

Older persons should be screened for DM annually; however, up to 30% of the diabetic elderly have an FBS of less than 126 mg/dL yet have a 2-hour oral glucose tolerance test (OGTT) of more than 200 mg/dL.[8] The vast majority of those who meet the OGTT criteria for diabetes, but not the FBS criteria, will have an HbA$_{1C}$ less than 7.0%.

Assessment of elderly diabetics is multisystemic and multidisciplinary, focusing on the complications:

1. Macrovascular complications of coronary, carotid, and peripheral atherosclerosis (patient interviews should focus on neurologic symptoms, syncope, chest pain—often atypical, exertional dyspnea or fatigue, and claudication); lipid profile and liver function tests and electrocardiogram are appropriate. However, there is limited evidence in support of treating hyperlipidemia in persons older than 75 years of age who have not had a recent myocardial infarction or stroke. There is no evidence to use high doses of statins.

2. A new systolic blood pressure goal of 140 or lower has been set for people with hypertension as well as diabetes. (A lower systolic target of 130 is to be considered in some individuals, such as younger people.) Blood pressure should be measured when not at the physician's office because "white coat" hypertension occurs in 25% of patients.

3. Microvascular renal complications are assessed by urinalysis, urinary microalbumin, and serum creatinine.

4. Retinal complications require an ophthalmologist for dilated retinal examination; glaucoma and cataracts should also be included in the screening.

5. Foot complications and vulnerability should be assessed at every visit. Neuropathy should be assessed by a monofilament test and examination for posterior column disease. If a posterior column is present then a vitamin B$_{12}$ test should be obtained.

BOX 41-2

CRITERIA FOR THE DIAGNOSIS OF DIABETES

Note: A$_{1C}$, FPG, or OGTT results should be confirmed by repeat testing unless unequivocal hyperglycemia is present. A$_{1C}$ 6.5% or greater*

OR

FPG 126 mg/dL or greater (7.0 mmol/L or greater)
Note: fasting = no caloric intake for at least 8 hrs

OR

2-hr PG during OGTT 200 mg/dL or greater (11.1 mmol/L or greater)
Note: Test as WHO describes, with glucose load equivalent to 75 g anhydrous glucose dissolved in water

OR

Random PG 200 mg/dL or greater (11.1 mmol/L or greater)

OR

When classic symptoms of hyperglycemia or hyperglycemic crisis are present

From ADA. Standards of Medical Care in Diabetes—2013. Diabetes Care 2013;36:S11-66.
DCCT, Diabetes control and complications trial; *FPG*, fasting plasma glucose; *OGTT*, oral glucose tolerance test; *PG*, plasma glucose; *NGSP*, National Glycohemoglobin Standardization Program; *WHO*, World Health Organization.
*Must be done in a lab using an NGSP-certified method, standardized to the DCCT assay.

BOX 41-1

CATEGORIES OF INCREASED RISK FOR DIABETES (PREDIABETES)*

Note: For all three tests, the increased risk of diabetes is continuous, extending below the lower limit of the ranges and becoming disproportionately greater at the higher ends of the ranges.
FPG 100-125 mg/dL (5.6-6.9 mmol/L)

OR

2-hr PG in OGTT** 140-199 mg/dL (7.8-11.0 mmol/L)

OR

A$_{1C}$ 5.7-6.4%

From ADA. Standards of Medical Care in Diabetes—2013. Diabetes Care 2013;36:S11-66.
FPG, Fasting plasma glucose; *OGTT*, oral glucose tolerance test; *PG*, plasma glucose.
*Previously called IFG (impaired fasting glucose) and IGT (impaired glucose tolerance).
**75-g oral glucose tolerance test.

6. Screening for mood and cognition should be considered annually (because of increased depression and dementia).

7. HbA$_{1C}$ should be assessed at the time of diagnosis and every 3 to 6 months thereafter because average blood glucose levels and microvascular complications are significantly related.

8. All diabetics need to have postural hypotension measured at every visit. Persons who complain of dizziness or falling within 2 hours of a meal should be screened for postprandial hypotension, which is present in 20% of patients with diabetes.

All diabetics should be referred for counseling. Certified diabetic educators (CDEs) are nurses, pharmacists, or dietitians who have passed a comprehensive national examination and can instruct patients about nutrition, home glucose monitoring, recognition and prevention of hypoglycemia, and other complications.

CDEs are central to the health care team; they develop great insight into their patients' functional capacity and compliance (most elderly diabetics require several drugs). Older persons with diabetes need annual assessment of pneumococcal and influenza immunization status.

CASE 1

Discussion

Maria Sweetly has multiple risk factors for DM, including age older than 65, Hispanic descent, body mass index greater than 25, hypertension, and use of a thiazide diuretic. Her physical examination and history are compatible with peripheral neuropathy, and diabetes is a leading cause of peripheral neuropathy in the elderly. Other nondiabetic considerations that cause peripheral neuropathy are metabolic disorders (e.g., hypothyroid, azotemia, vitamin B$_{12}$ deficiency), alcohol and other toxins, iatrogenic illness (e.g., isoniazid, chemotherapy, HIV drugs), infections (e.g., HIV), and malignancy (e.g., bronchogenic carcinoma). Although a single fasting plasma glucose of 130 exceeds the 126 mg/dL threshold for diabetes, the World Health Organization and American Diabetes Association require two fasting plasma glucose levels equal to or exceeding 126 mg/dL in order to establish the diagnosis of DM. Additional laboratory tests to consider would be a lipid panel, HbA$_{1C}$, urinalysis, and urine microalbumin. Should the repeat FBS be less than 126 mg/dL, then a couple of glucose levels 2 hours after her largest meal should be obtained. A 2-hour value of 200 mg/dL or more would be sufficient to diagnose DM. Mrs. Sweetly has one of the six common geriatric syndromes seen in diabetics, namely, persistent pain. Diabetics should be screened for pain, cognitive decline, depression, injurious falls, urinary incontinence, and polypharmacy. Diabetes is also a recognized risk factor for osteoporosis. ▣

CASE 1

Maria Sweetly (Part 2)

A repeat FBS was 127 mg/dL, and her HbA$_{1C}$ was 8.9; total cholesterol was 205 mg/dL, triglycerides 250 mg/dL, high-density lipoprotein (HDL) 34 mg/dL, low-density lipoprotein (LDL) 121 mg/dL, and urine microalbumin 40 mg/L.

1. What treatment goals should you establish for Mrs. Sweetly?

2. What changes would you make in her medications? ▣

MANAGEMENT

The management of older adults with type 2 diabetes requires consideration of the effects of aging, changes in health status, and the potential benefits from therapeutic interventions.

Goals of therapy for an elderly patient with diabetes often differ from goals for younger people. Life expectancy, other medical conditions, and the patient's willingness and ability to comply with treatment are important factors. Elderly patients range from limited cognitive and/or physical functioning to others who are much more active. Patient goals should be documented and reassessed regularly. A recent consensus panel suggested that the goal in an older person should be an HbA$_{1C}$ between 7.0% and 7.5%. For older diabetics receiving therapy the "not below 6%" rule should be followed to avoid hypoglycemia.[10]

Quality of life is an important issue in any elderly patient. Aggressive treatment plans may not be reasonable (complicated, costly, uncomfortable side effects). In nursing home residents HbA$_{1C}$ levels up to 8% are acceptable.

Some goals for elderly diabetic patients include:
1. Prevention of hypoglycemia and hyperglycemia and associated symptoms (Box 41-3).
2. Decreased morbidity from microvascular and macrovascular complications.

BOX 41-3

FACTORS THAT PREDISPOSE ELDERLY TYPE 2 DIABETIC PATIENTS TO HYPOGLYCEMIA

- Poor or erratic nutritional intake
- Changes in mental status that impair the perception or response to hypoglycemia
- Increased polypharmacy and noncompliance with medications
- Dependence or isolation that limits receipt of early treatment for hypoglycemia
- Impaired renal or hepatic metabolism
- Presence of comorbid conditions that can mask or lead to misdiagnosis of hypoglycemic symptoms (dementia, delirium, depression, sleep abnormalities, seizures, myocardial infarction, cerebrovascular accident)
- Presence of other endocrine disorders such as adrenal insufficiency

3. Maintenance or improvement in general health and quality of life.
4. Reduction or prevention of medication side effects.

Lifestyle Interventions

Diet

Medical nutrition therapy (MNT) must be individualized by patient size and energy requirements. Carbohydrate intake remains key to glycemic control. Extremely low carbohydrate diets (less than 130 g per day) are not recommended because carbohydrates are important for energy, water-soluble vitamins and minerals, and fiber. In fact, 45% to 65% of daily calories should be carbohydrates. Weight loss by diet should be avoided in older persons because it has been shown to increase mortality rate in diabetics.[11]

Exercise

Physical activity improves insulin sensitivity, glycemic control, and selected risk factors for cardiovascular disease (hypertension, dyslipidemia), and decreases the risk of coronary artery disease. Resistance exercise is particularly effective when coupled with aerobic exercise.

Pharmacologic Therapy

Simple, inexpensive medication and monitoring regimens that maximize compliance are recommended, started at the lowest dose and titrated gradually to targets or side effects (Table 41-2).

Biguanides

The primary mechanism of action of biguanides is to decrease hepatic glucose production and intestinal absorption of glucose, improving insulin sensitivity. Although sulfonylureas traditionally have been used as first-line pharmacologic therapy for type 2 diabetic patients, many experts and the United Kingdom Prospective Diabetes Study (UKPDS) data suggest that, in the absence of contraindications (see below), metformin is the agent of first choice for diabetic patients who are overweight. There is increasing evidence that a primary protective effect may be unassociated with lowering glucose.

Metformin

Metformin is used as monotherapy in type 2 DM, or concomitantly with a sulfonylurea, insulin, or other oral agents. As monotherapy, metformin typically does not cause hypoglycemia or long-term weight gain. Older diabetic patients with reduced renal function (serum creatinine greater than 1.4 mg/dL) should not use metformin because of the risk of lactic acidosis. Older patients on metformin should have creatinine checks at least annually and with dose increases. Patients older than 80 with reduced muscle mass should have cystatin-C measured instead of creatinine.

Maximum doses of metformin are not generally used in the elderly. Metformin can cause anorexia, weight loss, and gastric distress.[12] Metformin should be discontinued in situations of potential hypoxemia (cardiovascular collapse, respiratory failure, acute myocardial infarction, septicemia) because lactic acidosis is a rare but potentially severe consequence. Metformin should be avoided in patients with impaired liver function, congestive heart failure, and metabolic acidosis and withheld before contrast studies with reevaluation of kidney function afterwards.

Sulfonylureas

The primary mechanism of action of sulfonylureas is enhanced beta cell secretion of insulin from the pancreas causing a decrease in glucose output from the liver, and an increase in insulin sensitivity in the peripheral.

Second-generation agents include glimepiride, glyburide, and glipizide. Patients should be educated about hypoglycemia, a dangerous side effect (diaphoresis, rapid heart rate, shaking, and nausea). Older persons often have hypoglycemia unawareness. Chlorpropamide is never to be used in the old because it produces prolonged hypoglycemia.

TABLE 41-2	Pharmacokinetics of Common Insulin Preparations			
Class	**Drug**	**Onset (hours)**	**Peak (hours)**	**Duration (hours)**
Rapid acting	Humalog, Novolog, Apidra	0.25	0.5 to 3	2 to 5
Short acting	Humulin R, Novolin R	0.5 to 1	2 to 3	8 to 12
Intermediate acting	Humalog Mix 75/25, Humalog Mix 70/30	0.25	0.5 to 4	24
	Humulin 70/30, Novolin 70/30	0.5	4 to 8	24
	Humulin I, Novolin I	1 to 2.5	8 to 12	18 to 24
	Humulin N, Novolin N	1 to 1.5	4 to 12	24
Long acting	Lantus (glargine)	1	-	24
	Levemir (detemir)	1	-	20

Thiazolidinediones

The thiazolidinediones pioglitazone and rosiglitazone are indicated as monotherapy in type 2 diabetes as an adjunct to diet and exercise. They may be used with a sulfonylurea, metformin, or insulin. They lower glucose by improving target cell response to insulin, without increasing pancreatic insulin secretion (they require insulin for activity); thus they are unlikely to cause hypoglycemia. When used as monotherapy, they generally do not cause hypoglycemia. Liver functions should be monitored; exercise caution with active liver disease. Class III or IV heart failure is a contraindication because of potential fluid retention. These drugs accelerate bone loss and as such can increase fractures. There is some evidence that they may cause heart disease.

Meglitinides

Repaglinide and nateglinid are indicated in type 2 diabetes as monotherapy when hyperglycemia cannot be managed by diet and exercise alone or in combination with metformin or a thiazolidinedione in patients whose hyperglycemia cannot be controlled by exercise, diet, or a single agent. They need to be given before each meal and there is no reason to use them in older persons.

Alpha-Glucosidase Inhibitors

Acarbose and miglitol can be used as monotherapy, as an adjunct to diet and exercise, or in combination with a sulfonylurea, metformin, or insulin. They reversibly inhibit intestinal alpha-glucosidases, resulting in delayed glucose absorption and lowering of postprandial hyperglycemia and increased glucagon-like peptide (GLP-1). Flatulence and diarrhea are common; these side effects usually return to pretreatment levels with continued use. Acarbose and miglitol are not recommended if the serum creatinine is more than 2 mg/dL and are contraindicated in diabetic ketoacidosis, cirrhosis, and many intestinal diseases. They can be used to treat postprandial hypotension because increased GLP-1 slows gastric emptying.

Dipeptidyl Peptidase IV Inhibitors

Dipeptidyl peptidase IV inhibitors (DPPIV) block the breakdown of glucagon-like peptide I (GLP-I). They can be used as monotherapy and do not produce hypoglycemia. The three drugs of this class available in the United States are sitagliptin, linagliptin, and saxagliptin. These drugs can cause a severe skin rash. In combination with angiotensin-converting enzyme (ACE) inhibitors they can produce angioedema.

GLP-1 Agonists

GLP-1 agonists lower glucose and also produce anorexia, often gastrointestinal upset, and weight loss. As such, these drugs are not appropriate for older persons, although they can be excellent for overweight middle-aged persons. Agents available include exenatide and liraglutide.

Insulin

Insulin is indicated for diabetes that has been unresponsive to treatment with diet and/or oral hypoglycemic agents, but initiation of insulin in elderly people with type 2 diabetes should involve a multidisciplinary team. Insulin is often begun at a 10- to 15-unit dose, and as glucose control is achieved, some of the patient's oral diabetic medications can be withdrawn.

CASE 1

Discussion

The additional laboratory studies indeed confirm your suspicion of DM and suggest hyperlipidemia and the presence of Mrs. Sweetly's diabetes for at least 2 to 3 months. Mutual goal setting would be desirable, and because Mrs. Sweetly is otherwise healthy and presumably has good functional capacity, it would be reasonable to aim for blood pressures below 140/80 mmHg. Her elevated blood pressure should be confirmed on at least two home measurements and she should have a blood pressure measured standing. A low-dose angiotensin-converting enzyme (ACE) inhibitor would be preferred because of her diabetes with microalbuminuria. You should stop her hydrochlorothiazide and beta-blocker, because this will reduce polypharmacy. The theoretical problems with exacerbation of glucose intolerance with thiazides and the masking of hypoglycemic symptoms with beta-blockers are rarely clinically significant. It is reasonable to set a goal of getting her HbA_{1C} down to 7%, and for her total cholesterol to be below 200, triglycerides below 150, HDL above 45, and LDL below 120. We can wait a few months to see if exercise and improved glycemic control are able to bring the lipids to goal. Individualized MNT and diabetic education will be ordered, and self–glucose testing can be recommended. Should this prove ineffective after several months, then oral agents would be indicated. Metformin is a good choice because it is somewhat associated with weight loss and is proven to prevent macrovascular complications. ▣

CASE 1

Maria Sweetly (Part 3)

Twelve weeks later Mrs. Sweetly has substantial relief from her foot discomfort, and her blood pressure is 135/78 mmHg on a low-dose ACE inhibitor. Her HbA_{1C} is 7.5 on metformin. Her FBS is in the 110 to 130 mg/dL range.

What other measures can you recommend to her to reduce the macrovascular complications of coronary artery disease? ▣

LONG-TERM MANAGEMENT GUIDELINES

Smoking

Smoking is the most important modifiable cause of premature death associated with macrovascular and microvascular complications. Twelve percent of patients older than age 65 smoke.[7] Smoking cessation in the elderly may drop the risk of macrovascular and microvascular complications to presmoking levels. All diabetic patients who smoke should be assessed for willingness and offered counseling and pharmacologic interventions as appropriate.[13]

Hypertension Management

Hypertension is associated with stroke, coronary artery disease, peripheral vascular disease, retinopathy, nephropathy, and potentially neuropathy. Blood pressure control in diabetes is very important. A goal of less than 140/80 mmHg is recommended if tolerated: lowering below 130/80 mmHg has no extra benefit and may increase mortality. Gradual reduction is preferred. Systolic pressure should initially be lowered by no more than 20 mmHg; if this is well tolerated, further reduction is made. Patients with blood pressure greater than 160/100 mmHg should be offered pharmacologic and behavioral interventions within 1 month.[13] ACE inhibitors and angiotensin receptor blocking agents (ARBs) are preferred in diabetic hypertension because of their efficacy in lowering blood pressure and slowing the progression of proteinuria and nephropathy. Diabetes is not a barrier to the use of beta-blockers for hypertension and for cardioprotection in myocardial infarction or in hypertensive patients with diabetes and congestive heart failure. There is little evidence to justify withholding beta-blockers from diabetic patients because of metabolic concerns or fears of masking hypoglycemia. Because ACE inhibitors and ARBs are associated with renal impairment and hyperkalemia, renal function and serum potassium should be tested within 1 to 2 weeks of starting the drugs, once a year, and at dose increases.[13] Thiazide diuretics have been associated with hypokalemia in older persons; electrolytes should be checked within 1 to 2 weeks of starting, with dose increases, and once a year.[13] If the patient develops hypokalemia, hyporenin hyperaldosteronism should be considered. This is treated with spironolactone.[14]

Self-Monitoring of Blood Glucose

Frail, older patients with diabetes are more prone to hypoglycemia than are healthy older adults. Home blood glucose self-monitoring should thus be considered; it has been shown to decrease the likelihood of hypoglycemia.

Ability to self-monitor depends on functional and cognitive status. Patients with frequent or severe hypoglycemia may benefit from referral to a diabetes educator or endocrinologist, and should have more frequent contact with their primary clinician while therapy is being adjusted.[9] HbA_{1C} goals should be individualized: with good functional status and a longer life expectancy, 7% is appropriate. Short-term studies of adults 30 to 85 years who lowered their HbA_{1C} from 9.3% to 7.5% showed improved vitality, better cognitive functioning, better sleep, and decreased depression. A goal of 8% is appropriate with a life expectancy of less than 5 years or where the risk of hypoglycemia is a factor.[10] Patients who have met their HbA_{1C} goal and remain stable should be tested annually; before the HbA_{1C} goal is met, it should be tested at least every 6 months.[10]

Eye Care

Diabetic retinopathy is the most frequent cause of new cases of blindness among adults age 20 to 74 years.[15,16] The incidence of retinopathy is associated with the glycemic control over the past 6 years and elevated blood pressure; progression of retinopathy is linked to older age, male sex, and hyperglycemia. Early detection and treatment of diabetic retinopathy is paramount. Elderly patients with new-onset diabetes should have an initial screening, dilated-eye examination performed by an eye-care specialist, and a dilated-eye examination annually if they are at high risk for eye disease (e.g., those with symptoms of retinopathy, glaucoma, or cataracts; HbA_{1C} greater than 8%; type 1 DM; or blood pressure greater than 140/80 mmHg). At lower risk, the dilated-eye examination can be every 2 years.

Foot Care

Diabetic neuropathy is a microvascular complication of diabetes that can lead to foot ulcerations and even lower-limb amputation. Early recognition and management is key. At highest risk are persons with diabetes for more than 10 years, males, those with poor glycemic control, or those with cardiovascular, retinal, or renal complications. Patients should be educated on proper foot care and have a comprehensive foot examination at least once a year, more frequently if problems are already present. Diabetics are at greater risk for vascular foot ulcers, pressure ulcers, and amputation. Diabetics need special shoes and should be taught to protect their feet. A regular visit to the podiatrist to examine their feet and trim their toenails is important.

Osteoporosis

Although patients with type 2 diabetes have greater bone mineral density than those without diabetes, the bone is porous and more fragile; this puts patients with type 2 diabetes at increased risk for developing fractures.[17]

Hypogonadism

Male diabetics are at a higher risk of developing hypogonadism.

Nephropathy

Diabetic nephropathy is the leading cause of end-stage renal disease; it occurs in 20% to 40% of patients with diabetes. In the absence of previously demonstrated macroalbuminuria or microalbuminuria, an annual microalbumin screening test should be performed; it should also be done at the time of diagnosis of type 2 diabetes. Blood pressure and glucose control will slow the progression of nephropathy. ACE inhibitors delay the progression from microalbuminuria to macroalbuminuria and can slow the decline in the glomerular filtration rate in patients with macroalbuminuria.

Neuropathies

Peripheral neuropathy from diabetes affects up to 50% of older type 2 diabetic patients. Presentation is as an acute painful sensation, gradual onset numbness, or an asymptomatic foot ulcer. The monofilament pressure perception test, Achilles reflex, and 128-Hz tuning forks are tools useful in diagnosing peripheral neuropathy. Gabapentin and pregabalin are the two most widely used medications for neuropathic pain; gabapentin has given relief at much higher daily doses than were initially recommended. Other medications (including adjunctive use of antidepressants) may add to their effectiveness. Topiramate and alpha-lipoic acid are effective but are not yet labeled for this indication. Podiatry consultation for footwear and physical therapy consultation (for gait training and possible nerve stimulation, e.g., with a transcutaneous nerve stimulator [TENS] unit) should also be offered.

Falls and Syncope

Diabetes mellitus is a major cause of faints and falls in older persons. Diabetes has a number of effects that potentially increase falls: gait abnormalities, vision problems, orthostatic hypotension, foot deformities, vestibular abnormalities, altered vibration sense, neuropathy, a decrease in ankle dorsiflexion and step length, muscle weakness, and hypoglycemia.

Autonomic Neuropathy

Many persons with diabetes mellitus have autonomic neuropathy, which can be detected by examining the failure of the R-R interval to change during the Valsalva maneuver or by the squat test.[14] Persons with autonomic neuropathy often also have a prolonged QTc and this combination results in a markedly increased risk of arrhythmias, syncope, and sudden death. Many of these diabetics need to be investigated with an event monitor and may need insertion of an implantable loop recorder.

Cognition

Hyperinsulinemia and both hyperglycemia and hypoglycemia are directly related to declined memory-related cognitive scores. The risk of Alzheimer's dementia directly attributable to hyperinsulinemia or diabetes is as high as 39%.[18] Whether glycemic control decreases cognitive decline is speculative at present. Paradoxically, nasal insulin has been suggested as a treatment for dementia.

Diabetes Education

Elderly patients, as well as their caregivers, should complete comprehensive diabetes self-management education (DSME). It is a covered benefit under Medicare Part B. Patients should be advised that home blood glucose self-monitoring, when appropriate, has been associated with improved glycemic control. Monitoring technique should be routinely reviewed as functional ability may change over time. Education regarding medication use is vital; package inserts are often written in small print or on poor-quality paper. Language and health literacy may also be barriers to obtaining important information about medications. One study in older patients showed that 39% of patients stated that they could not read their medication labels, and 67% did not fully understand the labels. Physical activity combined with nutritional education can reduce weight and enhance blood pressure, and improve lipid and glycemic control.

Risk factors for foot ulcers and amputation should be discussed with the patient or a family member. Older adults may have cognitive and visual impairment, which can limit their ability to properly evaluate their feet on a regular basis. Patient education on foot care in middle-aged and older adults reduces rates of serious foot lesions and amputations of the foot. Recognition of hypoglycemia and hyperglycemia symptoms significantly improves glycemic control and adherence to medication regimens.

CASE 1

Discussion

Mrs. Sweetly should be encouraged to exercise. She has made great progress. Her A_{1C} has dropped from 8.8 to 7.5 with lifestyle modifications and a low-cost medicine. Overall morbidity and mortality will be prevented by achieving the blood pressure target, which has a greater impact on cardiovascular events than does glycemic control, and is a more powerful influence on microvascular complications. (She has achieved the target of lower than 140/80 mmHg.) Adding a dipeptidyl peptidase-IV (DPP-IV) inhibitor (e.g., sitagliptin) would be a consideration in the future because it could improve her HbA$_{1C}$ without producing hypoglycemia.

In addition, ongoing education and reinforcement, recognizing that her skills and even cognition may change over time, with close follow-up with laboratory tests and actual observations of foot and other aspects of her overall care, are crucial to maintaining the current success of her management. You—the primary care provider—will need to actively follow up, with scheduled visits to maintain observation for proteinuria and renal function, orthostasis, falling (often unreported), blood pressure control, and regular eye examinations. Her family members and other caregivers need to know about her illnesses and the need for professional care, because she will need more help with time. ◼

SUMMARY

Older persons have an increased incidence of diabetes and should be screened yearly for DM with a fasting venous plasma glucose level. Diabetes presents atypically in older individuals. Upon diagnosis of diabetes or prediabetes (formerly called impaired fasting glucose and impaired glucose tolerance), diabetic education, dietary education, exercise, and weight loss are appropriate interventions. Treatment goals for diabetes must often be balanced with the patient's expected life span and tolerance of side effects. Efforts to reduce diabetes-related mortality should be focused on macrovascular and cardiac complications with discontinuation of smoking, control of hypertension, and optimizing the lipid profile. Tight glycemic control has more impact on the microvascular complications. Elderly diabetics

are at particular risk for the geriatric syndromes of persistent pain, urinary incontinence, cognitive impairment, depression, injurious falls, and polypharmacy, and they should be screened for these syndromes within 3 to 6 months of initial diagnosis and regularly thereafter. Only through multidisciplinary efforts, including the primary care provider, geriatricians if available, diabetic educators, podiatrists, ophthalmologists, and pharmacists, as well as other specialists if indicated, will we truly optimize care of the elderly with diabetes, reduce their mortality, and preserve their functional capacity.

Web Resources

www.cdc.gov/diabetes/ndep. Centers for Disease Control National Diabetes Education Program.
www.diabeteseducator.org. American Association of Diabetes Educators.
www.diabetes.org. American Diabetes Association.

KEY REFERENCES

4. Mazza AD, Morley JE. Update on diabetes in the elderly and the application of current therapeutics. J Am Med Dir Assoc 2007; 8:489-92.
10. Sinclair A, Morley JE, Rodriguez-Manas L, et al. Diabetes mellitus in older people: Position statement on behalf of the International Association of Gerontology and Geriatrics (IAGG), the European Diabetes Working Party for Older People (EDWPOP), and the International Task Force on Experts in Diabetes. J Am Med Dir Assoc 2012;13:497-502.
13. Vijan S, Stevens DL, Herman WH, et al. Screening, prevention, counseling, and treatment for the complications of type 2 diabetes mellitus. J Gen Intern Med 1997;12:567-80.
14. Morley JE. Hypertension: Is it overtreated in the elderly? J Am Med Dir Assoc 2010;11:147-52.
16. Abrass IB, Schwartz RS. Special presentation of endocrine disease in the elderly. In: Fitzgerald FT, editor. Current practice of medicine. Vol. 1, No. 2. Philadelphia, PA: Current Medicine, 1998; p. 415-18.
18. Umegaki H. Neurodegeneration in diabetes mellitus. Adv Exp Med Biol 2012;724:258-65.

References available online at expertconsult.com.

Thyroid Disorders

James W. Campbell

OBJECTIVES

Upon completion of this chapter, the reader will be able to:

- Describe the presentations of hypothyroidism in an elderly population.
- Describe the presentations of hyperthyroidism in an elderly population.
- Define the euthyroid sick syndrome.
- Understand the risks and benefits of thyroid replacement therapy in an elderly population.

PREVALENCE AND IMPACT

Prevalence

Evidence of hyperthyroidism has a prevalence rate as high as 2.7%.[1] Hypothyroidism, including subclinical hypothyroidism, has a prevalence rate as high as 20% in the elderly population.[1] The reported prevalence of hypothyroidism is three times higher among women than men.[1] Abnormal thyroid-stimulating hormone (TSH) values are found in as many as 40% of acutely ill elderly patients.[2] It is important to note that there is a debate regarding clinical significance of elevations of TSH in the elderly population, particularly among the oldest old. Controversy exists about issues as critical as whether having mild thyroid dysfunction may actually have an improved mortality among older persons.

> Abnormal TSH does not mean thyroid disease.

CASE 1

Mary Peterson (Part 1)

Mary Peterson is an 84-year-old new patient to your office who presents for a complete evaluation. Initial history is remarkable for mild cognitive impairment, dysthymia, fatigue, and decline in instrumental activities of daily living (IADL) function. Physical examination is remarkable for slowing of deep tendon responses, bradycardia, and slowing of mobility as assessed by the "get up and go" test.

What would be appropriate initial screening laboratory test(s)? ▣

Impact

Thyroid dysfunction, in particular hypothyroidism, may have significant impact on the high rate of mental illness, particularly depression, among elderly persons. Thyroid dysfunction is also significantly related to lipid abnormalities, and lipid levels should be checked in all patients with thyroid underactivity; as well, thyroid activity should be checked in all patients with elevated cholesterol levels.[3] Thyroid disorders are more likely to go undiagnosed in patients over the age of 65 than in younger populations.[3] Hypothyroidism has been associated with a general slowing of mental and physical function, cold intolerance, weight gain, constipation, effects on blood pressure, and anemia. Although hyperthyroidism is associated with irregular heart rhythms, congestive heart failure, weight loss, and muscular weakness, these symptoms are common findings in numerous geriatric syndromes.[4]

> Thyroid dysfunction *must* be sought when evaluating depression (and other mental illness) in elders.

Additional online-only material indicated by icon.

RISK FACTORS AND PATHOPHYSIOLOGY

With age, the thyroid gland atrophies, fibrosis occurs, and there is accompanied lymphocytic infiltration as well as increasing colloid nodular production. Production of thyroxine (T_4) decreases with age; however, clearance is also reduced, leading to unchanged (T_4) levels. Triiodothyronine (T_3) levels remain unchanged in healthy older subjects.[5] The body's decreased use of thyroid hormone is felt to be related to a decline in lean body mass, including the metabolically active muscle, skin, bone, and viscera.

CASE 1

Mary Peterson (Part 2)

Ms. Peterson is screened for thyroid dysfunction with a serum TSH, and this reveals a TSH of 38 IU/mL. This was confirmed by a low T_4.

1. **Is this patient a clear candidate for thyroid placement?**

2. **Is this patient likely to have other identifiable symptoms of hypothyroidism on further review?** ▣

Hypothyroidism

The most common etiology of hypothyroidism is previous Hashimoto's disease (a cell-mediated autoimmune inflammatory process with the presence potentially of four different types of thyroid-directed antibodies), irradiation, surgical removal of the thyroid gland, or idiopathic hypothyroidism. Less common causes include pituitary and hypothalamic disorders leading to TSH deficiencies or iodine-induced hypothyroidism most commonly from medical agents, medications including amiodarone, potassium iodide, lithium, antithyroid drugs, or radio contrast agents.[6] Populations at high risk of thyroid dysfunction include people with high levels of radiation exposure, the elderly, and people with Down's syndrome.[7] People with diabetes are also felt to be at high risk of hypothyroid dysfunction.

See "Mary Peterson, Part 3: Discussion."

Hyperthyroidism

The prevalence of hyperthyroidism in older adults is 0.5% to 4%.[8] Hyperthyroidism is most likely due to Graves' disease with multinodular or uninodular active nodular goiter. Graves' disease is an auto-immune disorder with antibody formation to the TSH receptor and/or thyroid follicular cells. This antibody has TSH-like activity. Other etiologies include granulomatous or lymphocytic thyroiditis, in which there is leakage of thyroglobulin from the follicles. There are also iatrogenic sources of hyperthyroidism, including that induced by iodine or the use of amiodarone or from the over-ingestion of thyroid repletion agents.[6]

Thyroid Nodules/Thyroid Cancer

Prevalence of thyroid nodules increases with age. Radiation is a risk factor for thyroid cancer. However, in the very old, if that exposure was greater than 50 years ago, there is no indication of higher risk of cancer.[6] Papillary thyroid cancer is more common in older adults, as is anaplastic carcinoma, the most fatal histologic type of thyroid carcinoma. Thyroid cancer represents 1.5% of all cancers in women and 0.5% of all cancers in men.[1]

DIFFERENTIAL DIAGNOSIS AND ASSESSMENT

CASE 2

Barbara Simpson

Barbara Simpson is an 80-year-old woman evaluated in your office for mild dysthymia. She has a history of hypertension, glaucoma, and osteoarthritis. She has recently lost her husband of 46 years. As part of your evaluation, you check serum TSH, which is 9.7 IU/mL. You order a T_4 test, which is at the lower end of the normal range.

1. **Is Ms. Simpson suffering from hypothyroidism?**

2. **Would Ms. Simpson benefit from thyroid replacement?** ▣

CASE 2

Discussion

Ms. Simpson most likely is suffering from bereavement. The low-normal T_4 and the relatively mild elevation of TSH are consistent with subclinical hypothyroidism, and many of these patients do not progress to clinical hypothyroidism. Exposing her to thyroid replacement may not be beneficial. ▣

Subclinical Hypothyroidism

The syndrome of subclinical hypothyroidism is a relevant differential from symptomatic hypothyroidism in the elderly. Debate is currently ongoing regarding the benefits or possible risks of treating subclinical hypothyroidism. Subclinical hypothyroidism is defined by a normal serum-free T_4 level, combined with an elevation of the TSH level. The transition from subclinical to overt hypothyroidism is not inevitable and may only occur in 5% to 8% of the population with subclinical hypothyroidism on an annual basis.[1] Levels of TSH above 10 IU/mL are considered to be clearly abnormal, and those between 5 IU/mL and 10 IU/mL are considered to be of uncertain significance in the absence of any symptoms or signs of hypothyroidism.[1] Two recent studies have indicated potential detrimental effects of treatment of subclinical hypothyroidism by actually shortening survival.[9,10] Recent studies have also indicated a survival advantage in patients with higher TSH levels; studies indicate that patients with elevated TSH and low to normal T_4 levels have better survival.[11]

Hypothyroidism

There are a multitude of relatively nonspecific symptoms of hypothyroidism (Box 42-1). It is important to note that elderly patients have significantly fewer symptoms with hypothyroidism than do their younger counterparts. The complaints are often subtle and vague. Likewise, it is also important to be sensitive to the risk of attributing hypothyroidism symptomatology to an age-biased view of normal aging. Clearly, a high index of suspicion for hypothyroidism is indicated in evaluation of the geriatric patient.

Screening of the Asymptomatic Patient

The current recommendation for screening asymptomatic, well, elderly persons includes recommendations of the American Academy of Family Physicians and the American Association of Clinical Endocrinologists to measure thyroid function "periodically in all older women." The Canadian Task Force on Periodic Health Examination recommends maintaining a high index of clinical suspicion for nonspecific symptoms presenting with hypothyroidism (Box 42-2). The American College of Physicians recommends screening women over the age of 50 with one or more general symptoms that could be caused by thyroid disease. The American Thyroid Association recommends screening in elderly patients and all patients with autoimmune disease or with a strong family history of thyroid disease.[12] The American Thyroid Association recommends screening every 5 years for persons over the age of 35. In 1998, the American College of Physicians recommended screening in women over the age of 50. The U.S. Preventive Services Task Force did not find enough evidence to recommend screening in asymptomatic elderly women; however, they advised a high index of suspicion of low threshold for checking thyroid function in the at-risk population. Care must be used in the screening of patients who are otherwise ill, as a substantial portion will have abnormal thyroid function in the absence of true thyroid disease owing to euthyroid sick syndrome.[13-15]

Regarding screening for thyroid cancer, at this time there is no clearly defined screening mechanism that increases the benefit by providing early detection with significant differential treatment outcomes. Palpation of the thyroid gland remains part of good clinical practice and routine examination, although there is not high quality evidence to conclude that regular neck palpation could have a major effect on the natural history of this infrequent cancer.[1]

> Ill patients may have the euthyroid sick syndrome: abnormal thyroid function, but *not* true thyroid disease.

BOX 42-1

SYMPTOMS OF HYPOTHYROIDISM

Probably less common in elders[14]
Fatigue
Weakness
Depression
Dry skin

Significantly less common in elders
Weight gain
Cold intolerance
Muscle cramps
Parasthesias
　Libido
　Appetite
• Arthralgias
• Confusion
• Constipation
• Brittle nails
• Loss of hair
• Easy bruisability
• Low back discomfort

CASE 3

Oscar Madison

Oscar Madison is a long-term patient of yours and presents for his routine physical and well-adult care update in the fall. In addition to requesting his flu vaccination, he reports the following nonspecific symptoms: slowed mentation, diarrhea, and weight loss. His daughter reports as well that he has decreased appetite. On examination, he has a blood pressure of 142/86 mm Hg, pulse 88, respiratory 20, and

---

BOX 42–2

CLINICAL CONDITIONS WITH CLEAR INDICATION FOR THYROID DYSFUNCTION SCREENING

Depression
Down's syndrome
Postpartum depression
Women with family history of autoimmune disease
Hyperlipidemia

temperature 37.0°F. Testing reveals a mini-mental state examination (MMSE) of 22/30 and a global deterioration scale (GDS) of 5/15. The physical examination is otherwise unremarkable. Your evaluation includes a TSH of 0.2 IU/mL and an elevated T_4 on repeat examination; you suspect his thyroid gland may be enlarged without discrete nodule.

1. **What further studies would you consider?**

2. **Are his clinical findings consistent with hyperthyroidism?** ▣

CASE 3

Discussion

These findings are consistent with apathetic hyperthyroidism. Mr. Madison may have coexistent depression and/or mild dementia. However, in either case, he would benefit from a more euthyroid state. Evaluation with a radioactive thyroid scan would be appropriate to rule out the possibility of a "hot nodule." ▣

Hyperthyroidism

Prevalence in the elderly patient of overt hyperthyroidism is 0.2% to 2%, which is similar to that in the general population. Less than 35% of hyperthyroid patients over the age of 65 present with atypical symptoms.[6] As with younger patients, two thirds present with symptoms of tachycardia, goiter, and eye symptomology. Older patients are more likely than youth to present with relative tachycardia, weight loss, apathy, and fatigue as primary symptoms. Diarrhea and sweating are also far less common presenting symptoms in older individuals. Likewise, a sense of agitation or anxiety is less commonly reported in older persons. It has been reported that the tremor is as likely to appear in both age groups (Box 42-3).

Elderly patients are likely to have both heart failure as well as the possibility of angina at time of presentation, and as many as 27% will present with atrial fibrillation.[1] Hyperthyroidism in the elderly can be complicated by depression, myopathy,

---

BOX 42-3
SYMPTOMS AND SIGNS OF HYPERTHYROIDISM
This triad presents in more than 50%.[13]
Tachycardia*
Fatigue
Weight loss
Tremor
Atrial fibrillation
Anorexia
Nervousness
*Clinical suspicion should be raised at heart rates 90 or greater in older persons.

---

and osteoporosis. But the most dangerous complication is clearly thyroid storm. The elder person with thyroid storm may be at greater risk for death from the fever, tachycardia, nausea, vomiting, mental status changes, and heart complications. Assessment is still best done initially with the serum TSH.

CASE 4

Felix Unger

Felix Unger is a 78-year-old man who was recently admitted to hospital for an acute right middle cerebral artery distribution cerebrovascular accident complicated by congestive heart failure and acute renal insufficiency. He was noted to have a slowing of cognition and was assessed with a TSH test as well as other tests for reversible causes of functional decline.

1. **If the TSH is elevated, can you conclude Mr. Unger has hypothyroidism?**

2. **How long would it be reasonable to wait after his episode of acute illness before reassessment of TSH?** ▣

CASE 4

Discussion

Mr. Unger has an acute medical illness, and his thyroid laboratory abnormalities may be secondary to a euthyroid sick state. Repeating the laboratory test after resolution of his acute illness in 2 to 4 weeks will help determine if there is genuine thyroid deficiency. ▣

Euthyroid Sick Syndrome

Hypothyroidism should only be diagnosed in a patient with acute illness when there is an evaluation of T_4 and suppression of TSH which that does not normalize within 2 weeks after the resolution of the acute medical or psychiatric illness.[1]

MANAGEMENT

CASE 1

Mary Peterson (Part 3)

Ms. Peterson agreed to initiation or replacement therapy and has no significant coronary artery disease.

What would be a reasonable starting dose of 1-T_4? ▣

CASE 1

Discussion

Ms. Peterson has clinical hypothyroidism. TSH is the most appropriate screening test. As she has symptomatic hypothyroidism, she would benefit from replacement of thyroid hormone with low-dose Levo T$_4$. Once clinically suspected, more symptoms/signs attributable to hypothyroidism are likely to be appreciated. ▪

Hypothyroidism

Overt hypothyroidism with symptoms is treated by careful repletion of thyroid hormone with synthetic thyroid. It is important to assess for the possibility of coronary artery disease. In situations of high risk for coronary artery disease and potential for long-standing hypothyroidism, a stress cardiac imaging study is appropriate before reinitiating a normal metabolic rate. As with other geriatric pharmacology, starting low and going slow is clearly appropriate. A starting dose of 12.5 to 25 g per day is appropriate. The dosage should be increased every 6 weeks. It is rare to require doses greater than 75 to 125 g per day in an older person. Treatment goal is to restore T$_4$ to the normal range and TSH to the upper range of normal. These goals have to be tempered by coexisting cardiovascular disease. Over time, dosage may need to be decreased. Of particular note is the risk of overtreatment leading to osteoporosis in women.

> With a high CAD risk and potentially long-standing hypothyroidism, do a stress test before treatment; and always "start low, go slow."

Subclinical Hypothyroidism

As previously described, it is currently debated as to whether or not appropriate treatment should be instituted for levels between 5 and 10 without clear evidence of symptoms. Most important is to analyze and monitor for the appearance of true clinical hypothyroidism or an elevation into more clearly defined ranges of TSH. At this point in time, it does not appear that initially the treatment has a clearly proven benefit with subclinical hypothyroidism.

Hyperthyroidism

Cases owing to diffusely overactive thyroid or hyperfunctioning nodule or nodules are optimally treated with antithyroid medications propylthiouracil and methimazole. There is also a role for beta-blockade to improve symptomatic treatment, before the antithyroid medication restoring the patient to the euthyroid function. After a period of stabilization, radioactive iodine can be used for definitive treatment. After radioactive iodine treatment, the patient must be monitored for the appearance of hypothyroidism. In the case of possible underlying malignancies, surgical options may be entertained. In the case of inflammatory disease, the etiology of hyperthyroidism tends to spontaneously resolve over weeks to months but may require temporizing symptomatic treatment for relief. This is accomplished with a cautious use of beta-blockade. Of note in severe cases of inflammation, there may be a period of hypothyroidism after the acute event that may temporarily require thyroid replacement. Subclinical hyperthyroidism is estimated to occur in 3% to 8% of older individuals; this occurrence is thought to uncommonly lead to full-blown hyperthyroidism.[16]

KEY REFERENCES

1. Canadian Task Force on Preventive Health Care. Screening for thyroid disorders/cancer. Can Med Assoc J 2003.
2. Finucane P, Rudra T, Church H, et al. Thyroid function tests in the elderly patients with and without an acute illness. Age Ageing 1989;18:398-402.
3. American Association of Clinical Endocrinologists. Thyroid through the ages: The senior years. Aging 2001.
6. Diez JJ. Hyperthyroidism in patients older than 55 years: An analysis of the etiology and management. Gerontology 2003;49 (5):316-23.
16. Trivalle C, Doucet J, Chassagne P, et al. Differences in the signs and symptoms of hyperthyroidism in older and younger patients. J Am Geriatric Soc 1996;44:50-3.

References available online at expertconsult.com.

43

Osteoporosis

Heidi D. Nelson

OUTLINE

OBJECTIVES

Upon completion of this chapter, the reader will be able to:

- Differentiate primary and secondary osteoporosis and understand the medical conditions and medications associated with secondary osteoporosis.
- Understand how to determine individual fracture risk by identifying risk factors and secondary causes and determining bone mineral density.
- Interpret bone mineral density measurements and understand their use in predicting fracture risk and determining the need for drug therapy.
- Understand recommendations from the U.S. Preventive Services Task Force and the National Osteoporosis Foundation for bone density testing.
- Understand recommendations for calcium and vitamin D intake and how to determine if a patient requires supplementation.
- Describe the drugs currently approved for primary and secondary prevention, their effectiveness in preventing fractures, and potential adverse effects.

CASE 1

Harold Jackson

Harold Jackson is a 73-year-old widower who gets intermittent care from the local hospital emergency room and sometimes an urgent care office. His wife brings him to the walk-in clinic you cover occasionally because he has fallen "again." Mr. Jackson says he has emphysema but evidently he still smokes. They have lived in the old family farmhouse for many years, and don't get out much. He does not drive following an arrest for driving while intoxicated, his wife says. He takes a taxi home from the bar on his evenings out with his cronies. Last year Mr. Jackson fell at home and broke his wrist. It's still stiff and swollen. He did not follow up after his wrist was splinted in the emergency room. Tonight, he has dirty cuts up his arm and on his knee, and his back hurts. He looks dry and undernourished. He has a cough which is "nothing" he says; he has just come to get cleaned up because his hand is bleeding and to get a tetanus shot. He is unkempt, ill shaven, and has lost 11 pounds since his last visit to the same clinic 9 months ago. You ask about his wheezy cough, which he says is just his usual. "I used to take prednisone." Mrs. Jackson says, "He don't eat right." He says he has a bad stomach, and takes antacid pills and over-the-counter ranitidine, which relieves his symptoms. On examination he has some prolonged expiratory wheezes and basal crackles.

1. **What can you and Mrs. Jackson do to prevent Mr. Jackson from falling again and sustaining a more serious fracture?**

2. **What aspects of his history put him at risk of osteoporosis?**

3. **Does he already have osteoporosis?**

4. **What are his chances of dying after a hip fracture?**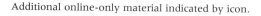

PREVALENCE AND IMPACT

Osteoporosis is a systemic skeletal condition characterized by low bone mass and microarchitectural deterioration of bone tissue that increases bone fragility and risk for fractures.[1] It is diagnosed on the basis of the presence of a fragility fracture or by bone mass measurement criteria. A fragility fracture results from forces that would not normally cause a fracture, such as a hip or wrist fracture from falling from standing height or a vertebral compression fracture. In the absence of a fracture, osteoporosis can be diagnosed by measuring bone mineral density (BMD). Results are expressed as a T-score, which is the difference between an individual's BMD measurement and normal values from a young healthy reference group. The World Health Organization developed definitions for normal, low, and osteoporotic levels of BMD based on T-scores for the spine, hip, or wrist for postmenopausal women and men age 50 and older.[2] By these criteria, bone density is normal for T-scores of −1.0 and higher; low for T-scores between −1.0 and −2.5 (also referred to as osteopenia), and osteoporotic for T-scores of −2.5 or lower (Box 43-1). However, T-scores identify only one aspect of the condition. Other important components, such as the rate of bone loss and quality of bone, are not currently measured.

Low bone density, osteoporosis, and related fractures are common in older adults. Estimates in 2012 indicated that as many as 50% of Americans older than age 50, or 12 million individuals, would be at risk for osteoporotic fractures during their lifetimes.[1] Fracture rates for women are higher than for men, and rates are highest in whites compared to other racial groups, although rates for all demographic groups increase with age.[3-5]

Osteoporosis-related fractures occur at many anatomic sites but are most common at the vertebrae, hip (proximal femur), and wrist (distal radius). All types of fractures are associated with increased mortality.[6-8] Approximately one third of men with hip fractures will die during the subsequent year, a higher rate than for women.[9] Nonfatal fractures at any site can impair function and quality of life, cause chronic pain and disability, and result in high costs for health care and lost productivity.

> All types of fractures are associated with increased mortality.

CASE 2

Georgia and Ann Pound (Part 1)

Georgia Pound is an 81-year-old woman whose only child, Ann, has cared for her for more than 20 years. Ann had always been there for her parents, seeing them Sundays and Fridays and holidays and staying over whenever either of them were ill. When Mr. Pound suddenly died when Ann was in her early 40s, she left her office job in a local bank and moved in to help her mother. Over the years they became a familiar sight, Mrs. Pound in her wheelchair and Ann bent over pushing her up the hill to the church and down again to the old family home. If you passed them on the street, two identical smiles looked up at you. They increasingly looked like sisters, Ann, 63, and Mrs. Pound, 81.

The two of them come to see you in your office. They had not been in for a long time. Mrs. Pound is in a bad mood. Ann is finding her mother more and more difficult; she complains by day and wakes confused in the night. "It's my back, I'm in pain goddammit!" says Mrs. Pound.

Mrs. Pound staggers out of her wheelchair that she has used constantly since breaking her hip 7 years ago. Her legs are edematous and her knees stiff from years of "resting." You examine her back, and it is tender around L2 to L4; standing, her kyphosis is more obvious and she says she has "shrunk."

1. **What is the first thing to do to help Mrs. Pound's mood?**

2. **Mrs. Pound's problem list includes previous hip fracture, hypertension, and osteoarthritic knees. What three chronic illnesses can already be added to her list?**

3. **What needs to be done for Ann?** ▣

RISK FACTORS AND PATHOPHYSIOLOGY

Bone mass is determined by genetic factors, nutrition, physical activity, and general health, and it peaks during early adulthood. Bone health is maintained by the process of bone remodeling, in which old bone is replaced by new. Bone loss occurs when bone removal outpaces replacement. This process also causes alterations

---

BOX 43-1

BONE DENSITY T-SCORES

T-score is the difference between an individual's bone density and the normal value of a reference group. It is expressed as the number of standard deviations above or below the mean of the normal values. T-score is used to classify bone density results into normal, low, and osteoporotic categories. These groupings were determined by the World Health Organization based on bone density measurements at the spine, hip, or forearm, and apply only to postmenopausal women and men age 50 and older.

If T-score is:	Bone density is:
−1.0 and higher	Normal
Between −1.0 and −2.5	Low (osteopenic)
−2.5 and lower	Osteoporotic

in the trabecular plates of bone, which further weakens bone structure (Figure 43-1). Bone loss progresses with aging and may be particularly active for women during menopause. Although bone loss and structural fragility are important causes of fracture, several others are contributory, such as the factors influencing falls (Figure 43-2).

DIFFERENTIAL DIAGNOSIS AND ASSESSMENT

Reassess risks for osteoporosis and fractures periodically; changes in health status influence the risk.

Osteoporosis and fractures may result from several contributing causes, and it is important to understand a patient's overall medical condition before planning interventions, particularly drug therapy. Individual risks for osteoporosis and fractures need to be reassessed periodically because changes in health status, such as the diagnosis of a new condition or initiation of a new medication, can influence a patient's risk profile.

Fracture History

Previously undetected vertebral fractures easily seen on x-rays are important in establishing the diagnosis of osteoporosis.

Patients with previous osteoporosis-related fractures are at high risk for subsequent fractures and are the most likely to benefit from osteoporosis drugs. Most patients are able to recall having had a previous fracture that required medical attention. Fractures are usually well documented in medical records and validated by radiographs. Tracking follow-up care is usually more difficult because it often occurs outside of the immediate care setting. As a result, evaluations for osteoporosis are often missed, drug therapy is frequently not prescribed, and rates of subsequent fractures are generally high.[10,11] Fractures that do not require immediate medical attention are often not recognized, particularly the majority of vertebral fractures with mild or no symptoms. Nonetheless, undetected vertebral fractures are also important in establishing the diagnosis of osteoporosis and determining needs for drug therapy, and can easily be seen on vertebral

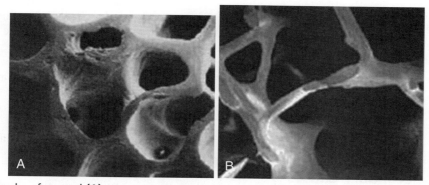

Figure 43-1   Micrographs of normal **(A)** versus osteoporotic **(B)** bone. (From National Osteoporosis Foundation. Physicians' guide to prevention and treatment of osteoporosis. http://www.nof.org.)

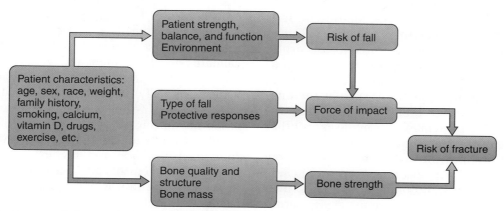

Figure 43-2   Fractures result from multiple contributing components relating to risk of fall, force of impact, and strength of bone.

x-rays. The National Osteoporosis Foundation (NOF) recommends vertebral imaging for older men and women.[12]

> Patients remember fractures and they are usually documented on x-ray films. However, bone density testing for osteoporosis is often not done, and avoidable fractures, disability, and even death can result.

CASE 2

Georgia and Ann Pound (Part 2)

For Mrs. Pound you prescribe acetaminophen, 650 mg, three times a day, as well as advising a heat-in-the-microwave pad.

Mrs. Pound allows you to x-ray her lumbar spine and, sure enough, the bones are thin, and the vertebral bodies of L2 and L3 are crushed, quite recently. Her vitamin D is at deficient levels. She agrees to take vitamin D so you start with 50,000 international units (IU) once a week.

You glance at quiet, worried Ann. Like mother, like daughter. Ann's back is also kyphotic even though she is only 63. Is it already too late to prevent her from breaking a hip one day and suffering vertebral fractures? You order BMD testing for Ann.

1. **What else is needed for Mrs. Pound? Should she be persuaded to take additional medication? What will you add first? Does she need more tests?**

2. **How can Ann prevent her own osteoporotic fractures?**

3. **What more should be done about Mrs. Pound's cognition?** ▣

Identification of Secondary Causes and Risk Factors

Osteoporosis may occur without a known cause (primary osteoporosis) or can occur as the result of another condition (secondary osteoporosis). It is important to identify potential secondary causes before determining the need for osteoporosis drugs. Common secondary causes include dietary deficiencies of calcium or vitamin D; medications (including glucocorticoids); health conditions such as rheumatoid arthritis; and several others that are often undetected (Box 43-2). Metabolic bone diseases other than osteoporosis, such as hyperparathyroidism or osteomalacia, may be associated with a low BMD. Tests to diagnose secondary causes include complete blood counts and blood chemistries, liver function, thyroid stimulating hormone (TSH), serum 25(OH)D, parathyroid hormone (PTH), and 24-hour

---

BOX 43-2

SECONDARY CAUSES OF OSTEOPOROSIS

Health Conditions
- Diabetes
- Hyperparathyroidism
- Gastric bypass; other gastrointestinal surgery
- Malabsorption
- Inflammatory bowel disease
- Hemophilia
- Lupus
- Rheumatoid arthritis
- Kidney disease
- Depression
- Multiple sclerosis
- Emphysema

Medications
- Aluminium antacids
- Anticoagulants
- Anticonvulsants
- Aromatase inhibitors
- Barbiturates
- Cancer chemotherapeutic drugs
- Cyclosporine A and tacrolimus
- Depo-medroxyprogesterone
- Glucocorticoids*
- Gonadotropin-releasing hormone agonists
- Lithium

U.S. Department of Health and Human Services. Bone health and osteoporosis: A report of the Surgeon General. Rockville, MD: U.S. Department of Hearth & Human Services. Office of the Surgeon General; 2004.

*At levels of 5 mg daily or more of prednisone or equivalent for 3 or more months.

---

urine calcium, as well as special studies in selected patients.

If a secondary cause is found, it is of course addressed. Bone density monitoring and osteoporosis treatment can be considered if the bone density is low or there is a fracture, depending on the underlying condition, the severity of osteoporosis, other aspects of the patient's health, and the patient's preferences.

Risk factors are also useful in determining needs for bone density testing and osteoporosis drugs. Several methods to calculate a patient's individual risk for fracture based on key risk factors derived from epidemiologic studies have been developed and tested. Although models vary, most are modest predictors of fractures, and the results of simple versus complex models are similar.[13] The Fracture Risk Assessment Model (FRAX), developed by the World Health Organization,[14] calculates a patient's 10-year probabilities of either a major osteoporotic fracture (spine, hip, or wrist) or, specifically, a hip fracture based on 11 risk factors (Box 43-3). FRAX has been validated for both men and women. Calculations can be made with and without bone density results using a publicly accessible web-based calculator.[15] The NOF has issued treatment recommendations based on specific 10-year risk thresholds calculated by FRAX (20% and higher risk for major osteoporotic fractures; 3% and higher risk for hip fracture).[12] However, this approach has not been tested in drug trials, and it is not yet known how effective these thresholds would be in reducing fractures in actual patients.

BOX 43-3

RISK FACTORS INCLUDED IN THE FRACTURE RISK ASSESSMENT MODEL (FRAX)

- Age
- Gender
- Low BMI (body mass index)
- Parent history of hip fracture
- Prior osteoporotic fracture
- Current smoking
- Current alcohol use of three or more drinks daily
- Femoral neck bone mineral density
- Oral glucocorticoids*
- Rheumatoid arthritis
- Presence of a secondary cause of osteoporosis

From FRAX calculator. http://www.shef.ac.uk/FRAX/tool.jsp.
*5 mg or more daily of prednisone for 3 or more months.

Bone Densitometry

> Bone density testing: test patients with osteoporosis-related fractures or secondary causes, all women age 65 and older, and postmenopausal women with key risk factors.

Bone measurement tests are used to predict fractures, diagnose osteoporosis, select patients for therapy, and monitor response to therapy. Current clinical guidelines recommend such testing in patients with osteoporosis-related fractures or secondary causes of osteoporosis, all women age 65 and older, and younger postmenopausal women with key risk factors.[12,16] Testing men age 70 and older is also recommended by the NOF.[12] Although data on appropriate testing intervals is limited, repeat testing is probably not useful for most patients until approximately 10 years after the initial measure.[17,18] Patients with BMD tests bordering the osteoporosis threshold may need a more frequent repeat test.

Bone density can be measured in a number of ways, although the most accepted method in the United States is by dual-energy x-ray absorptiometry (DXA, or DEXA) at the hip and spine. This test is usually conducted in a medical facility and uses a focused x-ray beam directed at a specific area of the bone. Its role in predicting fractures in men has only recently been evaluated in large studies. For each standard deviation reduction in femoral neck BMD, fracture risks at various anatomic sites are increased to similar levels for men and women.[13]

Several other types of bone measurement tests may be more easily available and less expensive, such as DXA of the wrist and other peripheral sites and quantitative ultrasound (QUS) of the calcaneus (heel). Large studies of postmenopausal women and men indicate that calcaneal QUS using various types of devices can predict fractures as well as DXA of the femoral neck, hip, or spine.[13] However, QUS is not a good predictor of DXA and it remains unclear how results of QUS can be used to select individuals for drug therapies that were proven effective based on DXA criteria. For these reasons, DXA measurements of the hip and spine are considered the gold standard.

CASE 2

Georgia and Ann Pound (Part 3)

Ann's BMD tests come through with the following T-scores: −3.2 hip; −2.0 wrist; −2.7 spine. These results fulfill the WHO criteria for osteoporosis. You recommend calcium and vitamin D for her too, and alendronate once a week. Without the wheelchair to support her, Ann's balance is unsteady, and you arrange physical therapy for balance and gait training. Ann starts to enjoy, for the first time in her life, the sense of energy that exercise gives.

Mrs. Pound's Mini-Mental State Exam (MMSE) score is 16/30. You start calcium supplements and donepezil.

1. **What else could be done for Mrs. Pound's osteoporosis?**

2. **What can be done about the stress on Ann?** ▣

MANAGEMENT

Universal Recommendations

Several factors can be modified to reduce the risk of osteoporosis and fractures (Box 43-4). These include

BOX 43-4

REDUCING RISK FACTORS FOR OSTEOPOROSIS AND FRACTURES

Modify secondary causes of osteoporosis
- Health conditions that cause or contribute to osteoporosis and fractures
- Medications

Adequate calcium and vitamin D intake
- 1200 mg daily of elemental calcium
- 800-1000 international units daily of vitamin D
- Supplements if diet is inadequate or other problems limit intake or absorption

Regular weight-bearing, muscle-strengthening exercise
- Increases bone density
- Reduces risk of falls

Prevent falls
- Correct vision and hearing
- Evaluate gait and balance
- Assess medication side effects
- Evaluate home safety
- Hip protectors if high fall risk

Discontinue tobacco

Avoid excess alcohol
- Three or more drinks per day adversely affects bone
- Increases fall risk

maintaining adequate calcium and vitamin D intake, performing regular weight-bearing and muscle-strengthening exercise, preventing falls, discontinuing tobacco use, and avoiding excessive alcohol intake (defined as three or more drinks daily).

Calcium and Vitamin D Intake

Current dietary recommendations for patients older than age 50 include 1200 mg of elemental calcium and 800 to 1000 IU of vitamin D per day.[19] Because the average American consumes only 800 mg of calcium per day and insufficient amounts of vitamin D, many patients are calcium deficient. As a result, they maintain calcium balance through bone absorption, exacerbating bone loss. Several medical conditions and medications common among older patients interfere with calcium absorption, such as gastric achlorhydria and use of H_2-receptor antagonists. These should be considered when evaluating calcium supplementation needs.

Vitamin D improves not only calcium absorption, bone health, and muscle function, but also balance and the risk of falling. Vitamin D deficiency is particularly common among elderly patients who are homebound or institutionalized, live at northern latitudes, or have gastrointestinal malabsorption or chronic renal insufficiency (CKD). The NOF recommends the same intake of vitamin D as other dietary guidelines (i.e., 800 to 1000 IU per day of vitamin D, specifically for all adults age 50 and older) and recommends increased doses for patients at risk of deficiency, to bring their serum 25(OH)D level to 30 ng/mL (75 nmol/L) or higher.[12]

A meta-analysis of randomized controlled trials (RCTs) enrolling older men and women indicated that combined vitamin D intake and calcium supplementation significantly reduced the risk for fractures compared to placebo.[19] However, this effect was statistically significant for only institutionalized elderly patients, not community-dwelling elderly or postmenopausal women, or community-dwelling postmenopausal women with previous fractures. A meta-analysis of trials of vitamin D supplementation alone versus placebo showed no reduction in fracture risk.[19] Adverse effects of supplementation were evaluated in the Women's Health Initiative (WHI) trial that reported an increase in risk for renal and urinary tract stones with vitamin D and calcium supplementation compared to placebo.[20] A separate trial of a single annual megadose of vitamin D_3 (500,000 IU) indicated increased risk for fall and fractures.[21]

> Combined vitamin D and calcium supplementation significantly reduces fracture risk in institutionalized elderly men and women, and vitamin D alone does not.

Exercise and Fall Prevention

Exercise increases bone density and reduces falls and fractures by improving agility, strength, posture, and balance. The NOF strongly endorses lifelong physical activity at all ages, both for osteoporosis prevention and overall health.[12] Falls may also be reduced by correcting vision and hearing deficits; evaluating balance, gait, and mobility; reviewing prescription medications for side effects that may affect balance; and reducing fall hazards at home. These are more fully described in Chapters 19, 20, and 21. The U.S. Preventive Services Task Force recommends exercise or physical therapy and vitamin D supplementation to prevent falls in community-dwelling adults aged 65 years or older who are at increased fall risk.[22]

Pharmacologic Therapy

> Clarify what the indications are for osteoporosis drugs before prescribing; is it primary prevention, secondary prevention, or both?

Osteoporosis drugs are approved by the U.S. Food and Drug Administration (FDA) specifically for primary prevention, secondary prevention, or both, and it is important to clarify these indications before initiating therapy (Box 43-5). All drugs improved bone density in RCTs; only some drugs demonstrated fracture reduction, a more clinically relevant measure.

Drugs for primary prevention are intended for patients without previous fractures who have bone density above the osteoporotic range (i.e., T-score > −2.5). Six drugs are FDA approved for primary prevention for postmenopausal women and none are approved for men (Table 43-1). These include four

---

BOX 43-5

INDICATIONS FOR OSTEOPOROSIS DRUGS

Primary prevention—postmenopausal women with:
- Low bone density (T-score −1.0 to −2.5) at hip or vertebra not related to other causes (such as medications, other health conditions, or other risk factors).
- Use estimates of 10-year probabilities of hip or major osteoporosis-related fractures based on bone density and risk factors to determine need for primary prevention drugs.

Secondary prevention—postmenopausal women and men age 50 and older with:
- Fracture likely from osteoporosis (e.g., hip or vertebral), or other fracture from minor trauma.
- Low bone density (T-score −2.5 or lower) at hip or vertebra, not related to other causes such as medications or other health conditions.

From Drugs//www.accessdata.fda.gov/scripts/cder/drugsatfda.

TABLE 43-1	Drugs Approved for Primary Prevention of Osteoporosis and Fractures in Postmenopausal Women			
	Reduces Fractures in RTCs			
Generic Name	**Vertebral**	**Nonvertebral**	**Route**	**Dose**
Bisphosphonate				
Alendronate	Yes	No	Oral*	5 mg daily
			Oral	35 mg weekly
Ibandronate	No trials	No trials		
			Oral	150 mg monthly
Risedronate	No	No	Oral	5 mg daily
			Oral	35 mg weekly
			Oral	75 mg for 2 days every month
			Oral	150 mg monthly
			Oral	35 mg weekly with 1250 mg calcium carbonate† for 6 days per week
Zoledronic acid	No	No	IV	5 mg once every 2 years
Estrogen				
Estrogen	Yes	Hip, combined‡	Oral and transdermal	Varies by type
Estrogen combined with progestin	Yes	Hip, combined	Oral and transdermal	Varies by type
Raloxifene	Yes	No	Oral	60 g daily

From Drugs//www.accessdata.fda.gov/scripts/cder/drugsatfda; Nelson HD, Haney EM, Dana T, et al. Screening for osteoporosis: An update for the U.S. Preventive Services Task Force. Ann Intern Med 2010;153:99-111.
(Drug information is frequently updated. Please check reliable current sources before prescribing.)
*Pill form unless otherwise indicated.
†Equivalent to 500 mg elemental calcium.
‡For all types of nonvertebral fractures combined such as hip, wrist, ankle, etc.

bisphosphonate drugs (alendronate, ibandronate, risedronate, and zoledronic acid); several forms of estrogen alone or combined with progestin; and raloxifene, an estrogen agonist/antagonist. For some of the drugs, such as alendronate, prevention doses are smaller than treatment doses. Alendronate, raloxifene, and estrogen reduced vertebral fractures in trials of women without previous fractures.[13] The Fracture Intervention Trial of alendronate stratified results according to baseline bone density and found that fractures were reduced only for women with baseline T-scores ≤ −2.5.[23] Estrogen also reduced nonvertebral fractures in the WHI trials, and bisphosphonates reduced primary nonvertebral fractures in a sensitivity analysis of a meta-analysis of trials.[13] No trials reported effects on fracture-related morbidity and mortality.

Drugs for secondary prevention are intended for individuals with previous osteoporosis-related fractures or T-scores ≤ −2.5. Eight drugs are FDA approved for secondary prevention for postmenopausal women and four for men (Table 43-2). For women, these include four bisphosphonate drugs: calcitonin, denosumab, raloxifene, and teriparatide. In trials of women with previous fractures, all of these drugs reduced vertebral fractures, and all except calcitonin and raloxifene reduced fractures at other sites.[13] For

men, approved drugs include three bisphosphonates (alendronate, risedronate, and zoledronic acid) and teriparatide. Men were included in trials that demonstrated reduced vertebral fractures for alendonate and zoledronic acid and reduced nonvertebral fractures for zoledronic acid.

In general, osteoporosis drugs are most effective in reducing fractures for patients with very low bone density, previous fractures, and multiple risk factors. Long-term data on benefits and adverse effects (Table 43-3) are limited and head-to-head trials are lacking.[13,24] To maximize their effectiveness and minimize their potential adverse effects, these drugs should be used selectively and for a limited period of time, generally 3 to 5 years.

A patient's response and potential adverse effects from the drug should be monitored by follow-up visits with the prescribing physician, appropriate laboratory tests, and bone density testing. The NOF recommends retesting with DXA of the hip and spine after 2 years of treatment.[12] Some physicians also monitor drug response by following biochemical markers of bone turnover. However, experts are divided about the usefulness of this approach because markers have a high degree of biological and analytical variability.

TABLE 43-2   Drugs Approved for Secondary Prevention of Osteoporosis and Fractures in Postmenopausal Women and in Men

Generic Name	Approved for men?	Reduces Fractures in RTCs		Route	Dose
		Vertebral	Nonvertebral		
Bisphosphonate					
Alendronate	Yes	Yes (M, W)	Hip (W), combined (W)*	Oral† Oral‡ Oral	10 mg daily 70 mg weekly 70 mg weekly with 2800 IU or 5600 IU of vitamin D3
Ibandronate	No	Yes (W)	No	Oral IV and injection	150 mg monthly 3 mg every 3 months
Risedronate	Yes§	Yes (W)	Hip (W), combined (W)	Oral Oral Oral Oral Oral	5 mg daily 35 mg weekly 75 mg for 2 days every month 150 mg monthly 35 mg weekly with 1250 mg calcium carbonate for 6 days
Zoledronic acid	Yes	Yes (M, W)	Hip (W), combined (M, W)	IV	5 mg once yearly
Calcitonin	No	Yes (W)	No	Nasal spray Injection	200 IU daily 100 IU every other day
Denosumab	Yes	Yes (W)	Hip (W), combined (W)	Injection	60 mg every 6 months
Raloxifene	No	Yes (W)	No	Oral	60 mg daily
Teriparatide	Yes	Yes (W)	Combined (W)	Injection	20 micrograms daily

From Drugs@FDA (www.accessdata.fda.gov/scripts/cder/drugsatfda); Nelson HD, Haney EM, Dana T, et al. Screening for osteoporosis: an update for the U.S. Preventive Services Task Force. Ann Intern Med 2010;153:99-111.
(Drug information is frequently updated. Please check reliable current sources before prescribing.)
M, Men; *W*, postmenopausal women.
*For all types of nonvertebral fractures combined such as hip, wrist, ankle, etc.
†Pill form unless otherwise indicated.
‡Comes in pill or oral solution.
§Risedronate 35 mg weekly.

Bisphosphonates

Bisphosphonates reduce fractures by inhibiting osteoclastic activity during bone remodeling. They are approved for primary and secondary prevention and for men as well as postmenopausal women. Bisphosphonates provide many different dosing options, including oral forms (alendronate, ibandronate, and risedronate) that can be taken daily, weekly, or monthly; and intravenous infusions that can be administered every 3 months (ibandronate), yearly (zoledronic acid treatment dose), or every other year (zoledronic acid prevention dose). Combinations with vitamin D or calcium are also available. Specific dosing schedules may be particularly useful for elderly patients with special needs and preferences. Bisphosphonates are recommended for patients using long-term glucocorticoid therapy.[25]

Oral bisphosphonates may cause irritation of the esophagus and should be avoided in patients with esophageal dysmotility, ulcers, or other problems. To reduce effects, drugs should be taken with a large glass of water first thing in the morning. After taking the drug, patients need to sit or stand upright for 30 to 60 minutes and should not eat or drink anything else during this time. Bisphosphonates should not be used by patients with low blood calcium levels or impaired kidney function. Additional adverse effects include atrial fibrillation, muscle and joint pain, midfemur fractures, and osteonecrosis of the jaw, although most cases of osteonecrosis occurred in patients with cancer using high doses of intravenous bisphosphonates. Major adverse effects are rare; however, patients need to be aware of them when deciding to use these drugs and physicians should monitor them.

Calcitonin

Calcitonin, a hormone naturally produced in the thyroid gland, reduces bone resorption. For osteoporosis

TABLE 43-3	Main Adverse Effects of Osteoporosis Drugs				
	Main Adverse Effects				
Medication	**Gastrointestinal**	**Cardiovascular**	**Musculoskeletal**	**Cancer**	**Other**
Bisphosphonates	Esophageal ulcers and other serious events Acid reflux, nausea, vomiting	Atrial fibrillation?	Severe reversible musculoskeletal pain	Esophageal cancer (rare)	Osteonecrosis of jaw (mostly in cancer patients on high-dose IV preparations), atypical femur fractures
Calcitonin	No increase	No increase	Not reported	No increase	Nasal irritation with spray
Denosumab	Not reported	Not reported	Not reported	Not reported	Hypocalcemia, cellulitis, osteonecrosis of jaw, atypical femur fractures
Estrogen alone	Not reported	Increases stroke Increases blood clots	Not reported	Increases endometrial cancer	Increases gallbladder disease, urinary incontenence
Estrogen combined with progestin	Not reported	Increases stroke Increases blood clots	Not reported	Increases breast cancer	Increases vaginal bleeding, gallbladder disease, uninary incontenence, dementia
Raloxifene	Not reported	Increases blood clots	Leg cramps	No increase Reduces breast cancer in postmenopausal women	Increases hot flashes
Teriparatide	No increase	Not reported	Leg cramps	No increase	Not reported

From Drugs@FDA (www.accessdata.fda.gov/scripts/cder/drugsatfda); Nelson HD, Haney EM, Dana T, et al. Screening for osteoporosis: an update for the U.S. Preventive Services Task Force. Ann Intern Med 2010;153:99-111.
(Drug information is frequently updated. Please check reliable current sources before prescribing.)

therapy, salmon calcitonin is used as a daily injection or nasal spray. It is FDA approved only for women with low bone density who are 5 years or more postmenopausal, although few trials have evaluated its effects on fractures. Its main adverse effects include nausea and effects related to its administration such as nasal irritation with the spray and skin inflammation with the injection.

Denosumab

Denosumab is a monoclonal antibody that inhibits bone resorption. It was approved for postmenopausal women at high risk for fractures or intolerant of other drugs, and is only available as an injection that is administered in a clinical setting every 6 months. Denosumab reduced fractures at several sites for postmenopausal women with previous fractures when compared with women taking placebo.[26] Few adverse effects have been reported to date, reflecting in part the recency of its availability for general use.

Estrogen

Many forms of estrogen are approved for primary prevention for postmenopausal women; however, package inserts indicate that when used solely for this purpose, estrogen should only be considered for women at high risk of osteoporosis and nonestrogen medications should be considered first.[25] Estrogen is not approved for secondary prevention or for men. Estrogen is most commonly used as a tablet taken daily, or as a skin patch replaced weekly. Several types of estrogen are available, although oral conjugated equine estrogen is most commonly prescribed in the United States and was used in the WHI trials. Women who have not had hysterectomies should use estrogen combined with progestin to avoid causing uterine bleeding or cancer.

Estrogen reduced vertebral and nonvertebral fractures compared to placebo for women in the WHI, although it was also associated with many important adverse effects,[27] including stroke, thromboembolic events, gallbladder disease, and urinary incontinence. Estrogen combined with progestin also increased breast cancer and vaginal bleeding. Estrogen may provide an osteoporosis benefit for women using it for short-term management of menopausal symptoms, but it is not considered a first-line choice because of these adverse effects.

Raloxifene

Raloxifene inhibits bone resorption and decreases bone turnover. As an estrogen agonist/antagonist, raloxifene provides some of estrogen's health benefits while avoiding some of its harms and is approved for primary and secondary prevention for postmenopausal women only. It reduces vertebral fractures for women with or without previous fractures, but does not reduce fractures at other sites. Raloxifene also reduces risk for breast cancer by 56%, an unexpected finding in trials designed for fracture and heart disease prevention,[28] providing an option for postmenopausal women with increased risks for both osteoporosis and breast cancer. Raloxifene causes thromboembolic events, although risks are lower than with estrogen. Whereas estrogen relieves hot flashes, raloxifene can cause them. Raloxifene also can cause leg cramps and other nuisance symptoms, but these vary widely among users.

Teriparatide

Teriparatide, recombinant human parathyroid hormone, increases bone density by stimulating bone formation, and reduced vertebral and nonvertebral fractures in clinical trials. It is approved for secondary prevention for postmenopausal women and men, but can only be taken for 2 years. Teriparatide is taken by a daily subcutaneous injection in the thigh or abdominal wall. Muscle pain, headaches, dizziness, nausea, and temporary hypotension are its most common adverse effects. Teriparatide caused osteosarcomas in laboratory rats and should not be used in humans

with increased risks for this type of tumor. It also interacts with the heart medication digoxin and the two drugs should not be used together.

Case 2

Discussion

Ann joins a weekly group meeting for caregivers at her church. Her exercise program has energized her. The group talks about the caregiver's health, end-of-life care, and life after the loved one is gone.

Mrs. Pound's dementia progresses quickly, and she is hospitalized with a dense left hemiplegia. She develops pneumonia and when intubation is imminent, Ann, as medical power of attorney, expresses her mother's wishes against life support, and Mrs. Pound never regains consciousness. Ann feels guilty, and—ever the caregiver—when a call comes in a few months later to "come down and help" Mrs. Pound's sister in Orlando after surgery, she feels she has to go. She continues her alendronate, exercise, calcium, and vitamin D under the care of a new doctor in Florida. ◧

SUMMARY

Osteoporosis is a common condition associated with aging that is characterized by low bone mass and weakening of bone tissue. Several strategies to screen, prevent, and treat osteoporosis are based on strong research evidence and are recommended by professional organizations (Table 43-4). These include determining individual risks for fracture by identifying risk factors and secondary causes and obtaining bone densitometry. Treating secondary causes and modifiable risk factors and providing osteoporosis drugs may be indicated for individual patients. Osteoporosis drugs reduce risk for osteoporosis-related fractures by increasing bone thickness, but differ by their mechanisms, effectiveness, how they are taken, and their adverse effects.

TABLE 43-4	Evaluation and Prevention of Osteoporosis and Fractures	
Indications	**Strategy**	**Level of Evidence**
Risk assessment and bone density screening	All women age 65 and older, and younger women with risk factors	B
Primary prevention in patients without previous fractures and T-scores > −2.5	Identify and treat secondary causes and risk factors	No studies
	Exercise and fall prevention if increased risk	B
	Calcium and vitamin D supplementation if insufficient	A*
	Drug therapy	A (women)
Secondary prevention in patients with fragility fractures or T-scores ≤ −2.5	Drug therapy	A (women; men)

A = supported by one or more high-quality randomized controlled trials (RCTs); B = supported by one or more high-quality nonrandomized cohort studies or low-quality RCTs; C = supported by one or more case series and/or poor-quality cohort or case-control studies.
*Significant fracture reduction in RCTs of institutionalized elderly patients.

Web Resources

www.accessdata.fda.gov/scripts/cder/drugsatfda. Drug approval reports from the U.S. Food and Drug Administration.

www.shef.ac.uk/FRAX/tool.jsp. World Health Organization fracture risk assessment tool (FRAX).

www.nof.org. National Osteoporosis Foundation.

www.uspreventiveservicestaskforce.org. U.S. Preventive Services Task Force.

KEY REFERENCES

1. U.S. Department of Health and Human Services. Bone health and osteoporosis: A report of the Surgeon General. Rockville, MD: U.S. Department of Hearth & Human Services. Office of the Surgeon General; 2004.

12. National Osteoporosis Foundation. Clinician's Guide to prevention and treatment of osteoporosis. Washington, DC: National Osteoporosis Foundation; 2013.

13. Nelson HD, Haney EM, Dana T, et al. Screening for osteoporosis: An update for the U.S. Preventive Services Task Force. Ann Intern Med 2010;153:99-111.

14. Kanis JA on behalf of the World Health Organization Scientific Group. Assessment of osteoporosis at the primary health care level. 2008 Technical Report. University of Sheffield, UK: WHO Collaborating Center; 2008.

16. U.S. Preventative Services Task Force. Screening for osteoporosis. U.S. Preventive Services Task Force Recommendation Statement. Ann Intern Med 2011; 154:345-364.

References available online at expertconsult.com.

Arthritis and Related Disorders

Yuri Nakasato and Melissa Christensen

OBJECTIVES

Upon completion of this chapter, the reader will be able to:

- Understand the differential diagnosis of common rheumatic conditions affecting the older population.
- Recognize that arthritis in later life is different from that in the younger population.
- Understand strengths, limitations, and adverse effects of medications used to treat musculoskeletal disorders in older people.

Additional online-only material indicated by icon.

CASE 1

Mrs. Montes (Part 1)

Mrs. Montes, a 90-year-old Hispanic woman, comes to the office with nonspecific "multiple joint aches and pains." She was brought by family members and is in a wheelchair. Her comorbidities include diabetes, hypertension, hypercholesterolemia, coronary artery disease, heart failure, atrial fibrillation, arthritis, and mild dementia. She states that the aches and pains are recent, but she cannot recall when they started. According to her family, 4 weeks ago she was able to do her basic activities of daily living (ADLs) and some instrumental ADLs. A week ago she started refusing to walk. She has early morning stiffness that lasts more than 1 hour. Her examination is notable for the presence of Heberden's and Bouchard's nodes.

1. **What is the likely cause of Mrs. Montes's complaints?**
2. **What treatment should be offered?**
3. **What is the significance of her Heberden's and Bouchard's nodes?** ▣

PREVALENCE

Arthritis is a common and prevalent condition that is acquiring more importance as the population ages. Models of care are proliferating to satisfy this demand through geriatric rheumatology or gerontorheumatology.[1-6]

Osteoarthritis (OA) is the most common arthritic condition among the elderly, affecting 13.9% of U.S. adults, or 26.9 million people (Table 44-1). Other rheumatic disorders prevalent among the elderly are rheumatoid arthritis (RA; 1.5 million cases in the United States), gout (6.1 million cases), pseudogout (10,000 to 40,000 people ages 65 to 85), polymyalgia rheumatica (PMR; approximately 450,000 cases, 90% of whom are 60 years and older), and giant-cell arteritis (GCA; 110,000 Americans, 90% of whom are older than 60 years).[6]

RISK FACTORS AND PATHOPHYSIOLOGY

Osteoarthritis

OA, although highly prevalent in later life, does not appear to be directly caused by aging. Predisposing factors include obesity, female sex, quadriceps weakness, major joint injury and/or instability, poor proprioception, heavy physical activity, and genetics. OA is manifest first by cartilage irregularity, followed by eburnation or ulceration of the cartilage surface, and eventually by frank cartilage loss.

TABLE 44-1 Differential Diagnosis of Prevalent Rheumatic Disorders in the Elderly

Disorder	Prevalence, etc.	Impact on Mortality	Pathophysiology and Risk Factors	Clinical Comparison	Laboratory	X-rays	Management
Osteoarthritis (OA)	13.9% of U.S. adults or 26.9 million people.[7,8,9]	Prevalence of coronary artery disease (CAD) in patients with OA is 27%[10]	Predisposing factors: age, obesity, female, inheritance, quadriceps weakness, major joint injury/instability, poor proprioception, heavy physical activity.	Insidious and chronic. Affects DIPs, PIPs, CMCs, hips, knees, back, and neck. Heberden's nodes (DIPs), and Bouchard's nodes (PIPs) are prevalent	ANA (−), RF (−); ESR normal; CRP normal.	Presence of osteophytes, loss of articular space, subchondral sclerosis.	Canes, braces, thermotherapy, exercise, narcotics, and knee and hip replacement
Younger-Onset Rheumatoid Arthritis (YORA)	About 1.5 million in U.S.: women more often than men. RA prevalence diminishes after menopause.	Prevalence of CAD is 50%. Cardiovascular mortality accounts for half of all deaths[10,11]	HLA-DR4 present in RF (+) patients and in some RF (−) patients	Insidious and chronic. Affects MCPs, PIPs, wrists, knees, and shoulders. Compared to EORA, Symptoms: >distal	ANA (±); RF (+) 80%, Anti-CCP (+), ESR and CRP can be elevated[12,13]	Loss of articular space, erosions, juxtaarticular osteopenia, ulnar deviation	Low-dose steroids
Elderly-Onset Rheumatoid Arthritis (EORA) >60 years	Unknown. Sex distribution 1:1	No data	HLA-DR4 is present in RF (+) and less likely in RF (−) patients	More acute and infectious like, Symptoms: >proximal Outcome: worse	ANA (±), RF (+) 32-89%, ESR higher at onset	As YORA	Low-dose steroid
Gout in Elderly	U.S. prevalence 5.1 million. Men more often than women. Most are men with onset at middle age. Elderly-onset gout is after age 60, sex distribution is 1:1. If onset after age 80, women are almost 100%	Hyperuricemia may produce HTN[14]	It is associated with diuretic use and renal disease. Other classic risk factors include obesity, hypertension, and heavy alcohol use (less common). Gout is an inflammatory response to MSU crystals.	Elderly-onset gout is still acute but more polyarticular, more likely to involve small joints and develop tophi more rapidly and in unusual locations	ANA (−), RF (−). High serum uric acid, MSU (negative birefringent) on synovial fluid	Overhanging edge, with erosions. Affects mainly the first MTP, but it is common in hands	NSAIDs, colchicines, allopurinol, steroids PA or intraarticular. Diet low in red meats and seafood[15]

Continued on following page

TABLE 44-1	Differential Diagnosis of Prevalent Rheumatic Disorders in the Elderly (Continued)						
Disorder	Prevalence, etc.	Impact on Mortality	Pathophysiology and Risk Factors	Clinical Comparison	Laboratory	X-rays	Management
Pseudogout in elderly	Age 65-75; 10,000 to 15,000. Age >80: 40,000 per 100,000 people	Unknown	Inflammatory reaction to CPPD crystals. With intraarticular calcification (chondrocalcinosis)	Affects mainly the elderly population, most commonly the knee. Concomitant OA.	CPPD crystals (positive birefringent on polarizing microscope) in synovial fluid	Chondrocalcinosis in hands, pelvis, and knees mostly.	NSAIDs, intraarticular steroids.
Younger-onset systemic lupus erythematosus (SLE)	SLE affects at least 239,000 Americans: 4,000 white men, 41,000 white women, 31,000 black men, and 163,000 black women	Premature atherosclerosis. Interval between onset and diagnosis is 32.5 months. Survival 97% at 5 years and 90% at 10 years	T-cell genetic susceptibility plus natural senescence; stress factors may tip the balance to clinic disease. Unspecified environmental stimuli, illness, and infection.	Insidious and chronic. Usually systemic affecting kidneys, brain, lungs, heart, blood, and skin. Renal failure is a common fear.	ANA, dsDNA, Sm, Ro/SSA (+); C3, C4 low; ESR and CRP high; APS ab (+). Pancytopenia.	Pericarditis changes, pleural effusion. Jaccoud's arthropathy.	High-dose steroids for flares.
Late-onset SLE (>50 years)	Female to male (6.9:1) Compared with younger-onset SLE, more common in whites	5-year survival rate is comparable to younger-onset SLE	Genetic factors, nongenetic, environmental, and life-style factors	Tend to be milder. Weight loss, muscular aches and pains, disturbances of cognition or affect. Arthritis and arthralgias of the hands and wrists, rash, Raynaud's phenomenon, vague central nervous system symptoms	ANA (weakly+) (up to 36% of healthy elderly people have nonspecific low titers of ANA), Anti dsDNA, Anti-SM, Anti-Ro/SSA (+), C3, C4 low. ESR/ CRP high	Same as younger-onset SLE	Same as younger-onset SLE. Careful with side effects

Disease	Epidemiology	Prognosis	Etiology	Symptoms	Labs	Imaging	Treatment
Polymyalgia Rheumatica (PMR)	600 cases/100,000 90% are over 60 years. Total 450,000 Americans, most of whom are white	Overall life expectancy is essentially identical to the general population	Unknown. Synovitis with T-cell and macrophage infiltration.	At least 1 month of aching and morning stiffness in at least two of the following three areas: shoulders and upper arms, hips and thighs, neck, and torso.	ESR/CRP high, RF (−), anti-CCP (−)	Negative	Steroids
Giant-Cell Arteritis (GCA, temporal arteritis)	200 cases/100,000 Americans	15-20% of patients with PMR will have GCA. 15% with GCA have visual loss	Related to PMR	Headache, jaw claudication, visual disturbances, scalp tenderness, fever, weight loss, and fatigue	ESR/CRP high Positive temporal artery biopsy (can be negative due to skip lesions)	Negative imaging, unless patient develops a stroke	Steroids, ASA to prevent strokes[16]
Idiopathic inflammatory myopathies (IIM), polymyositis (PM), dermatomyositis (DM), and sporadic inclusion body myositis (S-IBM)	Unknown prevalence. S-IBM is the most common after age 50.	Starting after age 50 is associated with an increased risk of mortality. The frequency of malignancy in patients with PM-DM increases with age.	Consider hypothyroidism, hyperthyroidism, osteomalacia, amyloid myopathy, drug-induced, corticosteroids, alcohol, colchicines, lipid-lowering agents	Weakness of limbgirdle and anterior neck flexors, progressive over weeks to months.	ESR/CRP high, CK high, aldolase high, AST/ALT high, LDH high, Anti-Jo antibodies positive (PM-DM). EMG/NCS usually positive. Muscle biopsy is the gold standard	None.	Steroids and DMARDs. Usually S-IBM is unresponsive to treatment. The response to therapy of elderly patients with PM-DM is poorer than in younger adults

ALT, alanine aminotransferase; *ANA*, antinuclear antibodies; *anti-CCP*, anti-cyclic citrullinated peptide; *APS*, antiphospholipid syndrome; *APS antibodies*, lupus anticoagulant and anticardiolipin antibodies; *ASA*, acetylsalicylic acid; *AST*, aspartate aminotransferase; *CAD*, coronary artery disease; *CK*, creatinine kinase; *CMC*, carpometacarpal joints; *CPPD*, calcium pyrophosphate dehydrated; *CRP*, C-reactive protein; *DIP*, distal interphalangeal joints; *DMARDs*, disease modifying anti-rheumatic drugs; *ds DNA*, anti-double-stranded DNA; *EMG/NCS*, electromyogram/nerve conduction studies; *EORA*, elderly-onset rheumatoid arthritis; *ESR*, erythrocyte sedimentation rate; *HLA*, human lymphocyte antigen; *HTN*, hypertension; *LDH*, lactate dehydrogenase; *MSU*, monosodium urate crystals; *NSAID*, nonsteroidal antiinflammatory drugs; *PIP*, proximal interphalangeal joints; *PMR*, polymyalgia rheumatica; *RF*, rheumatoid factor; and *Sm*, anti-Smith antibodies.

Rheumatoid Arthritis

RA prevalence increases with age but predisposing factors are unknown. There is inflammation of the synovium of the joints that extends to the cartilage (pannus formation) and then invades the adjacent bone, causing erosions.

Gout and Pseudogout

Gout, an inflammatory reaction to monosodium urate (MSU) crystals, is associated with hyperuricemia. Risk factors include diuretic use, renal disease, obesity, hypertension, and heavy alcohol use. Urate crystals initiate and sustain attacks of acute inflammation because they stimulate release of inflammatory mediators. Pseudogout, an inflammatory reaction to calcium pyrophosphate dehydrate (CPPD) crystals, is associated with disorders of phosphate, magnesium, parathyroid and thyroid hormone, and hemochromatosis. Attacks are provoked by trauma, acute diseases, or surgery.

Polymyalgia Rheumatica and Giant-Cell Arteritis

PMR and GCA are closely related. The disease-initiating triggering of the immune system in PMR is unknown. GCA is a chronic, systemic vasculitis that affects the elastic membranes of the aorta and its extracranial branches, particularly the external carotid artery with its superficial temporal division.[17,18]

DIFFERENTIAL DIAGNOSIS AND ASSESSMENT

The differential diagnosis and assessment for arthritic conditions in older people is similar to that of younger individuals. Table 44-1 provides laboratory and x-ray studies to assist with assessment. A component of assessment is determining whether the symptoms with which the patient presents are atypical manifestations of typical diseases, as indicated in Table 44-2.

Osteoarthritis

OA usually has an insidious onset and chronic course. It affects the distal interphalangeal (DIP) joints, causing characteristic Heberden's nodes, and the proximal interphalangeal (PIP) joints, causing Bouchard's nodes. In addition, there is frequent involvement of the hips, knees, back, and neck. OA is a progressive disorder that takes many years to cause significant disability. Unfortunately, there is no cure. The development of Heberden's and Bouchard's nodes may take 1 or 2 years; they may be painful and soft initially and later harden and calcify as pain subsides. Two thirds of patients older than 65 years have x-ray changes consistent

TABLE 44-2	Atypical Musculoskeletal Manifestations of Typical Diseases
Shoulder pain	Acute myocardial infarction, pneumonia, costochondral pain, intraabdominal bleeding, or perforation
Temporomandibular	Acute myocardial infarction joint pain
Hip pain	Pancreatitis, psoas muscle abscess or hematoma, hip fracture, hernia
Back or extremity pain	Bone metastasis, osteomyelitis, tumor, or deep venous thrombosis
Myalgias	Rhabdomyolysis

with OA.[8] Laboratory studies reveal a negative antinuclear antibodies (ANA) and RA factor, and normal erythrocyte sedimentation rate (ESR) and C-reactive protein (CRP). X-ray films show osteophytes, with loss of articular space and subchondral sclerosis.

> Osteoarthritis usually has an insidious onset and chronic course.

Rheumatoid Arthritis

RA tends to have a more acute presentation in older than in younger individuals, with more involvement of proximal joints. The diagnostic approach is similar to that used with younger individuals, with a positive rheumatoid factor (RF) in 80% of cases, positive anticyclic citrullinated peptide (anti-CCP), sensitivity of 80% and specificity of 98% to 100%, and high ESR and CRP.[12] A positive ANA is usually seen in patients with RA. X-ray studies show loss of articular space, multiple erosions, juxtaarticular osteopenia, and ulnar deviation.

> RA has a more acute presentation in older than in younger individuals, with more involvement of proximal joints.

Gout

Gout is acute in both older and younger individuals, but in older people tends to be more polyarticular and is more likely to involve small joints, particularly of the hands. It characteristically involves the metatarsal phalangeal joint (MTP). ANA and RF are negative, but uric acid is high. MSU crystals are found in the synovial fluid and are needle-shaped crystals that are bright yellow when parallel to the axis or negatively birefringent on a polarizing microscope. MSU crystals are inside the neutrophils in active inflammation owing to phagocytosis. X-ray studies show erosions that are usually slightly removed from the joint, which is atrophic and hypertrophic, leading to erosions with an "overhanging edge."

> Gout characteristically involves the MTP joint.

Pseudogout

Pseudogout affects mainly older people, primarily in the knee. It often accompanies OA and is confirmed by the finding of CPPD crystals in the synovial fluid. Crystals are rod-shaped and blue when parallel to the axis or positively birefringent on a polarizing microscope. X-ray studies show chondrocalcinosis primarily in the hands, pelvis, and knees.

> Pseudogout affects mainly older people, primarily in the knee.

Polymyalgia Rheumatica and Giant-Cell Arteritis

PMR is a clinical diagnosis with usually at least 1 month of aching and morning stiffness in at least two of three areas: shoulders and upper arms, hips and thighs, neck and torso. Characteristically there is a very high ESR and CRP and negative RA and anti-CCP. X-ray studies are negative. GCA is related to PMR and often has the presenting symptoms of headache, jaw claudication, visual disturbances, fever, weight loss, and fatigue. An involved temporal artery may be tender. GCA diagnosis is established by biopsy of a temporal artery, or angiographic appearance of large arteries (subclavian, axillary, or aorta). Most commonly visual failure is related to stenosis of a branch of the ophthalmic artery. Blindness is sudden and painless.

Role of Arthrocentesis

Arthrocentesis looks for three things in the synovial fluid: cell count, crystals, and culture. The information obtained will suffice in the differential diagnosis of most arthritic conditions. Noninflammatory fluids have less than 1000 white blood cells (WBC), whereas inflammatory fluids tend to have more than 2000 WBC. Fluids with more than 100,000 WBC indicate septic arthritis until proven otherwise. See Table 44-3 for conditions that cause inflammatory versus noninflammatory arthritides. Carefully selecting the kind of needle for this procedure is important. For instance, ordinarily, an 18-gauge needle can be used safely in the knee. If the patient is anticoagulated, a 22- or

TABLE 44-3	Classification of Arthritic Conditions Based on Inflammation	
Inflammatory	**Noninflammatory**
Rheumatoid arthritis	Osteoarthritis
Polymyalgia rheumatica	Fibromyalgia or
Myositis or	myofascial pain
dermatomyositis	Soft-tissue disorders
Crystal arthropathies	(e.g., tendonitis, bursitis)
Septic arthritis	Chronic low-back pain
Spondyloarthropathies	(gout and pseudogout)
and seronegative	Diabetic
oligoarthritis	cheiroarthropathy
Systemic lupus	Dupuytren's contracture
Vasculitis (giant-cell	Osteoporosis
arteritis and small-	Reflex sympathetic dys-
vessel vasculitis)	trophy erythematosus,
Paraneoplastic syndrome	Sjögren's (regional pain
	syndrome), tissue
	disorders and other
	connective tissue
	disorders

25-gauge needle minimizes risk of bleeding. There should be an attempt to obtain clean, blood-free fluid for accurate analysis. As much fluid as possible should be drained with one needle-stick to minimize discomfort. There is no need to stop anticoagulation if the procedure is properly done.

> Arthrocentesis looks for three things in the synovial fluid: cell count, crystals, and Gram stain/culture.

CASE 1

Mrs. Montes (Part 2)

You prescribed for Mrs. Montes acetaminophen up to 4 g a day. However, there was no subsequent improvement. Glucosamine and chondroitin were added with no further improvement. Mrs. Montes was anticoagulated with warfarin (Coumadin) so traditional nonsteroidal antiinflammatory drugs (NSAIDs) were contraindicated. Instead, cyclooxygenase (COX) 2 inhibitors were prescribed with mild improvement. The family discontinued the medications when informed that COX-2 inhibitors could cause heart attacks.

On a return visit, Mrs. Montes can stand and walk with one-person assistance. There is swelling, redness, and warmth of both wrists. There is tenderness in the PIP joints and metacarpal phalangeal (MCP) joints. The right knee is swollen, red, and painful.

What should be done to further manage Mrs. Montes's joint complaints? ▶

Discussion

You conclude that 6 months ago the diagnosis of OA was correct. The local doctor followed proper evidence-based medicine guidelines, but the patient did not get significantly better. The fact that this patient had baseline OA does not preclude her from having an inflammatory condition such as gout or RA. Given the polyarticular distribution, the most common explanation for Mrs. Montes's problems would be RA. It could also be a polyarticular gout or septic arthritis.

The next step is a knee arthrocentesis. The arthrocentesis reveals 25 mL of turbid yellowish fluid that shows negatively birefringent crystals under the polarizing microscope. They are uric acid crystals but they are not intracellular, suggesting an incidental finding. Concomitant studies include RF, ANA, ESR, CRP, blood cell count, comprehensive metabolic panel with uric acid, and x-ray examinations of the hands, wrists, and knees. Given that Mrs. Montes does not appear acutely ill, you send her home on tramadol for pain control and instructions to the family to contact you if symptoms worsen. You maintain concern about the possibility of a septic arthritis, given that elderly individuals can present with septic arthritis without a fever or the appearance of initially being acutely ill.

Subsequently laboratory results become available. The fluid is inflammatory at 40,000 WBC with no organisms in the Gram stain and negative culture. The RF is positive, ESR and CRP are high, anti-CCP is positive, and ANA is positive. The x-ray films show periarticular osteopenia of the hands and no changes of the knees. The uric acid is normal. The patient is diagnosed with RA and started on low-dose steroids for the acute flare. Subsequently she is tried on sulfasalazine and referred for rheumatology consult and treated with methotrexate.

The uric acid crystals confounded the clinical picture. This patient may have had intercritical gout. It is uncommon to find gout and RA simultaneously. Additionally, having a normal uric acid was sufficient justification not to start allopurinol. However, if a gout flare occurs, that would be sufficient grounds to start allopurinol despite a normal uric acid. ◾

MANAGEMENT

General Considerations

To develop appropriate management plans for an older patient, it is essential to assess impact of the musculoskeletal problem on the patient's overall functional status.[19,20] There is little correlation between symptoms and x-ray findings. Patients may have moderate to severe x-ray findings of arthritis but be asymptomatic and fully functional, or they may have absent or mild x-ray findings with severe pain and disability.[21,22] The approach to therapy will vary based on whether the patient is robust, frail, demented, or at the end of life.[23] Patients with rheumatic disorders are more likely to die from cardiovascular problems than from the musculoskeletal condition.[10]

Once the patient's functional status and overall prognosis are determined, there should be an assessment of whether there is a cure, rehabilitation, or a need for palliative interventions for the rheumatic condition. The goal is to improve the patient's well-being and quality of life.

In many cases, the first line of therapy for short-term therapy of arthritic conditions in the elderly is NSAIDs. Elderly patients with multiple comorbidities and who are anticoagulated are at higher risk of peptic ulcer disease and associated complications. If traditional NSAIDs or COX-2 inhibitors are to be used, then specific precautions should be taken (Table 44-4); otherwise other pain medications can be ordered until the etiology of the symptoms is determined and specific treatment is given.

The interprofessional team is important in care of older individuals with arthritis. Physical and occupational therapists are key in training patients to compensate for lost function, and to help select and use assistive devices. Social workers are invaluable in finding resources within communities particularly if patients have problems, such as severe arthritis and dementia. Pharmacists find ways to combine prescribed medications and ways to reduce cost and avoid interactions.

> The approach to therapy will vary based on whether the patient is robust, frail, demented, or at the end of life; patients with rheumatic disorders are more likely to die from cardiovascular problems than the musculoskeletal condition.

Osteoarthritis

Treatment options for OA, with the level of evidence that supports those options, are detailed in Table 44-5. The foundation for therapy is NSAIDs. The approach to the use of NSAIDs is presented in Table 44-4. Acetaminophen has not been found to be as effective but serves as a reasonable alternative for those patients who cannot tolerate NSAIDs. Failing NSAIDs and/or acetaminophen, narcotic analgesics are reasonable next steps. Exercise, particularly guided by a therapist, is essential for strengthening muscles around joints affected by OA, and relieving pain and instability. Often physical and occupational therapists will recommend assistive devices, such as canes and braces. Ultimately, for patients who are not responsive to these interventions, knee and hip replacements are considerations.

TABLE 44-4	Considerations for Use of Traditional Nonsteroidal Antiinflammatory Drugs (NSAIDs) and Cyclooxygenase (COX) 2 Inhibitors[24,25]

Traditional NSAIDs

Omit alcohol.

Take with food and water.

Watch for over-the-counter (OTC) NSAIDs adding to prescribed amount consumed.

Keep the dose low. Consider using OTC NSAID, in which the dose is lower than by prescription.

Consider stopping the medication if the patient is dehydrated.

Older patients should be monitored for gastrointestinal side effects, and serum creatinine should be checked periodically.

Consider combining NSAIDs with H_2-blockers, PPIs, or misoprostol (at least 800 micrograms units).

Salicylate levels should be measured in serum when more than 3600 mg per day are consumed.

Nonacetylated salicylates lack cardiovascular protective effect, but have less risk for peptic ulcers.

Combination of angiotensin-converting enzyme (ACE) inhibitors and NSAIDs may be nephrotoxic.

COX-2 Inhibitors

COX-2 inhibitors are no better at relieving pain than traditional NSAIDs.

Older patients are at risk of cardiovascular events with NSAIDs (traditional and COX-2 inhibitors).

COX-2 may increase blood pressure and edema, and cause more renal failure than traditional NSAIDs.

COX-2 has fewer gastrointestinal complications than traditional NSAIDs.

COX-2 can be combined with aspirin, but the risks of gastrointestinal problems increase.

Monitoring of COX-2 is more important in the elderly population, and side effects and recommendations are similar to that of traditional NSAIDs.

PPI, Proton pump inhibitor.

TABLE 44-5	Treatment of Osteoarthritis[26,27]
Treatment Method	**Systematic Review**
Acetaminophen (APAP) (up to 4 g/day)	Evidence suggests NSAIDs are superior to APAP for pain in OA but not superior in improving function. Daily doses of APAP <2000 mg/day are not associated with an increased risk for upper GI complications.
Nonaspirin, NSAIDs for OA of the knee and hip	There is no substantial evidence available related to efficacy to distinguish between equivalent recommended doses of NSAIDs.
Intraarticular viscosupplementation	A systematic study is ongoing. Evidence is conflicting about benefits compared to placebo.
Glucosamine	It is effective and safe in OA. Long-term toxicity is not known. There is no data about the many different preparations.
Plaquenil	A systematic study is ongoing. It may help with inflammatory (erosive) OA.
Thermotherapy	Cold packs seem to be better than hot packs applied to affected joint.
Electromagnetic fields	Electrical stimulation therapy may provide significant improvements for knee OA.
Herbal treatments	Avocado-soybean appeared effective. Most study participants <65 years.
Exercise	Therapeutic exercise reduces pain and improves function in knee OA.
Cyclooxygenase (COX) 2 inhibitors	COX-2 inhibitors reduce gastroscopically diagnosed ulcers compared to other NSAIDs, but the reduction in clinical effects was less marked, and all NSAIDs increase the risk of myocardial infarction.

APAP, Acetaminophen; *GI*, gastrointestinal; *NSAIDs*, nonsteroidal antiinflammatory drugs; *OA*, osteoarthritis.

Rheumatoid Arthritis

RA should be treated with one of the disease-modifying antirheumatic drugs (DMARDs) outlined in Table 44-6. Baseline therapy starts with low-dose steroids (e.g., 7.5 mg of prednisone daily). If this dose is exceeded, prophylaxis for glucocorticoid-induced osteoporosis should be initiated, including calcium, vitamin D, and bisphosphonates. Hydroxychloroquine is another option, started at the standard dose, with every 6-12 month follow-up by an ophthalmologist looking for reversible retinal deposits. Sulfasalazine, methotrexate, and leflunomide also help control inflammation. With these medications routine laboratory work is needed to monitor for potential side effects. Finally, biologicals (immunomodulators) can be added to other DMARDs for maximum benefit of preventing

TABLE 44-6	Disease-Modifying Antirheumatic Drugs (DMARDs)[28-30]	
Drug	**Usual Dose**	**Common Side Effects**
Azathioprine (Imuran)	50-150 mg per day in 1 to 3 doses orally	Myelosuppression, hepatotoxicity, lymphoproliferative disorders, nausea, hair loss
Methotrexate	7.5-25 mg per week in a single dose orally or SQ. Start low and increase by 5 mg every 1 to 2 months until effects are achieved	Myelosuppression, hepatotoxicity, hepatic fibrosis, cirrhosis, pulmonary infiltrates or fibrosis, mouth sores, nausea, hair loss
Sulfasalazine (Azulfidine, Azulfidine EC)	500-3000 mg per day in 2 to 4 doses orally	Myelosuppression, hepatotoxicity, nausea
Leflunomide (Arava)	10-20 mg per day in a single dose orally	Myelosuppression, hepatotoxicity, cirrhosis, diarrhea, hair loss
Hydrocychloroquine sulfate (Plaquenil)	200-400 mg per day in two doses orally	Retinal toxicity, rash
Etanercept (Enbrel)	25 mg SQ twice a week, or 50 mg SQ once a week	Increased risk of infections, tuberculosis, histoplasmosis or other; injection site reactions
Infliximab (Remicade)	3-10 mg/kg IV. Given at 0, 2, 6 weeks then every 8 weeks (usually taken with methotrexate)	Increased risk of infections, infusion reactions
Adalimumab (Humira)	40 mg SQ once a week or every 2 weeks	Same as etanercept
Golimumab (Simponi)	50 mg SQ once a month	Same as etanercept
Anakinra (Kineret)	100 mg SQ daily, 100 mg SQ every other day in severe kidney disease	Same as etanercept
Abatacept (Orencia)	500-1000 mg IV 0,2,4 weeks then every 4 weeks or 500-1000 mg IV one time, then 125 mg SQ weekly	Same as etanercept versus infliximab depending on SQ or IV
Tocilizumab (Actemra)	4-8 mg/kg IV every 4 weeks	Same as infliximab. Myelosuppression, hepatotoxicity, hyperlipidemia
Rituximab (Rituxan)	1000 mg IV 0,2 weeks and again when arthritis becomes active. On average every 6 months	Same as infliximab. Tumor lysis syndrome, progressive multifocal leukoencephalopathy (PML)

EC, enteric coated; *IV*, intravenous; *SQ*, subcutaneously.

erosions. However, before starting them, a tuberculosis (TB) skin test or quantiferon TB gold should be checked as well as hepatitis B and hepatitis C, because these medications may reactivate TB, and other infections. These tests need to be repeated every 1 to 2 years to monitor for these infectious diseases. It is also important to update pneumococcal and influenza vaccinations.

The more complex DMARDs should probably be deferred to the judgment of a rheumatologist. It is important that patients with RA be involved in physical and occupational therapy, to preserve function and to compensate for deformities. The physical and occupational therapists can be very helpful in determining appropriate assistive devices to compensate for diminished functional capacity.

Gout and Pseudogout

Gout is treated with NSAIDs and/or colchicine. Allopurinol should be initiated once the acute flare has been controlled. Oral or intraarticular steroids can be very helpful with a severe acute attack. Patients with gout should be instructed to consume a diet low in red meats and seafood. Pseudogout is treated with NSAIDs and, on occasion for severe attacks, with intraarticular steroids.

Polymyalgia Rheumatica and Giant-Cell Arteritis

PMR and GCA are treated with oral steroids. GCA patients should also be treated with low-dose aspirin to limit the likelihood of stroke (see Table 44-1).

SUMMARY

An interprofessional team can help significantly improve the quality of life of older individuals with arthritis. Exercise is essential because it minimizes pain and improves function in individuals suffering from arthritis. Lifelong physical activity maximizes the benefits of exercise in patients with rheumatic disorders and will often engage the individual in social activities. A coordinated approach to arthritis will help these older people achieve successful aging by modifying disability, maximizing physical and mental function, engaging the patient in social activities, and ultimately changing the patient's course to help attain maximum life potential.[31]

Web Resources

www.niams.nih.gov/hi/index.htm. National Institutes of Health's National Institute of Arthritis and Musculoskeletal Diseases.
www.arthritis.org. Arthritis Foundation.
www.rheumatology.org. American College of Rheumatology.
www.cdc.gov/arthritis. Centers for Disease Control and Prevention.

KEY REFERENCES

3. Nakasato YR, Yung R. Geriatric rheumatology: A comprehensive approach. New York: Springer; 2011.
6. Arthritis Foundation. Primer on the rheumatic diseases. 13th ed. (corrected). Atlanta: Arthritis Foundation; 2008.
13. Aletaha D, Neogi T, Silman AJ, et al. 2010 Rheumatoid arthritis classification criteria: An American College of Rheumatology/European League Against Rheumatism collaborative initiative. Arthritis Rheum 2010;62:2569-81.
26. Hochberg MC, Altman RD, April KT, et al. American College of Rheumatology 2012 recommendations for the use of nonpharmacologic and pharmacologic therapies in osteoarthritis of the hand, hip, and knee. Arthritis Care Res 2012;64:465-74.
28. EULAR recommendations for the management of rheumatoid arthritis with synthetic and biological disease-modifying antirheumatic drugs. Ann Rheum Dis 2010;69:964-75.

References available online at expertconsult.com.

45

Foot Problems

Arthur E. Helfand and Jeffrey M. Robbins

OBJECTIVES

Upon completion of this chapter, the reader will be able to:

- Recognize the primary clinical changes in the aging foot.
- Identify the primary systemic diseases associated with foot problems.
- Understand the important principles and protocols of podogeriatric and chronic disease assessment of the aging foot and its related structures.
- Identify the essential complicating foot problems in the older adult.
- Recognize the importance of diabetic, avascular, and neurosensory-related foot problems in the aging patient.

- Understand the primary need to manage foot and related problems in the older patients in order to maintain the quality of life.

PRIMARY CARE CONSIDERATIONS IN THE OLDER PATIENT

Diseases and disorders of the foot and its related structures represent some of the most painful, distressing, and disabling afflictions associated with aging, usually alter the patient's quality of life, and may contribute to institutionalization. As society considers the basic needs of the older population, it is recognized that health is but one of those needs, and not always given the highest in priority. There are two important catalytic factors in the older individual's ability to remain as a vital part of society. They are a keen mind and the ability to ambulate. Podiatric care is an essential service to foster mobility and independence among older persons and to protect their general health and a sense of well-being. The ability to remain ambulatory may be the only dividing line between institutionalization and remaining an active viable member of society.[1]

Foot and related pathologies in the older patient are a significant health concern, both from a standpoint of prevalence and incidence. The immobility that results from a focal foot problem or as the result of complications of a systemic disease, such as diabetes mellitus, peripheral vascular diseases, lower extremity arterial disease, and degenerative joint changes, can have a significant negative impact on the patient's ability to maintain a quality of life as a useful member of society.[2]

There are many systemic and/or life changes that contribute to high-risk foot problems. Some are as follows: agitation, compulsive activities, increased foot perspiration, neurologic and sensory deficits, neurotic excoriation, changes in mental status, self-mutilation, chronic constipation and incontinence, weakened muscle and bone structure, impaired cardiovascular function, diabetes mellitus, peripheral vascular and lower extremity arterial disease, foot deformities, reduced interest and/or participation in social activities, decreased and/or loss of mobility, pododynia dysbasia, sleep problems, undertreated and/or improperly treated hyperkeratosis, onychauxis, onychomycosis, ulcers, tinea pedis, xerosis, abrasions and/or lacerations, reduced interest and/or participation in social activities, and a reduction of independent and/or instrumental activities of daily living. Good foot care is an essential for the elderly who prize remaining independent.[3]

Additional online-only material indicated by icon.

The immobility that results from a local foot problem or as the result of complications of a systemic disease, such as diabetes mellitus, peripheral vascular diseases, lower extremity arterial disease, and degenerative joint changes, can have a significant negative impact on the patient's ability to maintain quality of life as a useful member of society.

Changes in the Foot in Relation to Age

There are many factors that contribute to the development of foot problems in the elderly. They include the aging process itself and the presence of multiple chronic diseases. Other significant factors include the degree of ambulation, the duration of prior hospitalization, limitation of activity, prior institutionalization and episodes of social segregation, inappropriate prior care, emotional adjustments to disease and life in general, multiple medications for multiple chronic diseases, and the complications and residuals associated with other diseases. The management of foot problems in the geriatric patient requires a comprehensive and team approach by those licensed to maximize the quality of care provided.

The skin of the foot is usually one of the first structures to demonstrate early change. There is usually a loss of hair below the knee and on the dorsum of the foot and toes.

Atrophy then follows with the skin appearing parchmentlike and xerotic. Brownish pigmentations are common and related to the deposition of hemosiderin. Hyperkeratosis when present may be resulting from keratin dysfunction, a residual to repetitive pressure, atrophy of the subcutaneous soft tissue, and/or as space replacement as the body attempts to adjust to the changing stress placed on the foot.[4]

The toenails undergo degenerative trophic changes (onychopathy); thickening and/or longitudinal ridging (onychorrhexis) related to repeated microtrauma, disease, and nutritional impairment. Deformities of the toenails become pronounced and complicated by xerotic changes in the periungual nail folds as onychophosis (hyperkeratosis) and tinea unguium (onychomycosis). These conditions are usually longstanding, chronic, and very common in the elderly and, in the case of onychomycosis (Figure 45-1), present a constant focus of infection.

Deformities of the toenails become pronounced and complicated by xerotic changes in the periungual nail folds as onychophosis (hyperkeratosis) and tinea unguium (onychomycosis). These conditions are usually longstanding, chronic, and very common in the elderly and, in the case of onychomycosis, present a constant focus of infection.

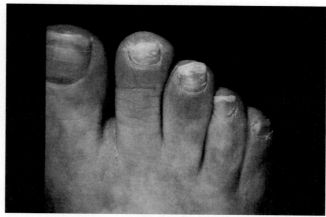

Figure 45-1   Marked ischemia and peripheral arterial disease related to diabetes mellitus.

There is a progressive loss of muscle mass and atrophy of tissue caused by disease, decreased function, and a lack of activity, which increases the susceptibility of the foot to injury; thus even minor trauma can result in a fracture and a marked limitation of activity.

CASE 1

Joel Berger

Joel Berger is a 70-year-old male with a history of mild congestive heart failure. Pedal pulses were present and there were early clinical symptoms and signs of peripheral arterial disease. Mr. Berger has pain and a small hematoma on the dorsum of his left second toe. He indicates that he dropped a can on his foot, but that he was wearing a soft slipper. The toe has continued to hurt, especially when walking. Mild hammertoes were noted and the patient indicated that he has had arthritis for some time.

What would be your initial steps? ▣

CASE 1

Discussion

Initial management would include radiographs to rule out a fracture. If there is a fracture in good position, a silicone mold can be fabricated or hypoallergenic tape with proper precautions to protect the web space from maceration can be used to immobilize the toe with the possibility of a surgical shoe for ambulation. Without evidence of fracture, a silicone mold can still be employed for a shorter period to splint the joint, followed by the use of a silicone protective tube. The patient should be instructed to take special care when moving heavy objects from cabinets and to consider a leather opera-type slipper for extra protection. Disruption of the vascular supply could precipitate necrotic changes distal to the trauma site so that reassessment and follow-up are important. ▣

PODOGERIATRIC ASSESSMENT

The initial evaluation of the older patient should include a comprehensive assessment and risk stratification process. A comprehensive podogeriatric and chronic disease assessment protocol (Helfand Index),[5] developed for the Pennsylvania Department of Health, enables practitioners to initiate a diagnostic and risk stratification procedure that includes multiple elements. The comprehensive assessment tool can be used to assess both pathology and risk factors. These elements include demographics, history of present illness, and past medical history. Current prescriptions and over-the-counter medications should be noted.[6]

The dermatologic evaluation should include but is not limited to the following: hyperkeratosis, bacterial infection, ulceration, cyanosis, xerosis, tinea pedis, verruca, hematoma, rubor, discoloration, and preulcerative changes. The foot orthopedic assessment includes but is not limited to the following: hallux valgus, hallux rigidus limitus, anterior imbalance, Morton's syndrome, digiti flexus (hammertoes), and bursitis.[7-9]

The peripheral vascular evaluation should include but is not limited to the following: coldness, trophic changes, palpation of the dorsalis pedis and posterior tibial pulses, the history of night cramps and/or claudication, edema, atrophy, varicosities, atrophy, and other findings. Amputation or partial amputation should be noted. The neurologic evaluation should include but is not limited to the following: Achilles and superficial plantar reflexes, vibratory sense (pallesthesia), response to a loss of protective sensation, sharp and dull reaction, joint position, burning, and other findings.[10]

Identifying Complicating Foot Problems

The primary manifestations in the foot include but are not limited to the following: plantar fasciitis, spur formation, periostitis, decalcification, stress fractures, tendonitis, tenosynovitis, residual deformities, pes planus, pes cavus, hallux valgus, digiti flexus (hammertoe), rotational digital deformities, joint swelling, increased pain (podalgia), limitation of motion, and pain and a reduced ambulatory status (pododynia dysbasia).[11]

Diabetes and Foot Care

The older diabetic patient presents a special problem in relation to foot health.[12] It has been projected that 50% to 75% of all amputations in the diabetic can be prevented by early intervention where pathology is noted, by improved foot care health education, and by periodic assessment prior to the onset of symptoms and pathology (secondary and tertiary prevention). The elderly diabetic is a patient with all of the problems related to the disease itself. These include vascular impairment, the degenerative changes of aging, neuropathy, dermopathy, and marked atrophy and deformity related to both diabetes mellitus and aging. These factors are also complicated by the social restrictions related to these multiple pathologies.[13,14]

> The older diabetic patient presents a special problem in relation to foot health. It has been projected that 50% to 75% of all amputations in the diabetic can be prevented by early intervention where pathology is noted, by improved health education, and by periodic evaluation prior to the onset of symptoms and pathology (secondary and tertiary prevention).

The older diabetic patient with neuropathy has insensitive feet that will usually exhibit some degree of paresthesia, sensory impairment to pain and temperature, motor weakness, diminished or lost Achilles and patellar reflexes, decreased vibratory sense, a loss of proprioception, xerotic changes, anhidrosis, neurotrophic arthropathy (Charcot), atrophy, neurotrophic ulcers, and the potential for a marked difference in size between two feet. There is a greater incidence of infection, necrosis, and gangrene.[15] Vascular impairment adds pallor, a loss, or decrease in the posterior tibial and dorsalis pedis pulse, dependent rubor, a decrease in the venous filling time, coolness of the skin, and trophic changes. Numbness and tingling as well as cramps and pain can be demonstrated. There is usually a loss of the plantar metatarsal fat pad that predisposes the patient to ulceration in relation to the existing bony deformities of the foot and repetitive microtrauma.[15-17]

Hyperkeratotic lesions form as space replacements and provide a focus for ulceration because of increased pressure on the soft tissues with an associated localized avascularity from direct pressure and counterpressure. Tendon contractures and claw toes (hammertoes) are common. A warm foot with pulsations in an elderly diabetic with neuropathy is not uncommon. When ulceration is present, the base is usually roofed by hyperkeratosis that retards and many times prevents healing. Necrosis and gangrene are associated with infection with eventual occlusion and gangrene. Foot drop and a loss of position sense may be present. Pretibial lesions are indicative of this change as well as microvascular infarction. Arthropathy gives rise to deformity (Charcot), altered gait patterns, and a higher risk for ulceration and limb loss.

Risk assessment models similar to one used in the Department of Veterans Affairs Prevention of Amputation and Treatment Program can identify patients at risk for foot wound and amputations and those at high risk. It involves assessment for disease procurers, in this case peripheral vascular disease, loss of protection sensation, and foot deformities, and assigning a risk level to each patient. A management and referral algorithm is used to quickly refer those patients at high risk for care and schedule those at lower risk for ongoing surveillance. This is always coupled with foot care health education and follow-up on adherence of those behaviors.[18-20]

> Hyperkeratotic lesions in the diabetic patient form as space replacements and provide a focus for ulceration because of increased pressure on the soft tissues with an associated localized avascularity from direct pressure and counterpressure.

Radiographic findings in the foot in older diabetics usually demonstrate thin trabecular patterns, decalcification, joint position changes, osteophytic formation, osteolysis, deformities, and osteoporosis. Pruritus and cutaneous infections are more common in the diabetic. Dehydration, trophic changes, anhidrosis, xerosis, and fissures are predisposing factors to calcaneal ulceration. The most commonly demonstrated nail changes are noted but not limited to the following: diabetic onychopathy (nutritional and vascular changes); onychorrhexis (longitudinal striations); onycholysis (shedding from the distal portion); onychomadesis (shedding from the proximal portion; Figure 45-2); subungual hemorrhage (bleeding in the nail bed); onychophosis (keratosis); onychauxis (thickening with hypertrophy); onychogryphosis (thickening with gross deformity); onychia (inflammation; Figure 45-3); onychomycosis (fungal infection); subungual ulceration (ulceration in the nail bed); deformity; hypertrophy; incurvation or involution (onychodysplasia); subungual hemorrhage (nontraumatic); onycholysis (freeing from the distal segment); onychomadesis (freeing from the proximal segment); and autoavulsion.[21-23]

CASE 2

Rita Harris (Part 1)

Rita Harris is a 75-year-old female, living in her home with her husband. She has a history of adult-onset (non–insulin-dependent) diabetes mellitus (NIDDM), with 12 years' duration of diabetes since initially diagnosed. Mrs. Harris remains diet controlled with adequate control, as reported by her endocrinologist. She reports noticing a

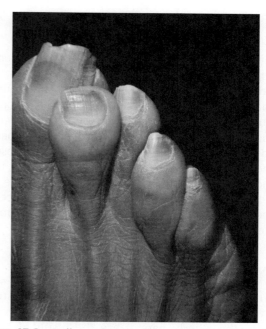

Figure 45-2 Hallux valgus, hammertoes, bowstring dorsal tendons, overriding second toe, onychodystrophy.

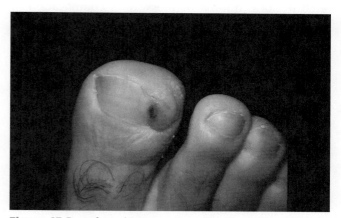

Figure 45-3 Infected ingrown toenail with periungual ulcerative granulation tissue, hallux.

dark spot under her left great toenail in recent months but with no pain. She has trophic changes and diminished pedal pulses. Doppler studies detect both pedal pulses. Testing with a monofilament demonstrates a loss of sensation distal to the metatarsal shaft area. All toenails demonstrate onychorrhexis, and xerosis was noted. No other significant clinical findings were noted. What are your primary considerations given Mrs. Harris's lack of pain?

What is the most important consideration in the differential diagnosis given the lack of pain?
1. **Subungual heloma**
2. **Subungual ulceration**
3. **Subungual hematoma**
4. **Subungual exostosis**
5. **Subungual spur**
6. **Subungual melanoma** ◼

CASE 2

Discussion

Initial management includes radiographs to rule out an exostosis or spur or other bony change. If the concern is related to a possible melanoma, biopsy should be completed with appropriate surgical referral. With a history of trauma, a subungual hematoma should be considered. Without trauma, a subungual diabetic ulcer should be considered. If there is an enlargement of the dorsal aspect of the tip of the distal phalanx on x-ray examination, a subungual heloma should be considered. Appropriate management depends on the diagnosis. A depth shoe, silicone tube, or lamb's wool can then be employed to help reduce pressure. ▫

ONYCHIA

Onychia is an inflammation involving the posterior nail wall and nail bed. The onychial changes that occur in the elderly patient are the result of a new disease or are the residual of long-term disease, injury, and/or functional modification. It is usually precipitated by local trauma or pressure, a complication of systemic diseases such as diabetes mellitus, and is an early sign of a developing infection. Mild erythema, swelling, and pain are the most prevalent findings. Treatment should be directed to removing all pressure from the area and the use of tepid saline compresses for 15 minutes, three times per day. With systemic complications, systemic antibiotics should be instituted early along with radiographs and scans to detect bone change at its earliest sign. Lamb's wool, tube foam, or shoe modification should also be considered to reduce pressure to the toe and nail. If the onychia is not treated early, paronychia may develop with significant infection and abscess of the posterior nail wall. The infection progresses proximally and deeper structures may become involved. The potential for osteomyelitis is greater in the presence of diabetes mellitus and vascular insufficiency. Necrosis, gangrene, and the potential for amputation become reality. Management includes establishing drainage, culture and sensitivity, radiographs and scans as appropriate, the use of saline compresses, and appropriate systemic antibiotics. Always advise against maceration of tissue. Early follow-up is essential because these conditions can result in significant problems in management.[24]

Treatment of onychia should be directed toward removing all pressure from the area and the use of tepid saline compresses for 15 minutes, three times per day, continuing surveillance, and appropriate antibiotics, as indicated. Note: Foot soaking is not recommended.

Deformities of the toenails are the result of repeated microtrauma, degenerative changes, or disease. For example, the continued rubbing of the toenails over the years against the inferior toe box of the shoe is sufficient trauma to produce change. The initial thickening is termed onychauxis. Onychorrhexis with accentuation of normal ridging, trophic changes, and longitudinal striations are onychopathic when related to disease and/or nutritional etiology. When debridement is not completed on a periodic basis, the nail structure elongates, continues to thicken, and becomes deformed with shoe pressure. Onychogryphosis or "ram's horn nail," is usually complicated by fungal infection. The resultant disability can prevent the elderly person from wearing shoes. Pain is usually associated with shoe pressure and the deformity. In addition, a traumatic avulsion of the nail is more frequent with this condition. The exaggerated curvature (onychodysplasia; Figure 45-4) may even penetrate the skin, with resultant infection and ulceration. Management should be directed toward periodic debridement of the onychial structures both in length and thickness, with as little trauma as possible. The degree of onycholysis (freeing of the nail from the anterior edge) and onychoschizia (splitting) helps determine the level of debridement. With the excess pressure of deformity, the nail grooves tend to become onychophosed (keratotic). When this occurs, debridement and the use of mild keratolytics and emollients, such as Keralyt Gel and 42% urea preparations, provide some measure of home care for the patient. With onycholysis, subungual debris and keratosis develop, which increases discomfort and may generate pain. However, the patient may not complain of pain and discomfort, and care should be provided with the deformity. In addition, with degenerative changes, the loss of protective sensation in the form of sensory neuropathy may be present, which tends to defer care

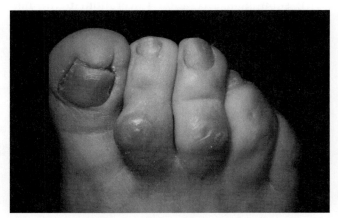

Figure 45-4 Hallux valgus, multiple hammertoes, heloma related to contractures and pressure, and onychodystrophy.

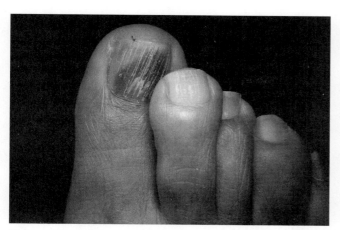

Figure 45-5 Subungual hematoma and onychorrhexis of hallux with onychomycosis, deformity of second toe with early onychia.

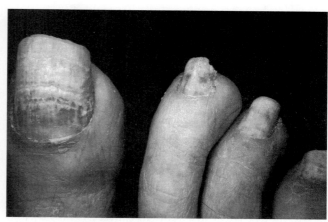

Figure 45-6 Onychauxis, onychomycosis, onychodystrophy, xerosis, and distal digital deformity.

by the patient until a complicating condition occurs (Figure 45-5).[25,26]

ONYCHOMYCOSIS

The most common nonbacterial infection of the toenails is onychomycosis. It is a chronic and communicable disease and clinically it may appear as distal subungual, white superficial, proximal subungual, total dystrophic, or candida onychomycosis. In the superficial variety, the changes appear on the superior surface of the toenail and generally do not invade the deeper structures. In both the distal, proximal, and total dystrophic manifestations, the nail bed, as well as the nail plate, are infected. There is usually some degree of onycholysis (freeing of the nail from the distal edge) and subungual keratosis. In the elderly, because of the long-standing chronic nature of this condition, the posterior nail wall and eponychium demonstrate xerotic changes and hypertrophy, as does the nail plate. Candida is most common in patients with some form of chronic mucocutaneous manifestation. Patients with AIDS may demonstrate subungual white onychomycosis.[27]

> The most common nonbacterial infection of the toenails is onychomycosis. It is a chronic and communicable disease and clinically it may appear as distal subungual, white superficial, proximal subungual, total dystrophic, or candida onychomycosis.

The elderly patient with this condition usually has the presenting symptom of chronic infection, involving one or more of the nail plates. The entire thickness of the nail plates is usually involved with resultant hypertrophy and deformity. Pain is usually not a significant factor because of the normal lessening of sensation in the elderly but can be present when the deformity becomes excessive and is related to external pressure. Mycotic onychia; autoavulsion; subungual hemorrhage; a foul, musty odor; and degeneration of the nail plate are common findings. The most practical form of treatment in the elderly is one of management. Because of the chronicity of the condition and the fact that once the matrix of the nail is involved and hypertrophy and deformity occur, the residuals cannot be reversed. In addition, multiple drug use for systemic diseases and vascular impairment limits systemic management. Periodic debridement, the use of 35% to 50% urea to aid in debridement, and the use of a topical fungicide in an alcoholic base to permit penetration, provide a conservative approach to management. Systemic antifungals can also be employed as indicated. Onychomycosis must be viewed as a chronic infectious disease, deserving management as any other chronic condition, such as hypertension and/or diabetes mellitus (Figure 45-6).

INGROWN TOENAILS (ONYCHOCRYPTOSIS)

Ingrown toenails in the elderly are usually the end result of deformity, improper care, and long-standing onychodysplasia. When the nail penetrates the skin, an abscess and then infection result. If not managed early, periungual granulation tissue may form, which complicates treatment. Deformity and involution also provide a complicating factor. In the early stage, a segment of the nail can easily be removed using a nail splitter (English or anvil type) and an onychotome, then drainage established, saline compresses employed for 15 minutes three times a day, and antibiotics used as indicated. It should be noted that providing antibiotics without removing the offending portion of toenail will not resolve the problem. Measures should be taken to prevent the problem in the future. When granulation tissue is present, excision, fulguration, desiccation, or the use of caustics (such as silver nitrate [75%]) and astringents are employed to reduce the granulation tissue. In all cases, removal of the penetrating nail is primary. Partial excision of the nail plate and matrix can be completed using regional anesthesia followed by chemical cautery of the matrix area with liquefied phenol, for example. With this procedure, postoperative management includes isopropyl alcohol compresses and topical steroid solutions, three times per day to healing. Surgical excision of the matrix without chemical cautery is also a valid option.

With aging, we also find changes in the nail plate, which when viewed distally appears C-shaped. This abnormal curvature is incurvation or involution. When present, the pressure of the nail plate on the nail bed and folds produces onychophosis (hyperkeratosis in the nail folds) and discomfort, with complaints similar to an ingrown toenail. The condition may precipitate pressure ulcerations and infection. When this condition is severe, early and total removal of the nail plate and matrix should be considered to avoid complications as the patient ages.[28]

DRYNESS AND XEROSIS

Dryness of the skin and xerosis are common problems in the older patient. They result from a lack of hydration and lubrication, and to some degree are part of the normal aging and degenerative process. There is usually some evidence of keratin dysfunction that can be associated with xerosis. Fissures develop as a result of dryness and when present on the heel, with associated stress, present a potential hazard for the development of ulceration. Initial management includes the use of an emollient following hydration of the skin; 42% urea is helpful to aid as a mild and safe keratolytic. A plastic or Styrofoam heel cup can be of assistance in minimizing trauma to the heel, thus reducing the potential for complications. Pruritus is a common complaint of the elderly and is usually more severe in the colder weather. It is related to dryness, scaliness, decreased skin secretions, keratin dysfunction, environmental changes, and defatting of the skin that is usually precipitated by the constant use of hot foot soaks. The patient will scratch with excoriations noted on examination. Chronic tinea, allergic, neurogenic, and/or emotional dermatoses should be considered as part of the differential diagnosis and treated accordingly. Management consists of hydration, lubrication, protection, topical steroids if indicated, and judicious use of antihistamines in minimal doses to control the itching, which is usually the primary complaint, unless medically contraindicated.

If excoriations are infected, proper antibiotic therapy should be instituted.

> Initial management of fissures that are a result of dryness on the heel includes the use of an emollient following hydration of the skin; 42% urea is helpful to aid as a mild and safe keratolytic. A plastic or Styrofoam heel cup can be of assistance in minimizing trauma to the heel, thus reducing the potential for complications.

TINEA PEDIS

Tinea pedis in the elderly patient is many times an extension of onychomycosis, which serves as a focus of infection. It is more common in warmer weather with the chronic keratotic type more common clinically in the elderly. Poor foot hygiene in many older patients and the inability to see their feet may motivate the patient to seek care only when the condition becomes clinically significant. Proper foot health education is also an important element of care. The variety of topical medications available can usually control this condition. Solutions and/or creams (water washable or miscible) should be used when the patient is unable to easily remove an ointment base.

HYPERKERATOTIC LESIONS

Common complaints of most elderly are the many forms of hyperkeratotic lesions, such as tyloma (callus) and heloma (corn) and their varieties, which include hard, soft, vascular, neurofibrous, seed, and subungual. Intractable keratoma, eccrine poroma, porokeratosis, and verruca must be differentiated from these keratotic lesions, although each may present initially as a hyperkeratotic area. The biomechanic and pathomechanic factors that help create these problems are those associated with stress (i.e., compressive, tensile, and/or shearing). The loss of soft tissue as part of the aging process and atrophy of the plantar fat pad increase pain and limit ambulation. Contractures, gait changes, deformities, and the residuals of arthritis are all additional factors that need to be considered in management. The incompatibility of the foot type (inflare, straight, or outflare) to the shoe last is another factor to be considered. It is important to recognize that there is usually not one factor, but a multiplicity of conditions including skin tone and elasticity, which result in the development of keratotic lesions in the elderly. Their management is not routine and the term management signifies a period of continuing care, as with any other chronic condition in the elderly, to provide for ambulation and comfort.

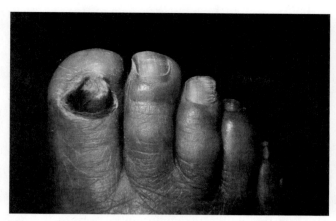

Figure 45-7 Onychodysplasia—incurvated hallux toenail, onychomycosis, multiple hammertoes.

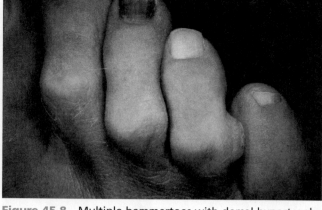

Figure 45-8 Multiple hammertoes with dorsal hypertrophy and heloma molle, fourth toe.

The common sites for the development of hyperkeratotic lesions (calluses and corns) include but are not limited to dorsal or distal digital, plantar metatarsal heads, marginal calcaneal, and with deformities such as hammertoes (Figure 45-7), digital rotations, contractures, hallux valgus, bunion, and/or tailor's bunion. These deformities are precipitating factors to foot-to-shoe-last incompatibilities that produce excessive pressure and friction on segments of the foot. Management and treatment should be directed toward the functional needs of the patients and on their activity needs for daily living. Considerations include debridement, padding, emollients, shoe modifications, and shoe last changes, orthoses, and surgical revision as indicated. Materials to provide soft tissue replacement, weight dispersion, and weight diffusion are also indicated. It is important to recognize that keratotic lesions of long standing represent a hyperplastic and hypertrophic pathology and that even when weight bearing is removed, they tend to persist. In a sense, hyperkeratotic lesions are a form of body protection to pressure and friction and are symptoms of an abnormal state. If permitted to persist, enlarge, and condense, they become primary irritants. With pressure such as weight bearing and ambulation, they produce local avascularity, which can precipitate ulceration and their resultant sequelae. Pressure ulcers in the foot usually begin with subkeratotic hemorrhage (Figures 45-8 and 45-9). Once debrided and managed properly, they usually heal but may be repetitive unless adequate measures are instituted to reduce the pressure to the localized areas of ulceration. Even with all measures, the problem may persist because of residual deformity and systemic diseases such as diabetes mellitus. Thus management and monitoring are similar to any other chronic condition in the elderly and can have a significant impact on the social elements of society, for without ambulation, the elderly patient often needs to be institutionalized.[29,30]

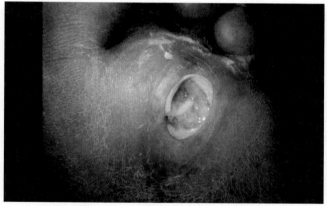

Figure 45-9 Plantar diabetic ulcer, metatarsal prolapse, anterior metatarsal fat pad displacement.

The common sites for the development of hyperkeratotic lesions (calluses and corns) include but are not limited to dorsal or distal digital, plantar metatarsal heads, marginal calcaneal, and with deformities such as hammertoes, digital rotations, contractures, hallux valgus, bunion, and/or tailor's bunion.

FOOT DEFORMITIES

There are a variety of residual foot deformities that can be present in multiple combinations in the elderly. These include but are not limited to hallux valgus, hallux varus, splay foot, hallux flexus, digiti flexus (hammertoe), digiti quinti varus, overlapping toes (Figure 45-10), underriding toes, prolapsed metatarsals, pes cavus, pes planus, pronation, hallux limitus, and hallux rigidus.

Biomechanic, pathomechanic, and stress-related pathologies such as plantar fasciitis, spur formation, periostitis, decalcification, stress fractures, tendonitis,

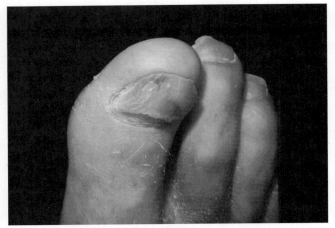

Figure 45-10 Onychomadesis, onychomycosis, hallux toenail.

tenosynovitis, residual deformities, pes planus, pes cavus, hallux valgus, digiti flexus (hammertoes), rotational digital deformities, joint swelling, pain, limitation of motion, and painful and limited ambulatory function (pododynia dysbasia—ambulatory dysfunction) create functional problems in relation to gait and obtaining adequate footwear. Treatment consists of both nonsurgical and surgical considerations. Age itself should not be the final determining factor in considering surgery. What is important is to determine what can be planned to maintain a quality of life for the patient. Consideration should also be given to the patient's ability to adapt to change in relation to ambulation, for to have an anatomically corrected joint and a patient who cannot ambulate without pain defeats the purpose of treating the elderly.

Conservative modalities include shoe last changes, shoe modifications, orthoses, digital braces, physical medicine, exercises, and mild analgesics for pain. The residuals of deformity limit the ability of the patient to maintain a good quality of life.

The residuals of these deformities can produce inflammatory changes such as periarthritis, bursitis, myositis, synovitis, neuritis, tendonitis, sesamoiditis, and plantar myofascitis, for example, which should be managed medically, physically, and mechanically to keep the patient ambulatory and pain free.[31]

> Conservative modalities to treat biomechanic and pathomechanic abnormalities include shoe last changes, shoe modifications, orthoses, digital braces, physical medicine, exercises, and mild analgesics for pain.

SUMMARY

Much of the ability to remain ambulatory in the period of aging is directly related to foot health. In order to maintain foot health, and thus ambulation, practitioners must think comprehensively, and recognize that team care must be an essential part of geriatrics and gerontology. Foot health education, such as programs developed by Feet First and If the Shoe Fits, are available to both patients and professionals, and should be employed as a part of all geriatric patient education programs. With the high prevalence and incidence of foot problems in the elderly, much of their quality of life will depend on their ability to remain mentally alert and ambulatory.[32]

KEY REFERENCES

5. Banks A, Downey MS, Martin DE, Miller SJ. McGlamry's forefoot surgery. Philadelphia: Lippincott, Williams & Wilkins; 2004.
11. Foster AVM. Podiatric assessment and management of the diabetic foot. Edinburgh, Scotland: Churchill-Livingstone-Elsevier; 2006.
15. Ham RJ, Sloane PD, Warshaw GA, et al. Primary care geriatrics—a case based approach. 5th ed. Philadelphia: Mosby/Elsevier; 2007.
24. Helfand AE. Clinical assessment of peripheral arterial occlusive risk factors in the diabetic foot [editorial]. Int J Clin Pract 2007;61(4):540-1.
28. Merriman LM, Turner W. Assessment of the lower limb. 2nd ed. New York: Churchill Livingstone–Elsevier; 2002.
32. Yates B. Merriman's assessment of the lower limb. 3rd ed. Edinburgh, Scotland: Churchill Livingstone–Elsevier; 2009.

References available online at expertconsult.com.

Cancer

Miriam B. Rodin, James A. Wallace, and Tanya M. Wildes

OBJECTIVES

Upon completion of this chapter, the reader will be able to:

- Be aware of age-related differences in cancer biology that affect age-related decisions for the management of specific cancers.
- Summarize general principles of cancer management applied to the elderly.

- Be prepared to apply geriatric principles to maintaining functional status of elderly cancer patients.
- Be familiar with disease-specific treatment guidelines for several common cancers in the elderly.
- Apply current cancer prevention and cancer screening guidelines appropriately to the elderly.
- Understand special issues in the care of cancer survivors.

CANCER IN THE ELDERLY

Cancer is the second leading cause of death and a major cause of morbidity for persons age 65 and older. More than 50% of all new solid tumor diagnoses are made among people over age 65.[1,2] In addition there are now more than 11 million cancer survivors in the United States, 6.5 million of whom are of Medicare age.[3] Cancer control in older individuals includes early diagnosis, prevention, individualized treatment plans, supportive care, end-of-life care, and survivor care. The primary care physician (PCP) plays a key role in each stage of cancer care and it is increasingly clear that patients benefit from having a multidisciplinary team.

Frequently it is the PCP who first detects the cancer. It is important that geriatricians and other primary care providers have a good understanding of the risks and benefits of current therapies for various cancers in order to interpret specialist recommendations and assist patients and families to make realistic, that is, neither irrationally optimistic nor pessimistic, decisions. Furthermore, an informed PCP can often be the best advocate for a patient who is also encountering oncologists with overly optimistic or pessimistic biases with respect to older adults. Referral to an oncologist sometimes results in differing perspectives on treatment; having the specialist and PCP involved and on the same page helps patients with difficult decisions and complex treatments.

CASE 1

Jane Thompson (Part 1)

Jane Thompson, an 81-year-old woman, is brought to the hospital semicomatose by an ambulance. Two weeks earlier, she was reported by her daughter to be in excellent general health, with the exception of osteoarthritis. She was independent in her activities of daily living (ADLs) and in her instrumental ADLs (IADLs). She had lived alone for 12 years, since the death of her husband. After fluid resuscitation in the emergency department and correction of her electrolytes on the inpatient service, the patient becomes responsive but is still confused. She is unable to tolerate oral fluids or food. An esophagogastroscopy shows gastric outlet obstruction by a mass. The biopsy reveals it is a diffuse large B-cell lymphoma (DLBCL). By computed tomography (CT) scan the tumor appears unresectable. You initiate intravenous total parenteral nutrition (TPN) and call an oncologist for consultation.

1. **Who will make decisions regarding how aggressive Mrs. Thompson's medical care will be?**

2. **What options are available to provide nutritional support to Mrs. Thompson?**

3. **What cancer-directed treatment options are available to provide treatment for Mrs. Thompson's tumor?**

4. **Prior to this event, what was Mrs. Thompson's estimated remaining life expectancy?**

5. **If Mrs. Thompson is treated with standard chemotherapy what is the likelihood of complete remission?**

6. **What is the likely duration of that remission?**

7. **What are her risk factors for severe treatment toxicity?**

8. **What can/should be done to control the risks of treatment?** 🔊

Cancer Biology and Aging

More than half of new diagnoses of the common solid tumors including lung, breast, colon, prostate, and ovarian cancers occur in those aged 65 and older. For most of these cancers, incidence increases with age at least to age 85, after which the rate of increase levels off. However, the biological behavior of most common solid tumors changes with the age of the patient as a result of mechanisms shown in Table 46-1.[4]

Poorer survival of elderly cancer patients is partly because of differences in the cancer biology and possibly because of the choices made about their treatment. Examples of neoplasms of older people that are less responsive to chemotherapy include osteosarcomas, glioblastomas, and several hematologic and lymphatic malignancies. Acute myelogenous leukemia (AML) and Hodgkin's and non-Hodgkin's lymphomas have different genetics and different prognostic characteristics in the elderly. Age itself should not determine the treatment of cancer. Sixty-seven percent of older persons with AML have a poor prognosis biology that is multidrug resistant, but 33% have a disease responsive to current chemotherapy. Although 80% of older women have an indolent form of breast cancer that is hormone sensitive, 20% of older women breast cancer patients have an aggressive disease that may benefit from adjuvant chemotherapy and radiotherapy.[11]

Recent advances in genetic analysis of tumor cells promise to improve chemotherapy targeting. That is, for some malignancies, oncologists can predict which cancers will respond to available chemotherapy agents and which will not. In the elderly this is especially useful because the decision to accept highly toxic treatment should be conditioned by the probability of response. Examples of cancer cell markers effectively selected by newer targeted chemotherapy agents include HER2/neu, which indicates responsiveness to trastuzumab; KRAS in colon cancer predicts sensitivity to cetuximab. Other genetic markers are BRAF and mTOR. Molecular profiling of tumors is rapidly emerging as an exciting modality and testing has greatly grown in availability.[12]

In addition to tumor biology, aspects of host resistance may account for poorer survival in the elderly. This includes both systemic responses and age-related differences in the tumor microenvironment. Immune senescence impairs surveillance for abnormal cells.[9] Microenvironmental factors such as angiogenesis and tissue growth factors differ with age as do whole organism characteristics such as renal function and cardiovascular fitness. One well-studied example is the inflammatory response. For example, the concentration of interleukin (IL) 6 in the circulation increases with age. Some cancers also stimulate the inflammatory response. Chronic inflammation may play a role in tumor formation, for

TABLE 46-1	Selected Age-Related Changes in Tumor Biology[5-7]	
Disease	**Prognosis**	**Mechanism**
Acute myelogenous leukemia	Worse	Increased multiple drug resistance. Increased incidence of stem cell leukemia[8]
Large cell non-Hodgkin lymphoma	Worse	Increased circulating IL-6 stimulates lymphoid proliferation[9,10]
Breast cancer	Better	Increased expression of hormone receptors, well differentiated, slowly proliferating; reduced production of tumor growth factors by host
Non–small cell lung cancer	Better	Less chemotherapy responsive but more indolent for unknown reasons
Celomic ovarian cancer	Worse	Unknown

Data from Dendaluri N, Ershler WB. Aging biology and cancer. Semin Oncol 2004;31:3580-7; Irminger-Finger I. Science of cancer and aging. J Clin Oncol 2007;25:1844-51; and Hornsby PJ. Senescence as an anticancer mechanism. J Clin Oncol 2007;25:1844-51.

example in some gastrointestinal (GI) malignancies such as colon cancer. Blunted T-cell and natural killer (NK) cell immune surveillance has been thought to undermine host response to neoplastic cells.[9,10] Clinical applications of these observations include the following: Contrary to expectations, some cancers such as myeloid and lymphoid malignancies may become more aggressive with age. Some, such as non–small cell lung adenocarcinoma, estrogen/progesterone responsive positive breast cancers, and prostate adenocarcinomas, are more indolent because the microenvironment does not stimulate growth.

> More than half of new diagnoses of the common solid tumors including lung, breast, colon, prostate, and ovarian cancers occur in those aged 65 and older.

Evidence-Based Treatment

Applying clinical trials findings to practice always involves comparing the trials population with the local clinical population. In cancer treatment the clinical trials conducted by the cooperative groups rarely include patients older than age 70. One factor for the low inclusion rate is that older adults are rarely asked to participate even though they are just as willing, all things being equal, as younger patients.[13] If clinical trials require considerable travel elderly patients may be reluctant to drive or may lack a household driver.

Trials are also typically sponsored by the drug manufacturers who may set recruitment criteria that exclude the elderly specifically because of age, coexisting conditions, and burden of travel. Nonetheless, a few trials have included significant numbers of patients older than age 70; secondary analyses of cooperative group trials databases have attempted to pool or perform meta-analysis to extract age-related treatment data; and the National Cancer Institute–Medicare merged database has been productively explored for population level experience.

The subgroup analyses of clinical trials of adjuvant chemotherapy for breast and colon cancers have shown equal benefit from equal treatment in terms of standard oncology endpoints of tumor response and disease free survival. However, population-based data demonstrate that elderly patients do more poorly than younger patients and receive less treatment even when adjusted for stage of disease and inferred performance status.[14] The reasons for differences between the clinical trial results and community results include referral bias of the most fit patients to the trial centers, better adherence to standards of cancer-directed care including choice of agents, dose-density and toxicity monitoring at referral centers, and better

quality of supportive and follow-up care through the trial centers.

At least two oncology professional societies have studied these data and offered recommendations for the treatment of specific cancers in elderly patients. The International Society for Geriatric Oncology (SIOG) and the National Comprehensive Cancer Network (NCCN) maintain updated treatment recommendations and online links to current literature for the elderly on their websites. The cooperative trials groups have shown heightened awareness of the need for age-representative trials design and enrollment, and more patient-centered rather than disease-centered outcomes.[15]

The overall goal is to avoid undertreating curable and controllable disease in consenting patients, and to avoid overtreating both indolent and poor prognosis disease. Finding the "just right" approach requires experience, collaboration, and expertise. Principles for cancer treatment in older adults have been endorsed by SIOG and NCCN (Box 46-1).

BOX 46-1

PRINCIPLES OF CANCER TREATMENT IN OLDER ADULTS

- Treatment should be based on the extent and biology of the tumor not the age of the patient.
- Healthy elderly derive equal benefit from equal treatment for their cancers.
- Vulnerable elderly require weighing the risks and benefits of treatment in terms of both risk and quality of life during treatment as the "down payment" for extension of life after active treatment. (Especially true when the goal of cancer treatment is not cure but an estimated likelihood of surviving 1, 2, or 5 years without symptomatic cancer progression or recurrence. If the likelihood of early recurrence is high relative to estimated remaining life expectancy, the calculus changes to time spent with poor quality of life due to treatment vs. due to cancer.)
- Geriatric principles accurately identify fit, vulnerable, and frail patients, that is, staging the aging.
- Standard geriatric assessments predict cancer treatment intolerance because they identify specific vulnerabilities that can be remediated to improve treatment tolerance.
- Excellent supportive care, symptom management, and attention to maintaining functional status may improve treatment tolerance and prevent toxicity-related hospitalizations.
- Elective cancer surgery poses no greater risk than non-cancer surgery.
- Many radiotherapy protocols are well tolerated by the elderly. Newer technology has improved efficacy for selected cancers with reduced total body tissue exposures.
- Treatment decisions should be guided by the patient's treatment goals.

From National Comprehensive Cancer Network. http://www .nccn.org/professionals/physician_gls/f_guidelines.asp.

Staging the Aging

Oncologists typically assess patients as fit or unfit for standard therapy (Figure 46-1). If they feel a patient will not tolerate standard therapy they may attempt dose-reduced therapy or treatment with a single agent as opposed to combination therapy. This approach is flawed because it is not evidence-based, and because for reasons previously explained, the evidence base is limited with regard to older patients. International data reveal that elderly patients receive less cancer-directed therapy, so the lessened toxicity is also accompanied by less efficacy.[16]

Global functional/fitness-for-treatment assessments do not make explicit the clinician's subjective biases. The most commonly used functional assessments in the United States are the Eastern Cooperative Group Performance Status (ECOG-PS) and the Karnovsky Performance Status (KPS) scales. Both are subjective but nonetheless have withstood the test of time and continue to be highly predictive of early mortality.[17] These scales are used to track treatment tolerance not to predict it. They do not identify specific risk factors for treatment intolerance that may be remediable.

There are differences in practice style. Some oncologists choose to front load the treatment to give as much chemotherapy as possible before the patient needs a break. Some choose to test tolerance by lowering doses and spreading them out to lessen toxicity, but that also lessens tumor cell killing. Neither approach has clinical trial–based evidence. For example, in breast cancer, single agents, either alone or as a sequential regimen in metastatic disease, are better tolerated than combination therapies. The combination therapies produce better results in terms of tumor shrinkage but survival does not seem to differ between the approaches. The current weight of opinion among oncologists specializing in treating older adults is to try to give standard protocols for which there is evidence if the patient is fit and willing.[18]

Over the past several years there have been increasing numbers of studies in which geriatric screening tools are used to describe clinical samples of elderly cancer patients. As yet there are limited data showing that geriatric screening tests incorporated into cancer treatment affect decisions or outcomes.[19] However, there are a few preliminary studies, mainly from France, that may soon yield results.[20] A source of resistance to routine geriatric assessment has been that oncologists are concerned that performing many screening tests will be too time consuming for their practices and that the screening tests will generate information that they cannot use.[21] Several studies have tested short screens to identify only those patients who should be comprehensively evaluated and to quantify the amount of time it takes to gather the data.[22-24]

The various components of a comprehensive geriatrics assessment include functional status (ADLs and IADLs), cognitive screening, review of medications for potentially harmful or just unnecessary polypharmacy, nutritional status, vision and hearing, gait and fall risk assessment tools, depression, and delirium. There is no reason to choose one specific validated screening tool over another with which the clinician is familiar or has comparative data in the medical record

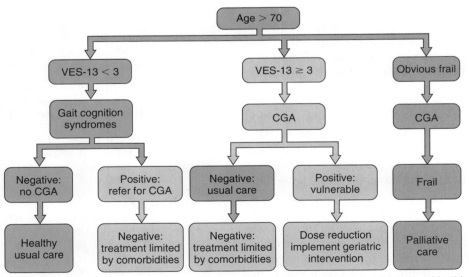

Figure 46-1   A decision tree for staging the aging. *CGA*, comprehensive geriatric assessment ; *VES*, Vulnerable Elders Survey. (Data from Rodin MB, Mohile SG. A practical approach to geriatric assessment in oncology. J Clin Oncology [Review] 2007;25(14):1936-44; and Mohile SG, Bylow K, Dale W, et al. A pilot study of the Vulnerable Elders' Survey-13 as compared to comprehensive geriatric assessment for identifying disability in older prostate cancer patients receiving androgen ablation. Cancer 2007;109:802-10.)

for the patient. It is important to recognize that these tools were devised to determine intermediate- to long-term outcomes including loss of independence (nursing home placement) and longevity over a range of several years.[25]

Remaining life expectancy (RLE) is a prognostic indicator, obviously not an absolute prediction of the future. For an older person with a long RLE, a new cancer diagnosis may shorten RLE. The value of having an estimate is to draw a frame around the expected course of the disease within a realistic span of time (Table 46-2).[26] A highly treatable cancer may have a low probability of recurrence within the patient's RLE, even if it is not completely "cured." The mirror image of this assessment is whether the treatment poses a higher risk than the cancer or whether the cancer is likely to progress during the patient's RLE or not. Heuristically, is the patient's precancer life expectancy less than 5, 5 to 9, or 10 or more years? With successful treatment, what is the probability of symptomatic progression within 5 years? Is it less than 10%, less than 50%, less than 80%? Do the risks of standard treatment— including surgical risk, serious toxicity, or suffering or death—outweigh any theoretical benefit? Several studies have specifically examined the performance of common functional scales for chemotherapy tolerance.[27-30]

Low-risk asymptomatic cancers can be watched in frail patients; cancers that are likely to become symptomatic during a short time and that are responsive to low-toxicity therapy can be treated in frail patients. Treatment for high-risk tumors requiring highly toxic therapy should be offered only to the most fit patients where RLE will allow them to enjoy their survival. Extreme frailty is usually recognized without difficulty. Because oncologists generally see a selected group of reasonably healthy older patients, geriatricians' greatest contribution is in decision making for the apparently fit but "vulnerable" or "subclinical frail" patients.[23]

The National Cancer Center Network recognizes that some form of geriatric assessment provides information essential to the treatment of persons 70 years old or older.[31] These guidelines also recognize the importance of caregiver support, out-of-pocket costs for people on fixed income, access to care, depression, malnutrition, and polypharmacy. Patients who are dependent in IADLs, especially in the use of transportation, ability to take medications, and money management, are at increased risk for complications.

It is important to lay out in a clear and systematic manner the likely course of the cancer if not treated or with best possible treatment and best expected outcome based on the cancer alone. Then the individual's life expectancy based on stable comorbidities and functional status needs to be measured against the likely duration of toxic therapy and duration of remission to be gained. Then it makes sense to let the patient weigh the balance and set his or her goals.[32,33]

> Geriatric assessment provides information essential to the treatment of cancer in persons aged 70 years or older.

Recently, two important studies have shown a role for geriatric consultation. One trial involved randomizing advanced lung cancer patients to usual care or to proactive palliative care assessments. The palliative care group lived longer and terminated active treatment earlier.[34] In an observational study in the context of a clinical trial, advanced lung cancer patients who had previously documented IADL dependencies were 50% more likely, patients who could not walk a block outside their homes were 75% more likely, and patients who had a previous fall were 2.5 times more likely to experience serious chemotherapy toxicity.[27] Geriatricians have been careful to separate the patient's functional status from comorbidity burden. This separation appears to hold with cancer patients, because studies confirm that toxicities are independently predicted by functional variables and by summary comorbidity variables. Simply doing assessments will not change outcomes. However, the geriatric model of multidisciplinary continuity of care may improve outcomes as demonstrated in a multicenter Veterans Administration trial showing that among functionally impaired veterans randomized to geriatric outpatient care, those with cancer benefitted the most with

TABLE 46-2	Remaining Life Expectancy (RLE) in Years by Age (5 yrs), Sex, and Quartile (Lowest, Middle 2, Highest)														
	70 yrs			**75 yrs**			**80 yrs**			**85 yrs**			**90 yrs**		
Sex	L	M	H	L	M	H	L	M	H	L	M	H	L	M	H
Men	6.7	12.4	18.0	4.9	9.3	14.2	3.3	6.7	10.8	2.2	4.7	7.9	1.5	3.2	5.8
Women	9.5	15.7	21.3	6.8	11.9	17.0	4.6	8.6	13.0	2.9	5.9	7.9	1.8	3.9	6.8

LE, Life expectancy; *L*, low quartile of LE; *M*, middle quartile of LE; *H*, high quartile of LE.
Adapted from Walter LC, Covinsky KE. Cancer screening in elderly patients: A framework for individualized decision-making. JAMA 2001;285:2750-6.

respect to quality of life.[35] Adverse events beyond direct drug toxicity should be considered in future studies when additional outcomes can be built into the trial protocols.

Oncologists know the direct toxic effects of the agents they use including emetogenicity; bone marrow suppression; and acute renal, neurologic, cardiac, and pulmonary toxicities. With the introduction of new biological agents, the more common toxicities of the cytotoxic agents such as mucositis, nausea and vomiting, neutropenia, neuropathy, and hair loss, are somewhat mitigated. Oncologists are also aware of subjective symptoms such as depression and fatigue but they have a relatively limited armamentarium for effective intervention. Furthermore, delirium is common on inpatient oncology units but there are little to no data on low-grade delirium in oncology outpatients. Geriatric assessments and geriatric interventions may prove to be effective for maintaining functional status in elderly cancer patients.

Chemotherapy is largely an outpatient procedure and oncology nurses are skilled in administering preventive protocols to reduce immediate nausea and vomiting, cutaneous itching and burning, and anxiety. However, elderly patients who experience less immediate chemotherapy induced nausea (CIN) are more subject to delayed toxicities including nausea, bone marrow suppression, neutropenia, anorexia, fatigue, and diarrhea.[36] The impact of known late toxicities may be more serious in the elderly because of preexisting vulnerabilities. At some institutions out-of-town patients may be kept close by in dedicated housing near the hospital or admitted to skilled nursing facilities (SNFs) to carry them through chemotherapy. Thus nursing homes need to be aware and prepared to manage predictable delayed toxicities.[37] SNF-level care anticipates functional problems. An elderly patient at home, especially alone at home, who is suffering from fatigue, anorexia, or low-grade delirium may not be able to recognize, report, and self-manage toxicities. Recognizing mild mobility problems, mild cognitive impairment, or dementia is crucial for an elderly patient's ability to maintain nutrition and hydration, and avoid falls. Minor mobility problems may get worse as a result of orthostatic hypotension, fatigue, anorexia, and sleep dysfunction. Nausea, vomiting, diarrhea, anorexia, and mucositis require adequate supports in the home to manage medications, fluids, and toileting. Active supportive symptomatic management is crucial.

GENERAL PRINCIPLES OF CANCER MANAGEMENT

Cancer treatment includes local and systemic treatment. Local treatment includes surgery and radiation therapy. Systemic treatment includes several classes of drugs: cytotoxic chemotherapy, hormonal therapy, biologic therapy, and targeted therapy. Each treatment modality has predictable potential side effects.

Local Therapy

Elective surgery for cancer is reasonably safe throughout the ninth decade of age.[38,39] The major differences in surgical mortality between younger and older individuals are seen in emergency surgery of the GI tract. Standard screening for cancer of the large bowel may substantially reduce the need for emergency surgery. Elective cancer surgery poses no greater risk than noncancer surgery. The usual perioperative risk stratification and monitoring for delirium and early nutritional support should be performed. Early mobilization and referral for rehabilitation should also be encouraged.

Surgical practice with respect to breast cancer has trended toward less extensive procedures. For example in breast cancer, radical and modified radical mastectomies are now rarely performed. Lumpectomy with sentinel lymph node dissection has for many patients obviated the need for axillary dissection, given the low risk for extended axillary involvement (if less than three lymph nodes) and high morbidity (lymphedema, pain, shoulder weakness, and contractures.)

By contrast, surgical debulking of ovarian cancers is trending toward longer procedures to achieve more complete excisions. Improved radiation technology, such as cyberknife, may in some cases eliminate the need for surgical excision of isolated small tumors.[40]

Several studies attest to the safety of radiation therapy in older patients, even those aged 80 or older.[41] Radiation therapy can sometimes be used in lieu of surgery for curative purposes in selected patients and for palliation of pain and obstruction. The combination of chemotherapy and radiation for cancer of the larynx, esophagus, and small rectal tumors produces results comparable to surgery with the advantage of organ preservation.[42] Radiation and surgery remain effective strategies for curative prostate cancer therapy, but the best use of these interventions is actively under discussion.[43]

> Studies attest to the safety of radiation therapy in older patients, even those aged 80 or older.

Systemic Therapy

Systemic therapy involves oral and intravenous agents of several classes (Box 46-2).

Hormonal Therapy

The aromatase inhibitors (AIs) have proven more effective than the older selective estrogen receptor modulators (tamoxifen and toremifene) in the management

BOX 46-2

CLASSES OF SYSTEMIC ANTINEOPLASTIC TREATMENT

Hormonal Therapy
Selective estrogen receptor modulators (SERMs)
Aromatase inhibitors
Progestins
Luteinizing hormone-releasing hormone (LHRH) analogs
LHRH antagonists
Estrogens
Androgens
Androgen antagonists
Adrenal antagonists
Corticosteroids

Biologic Therapy
Interferons
Interleukin-2

Tumor Vaccines (Mostly in Clinical Trials)
HPV is given for prevention of cervical cancer. Future uses include likely penile and possibly oropharyngeal cancers.

Cytotoxic Chemotherapy
Alkylating agents
Antimetabolites
Antibiotics
Plant derivatives

Targeted Therapy
Monoclonal antibodies
Immune-destruction of the tumor
Carriers of cytotoxic material inside the tumor
Inhibitors of the action of tumor growth factors

Tyrosine kinase inhibitors
Farnesyl transferase inhibitors
Angiogenesis inhibitors

HPV, Human papillomavirus.

receptor modulators (SERMs) are generally ineffective. The risk of endometrial cancer, thrombosis, and cataracts is lower with AIs compared with SERMs. Despite this advantage, AIs are known to increase osteoporosis and that raises the risk for subsequent bone fractures. Additionally, letrozole has been shown to increase the levels of circulating low-density lipoprotein and has been associated with an increased risk for cardiovascular deaths in a European study. A bone density study prior to AI therapy should be done. With osteopenia or osteoporosis it is prudent practice to also give bisphosphonates and replete vitamin D.[44]

A new SERM, fulvestrant, is a pure estrogen antagonist that has recently become available. Its activity may be comparable to that of AIs. This agent is administered by intramuscular injections. Poor adherence to oral antiestrogens has made this attractive in some circumstances. Progestins, whose activity is inferior to that of AIs, are used occasionally as third-line agents in metastatic breast cancer.

Gonadotropin-releasing hormone (GnRH) analogs cause medical castration and are currently preferred in the management of prostate cancer. Treatment with GnRH analogs may be given along with oral androgen antagonists (e.g., bicalutamide, flutamide) during the first 2 weeks of treatment to counteract the burst of testosterone after the first dose of analogs. As single agents, the androgen antagonists are inferior to luteinizing hormone-releasing hormone (LHRH) analog therapy. Adrenal suppressors including aminoglutethimide and ketoconazole at high doses have some activity as second- or third-line hormonal treatment of relapsed prostate cancer.[43]

Cytotoxic Chemotherapy

Cytotoxic chemotherapy includes diverse groups of drugs that preferentially kill proliferating cells and spare resting-phase cells. The common toxicities of cytotoxic chemotherapy are listed in Table 46-3. Age is a risk factor for most of these complications because the reserves of progenitor cells are lower. The timing

of breast cancer. For the majority of practitioners, these compounds are now the initial treatment of choice, both in the adjuvant setting and in metastatic disease.[44] The AIs are active even in tumors that overexpress the HER2neu (human epidermal growth factor receptor 2) protein, for which selective estrogen

TABLE 46-3	Chemotherapy-Related Toxicity in Older Individuals[45]
Type of Toxicity	**Agents Involved**
Myelodepression	All agents, except vincristine, bleomycin, L-asparaginase, streptozotocin
Alopecia	Most agents except gemcitabine (oral fluorinated pyrimidine, 5-FU)
Mucositis (diarrhea)	Fluorinated pyrimidines, methotrexate, anthracyclines (doxorubicin, daunorubicin, idarubicin, epirubicin)
Cardiotoxicity	Anthracyclines (doxorubicin, daunorubicin, idarubicin, epirubicin), mitomycin C
Peripheral neurotoxicity	Alkaloids (vincristine, vinblastine, vinorelbine), cisplatin, podophyllotoxins (etoposide, teniposide), taxanes (taxotere, paclitaxel)
Central neurotoxicity	All agents (delirium, "chemo brain," possibly dementia), high dose cytarabine and 5-FU (cerebellar toxicity)
Anemia	Nearly all antineoplastics
Fatigue	Nearly all antineoplastics
Depression	Interferons

of the toxicities is related to the mechanisms of the drugs. For example nausea may be an acute reaction to drug crossing the blood–brain barrier or it may be delayed and a result of depression of GI motility. Mucosal injury and hair loss peak within the normal turnover cycle of rapidly dividing endothelial cells. Knowing the drugs and their toxicity profiles helps to anticipate potential problems.

A number of steps may ameliorate the toxicity of chemotherapy in older individuals:[45]

- Adjust the dose to the renal function. In particular for patients older than age 65, the dose of chemotherapy should be adjusted to the calculated glomerular filtration rate from a measured 24-hour urine sample.
- Reducing the dose to test tolerance with the intent that doses may be escalated in subsequent cycles if the drugs are tolerated. This strategy is ill advised in situations in which chemotherapy is administered for cure, because the full dose is based on clinical trials and improves the chances of achieving a cure.
- Older patients are more likely to experience severe bone marrow suppression, including anemia, thrombocytopenia, and neutropenia. Support with hematopoietic growth factors. NCCN and SIOG guidelines recommend routine preventative use of agents to prevent neutropenia.[31] Pegfilgrastim prevents neutropenic infections in approximately 50% of cases and has largely replaced granulocyte colony stimulating factor (G-CSF) because it can be administered once for each cycle of chemotherapy (with a minimum of 14 days between treatments), whereas G-CSF requires daily administrations for 7 to 10 days.
- Anemia may be caused by the cancer or by the treatment, and initially it was hoped that treating anemia aggressively would also relieve the burden of fatigue many cancer patients feel. Epoetin A and darbepoetin A will raise hemoglobin levels in approximately 75% of patients. Management of anemia during cytotoxic chemotherapy has two goals: prevention of functional decline caused by fatigue, and treatment of fatigue itself if it is caused by profound anemia. Clinical trials have failed to support the goal of normalizing hemoglobin as effective treatment of cancer fatigue.[46] Current guidelines advise against using these agents either in patients being treated for cure or for patients in palliative care because of excess thrombotic events and the potential for stimulating tumor growth, especially with head and neck and non–small cell lung cancer.
- Cardiotoxicity occurs as early (reversible) congestive heart failure with trastuzumab and a late-onset restrictive form associated with anthracyclines. Anthracycline cardiotoxicity is not dose related; it occurs several years after completion of treatment and may contribute to congestive heart failure in long-term survivors. There appear to be individual susceptibilities but these have not yet been identified so many oncologists are reluctant to give anthracyclines to elderly patients who may already have cardiomyopathy. Cardioprotective strategies including giving anthracyclines as continuous infusions rather than bolus; concomitant administration of doxorubicin and dexrazoxane, which prevents the formation of free radicals in the myocardium; and administration of pegylated liposomal doxorubicin in lieu of doxorubicin have been adopted.[47]

- Severe mucositis is miserable. The dysphagia contributes to severe fluid and nutritional deficits. Mucositis is a severe problem for patients receiving "chemorads" treatment for head and neck cancers. It is sometimes not possible for patients to take oral nutrition and they are temporarily tube fed. Although the treatment is debilitating and painful, the cure rate is high for those who can tolerate the toxicity. Palliative agents include oral anesthetics and coating agents, "magic mouth wash." A newer oral solution of glutamine (AES12) is a keratinocyte growth factor that reduces incidence and severity of mucositis from high-dose chemotherapy. The substitution of capecitabine, an oral prodrug activated into fluorouracil inside the neoplastic tissue for intravenous fluorinated pyrimidines (fluorouracil and floxuridine), minimizes the exposure of the normal mucosa to fluorouracil.[48]
- In addition to capecitabine and pegylated liposomal doxorubicin, a number of new drugs with favorable toxicity profiles are useful in older individuals. These include taxanes in low weekly doses, vinorelbine, and gemcitabine.

Targeted Therapy

New insights in cancer cell biology have allowed the development of drugs that target specific components or specific metabolic processes of the tumor. Theoretically, targeted therapy would spare normal tissues that do not express the intracellular machinery or cell surface markers of the malignant cells.

Monoclonal antibodies may target either tumor surface antigens or intercept growth factors or growth factor receptors. They may destroy the tumor by an immune mechanism, by using cell surface receptors to carry the cytotoxic substance into the tumor, or by interfering with the vital processes of the tumor. Rituximab and alemtuzumab target respectively the CD 20 and the CD 52 antigens and are effective in lymphoid malignancies. Trastuzumab and cetuximab target different components of the epithelial growth factor receptors and are effective in cancer of the breast and of the large bowel, respectively. Bevacizumab is a monoclonal antibody directed to the vascular endothelial growth factor (VEG-F) and is used in several solid tumor cancers.[45]

All monoclonal antibodies may cause anaphylactic reactions. Alemtuzumab may cause severe, prolonged myelosuppression and immune deficiency (neutropenia.) Trastuzumab may cause reversible heart failure by a different mechanism than the anthracyclines, which is irreversible. Cetuximab causes a severe acne-like reaction. Bevacizumab is used only with caution in the elderly because of associated hypertension, bleeding, and visceral perforation.[45]

Rituximab and similar antibodies have been tagged with radioisotopes (radioimmunotherapy) to deliver high radiation doses to the tumor. Although highly effective, radioimmunotherapy may still be associated with severe myelosuppression. Thalidomide and recently developed congeners (lenalidamide) have substantial activity in multiple myeloma with relatively little toxicity. Side effects include somnolence, constipation, and thromboembolism.[45]

A relatively new group of drugs are the tyrosine kinase inhibitors (TKIs). Tyrosine kinase is a key enzyme of intracellular signal transduction. A number of small ATP-like molecules inhibit this enzyme and consequently tumor growth. Imatinib inhibits the soluble TK and is effective in chronic myelogenous leukemia (CML), in the acute lymphoblastic leukemias (ALL) with Ph chromosome, in stromal tumors of the stomach, and in hypereosinophilia. Gefitinib (unavailable in the United States) and erlotinib inhibit the TK associated with growth factor receptors and are sometimes effective with little toxicity in non–small cell lung cancer, particularly tumors with certain epidermal growth factor receptor (EGFR) mutations. In general monoclonal antibodies and antiangiogenic factors represent an alternative to cytotoxic chemotherapy for older patients because they are less symptomatically toxic. Several are oral drugs so travel is reduced and some patients experience strong tumor response.[45]

CASE 1

Jane Thompson (Part 2)

Mrs. Thompson's three children disagree on what they believe that their mother would prefer. You review the options for therapy with the oncologist, and after 3 days, the family agrees to a trial of therapy. Mrs. Thompson, now fully awake and in agreement, will be treated with cyclophosphamide, vincristine, doxorubicin, and prednisone (CHOP regimen) with rituximab at reduced doses because of her recent kidney injury. She is given one round of reduced CHOP-R and discharged to an SNF on TPN. After 20 days Mrs. Thompson returns to the oncologist's office able to eat on her own. She has also regained her independence with ADLs. TPN is discontinued, and the patient receives five more courses of chemotherapy at full doses with G-CSF support (pegfilgrastim, a hemopoietic growth factor). After 4 years she is still independent and in complete remission. ■

CASE 1

Discussion

The specific disease and Mrs. Thompson's health status are both important aspects of this case. This disease, DLBCL, is highly responsive to chemotherapy. Although age is a poor prognostic factor, more than 50% of persons older than age 60 will have a complete response to chemotherapy, and 30% are curable (defined as 5 years with no recurrence). Although Mrs. Thompson had a poor performance status when she was brought to the hospital, she had been totally independent 2 weeks before. Her poor condition was the result of an acute change that was reversed with fluid resuscitation and treatment of the gastric obstruction. Given their diminished organ reserve, older individuals' general condition may deteriorate more quickly in response to stress. To judge the fitness of older individuals for chemotherapy, their condition should be judged from the patient's functional status before the acute event and his or her response to treatment of the acute problem. ■

CASE 2

Mary Davis (Part 1)

A nursing aide finds a 1.5-cm nodule on the right breast of your patient, Mary Davis. She is a 90-year-old woman confined to a wheelchair by arthritis. She is quite conversational and her last documented Mini-Mental State Exam (MMSE) was 20/30. She has a history of congestive heart failure but has never been symptomatic over the 2 years you have cared for her. You are aware that independently of age, her ADL dependence and dementia are risk factors for toxicity of cytotoxic chemotherapy and for postoperative delirium if surgery is attempted. Mrs. Davis defers decisions to her family.

After discussion with the patient's family and a medical oncologist, you recommend that a fine-needle aspiration biopsy be performed in radiology. Mrs. Davis becomes agitated, and the procedure is aborted. Her son refuses to consent to reattempting the procedure. The nodule is watched and does not seem to be changing over the next 6 months.

1. **What is the natural history of untreated breast cancer in women aged 70? 80? 90?**

2. **What diagnostic steps are appropriate for a woman with RLE less than 5 years, 5 to 9 years, more than 10 years? Mammography? Needle biopsy? Excisional biopsy? Observation?**

3. **Should you empirically treat with a SERM or AI? Or do nothing?** ■

BREAST CANCER

Carcinoma in Situ

Stage migration has affected the presentation of breast cancer in the elderly. Approximately 20% of newly diagnosed breast cancers are in situ, found on mammograms and often not palpable. This is an increase from 1% in 1970. The most common form is ductal carcinoma in situ (DCIS), which is treated with simple or partial mastectomy. With a disease as heavily screened for as breast cancer, interpreting treatment results should take account of the so-called "Will Rogers effect." That is, with discovery and treatment of early stage disease that includes disease with both indolent and aggressive potential, treatment effectiveness will likely be overestimated. Because of this effect, treatment outcomes should be interpreted by both biological and stage criteria. Thus the need for radiotherapy, especially in older women, is in doubt and is reserved for excisions with affected margins and higher grade tumors. Taking tamoxifen for 5 years decreases the risk of local recurrence after partial mastectomy by 80%.[49,50]

> Stage migration has affected the presentation of breast cancer in the elderly; approximately 20% of newly diagnosed breast cancers are in situ, found on mammograms and often not palpable.

Localized Carcinoma of the Breast

Localized carcinoma of the breast (stages I to IIIA) is a surgically curable disease. The decision tree for management has grown more complex as less invasive treatments have been shown to be effective. Examples are simple or partial mastectomy (lumpectomy) alone or with radiotherapy for larger tumors, if the surgical pathology shows infiltrated margins or tumors have aggressive histology. Postoperative irradiation has no impact on freedom from distant metastases and overall survival. It only affects the likelihood of local recurrence. Irradiation of the breast has minimal complications in older women but it is inconvenient and expensive. The risk of local recurrence after partial mastectomy declines with the age of the patient.[50] If the risk of local recurrence within 5 years is 10% or less and this risk is acceptable to the patient, postoperative radiation probably offers no advantages to an older woman.

Axillary lymph node dissection is a complicated subject. The options are sentinel node sampling, partial dissection, and complete dissection. Axillary lymph node dissection is associated with substantial morbidity, including chronic lymphedema and functional limitations of the upper extremity. Lymph node mapping may obviate the need of this procedure in the majority of patients. After the injection of a radioactive tracer, it is possible to identify the so-called sentinel lymph node. If this lymph node is clear of metastases, axillary dissection is unnecessary. Also a localized stage I or small stage II tumor might not require axillary sampling at all in an older woman with good histology in the initial biopsy.[51]

Adjuvant chemotherapy should be reserved for women who are similar to the women who participated in the clinical trials and should be based on likelihood of recurrence during the woman's RLE. A node-negative simple mastectomy requires no radiation or adjuvant cytotoxic therapy. All mastectomy specimens should be tested for hormone receptors, proliferation rate, and HER2/neu antigens (the antigen for the epithelial growth factor receptor). This provides important prognostic information as well as data for treatment. More centers are offering genomic profiling of other genetic markers of biological behavior and drug susceptibility to match tumor, drugs, and patients with the greatest chance of benefit. Oncotyping allows patients to think about the likelihood of recurrences for the type of breast cancer they have (or other cancers for which prognostic markers are available). They can decide how to balance their likelihood of recurrence with their willingness to take adjuvant chemotherapy. The benefits of adjuvant chemotherapy decline with age. In aggregated data, based on randomized controlled trials (RCTs) completed before the era of widely available oncotyping, there appears to be no benefit beyond the age of 70. Cytotoxic therapy is usually reserved for locally advanced stage II and III tumors with biologically aggressive histology and positive lymph nodes or for metastatic disease.

If it is the woman's choice, chemotherapy should be reserved for fit women with negative hormone receptors and overexpression of HER2neu. Anthracyclines are very effective against these tumors, doubling the cure rate.[11]

Adjuvant treatment with AIs delays the recurrence of breast cancer more effectively than do SERMs in hormone receptor–rich tumors and is preferred by the majority of practitioners.[52] Current practice suggests that SERMS and AIs be used for 5 years, and then stopped.

Metastatic Carcinoma of the Breast

All management of metastatic breast cancer is palliative. The goal of palliative chemotherapy is to reduce tumor burden and delay progression to symptomatic disease or to lessen symptoms that are caused by the cancer itself, such as bone pain. The choice depends on the patient's overall performance status, biology of the tumor, the specific symptoms to be palliated, and the woman's wishes with regard to quality of life. It is important to clarify advance directives if they have not yet been documented.

Cytotoxic chemotherapy is indicated for (apparently) hormone receptor–rich tumors that have failed at least two forms of hormonal treatment, or for tumors that lack hormone receptors. Isolated brain metastases may be managed with surgery or radiotherapy, but multiple brain metastases will require a decision about hospice or whole brain radiation therapy. Isolated bone metastases involving weight-bearing bones such as the femur, the tibia, or the humerus should undergo surgical fixation to prevent pathologic fractures in otherwise functionally intact women. Such findings in a previously nonambulatory patient would suggest early referral for palliative care. It is important to remember that, in general, with symptomatic metastatic disease in a chronically ill, debilitated patient, treatment has little or no impact on survival. However, some women may live several years with stable metastatic disease, as shown in Table 46-4. The risks, costs, and benefits of tumor-directed palliation should be assessed and reassessed.[11]

Several forms of chemotherapy with limited toxicity are available. For patients with tumors that overexpress the HER2/neu antigen, a combination of trastuzumab and weekly taxane is the treatment of choice. For the other patients, weekly Taxol, Taxotere, or vinorelbine (Navelbine); oral capecitabine; or pegylated liposomal doxorubicin every 4 weeks are well tolerated and of similar efficacy.

CASE 2

Discussion

We do not know how long Mrs. Davis's tumor was there before it was discovered so we do not know if it is growing rapidly or slowly. No change over 6 months, however, suggests slower growth. The recommendation of a biopsy for Mrs. Davis was reasonable because the procedure has negligible morbidity and might have provided prognostic information about the aggressiveness of the tumor, use of SERMs or AIs, and the value of simple excisional biopsy. If Mrs. Davis's fine needle aspiration (FNA) revealed ductal carcinoma in situ (DCIS), observation alone would be acceptable in view of her estimated RLE; DCIS is unlikely to cause local symptoms or metastasize. The patient's

TABLE 46-4	Median Survival in Months of Patients with Metastatic Breast Cancer by Location of Metastases
Location	Survival (Months)
Liver (>than 30% replacement	3
Lung (lymphangitic)	3
Lung (nodular)	22
Skin	27
Bones	36+

reaction, however, and the denial of permission to try again prevented the biopsy.

The suspicion of metastatic disease was low, so further imaging with bone scans and CT did not appear necessary. A chest radiograph could show lung metastasis and possible humerus, rib, and thoracic spine lytic lesions. Basic blood work including a complete blood count, to exclude significant anemia, and a metabolic blood panel could show significant liver and bone metastasis by transaminases, albumin, alkaline phosphatase, and calcium levels.

In a 90-year-old woman, a breast nodule should be considered cancer unless proved otherwise. There is an 80% chance the tumor was hormone receptor positive. A number of approaches were reasonable in this case. A local resection under local anesthesia would be diagnostic and curative and prevent local complications such as fungating, painful, and ulcerating masses. However, Mrs. Davis's reaction to the biopsy precludes a local anesthesia approach. Empiric treatment with tamoxifen would have had a 60% to 80% chance of a measureable response. The chief disadvantage of tamoxifen is risk of deep vein thrombosis, which is increased for an older woman immobilized by arthritis. An AI could worsen her osteoporosis and she would have to be treated with either oral or IV bisphosphonate. Close observation was reasonable because the average life expectancy of this woman with moderate dementia and functional impairment was probably less than 2 years. The median time for her tumor to metastasize or cause local problems such as erosion through the skin is more than 3 years based on observational studies of local breast cancer. Because breast masses are superficial it is easy enough to follow with observation alone. ◼

CASE 3

Chao Min Xi (Part 1)

Zhao Min Xi comes to your office with his son as an interpreter. He is a 79-year-old man who has been losing weight and suffering from sweats at night since his arrival from China several months back. He is otherwise independent around the house. Mr. Chao does little outside the home because he does not speak English and the family operates a small factory in a small town with few other Chinese people. You discover that he has enlarged lymph nodes in both axillae. You exclude active tuberculosis infection. After referral for biopsy, the pathologist confirms peripheral T-cell lymphoma (PTCL). CT scans of the chest and abdomen and a bone marrow biopsy are negative for lymphoma. During the workup of the lymphoma, the patient went to a urologist because of difficulty urinating. As a result of this consultation Mr. Chao's PSA was found to be 82 ng/mL. Transrectal prostatic biopsy reveals a Gleason 8 (aggressive) prostatic adenocarcinoma. The patient's hemoglobin is 10.2, serum creatinine is 1.7, and BUN is 26. Serum erythropoietin levels are 3 mg/mL, low. You are unable to formally assess cognition and depression but he appears to be quite conversational with his son; he asks questions through his son and otherwise appears to be quite lively. ◼

PROSTATE CANCER

Prostate cancer is the most common cancer and the second most common cause of cancer death for American men. Incidence in Asian men is somewhat lower on a population level. The widespread use of prostate-specific antigen (PSA) for screening asymptomatic men has led to a doubling of the reported incidence of prostate cancer in the last decade.[53] There is no conclusive evidence that screening has reduced the risk of death from prostate cancer, especially for men older than 65. Much of the current debate has to do with the contribution of radical prostatectomy and of radiation to survival of men after diagnosis.[54] The current staging and treatment of prostate cancer are summarized in Table 46-5.

Close observation (active surveillance) for patients with localized disease is a reasonable approach for men age 70 or older with well-differentiated tumor (Gleason score of 7 or lower). In all other cases, some form of local treatment is reasonable. Brachytherapy (radiation by internal implant) may have fewer complications than external beam radiation therapy (EBRT). In younger men there is increased risk for a second, radiation-induced cancer. Early symptoms of fatigue generally worsen over the course of radiotherapy but resolve when therapy is completed. Late complications of radiation include chronic cystitis and proctitis that can only be managed symptomatically.

Poor prognostic factors for localized disease (stages A, B, and C) include a poorly differentiated tumor Gleason grade 8 or higher, extracapsular involvement beyond the seminal vesicles, and a PSA level greater than 30 ng/mL.

The role of androgen ablation for asymptomatic lower Gleason grade tumors is debatable because castration levels of testosterone induce secondary morbidities including increased cardiovascular risk, osteoporosis, muscle wasting, weight gain, and subjective symptoms of hot flashes, loss of libido, and subsyndromal depression. Only one third of these patients will develop clinical metastases within 10 years.[55]

Hormonal treatment is the mainstay of management of metastatic prostate disease. It has been demonstrated that hormonal treatment initiated immediately upon diagnosis of asymptomatic metastases is superior to delaying hormonal treatment until symptoms develop.[37] It is unclear, however, whether hormonal treatment should be instituted for biochemical progression, that is, rising PSA after radical prostatectomy (stage D1.5 disease) without evidence of metastasis. The role of cytotoxic chemotherapy is limited to treating symptomatic metastatic disease that has become resistant to hormonal agents. Treatment is not curative. Spot radiation may help pain from bone metastasis; some centers use intravenous heavy particle isotopes such as strontium 89, which produces more prolonged responses but also more severe myelosuppression. Most centers will use zoledronate prophylactically or symptomatically to prevent or treat the pain and delay the progression of bony metastases.

CASE 3

Chao Min Xi (Part 2)

Mr. Chao and both sons arrive for a family meeting in which the oncologist proposes CHOP (rituximab, cyclophosphamide, doxorubicin, vincristine, and prednisone) given every 3 weeks and G-CSF daily injections for a week following chemotherapy. If he becomes symptomatically anemic, transfusion would be considered. The prostate cancer will be treated simultaneously with goserelin, an LHRH analog, and anastrozole (Casodex), an antiandrogen. Any further treatment of the prostate cancer would be deferred until the lymphoma is addressed. In any case, the survival benefit of additional radiation to the prostate is debatable.

TABLE 46-5	Clinical Staging of Prostate Cancer	
Stage	**Clinical Description**	**Treatment**
A	No palpable lesion, biopsy only	Observation
B1	Palpable nodule 1 lobe	Radical prostatectomy, EBRT or brachytherapy
B2	Palpable nodule both lobes or one dominant nodule >1.5 cm	Same
C	Locally advanced, invading the capsule	Radiation and hormonal therapy
D1	Extracapsular involves pelvic lymph nodes	Lymph node dissection and hormonal therapy
D1.5	Chemical recurrence, rising PSA after prostatectomy	Hormonal therapy if PSA doubling time is <10 months, occurs within 2 years of prostatectomy, or if the primary was Gleason 8 or higher
D2	Extensive retroperitoneal lymph node involvement, distant metastasis	Hormonal therapy
D2.5	Rising PSA after definitive treatment	Consider cytotoxic therapy if second- and third-line hormonal therapy fails or treat only if symptomatic metastasis occurs.

EBRT, External beam radiation therapy; *PSA,* prostate-specific antigen.

The more immediate problem is how to support Mr. Chao through the next few months of chemotherapy for lymphoma. As an immigrant Mr. Chao did not have Medicare; nor did he have a privately paid major medical policy. His family had sufficient funds to cover his treatment and to house him in an SNF located on the campus of the hospital and cancer center. On admission to the SNF his weight was 92 lbs, which declined to 89 lbs. However, his son said Mr. Chao never weighed as much as 100 lbs. He refused restorative physical therapy largely because he did not speak English and he found it tiring to try to comply with instructions he did not understand. He tended to stay in his room and sleep most of the day. You are concerned about his apparent decline in functional status. The evening nurse reported he got up in the early evening and walked independently in the hall while other residents were at dinner or asleep. A problem was that he missed scheduled meals. Once a month his out-of-town daughter came for a week and he went home with her until his next cycle of chemotherapy. Mr. Chao's standing orders in the nursing home covered follow-up labs, GI toxicity, fluids, and nutrition. Pegfilgrastim (granulocyte colony–stimulating factor) was prescribed. He ultimately received six cycles of CHOP with complete remission. He was briefly hospitalized overnight for an episode of neutropenic fever. His PSA declined to 0.3 mg/mL and further prostate cancer–directed therapy was deferred indefinitely.

Discussion

Mr. Chao's case allows examination of common problems related to cancer and age. First, Mr. Chao lives in a small town more than an hour away from the cancer center and is dependent on his son for transportation because neither he nor his wife can drive and his daughter-in-law does not feel safe with highway driving. Mr. Chao is socially isolated by language even though he has no ambulatory problems.

Geriatric assessment for this elderly man with two cancers was limited by the language barrier; however, close observation of family interactions and gait assessment performed by the evening shift nurse indicated that although he was very thin by Western standards Mr. Chao was in good physical condition and his functional limitations were not caused by physical or cognitive impairments. Care planning was designed to minimize the stress on his support system. The nursing home relieved the patient and the family of tiring long-distance drives. Coordination of care between the physician at the SNF and the oncologist at the cancer center allowed standing orders to anticipate chemotoxicity in a safe environment where his nutrition, ambulation, and fluid status could be monitored.

Multiple neoplasms are common in older individuals. The management should start with the neoplasm that most immediately threatens the patient's life. Median survival of PTCL is approximately 18 months without treatment. Mr. Chao's very high PSA suggests a more advanced cancer, but no metastatic disease was identified so it is prostate cancer stage C, which has an approximately 5-year survival expectation. First attention should be directed to the lymphoma.

Mr. Chao has an aggressive disease. The treatment of diffuse large B-cell non-Hodgkin's lymphoma (the most common form of intermediate-grade lymphoma) involves a combination of an alkylating agent, an anthracycline, a glucocorticoid, and rituximab. The most popular of these combinations is R-CHOP (rituximab, cyclophosphamide, doxorubicin, vincristine, and prednisone). In early disease (stages I and II), three courses of R-CHOP followed by radiation therapy produce a cure rate of 60% to 80%.[56,57] In more advanced disease, six cycles of chemotherapy are administered with a cure rate of 60% to 80%.[57]

Although he had a complete response to his treatment for non-Hodgkin's lymphoma, Mr. Chao has a high likelihood of recurrence within 5 years. Attention is turned to his prostate cancer. The survival advantage attributed to radical prostatectomy is experienced by men who have an RLE of more than 10 years. Mr. Chao has a high likelihood of recurrent PTCL early in this period so his estimated RLE is less than 10 years. Furthermore, the subjective harms of surgery include incontinence and impotence. Delayed risks from radiation include proctitis, cystitis, second cancers, and impotence. This should be balanced against the risk of accelerated frailty caused by androgen ablation in this small man. ◉

CASE 4

Geraldine Brown (Part 1)

Geraldine Brown is a 72-year-old woman who came to your office for follow-up of a newly discovered microcytic anemia. You are following her for uncomplicated hypertension and mild hypothyroidism. You are concerned about her memory because her MMSE was recently 23/30. She had not finished high school and had been a domestic worker and hotel maid during her working years. Mrs. Brown lives alone, drives a car locally, and has a daughter nearby. You ordered a diagnostic colonoscopy, which reveals an apple core lesion of the ascending colon. She subsequently underwent surgical resection without incident. Surgical pathology revealed stage III disease. She was able to return home with home health care and help from her daughter a week after surgery. She did not experience hospital-acquired delirium.

Should Mrs. Brown receive adjuvant chemotherapy? ◉

COLON CANCER

Cancer of the large bowel is the second leading cause of cancer death in women and the third leading cause in men. Incidence of this neoplasm increases with age, at least until age 95. The staging of colon cancer follows the tumor size, nodes involved, metastasis present (TNM) system. TNM stage I, T1-2, is limited to mucosa and submucosa; stage IIA, T3-3, invades muscularis propria; Stage IIB invades the outer layer of colon proper, the serosa. Stage III is any lymph node involvement. Stage IV involves distant metastases, typically the liver, regional abdominal lymph nodes, or lung because of the lymphatic drainage of the large bowel. The clinical workup of cancer of the large bowel includes a full colonoscopy and a CT scan of the chest, abdomen, and pelvis, or a positron emission tomography (PET) scan to evaluate for metastases. The serum carcinoembryonic antigen (CEA) should not be used as a diagnostic serum marker because a number of different conditions can cause false positives. It is useful to draw the CEA level prior to surgery because if it is elevated, return to low levels implies that the surgery was effective; and elevated levels suggest recurrence or incomplete resection.

Resection of stage I and IIA colorectal cancer results in a cure rate as high as 90%. Several studies have demonstrated the benefits of adjuvant treatment in stage III cancer and in some subsets of stage IIB cancer. Adjuvant treatment consists of a combination of fluorouracil and leucovorin administered over 6 months. The addition of oxaliplatin to a multiagent protocol improves the cure rate by 5% but it is associated with significant toxicity, especially painful neuropathy and thrombocytopenia.[58] In metastatic disease, the combination of fluorouracil, leucovorin, and irinotecan or oxaliplatin produces a response rate of approximately 40% with a median duration response of 8 months.[58] The addition of bevacizumab (Avastin), cetuximab (Erbitux), and aflibercept (Zaltrap) further improve response and survival but they have not been specifically studied in the elderly.[58] Bevacizumab has been associated with adverse cardiovascular events and colonic perforation, especially in the elderly.

> Cancer of the large bowel is the second leading cause of cancer death in women and the third leading cause in men; incidence increases with age, at least until age 95 years.

CASE 4

Geraldine Brown (Part 2)

Mrs. Brown has several comorbidities including mild dementia but none affecting her physical functional status. Her surgical risk for abdominal surgery was acceptable and she did well after surgery. She and her daughter agreed to adjuvant therapy, which she tolerated very well, and she continued to drive her car. Her 1-year follow-up colonoscopy was clear.

About 3 years later, however, Mrs. Brown complained of feeling tired and had lost 10 pounds. Her MMSE was now 20/30. Abdominal CT revealed several small metastatic lesions. The oncologist recommended a second course of multiagent chemotherapy which she and her daughter agreed to; however this time the toxicities were

severe enough that despite shrinkage of the tumors, they elected to stop multiagent therapy.

Mrs. Brown was continued on single-agent treatment, capecitabine, without apparent side effects. Follow-up imaging revealed stable liver disease. The situation remained as such for over a year and then Mrs. Jackson began to develop worsening cognitive performance. Her daughter took over transportation, medication and money management, and reported that sometimes when she came over in the afternoon Mrs. Brown had not yet been out of bed or eaten. Her weight began to decline again and she looked gaunt. Imaging of her liver remained unchanged. Her MMSE was now 13/30. The oncologist wished to continue capecitabine but the patient deferred to her daughter, who chose to stop active treatment. Hospice was initiated and Mrs. Brown passed away without discomfort 8 months later in her own home.

1. **What caused Mrs. Brown's weight loss?**

2. **Was her cognitive decline a result of cancer, cancer treatment, or progression of dementia unrelated to cancer?**

3. **Do you agree with Mrs. Brown's daughter's decision?** ▣

In approximately 50% of patients with colon cancer, the only site of metastatic disease is the liver. When feasible, local management of liver metastases may prolong survival and may even result in cure. Surgical resection of liver metastases followed by infusional chemotherapy with floxuridine in the hepatic artery results in prolonged remission in approximately 40% of patients.[46] Thermoablation of metastases with ultrasound is an alternative to surgery suitable for older individuals at poor surgical risk but cure is rare.

All patients who have had a curative resection of cancer of the large bowel should undergo surveillance colonoscopy. The first examination is generally performed 1 year after surgery; the other examinations are performed at 3- to 5-year intervals. Yearly abdominal CT and periodic determinations of CEA for 5 years are also indicated.

CASE 4

Discussion

Mrs. Brown lived about 5 years after her first diagnosis, most of it with good quality of life. The single-agent therapy probably did effectively control her cancer but the progression of her dementia was the chief threat to her quality of life. Although her daughter was able to provide some in-home care once Mrs. Brown's dementia had progressed, she was at high risk for nursing home placement. Her daughter made the substituted judgment that staying home was her mother's first priority. With hospice, her daughter, and her granddaughter, Mrs. Brown was able to stay home. ▣

CANCER SCREENING AND CHEMOPREVENTION OF CANCER

Cancer screening remains highly controversial and emotional in the public and in general. Medical specialties exhibit cultural differences in their acceptance of the U.S. Preventive Services Task Force recommendations[59] (see Chapter 4).

Chemoprevention of cancer involves administration of substances that block or offset the late stages of carcinogenesis, where the gradual accumulation of transcriptional errors over time may impair naturally occurring apoptosis. Although chemoprevention of cancer is an enticing strategy of tumor control in the older person, the general use of drugs and dietary supplements cannot be recommended for the following reasons:

- No proof yet exists that chemoprevention reduces cancer-related morbidity and mortality. For example, finasteride reduced the total incidence of prostate cancer but appeared to increase the risk of the most aggressive forms of the disease.
- Medications used for chemoprevention may have serious complications. For example, tamoxifen has been associated with cerebrovascular accidents, deep vein thrombosis, and endometrial cancer. Cyclooxygenase 2 inhibitors may also be associated with cardiovascular and renal complications and for that reason alone are off many pharmacy formularies.

At least four groups of substances have demonstrated chemopreventive activity in humans:

Hormonal Agents

SERMs, including tamoxifen and raloxifene, and aromatase inhibitors, including anastrozole, letrozole and exemestane, may prevent breast cancer. The SERMs may also prevent osteoporosis but are associated with increased risk for venous thromboembolism. The aromatase inhibitors that are currently considered first line for adjuvant therapy of hormone-sensitive breast cancer also are known to cause osteoporosis and should not be given without bisphosphonate therapy. If there is a contraindication to bisphosphonates other considerations should be taken on an individualized basis.

The 5-a reductase inhibitor finasteride, which is often used in conjunction with alpha-1 blockers for symptomatic management of benign prostatic hyperplasia (BPH) with lower urinary tract symptoms (LUTS), may prevent prostate cancer.[15] Other 5-a reductase inhibitors have been developed for BPH with LUTS but have not been studied for prostate cancer effect. Stronger androgen deprivation therapies (ADTs) are used for treatment of confirmed prostate cancer.

Retinoids

Retinoids may prevent cancer of the upper airways in smokers. The current recommendation, however, is to avoid such use because of the apparent adverse effects found in the one clinical trial.

Nonsteroidal Antiinflammatory Drugs

Specific nonsteroidal antiinflammatory drugs, the COX-2 inhibitors, and aspirin may prevent cancer of the large bowel and of the breast. Colon cancers in the elderly more often express COX-2 receptors than those in younger patients. Aspirin use has been associated with better outcomes of diagnosed colon cancer but a causal link is not established.

HMG-CoA Reductase Inhibitors

Recent studies indicate that the cholesterol-lowering drugs HMG-CoA reductase inhibitors may prevent different cancers, including cancers of the large bowel and of the breast. There is no recommendation to prescribe statins for this indication.

SUMMARY

Cancer is the second leading cause of death and a major cause of morbidity for older adults. The biology of some cancers is age-associated. Specifically, some common cancers are more indolent, such as breast and prostate cancer, non–small cell lung cancer, and some subtypes of lymphoma and ovarian cancer. However, several are more aggressive, including several acute leukemias and lymphomas. Therefore age alone should not determine the treatment of cancer. The cancer and the patient must be staged separately and the treatment must be grounded in evidence-based expectations. Often there is limited evidence for cancer treatment in the elderly. A geriatric assessment should be used to determine how well or poorly the evidence fits the patient. This calculation should take into account the patient's goals in terms of survival and quality of life, and the probability of achieving them. All geriatric cancer patients should be provided with best supportive and symptomatic care regardless of prognosis, good or bad. Continuous communication between the oncologist and the geriatrician should improve treatment tolerance and thus treatment effectiveness.

Web Resources

www.cancer.org. American Cancer Society.
www.nci.nih.gov. National Cancer Institute.
www.guidelines.gov. Agency for Healthcare Research and Quality's National Guideline Clearinghouse.
www.uspreventiveservicestaskforce.org/adultrec.htm. U.S. Preventive Services Recommendations for Adults.
www.adjuvantonline.com. Decision-making tools for health care professionals.
www.nccn.org/professionals/physician_gls/f_guidelines.asp. National Comprehensive Cancer Network.
www.siog.org. International Society of Geriatric Oncology.

KEY REFERENCES

16. Aapro M, Köhne C-HS, Cohen HJ, Extermann M. Never too old? Age should not be a barrier to enrollment in cancer clinical trials. Oncologist 2005;10(3):198-204.

19. Biganzoli L, Wildiers H, Oakman C, et al. Management of elderly patients with breast cancer: Updated recommendations of the International Society of Geriatric Oncology (SIOG) and European Society of Breast Cancer Specialists (EUSOMA) [review]. Lancet Oncology 2012;13(4):e148-60.

22. Rodin MB, Mohile SG. A practical approach to geriatric assessment in oncology [review]. J Clin Oncol 2007;25(14):1936-44.

28. Hurria A. Communicating treatment options to older patients: Challenges and opportunities. J Nat Comprehensive Cancer Network 2012;10(9):1174-6.

36. Rodin M. Cancer patients in nursing homes: What do we know? J Am Med Directors Assoc 2008;9(3):149-56.

55. Droz JP, Balducci L, Bolla M, et al. Background for the proposal of SIOG guidelines for the management of prostate cancer in senior adults. Crit Rev in Oncol-Hem 2010;73:68-91.

References available online at expertconsult.com.

47

Anemia

Lodovico Balducci

OBJECTIVES

Upon completion of this chapter, the reader will be able to:

- Define anemia in the older aged person.
- List the causes of anemia.
- Discuss the medical consequences of anemia.
- Outline the treatment of anemia, and explain how to address the medical consequences of the disease.

As is the case with the majority of diseases, the incidence and prevalence of anemia increase with age.[1-8] The prevalence of anemia is higher among institutionalized than among home-dwelling older individuals.[9-12] With the aging of the population one may expect anemia to become an increasingly common problem.

CASE 1

George Cooper (Part 1)

George Cooper is a 91-year-old recently widowed gentleman who has been a longtime patient in your practice. He has a history of blood loss anemia from an upper gastrointestinal hemorrhage 10 years ago; the source was diagnosed as acute esophageal ulceration. He has been on long-term proton pump inhibitor therapy. After iron replacement his hemoglobin remained at 11 g/dL. He also has chronic renal

insufficiency and received epoetin alpha monthly for a few years until his hemoglobin stabilized at 10.5, and epoetin alpha was discontinued 2 years ago. Mr. Cooper visits your office today for an annual physical examination, and laboratory studies drawn yesterday show the following: white blood count (WBC), 2.9 X10^3/μL (normal differential); hemoglobin, 8.6 g/dL; hematocrit, 26.3%; mean cell volume (MCV), 97.4 fL; Mean corpuscular hemoglobin concentration (MCHC), 32.7%; platelet count, 97,000 × 10^3 μL. Blood urea nitrogen (BUN) and creatinine are stable at 34 mg/dL or milligrams per deciliter and 1.54 mg/dL. He has been feeling more fatigued lately, but otherwise Mr. Cooper has no other constitutional or focal symptoms.

1. **What is the differential diagnosis of Mr. Cooper's anemia?**

2. **What are your next steps in evaluation?** ◘

DEFINITION OF ANEMIA

Normal hemoglobin values may be defined as the average values of hemoglobin in a large population of apparently normal individuals. This is the approach taken by the World Health Organization (WHO). An alternative approach defines as normal values those at which the lowest risk of medical events is seen. For this purpose, the medical events of interest in an older population include death, loss of independence, and reduction of active life expectancy.

The WHO defines anemia as hemoglobin concentrations less than 13.5 g/dL for men and less than 12.0 g/dL for women.[13] According to this definition the prevalence of anemia is higher in men than in women after age 65 and is higher in black than in white people for any age group.

A number of recent studies have questioned the WHO definition of anemia in older women. The Women's Health and Aging Study (WHAS), a prospective study of 1003 women 65 and older living in the Baltimore area, showed that hemoglobin levels lower than 13.4 g/dL represented a risk factor for mortality and values lower than 13.0 g/dL a risk factor of disability and functional dependence.[14,15] Likewise, the Cardioascular Health Study (CHS) found that hemoglobin levels below 12.6 g/dL were an independent risk factor for mortality in women 65 and older.[16] Based on these findings it would appear reasonable to consider the lowest normal hemoglobin levels in older women to be between 12.5 and 13.0 g/dL. When these levels are adopted, the difference in incidence and prevalence of anemia between older men and women disappears.

The issue of whether African Americans should be considered anemic at lower hemoglobin levels than individuals of other races is still controversial. A recent study of the population aged 70 to 79 in Memphis, Tenn., revealed that the risk of mortality and functional disability for older blacks increased only for hemoglobin levels 2 g lower than the WHO standard, over a 2-year observation time.[7] At the same time, a longitudinal study of older African Americans at Duke University showed that the risk of mortality and disability was higher when levels of hemoglobin were below the WHO standards.[17] Similar finding were reported in a longitudinal study of individuals 65 and older in Chicago, over 13 years.[18] For the present time it appears prudent to consider older African Americans with hemoglobin levels lower than the WHO standards to be anemic.

CAUSES OF ANEMIA (BOX 47-1)

> In more than 50% of cases, anemia in people older than 65 years has a treatable cause and therefore even mild anemia warrants evaluation.

The causes of anemia in older individuals in the outpatient setting are shown in Table 47-1.[1,4,5,6] Two recent studies conducted in specialized anemia clinics explored the causes of anemia in the older aged person. The variation between different studies may be partly explained by the fact that they were conducted at different times and in different populations. Patients in the Biella[5] and the Chicago[6] studies underwent an intensive evaluation of the causes of anemia as they were followed in a specialized anemia clinic. The causes of anemia were not consistently investigated in either the National Health and Nutrition Examination Survey (NHANES)[1] or the Olmstead county studies.[4] Despite these differences some common trends are recognizable:

- In more than 50% of cases anemia has a cause that is both recognizable and treatable. Thus a thorough investigation of the causes of anemia, even of mild anemia, in older individuals is warranted.
- In at least a third of cases the cause of anemia remains unexplained, even after an intensive workup. In the Biella study eventually one fourth of the patients with anemia of unknown causes developed myelodysplasia during the follow-up period.

The Biella study highlighted that more than half of the patients with anemia had more than one cause for their anemia.

> More than half of older patients with anemia have more than one cause for their anemia.

The main cause of iron deficiency in older age is blood loss, especially from the gastrointestinal tract,[19-22] which should be thoroughly evaluated even in the absence of symptoms and in the presence of negative hemoccult stool test. At the same time it is important to remember that in 30% to 50% of adults a cause of blood loss is not identified and iron malabsorption may be the main cause of iron deficiency. Causes of iron malabsorption may include atrophic gastritis, *Helicobacter pylori* infection, and celiac disease. In the presence of iron malabsorption, oral iron therapy may be ineffective.

> The main cause of iron deficiency in older people is blood loss, even when the heme test of the stool is negative.

The incidence and prevalence of B_{12} deficiency increase with age.[23,24] The most common cause of B_{12}

BOX 47-1

POSSIBLE CAUSES OR CONTRIBUTORS TO ANEMIA OF UNKNOWN CAUSE

- Early cases of myelodysplasia
- Glomerular filtration rate lower than 60 mL/minute
- Hypogonadism in both older men and women
  - Androgen deprivation
  - Aromatase inhibitors
- Nutrition
- Relative erythropoietin deficiency

TABLE 47-1	Causes of Anemia in Older Individuals			
	NHANES III[1]	**Olmsted County[4]**	**Biella[5]**	**Chicago[6]**
Iron deficiency	16%	15%	16%	25%
Anemia of chronic inflammation (ACI)	33.6%	36%	17%	10%
B_{12} and/or folate deficiency	14.3%	NA	10%	3.4%
Renal insufficiency	12%	8%	15%	3.5%
Hematologic malignancies	NA	NA	7.4%	NA
Thalassemia	NA	NA	4.5%	7.5%
Unknown cause	24%	33%	26%	44%

NHANES, National Health and Nutrition Examination Survey.

deficiency is the inability to digest B_{12} in food because of decreased gastric secretion of hydrochloric acid and pepsin; people with this condition may respond to oral crystalline B_{12}.[23,24] Drug-induced B_{12} deficiency is increasingly common,[25] especially with the use of proton pump inhibitors and metformin. In addition to anemia, B_{12} deficiency may be a cause of neurologic disorders including dementia, and posterior column lesions.

The anemia of unknown causes represents a special diagnostic challenge. Some of these patients may represent early cases of myelodysplasia or unrecognized chronic renal insufficiency. In some studies, as many as 75% of patients develop anemia when glomerular filtration rate is lower than 60 mL/minute.[26,27] These values are common in individuals 65 and older and are almost universal after age 80. Hypogonadism may account for some of these cases.[28] The role of hypogonadism was highlighted in the Chianti study, which found low levels of circulating testosterone in three fourths of older men and women with anemia. In addition, low testosterone levels were highly predictive of future development of anemia in nonanemic subjects. The possibility of preventing or reversing anemia with testosterone replacement needs study. After aromatization to estrogen, androgens stimulate the proliferation of hematopoietic stem cells through estrogen receptor alpha that activates the ten-eleven-translocation (TET) gene and leads to increased telomerase synthesis.[29] It is worth remembering that hormonal treatment of cancers, such as androgen deprivation for prostatic cancer and aromatase inhibitors for breast cancer, may cause anemia through this mechanism.

Nutrition may play an important role in anemia of unknown causes.[30] In addition to protein/calorie malnutrition that becomes more common with aging, a lack of specific nutrients may be important. Recent studies identified deficiency of vitamin D[31] and copper[32] as potential causes of anemia in older individuals.

Relative erythropoietin deficiency appears central to most cases of anemia of unknown cause in the elderly. In the anemia clinic of the University of Chicago,[6] older patients with anemia of unknown causes failed to show an increase in erythropoietin with a drop in hemoglobin levels, unlike patients with iron deficiency in whom an inverse relationship existed between circulating levels of erythropoietin and hemoglobin. Ferrucci et al. found that the levels of erythropoietin were more elevated in the presence of normal hemoglobin levels, but failed to increase appropriately when hemoglobin levels dropped, in patients with increased concentrations of inflammatory cytokines in the circulation.[33] Inflammatory cytokines may both reduce the sensitivity of erythropoietic precursors to erythropoietin and inhibit erythropoietin secretion. In other words, most cases of anemia of unknown origin would represent a form of anemia of inflammation. This is reasonable because aging is seen as a form of chronic and progressive inflammation.[34] This hypothesis, however, is questioned by a recent study showing that no relation exists between the excretion of hepcidin in the urines of older individuals and their hemoglobin levels.[35] Hepcidin is key to the pathogenesis of anemia of inflammation.[36] This enzyme shuts down the transport of iron from the gastrointestinal tract and from bone marrow stores by destroying the iron-transporting protein ferroportin. The production of hepcidin occurs in the liver and is stimulated by inflammatory cytokines, and in particular interleukin 6.

An area of controversy is whether anemia may develop in older individuals in the absence of a specific disease from exhaustion of hematopoietic reserves, which may include numeric as well as functional abnormalities of the hematopoietic stem cells and failure of the hematopoietic microenvironment to support the viability of these elements. In some cross-sectional studies the average hemoglobin levels appeared consistent in all age groups at least up to age 85, though the prevalence of anemia increased with age.[37-40] These data suggested that anemia is not a necessary consequence of age. Two longitudinal studies, one from Japan[41] and the other from Sweden,[42] revealed a small but progressive decline in hemoglobin concentration with age. Such findings suggest that a progressive erythropoietic exhaustion of low degree may occur with aging. It may become significant under conditions of erythropoietic stress, such as blood loss with a delayed and incomplete correction of anemia.

> An important diagnostic issue is recognition of iron deficiency in the presence of anemia of inflammation.

Because anemia may have multiple causes in up to 50% of anemic older people,[5] the diagnosis of the causes of anemia in the older person involves some unique problems. Perhaps the most important diagnostic issue is the recognition of iron deficiency in the presence of anemia of inflammation (Table 47-2). A foolproof diagnostic test does not exist, but elevated levels of soluble transferrin receptors and low circulating levels of hepcidin suggest some degree of iron deficiency. In this situation an improvement of anemia following iron treatment confirms the diagnosis of iron deficiency. The distinction is important not only for therapeutic reasons. A diagnosis of iron deficiency should trigger investigations for occult bleeding.[20]

An algorithm to investigate anemia in the older person is presented in Figure 47-1. The reticulocyte count generally differentiates between anemia related to increased blood loss and anemia related to decreased

TABLE 47-2	Differentiating the Anemias of iron Deficiency and Chronic Inflammation	
	Anemia of Inflammation	**Iron-Deficiency Anemia**
Serum iron	Low	Low
Total iron-binding capacity	Decreased	Increased
Ferritin levels	Increased	Decreased
Soluble transferrin receptor	Decreased	Increased
Hepcidin levels	Increased	Decreased

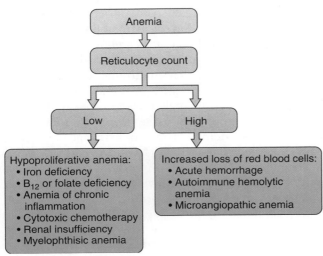

Figure 47-1 Anemia workup.

production of red blood cells. Increased blood cell loss includes both hemorrhage and hemolysis. Anemia caused by decreased production of red blood cells is the most common type, and the size of the red blood cells (mean cellular volume [MCV]) may provide a clue to the cause:

• Microcytosis (i.e., smaller red blood cells) is generally a sign of decreased production of hemoglobin. The main causes in older people include iron deficiency or chronic inflammation. Hemoglobinopathy such as thalassemia may contribute to microcytosis as well.

• Macrocytosis or enlarged red blood cells is generally caused by reduced synthesis of DNA. The cells are overgrown because they cannot reproduce. Currently the most common cause is cytotoxic chemotherapy of cancer or of autoimmune diseases. Other causes include B_{12} and folate deficiency. Hypothyroidism, copper deficiency, and myelodysplasia may also lead to macrocytosis. Macrocytosis may be rarely seen in conditions in which the red blood cell membrane is overexpanded because of accumulation of cholesterol as

it is seen in liver failure with L-CAT (lysolecithin-cholesterol acetyl transferase).

• Normocytosis is an indication of erythropoietin deficiency (renal insufficiency, chronic inflammation) or of deceased production of red blood cells resulting from exhaustion of red blood cell precursors (aplastic anemia).

> One fourth of patients with anemia of unknown cause develop myelodysplasia during the follow-up period.

The MCV may not be a reliable indicator in older individuals because multiple causes of anemia have different effects on MCV. For example, the combination of iron and B_{12} deficiency may lead to normocytosis. When B_{12} levels are borderline (between 150 and 300 μg/dL), one should also check the methylmalonic acid and cystein levels. An increased concentration in either of these substances suggests functional B_{12} deficiency.

A bone marrow examination is generally not necessary for the diagnosis of anemia from iron, B_{12}, folate, or copper deficiency because the assessment of the concentration of these substances in the blood allows diagnosis. Bone marrow examination is necessary when one suspects the diagnosis of myelodysplasia or of marrow-occupying diseases (myelofibrosis, cancer, infections). If myelodysplasia or a neoplastic disorder of the marrow is suspected, cytogenetics and flow cytometry of the marrow should be obtained

> The MCV may not be a reliable indicator in older individuals because multiple causes of anemia have different effects on MCV.

CONSEQUENCES OF ANEMIA

The clinical consequences of anemia are listed in Box 47-2.[3] A number of studies demonstrate that anemia is an independent risk factor for mortality in older individuals.[16-18, 43-49] Of these, the WHAS is the most

---

BOX 47-2

CONSEQUENCES OF ANEMIA IN OLDER INDIVIDUALS

• Decreased survival
• Fatigue and functional dependence
• Increased risk of therapeutic complications, including chemotherapy-related toxicity
• Increased risk of coronary death
• Increased risk of congestive heart failure
• Increased risk of dementia

provocative. The risk of mortality for home-dwelling women older than age 65 was increased for those with hemoglobin levels lower than 13.4 g/dL.[45]

Perhaps the most serious consequence of anemia in older individuals is functional dependence and inability to live alone.[50-53] The WHAS,[50] the EPESE,[51] and the Chianti study[53] all demonstrated that anemia after age 65 was associated with decreased ability to perform instrumental activities of daily living and with mobility impairments. Of interest, in all these studies, there was an inverse linear relation between hemoglobin levels lower than 13.5 g/dL and risk of functional dependence and mobility impairment, indicating that even mild anemia may have serious health and social consequences.

Anemia is associated with increased risk of therapeutic complications. At least four studies showed that anemia was an independent risk factor for the complications of cytotoxic chemotherapy.[54-57] Because the majority of antineoplastic agents are bound to red blood cells, one may expect that the concentration of free drug in the circulation, and the risk of toxicity, may increase with anemia.[54] At the same time, the condition of chronic hypoxia caused by anemia may enhance the vulnerability of normal tissues to treatment complications. Cerebral hypoxia is a likely explanation for the increased risk of postoperative delirium associated with anemia.[58]

The association of chronic anemia and heart failure is well known. A review of Medicare records showed that individuals 65 and older with myocardial infarction and hematocrit lower than 30% were more likely to die if they did not receive blood transfusions.[59]

One of the most titillating possibilities is that anemia may cause cognitive impairment. A study of patients with chronic renal failure showed that cognitive decline was more common among patients whose anemia had not been corrected with erythropoietin.[60] Jacobsen et al. showed a correlation between hemoglobin levels and performance on three cognitive tests in women with cancer receiving chemotherapy.[61] And a systematic review of three longitudinal studies showed that anemia was an independent risk factor for dementia.[62] In addition, the prevalence of other geriatric syndromes was increased in the presence of anemia. In particular, anemia is frequently identified as an independent risk factor for falls.[10,63]

ANEMIA: A CROSSROAD OF AGING

After reviewing the causes and the complications of anemia in older persons, one may see anemia as a crossroad of several aging-related events. These include the following:

- Hematopoietic exhaustion. This may result from a reduction in the concentration of hematopoietic stem cells as well as in functional abnormalities of these elements.[64-66] Pang et al. recently reported that with age hematopoietic stem cells tend to differentiate into myeloid rather than erythroid elements.[66] This phenomenon could lead to anemia through a so-called stem-cell steal. Hematopoietic exhaustion may also be influenced by external factors including drugs or exposure to radiation. It is well known that older individuals are more susceptible than younger ones to develop myelodysplasia after exposure to cytotoxic chemotherapy.[67]
- Chronic and progressive inflammation appears as a universal characteristic of aging. Chronic inflammation is associated with anemia through a number of mechanisms already described,[6,33,34] which include reduced iron mobility and relative erythropoietin deficiency.
- A reduction in glomerular filtration rate is universal with age, and is associated with reduced erythropoietin production.[26,27]
- Geriatric syndromes, including cognitive decline, falls, and functional dependence, are associated with anemia.
- The risk of mortality is increased among elderly anemic individuals.

It is reasonable to ask whether the correction of anemia may prevent death or the common complications of aging. Unfortunately the answer to this critical question is still not known.

TREATMENT OF ANEMIA

Treatment must be based on the specific causes of anemia (see Box 47-1). Replenishment of nutritional deficiencies including iron, cobalamin, and copper, and treatment of underlying conditions such as hypothyroidism are indicated. Because iron absorption may be compromised, many authors recommend intravenous iron replacement. In the United States low molecular weight iron dextran is the most common preparation used. The advantage of this preparation includes the ability to administer the full amount of iron over a single session. The disadvantages include the risk of anaphylactoid reaction and the need for administration over several hours. Ferumoxytol (FeraHeme) is approved in the United States for the treatment of iron deficiency in patients with chronic renal insufficiency. The advantages include the administration over a few minutes and the absence of immediate adverse reactions. Disadvantages include the high cost and the fact that only 510 mg can be administered during a single session. Other preparations of iron available in Europe include ferric carboxymaltose and ferumoxytol. Both appear free of immediate reaction and may be administered over a few minutes.[68]

Vitamin B$_{12}$ (cobalamin) is effective orally at high doses in patients with pernicious anemia.[69] It is reasonable, albeit unproven, to assume that oral preparation may be effective in older individuals without pernicious anemia, whose major problem appears to be inadequate digestion of food B$_{12}$. Indefinite B$_{12}$ replacement was considered desirable until recently. This assumption was questioned by a recent article showing a direct relationship between vitamin B$_{12}$ levels and mortality among older hospitalized patients.[70] Until the meaning of this association is clarified it is reasonable to limit the replacement treatment until normal blood levels of B$_{12}$, methylmalonic acid, and cystein (markers of B$_{12}$ deficiency) are achieved.

The biggest controversy concerns the management of anemia of inflammation (the most common form of anemia in older individuals) with erythropoietic-stimulating agents (ESAs) such as epoetin α or β and darbepoetin α.[71-73] These compounds were effective in improving fatigue and quality of life of cancer patients, but a number of recent studies suggest that they may cause deep vein thrombosis and stimulate the growth of some tumors, especially cancer of the breast and of the head and neck. It should be underlined that these complications were observed mainly in patients not receiving chemotherapy for their cancer and almost exclusively when hemoglobin levels were raised about 12 g/dL. Also, a meta-analysis of studies using exclusively darbepoetin in patients receiving chemotherapy failed to show any increase in tumor growth.[73]

These findings led to a halt of all attempts to treat anemia of inflammation in older individuals with ESAs. Hopefully these studies may be resumed in the future, once the risks of ESAs are clarified.

CASE 1

Discussion

The fact that Mr. Cooper has all three cell lines (red cells, white cells, and platelets) below normal levels is concerning for global bone marrow dysfunction. This is of special concern because he has had a chronic anemia for several years, a fact which increases his risk of developing a myelodysplastic syndrome. His MCV is elevated and you order thyroid-stimulating hormone, fasting serum folate, and B$_{12}$ levels. You know that frequently there is more than one contributor to anemia in older people, and because of Mr. Cooper's history of gastrointestinal bleeding you are concerned about an element of iron deficiency and obtain iron, total iron-binding capacity, and ferritin levels. You also need to determine if this is a hypoproliferative process, and a reticulocyte count will be helpful. When these studies return showing B$_{12}$, folate, and iron stores and a low absolute reticulocyte count, you refer Mr. Cooper for a bone marrow biopsy. Results of the biopsy are consistent with a myelodysplastic syndrome. He restarts erythropoietin injections, which raises his hemoglobin to between 10.5 and 11, and his energy improves. The white cell and platelet lines remain stable and you follow him closely with a consulting hematologist. ■

SUMMARY

Anemia, even mild anemia, has a negative influence on survival, function, and health of older individuals. Anemia should be considered present with hemoglobin levels lower than 13 g/dL in older women and 13.5 g/dL in older men. There are no good reasons at present to use different standards for the definition of anemia in African American and Caucasian patients. Anemia is associated with increased mortality, increased risk of functional dependence, geriatric syndromes, and therapeutic complications in older individuals, but it is not clear whether reversal of anemia will reverse these risks. Frequently, anemia in older individuals has more than one cause and in approximately 50% of cases the causes of anemia are treatable. The major area of controversy concerns the treatment of anemia of inflammation with ESAs. More studies are urgently needed in this area.

KEY REFERENCES

1. Guralnik JM, Eisenstaedt RS, Ferrucci L, et al. Prevalence of anemia in persons 65 years and older in the United States: Evidence for a high rate of unexplained anemia. Blood 2004;104: 2063-8.
2. Ferrucci L, Balducci L. Anemia of aging: Role of chronic inflammation and cancer. Semin Hematol 2008;45:242-9.
5. Tettamanti M, Lucca U, Gandini F, et al. Prevalence, incidence and types of "mild anemia" in the elderly: The "Health and Anemia" population bases study. Hematologica 2010;95:1849-56.
8. Pang W, Schrier SL. Anemia in the elderly. Curr Opin Hematol 2012;19:133-40.
20. Vannella L, Aloe Spiriti MA, DiGiulio E, at al. Upper and lower gastrointestinal causes of iron deficient anemia in elderly compared with adult outpatients. Minerva Gastroenterol Dietol 2010;56:397-404.

References available online at expertconsult.com.

48

Pulmonary Disease

Priyal Amin and Andrew M. Smith

Additional online-only material indicated by icon.

OBJECTIVES

Upon completion of this chapter the reader will be able to:

● Recognize and describe the changes in pulmonary physiology among the aging population.

● Identify and differentiate the signs and symptoms of pulmonary diseases in the geriatric population with multiple comorbidities.

● Define the differences between asthma, chronic obstructive pulmonary disease (COPD), and restrictive lung diseases in terms of diagnosis and management.

● Demonstrate the understanding of interpretation and the value and limitations of diagnostic tests for pulmonary diseases.

ABBREVIATIONS

Spirometry
PEFR: peak expiratory flow rate
FEV_1: forced expiratory volume in 1 second
FVC: forced vital capacity
TLC: total lung capacity
DLCO/VA: diffusing capacity of the lung for carbon monoxide corrected for alveolar volume
(E)RV: (end) residual volume
FRC: functional residual capacity
LLN: lower limit of normal

Medications
SABA: short-acting $beta_2$ agonist
LABA: long-acting $beta_2$ agonist
ICS: inhaled corticosteroid
LTRA: leukotriene receptor antagonist

PULMONARY PHYSIOLOGY AND AGING

The respiratory system, induced by chronic low-grade inflammation and stress-mediated imbalances, undergoes anatomic, physiologic, and immunologic changes with age. Studies have shown that the rapid rate of decline of peak aerobic capacity has significant repercussions with regard to functional independence and quality of life, in both healthy older persons and in those with disease-related deficits.[1] With the number of people in the United States older than age 65 years estimated to reach 71 million by 2030, a thorough understanding of the natural progression of age-related changes in the respiratory system is necessary.[2]

The respiratory system comprises mainly the rib cage, diaphragm, and lungs. Osteoporosis may result in reduced height of the thoracic vertebrae with subsequent kyphosis. Kyphosis reduces the ability of the thoracic cage to expand during inspiration and places the diaphragm at a mechanical disadvantage to generate effective contraction.[2] Similarly, age-related decline in diaphragmatic strength related to muscle atrophy and reduction in the fast-twitch fibers can result in respiratory fatigue and eventual ventilatory failure.[3] In addition, degradation of the elastic fibers around alveolar ducts, and loss of elastic recoil of the lungs and the supporting lung parenchyma, lead to air trapping from early closure of the small airways and can cause hyperinflation with increased residual volume and functional residual capacity.[4,5]

Age-related decreased ability of the respiratory center in the medulla oblongata to detect hypoxia or hypercapnia results in a diminished ventilatory response in cases of aggravated airway obstruction.[5] Furthermore, decreased perception of bronchoconstriction and diminished physical activity with age can result in a reduced awareness of respiratory disease and thus delayed diagnosis and treatment initiation. Given these changes a heightened awareness of pulmonary disease is necessary among primary care physicians to diagnose and initiate treatment early.

> Differentiating a disease state from normal aging is important when evaluating the elderly population in a clinical setting.

ASSESSMENT OF PULMONARY DISEASES BASED ON SIGNS AND SYMPTOMS

As in any other age group, the presence of episodic symptoms of airflow obstruction or airway hyperresponsiveness must be documented to establish a diagnosis of obstructive lung diseases in the geriatric population.[6] These symptoms include but are not limited to the presence of wheezing, chest tightness, cough with or without mucus production, or shortness of breath with or without exertion. Such information can be obtained via a detailed medical history and a physical examination focusing on the upper and lower respiratory tract and the chest. Table 48-1 lists the most commonly seen differential diagnosis of pulmonary diseases in older adults with these symptoms.

When evaluating a patient with wheezing, the diagnoses of asthma and chronic obstructive pulmonary disease (COPD) must be considered. Risk factors associated with each disease should be evaluated.

TABLE 48-1	Differential Diagnosis for Pulmonary Diseases in Older Adults
Congestive heart failure
Coronary artery disease
Pulmonary embolus
Mechanical obstruction caused by mass or enlarged lymph nodes
Pulmonary infiltrated with eosinophilia/eosinophilic bronchitis
Allergic bronchopulmonary aspergillosis (ABPA)
Churg-Strauss vasculitis
Obliterative bronchiolitis
Post-nasal drip
Vocal cord dysfunction
Gastro-esophageal reflux disease (GERD)
Mechanical aspiration
Tracheomalacia (as a result of underlying rheumatologic diseases [e.g., relapsing polychondritis])

Modified from Expert Panel Report 3 (EPR-3): Guidelines for the diagnosis and management of asthma-summary report 2007. J Allergy Clin Immunol 2007;20(5 Suppl):S94-138.

Because congestive heart failure with or without ischemic heart disease could cause wheezing it is important to consider cardiac causes of wheezing as well as when a patient has concomitant chest pain, palpitations, lower extremity edema, or jugular venous distention. Other causes of bilateral wheezing include mechanical obstruction caused by mass or enlarged lymph nodes, which may also produce unilateral wheezing. Allergic bronchopulmonary aspergillosis (ABPA) is diagnosed based on the presence of an Immunoglobin E >1000 ng/mL, presence of central bronchiectasis on chest computed tomography (CT), a serum IgE and/or Immunoglobin G positive for *Aspergillus fumigatus*, and immediate hypersensitivity skin testing positive to *Aspergillus fumigates*. Churg-Strauss vasculitis is a small and medium vessel diagnosed by the presence of any four of the following criteria: asthma, peripheral eosinophilia greater than 10%; presence of mononeuropathy or polyneuropathy, nonfixed pulmonary infiltrates, presence of paranasal sinus abnormalities, and histologic evidence of extravascular eosinophils.

When evaluating a patient with a chronic cough (lasting more than 6 weeks), the obstructive and restrictive pulmonary diseases and cough variant asthma must be considered. In addition, the differential includes cough caused by postnasal drip, medications such as angiotensin-converting enzyme (ACE) inhibitors, and gastroesophageal reflux disease. Coughing with hoarseness of the voice may also be a sign of vocal cord dysfunction (VCD). VCD, also referred to as paradoxical vocal cord motion (PVCM), is a condition where there is paradoxical adduction of the anterior portion of the vocal cords during inspiration. VCD can be diagnosed based on videostroboscopy. Flattening of the inspiratory loop on spirometry may also be seen in VCD.

CASE 1

Harold Walker (Part 1)

Harold Walker, a 77-year-old male, visits your office with sputum production and profuse rhinorrhea, ongoing for years. Sputum is grayish, sometimes yellow a few times per year. He reports intermittent wheezing. He reports no known triggers. Mr. Walker smokes a pipe only socially. He used an inhaler a few weeks ago and felt that it possibly helped. Mr. Walker reports no problems with walking on level ground. He does report dyspnea when walking uphill. He has never been hospitalized or been to urgent care for dyspnea. His Asthma Control Test score is 9 (poor control). Vital signs and physical examination are essentially normal except for a peak expiratory flow rate of 110. Spirometry with prebronchodilator and postbronchodilator measurements, lung volumes, and diffusion studies were performed (Table 48-2).

After reviewing the test results, you start Mr. Walker on a medium dose inhaled corticosteroid (ICS). His respiratory symptoms completely disappear over 6 weeks and baseline spirometry returns to normal.

What is Mr. Walker's likely diagnosis? ▣

COMMON OBSTRUCTIVE PULMONARY DISEASES IN THE OLDER ADULT

Asthma

Definition and Epidemiology

Asthma is a chronic inflammatory disorder characterized by variable and recurring symptoms of airway hyperresponsiveness, bronchoconstriction, and airway inflammation. More than 22 million Americans have asthma, with the incidence being 1 in 1000 per year among adults and older adults.[6,7] The prevalence of asthma in the geriatric population is estimated to be 10%. Approximately 3.1 million Americans older than age 65 years have asthma.[6,7]

Asthma in the elderly can present as a heterogeneous disease at any age with varying degree of severity. Unlike in the young, when asthma begins later in life it is rarely an extrinsic (i.e., an IgE-mediated process) or familial.[7] Triggers may include indoor and outdoor allergen exposure, pollutants, molds, endotoxin, and latent viral and bacterial infections. These triggers may induce bronchoconstriction, airway inflammation, and edema, which are hallmark features of the airway obstruction that causes asthma.[6,7] Approximately 15% of U.S. adults with asthma have asthma attributable to occupational exposures and this number continues to rise.[8,9]

Asthma in the elderly may often have an irreversible component owing to three main factors, unrelated to the pack-years of smoking.[10] The first factor is that more severe disease can lead to airway remodeling causing diffuse thickening of the basement membrane. This remodeling and hypertrophy of smooth muscles and submucosal glands in some bronchial segments results in irreversible obstruction. The second factor leading to fixed obstruction is the time and age of onset of disease. Asthma may begin as early as the fourth or fifth decades of life. Asthma can go undetected and untreated for several years, leading to an accumulation of pulmonary damage. A third factor is the coexistence of underlying COPD or pulmonary fibrosis.[7] Patients may have more than one pulmonary disease; therefore a mixed defect or partial reversibility may be a clue.

Diagnosis

The later section of this chapter that discusses objective evaluation of pulmonary diseases gives detailed information on how to evaluate a patient with signs and symptoms suggestive of asthma. Briefly, all patients with suspected asthma should be evaluated to confirm the objective diagnosis of asthma. Because

TABLE 48-2	Case 1 Spirometry Results						
	Baseline				**Post**		
	Actual	Predicted	% Predicted	LLN	Actual	% Change	% Predicted
SPIROMETRY							
FVC (L)	2.54	3.03	84	2.27	2.80	10	92
FEV$_1$ (L)	1.48	2.14	69	1.50	1.76	19	82
FEV$_1$/FVC (%)	58	72	81	62	63	8	87
LUNG VOLUMES							
TLC (L)	6.61	5.71	116	4.31			
DIFFUSION							
DLCO/VA	4.00	4.12	97	2.66			

DLCO, Carbon monoxide diffusing capacity; *FEV$_1$*, forced expiratory volume in 1 second; *FVC*, forced vital capacity; *LLN*, lower limit of normal; *TLC*, total lung capacity; *VA*, alveolar volume.

asthma is a disease of reversible airflow limitation, confirmatory tests would include spirometry with a reversible obstructive defect or methacholine bronchoprovocation challenge test with a drop in forced expiratory volume in 1 second (FEV_1) of 20% or more from baseline at any concentration of methacholine less than 4 mg/mL.

> Asthma in the older adult is more severe, progressive, and may often have an irreversible component owing to three main factors—airway remodeling, age of onset, and coexistence of COPD or pulmonary fibrosis.

Treatment

The Global Initiative for Asthma (GINA) guidelines identify four components of asthma care: (1) development of doctor–patient relationship; (2) identification and reduction of exposure to risk factor; (3) assessment, treatment, and monitoring of asthma; and (4) managing asthma exacerbations.[11,12] Development of a partnership between the physician and patient leads to effective management of asthma that provides comprehensive education in terms of proper use of medications. Education should include monitoring of skills needed to use aerosol medications, understanding differences between controller and reliever medications, recognizing worsening of asthma symptoms with or without peak

expiratory flow rate (PEFR) monitoring, Asthma Action Plan (see Web Resources), and seeking medical advice when appropriate.[11] Physicians should also address any patient concerns regarding asthma, the medications, or management.

The second component of comprehensive asthma care involves identification of and then control of exposure to risk factors, such as cigarette smoke (active and passive), drugs (nonsteroidal antiinflammatory drugs [NSAIDs], beta-blockers, etc.), occupational sensitizers (diisocyanates, trimellitic anhydride, sulfur dioxide fumes, etc.), and sensitization to aeroallergens. Patients with moderate to severe asthma should be advised to receive the influenza vaccine yearly.[12] Avoidance measures improve control of asthma and reduce the need for medications.

The third component of asthma care is assessing asthma severity and control, treating to achieve control, and monitoring to maintain control. The distinction between severity and control represents a major change in the National Heart, Lung, and Blood Institute (NHLBI) guidelines updated in 2007. Assessment of asthma severity is based on frequency of asthma-type symptoms, nocturnal awakening, and use of a short-acting beta$_2$-agonist ($SABA_2$) along with degree of interference with daily activity, and lung function measurements (using FEV_1 and FEV_1/FVC [forced vital capacity]) (Figure 48-1). Asthma severity grading should be used to initiate asthma therapy. Based on the level of severity, asthma can be categorized into

Components of severity		Classification of asthma severity (youths ≥ 12 years of age and adults)			
		Intermittent	Persistent		
			Mild	Moderate	Severe
	Symptoms	≤ 2 days/week	> 2 days/week but not daily	Daily	Throughout the day
	Nightime awakenings	≤ 2x/month	3–4x/month	> 1x/week but not nightly	Often 7x/week
Intermittent Normal FEV_1/FVC: 8–19 yr 85% 20–39 yr 80% 40–59 yr 75% 60–80 yr 70%	Short-acting beta$_2$-agonist use for symptom control (not prevention of EIB)	≤ 2 days/week	> 2 days/week but not > 1x/day	Daily	Several times per day
	Interference with normal activity	None	Minor limitation	Some limitation	Extremely limited
	Lung function	• Normal FEV_1 between exacerbations • FEV_1 > 80% predicted • FEV_1/FVC normal	• FEV_1 ≥ 80% predicted • FEV_1/FVC normal	• FEV_1 > 60% but < 80% predicted • FEV_1/FVC reduced 5%	• FEV_1 < 60% predicted • FEV_1/FVC reduced > 5%
Risk	Exacerbations requiring oral systemic corticosteroids	0–1/year	≥ 2/year —————————————→		
		←——— Consider severity and interval since last exacerbation. Frequency and severity may fluctuate over time for patients in any severity category. ———→			
		Relative annual risk of exacerbations may be related to FEV_1			

Figure 48-1 Classification of asthma severity. (Reproduced from Expert Panel Report 3 [EPR-3]: Guidelines for the diagnosis and management of asthma-summary report 2007. J Allergy Clin Immunol 2007;120[5 Suppl]:S94-138.)
EIB, exercise induced bronchoconstriction.

intermittent, mild-persistent, moderate-persistent, or severe-persistent.[6,11,12] Asthma control should then be assessed at all subsequent visits to minimize risk and maximize function (Table 48-3). Assessment of asthma control is also based on the aforementioned factors, and is categorized into well controlled, not well controlled, and very poorly controlled.[6,11,12]

As an aid in the assessment of control, an asthma control questionnaire such as the Asthma Control Test (ACT) can be used on follow-up visits for evaluation of asthma control. The ACT is a valid and reliable measure of changes occurring in asthma control. A score lower than 19 out of 25 is considered a marker of poor control. (The Preventive Maintenance section later in the chapter discusses the medications used in the management of chronic asthma.)

The fourth component of asthma care is managing asthma exacerbations, acute or subacute episodes of worsening of asthma-related symptoms characterized by decreases in expiratory flow. Risk factors for asthma-related death from exacerbations include previous history of severe exacerbation needing intubation or an intensive care unit admission, two or more hospitalizations or three or more emergency room visits in the past year, difficulty perceiving airway obstruction, lower socioeconomic status, and the presence of other comorbid conditions. Worsening PEFR at home can help identify early signs of an exacerbation and can help monitor response to

therapy used to treat an exacerbation. Adjusting medications, by increasing the short-acting beta agonist (SABA) or adding a short course of oral systemic corticosteroids, is recommended. Doubling the dose of inhaled corticosteroids (ICSs) is generally not effective. A drop in the PEFR of 40% to 69% from the patient's personal best is a marker of a moderate-severity asthma exacerbation that requires an in-office visit or emergency department visit and the use of an oral steroid. A drop in the PEFR of more than 40% from the patient's personal best will likely require hospitalization.

Ongoing therapy for asthma can be tailored accordingly to the NHLBI guideline's six-step treatment approach for all patients 12 years of age or older with asthma (Figure 48-2).[6] Intermittent asthma can be managed with the use of a SABA as needed. For all categories of persistent asthma, ICS is the preferred first line of therapy for the long-term control, especially in those with more severe asthma.[11,13] Additional therapies include long-acting beta agonist (LABA), leukotrine receptor antagonist (LTRA: montelukast, zileuton), methylxanthine derivatives (theophylline), anticholinergic agents (ipratropium or tiotropium), cromones (cromolyn), or anti-IgE therapy (omalizumab). Addition of these therapies to ICS treatment can be considered on a case-by-case basis based on severity, lack of control, and presence of other comorbid conditions (Table 48-4). However it

TABLE 48-3	Assessment of Asthma Control			
Components of Control		**Classification of Asthma Control (Youths ≥12 years of age and adults)**		
		Well-Controlled	*Not Well-Controlled*	*Very Poorly Controlled*
Impairment	Symptoms	≤2 days/week	>2 days/week	Throughout the day
	Nighttime awakening	≤2x/month	1-3x/week	≥4x/week
	Interference with normal activity	None	Some limitation	Extremely limited
	Short-acting beta₂-agonist use for symptom control (not prevention of EIB)	≤2 days/week	>2 days/week	Several times per day
	FEV₁ or peak flow	>80% predicted/ personal best	60-80% predicted/ personal best	<60% predicted/ personal best
	Validated Questionnaires			
	ATAQ	0	1-2	3-4
	ACQ	≤0.75*	≥1.5	N/A
	ACT	≥20	16-19	≤15
Risk	Exacerbations	0-1/year	≥2/year	
		Consider severity and interval since last exacerbation.		
	Progressive loss of lung function	Evaluation requires long-term follow-up care.		
	Treatment-related adverse effects	Medication side effects can vary in intensity from none to very troublesome and worrisome. The level of intensity does not correlate to specific levels of control but should be considered in the overall assessment of risk.		

Modified from Expert Panel Report 3 (EPR-3): Guidelines for the diagnosis and management of asthma-summary report 2007. J Allergy Clin Immunol 2007;20(5 Suppl):S94-138.

ACQ, Asthma Control Questionnaire; *ACT,* Asthma Control Test; *ATAQ,* Asthma Therapy Assessment Questionnaire; *EIB,* exercise induced bronchoconstriction

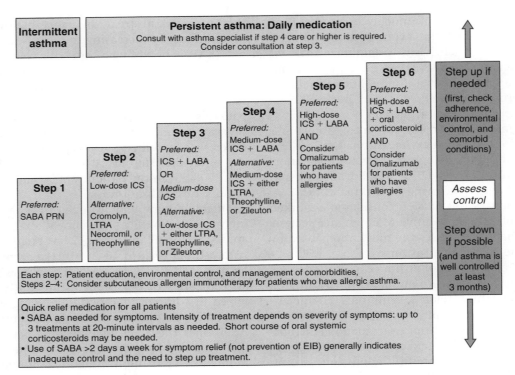

Figure 48-2 **Stepwise approach for managing asthma.** (Reproduced from Expert Panel Report 3 [EPR-3]: Guidelines for the diagnosis and management of asthma-summary report 2007. J Allergy Clin Immunol 2007;120[5 Suppl]:S94-138.) EIB, exercise induced bronchoconstriction.

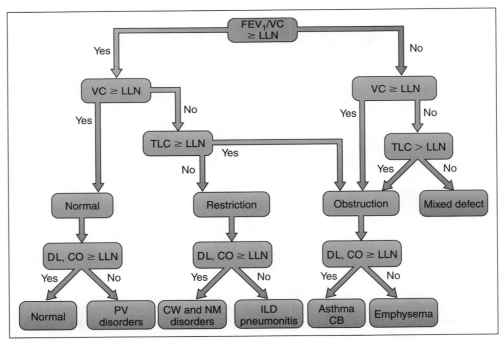

Figure 48-3 Patients may or may not present with the classic patterns, depending on co-morbidity, severity, and lung function prior to the disease onset. The decisions about how far to follow this diagram are clinical and will vary depending on the questions being asked and the clinical information available at the time of testing.

The forced expiratory volume in one second (FEV1)/ VC ratio and VC should be considered first. Total lung capacity (TLC) is necessary to confirm or exclude the presence of a restrictive defect when VC is below the lower limit of normal (LLN). The algorithm also includes diffusing capacity for carbon monoxide (DL,CO) measurement with the predicted value adjusted for hemoglobin. In the mixed defect group, the DL,CO patterns are the same as those for restriction and obstruction.

CB, chronic bronchitis; CW, chest wall; ILD, interstitial lung diseases; NM, neuromuscular; PV, pulmonary vascular. Modified from Pellegrino, R., et al., Interpretative strategies for lung function tests. Eur Respir J, 2005. 26(5): p. 948-68.

TABLE 48-4	Medications for the Management of Asthma in the Older Adult		
Medication	**Common Side Effects**	**Safety/Monitoring**	**Level of Evidence for Effectiveness***
Inhaled corticosteroids (ICS)	Oral or esophageal candidiasis, dysphonia, cough, skin thinning, osteopenia/osteoporosis(level C) and possible glaucoma	N/A	A
Long-acting bronchodilators (LABA)	Tremors, arrhythmia, and hypokalemia	Must be used in combination with ICS in asthma due to increased risk of deaths and severe exacerbations otherwise	B[‡]
Leukotrine receptor antagonist (LTRA; e.g., montelukast)	Neuropsychiatric side effects including suicidal behavior	N/A	A[§]
Zileuton	Jaundice, neuropsychiatric side effects including suicidal behavior	Liver function test monitoring	D
Methylxanthines (e.g., theophylline)	Multiple drug–drug interactions, arrhythmias, grand mal convulsions, hypercalcemia	Serum concentration levels	B
Anticholinergic agents (e.g., ipratropium and tiotropium)	Urinary retention, tachycardia, dry mouth, blurry vision, constipation	N/A	B
Inhaled cromolyn/nedocromil	None significant	N/A	B
Systemic corticosteroids	Increased appetite, weight gain, mood and behavior changes, insomnia, diabetes, osteoporosis/osteopenia, glaucoma, CHF exacerbation, immunosuppression, hypertension, GERD, myopathy	Diabetes screening, bone densitometry, and evaluation for glaucoma	A
Omalizumab[†]	Anaphylaxis (frequency 0.09%-0.2%)	N/A	B
Allergen immunotherapy (AIT)[†]	Asthma exacerbation, anaphylaxis	FEV_1 must be >70% of predicted with good asthma control prior to initiation of AIT	B

Table modified from: Expert Panel Report 3 (EPR-3): Guidelines for the Diagnosis and Management of Asthma-Summary Report 2007. J Allergy Clin Immunol, 2007. 120(5 Suppl): p. S94-138.

N/A, Not applicable.

[*]A = supported by one or more high quality randomized control trials; B = supported by one or more high-quality nonrandomized cohort studies or low-quality randomized control trials; C = supported by one or more case series and/or poor-quality cohort and/or case-control studies; D = supported by expert opinion and/or extrapolation from studies in other populations or settings; X = evidence supports the treatment being ineffective or harmful.

[†]AIT is used during steps 2-4 of the NHLBI's Stepwise Approach on Asthma Management guidelines for those patients with evidence of allergic asthma only. Omalizumab is used during steps 5-6 of the NHLBI's Stepwise Approach on Asthma Management guidelines for those patients with evidence of allergic asthma only. Clinicians who administer AIT or omalizumab must be equipped and prepared to recognize and manage anaphylaxis that may occur.

[‡]Level A when used in combination with ICS for steps 1-3 of the NHLBI's Stepwise Approach on Asthma Management guidelines.

[§]Level B for step 4 of the NHLBI's Stepwise Approach on Asthma Management guidelines.

should be noted that in 2010 the U.S. Food and Drug Administration indicated that the addition of LABAs to the therapeutic regimen of patients with poorly controlled asthma could worsen outcomes, particularly in African Americans and those not using ICSs. Therefore, a LABA should not be added until the patient has tried a medium-dose ICS first. Patients with severe asthma whose symptoms are not well controlled with high-dose ICS or combination therapy may require oral corticosteroids for maintenance of asthma control. If possible, an alternate day regimen may help reduce the systemic risks of oral corticosteroids as listed in Table 48-4 while still maintaining control (referred to as the minimal effective dose).

If asthma is not adequately controlled on the current regimen, then a stepping-up of therapy after ensuring medication compliance, proper technique, and avoidance of risk factors should be considered. Usually improvement should be noted in 1 month of therapy initiation. Risk and benefits, costs, and the patient's satisfaction with the level of control should also be discussed. Once asthma control is achieved for 3 months, a gradual step-down of therapy to the threshold amount of medications needed to maintain control should be considered. It is important to keep in mind that patients with cough variant asthma may have negative objective testing for asthma but will show improvement of symptoms with use of an ICS.

Preventive Maintenance

Asthma is a dynamic disease and ongoing monitoring is required. The goal of asthma therapy is to reduce the functional impairment in performing daily activities, maintain normal lung function, and prevent frequent use of SABA. Spirometry should be performed on at least a yearly basis to monitor control of asthma and, in some cases, may need to be done as frequently as once every 3 to 6 months. In addition, therapy should be targeted to reduce risk of future exacerbations, emergency room visits, or hospitalizations, and provide optimal pharmacotherapy with minimal or no adverse side effects.[11,12] For patients on ICS with increased risk of osteopenia or osteoporosis, daily supplementation with calcium and vitamin D may be recommended.[6] The Centers for Disease Control recommends that patients with asthma should receive an influenza vaccine annually to prevent complications from influenza.[6]

CASE 2

Jennifer Johnson (Part 1)

Jennifer Johnson, a 70-year-old woman, comes to your office for increasing shortness of breath on exertion, which she has had for more than 2 years. She states that she used to walk 1 mile daily. However, over the last 6 months, she has reduced routine exercise and needs to stop to catch her breath frequently. She has attributed this change to getting old. She was told 2 years earlier that she had "slight bronchitis" and was given an inhaler to use only when she was symptomatic, which helped minimally. In the last 6 months, she had three trips to the emergency department for recurrent bronchitis. She smoked one pack of cigarettes a day for the past 35 years, but stopped 6 months ago when she started to get worse. Spirometry performed in your office showed an FEV_1/FVC of 58% (below the lower limit of normal) and an FEV_1 of 62% of predicted. FVC was essentially normal. There was no significant change in her FEV_1 after the use of a SABA. Her diffusing capacity of the lung for carbon monoxide

corrected for alveolar volume (DLCO/VA) was below the lower limit of normal.

What is Mrs. Johnson's diagnosis and how would you manage her symptoms? ▣

Chronic Obstructive Pulmonary Disease (COPD)

Definition and Epidemiology

COPD is a common disease characterized by chronic, persistent, and progressive inflammation and irreversible airflow limitation. COPD is the fourth leading cause of death worldwide among both men and women.[14] The prevalence of COPD in the United States is approximated to be between 15 and 17 million.[15,16] COPD is thought to be equally prevalent in men and women in developed nations because of trends in tobacco smoking.[16] The BOLD study has estimated the worldwide prevalence of COPD among never-smokers to be 3% to 11%.[17] In addition to alpha-1-antitrypsin deficiency, which is the best known genetic risk factor for COPD, environmental tobacco smoke (ETS), age older than 40 years, cumulative exposure to ambient air pollutants including biomass fuels, occupational exposures to organic and inorganic dust and chemical particles, and tuberculosis are all risk factors for COPD.[14] In the longitudinal cohort of the Tucson Epidemiological Study of Airway Obstructive Disease, adults with asthma had a twelvefold higher risk of acquiring COPD than those without asthma.[18] Despite being a preventable and treatable disease, the morbidity and mortality of COPD is projected to dramatically increase over the next few years owing to chronic exposure to risk factors and the aging population.[14,19]

COPD is made up of a collection of three different processes that contribute to the disease pathology and symptomatology: chronic or recurrent bronchitis (presence of cough or sputum production for 3 months or longer for 2 consecutive years), emphysema (caused by parenchymal destruction and loss of elastic recoil), and airway responsiveness (caused by chronic inflammation leading to structural changes and airway narrowing). Chronic inflammation leads to narrowing of the peripheral airways, which in turn leads to a decrease in FEV_1 and FEV_1/FVC ratio and an increase in air trapping with resultant hyperinflation (measured by an increase in the functional residual capacity). These changes cause dyspnea and limited exercise capacity. Parenchymal destruction (along with a depressed ventilator drive) leads to decreased gas exchange, manifested as hypoxia, hypercapnia, and a depressed diffusing capacity of the lung for carbon monoxide (DLCO). Pulmonary hypertension may develop late in the course of COPD because of hypoxic vasoconstriction of pulmonary arteries and vascular smooth muscle hyperplasia, and if uncontrolled may lead to signs and symptoms of cor pulmonale.

Diagnosis

The section later in the chapter on evaluation of pulmonary disease discusses detailed information on how to evaluate a patient with signs and symptoms suggestive of COPD. Briefly, all patients with suspected COPD should be evaluated to confirm the objective diagnosis of COPD. Because it is a disease of irreversible airflow limitation, confirmatory tests would include spirometry with an irreversible obstructive defect. Hyperinflation and changes in diffusing capacity can also be measured if lung volumes and diffusion studies are ordered.

TABLE 48-5	Staging of COPD Based on Severity of Airflow Obstruction (for All Patients with Postbronchodilator $FEV_1/FVC < 70\%$)	
COPD Stage/Grade	**Severity**	**FEV_1 (% predicted)**
I	Mild	$\geq 80\%$
II	Moderate	$50\% \leq FEV_1 < 80\%$
III	Severe	$30\% \leq FEV_1 < 50\%$
IV	Very Severe	$30\% \leq FEV_1$

Table modified from Global Initiative for Chronic Obstructive Lung Disease. Global strategy for the diagnosis, management, and prevention of chronic obstructive pulmonary disease, 2011 guidelines. http://www.goldcopd.org.

> A diagnosis of COPD made in the clinical context of patients who have dyspnea and chronic cough with sputum production in setting of exposure to risk factors (including but not limited to tobacco smoke exposure) needs to be confirmed by spirometry.

Treatment

The goals of COPD assessment are to determine the severity of airflow limitation using the objective tests mentioned below, determine the impact of disease on the quality of life, and determine the risk of future exacerbations, hospital admissions, or death. Weighing the risks and benefits these factors can then be used to guide COPD therapy and help with the management of risk factors and comorbidities, such as cardiovascular disease, lung cancer, sarcopenia, osteoporosis, and depression. Criteria for staging of COPD are based on airflow limitation (Table 48-5). The COPD Assessment Test (CAT) is a validated questionnaire that can assess COPD symptoms on follow-up visits. A score of 10 or higher on the CAT indicates

poor control of symptoms. Up to 20% of patients with stage II COPD will have frequent exacerbations needing treatment with systemic steroids and antibiotics. The risk of exacerbations goes up with each stage. Patients with two or more exacerbations, regardless of their stage, are considered high risk for future exacerbations. The 2011 GOLD guidelines recommend using severity based on airflow limitation, the risk of exacerbations, and the CAT score to divide patients into four categories based on low versus high risk and less versus more symptoms (Table 48-6).[14,19] This approach then helps tailor management with therapy. In addition to these measures, the risks and benefits, costs, the patient's ability to physically use an inhaler, and inhaler technique should be evaluated at each visit as part of the treatment plan.

Table 48-7 outlines the treatment of COPD. Bronchodilator medications are central to symptom management in COPD. Regular use of LABA or as-needed use of SABA improves FEV_1, dyspnea, and reduces exacerbation rates. The use of LABA and long-acting anticholinergics is preferred over short-acting formulations of both.[14] Multiple studies have shown that the

TABLE 48-6	Categorization of COPD Patients Based on Symptoms, Airway Limitation, and Risk of Exacerbation		
Category	**Symptom Score**	**Risk of Exacerbation (No. per year)**	**Airway limitation (Stage)**
A (Low risk, Less symptoms)	CAT <10	0, 1	I, II
B (Low risk, More symptoms)	CAT ≥10	0, 1	I, II
C (High risk, Less symptoms)	CAT <10	≥2	III, IV
D (High risk, More symptoms)	CAT ≥10	≥2	III, IV

Table modified from Global Initiative for Chronic Obstructive Lung Disease. Global strategy for the diagnosis, management, and prevention of chronic obstructive pulmonary disease, 2011 guidelines. http://www.goldcopd.org.
When assessing choose the highest risk according to stage or exacerbation history.
CAT, COPD Assessment Test.

TABLE 48-7	Medications for the Management of COPD in the Geriatric Population			
Medication	**Used for COPD Category (in order of preference)**	**Common Side Effects**	**Safety/ Monitoring Needed**	**Level of Evidence for Effectiveness***
Short-acting beta$_2$-agonist (SABA)	A, B, C, D	Tremors, arrhythmia, hypokalemia	N/A	A, B
Long-acting beta$_2$-agonist (LABA)	B, A			
Short-acting anticholinergics	A, B, C, D	Urinary retention, tachycardia, dry mouth, blurry vision, constipation	N/A	A, B
Long-acting anticholinergics	B, C, D, A			
Combination bronchodilator therapy (e.g., combi-vent)	A, B, C, D	See above	N/A	B
Methylxanthines (e.g., theophylline)	A, B, C, D†	Multiple drug–drug interactions due to metabolism by CYP450, arrhythmias, grand mal convulsions, hypercalcemia	Serum concentration levels	B
Combination ICS and LABA	C, D	See above and pneumonia	N/A	A (in severe COPD), B
Mucolytics/antitussives/ antioxidants	Used as adjunct therapy during exacerbations	N/A	N/A	D, B‡
Systemic corticosteroids	Used during exacerbations	Increased appetite, weight gain, mood and behavior changes, insomnia, diabetes, osteoporosis/ osteopenia, glaucoma, CHF exacerbation, immunosuppression, hypertension, GERD, myopathy	N/A	A
Antibiotics	Used in treatment of COPD exacerbations due to an infectious cause	Specific to type of antibiotic used	Specific to type of antibiotic used	B

Table modified from Global Initiative for Chronic Obstructive Lung Disease. Global strategy for the diagnosis, management, and prevention of chronic obstructive pulmonary disease, 2011 guidelines. http://www.goldcopd.org.
CHF, Congestive heart failure; *CYP450*, cytochrome P450; *GERD*, gastroesophageal reflux disease; *ICS*, inhaled corticosteroid.
Long-term monotherapy with ICSs is never used in the treatment of COPD.
*A = supported by one or more high-quality randomized control trials; B = supported by one or more high-quality nonrandomized cohort studies or low-quality randomized control trials; C = supported by one or more case series and/or poor-quality cohort and/or case-control studies; D = supported by expert opinion and/or extrapolation from studies in other populations or settings; X = evidence supports the treatment being ineffective or harmful.
†Third line of treatment in addition to other classes of medications being used.
‡For the use of N-acetylcysteine.

use of combination SABA or LABA with short- or long-acting anticholinergics has been shown to produce a greater improvement in FEV$_1$ than either class alone, with an added benefit of lower tachyphylaxis. The benefits of ICSs in COPD are controversial. Their role in the management of stable COPD is recommended in those patients with an FEV$_1$ less than 60%. Use of ICS in this group significantly improves symptoms, quality of life, FEV$_1$, and lowers the risk of exacerbations.[14] Similarly, combination ICS with a LABA

is recommended for those with moderate-severe COPD. Regular use of mucolytics and antitussives in stable COPD has very small benefit. Hence widespread use of these agents is not recommended. Prophylactic use of antibiotics other than for treating infectious causes of COPD exacerbations is not recommended.[14]

Management of COPD also involves recognizing and treating exacerbations, which are precipitated most commonly by viral upper respiratory infections or bronchitis. The goal of treatment of acute exacerbations is to minimize their impact and to reduce the risk of future exacerbations. SABA and short-acting anticholinergic agents are the preferred bronchodilators for treatment of COPD exacerbations. Use of systemic steroids and antibiotics can shorten the hospital stay and improve FEV_1 and hypoxia. Indications for hospital admissions include older age, a marked increase in intensity of symptoms (with worsening resting dyspnea), severe underlying COPD or frequent exacerbations, new onset of cyanosis or peripheral edema, altered mental status, failure of symptoms to respond effectively to home medications, or the presence of serious comorbid conditions.

In addition to pharmacotherapy, patients with an FEV_1 less than 35% or with clinical signs of respiratory or right-sided heart failure should have pulse oximetry to evaluate for hypoxia. Long-term oxygen therapy should be initiated in those who have a SaO_2 88% or lower, with or without hypercapnia, and those with pulmonary hypertension, polycythemia, or congestive heart failure (CHF). A minimum of 6 weeks of pulmonary rehabilitation has been shown to improve exercise capacity, strength, endurance, quality of life, and overall survival with reduced hospitalizations and the intensity of breathlessness in COPD patient categories B to D (see Table 48-6).[14]

> Smoking cessation has the greatest longitudinal impact on the outcome of COPD; hence smoking cessation counseling should be provided at every health care visit.

Preventive Maintenance

Identification and reduction of exposure to risk factors is necessary for reduction of symptoms and risks of COPD. Smoking cessation has the greatest longitudinal impact on the outcome of COPD. Smoking cessation counseling should therefore be provided at every

health care visit.[20] Routine follow-up is essential in the care of COPD. At each visit, one should discuss monitoring symptom control, address management of comorbid conditions, and discuss use of medications and side effects, as well as avoidance of exposure to risk factors including smoking cessation. In those with stable COPD, spirometry should be performed at least once a year. Yearly influenza vaccine is recommended in all patients with COPD and pneumococcal vaccine in those older than 65 years to reduce the risk of pneumonia, hospitalization, and death.

CASE 3

Fred Barnes (Part 1)

Fred Barnes, a 65-year-old male with hypertension, hyperlipidemia, diabetes, coronary artery disease, hypothyroidism, and reflux comes to your office for the evaluation of dyspnea (Table 48-8). His dyspnea started 2 years ago with some worsening over time. He reports no wheezing but has coughing. He denies chest pain, palpitations, dizziness, and hospital visits for dyspnea. Mr. Barnes quit smoking 25 years ago and has a 30 pack-year tobacco history. Cardiac evaluation to date, including echocardiogram and nuclear stress test, has not revealed acute cardiac disease. Except for obesity, his exam is essentially normal. Pulmonary function testing is performed.

What major pattern of respiratory disease do you see in this patient? ◘

RESTRICTIVE PULMONARY DISEASES IN THE OLDER ADULT

Restrictive lung diseases are a category of respiratory diseases in which there is a restriction of lung expansion. This restriction results in decreased lung volume, increased work of breathing, and inadequate ventilation and/or oxygenation. Two examples of restrictive lung disease in the geriatric population are obesity and idiopathic pulmonary fibrosis.

TABLE 48-8	Case 3 Spirometry Results						
	Baseline				**Post**		
	Actual	*Predicted*	*% Predicted*	*LLN*	*Actual*	*% Change*	*% Predicted*
Spirometry							
FVC (L)	2.45	5.03	49	4.02	2.52	3	50
FEV_1 (L)	1.85	3.76	49	2.92	1.93	4	51
FEV_1/FVC (%)	75	75	100	65	77	2	102
Lung Volumes							
TLC (L)	4.83	7.63	63	6.23			
Diffusion							
DLCO/VA	4.99	3.95	126	2.49			

DLCO/VA, diffusing capacity of the lung for carbon monoxide corrected for alveolar volume; *FEV1,* forced expiratory volume in 1 second; *FVC,* forced vital capacity; *LLN,* lower limit of normal; *TLC,* total lung capacity; *VA,* alveolar volume.

Obesity

Definition and Epidemiology

The prevalence of obesity (body mass index [BMI] above 30) in older adults in the United States is increasing, with an estimated 37% of men and 42% of women older than age 60 being obese in 2010.[21] Adults aged 60 years and over and older women were more likely to be obese than younger adults and older men. Men tend to have central obesity (with increased adipose tissue in the anterior chest wall, anterior abdominal wall, and visceral organs), whereas women tend to have peripheral obesity.

Pathophysiology

The effects of obesity on pulmonary function are complex. Besides the physical changes, obesity also leads to mechanical changes in the lungs. Many obese patients have breathlessness on exertion along with wheezing. Weight gain causes reduced FEV_1 and FVC, increased FEV_1/FVC ratio of more than 70%, and reduced end residual volume (ERV). Central obesity lowers chest wall compliance, limits lung and diaphragmatic movement, and increases airway resistances, hence increasing the work of breathing and airway resistance.[22] These changes lead to ventilation–perfusion abnormalities and arterial hypoxemia, particularly on exertion and in the supine position.

Obesity results in increased morbidity and mortality from asthma and COPD. Studies have shown that an elevated BMI in older asthmatic patients is strongly associated with poorer asthma symptom control and increased asthma exacerbations. Moreover, obese asthmatics are more than 5 times as likely to have poorly controlled asthma as nonobese asthmatic adults.[22,23] In addition, this obese asthmatic subset of patients may represent a distinct asthma phenotype whose symptoms may be poorly responsive to corticosteroids because of a characteristically unique inflammatory pathophysiology. The risks of developing obstructive sleep apnea (OSA) and obesity hypoventilation syndrome are significantly higher with higher BMI. OSA is characterized by repeated obstructive apneas caused by a collapsible upper airway from failure of neuromuscular control of the pharyngeal dilatory muscles while asleep.

Treatment

Weight loss in obese persons of any age has been shown to improve obesity-related complications, physical function, and the quality of life. Lifestyle interventions, including a low calorie diet, increased physical activity, goal setting, and providing the necessary social support, are just as effective in older subjects as younger ones. At the present time there is insufficient data from clinical studies to support the use of weight loss medications or surgeries in patients older than 60 years.[24]

Idiopathic Pulmonary Fibrosis

Definition and Epidemiology

Idiopathic pulmonary fibrosis (IPF) is defined as a specific form of chronic, progressive fibrosing interstitial pneumonia of unknown cause, primarily occurring in older adults, limited to the basilar lungs, that is associated with dyspnea, progressive decline in lung function, and radiologic pattern of interstitial infiltrates.[25] IPF generally presents in the fifth and sixth decades of life and is more common in older men than women. The annual incidence is estimated at 27 to 76 per 100,000 in those older than 75 years of age.[26] The prevalence in adults older than 65 years of age is estimated to be 29 to 277 per 100,000.[26]

Pathophysiology

The unique histopathology of IPF is characterized by lesions of varying age, comprised of areas of acute lung injury that then sequentially progress to chronic areas of fixed parenchymal fibrosis with honeycombing and foci with proliferating fibroblasts and myofibroblasts. In large epidemiologic studies, environmental factors such as exposure to tobacco smoke may be important in the pathogenesis of idiopathic pulmonary fibrosis. In most reported case series, up to 75% of index patients with IPF were noted to be current or former smokers.[25] In addition, association between IPF and exposure to latent viral infections, especially the herpes virus family, has been reported. Even though no occupational exposures (such as silica, asbestosis, etc.) have been linked strongly as a cause of IPF, a detailed history regarding possible occupational exposures should be obtained to rule out pneumoconiosis.

Diagnosis

The typical symptoms of IPF are dyspnea on exertion and a nonproductive cough.[25] The physical examination in most patients reveals fine bibasilar inspiratory crackles. Clubbing is seen in up to 50% of patients. Later in the disease process, signs of severe pulmonary hypertension and cor pulmonale may become apparent in patients with progressing IPF. Spirometry typically reveals a restrictive ventilatory defect with an increased FEV_1/FVC ratio of more than 70%, and a reduction in total lung capacity (TLC) to less than 80%; decreased lung compliance also leads to diminished functional residual capacity (FRC) and residual volume (RV). However, patients who smoke may also have a concurrent obstructive ventilatory defect.[25] Impairments in gas exchange may be demonstrated by a decrease in the DLCO or by hypoxemia during graded exercise testing. A chest radiograph or chest CT in IPF will show bilateral patchy reticular opacities most prominent in the periphery and in the lower lobes, irregular septal thickening, subpleural honeycombing caused by fibrosis, and bronchiectasis. Lung biopsy remains the standard for diagnosing IPF, and optimal evaluation requires biopsies from several sites, necessitating referral to a pulmonologist.

Treatment

At present the treatment of IPF remains largely supportive, with evidence that the patient's survival may be improved by referral to a pulmonologist or centers specializing in the evaluation of interstitial lung diseases.[25] Median survival after diagnosis of IPF is 3 years. Therefore, after diagnosis a prompt evaluation for lung transplantation should be obtained, especially in patients younger than 55 years of age and without complicating comorbid conditions. The incidence of bronchogenic carcinoma is increased in patients with IPF.

OBJECTIVE EVALUATION OF PULMONARY DISEASES

When evaluating a patient with complaints involving the pulmonary system, in addition to a detailed history and physical examination, objective tests must show the presence of airflow obstruction (with or without reversibility) or restriction. This evaluation can be done with the use of spirometry or methacholine provocation testing. The use of home peak flow monitoring or in-office fraction exhaled nitric oxide measurement may offer additional benefit not only in diagnosing disease but in monitoring control or loss of control of pulmonary symptoms specifically related to asthma. Last but not least, in the absence of objective evidence for obstructive or restrictive lung disease, additional studies and imaging modalities may be needed for evaluating other possible diagnoses that manifest with pulmonary symptoms (as listed in Table 48-1).

Spirometry

Spirometry is a pulmonary function test (PFT) that measures lung function, specifically the flow and volume of air that can be exhaled and inhaled. Airflow limitation in both asthma and COPD can be best be measured by spirometry, the most widely available test of lung function. With consistent patient effort, spirometry is also the most reproducible test of lung function. Spirometry is used to demonstrate obstruction and assess reversibility of the underlying lung pathology. The routine use of spirometry in the diagnosis of obstructive diseases is considered a clinical standard of practice. Office spirometers are now widely available for use in primary care offices, and several studies emphasized the importance of using spirometry in a primary care setting as a screening tool for the early detection of obstructive or restrictive lung disease. Because spirometry is used as a screening and a confirmatory test, the precise sensitivity and specificity for the test do not exist.

Spirometry should measure the volume of air forcibly exhaled for at least 6 seconds from the point of maximal inspiration (forced vital capacity, FVC) and the volume of air exhaled during the first second of this maneuver (forced expiratory volume in 1 second, FEV_1). The ratio of FEV_1 to FVC is calculated. The reference values for these are based on age, height, sex, and race. Simplified algorithms are available to aid in the interpretation of spirometric measures (Figure 48-2).[27]

Guidelines for the diagnosis of asthma and reversibility are determined by an increase in FEV_1 of 12% and 200 mL from baseline after inhalation of a short-acting bronchodilator.[6] When the pretest probability of asthma is high and the use of a SABA does not demonstrate reversibility in FEV_1, a short course of steroids followed by repeat spirometry can be used to demonstrate reversibility.

To make the diagnosis of COPD in the appropriate clinical context, a postbronchodilator FEV_1/FVC ratio of less than 70% is necessary.[14] The use of this ratio versus the cutoff based on the lower limit of normal (LLN) may result in more frequent diagnosis of COPD in the elderly population compared to those 45 years of age and younger. The postbronchodilator FEV_1 can then be used to grade the severity of COPD (see Table 48-5).

When diagnosis is restrictive lung disease such as that caused by obesity or IPF, spirometry will reveal a restrictive ventilatory defect with an increased FEV_1/FVC ratio and reduction in TLC of less than 80% predicted.

> The use of spirometry is essential in the diagnosis and management of obstructive lung diseases such as asthma and COPD.

Methacholine Bronchoprovocation Challenge Test

Methacholine bronchoprovocation challenge test (MCCT) is a method of evaluating airway hyperresponsiveness. MCCT is most useful in excluding a diagnosis of asthma; this is because the test has a higher negative predictive value and sensitivity than positive predictive value.[28] An MCCT can also be used when the pretest probability of asthma is high and results of spirometry are inconclusive.

A positive MCCT test is considered to be a drop in FEV_1 of 20% or more from baseline at any concentration of methacholine less than 4 mg/mL. This dose is defined at the PC_{20} (provocation concentration). Bronchial responsiveness may be decreased by certain factors such as use of SABA, LABA, anticholinergic inhaler, theophylline, antihistamines, antileukotriene agents, or the consumption of caffeine in the past 8 to 48 hours before testing.

Absolute contraindications for performing an MCCT are severe airflow limitation with FEV_1 below 50% of predicted or less than 1 L, history of a heart attack or stroke in the last 3 months, uncontrolled hypertension (systolic blood pressure above 200 and diastolic blood pressure above 100), or a known aortic aneurysm. Relative contraindications to performing an MCCT are moderate airflow limitation with FEV_1 less than 60% predicted or less than 1.5 L, inability to perform acceptable quality spirometry, or current use of cholinesterase inhibitor medications such as for myasthenia gravis. Also, patients who are concurrently receiving beta-blockers may have exaggerated or prolonged responses (i.e., bronchoconstriction) to methacholine challenge and may not respond readily to treatment; therefore use of beta-blockers is contraindicated for performing MCCT.

Peak Expiratory Flow Rate Monitoring

A peak expiratory flow rate (PEFR) is the maximum airflow rate measured during forceful exhalation starting from full inhalation using a peak flow meter device readily available by prescription at pharmacies. PEFR is measured in liters per minute. Standard values are based on sex, age, and height. Self-monitoring at home can be used to assess the level of asthma control and signs of worsening asthma. Home PEFR monitoring is particularly helpful for patients who have difficulty perceiving symptoms, a history of severe exacerbations, or moderate or severe asthma.

PEFR can categorize patients into the green (PEFR 80% to 100% of personal best), yellow (PEFR 50% to 80% of personal best), or red zone (PEFR less than 50% of personal best), and thereby guides appropriate treatment actions. A greater than 20% (or 60 L/min) improvement in the postbronchodilator PEFR or a diurnal variation in the PEFR of more than 20% or more than 10% with twice daily reading over a 2- to 4-week period suggests a diagnosis of asthma.[12] Peak flow monitoring cannot be used reliably to diagnose COPD.[14]

Fractional Exhaled Nitric Oxide Measurement

Fractional exhaled nitric oxide (FeNO) measurement is a complementary, standardized, noninvasive, and quantitative tool for diagnosing and monitoring airway inflammation (specifically asthma) that can be easily performed in an office setting. During an inflammatory state, such as asthma, several cell types including eosinophils upregulate *inducible* nitric oxide synthase (*i*NOS) that synthesizes nitric oxide. Measurement of fractional nitric oxide concentration in exhaled breath therefore provides a good measure of airway inflammation. FeNO is generally elevated in patients with asthma who are not on ICS.[29]

Evidence-based guidelines for the interpretation of FeNO measurements are listed in Table 48-9. In addition, FeNO measurements can be used to diagnose eosinophilic airway inflammation, to determine the likelihood of responsiveness of individuals with chronic respiratory symptoms possibly caused by airway inflammation related to ICS, and to unmask nonadherence to corticosteroid therapy. The role of FeNO measurements in COPD is still unclear.

Pulmonary Imaging

Radiographic imaging may show structural changes, such as hyperinflation of the lungs with flattening of the diaphragm or increase in the volume of the retrosternal air space, that may occur as a result of the underlying disease pathology. The routine use of a chest x-ray study or computed tomography (CT) of the lungs is not recommended in making the diagnosis of asthma or COPD.[14] Such imaging techniques may be useful for establishing the presence of comorbid conditions such as pneumonia, pulmonary fibrosis, bronchiectasis, allergic bronchopulmonary aspergillosis (ABPA), lung cancer, and cardiac disease. A chest CT is also helpful in determining the distribution of emphysematous changes if lung volume reduction surgery is planned. Such imaging techniques should be considered in patients with acute changes

TABLE 48-9	Interpreting Fractional Exhaled Nitric Oxide (FeNO) Levels
FeNO level	**Implications**
< 25 ppb	Eosinophilic inflammation and responsiveness to corticosteroids are less likely.
25-50 ppb	Implications unclear and should be interpreted cautiously with reference to clinical context.
> 50 ppb	Eosinophilic inflammation and in symptomatic patients responsiveness to corticosteroids are likely.

Table modified from Dweik RA, et al. An official ATS clinical practice guideline: Interpretation of exhaled nitric oxide levels (FeNO) for clinical applications. Am J Respir Crit Care Med 2011;184(5):602-15.
ppb, Parts per billion.

in symptoms that do not fit the clinical picture of asthma or COPD and those who are at risk for the mentioned comorbidities.

SUMMARY

Asthma, COPD, and restrictive lung diseases are common in older adults. Standards for diagnosis, acute symptom management, and preventive maintenance are outlined in validated clinical guidelines.

Web Resources

www.nhlbi.nih.gov/health/prof/lung/asthma/naci/discover/action-plans.htm. A written Asthma Action Plan from the National Heart, Lung, and Blood Institute.

www.ginasthma.org. Global Initiative for Asthma.

www.goldcopd.org. Global Initiative for Chronic Obstructive Lung Disease.

www.aaaai.org. American Academy of Allergy, Asthma and Immunology.

KEY REFERENCES

6. Expert Panel Report 3 (EPR-3). Guidelines for the Diagnosis and Management of Asthma-Summary Report 2007. J Allergy Clin Immunol 2007;120(5 Suppl):S94-138.

7. Reed CE. Asthma in the elderly: Diagnosis and management. J Allergy Clin Immunol 2010;126(4):681-7; quiz 688-9.

11. Attaining optimal asthma control. A practice parameter. J Allergy Clin Immunol 2005;116(5):S3-11.

12. Global Initiative for Asthma. Global Strategy for Asthma Management and Prevention, Global Initiative for Asthma (GINA) 2012. Available from: http://www.ginasthma.org/. Accessed July 5, 2013.

14. Global Initiative for Chronic Obstructive Lung Disease. Global Strategy for the Diagnosis, Management and Prevention of COPD, Global Initiative for Chronic Obstructive Lung Disease (GOLD) 2013. Available from: http://www.goldcopd.org/. Accessed July 5, 2013.

References available online at expertconsult.com.

49

Infectious Diseases

Suzanne F. Bradley

OBJECTIVES

*Upon completion of this chapter, the reader
will be able to:*

- Recognize the most common causes of
  infection in older adults.
- Understand how the causes of infections
  in older adults vary with the place of
  acquisition.
- Understand how the clinical presentation
  of infection differs with increasing age.
- Understand how to manage, treat, and
  prevent the most common infectious syndromes found in the older adult.

GENERAL PREVALENCE AND IMPACT

Despite medical advances, infection remains a major
cause of morbidity and mortality in the aged. When
considering causes of infection in older adults, it is
important to know where the infection was acquired, what infections are most common in those
settings, and what microorganisms cause those infections. Urinary tract infection (UTI), lower respiratory tract infection (LRTI), and skin and soft tissue
infection (SSTI) are the most common infectious

Additional online-only material indicated by icon.

syndromes seen among older adults regardless of whether the infection was acquired in the community, in a nursing home, or in a hospital. Bloodstream infections (BSI) are reported more frequently among older adults who are in hospital, whereas a wider variety of gastrointestinal (GI) infections are found among community-dwelling elderly and nursing home residents. Overall rates of infection in nursing homes and hospitals are similar, but those in chronic care settings are generally thought to be less severe.[1-5]

Microorganisms vary with the setting in which the infection is acquired. Infections are generally defined to be nursing home acquired or hospital acquired if the patient has been in the facility for at least 72 hours. Older adults may also acquire health care-associated infections even if they have not been hospitalized recently through contact with outpatient clinical settings such as a dialysis unit or outpatient intravenous therapy center.

Delayed recognition that an older patient is infected can result in delayed treatment. As a consequence, the elderly are more likely to die from their infections; their mortality is twofold to twentyfold higher than in young adults.[6-9]

GENERAL PATHOPHYSIOLOGY AND RISK FACTORS

Why the elderly are at increased risk of infection with poor outcome is a complex question. Predisposing risk factors for infection include immunosenescence, frailty with impaired functional status, increased prevalence of predisposing comorbid illnesses, exposure to pathogens within institutional settings, and complications of medical treatment.[10]

Changes in the immune system are found with normal aging. However, all aspects of the immune system of the older adult are not necessarily affected or depressed to the same degree. The most prominent impact of age is seen on the acquired or adaptive immune system. The adaptive immune system recognizes new infections through generation of specific T-lymphocytes and antibody-producing B-lymphocytes. Age-related defects have been described predominantly in T-cells. Other acquired conditions in the elderly, such as malnutrition, can contribute to further decline in T-cell function. T-cells are important for host defenses against pathogens that can reside within cells. Antibody production is essential to facilitate uptake and killing of encapsulated bacteria by phagocytic cells (Box 49-1). Neoplasms seen with increasing frequency in older adults can contribute to depressed antibody production and function. Defects in antibody response may explain why some responses to vaccinations and outcomes from infections are often poor in the aged.[11]

> **BOX 49-1**
>
> **INFECTIONS ASSOCIATED WITH AGE-ASSOCIATED CHANGES IN HOST DEFENSES**
>
> 1. Intracellular pathogens—T-cell mediated defects
>   *Listeria monocytogenes*
>   *Salmonella* spp.
>   *Legionella* spp.
>   Mycobacterial infections
>   Herpes zoster
> 2. Encapsulated bacteria—B-cell mediated defects/antibody production
>   *Streptococcus pneumoniae*

GENERAL PRINCIPLES OF DIAGNOSIS, ASSESSMENT, AND MANAGEMENT

Recognition that the older patient has an infection may be delayed in part because his or her symptoms and signs of infection are atypical. Clinicians may also ascribe complaints or abnormal physical findings or complaints to preexisting illnesses and not consider infection as the cause. In addition, cognitively impaired older adults may not be able to perceive symptoms of infection or communicate them to their healthcare provider.[12,13]

> Infections are not recognized in the elderly because their clinical presentation may be atypical.

The febrile response may be blunted or the onset delayed. Furthermore, appropriate increases in body temperature of 2° F or 1° C diagnostic of fever may not be recognized because the normal temperatures of older adults are lower at baseline. In addition, other markers of inflammation such as leukocytosis may be lacking. In one study, 48% of infected older adults were afebrile and 58% did not demonstrate significant leukocytosis. Because of a lack of an inflammatory response, more than half of older adults may not have localizing symptoms of infection, and focal findings for infection may be minimal or absent on physical examination.[13-24]

> Approximately half of infected older adults will not have localizing symptoms or findings on physical examination.

> Approximately half of infected older adults will not have a fever or have inflammation on laboratory examination.

Many older adults take medications with antiinflammatory effects, such as aspirin, acetaminophen, nonsteroidal antiinflammatory agents, corticosteroids, cytokine inhibitors, and antineoplastic agents that may further cloud the interpretation of the patient's history, physical examination, and laboratory findings. Therefore, it is not surprising that the diagnosis of infection is often missed or delayed in the elderly. Therefore, it is essential to consider infection in the older patient even if typical signs and symptoms are absent.[12-24]

Diagnosis of infection in older adults is further compromised by limited access to laboratory and diagnostic procedures in some settings. There is also a lack of diagnostic algorithms that have been specifically validated for use in the elderly. Recently, the McGeer Criteria were updated following a rigorous systematic review of the scientific literature related to the diagnosis of infectious syndromes in older adults.[25] Although these criteria are intended for the retrospective detection of infections acquired in nursing-home residents, they may provide a useful evidence-based conceptual framework for the clinician who is trying to diagnose infections in the elderly (Tables 49-1 to 49-4).

The following sections discuss a few aspects of the general diagnostic approach that have been shown to be of potential use in the assessment for infection in older adults.[13-29]

General Symptoms

Changes in Functional Status

An acute change in the ability to perform basic activities of daily living (ADLs) has been shown to be predictive of infection 77% of the time in nursing home residents. Acute change in functional status is a simple and potentially important clue that infection might be present.[12,13]

Confusion

The symptom of confusion or altered mental status has traditionally been closely associated with presence of infection in older people. Unfortunately, this terminology is vague and does not differentiate between new symptoms (delirium) that might herald the presence of a new problem such as infection versus more chronic conditions that alter mental status such as dementia, depression, and other psychiatric disorders. In addition, confusion and altered mental status do not provide any indication whether these chronic symptoms are stable or have acutely worsened.

General Signs and Laboratory Findings

Fever

A temperature of 101° F or higher is a highly specific indication of infection, but many older adults will not achieve this definition for fever. Alternative definitions for fever have been recommended as more sensitive means to detect infection in older adults. It has been shown that a fever threshold of 100° F or higher detects 70% of infections in nursing home residents with a specificity of 90%. Other definitions of fever in the elderly include a 2.4° F increase over baseline temperature or higher than 99° F orally or 99.5° F rectally.[13,25]

Dehydration

Dehydration may accompany fever and suggest possible infection in this population. Nonspecific findings of decreased oral intake, dry mucous membranes, or furrowed tongue could be important clues that fever and infection are present.[13,27-29]

Delirium

The Confusion Assessment Method can be performed rapidly to differentiate delirium from other chronic psychiatric conditions with high interobserver reliability, high sensitivity (>94%), and high specificity (90%-100%) (see Chapter 16).[13,25,26]

Complete Blood Count

A complete blood count is one laboratory test that has been shown to be highly predictive of infection in older adults. Presence of leukocytosis, neutrophilia, and left shift may be useful if present when evaluating the elderly patient with suspected infection (neutrophilia is present with >14,000 leukocytes/mm^3; left shift is present with >6% bands or ≥1500 bands/mm^3).[13,24,25]

Management

Empiric Therapy versus Culture-Based Treatment

The decision to start antibiotic therapy should be based on the patient's clinical condition. All patients with possible infection do not require urgent treatment. If urgent treatment is needed, then the choice of antibiotic should be based on the most likely clinical syndrome, the common organisms causing that condition, and knowledge of local antibiotic resistance patterns. Decision algorithms for when to begin treatment have been developed for nursing home residents (Table 49-5).[30-32]

The optimum route of antibiotic administration may be influenced by the severity of the patient's clinical condition and access to health care resources. Intravenous or intramuscular therapy may be preferred in the patient with an ileus in whom absorption of an oral antibiotic is not guaranteed. If intravenous therapy is preferred, broad-spectrum penicillins plus a beta-lactase inhibitor, second generation cephalosporins, and carbapenems generally treat a variety of

TABLE 49-1	Criteria For Urinary Tract Infection (UTI)
Criteria	**Comments**

A. Without an indwelling catheter:
Both criteria 1 and 2 present:
1. At least **one** of the following sign/symptom subcriteria (a-c) present:
  a. Acute dysuria or acute pain, swelling, or tenderness of the testes, epididymis, or prostate
  b. Fever or leukocytosis
and
At least **one** of the following localizing urinary tract subcriteria:
    i. Acute costovertebral angle pain or tenderness
    ii. Suprapubic pain
    iii. Gross hematuria
    iv. New or marked increase in incontinence
    v. New or marked increase in urgency
    vi. New or marked increase in frequency
  c. In the absence of fever or leukocytosis, then at least **two** or more of the following localizing urinary tract subcriteria:
    i. Suprapubic pain
    ii. Gross hematuria
    iii. New or marked increase in incontinence
    iv. New or marked increase in urgency
    v. New or marked increase in frequency
	UTI should be diagnosed when there are localizing genitourinary signs and symptoms and a positive urine culture.
	A diagnosis of urinary infection can be made without localizing symptoms if a blood culture isolate is the same as the organism isolated from the urine, and there is no alternate site of infection.
	In the absence of a clear alternate source, fever or rigors with a positive urine culture in the noncatheterized resident or acute confusion in the catheterized resident will often be treated as urinary tract infection. However, evidence suggests most of these episodes are likely not from a urinary source.
	Pyuria does not differentiate symptomatic UTI from asymptomatic bacteriuria.
	
	Absence of pyuria in diagnostic tests excludes symptomatic UTI in residents of long-term care facilities.

2. **One** of the following microbiologic subcriteria:
  a. $\geq 10^5$ cfu/mL of no more than two species of microorganisms in a voided urine
  b. $\geq 10^2$ cfu/mL of any number of organisms in a specimen collected by in and out catheter
	Urine specimens for culture should be processed as soon as possible, preferably within 1 to 2 hours. If urine specimens cannot be processed within 30 minutes of collection, they should be refrigerated. Refrigerated specimens should be cultured within 24 hours.

B. With an indwelling catheter:
Both criteria 1 and 2 present:
1. At least **one** of the following sign/symptom subcriteria (a-d) present:
  a. Fever, rigors, or new onset hypotension, with no alternate site of infection
  b. Either acute change in mental status or acute functional decline with no alternate diagnosis and leukocytosis
  c. New onset suprapubic pain or costovertebral angle pain or tenderness
  d. Purulent discharge from around the catheter or acute pain, swelling, or tenderness of the testes, epididymis, or prostate
	Recent catheter trauma, catheter obstruction, or new onset hematuria are useful localizing signs consistent with UTI, but not necessary for diagnosis.

2. Urinary catheter culture with $\geq 10^5$ cfu/mL of any organism(s)	Urinary catheter specimens for culture should be collected following replacement of the catheter (if current catheter has been in place >14 days).

Adapted from Stone ND, Ashraf MS, Calder J, et al. and the Society for Healthcare Epidemiology Long-Term Care Special Interest Group. Definitions of infection for surveillance in long-term care facilities: Revisiting the McGeer criteria. Infect Control Hosp Epidemiol 2012;33:965-77.
cfu/mL, colony forming units per microliter.

gram-positive cocci and gram-negative bacilli including methicillin-susceptible staphylococci (MSSA) and penicillin-susceptible enterococci. Penicillins cannot be given intramuscularly and many of the beta-lactam antibiotics are limited by their frequent dosing intervals.

If the patient is penicillin-allergic or if antibiotic resistance is a concern, combination therapy with several antibiotics may be necessary.

Ideally treatment should be based on results of cultures and antimicrobial susceptibilities. Duration of

TABLE 49-2	Criteria for Lower Respiratory Tract Infection (LRTI)
Criteria	**Comments**

A. Influenza-like illness:
Both criteria 1 and 2 present:
1. Fever
2. At least **three** of the following symptom subcriteria (a-f) present:
  a. Chills
  b. New headache or eye pain
  c. Myalgias or body aches
  d. Malaise or loss of appetite
  e. Sore throat
  f. New or increased dry cough
	If criteria for influenza-like illness and another upper or lower respiratory tract infection are met at the same time, only the diagnosis of influenza-like illness should be recorded.
	Because of increasing uncertainty surrounding the timing of the start of influenza season, the peak of influenza activity, and the length of the season, "seasonality" is no longer a criterion to define influenza-like illness.

B. Pneumonia:
All criteria 1-3 present:
1. Interpretation of a chest radiograph as demonstrating pneumonia or the presence of a new infiltrate
2. At least **one** of the following respiratory subcriteria (a-f):
  a. New or increased cough
  b. New or increased sputum production
  c. O_2 saturation < 94% on room air or a reduction in O_2 saturation of more than 3% from baseline
  d. New or changed lung exam abnormalities
  e. Pleuritic chest pain
  f. Respiratory rate of ≥25/min
3. At least **one** constitutional criterion
	For both pneumonia and lower respiratory tract infections, presence of underlying conditions that could mimic a respiratory tract infection presentation (e.g., congestive heart failure or interstitial lung diseases) should be excluded by a review of clinical records and an assessment of presenting symptoms and signs.

C. Lower respiratory tract (bronchitis or tracheobronchitis): **All** criteria 1-3 present: 1. Chest radiograph not performed, or negative for pneumonia or new infiltrate 2. At least **two** of the respiratory criteria (B. 2. a-f) listed above 3. At least **one** constitutional criterion	

Adapted from Stone ND, Ashraf MS, Calder J, et al. and the Society for Healthcare Epidemiology Long-Term Care Special Interest Group. Definitions of infection for surveillance in long-term care facilities: Revisiting the McGeer criteria. Infect Control Hosp Epidemiol 2012;33:965-77.

therapy should be based on the presumed clinical syndrome to be treated and the organism isolated. Oral therapy can be considered for some severe infections if the medication is 100% bioavailable, the patient is clinically stable, and he or she has a functional GI tract. Other considerations when choosing an antibiotic include cost, drug interactions, and toxicity. Appropriate adjustments in dose and frequency of administration should also be made for renal and hepatic dysfunction if present.

Antibiotic Resistance

In the past, we could assume that antimicrobial-resistant bacteria were found primarily in health care settings where antibiotic use is most intense. Methicillin-resistant *Staphylococcus aureus* (MRSA), vancomycin-resistant enterococci (VRE), multidrug-resistant *Streptococcus pneumoniae* (DRSP), and multidrug-resistant gram-negative bacilli are still found primarily in hospitals, nursing homes, and in patients recently discharged from those facilities. However, emergence of community-acquired MRSA (CA-MRSA) and multidrug-resistant gram-negative infections in healthy older people has become an increasing problem. Some strains of gram-negative bacilli, particularly *Escherichia coli* and *Klebsiella pneumoniae*, have become increasingly resistant to beta-lactam antibiotics because of the production of extended-spectrum beta-lactamases (ESBLs) and carbapenemases. These strains are typically resistant to all third- and fourth-generation cephalosporins (ceftazidime and cefepime), extended-spectrum penicillins (piperacillin), monobactams (aztreonam), and many other antibiotic classes (quinolones, sulfonamides). Dependence on the carbapenems (imipenem, meropenem, ertapenem) as the last resort to treat severe gram-negative infections is greatly threatened by the emergence of carbapenemase-producing strains.[33-37]

TABLE 49-3   Criteria for Skin and Soft Tissue Infection (SSTI)

Criteria	Comments

A. Cellulitis/soft tissue/wound infection
At least **one** of the following criteria present:
1. Pus present at a wound, skin, or soft tissue site
 	
2. New or increasing presence of at least **four** of the following sign/symptom subcriteria:
  a. Heat at the affected site
  b. Redness at the affected site
  c. Swelling at the affected site
  d. Tenderness or pain at the affected site
  e. Serous drainage at the affected site
  f. **One** constitutional criterion
	More than one patient with streptococcal skin infection from the same serogroup (e.g., A, B, C, G) in a health care institution may suggest an outbreak.
	For wound infections related to surgical procedures use the Centers for Disease Control and Prevention's National Healthcare Safety Network Surgical Site Infection criteria.
	Presence of organisms cultured from the surface (e.g., superficial swab culture) of a wound is not sufficient evidence that the wound is infected.

B. Scabies
Both criteria 1 and 2 present:
1. A maculopapular and/or itching rash
2. At least **one** of the following subcriteria:
  a. Physician diagnosis
  b. Laboratory confirmation (scraping or biopsy)
  c. Epidemiologic linkage to a case of scabies with laboratory confirmation
	Care must be taken to rule out rashes related to skin irritation, allergic reactions, eczema, and other noninfectious skin conditions.
	An epidemiologic linkage to a case can be considered if there is evidence of geographic proximity, temporal relationship to the onset of symptoms, or evidence of common source of exposure (e.g., shared caregiver).

C. Fungal oral/perioral and skin infections Oral candidiasis: **Both** criteria 1 and 2 present: 1. Presence of raised white patches on inflamed mucosa, or plaques on oral mucosa 2. A medical or dental provider diagnosis Fungal skin infection: **Both** criteria 1 and 2 present: 1. Characteristic rash or lesions 2. Either a medical provider diagnosis or laboratory-confirmed fungal pathogen from scraping or biopsy medical	Mucocutaneous candida infections are usually caused by underlying clinical conditions such as poorly controlled diabetes or severe immunosuppression. Although not transmissible infections in the health care setting, they can be a marker for increased antibiotic exposure. Dermatophytes have been known to cause occasional infections, and rare outbreaks, in the LTC setting.
D. Herpes viral skin infections: Herpes simplex infection: **Both** criteria 1 and 2 present: 1. A vesicular rash 2. Either physician diagnosis or laboratory confirmation Herpes zoster infection: **Both** criteria 1 and 2 present: 1. A vesicular rash 2. Either physician diagnosis or laboratory confirmation	Reactivation of herpes simplex ("cold sores") or herpes zoster ("shingles") is not considered a health care–associated infection. Primary herpes viral skin infections are very uncommon in an LTCF, except in pediatric populations where it should be considered health care–associated.
E. Conjunctivitis At least **one** of the following criteria present: 1. Pus appearing from one or both eyes, present for at least 24 hours 2. New or increased conjunctival erythema, with or without itching 3. New or increased conjunctival pain, present for at least 24 hours	Conjunctivitis symptoms ("pink eye") should not be caused by allergic reaction or trauma.

Adapted from Stone ND, Ashraf MS, Calder J, et al., and the Society for Healthcare Epidemiology Long-Term Care Special Interest Group. Definitions of infection for surveillance in long-term care facilities: Revisiting the McGeer criteria. Infect Control Hosp Epidemiol 2012;33:965-77.

LTC, Long-term care; *LTCF*, long-term care facility.

Because of increasing antibiotic-resistant strains in hospitals, nursing homes, and in the community, it is imperative that providers ask themselves if patients with positive cultures, particularly for MRSA, VRE, or ESBL-positive bacteria have significant symptoms and signs of infection that warrant antimicrobial therapy rather than observation. In general, treatment of asymptomatic colonization with these bacteria will not permanently eradicate the organism, prevent infections, or improve patient outcomes.

TABLE 49-4	Criteria for Gastrointestinal (GI) Infection	
Criteria	**Comments**	
A. Gastroenteritis At least **one** of the following criteria present: 1. Diarrhea, three or more liquid or watery stools above what is normal for the resident within a 24-hour period 2. Vomiting, two or more episodes in a 24-hour period 3. **Both** of the following sign/symptom subcriteria present: 　a. A stool specimen positive for a pathogen (such as Salmonella, Shigella, *Escherichia coli* O157:H7, Campylobacter species, rotavirus) 　b. At least **one** of the following GI subcriteria present: 　　i. Nausea 　　ii. Vomiting 　　iii. Abdominal pain or tenderness 　　iv. Diarrhea	Care must be taken to exclude noninfectious causes of symptoms. For instance, new medications may cause diarrhea, nausea, or vomiting; initiation of new enteral feeding may be associated with diarrhea; nausea or vomiting may be associated with gallbladder disease. Presence of new GI symptoms in a single resident may prompt enhanced surveillance for additional cases. In the presence of an outbreak, stool specimens should be sent to confirm the presence of norovirus, or other pathogens (such as rotavirus or *E. coli* O157:H7).	
B. Norovirus gastroenteritis: **Both** criteria 1 and 2 present 1. At least **one** of the following GI subcriteria present: 　a. Diarrhea, three or more liquid or watery stools above what is normal for the resident within a 24-hour period 　b. Vomiting, two or more episodes in a 24-hour period 2. A stool specimen positive for detection of norovirus either by electron microscopy, enzyme immunoassay, or by a molecular diagnostic test such as polymerase chain reaction (PCR).	In the absence of laboratory confirmation, an outbreak (two or more cases occurring in the long-term care facility [LTCF]) of acute gastroenteritis due to norovirus infection in an LTCF may be assumed to be present if **all** of the following criteria are present ("Kaplan criteria"): 　a. Vomiting in more than half of affected persons 　b. A mean (or median) incubation period of 24-48 hours 　c. A mean (or median) duration of illness of 12-60 hours 　d. No bacterial pathogen is identified in stool culture	
C. *Clostridium difficile* infection: **Both** criteria 1 and 2 present 1. **One** of the following GI subcriteria present: 　a. Diarrhea, three or more liquid or watery stools above what is normal for the resident within a 24-hour period 　b. The presence of toxic megacolon (abnormal dilatation of the large bowel documented radiologically) 2. **One** of the following diagnostic subcriteria present: 　a. The stool sample yields a positive laboratory test result for *C. difficile* toxin A or B, or a toxin-producing *C. difficile* organism is identified in a stool culture or by a molecular diagnostic test such as PCR. 　b. Pseudomembranous colitis is identified during endoscopic examination or surgery, or in histopathologic examination of a biopsy specimen.	A "primary episode" of *C. difficile* infection is defined as one that has occurred without any previous history of *C. difficile* infection, or that has occurred more than 8 weeks after the onset of a previous episode of *C. difficile* infection. A "recurrent episode" of *C. difficile* infection is defined as an episode of *C. difficile* infection that occurs 8 weeks or less after the onset of a previous episode, provided that the symptoms from the earlier (previous) episode resolved. Individuals previously infected with *C. difficile* may continue to remain colonized even after symptoms resolve. In the setting of a GI outbreak, individuals could test positive for *C. difficile* toxin because of ongoing colonization and also be coinfected with another pathogen. It is important that other surveillance criteria are used to differentiate infections in this situation.	

Adapted from Stone ND, Ashraf MS, Calder J, et al., and the Society for Healthcare Epidemiology Long-Term Care Special Interest Group. Definitions of infection for surveillance in long-term care facilities: Revisiting the McGeer criteria. Infect Control Hosp Epidemiol 2012;33:965-77.

CASE 1

Florence Rowe (Part 1)

Florence Rowe is a 97-year-old woman who resides in a senior apartment. She lives alone with minimal assistance, but has had mild short-term memory deficits for many years. A friend who visits several times a week has noted that Mrs. Rowe has been sleeping more than usual for the past month. The visitor urges Mrs. Rowe to go to an urgent care center. A urinalysis is obtained and shows white blood cells in her urine too numerous to count. A culture of urine grew greater than 100,000 colony-forming units of *Escherichia coli*. Mrs. Rowe is told that she has an obvious urinary tract infection and she is given a prescription for cephalexin for 3 days. She sees

TABLE 49-5	Minimum Criteria for the Initiation of Antibiotics in Residents of Long-Term Care Facilities

Urinary Tract Infection	Categories	Minimum Criteria
Fever*	No catheter	One or more of the following: new or worsening urgency, frequency, suprapubic pain, gross hematuria, CVA tenderness, urinary incontinence
Fever	Chronic indwelling catheter	New CVA tenderness *and* rigors without cause *or* new onset delirium**

Respiratory Tract Infection	Categories	Minimum Criteria
High fever	>102° F (>38.9° C)	Respiratory rate >25 breaths/minute *or* productive cough
Fever	≦102° F (≦38.9° C)	Cough *plus one* of the following: tachycardia >100 beats/minute, delirium, rigors, respiratory rate >25 breaths/minute
Afebrile	COPD	New or increased cough and purulent sputum production
Afebrile	No COPD	New cough with purulent sputum and one of the following: respiratory rate >25 breaths/minute *or* delirium

Skin/Soft Tissue Infection	Categories	Minimum Criteria
Applies to intact skin, devices, or ulcers		Fever or new or increasing redness, tenderness, warmth or swelling at the affected site***

Fever/Focus Unknown		Minimum Criteria
		Fever *and one* of the following: new onset delirium *or* rigors

Adapted from Loeb M, Bentley DW, Bradley S, et al. Development of minimum criteria for the initiation of antibiotics in residents of long-term-care facilities: Results of a consensus conference. Infection Control Hosp Epidemiology 2001;22:120-4.

COPD, chronic obstructive pulmonary disease; *CVA*, costovertebral angle.

*Fever is defined as a single temperature of >100° F (>37.9° C) or >2.4° F (>1.5° C) unless otherwise stated.

**Delirium is defined by the *Diagnostic and Statistical Manual of Mental Disorders*, 4th edition.

***Does not include nonbacterial infections (herpes), deep tissue, or bone infection; noninfectious causes such as burns, thromboembolic disease, and gout can be mistaken for skin/soft tissue infection.

you in follow-up 1 week later. You find that Mrs. Rowe is alert and attentive. She is oriented to place, person, and time and answers questions appropriately. She recalls that she has felt well recently but has been staying up late watching old movies on her new television. She denies having had fever, frequency, urgency, or dysuria or pain over her flanks and bladder.

1. **Did Mrs. Rowe have a urinary tract infection?**

2. **Was treatment with cephalexin appropriate?** ■

URINARY TRACT INFECTION (UTI)

Prevalence and Impact

UTI is the most common infection seen in older adults in the community, nursing home, or hospital. Overdiagnosis is common. Many clinicians erroneously assume that only a positive urinalysis and culture are required for diagnosis. It is well established that significant but asymptomatic bacteriuria ($\geq 10^5$ colony-forming units [cfu] per mL) increases with age and debility.[25,38-43]

Pathophysiology and Risk Factors

Why are bacteriuria and UTI so common in older adults? Conditions or diseases that lead to alterations in normal flora and urinary stasis and obstruction are associated with increased risk of bacteriuria. Shifts in normal perineal flora may occur as a consequence of estrogen deficiency with a shift in the normal acidic vaginal pH to a more alkaline environment. With that shift in the local vaginal environment, potentially more pathogenic enteric gram-negative bacilli emerge and normal gram-positive flora is suppressed. Functional dependency in toileting and need for assistance by health care personnel can lead to contamination of the urethral orifice with pathogenic bacteria. Bacteria can be introduced into the bladder with introduction of a urinary device.

Urinary obstruction and stasis can also occur as a consequence of normal aging and local or systemic comorbid disease. In males, prostatic hypertrophy that occurs with normal aging can lead to obstruction, urinary stasis, and increased frequency of UTI. Neoplasms and stones that occur with increasing age may lead to obstruction and infection throughout the urinary tract. Cystocele, cerebrovascular accident, and diabetic neuropathy may impair bladder emptying and encourage the development of urinary stasis and bacteriuria.[44,45]

Differential Diagnosis, Assessment, and Management

Asymptomatic Bacteriuria

A major dilemma for clinicians is differentiating UTI from asymptomatic bacteriuria. Presence of significant pyuria (≥10 white blood cells per low-power field) in older adults is not a useful indicator of urinary tract infection. A significant proportion of asymptomatic older adults (30%) will have significant and persistent pyuria. Pyuria can be found in conditions such as nephrolithiasis and primary diseases of bowel found adjacent to the urinary tract such as diverticulitis, inflammatory bowel disease, and intraabdominal abscess. Absence of pyuria is useful, however. A negative urinalysis for pyuria is 99% predictive that bacteriuria, and hence UTI, is not present. Alternate diagnoses should be pursued.[43-45]

Symptomatic UTI

The diagnosis of UTI rests principally on patient history of symptoms and physical signs referable to the urinary tract (see Table 49-1).[25] The symptoms and signs must be new or worsening of chronic symptoms. Symptoms of lower UTI or cystitis include suprapubic pain, dysuria, frequency, and urgency. Flank pain and fever are more typical of upper tract infection or pyelonephritis. Odiferous or cloudy urine indicate the presence of metabolites, urine concentration, crystals, and sediment and are not useful indicators for the presence of a UTI.[44,45]

Even in the cognitively impaired nursing home resident, physical signs referable to the urinary tract can be helpful especially if they resolve with treatment. Reproducible pain over the external genitalia (in a male), bladder, or flanks in the presence of significant bacteriuria and pyuria provides presumptive evidence that a UTI is present. In nursing homes, only 10% of fevers are caused by a urinary source. As a result, fever associated with change in mental status is rarely the result of a UTI and another cause should be sought. Special consideration might be given to patients with urinary catheters; 50% who have fever will have secondary bacteremia with the same organism present in urine.[25,44-49]

Management and Treatment

Asymptomatic Bacteriuria. If an older adult has significant bacteriuria, pyuria, and symptoms, then treatment for UTI is appropriate. However, treatment of asymptomatic bacteriuria does not permanently eradicate the organism and, with rare exception, no benefit of treatment for the older adult has been demonstrated in terms of improved well-being, relief of chronic symptoms, or survival. Change to One exception is the treatment of patients with asymptomatic bacteriuria who undergo a prostatic resection; postoperative bacteremia is substantially reduced in that population. Otherwise, treatment of asymptomatic bacteriuria is a major cause of inappropriate antibiotic use and emergence of antibiotic resistance. Education of clinicians regarding the importance of this problem poses a major challenge for antimicrobial stewardship programs.[25,43]

> Treatment of "dirty urine" in the elderly with asymptomatic bacteriuria is not beneficial.

Uncomplicated UTI. Predictability of the infecting organism and its response to treatment relates in part to gender, general health, and anatomy of the genitourinary tract. Many postmenopausal women have had a history of UTI throughout their lives that responds predictably to empiric treatment directed against *Escherichia coli* (uncomplicated UTI) (Table 49-6). Uncomplicated UTI requires that the woman be healthy without diabetes and immunosuppression. In addition, there are not functional or anatomic abnormalities of the urinary tract or the need for catheter use. An uncomplicated UTI cannot be nosocomially acquired.[44,45,50]

Women with an uncomplicated cystitis do not necessarily require culture prior to initiation of treatment unless they have symptoms of pyelonephritis, they have recurrence of symptoms, or if local antibiotic resistance is a concern (Table 49-7). Otherwise, the optimum antibiotic treatment of urinary symptoms in older adults should be based on culture results and antimicrobial susceptibilities. In the event that symptoms are severe with impending sepsis, then empiric antibiotic choices can be initiated based on local epidemiology data and antimicrobial susceptibility patterns. Use of nitrofurantoin may be limited in older adults because of contraindications in patients with renal insufficiency (creatinine clearance <40 cc/min). Fosfomycin and nitrofurantoin are not indicated for pyelonephritis. The duration of treatment for cystitis and pyelonephritis is dependent on the antibiotic chosen (see Table 49-7).[50]

Topical estrogen use may reduce recurrent episodes of UTI in healthy older women by normalizing vaginal pH and restoring normal flora. Cranberry juice may reduce significant bacteriuria in older women by inhibiting binding of gram-negative bacilli to uroepithelial cells. Prophylaxis with postcoital or once-daily low doses of trimethoprim-sulfamethoxazole, quinolones, or nitrofurantoin may be considered on older women as well as younger women with uncomplicated and recurrent UTI.[44,45]

TABLE 49-6	Bacterial Etiologies Vary with Residence among Older Adults with Urinary Tract Infection (UTI)				
	Community-Based		Long-Term Care Facility		
Bacteria (%)	Women	Men	Women	Men	CIC
Escherichia coli	75	44	54	25	10-37
Klebsiella spp.	5.3	6.3	11	8.3	3-21
Enterobacter spp.	3.5	13	3.6	2.7	——
Proteus mirabilis	11	19	25	67	9-36
Providencia spp.	—	—	—	28	5-61
Pseudomonas spp.	2	19	3.6	33	5-30
Enterococcus spp.	—	—	1.8	5.6	7-28
Coagulase-negative STAPHYLOCOCCUS	—	—	—	2.7	1-9

Adapted from Nicolle LE. Urinary tract infection. In: Yoshikawa TT, Rajagopalan S, editors. Antibiotic therapy for geriatric patients. New York: Taylor & Francis Group; 2006, p. 487-501; and Nicolle LE. In: Yoshikawa TT, Norman DC, editors. Infectious diseases in the aging: A clinical handbook. 2nd ed. New York: Humana Press; 2009, p. 165-180.

CIC, Chronic indwelling catheter.

TABLE 49-7	Treatment of Woman with Uncomplicated Urinary Tract Infection (UTI)
Cystitis	**Pyelonephritis**
Able to tolerate medication **Absence of:** <ul><li>pyelonephritis symptoms</li><li>fever, flank pain</li><li>allergy history</li></ul> **First-Line Oral Treatment Options** Nitrofurantoin 100 mg bid × 5 days* TMP/SMZ DS bid × 3 days (avoid if prior UTI in 3 months, or 20% resistance to sulfas in the community) Fosfomycin 3 gm single dose* (lower efficacy) Pivmecillinam 400 mg bid × 5 days* (lower efficacy) **Second-Line Treatment Oral Options** Quinolones	**Obtain a urine culture** **Hospitalized—give IV dose initially** <ul><li>ceftriaxone</li><li>aminoglycoside</li><li>quinolone (unless resistance >10%)</li></ul> **First-Line Oral Treatment Options** Ciprofloxacin 500 mg bid × 7 days Levofloxacin 750 mg qd × 7 days TMP/SMZ DS bid × 14 days Beta-lactam 10-14 days (less efficacious)

Adapted from Gupta K, Hooton TM, Naber KG, et al. International clinical practice guidelines for the treatment of acute uncomplicated cystitis and pyelonephritis in women: A 2010 update by the Infectious Diseases Society of America and the European Society for Microbiology and Infectious Diseases. Clin Infect Dis 2011;52:e103-20.

IV, Intravenous; TMP/SMZ DS, trimethoprim-sulfamethoxazole double-strength.

*Avoid if early pyelonephritis suspected.

Complicated UTI. For the remainder of the elderly with UTI symptoms who have abnormal urinary tract anatomy, require a urinary device, or are exposed to antibiotic-resistant pathogens in hospitals and nursing homes (complicated UTI), appropriate management requires obtaining a urine sample for culture and antimicrobial susceptibilities because their infecting organisms and treatment responses are not predictable (see Table 49-6). Most of these patients have reinfection with a new organism rather than relapse with the same organism.[44-46]

> The optimal treatment of complicated UTI in the older adult must be based on results of the urine culture; the organisms causing the infection and their resistance patterns are not predictable.

By definition, when UTIs in men occur, they have a complicated UTI because urinary tract abnormalities or catheter use is invariably present. In contrast with uncomplicated UTI in healthy older women, bacteriuria in healthy men is most commonly the result of not only *E. coli*, but also of *Proteus mirabilis* and enterococci. In hospitalized elderly patients with complicated UTI, *E. coli* is still the predominant pathogen, but *Pseudomonas aeruginosa* occurs with increasing frequency, followed by *Candida albicans* and other antibiotic-resistant gram-negative bacilli. Chronic catheter-use has been associated with infections resulting from *Providencia stuartii* and coagulase-negative staphylococci. True polymicrobial infection can occur in elderly institutionalized patients even in the absence of an indwelling catheter.[44-46]

In the clinically stable patient, therapy can be withheld until culture results are known. When the diagnosis of UTI is uncertain, empiric antibiotic use may obscure the true diagnosis. Empiric treatment of complicated UTI should be based on the place of acquisition and primarily directed against gram-negative bacilli. For patients with complicated UTI, therapy must be reevaluated once culture and antimicrobial susceptibilities are available given the high prevalence of antibiotic resistance within and outside health care settings.[44,45]

Duration is based on response to symptoms and predisposing factors. For patients with short-term catheters in whom the catheter is removed and there are no upper tract symptoms, 3 days of antibiotic treatment may be sufficient. Some recommend 5 to 7 days if the patient is not severely ill and the clinical response is prompt. Longer therapy of 10 to 14 days is recommended for a delayed response (Box 49-2). If there is a relapse of symptomatic bacteriuria, a longer course of antibiotics may be needed to eradicate a chronic bacterial prostatic focus. Use of antimicrobial agents that penetrate prostatic tissue (quinolones, trimethoprim-sulfamethoxazole, cephalexin) is required for 6 to 12 weeks.[44-46]

Management of patients who do not have symptoms localized to the urinary tract or cannot report them present a particular problem, particularly in nursing homes. Febrile nursing home residents that meet criteria for fever and delirium could receive empiric therapy with close reevaluation. For a patient with frequent and transient episodes of mental status that do not meet criteria for delirium, a trial of intravenous fluids to treat dehydration and promote urinary tract flushing could be considered. Alternatively, a trial of empiric antibiotics could be started, but stopped at 72 hours if the evaluation is negative for urinary abnormalities, the patient does not improve on empiric therapy, or another diagnosis becomes evident. UTI can be excluded if improvement is seen but the bacterial isolates found are not susceptible to empiric antibiotic choices. Treatment of bacteriuria

---

BOX 49-2

INDWELLING URINARY CATHETERS: APPROPRIATE CARE, TREATMENT, AND PREVENTION OF URINARY TRACT INFECTION (UTI)

Indwelling catheters should:
  Be used only for appropriate indications.
  Be removed immediately when they are no longer needed.
  Be inserted using aseptic technique and sterile equipment.
  Be used only in conjunction with a closed drainage system.
Indwelling urinary catheters should not be used for incontinence except when all other approaches have failed.
Catheter care *not* recommended:
  Enhanced meatal care
  Routine catheter changes
  Routine irrigation of catheters
  Routine use of antimicrobial prophylaxis
Urine Cultures
  A urine culture should be obtained prior to initiating antimicrobial treatment.
  A urinary catheter should be changed or removed prior to obtaining a urine culture.
Duration of Appropriate Treatment
  Prompt resolution of symptoms: 7 days
  Delayed resolution of symptoms: 10-14 days

Adapted from Hooton TM, Bradley SF, Cardenas DD, et al. International clinical practice guidelines for the diagnosis, prevention, and treatment of catheter-associated urinary tract infection. Clin Infect Dis 2010;50:625-63.

---

related to chronic indwelling urinary devices should be considered only when typical symptoms are present or fever is present without another focus evident. A randomized trial found that nursing homes that used this algorithm had similar outcomes and reduced antibiotic use compared with nursing homes that were randomized to usual care.[30,31,46]

> **Urinary tract infection in the patient with a chronic indwelling catheter is a diagnosis of exclusion.**

Follow-up samples of urine for culture should be obtained only if symptoms of infection persist or recur to verify if a secondary infection with a new organism resistant to therapy has emerged during treatment. In addition, ultrasound or computerized tomography (CT) should be considered if fever or bacteriuria fails to improve on appropriate therapy or if the patient has recurrent UTI to rule out the presence of obstruction or abscess. Surgical or pharmacologic relief of obstruction or stasis may be effective, particularly if the patient has relapsing episodes of UTI with the same organism.[44,45]

Recurrent UTI with the same organism should prompt a search for anatomic defects that can be remediated.

Indications for urinary catheter use and alternative means of toileting should be reviewed, especially if incontinence and convenience are the only indications. Intermittent urethral catheterization may be associated with fewer infections. Routine catheter changes or irrigation with antimicrobial agents is not effective in preventing infection. Suppressive antibiotics can reduce the frequency of recurrent UTIs in spinal cord patients with chronic catheters, but resistance rapidly emerges.[46]

CASE 1

Discussion

Mrs. Rowe has significant pyuria and bacteriuria. She has had no new or worsening symptoms referable to the urinary tract that suggest infection. Sleepiness of weeks' duration is not indicative of a urinary tract infection. Asymptomatic bacteriuria and pyuria is a very common and benign condition in older adults. The degree of pyuria does not help differentiate infection from asymptomatic bacteriuria.

Treatment of asymptomatic bacteriuria does not benefit the patient; it does not prevent recurrence of bacteriuria, prevent future episodes of symptomatic urinary tract infection, or improve the patient's well-being or mortality. Treatment is only warranted when urinary tract symptoms are present. Mrs. Rowe did not have urinary symptoms so treatment with antibiotics was not warranted. ▣

LOWER RESPIRATORY TRACT INFECTION (LRTI)

Prevalence and Impact

Pneumonia and bronchitis are common causes of hospitalization among older adults. They comprise the second most common cause of infection in nursing homes; rates of pneumonia range from 33 to 114 cases per 1000 residents per year or 0.3 to 2.5 episodes per 1000 days of resident care.[51-54] Despite advances in antibiotics, vaccines, and other treatments, LRTI remains one of the top ten causes of death in older adults.[51-54]

Tuberculosis (TB) continues to be a problem in the United States; approximately 15,000 cases of illness are diagnosed each year and a disproportionate number of infections are found among the elderly. Most cases of TB disease occur in community-dwelling elderly persons, but nursing home residents are at greatest risk for poor outcomes.[55,56]

Pathophysiology and Risk Factors

Risk factors for LRTIs are particularly common in older adults either because of the consequences of aging, acquired conditions, or treatment of those illnesses. Microaspiration and inhalation of potential oral flora pathogens is an everyday occurrence. Multiple host defenses reduce the likelihood that pneumonia will develop in the normal host. Pathogens are contained by respiratory tract mucus, local inflammatory responses, and secretory antibodies. Pathogens are removed by expectoration of sputum through the actions of ciliated respiratory epithelium and cough reflexes. Swallowed pathogens are killed by gastric acid.[51-54,57]

Handling respiratory secretions appropriately is a major barrier to the development of pneumonia. Common neurologic and psychiatric conditions or sedating medications can impair recognition that aspiration is occurring or result in a swallowing disorder.[51-54] Achlorhydria may result as a consequence of aging itself or from the use of medications that neutralize or block the production of stomach acid. Age-related declines in lung elasticity, respiratory musculature, and kyphosis contribute to diminished cough reflexes. Common conditions such as obstructive airways disease, emphysema, bronchiectasis, and presence of neoplasms can also reduce mucociliary clearance.[51-54]

Normal aging, age-associated conditions, and their treatments also result in changes in oropharyngeal flora. Alterations in oropharyngeal environment allow the flora to change from predominantly gram-positive cocci to carriage with gram-negative bacilli.[51-54,58] Older adults also have more exposure to pathogens that cause respiratory disease through more frequent interactions with health care settings.[58]

Acquisition of respiratory pathogens via inhalation of droplets (influenza) or airborne pathogens (*Mycobacterium tuberculosis*) is less common. Older adults generally acquired asymptomatic latent TB infection (LTBI) when they were young and the infection was prevalent. Aging and conditions that lead to waning cell-mediated immunity increase the likelihood that reactivation of symptomatic TB disease will occur.[55,56]

Differential Diagnosis, Assessment, and Management

Although LRTI is common in older adults, making a definitive diagnosis can be difficult. The symptoms of cough and dyspnea are common among older adults with underlying cardiopulmonary disease and are not specific for LRTI. The diagnosis of LRTI is easily missed if one relies only on the presence of inflammatory signs such as fever and leukocytosis; many frail elderly adults may lack a typical presentation. Only 56% of nursing home residents with pneumonia will have the symptom triad of cough, dyspnea, and fever; 60% will have isolated cough, and 40% will have dyspnea alone.[51-54,59] Presence of rales on physical examination is lacking in 45% of residents with pneumonia. It is, therefore, important that the clinician have a low threshold to evaluate elderly patients for pneumonia with careful attention to new or worsening symptoms and signs, both typical and atypical for pneumonia (see Table 49-2).[13,25,51-54]

New or worsening dyspnea seems to be a particularly important clue that LRTI is present. Tachypnea with tachycardia was noted in 66% of older adults with pneumonia, and may be one of the earliest clues that LRTI is present. A strong association between respiratory rates 25 breaths per minute or faster and the presence of pneumonia has been made in the elderly. This elevated respiratory rate coupled with a pulse oximetry below 90% is an accurate predictor of impending respiratory failure.[13,25,59,60]

Chest radiographs, regardless of quality, technical difficulties, or lack of prior films for comparison, are helpful to confirm LRTI in more than 90% of nursing residents. Chest radiographs can provide useful prognostic information (multilobar disease) as well as detect issues that might alter how the patient is evaluated and treated, such as empyema or possible neoplasms.[13,25,61]

patients in hospital, hospital-acquired pneumonia (HAP) caused by resistant gram-negative bacilli, especially *P. aeruginosa* and *S. aureus*, are more likely. Patients with prior health care exposure and less-debilitated nursing home residents tend to have causes of pneumonia that overlap with those found in patients with CAP and HAP, so-called health-care associated pneumonia (HCAP). Gram negative bacillary LRTIs are less common in nursing homes when compared with hospitals; *Klebsiella* is the most common organism when they occur (Table 49-8).[51-54,62-65]

Atypical Pneumonia

Legionella pneumophila, other *Legionella* species, *Chlamydophlia (Chlamydia) pneumoniae*, and *Mycoplasma pneumoniae* may cause atypical pneumonitis in the elderly. *Legionella* occurs predominantly in older persons with underlying illness. Parainfluenza, respiratory syncytial virus (RSV), rhinovirus, metapneumovirus, coronaviruses, influenza, and adenovirus are increasingly recognized as causes of atypical pneumonia in older adults.[66-71] Identification of atypical causes of pneumonia is more difficult than identification of typical causes. Outbreaks of RTI, particularly during winter months, generally favor a viral etiology. Newer rapid antigen and molecular diagnostic testing of nasopharyngeal specimens are increasingly favored over more labor intensive and less

---

CASE 2

Evelyn Rafferty (Part 1)

Evelyn Rafferty is an 85-year-old woman who had a subdural hematoma following a fall several years ago with residual expressive aphasia. She requires assistance with many of her ADLs. Mrs. Rafferty recently moved to a long-term care facility and had been doing well. Today, the nurse's aide reports that Mrs. Rafferty has a new cough and shortness of breath. The charge nurse verifies that her temperature is 100° F with a respiratory rate of 25 breaths per minute and a pulse oximetry of 90% on room air. You are called and verify that the patient appears to be lethargic and has new crackles on lung examination.

1. **What is Mrs. Rafferty's most likely diagnosis?**

2. **What are the next most appropriate steps in the management of her respiratory problem?** ▶

Typical Pneumonia

Sputum gram stain and cultures of sputum and blood can be useful in establishing the cause of typical bacterial pneumonia; however, collection of clinical specimens from older patients who cannot cooperate or cough is difficult, and contamination with upper airway secretions is frequent.[51-54,62,63]

In community-acquired pneumonia (CAP) in the elderly, LRTI resulting from *S. pneumonia, Haemophilus influenzae,* and *Moraxella* is most common. In debilitated

TABLE 49-8	Common Etiologies of Community-Acquired Pneumonia (CAP)	
Patient Type	**Etiology**
Outpatient	*Streptococcus pneumoniae*
	Mycoplasma pneumoniae
	Haemophilus influenzae
	Chlamydophila (Chlamydia) pneumoniae
	Respiratory viruses
Inpatient (non-ICU)	*S. pneumoniae*
	M. pneumoniae
	C. pneumoniae
	H. influenzae
	Legionella species
	Aspiration
	Respiratory viruses
Inpatient (ICU)	*S. pneumoniae*
	Staphylococcus aureus
	Legionella species
	Gram-negative bacilli
	H. influenzae

Adapted from Mandell LA, Wunderink RG, Anzueto A, et al. Infectious Diseases Society of America/American Thoracic Society consensus guidelines on the management of community-acquired pneumonia in adults. Clin Infect Dis 2007;44:S27-72.
Respiratory viruses = influenza A and B, adenovirus, respiratory syncytial virus, parainfluenza.
ICU, intensive care unit.

available tissue culture and acute and convalescent serology. In health care facilities, the presence of influenza would prompt initiation of antiviral prophylaxis and more intensive infection control measures. Diagnosis of influenza in individual patients still should rely on history and symptoms. Knowledge that influenza is in the community with fever and new respiratory symptoms of less than 48 hours' duration is just as sensitive as current antigen-based testing and at less expense.[64-71]

> Consider atypical respiratory pathogens if a similar illness occurs in multiple patients, health care personnel, and visitors.

Mycobacterial Infection

Failure of an infiltrate to respond to reasonable antibiotic therapy for common pathogens suggests that other infectious and noninfectious etiologies should be considered. Tuberculosis should be considered particularly if there is a history of familial or occupational exposures or other risk factors such as residence in an endemic geographic area, prison, or in a nursing home.[55,56] Pulmonary TB is found most commonly in the elderly, whereas extrapulmonary disease may be seen more often in younger persons. Negative TB screening tests such as the tuberculin skin test (TST) or interferon gamma-based assays (Quantiferon Gold in Tube or T-SPOT) do not exclude the diagnosis of TB disease. In older patients with active TB infection, 25% of TSTs will be negative.

Chest roentgenographic findings that are often seen with TB infection are frequently misinterpreted in older adults because of lack of clinical suspicion. Although reactivation disease seen in the upper lobes is most typical for TB, lower lobe infiltrates, adenopathy, and pleural effusions can occur. Evaluation for TB disease should be directed by abnormalities noted on physical and laboratory examinations; body fluids and tissues should be sent for culture and smear for acid-fast bacilli (AFB). Some specimens found to have AFB on smear may be probed directly to rapidly identify these organisms as related to TB.[55,56]

> Negative screening tests for latent tuberculosis do not exclude the possibility of TB disease in the symptomatic patient with suspected infection.

Management and Treatment

Several factors influence how LRTI should be managed in the elderly. Severity of illness should be assessed using scores, such as CURB-65 Criteria, that predict short-term mortality and help with decisions regarding inpatient versus outpatient care (Box 49-3).[62] The site of acquisition of the LRTI also helps predict whether antibiotic-resistant bacteria may be causing the infection (Box 49-4).[63] For elderly with CAP, empiric treatment should be based on the most likely organisms as well as the severity of illness (see Table 49-8). Empiric treatment with penicillin or ampicillin alone should be avoided, until cultures are back, because of high rates of beta-lactamase-producing *H. influenzae* and

---

BOX 49-3

COMMUNITY-ACQUIRED PNEUMONIA (CAP) SEVERITY OF ILLNESS SCORE (CURB-65 CRITERIA)

Factor	Criteria
Confusion	disoriented person, place, time
Uremia	≥20 mg/dL
Respiratory rate	>30 breaths/minute
Low Blood pressure	systolic/diastolic 90/60 mmHg
Age 65 years or greater	increased age

Number of factors	30-Day Mortality (%)	Recommended Treatment Site
0	0.7	Outpatient
1	2.1	Outpatient
2	9.2	Inpatient Ward
3	14.5	ICU
4	40.0	ICU
5	57.0	ICU

Adapted from Mandell LA, Wunderink RG, Anzueto A, et al. Infectious Diseases Society of America/American Thoracic Society consensus guidelines on the management of community-acquired pneumonia in adults. Clin Infect Dis 2007;44:S27-72.

BOX 49-4

RISK FACTORS FOR RESISTANT PATHOGENS CAUSING HOSPITAL-ACQUIRED PNEUMONIA (HAP) AND HEALTHCARE-ASSOCIATED PNEUMONIA (HCAP)

- Immunosuppressive disease and/or therapy
- Antimicrobial treatment within the past 3 months
- Rates of antibiotic resistance high in the community or within the institution
- Currently hospitalized for ≥5 days
- Risk factors for HCAP:
  Hospitalization for ≥48 hours within the past 3 months
  Residence in a long-term care facility
  Home infusion therapy (including antibiotics)
  Chronic dialysis within 1 month
  Home wound care
- Family member with known multidrug-resistant pathogen

Adapted from American Thoracic Society, Infectious Diseases Society of America. Guidelines for the management of adults with hospital-acquired, ventilator-associated, and healthcare-associated pneumonia. Am J Respir Crit Care Med 2005;171: 388-416.

multidrug-resistant pneumococci in this population. Currently in the United States, use of a penicillin/beta lactamase inhibitor combination (ampicillin plus sulbactam or clavulanic acid, or piperacillin plus tazobactam), beta-lactamase-resistant cephalosporins (ceftriaxone), or quinolones with activity against *S. pneumoniae* (gatifloxacin, moxifloxacin) are effective in treating resistant pneumococci.[62]

In addition, empiric initial therapy for atypical bacterial pathogens has been recommended for CAP or HCAP treated with beta lactam–beta lactamase combinations. Macrolides and quinolones have activity against atypical bacteria. For healthy elderly with CAP who are clinically stable, therapy with oral agents may be appropriate. For HAP, therapy should target resistant gram-negative bacilli, *S. aureus,* and *Legionella* when present in a given geographic area. If influenza is in the community, prompt initiation of neuraminidase inhibitors, such as oseltamivir, should be considered.[62-64]

In the patient with positive TB smears or a clinically compatible illness, empiric four-drug RIPE (rifampin, isoniazid, pyrazinamide, and ethambutol) therapy is generally given until culture and susceptibility results are known. Experts in the management of TB disease should be consulted especially if the patient has a history of prior therapy for TB or has resided in a part of the world where multidrug-resistant or extremely resistant drug strains are found.[55,56]

Prevention of pneumonia in older adults should focus on reduction of individual risk factors and vaccination. Medications that are sedating, contribute to dry mouth, or cause achlorhydria should be minimized or avoided. Use of feeding tubes should be avoided if feasible. Oral hygiene to reduce colonization with pathogens and techniques to minimize aspiration can be considered, but data regarding efficacy are limited. Vaccination of older adults has been effective in reducing the complications of influenza and the prevention of invasive pneumococcal disease. Recent recommendations suggest that some immunocompromised adults be immunized with the 13-valent pneumococcal in addition to the 23-valent vaccine.[72,73] Screening for LTBI and its treatment should be considered for all older adults.[55,56] Health care workers also play an important role in reducing LRTI rates in their patients by adhering to hand hygiene and isolation procedures, receiving influenza vaccines annually, and participating in TB screening programs.[55,56,64,65]

CASE 2

Discussion

A temperature of 100° F is indicative of significant fever in older adults. Mrs. Rafferty also has symptoms of new or worsening cough and tachypnea with rales on examination that are commonly associated with LRTI in nursing home residents. The respiratory rate of 25 breaths per minute is clearly abnormal; this degree of tachypnea has been strongly associated with the presence of pneumonia in older adults. Mrs. Rafferty's oxygen saturation of 90% in the face of a high respiratory rate and worsening lethargy are indicators that she has impending respiratory failure related to pneumonia.

Mrs. Rafferty is critically ill, so it is essential that the health care provider rapidly establish what the goals of care are based on the patient's and family's wishes and where those care goals can optimally be met. While oxygen is administered and venous access established, decisions must be made either to transfer the patient to an acute care setting where respiratory support and intensive monitoring are available or to treat the patient in the nursing home setting. If the patient remains in the nursing home, then attention can rapidly turn to decisions regarding comfort care and antibiotic treatment. ■

SKIN AND SOFT TISSUE INFECTION (SSTI)

Prevalence and Impact

SSTIs are the third most common infection seen in older adults. In nursing homes, rates of 1% to 9% have been reported with a prevalence of 0.9 to 2.1 per 1000 patient days.[3,74,75] Primary infection of soft tissue and secondary infection of preexisting wounds are some of the most common manifestations of SSTI. Primary SSTIs range from common, superficial, and less severe pyodermas involving skin and mucous membranes to less common life-threatening infections extending to fascia (fasciitis), muscle (myositis), and bone (osteomyelitis).[76-80] Secondarily infected ulcers and postoperative wound infections are particularly common among nursing home residents and hospitalized elderly. Approximately 6% of pressure ulcers in nursing home residents will become infected at a rate of 1.4 infections per 1000 resident days.[81-83]

Pathophysiology and Risk Factors

Intact skin and mucous membranes are major barriers to invasion by microorganisms. Even small breaks in mucocutaneous barriers can facilitate the introduction of many different pathogens including bacteria, fungi, and viruses. Thinning of skin, decreased mobility, maceration related to incontinence, edema, reduced blood flow, medications, and devices are some of the many factors that alter the integrity of mucocutaneous barriers and contribute to the development of SSTIs in the older adult.[84] Other risk factors involved in the development of SSTIs include waning immunity, exposures to potential pathogens, and conditions that promote overgrowth of the patient's flora. Reactivation of latent viral mucocutaneous infections is common; 10,000 to 20,000 cases of herpes zoster occur annually in nursing home residents.[79,85]

Older adults who reside in shared living quarters are more likely to be exposed to potential pathogens that cause SSTIs. Ectoparasitic infections such as scabies (*Sarcoptes scabiei*), lice (*Pediculus humanus capitis* [head lice], *P. humanus corporis* [body lice], and *Phthirus pubis* [pubic lice]), and bed bugs (*Cimex lectularius*) through direct exposure to another infected person or from contaminated fomites.[79,86-90]

Preexisting wounds can become secondarily infected by contamination from the hands of health care personnel and from contact with the environment (exogenous acquisition) or from the patient's own flora (endogenous acquisition). Other factors contribute to overgrowth of endogenous flora, such as fungi, including antibacterials and corticosteroids.[91-93]

Differential Diagnosis, Assessment, and Management

Primary SSTI

Clinical Manifestations. Primary bacterial SSTIs are most often caused by beta-hemolytic streptococci (*S. pyogenes*) and *S. aureus*, and common and superficial manifestations of these infections include cellulitis, erysipelas, impetigo, paronychia, and conjunctivitis (see Table 49-3).[25,79] Conjunctivitis is defined as the presence of purulence or new or worsening erythema in one or both eyes for more than 24 hours. Associated pain and pruritus are frequent, and allergy and trauma should be excluded. A cause of conjunctivitis may be established in fewer than 40% of cases; most are the result of *S. aureus*, *Moraxella catarrhalis*, and *Hemophilus* spp.[80]

Primary infections of fascia and muscle do occur, but are much less frequent; outbreaks of deep infection have been reported in the community and in health care settings. In older adults that have cellulitis, increasing pain and worsening symptoms out of proportion with physical findings should immediately raise suspicion for deeper infection and prompt emergent evaluation.[79]

> **Increasing pain and worsening symptoms out of proportion with findings on skin exam must prompt urgent evaluation for deeper soft tissue infection.**

Nonbacterial causes of primary SSTI also occur. Candida infection, primarily *C. albicans*, involves skin and mucosa resulting in many clinical manifestations including thrush, denture stomatitis, chelitis, paronychia, and intertrigo. Dermatophyte infections involving various body sites include tinea corporis, tinea pedis, tinea cruris, and tinea unguium (onychomycosis) (see Table 49-3).[91-93]

Herpes infections are typically painful or pruritic. Mucocutaneous vesicles or ulcerations due to herpes simplex typically involve nasolabial, genital, or rectal skin and mucosa. A vesicular rash located in a dermatomal distribution is diagnostic for herpes zoster infection (see Table 49-3).[79,85]

> **Consider the diagnosis of herpes zoster infection if a rash does not cross the midline.**

Scabies infection can manifest atypically in the debilitated older nursing home resident or hospital patient where efficient person-to-person transmission occurs. The typical inflammatory response with resulting pruritus may be lacking in these patients. Burrows and rash in intertriginous areas are often absent and hyperkeratotic or crusting may be more typical (Norwegian scabies). The diagnosis is frequently made when pruritus and more typical rash are seen in family members, visitors, or health care workers (see Table 49-3).[79,86-89] Bed bugs are generally a community-associated infection. Acquisition of bed bugs in the health care setting is unusual because furniture must be readily cleanable. Red pruritic nodules are noted in a linear distribution.[90]

> **Consider the diagnosis of scabies if rashes occur in health care personnel and visitors.**

Diagnosis. The diagnosis of primary SSTIs is generally based on the clinical appearance and location of the lesion. When the presentation is atypical or the patient is not responding to treatment, appropriate samples of pus, blister fluid, or skin scrapings can be useful to verify the diagnosis.[91-93] Presence of giant cells on Tzanck smear is pathopneumonic for herpes infection. Speciation of herpes viruses as simplex or zoster can be confirmed by obtaining vesicle fluid for immunofluorescence antigen and culture. Differentiation between the two viral species is important because of infection control issues and the higher doses of antivirals required for herpes zoster.[79,85]

> **Swabs of superficial wounds do not predict what bacteria are invasive and causing infection; only send deep specimens such as tissue and bone for culture.**

Frail older adults are often heavily infested with scabies; examination of deep skin scrapings under immersion oil readily detects mites, ova, and feces. Lice are typically found crawling at the base of hair follicles (nits), in the scalp (head lice), or in the seams of clothing (body lice). Adult bed bugs run rapidly; they are flat, red brown, and the size of an apple seed. Bed bugs are rarely found on the patient; they infest clothing and furniture. Remnants of bugs and blood are typically found along the seams of mattresses and overstuffed furniture.[79,86-90]

Management and Treatment. Treatment for primary SSTIs of presumed bacterial etiology may be started empirically if the patient has significant signs of systemic illness or deferred pending the results of cultures if the patient is clinically stable. Empiric treatment should be based on the place of acquisition and directed against the most likely causative organisms, generally *S. aureus* and beta-hemolytic streptococci. For severe infection, empiric intravenous therapy would be appropriate. For less severe symptoms, oral antibacterial agents may be considered.[76-78]

Unfortunately, MRSA is no longer confined to hospitals and now accounts for more than 50% of primary bacterial SSTIs seen in the community, and decisions regarding empiric treatment of less severe infections with oral agents are no longer simple. Some experts recommend that all community-associated primary SSTIs be treated with clindamycin, a drug that treats many CA-MRSA strains as well as beta-hemolytic streptococci. Others note that the risk for CA-MRSA is increased if the primary SSTI has evidence for abscess formation or drainage when compared with cellulitis alone. In that instance, a beta-lactam antibiotic is recommended for cellulitis alone and clindamycin or trimethoprim-sulfamethoxazole when abscesses or drainage are present. Still others note that the choice of antibiotic has little impact on CA-MRSA and surgical incision and drainage is most important.[94]

> A scalpel is the best treatment for large MRSA skin abscesses.

For treatment directed against MSSA and streptococci, including oral treatment with first-generation cephalosporins (cephalexin) and antistaphylococcal penicillins (dicloxacillin, amoxicillin-clavulanate) are appropriate. For penicillin-allergic patients, clindamycin or a quinolone with activity against streptococci (moxifloxacin) can be used. For severe bacterial SSTIs, empiric treatment should be directed against MRSA until results of cultures are known; vancomycin, daptomycin, tigecycline, or oral linezolid could be considered.[78]

Oral acyclovir, famciclovir, or valacyclovir are effective for herpes simplex and localized herpes zoster infections; herpes zoster requires higher doses of these agents. Antiviral treatment is recommended for older adults to reduce postherpetic neuralgia and if they have ophthalmic involvement or disseminated disease. Disseminated herpes zoster should be treated intravenously. Patients should also receive appropriate treatment for acute pain and management of postherpetic neuropathic pain.[79,85] Herpes zoster can be prevented and postherpetic neuralgia attenuated in older adults given a live virus vaccine.[95]

Topical treatments with nystatin or clotrimazole troches or systemic treatment with oral fluconazole are effective for oral candidosis. Topical clotrimazole or oral fluconazole is also effective for cutaneous candidosis. For dermatophyte infection, oral itraconazole or terbinafine is most beneficial. Drug interactions and hepatotoxicity are significant issues with systemic azoles and terbinafine; careful monitoring is essential during therapy. Onychomycosis typically requires months of therapy with an effective oral agent.[91-93]

Treatment of scabies can be difficult in the debilitated patient. To avoid lindane-associated central nervous system toxicity, permethrin 5% cream is preferred. The cream should be applied from the neck to toes and left in place for up to 12 hours, and nails should be trimmed. Oral ivermectin should be considered for patients with crusted scabies. Antipruritic therapy should also be given as needed. For head and pubic lice, permethrin or lindane shampoo is applied to the affected area followed by frequent combing to remove nits. Patients should be reexamined weekly to assure that the scabies and lice have been eradicated.[79,86-89]

Empiric treatment for conjunctivitis should be directed against *S. aureus* and beta-hemolytic streptococci until results are known. Appropriate topical ophthalmic antibiotic drops or ointments are erythromycin, quinolones, sulfonamides, and tetracyclines. There are no specific treatments for viral conjunctivitis. Treatment should focus on symptomatic relief with the use of cool compresses, analgesia, and artificial tears. Patients should be monitored closely for bacterial superinfection.[80]

Secondary SSTI

Clinical Manifestations. Secondary infections of wounds (e.g., pressure ulcers, diabetic ulcers) can range from localized involvement of skin to extension into subcutaneous tissue, muscle, and bone associated with bacteremia and severe systemic infection. Secondary infection of wounds is diagnosed primarily by the presence of localized clinical signs and symptoms; local findings may range from nonhealing to erythema, warmth, tenderness, and purulence to presence of necrotic tissue and crepitus. Systemic inflammatory signs of fever and leukocytosis may be absent (see Table 49-3).[25,78]

Diagnosis. Wound assessment should include its location and measurement of its circumference and depth using a probe or at the time of surgery. Involvement of underlying structures such as bone should be noted. Superficial bacterial colonization of wounds is universal. Superficial swab culture of the exposed surface of the wound does not reflect the cause of infection. Cultures of deep pus, tissue, and blood are required for accurate diagnosis and optimum treatment of infected open wounds. Debridement of superficial necrosis and fibrinous tissue should be performed prior to obtaining tissue for deep culture.[78,81-83,96]

Many secondary wound infections are polymicrobial. Aerobic gram-negative bacilli (*E. coli, Proteus, Pseudomonas*) and gram-positive cocci (streptococci and staphylococci) and anaerobic flora (*Bacteroides, Peptostreptococci, Clostridium perfringens*) commonly infect perineal and lower extremity wounds. Culture of obligate anaerobes from tissue requires special handling by the microbiology laboratory.[78,81-83,96]

If the wound is contiguous with bone, osteomyelitis may be present. In the diabetic foot, palpable bone on the probe-to-bone test (PTB) correlates well with the presence of bone infection. In the pressure ulcer, confirmation of osteomyelitis by histopathology on bone biopsy is the gold standard, but sampling error is an issue. The most sensitive and specific imaging study for the diagnosis of osteomyelitis is magnetic resonance imaging (MRI). MRI is also useful to choose an optimal site for bone biopsy, histopathology, and culture. In the patient with a pressure ulcer, radiography and radionucleotide scintigraphy are not helpful because they cannot differentiate osteomyelitis from pressure-related heterotopic bone formation. In contrast, CT is relatively insensitive to detect osteomyelitis and its use should be limited to evaluation of the soft tissues.[78,81-83]

> Proper evaluation of the diabetic foot requires debridement and exploration of all wounds with a probe; palpable bone is diagnostic for osteomyelitis.

Management and Treatment. Initial treatment of secondary wound infection should focus on remediation of the underlying cause and local wound care in addition to antibiotic treatment. Improvement in mobility, relief of pressure, control of diabetes, incontinence, and edema, and improvement in arterial flow are just a few of the issues that need to be addressed if successful wound healing is to occur. Use of negative pressure occlusive dressings have substantially shortened the time to healing for some patients with large wounds that are not located over major vessels.[78,96]

For severe systemic infection, empiric therapy should be given based on community or nosocomial acquisition and knowledge of local resistance patterns.

Initial empiric treatment for serious infection is typically intravenous and directed against MRSA with antibiotics that treat aerobic and anaerobic pathogens. Single agents such as cefoxitin or cefotetan, broad-spectrum penicillin-beta-lactamase combinations such as ticarcillin-clavulanate or piperacillin-tazobactam, or carbapenems are appropriate choices. Ciprofloxacin and levofloxacin do not have anaerobic activity, but can be combined with clindamycin or metronidazole.[78,96]

Definitive therapy is based on the results of deep tissue and blood cultures. Acute wound infections that involve bone or bacteremia with *S. aureus* generally require prolonged intravenous therapy for 6 weeks or more. Otherwise, the duration of intravenous therapy is based on clinical experience. Serial measurement of a number of parameters may be helpful in making this decision, including the following: improvement in pain, resolution of fever, erythema, drainage, tissue necrosis, reduction in the size of the wound, clearance of bacteremia, and improvement in elevated inflammatory markers such as leukocytosis, neutrophilia, thrombocytosis, erythrocyte sedimentation rate, and C-reactive protein (CRP). Once the patient's clinical status and wound have substantially improved, transition from intravenous to oral therapy can be considered based on culture results.[78,96]

Prevention of secondary SSTI should focus on prevention of wounds and alleviation of the underlying cause. Health care providers should always adhere to infection control procedures, such as hand hygiene and glove use, when examining patients with wounds.[78,96]

GASTROINTESTINAL (GI) INFECTION

Prevalence and Impact

Manifestations of intraabdominal infection in older adults include infectious diarrhea, gastroenteritis, and intraabdominal abscesses. Infectious diarrhea with or without the nausea and vomiting of gastroenteritis is very common in older adults.[97,98] Although precise rates of GI infection are not known, approximately one third of nursing home residents will have an episode of diarrhea each year. More than 50% of all deaths caused by diarrhea in the United States occur in adults aged 75 years and older.[74,99-104] One third of diarrheal deaths occur in nursing home residents. Infections with *Salmonella* may be particularly severe. Complications and fatality rates from enteric (typhoid) fever are greatest in persons aged 50 years and older. Salmonella gastroenteritis outbreaks in nursing homes have been associated with mortality rates of 10% or more.[105,106]

Intraabdominal abscesses, although less common, pose major problems for older adults.[98] Intraabdominal abscess is a leading consideration in the older adult with fever of unknown origin. Cholecystitis and diverticulitis are common; 10% to 20% of patients with diverticulitis will have the complication of diverticular abscess. Appendicitis is rare in older adults; only 5% to 10% of cases will be in this age group. A disproportionate number of elderly patients will die of appendicitis and diverticular abscess; mortality in this group exceeds 50% for both infections.[97,98,101,102] It is critical that clinicians consider these uncommon but deadly infections when evaluating the older patient with suspected infection.

Pathophysiology and Risk Factors

For *C. difficile*, aging and debility have been associated with increased frequency of colonization and infection in the elderly. Increased predisposition to *C. difficile* in the aged is also thought to be related in part to defects in the innate immune system, inadequate production of toxin A antibody, or inadequate neutralization of toxin A by antibody. Even so, most elderly persons who carry toxin-producing *C. difficile* strains will not develop symptomatic infection until they receive an antibiotic. It is thought that *C. difficile* emerges because it is resistant to the antibiotic prescribed and not because other bacteria are suppressed or killed by the drug.[104]

More than one third of nursing home residents will acquire *C. difficile* within 2 weeks of receiving antibiotic therapy, illustrating how pathogens that cause diarrhea easily spread in closed environments of group homes and chronic health care facilities. Devices such as feeding tubes and thermometers have been shown to provide effective means of introducing *C. difficile* and other organisms into the GI tract. *C. difficile* spores readily survive in the health care environment and can contaminate devices and the hands of personnel.[104,107] Outbreaks of diarrhea have also occurred because of contaminated food or water, or by pets.[74,103]

Age-related changes in the GI tract contribute to the development of abscesses in older adults. For example, 50% of the population will have diverticulosis by age 80. Increased rates of cholelithiasis and intraabdominal malignancy are seen in the aged.[97,98]

Differential Diagnosis, Assessment, and Management

Classification and Clinical Manifestations

Inflammatory signs of pain, fever, and leukocytosis may be lacking in patients with intraabdominal abscess. Clinical suspicion and early imaging by CT scanning and radionucleotide scintigraphy are critical to diagnosing appendicitis and finding abscesses involving the liver, biliary tract, spleen, and gut.[97,98,108]

Diarrhea is typically defined as more than three watery, loose, or unformed stools per day for 48 hours or more. Symptoms can be mediated by direct invasion of the GI tract by the organism or by the elaboration of toxins. The causes of diarrhea are generally deduced by place of onset, exposure history, the presence or absence of inflammatory signs, and bloody stool, and if an outbreak is present (see Table 49-4).[25,104,107,109]

Invasive Bacterial Diarrheas. Invasive bacterial diarrheas, caused by *Salmonella, Shigella, Campylobacter,* and others, can be characterized by symptoms and signs of inflammation. Pain, fever, and leukocytosis, with blood found on occasion in stool, are prominent findings. Diagnosis of bacterial diarrhea may be suspected if fecal leukocytes are present. Elevated peripheral leukocyte counts may be seen with invasive diarrheas. Diagnosis of invasive bacterial diarrhea is made by culture of stool.[109]

Toxin-Mediated Diarrheas. Some bacterial diarrheal illnesses are mediated by the effects of toxin on the GI tract rather than by direct invasion. Shiga toxin–producing strains of enterohemorrhagic *E. coli* (EHEC) are associated with outbreaks of foodborne disease and hemolytic uremic syndrome. This noninvasive infection is not associated with inflammatory signs but bloody diarrhea can be impressive because of the effects of the toxin on the GI tract. Shiga toxin–producing *E. coli* can be detected by stool culture using special media. Molecular assays are also available that detect specific Shiga toxin–producing strains of *E. coli,* such as 0157:H7.[109,110]

Clinical manifestations of another toxin-mediated bacterial diarrhea, *C. difficile,* range from asymptomatic to mild diarrhea, pseudomembranous colitis, and toxic megacolon. Symptoms can vary from fever with mild crampy abdominal pain to ileus and peritonitis. More recent *C. difficile* strains appear to cause more severe manifestations in the elderly and immunosuppressed with increased risk of toxic megacolon and death. Very high peripheral leukocyte counts ($>$30,000 cells/mm^3) are suggestive, but not specific, for *C. difficile* infection.

The laboratory diagnosis of *C. difficile* now requires a multistep procedure. A stool assay for glutamine dehydrogenase (GDH) antigen is performed first as a marker that the *C. difficile* bacterium is present in stool and possible infection. Assays for the presence of toxin A and B are performed on GDH-positive specimens using an antigen-based method or by a less commonly available molecular method. Antigen-based tests for toxin A and toxin B are easily performed and rapid, but false negative tests occur. The more sensitive molecular test for both toxins A and B is done on those GDH-positive/toxin-negative tests. This approach eliminates toxin testing of all stools that do not contain the *C. difficile* bacterium. Detection of toxins A and B is more sensitive, thus eliminating the need to send more than one stool specimen for diagnosis.[104,108]

> **Consider the diagnosis of *C. difficile* infection in any patient with a white blood cell count greater than 30,000 cells/mm³.**

Carriage of toxin-producing *C. difficile* in older adults without diarrhea is common, and treatment of this asymptomatic colonization does not alter outcome. Thus submission of nondiarrheal stools that do not conform to the shape of the container will not be tested. Endoscopy is not a substitute for stool toxin assays because few *C. difficile* infections are associated with presence of pseudomembranes and isolated right-sided disease can be missed.[104,108]

> **Patients who no longer have diarrhea but had stools positive for *C. difficile* toxin do not benefit from treatment.**

Non-Invasive Diarrheas. Acute gastroenteritis caused by noninvasive pathogens is characterized by nausea and vomiting associated with watery, non-bloody stools, with absence of fever and other signs of inflammation. Outbreaks of watery diarrhea are typically caused by viruses such as norovirus, calciviruses, adenoviruses, enteroviruses, and rotavirus.[74,111-113] Food poisoning or intoxications caused by ingestion of preformed toxins made by *Bacillus cereus*, *C. perfringens*, and *S. aureus* may mimic outbreaks of viral gastroenteritis.[74,103] The onset of food poisoning occurs within hours of ingesting food. Outbreaks of chronic diarrhea caused by *Giardia lamblia* and *Cryptosporidia* have been reported in nursing homes related to contaminated water and food, and in child-care programs.[113-117] Specific diagnosis of noninvasive gastroenteritis is generally not warranted unless an outbreak is suspected.

In health care facilities, infection control procedures for enteric precautions should be initiated and hand washing emphasized. Laboratories increasingly rely on antigenic detection for *Giardia* and *Cryptosporidia* and molecular methods for the diagnosis of some viruses.

Management and Treatment of Diarrhea

Early identification and treatment of dehydration are important for treatment of all diarrheal illnesses.

Management and Treatment of Invasive Diarrheas. For invasive diarrheas, the decision to treat should be based on the patient's clinical condition and results of cultures and antibiotic susceptibilities. For empiric therapy of severe infection, most invasive pathogens remain susceptible to the quinolones. The elderly with *Shigella* infection are at greater risk of bacteremia and death. They should be treated given the potential severity of illness and to eradicate the organism and prevent transmission to others. Treatment of nontyphoidal *Salmonella* infections is generally not recommended in younger patients. However, metastatic seeding to extraintestinal sites such as vascular and musculoskeletal systems has been reported following gastroenteritis with *Salmonella* in the elderly; many experts recommend treatment for this age group.[109]

Management and Treatment of Toxin-Mediated Diarrheas. For Shiga toxin–producing strains of *E. coli*, antibiotic treatment is not recommended because of increased risk of development of hemolytic uremic syndrome. Avoid administering antimotility agents with bloody diarrhea and proven infection with Shiga toxin–producing *Escherichia coli*.

For the treatment of *C. difficile* infection, all antibiotics that precipitated the episode should be stopped (Table 49-9).[108] Recent studies suggest that patients who meet criteria for severe infection may benefit from treatment with vancomycin. Intravenous vancomycin solution has been given orally as a substitute for

TABLE 49-9	Recommendations for the Treatment of *Clostridium difficile* Infection	
Clinical Definition	**Supportive Clinical Data**	**Recommended Treatment**
Initial episode, mild or moderate	wbc <15,000 cells/mL Cr <1.5 × baseline	Metronidazole, 500 mg 3× daily 10-14 days
Initial episode, severe	wbc ≥15,000 cells/mL	Vancomycin 125 mg 4× daily 10-14 days
Initial episode, severe, complicated	hypotension, shock Ileus, megacolon	Vancomycin 500 mg 4× daily po or IV *and* metronidazole 500 mg 3× daily IV Consider vancomycin enema
First recurrence		Same as for initial episode
Second recurrence		Vancomycin taper and/or pulsed regime

Adapted from Cohen SH, Gerding DN, Johnson S, et al. Clinical practice guidelines for *Clostridium difficile* infection in adults: 2010 Update by the Society for Healthcare Epidemiology of America (SHEA) and the Infectious Diseases Society of America (IDSA). Infect Control Hosp Epidemiol 2010;31:431-55.
Cr, Serum creatinine; *wbc*, white blood cells.

vancomycin capsules at significantly lower cost. Treatment should continue for 10 days. Relapses are common and a second course of the same drug given for initial therapy is generally effective. Initial treatment with fidaxomicin has been associated with fewer relapses in randomized studies when compared with vancomycin, but at greater cost.[108] Older adults are more likely to have recurrence of symptoms, and consultation with a specialist should be sought. Vancomycin tapered over weeks, vancomycin followed by rifaximin, nitazoxinide, intravenous immunoglobulin, probiotics, and even stool transplants have been tried.[108]

Management and Treatment of Noninvasive Diarrheas. For patients with noninvasive viral gastroenteritis, no specific treatment is available and symptomatic treatment is sufficient. Chronic diarrheas caused by *Giardia* should be treated with metronidazole. There is no specific therapy for *Cryptosporidia* infection; most patients improve with supportive therapy. Persistent infection tends to occur in the immunosuppressed and HIV patients; no specific therapy is available. These patients should be referred to a specialist.[109]

BLOOD STREAM INFECTION (BSI)

Prevalence and Impact

Primary versus Secondary BSI

Most bloodstream infections occur as a secondary consequence of infection at another site or source such as the urinary or respiratory tracts (secondary BSI). Most are associated with the presence of a device such as a urinary or intravenous catheter or a surgical procedure. *E. coli* and *Klebsiella* account for the majority of secondary BSIs occurring in community-dwelling elderly and nursing home residents. In hospitalized elderly, *E. coli* and *S. aureus* are the most common causes of secondary BSI.[118-128]

There are some BSIs without an obvious source (primary BSI) that are found predominantly in older adults; these include *L. monocytogenes*, miliary TB, and extraintestinal nontyphoidal salmonellosis.[55,56,105,106,129] These uncommon disseminated infections have been associated with increasing debility, achlorhydria, and waning cell-mediated immunity and comorbid diseases. Extraintestinal salmonellosis has also been related to the presence of vascular disease, gallstones, malignancy, and cirrhosis.[105,106]

The source of BSI has important prognostic implications in older adults. The best survival rates occur following intravascular catheter-related, genitourinary, and GI tract infections. The poorest survival is found among elderly patients with pneumonia complicated by BSI. Poor outcome following bacteremia is particularly great in elderly persons who are afebrile, have few localizing symptoms, and have multiorgan system failure. Poor outcome is typically related to delayed or inappropriate treatment.[1,2,118-128]

Complications of BSI

Unrecognized or inadequately treated BSI can also lead to complications and metastatic infection at other sites seeding native structures such as heart valves (infective endocarditis) and vertebrae (vertebral osteomyelitis) and implanted devices. Infective endocarditis (IE) and vertebral osteomyelitis are uncommon but serious complications of BSI that are found with increasing frequency among older adults. Older adults are almost fivefold more likely to acquire IE than younger patients. Older adults are more likely to have IE associated with degenerative valvular disease and less commonly related to rheumatic or congenital valvular disease. IE caused by enterococci and *S. bovis* are also seen more often in the elderly related to increased genitourinary and gastrointestinal disorders, such as neoplasms. The elderly are also twice as likely to die from their infection as younger persons, with an overall infection-related mortality rate in the elderly of 25%.[130-132]

Infection infrequently complicates the placement of 1% to 2% of hip and knee arthroplasties caused by inoculation of the implantation site at the time of surgery or hematogenous seeding. Hematogenous seeding may occur at any time after implantation. In older adults, greater than 60% of prosthetic hip infections are caused by staphylococci. It is estimated that 8% of older adults die as a consequence of this infection.[133-135]

Differential Diagnosis, Assessment, and Management

In the elderly patient with systemic illness, BSI must be suspected because the consequences of nontreatment are grave. A minimum of two blood samples should be obtained for culture at separate times before starting antibiotics to document that BSI is present. A secondary source of suspected BSI should be sought based on history of predisposing factors and presence of focal symptoms and signs. Appropriate cultures of those secondary sites and imaging should be obtained.

Recognition of the diagnosis of IE, in particular, can be very difficult. Although older adults are at the greatest risk of acquiring IE, they are also the group most often misdiagnosed. Older adults are significantly less likely to have the diagnosis of IE made by physical examination alone. Fever (55%), leukocytosis (25%), and splenomegaly (20%) may be lacking. Embolic complications are found less often. Obtaining multiple sets of blood cultures before beginning antibiotics is essential to make the diagnosis of IE. In addition, transthoracic echocardiography may be more difficult to interpret in the patient with mitral annular disease or presence of prosthetic valve. Use of transesophageal echocardiography is recommended in those instances to confirm the presence of vegetations.[130,131,132]

Empiric therapy for BSI and its complications should be based on the place of acquisition, likelihood of antibiotic resistance, and the most likely source. Definitive therapy should be based on results of cultures obtained from blood and suspected secondary sources (Table 49-10). Isolation of the same organism and identical antimicrobial susceptibility patterns suggests that a secondary BSI is present.

Given the severity of BSIs, most treatment will be given intravenously, and the duration of treatment will depend on the source of the infection, the organism, the response of the patient to treatment, and the presence of devices. Abscesses should be drained, particularly if the patient remains symptomatic and particularly if BSI persists despite appropriate antibiotic treatment. Devices associated with the infection should be removed when feasible to facilitate clearance of the infection. Consultation for management of BSI is recommended.[130-135]

HUMAN IMMUNODEFICIENCY VIRUS (HIV) INFECTION

Prevalence and Impact

Rates of HIV infection are rising most rapidly in adults aged 50 years and older. Older women and minority populations account for most of the new cases. By 2015

TABLE 49-10	Prevalence of Major Causes of Infective Endocarditis According to Age		
All Causes (%)	<65 Years n=1703	≥65 Years n=1056	*p* Value
Gram positive	81.1	88.1	<.001
Gram negative	4.1	2.7	
Fungal	1.5	1.5	
Other/culture negative	13.2	7.5	
Bacteria (%)			
Staphylococcus aureus	33.2	28.3	<.001
MRSA	21.1	35.8	<.001
Coagulase-negative staphylococci	9.1	14.0	<.001
Viridans streptococci	18.6	14.2	<.001
Streptococcus bovis	4.4	8.3	<.001
Enterococci	6.3	16.5	<.001

Adapted from Durante-Mangoni E, Bradley S, Selton-Suty C, et al. Current features of infective endocarditis in elderly patients: Results of the International Collaboration on Endocarditis Prospective Cohort Study. Arch Intern Med 2008;168:2095-103.
MRSA, Methicillin-resistant *Staphylococcus aureus*.

more than 50% of all HIV-positive patients will be aged 50 years and older. In spite of these findings, the diagnosis of HIV is made relatively late in older adults. As a consequence, more elderly patients progress to acquired immunodeficiency or death (53%) within 12 months of diagnosis compared with younger patients (39%).[136,137]

Pathophysiology and Risk Factors

Many older adults are sexually active, but few patients use methods to protect themselves against sexually transmitted diseases. Thus the older patient is more likely to acquire HIV from sexual contact. A significant proportion of older men will have HIV risk factors such as men having sex with men (69%) and injection drug use (19%).[136,137]

Delayed diagnosis in the older adult contributes to lower CD4+ T-cell counts at baseline and more advanced HIV infection than in younger patients. Acquired immunodeficiency syndrome, defined in part by a CD4+ T-cell count of ≤200 cells/mm³, is associated with development of opportunistic infections, neoplasms, and increased risk of death.

In addition to the direct effects of HIV on the immune system, older adults with HIV frequently have a wasting syndrome suggestive of frailty. Cognitive dysfunction, bone loss, and vitamin D deficiency, commonly found in older HIV patients, are also associated with frailty, leading some to postulate that aging and HIV may have sarcopenia, inflammation with elevated cytokine levels, and insulin resistance as common pathways. It is known that untreated HIV also has a detrimental effect on commonly found comorbid conditions in the elderly such as cardiovascular disease, hepatitis, and metabolic syndrome.[138]

Management and Treatment

Many clinicians (78%) never ask their older patients whether they have risk factors for HIV or counsel their patients about how to prevent the disease. Few older adults know how to protect themselves or ask to be tested. It is essential that geriatricians consider HIV infection in their patients because early diagnosis is essential to improve survival. HIV must be excluded in older adults with wasting syndrome or encephalopathy rather than assuming these are complications of aging.[136-138]

> HIV should be considered in older adults who have dementia or wasting syndrome.

Referral of HIV-positive patients to clinicians with expertise in administration of highly active antiretroviral therapy (HAART) and monitoring of HIV infection is also crucial. Older patients are just as likely to tolerate their medications, with better compliance than younger patients. However, because older patients are on many more medications than the young, the potential for serious drug interactions is great. Geriatricians should consult with the HIV expert whenever a change in medications is contemplated to assure that drug interactions are minimized.[139]

HAART leads to increases in numbers of CD4+ cells and suppression of viral replication with reduced risk of opportunistic infections. Once CD4+ counts exceed 200 cells/mm^3 for approximately 12 months, the risk of opportunistic infections, such as *Pneumocystis jiroveci (carinii)* pneumonia, candidosis, *M. avium* complex (MAC) infection, toxoplasmosis, and others, declines significantly, and preventative medications can be stopped.[139]

Older adults who adhere to an effective HAART can generally expect that they will not die as a direct consequence of their HIV infection, and prevention of disease becomes a major focus of their care. HAART benefits HIV patients in other ways; cardiovascular and metabolic disease remains a bigger threat to their survival. Suppression of viral replication improves control of hyperlipidemia and progression of coronary artery disease.[139]

In addition to routine screening for colon carcinoma and immunizations, other challenges ensue in the surviving HIV patient. Chronic hepatitis C and hepatitis B infection may require additional treatment and close monitoring for cirrhosis and hepatocellular carcinoma. Papillomavirus associated with the presence of condyloma has been associated with squamous cell carcinoma of the rectum. HAART has been associated with aseptic necrosis of the hip; routine screening for osteopenia is recommended.[136-139]

SUMMARY

Diagnosis and management of infectious diseases in older adults poses a significant challenge for health care providers. Attention to the history with attention to risk factors and exposures may yield important clues about the causes of infection in complicated patients. Individual physical findings can be subtle and laboratory findings may be atypical. The astute clinician must make diagnostic and treatment decisions by focusing first on the most common infectious syndromes and the pathogens that cause them. Broad empiric treatment alone is not a substitute for a careful and thorough clinical assessment and systematic evaluation of the evidence for or against a diagnosis.

As one infectious diseases specialist once put it: "You just figure out what the problem is, what bug that is causing it, and treat it. Infectious Diseases really is that simple!"

Web Resources

www.idsociety.org. Infectious Diseases Society of America.
www.shea-online.org. Society for Healthcare Epidemiology of America.
www.apic.org. Association for Practitioners in Infection Control and Epidemiology.
www.thoracic.org. American Thoracic Society.
www.cdc.gov. Centers for Disease Control and Prevention.

KEY REFERENCES

9. Yoshikawa TT. Epidemiology of aging and infectious diseases. In: Yoshikawa TT, Norman DC, editors. Infectious diseases in the aging: A clinical handbook. 2nd ed. New York: Humana Press; 2009, p. 3-9.
10. Castle SC, Rafi A, Uyemura K, et al. In: Yoshikawa TT, Rajagopalan S, editors. Antibiotic therapy for geriatric patients. New York: Taylor & Francis Group; 2006, p. 19-35.
13. High KP, Bradley SF, Gravenstein S, et al. Clinical practice guideline for the evaluation of fever and infection in long-term care facilities 2008: Update by the Infectious Diseases Society of America. J Am Geriatr Soc 2009;57:375-94.
25. Stone ND, Ashraf MS, Calder J, et al. and the Society for Healthcare Epidemiology Long-Term Care Special Interest Group. Definitions of infection for surveillance in long-term care facilities: Revisiting the McGeer criteria. Infect Control Hosp Epidemiol 2012;33:965-77.
44. Nicolle LE. Urinary tract infection. In: Yoshikawa TT, Rajagopalan S, editors. Antibiotic therapy for geriatric patients. New York: Taylor & Francis Group; 2006, p. 487-501.
45. Nicolle LE. In: Yoshikawa TT, Norman DC, editors. Infectious diseases in the aging: A clinical handbook. 2nd ed. New York: Humana Press; 2009, p. 165-80.
71. Dumyati G. Influenza and other respiratory viruses. In: Yoshikawa TT, Ouslander JG, editors. Infection management for geriatrics in long-term care facilities. New York: Informa Healthcare; 2007, p. 191-214.
79. Schmader K, Twersky J. Herpes zoster, cellulitis, and scabies. In: Yoshikawa TT, Ouslander JG, editors. Infection management for geriatrics in long-term care facilities. New York: Informa Healthcare; 2007, p. 277-96.
83. Reynolds SC, Chow A. Infected pressure ulcers. In: Yoshikawa TT, Ouslander JG, editors. Infection management for geriatrics in long-term care facilities. New York: Informa Healthcare; 2007, p. 251-76.
92. Kauffman CA, Hedderwick SA. Fungal infections. In: Yoshikawa TT, Ouslander JG, editors. Infection management for geriatrics in long-term care facilities. New York: Informa Healthcare; 2007, p. 445-64.
97. Carson JG, Patterson RW, Wilson SE. Medical and surgical treatment of intra-abdominal infections. In: Yoshikawa TT, Rajagopalan S, editors. Antibiotic therapy for geriatric patients. New York: Taylor & Francis Group; 2006, p. 453-71.
98. Campbell BS, Wilson SE. Intraabdominal infections. In: Yoshikawa TT, Ouslander JG, editors. Infection management for geriatrics in long-term care facilities. New York: Informa Healthcare; 2007, p. 91-8.
135. Marculescu CE, Berbari EF, Osmon DR. Prosthetic joint infections in elderly patients. In: Yoshikawa TT, Norman DC, editors. Infectious diseases in the aging: A clinical handbook. 2nd ed. New York: Humana Press; 2009, p. 307-25.
139. Kirk JB, Goetz MB. Human immunodeficiency virus/acquired immunodeficiency syndrome. In: Yoshikawa TT, Norman DC, editors. Infectious diseases in the aging: A clinical handbook. 2nd ed. New York: Humana Press; 2009, p. 479-96.

References available online at expertconsult.com.

50

The Acute Abdomen

Marcia M. Russell

OUTLINE

OBJECTIVES

Upon completion of this chapter, the reader will be able to:

- Appreciate the special problems of the increasing numbers of older patients undergoing emergency abdominal surgery.

- Characterize the medical and surgical causes of acute abdominal pain in the older patient.

- Explain the approach to an older patient with acute abdominal pain including history and physical examination, laboratory tests, and radiographic imaging.

- Discuss the rationale for the management options for an older patient with acute abdominal pain, including emergent operation, serial abdominal examinations, observation, and nonoperative management.

Additional online-only material indicated by icon.

Alan Smith (Part 1)

Alan Smith, an 86-year-old man, visits your primary care office complaining of 24 hours of left lower quadrant abdominal pain. He is nauseated and does not feel like eating. He has not had pain like this before. He has a low grade fever (99.6° F) and his heart rate is 100.

1. **What elements of the physical examination are essential?**

2. **What tests should be ordered in your office?** ▫

PREVALENCE AND IMPACT

The definition of an acute abdomen is "signs and symptoms of acute intraabdominal pathology requiring treatment by surgical intervention."[1] However, it should be noted that not all episodes of acute abdominal pain require surgery but rather prompt diagnosis and treatment.[2] Acute abdominal pain is a common chief complaint for older patients seen in the emergency department (ED),[3] and this population consumes a disproportionate amount of time and resources in the ED in comparison to younger patients.[4] In addition, approximately 50% of older patients going to an ED with abdominal pain will require hospital admission, and 30% to 40% of these patients will eventually require surgical intervention.[5]

Not only does acute abdominal pain in the older population impact the ED, but the aging population has also been predicted to have a significant impact on the field of general surgery. The amount of procedure-based workload in general surgery is expected to increase 31% by 2020.[6] The aging population will significantly affect not only the number of procedures performed on older patients but also the percentage of emergency operations, because the risk of emergency surgery increases with age.[7] Previous research demonstrates significant variability in the percentage of emergency operations in the older population, ranging from 14% in a cohort of patients older than 80 years of age who had noncardiac surgery at Veterans Affairs hospitals,[8] 56% in a cohort of octogenarians undergoing major abdominal surgery,[9] and 69% to 72% in two cohorts of nonagenarians.[10,11]

RISK FACTORS AND PATHOPHYSIOLOGY

The workup of acute abdominal pain in the older patient is challenging for the following reasons: (1) older patients may have vague or nonspecific symptoms that are not suggestive of a specific pathophysiologic process; (2) older patients often lack the systemic (e.g., fever) or clinical signs (e.g., right lower quadrant tenderness) suggestive of acute intraabdominal pathology; (3) older patients are poor historians, or there is often difficulty obtaining an accurate history owing to memory loss or dementia; (4) older patients may delay seeking treatment or be dependent on others to be sent to a hospital for evaluation (e.g., nursing home residents); and (5) presence of comorbid disease may alter both the clinical presentation as well as the diagnostic evaluation.[4,12-15]

Misdiagnosis of acute abdominal pain is common in the older patient for all of the aforementioned reasons, so it is important to maintain a high index of suspicion.[16] Previous research has suggested a higher mortality for older patients with abdominal pain where the diagnosis occurred after admission to the hospital (19%) versus those patients with a correct preliminary diagnosis in the ED (8%).[17] Kizer et al. demonstrated that the sensitivity/specificity of a provisional ED diagnosis was lower for patients older than 65 (82% sensitivity and 86% specificity). In contrast, there was no difference in mortality based on agreement between the provisional ED diagnosis and the hospital discharge diagnosis, although there was a significant increase in disease-related morbidity.[14]

Age itself is a risk factor for some causes of an acute abdomen. Not only does the incidence of peptic ulcer disease increase with age, but in a series of 136 patients treated surgically for bleeding or perforated peptic ulcer, 80% of the deaths occurred in patients older than 70 years of age.[18] In addition, it is estimated that 30% to 50% of older patients have underlying cholelithiasis, and 50% to 80% have colonic diverticulosis. The incidence of abdominal aortic aneurysm also increases with age and is present in an estimated 5% of men older than age 65.[5] The incidence of colorectal cancer also increases with age. The median age of diagnosis for colorectal cancer is 69 years, with 61% of colorectal cancer cases diagnosed in patients 65 years of age or older from 2005-2009 using the National Cancer Institute Surveillance Epidemiology and End Results Program.[19] Previous research has also shown that elderly patients are more likely to have advanced stage colorectal cancer as well as require emergency surgery for complications of advanced colorectal cancer such as obstruction or perforation.[20]

Advanced age also contributes to mild immunosuppression, which may make the diagnosis of an acute abdomen more difficult in an older patient. The decline in immune competence impairs the ability of the older patient to increase neutrophil production in response to infection, which explains why older patients with acute intraabdominal pathology may have a normal white blood cell count.[21] A retrospective review of octogenarians with an acute abdomen demonstrated that 30% had a temperature lower than 99.5° F and a normal white blood cell count.[22] Comorbid medical disease such as diabetes mellitus, malignancy, or end-stage renal disease may also increase the degree of immunosuppression in an older patient.[5]

> Diagnosis of acute abdominal pain is challenging in the older patient—maintain high index of suspicion, and be ready for surgery!

DIFFERENTIAL DIAGNOSIS AND ASSESSMENT

The potential causes of acute abdominal pain in the older patient are numerous. One approach to classification of abdominal pain consists of determining which of the following four categories the cause of the pain falls into: (1) peritonitis, (2) bowel obstruction, (3) vascular catastrophe, or (4) nonspecific abdominal pain.[23] The differential diagnosis for both surgical and medical causes of acute abdominal pain in an older patient is shown in Box 50-1.

Several retrospective reviews have categorized the most common reasons for emergency abdominal surgery in the older patient. Arenal et al. performed a retrospective and prospective review of factors affecting mortality after emergency abdominal surgery in the older patient. The most common reasons for emergent exploration were intestinal obstruction (41%), peritonitis (29%), other etiology (21%), gastrointestinal (GI) bleeding (5%), and vascular mesenteric

---

BOX 50-1

DIFFERENTIAL DIAGNOSIS OF ACUTE ABDOMEN IN THE OLDER PATIENT

Surgical Causes of Acute Abdomen
Bowel obstruction: large bowel—incarcerated hernia, malignancy, volvulus (cecal or sigmoid); small bowel—adhesions, incarcerated hernia
Peritonitis: appendicitis, cholecystitis, diverticulitis
Perforated viscus: diverticulitis, duodenal or gastric ulcer, large-bowel obstruction with perforation
Vascular: aortic dissection, gastrointestinal hemorrhage, mesenteric ischemia/infarction, ruptured or symptomatic abdominal aortic aneurysm

Medical Causes of Acute Abdomen
Endocrine: diabetic ketoacidosis
Gastrointestinal: constipation, gastroenteritis, gastroesophageal reflux disease, inflammatory bowel disease (e.g., ulcerative colitis, Crohn's disease), malignancy, peptic ulcer disease
Genitourinary: adnexal mass, cystitis, pyelonephritis, renal calculi, other gynecologic pathology
Hepatobiliary: ascending cholangitis, choledocholithiasis, cholelithiasis, other causes of acute pancreatitis
Pulmonary: empyema, pneumonia, pulmonary embolus, pulmonary infarction
Other: myocardial infarction

disorder (4%).[24] Zerbib et al. performed a retrospective review of 45 patients older than 85 years of age who underwent emergency abdominal surgery. The most common causes of an acute abdomen were peritonitis secondary to cholecystitis or appendicitis (31%), small-bowel obstruction (SBO) (13%), mesenteric ischemia (13%), perforation secondary to diverticulitis or duodenal ulcer (13%), large-bowel obstruction secondary to sigmoid volvulus or obstructing colon cancer (11%), and other etiology.[25] Potts et al. performed a retrospective review of surgical abdomens in patients 80 years and older. The three most common diagnoses were acute cholecystitis (25%), hernia (21%), and bowel obstruction (16%).[22] More recent data from the 2005-2009 American College of Surgeons (ACS) National Surgical Quality Improvement Program (NSQIP) identified 37,553 patients undergoing emergency laparotomy.[26] The most common indications for surgery were obstruction (34%), perforation (24%), other (18%), neoplasm (8%), vascular insufficiency (7%), GI bleeding (4%), GI inflammation (3%), pancreatitis (1%), and fistula (1%).

> In general, there are four main categories of a surgical acute abdomen: (1) peritonitis, (2) perforated viscus, (3) bowel obstruction, and (4) vascular.

CASE 1

Alan Smith (Part 2)

The abdominal examination demonstrates tenderness to palpation in the left lower quadrant with mild guarding. Mr. Smith has a past medical history of chronic obstructive pulmonary disease (COPD) on home oxygen, coronary artery bypass graft for coronary artery disease, end-stage renal disease, and radical prostatectomy for prostate cancer. He was hospitalized 1 week ago for a COPD exacerbation and worsening renal function requiring initiation of hemodialysis. He was discharged home on a steroid taper for the COPD exacerbation. ◼

History and Physical Examination

Critical elements of the history and physical examination when evaluating an older patient with acute abdominal pain are outlined in Box 50-2. Careful attention must be paid to a thorough history and physical examination because the presentation of an older patient with an acute abdomen may be quite varied, ranging from mild abdominal pain to a change in mental status.[5] One distinction between medical and surgical causes of abdominal pain may be the temporal relation between the onset of pain and vomiting. Abdominal pain requiring an operation often

---

BOX 50-2

PERFORMING A HISTORY AND PHYSICAL EXAMINATION IN AN OLDER PATIENT WITH ACUTE ABDOMINAL PAIN

Patient History

Pain: Time of onset, location, radiation, quality, severity, palliating and provoking factors.
Gastrointestinal function: Anorexia, nausea, vomiting, bowel habits, characterization of emesis (e.g., bilious, bloody) and stool (e.g., diarrhea versus constipation, presence of blood, melena), and last time the patient ate, passed flatus, or had a bowel movement.
Associated symptoms: Generalized symptoms, including fever, chills, and fatigue, as well as organ-specific symptoms (e.g., chest pain, shortness of breath, cough with productive sputum, dysuria, hematuria).
Other medical problems: May elicit clues to the etiology of abdominal pain, especially prior history of diabetes, cardiac, pulmonary, or gastrointestinal disease.
Surgical history: Ask about all previous operations (especially abdominal procedures).
Current medications: Ask about all current medications, especially nonsteroidal antiinflammatory drugs (known association with gastrointestinal hemorrhage), warfarin or dabigatran (Pradaxa) (increased risk for bleeding or thrombotic/embolic event), steroids (immunosuppression), and beta-blockers (may blunt tachycardia).

Physical Examination

Vital signs: Monitor for tachycardia, hypotension; older patients are often normothermic or hypothermic.
Abdomen: Inspect for prior abdominal scars; *auscultate* for absence (e.g., ileus) or presence of bowel sounds (e.g., high pitched may be associated with bowel obstruction); *percuss* for presence of tympany (bowel obstruction) or pain (peritonitis) or dullness from fluid (ascites); *palpate* for presence of mass (e.g., phlegmon, malignancy, abdominal aortic aneurysm if pulsatile); and *evaluate* for hernia in umbilicus, groin, and prior abdominal incisions.
Rectal: Always do rectal to evaluate for tenderness, impaction, rectal mass, and presence of gross or occult fecal blood.
Genitourinary: Assess for costovertebral angle tenderness; evaluate testicles/scrotum for presence of hernia; or do pelvic exam to assess for ovarian/uterine pathology.

---

precedes vomiting (e.g., acute appendicitis), whereas vomiting often precedes the abdominal pain secondary to a medical condition (e.g., gastroenteritis).[1]

> Vomiting before abdominal pain think medical; pain before vomiting think surgical; be prepared for either and both.

Laboratory Testing

The initial diagnostic workup of an older patient for an acute abdomen should include standard laboratory tests such as complete blood count with differential, electrolytes, and renal function. Liver function tests, as well as amylase and lipase, should be sent if the differential diagnosis includes hepatobiliary pathology or pancreatitis. A urinalysis and urine culture should be sent if the history and physical examination suggests a urologic cause (e.g., nephrolithiasis, pyelonephritis). Blood cultures may be useful when abdominal pain is associated with fever or there is a high index of suspicion for sepsis. Coagulation tests should be sent for any patient taking warfarin or other anticoagulant, as well as those with GI hemorrhage or known severe liver disease. Type and cross-match should be sent for any patient with a source of active bleeding or a high likelihood of undergoing operative intervention with significant blood loss. Arterial blood gas or serum lactate may be useful when considering the diagnosis of mesenteric or bowel ischemia.

Radiographic Imaging

Radiographic imaging often provides useful information regarding the etiology of the acute abdominal pain. A chest x-ray examination could demonstrate pulmonary pathology as the source of the abdominal pain. Free air under the diaphragm is diagnostic for a perforated viscus, and will require an emergency exploratory laparotomy. An upright abdominal x-ray examination may demonstrate dilated loops of small or large intestine and/or air-fluid levels, which could confirm small- or large-bowel obstruction. Other diagnostic findings on plain films include abnormal calcifications (e.g., 10% of gallstones, 90% of kidney stones, and 5% of appendicoliths are radioopaque) and gas in the portal venous system (pneumobilia) or wall of the GI tract (pneumatosis intestinalis).[1]

> **Look for air under the diaphragm on x-ray films or CT; it means something is perforated and emergency surgery is literally vital.**

Alternative radiographic images include ultrasound (US) and computed tomography (CT). Abdominal US can often be performed at the bedside and provides information on the presence or absence of gallstones, abdominal aortic aneurysm, and hydronephrosis. A common radiologic investigation for an older patient complaining of abdominal pain in the ED is CT (90% of attending physicians in emergency medicine at a single residency program responded that it was their standard practice to order an abdominal CT scan for an older patient complaining of abdominal pain[27]). A prospective, observational, multicenter study assessed the use of abdominal CT in older ED patients with acute abdominal pain. Thirty-seven percent of older patients with acute abdominal pain were evaluated with abdominal CT scan, and of the patients receiving CT scans, 57% were diagnostic for the etiology

of the pain, 31% had nonspecific findings, and 12% were read by a radiologist as normal. The diagnostic ability of CT was significantly higher for patients requiring urgent surgical intervention at 85% (versus 71% for patients requiring acute medical intervention and 34% for patients requiring no acute intervention). The most common diagnostic CT findings were SBO (subacute bowel obstruction) or ileus (18%), diverticulitis (18%), urolithiasis (10%), cholelithiasis or cholecystitis (10%), abdominal mass/neoplasm (8%), pyelonephritis (7%), and pancreatitis (6%).[13] Similarly, a prospective observational cohort study evaluated the ability of CT to change decision making in older patients going to the ED with acute abdominal pain. Abdominal CT altered the decision for admission in 26%, altered the decision for surgery in 12%, and altered the suspected diagnosis in 45% of cases.[27]

> Radiographic imaging options for workup of an acute abdomen include chest x-ray examination, abdominal series, ultrasound, and CT scan.

CASE 1

Alan Smith (Part 3)

Chest x-ray study shows hyperinflated lungs consistent with COPD. There is no free air under the right hemidiaphragm. Laboratories are significant for an elevated white blood cell count of 14,000, hematocrit of 54%, and grossly abnormal electrolytes: sodium of 127 mmol/L, potassium of 6.5 mmol/L, chloride of 87 mmol/L, bicarbonate of 16 mmol/L, blood urea nitrogen (BUN) of 85 mg/dL, and creatinine of 5.5 mg/dL. While you are discussing these results with the patient, he has an episode of large bilious emesis. You repeat the vital signs: his pulse is now 120 with blood pressure of 90/50 mmHg. You have recommended the patient be transferred to the local hospital ED for additional workup.

1. **What are some potential causes of acute abdominal pain in Mr. Smith?**

2. **What is the most appropriate next step in Mr. Smith's management?** ▣

MANAGEMENT

Management of the older patient with an acute abdomen who appears seriously ill should initially follow the ABCs: First, the patient's *airway* and *breathing* should be assessed. If there is any concern about the adequacy of the airway or the ability of the patient to maintain oxygenation and ventilation, then the patient should be intubated. *Circulation* should be evaluated, including blood pressure, presence of active bleeding, and intravenous access. If peripheral intravenous access cannot easily be obtained, then a central line should be placed for fluid resuscitation with normal saline or lactated Ringer's. A surgical consultation should be obtained immediately for patients with a suspected diagnosis of ruptured abdominal aortic aneurysm, mesenteric ischemia, or for the presence of free air on plain x-ray studies. In addition, if the diagnosis remains unclear after initial laboratories and x-ray examination, surgical consultation should be obtained.[5]

CASE 1

Alan Smith (Part 4)

Fluid resuscitation is initiated in your office by the paramedics, prior to transfer of Mr. Smith to the ED at the local hospital. On arrival at the ED, he continues to be tachycardic with a systolic blood pressure of 90 mmHg. He is resuscitated with 2 liters of normal saline with improvement in the vital signs and is now stable enough to go for a CT scan.

What other specialties should be consulted in the care of Mr. Smith? ◉

Preparing for Potential Surgery

All older patients with acute abdominal pain should be maintained on nothing by mouth until a decision is reached regarding (1) the need for urgent surgery and (2) whether the probable etiology of the acute abdominal pain is medical or surgical. A nasogastric tube should be considered if there is a large volume of emesis and/or a diagnosis of bowel obstruction. A Foley catheter should be considered to monitor urine output, especially if a significant amount of volume resuscitation is required. Broad-spectrum antibiotics should be administered (with blood cultures drawn first if possible) if there is evidence of peritonitis or perforation. Blood should be sent for type and screen/cross-match if need for blood transfusion *or* surgical intervention is anticipated.

A best practices guideline on the optimal preoperative assessment of the geriatric surgical patient has been published by the ACS NSQIP and the American Geriatrics Society.[28] Although it may not be possible to perform all of the items suggested in the guideline for an elderly patient undergoing emergency abdominal surgery, the guideline does provide a useful preoperative checklist to help assess the elderly patient's risk of perioperative morbidity and mortality including areas unique to the geriatric patient such as cognitive status, risk for postoperative delirium, frailty, and history of falls.

Patient–Clinician Discussions

Postoperative complications for older patients undergoing emergency abdominal surgery are significant, with estimated rates of 30% to 68% morbidity and 5% to 31% mortality.[7,9-11,24,25,29] Given the known risks of perioperative morbidity and mortality in the older patient requiring emergency abdominal surgery, the surgeon should discuss the role of surgery with the patient and/or family members, the likelihood of complications and/or death, do not resuscitate (DNR) status, and the patient's preferences regarding cardiopulmonary resuscitation (CPR) and other life-sustaining measures. Before surgery, attempts must be made to discuss the patient's advance directive for medical decision making and to identify the surrogate decision maker. Previous research has demonstrated that clinicians often underestimate a patient's desire to withhold CPR.[30] The decision to withhold life-sustaining treatments increases with each decade of age by 19% for surgery, 15% for ventilator support, and 12% for dialysis.[31] Patient decisions to pursue aggressive treatments (such as surgery) are also influenced by the likely outcomes. For example, if the outcome was survival, but with severe functional or cognitive impairment, 74.4% and 88.8%, respectively, of participants would not choose to undergo treatment.[32] A recent study by Scarborough et al. described the outcomes of elderly patients with preoperative DNR status who underwent emergency general surgery.[33] Patients with a preoperative DNR order had higher mortality, were less likely to undergo reoperation, and were more likely to die when they experienced major postoperative complications in comparison to patients without a preoperative DNR. The authors hypothesize that one potential reason for higher mortality rates in the patients with a preoperative DNR is a failure to pursue rescue when postoperative complications occur.

> Clinicians (still) often underestimate a patient's desire to withhold CPR; document patient preferences before surgery!

It is also beneficial to quickly assess the patient's baseline functional status before surgery. A prospective cohort study demonstrated that seriously ill patients are more accurate in their estimates of future physical functioning than are either family members or physicians.[34] Also, a prognostic model for prediction of future functional status identified functional status 2 weeks before hospitalization as the single most important predictor of serious functional decline after hospitalization.[35]

> Clarify the functional status as it was 2 weeks ago; it is the real baseline and helps predict decline after hospitalization.

Discussion

CT scan shows perforated diverticulitis with a large pericolic abscess and a surgical consultation is obtained. Given Mr. Smith's multiple medical comorbidities, it is recommended that he undergo percutaneous drainage of the pericolic abscess in addition to medical management with bowel rest and broad spectrum antibiotics. A nephrology consultation for hemodialysis is also obtained, given the electrolyte abnormalities (especially the potassium of 6.5 mEq/dL and bicarbonate of 16 mmol/L) and the large volume of fluid resuscitation that will be needed (based on the patient's tachycardia, hypotension, and hemoconcentration with hematocrit of 54%). The patient's hemodynamic status and electrolytes are optimized, in anticipation of the possible need for surgical intervention. The following day, the patient's white blood cell count has increased to 24,000 and he is complaining of more abdominal pain. Repeat upright chest x-ray examination shows a large amount of free air under the right diaphragm. The patient is taken to the operating room for exploratory laparotomy. Intraoperative findings include feculent peritonitis and the patient undergoes sigmoid colectomy with end colostomy and Hartmann closure of the rectum. ◙

Nonoperative Management

If the patient does not require urgent operative intervention and a definitive diagnosis has not been reached, *observation* of the patient with serial abdominal examinations should be considered. Severe abdominal pain that lasts more than 6 hours increases the likelihood of surgical disease, whereas abdominal pain that improves with time decreases the probability of needing surgery.[1] Repeat laboratory tests and x-ray studies should be ordered for the following day to assess for changes in white blood cell count, degree of bowel obstruction, etc. Nonoperative management plays an important role in, for example, the conservative management of SBO, percutaneous drainage of an abscess from perforated appendicitis or diverticulitis, or endoscopic decompression of sigmoid volvulus.

Watchful waiting with serial abdominal x-ray studies and repeated clinical examinations and laboratory tests is reasonable if the pain is not worsening and the diagnosis is not clear or if death is a strong possibility in a frail, septic, shocked, very old person.

Consideration of nonoperative management may also be appropriate for elderly patients who are unlikely to survive emergency surgery or do not desire aggressive intervention but rather prefer comfort measures for pain management or control of symptoms. Al-Temimi et al. addressed this important issue of when death may be inevitable after emergency abdominal surgery using data from the ACS NSQIP.[26]

Mortality was 14% for patients undergoing emergency exploratory laparotomy and the variables of age, American Society of Anesthesiologists (ASA) class, functional status, and sepsis were most associated with mortality. In addition, patients with the following six characteristics had a probability of survival of less than 10%: older than 90 years, ASA class 5, septic shock, dependent functional status, and abnormal white blood cell count. This data is important to assist surgeons and patients and their families with decision making about end-of-life care versus potentially futile surgical intervention.

Outcomes After Operative Management

With respect to Mr. Smith's case study about perforated diverticulitis, previous research has shown that advanced age is an independent predictor of both morbidity and mortality after emergency surgery for diverticulitis.[36] Lidsky et al. used the ACS NSQIP data from 2005-2009 to identify 2264 patients undergoing emergency surgery for diverticulitis. Mortality rates increased with age, with observed postoperative mortality rates of 1.6% for nonelderly, 9.7% for elderly (age 65-79), and 17.8% for super elderly (age ≥80). Using multivariate logistic regression, age ≥80 increased the odds of death 2.7-fold while adjusting for other preoperative, intraoperative, and postoperative variables. In addition, the authors identified several postoperative complications with extremely high mortality rates in elderly patients such as stroke (50% mortality), acute renal failure (60% mortality), cardiac arrest (70% mortality) and coma lasting more than 24 hours (100% mortality). These results suggest that in order to improve the outcome of mortality for elderly patients undergoing emergency surgery, the focus should be on preventing postoperative complications.

> Emergency surgery (for diverticulitis): postop mortality compared to nonelders is 6 times greater for ages 65 to 79, 11 times greater for ages 80 and older.

Multiple studies have demonstrated increased risk of morbidity and mortality in elderly patients undergoing emergency abdominal surgery. A common complication that occurs after surgery in elderly patients is delirium. Engelberger et al. reviewed the frequency of postoperative delirium at their hospital in patients undergoing emergency colorectal surgery for peritonitis (the majority of the patients underwent surgery for perforated diverticulitis).[37] Postoperative delirium occurred in one third of patients and had a trend toward experiencing higher postoperative morbidity when compared to patients who did not experience postoperative delirium. This research is important because it highlights the frequency of postoperative delirium as well as the need for additional research to identify interventions to prevent delirium or improve outcomes in elderly patients who do experience post-operative delirium. With respect to the outcome of mortality, Mamidanna et al. evaluated 36,767 non-elective colorectal resections in patients aged 70 and older in England.[38] Thirty-day mortality rates increased with increasing age (17% for 70-75 years, 23% for 76-80 years, and 31% for ≥80 years). Long-term follow-up demonstrated that 51% of patients age 80 or older died within 1 year after surgery. This research is important because it highlights the dramatic increase in mortality by age group as well as the poor long-term survival in the elderly cohort. Finally, Duron et al. performed a multicenter prospective study in order to identify risk factors for mortality in major digestive surgery in the elderly. Similar to previous research, mortality rates increased exponentially with age and were significantly higher in the emergency surgery group (24% vs. 4% for elective surgery).[39] The authors identified six independent risk factors for mortality within the elderly: age ≥85 years (odds ratio [OR] 2.6), emergency surgery (OR 3.4), anemia (OR 1.8), white blood cell count above 10,000/mm^3 (OR 1.9), ASA class 4 (OR 9.9), and palliative cancer operation (OR 4.0). This research is important in order to identify patients at high risk of death after surgery, which may impact patient–provider discussions about the goals of surgery as well as potential outcomes.

SUMMARY

The population is aging, and increasing numbers of older patients are undergoing surgery. The risk for emergency abdominal surgery increases with age; some of the most common causes of acute abdomen in the older patient are obstruction, perforation, and peritonitis secondary to appendicitis, cholecystitis or diverticulitis. Diagnosis of an acute abdomen can be difficult, because older patients are less likely to have fever, leukocytosis, severe abdominal pain, or other classic signs and symptoms of acute abdominal pathology. The approach to an older patient with acute abdominal pain should be methodical and include a thorough history and physical examination, laboratory data, and x-ray studies if indicated. Surgical consultation should always be obtained if the diagnosis is unclear. Stabilization should be attempted before surgery. The management options for an older patient with acute abdominal pain are varied and include urgent operation, observation with serial abdominal examinations, and nonoperative management. The patient's wishes regarding CPR and other life-sustaining interventions should be established early in the course of the illness. The risks and potential outcomes of surgical intervention must also be explained to the patient or surrogate.

Web Resources

http://seer.cancer.gov/statfacts/html/colorect.html. National Cancer Institute's Surveillance Epidemiology and End Results (SEER) Stat Fact Sheet: Colon and Rectum.

KEY REFERENCES

14. Kizer KW, Vassar MJ. Emergency department diagnosis of abdominal disorders in the elderly. Am J Emerg Med 1998;16: 357-62.
26. Al-Temimi MH, Griffee M, Enniss TM, et al. When is death inevitable after emergency laparotomy? Analysis of the American College of Surgeons National Surgical Quality Improvement Program Database. J Am Coll Surg 2012;215:503-11.
28. Chow WB, Rosenthal RA, Merkow RP, et al. Optimal preoperative assessment of the geriatric surgical patient: A best practices guideline from the American College of Surgeons National Surgical Quality Improvement Program and the American Geriatrics Society. J Am Coll Surg 2012;215:453-66.
31. Hamel MB, Teno JM, Goldman L, et al. Patient age and decisions to withhold life-sustaining treatments from seriously ill, hospitalized adults. SUPPORT Investigators. Study to Understand Prognoses and Preferences for Outcomes and Risks of Treatment. Ann Intern Med 1999;130:116-25.
34. Wu AW, Young Y, Dawson NV, et al. Estimates of future physical functioning by seriously ill hospitalized patients, their families, and their physicians. J Am Geriatr Soc 2002;50:230-7.

References available online at expertconsult.com.

51

Benign Prostate Disease

Lisa J. Granville and Niharika Suchak

INCIDENCE AND PREVALENCE

This chapter reviews the two common benign conditions of the prostate gland: benign prostatic hyperplasia (BPH) and prostatitis. With advancing age, the prevalence of prostate diseases increases dramatically. Self-reported prostate disease affects about 3 million American men. BPH develops in more than half of men age 65 or older and affects the overwhelming majority of men older than age 85. The prevalence of prostatitis is similar to that of ischemic heart disease or diabetes mellitus.

CASE 1

Paul Phillips (Part 1)

Paul Phillips is a 67-year-old man who comes to your office asking for "something to stop me from going so often." He notes being unable to hold his urine for very long once he has an urge to void and arising three to four times each night to urinate. Some days he notes he is tired because voiding interferes with his sleep. He is concerned that the problem is interfering significantly with his daily golf game. He drinks diet cola about three times a day and has an evening cocktail four or five times a week.

His past medical history is remarkable for occasional constipation (he uses a stool softener two to three times a month), osteoarthritis of the knee which he manages with Tylenol extra strength two to three times a week, and bilateral cataracts for which he limits night driving. He takes a daily multivitamin and uses NoDoz alertness pills about four times a month when his sleep has been significantly interrupted.

What initial evaluation and management would you recommend for Mr. Phillips's lower urinary tract symptoms? ▣

Additional online-only material indicated by icon.

RISK FACTORS AND PATHOPHYSIOLOGY

Overview of Anatomy and Physiology Including Age-Related Changes

The male lower urinary tract is composed of the urinary bladder, prostate, and urethra. The prostate gland is an accessory gland of the male reproductive system. The retroperitoneal organ is located anterior to the rectum and encircles the neck of the urinary bladder and part of the urethra. Its main function is to produce fluid for semen, which transports sperm. A healthy adult prostate is walnut shaped with an average size of 20 g.

Upon gross appearance, the prostate includes a base and an apex. The base of the prostate is near the inferior surface of the bladder and a large part of the base is continuous with the bladder wall. The apex or lower end of the prostate is adjacent to the external urethral sphincter.

The prostate is a collection of 30 to 50 irregularly shaped tubuloalveolar glands that open into the prostatic urethra via separate branching ducts. These glands are embedded in fibromuscular stroma, dense with collagen and irregularly arranged smooth muscle. The outer layer of the prostate is a thin, indistinct fibroelastic capsule mixed with smooth muscle. Age-related changes in the prostate, such as glandular enlargement, increased smooth muscle tone, and decreased compliance secondary to altered collagen deposition, can lead to urinary symptoms.

The prostate is divided into four lobes. The anterior lobe lies in front of the urethra and consists of fibromuscular tissue. The median lobe is situated between the two ejaculatory ducts and the urethra. The right and left lateral lobes make up the bulk of the prostate and are separated by the prostatic urethra. The posterior lobe is the medial part of the lateral lobes and can be palpated through the rectum during digital rectal examination (DRE).

The prostate can be divided histologically into three concentric zones: the peripheral zone (the outermost area of the prostate that constitutes 70% of the glandular tissue), the central zone (that represents 25% of the glandular tissue), and the transitional zone (the innermost area that rests next to the urethra and constitutes 5% of the glandular tissue). This distribution of zones has clinical significance. The peripheral zone is the area that is palpated on DRE, is most commonly affected by chronic prostatitis, and is where 70% of adenocarcinomas are found. Benign prostatic hyperplasia commonly arises in the transitional zone.

The white serous prostatic fluid contains acid phosphatase, citric acid, zinc, prostate-specific antigen (PSA), and other protease and fibrolytic enzymes involved in liquefaction of semen. With aging, there is an increase in the number and calcification of prostatic concretions (mixture of prostatic secretions and debris from degenerated epithelial cells). It is postulated that prostatic concretions serve as a nidus for development of chronic bacterial prostatitis.

The prostate is under neurohormonal influence; alpha-1 adrenergic receptors are the predominant type of adrenergic receptors present in the smooth muscle of the prostate and help maintain urethral tone and intraurethral pressure. Testosterone is converted to dihydrotestosterone (DHT) by 5-alpha-reductase in prostatic stromal cells. Androgen stimulation of glandular tissue via DHT contributes to the development and growth of the prostate gland and may lead to benign prostatic hyperplasia. The prostate gland enlarges during a man's life via multiple growth spurts, with the last growth phase starting when a man is in his 50s. Problems with urinary flow usually appear only after the age of 50 as a consequence of the final growth phase. There is some evidence to suggest that the relative increase in circulating estrogen associated with aging may strengthen the effect of DHT on the prostate with promotion of cellular growth and glandular enlargement.

The pathophysiology of urinary symptoms associated with BPH can be attributed to both static and dynamic factors. The static component is a result of the enlargement of the prostate impinging upon the prostatic urethra and bladder outlet, whereas the dynamic component is related to the tension of prostatic smooth muscle. The static component may cause urinary symptoms because of excessive growth of the glandular tissue in the periurethral zone or stromal tissue in the transition zone. The direction of growth of glandular tissue can affect urinary flow. Growth toward the inside will probably cause direct urinary flow obstruction. The beginning phase of an outward growth of glandular tissue is less likely to cause urinary flow obstruction. The prostatic capsule may prevent progressive outward expansion of the prostate. Therefore, ongoing outward growth may ultimately result in compressive forces on the prostatic urethra. If the prostate can be thought of as a doughnut, then the hole in the middle of the doughnut becomes smaller by inward growth of tissue and/or inward compression when the capsule restricts outward expansion. Thus the size of the prostate as detected by a DRE, which correlates with outward growth, may not correlate with urinary flow symptoms. In addition, an increase in the tone of prostatic smooth muscle may lead to obstructive urinary symptoms without any prostate enlargement.

Voiding of urine is a synchronized action between the bladder and urethra. The bladder is innervated by parasympathetic nerves and their stimulation causes bladder muscle contraction leading to voiding of urine. Stimulation of sympathetic nerves that innervate the bladder neck and prostate causes closure of the bladder outlet. A voluntary sphincter in the bladder neck, supplied by the pudendal nerve and controlled by the higher cortical centers and diencephalons, enables conscious control of urine voiding. Multiple factors, including changes in the bladder, prostate, and/or urethra, can lead to voiding dysfunction in an aging male.

> Lower urinary tract symptoms can occur from a variety of conditions within and outside of the urinary tract; a diagnostic evaluation is necessary to determine etiology.

CLINICAL MANIFESTATIONS

Historically, the terms *prostatism* and *symptoms of benign prostatic hyperplasia* have been used to describe lower urinary tract symptoms (LUTS) in men. Although the term prostatism implies a prostatic cause for urinary symptoms, frequently no evidence exists for such an implication. LUTS are very common both in elderly men and women. BPH is a precise histological term, yet many older men with LUTS are described as suffering from the symptoms of BPH or from clinical BPH without this level of diagnostic evaluation. The use of the specific histological term is confusing in routine clinical practice.

The preferred term, *lower urinary tract symptoms (LUTS)*, describes patients' complaints without implying their cause. This is important because the symptoms are not gender, age, or disease specific. Transient causes of LUTS include drugs, dietary factors, restricted mobility, constipation, infection, inflammation, polyuria, and psychological causes. Stimulation of the alpha-1 adrenergic receptors in the smooth muscle of the stroma and capsule of the prostate, as well as in the bladder neck, can cause an increase in smooth-muscle tone, which can worsen LUTS.

Diseases that originate from the lower urinary tract (prostatic and nonprostatic diseases) and diseases that do not originate from the lower urinary tract (such as those that can affect the neural control of voiding mechanisms—for example, diabetes mellitus, cerebrovascular accident, Parkinson's disease, multiple sclerosis, and spinal cord injury) can affect the primary structures and systems involved with voiding and lead to LUTS.

Histologically, BPH is categorized as a hyperplastic process that results in enlargement of the prostate that may cause restriction in the flow of urine from the bladder. Subsequently obstruction induces bladder wall changes, such as thickening, increase in trabeculations, and irritability, that contribute to LUTS. Increased bladder sensitivity (detrusor overactivity [DO]) occurs even with small volumes of urine in the bladder. The bladder may gradually weaken and lose the ability to empty completely, leading to increased

residual urine volume and, possibly, acute or chronic urinary retention.

The International Continence Society has published standard terminology to define symptoms, signs, urodynamic observations, and conditions associated with lower urinary tract dysfunction.[1] LUTS are divided into three groups: storage, voiding, and postmicturition symptoms. Storage (irritative) symptoms include increased daytime frequency (voiding too often during the day), nocturia (to wake at night one or more times to void), urgency (sudden urge to urinate that is difficult to defer), incontinence (complaint of any involuntary leakage of urine), and bladder sensation (defined by five categories: normal, increased, reduced, absent, and nonspecific). Voiding (obstructive) symptoms are experienced during the voiding phase and include a slow stream (perception of reduced urine flow), splitting or spraying (character of stream), intermittent stream (urine flow that starts and stops), hesitancy (difficulty in initiating micturition), straining (muscular effort used to initiate, maintain, or improve the urinary stream), and terminal dribble (prolonged final part of micturition, when flow has slowed to a trickle/dribble). Postmicturition symptoms are experienced immediately after micturition and include a feeling of incomplete emptying (sensation of not emptying the bladder completely after finishing urinating) and postmicturition dribble (involuntary loss of urine immediately after completion of urination, usually after leaving the toilet in men, or after rising from the toilet in women).

CASE 1

Paul Phillips (Part 2)

Mr. Phillips's initial assessment reveals urinary frequency, urgency, nocturia, and straining with an IPSS (International Prostate Symptom Score) of 12. DRE reveals normal sphincter tone, prostate about 20 g with no asymmetry or nodules. Urinalysis is unremarkable. You educate Mr. Phillips about LUTS, discuss transient causes including caffeine and alcohol, and recommend discontinuation of NoDoz, avoidance of fluids 2 hours before bedtime, and dietary modifications with use of a bladder diary to help him identify triggers.

Two months later at a follow-up visit Mr. Phillips reports his frequency, urgency, and nocturia are much improved, with an IPSS of 5. He notes, "Now I can spend time with my friends and play a round of golf without worrying."

How frequently will Mr. Phillips need to be monitored for his BPH? When would it be appropriate to initiate BPH medication? ▣

> Medications should always be considered in the differential diagnosis as a cause of LUTS or worsening BPH symptoms.

BPH: DIFFERENTIAL DIAGNOSIS AND ASSESSMENT

The diagnosis of BPH in men is typically clinical, and one of exclusion. When a urinary symptom is noted, a standardized questionnaire, such as the IPSS, is used to quantify the severity of LUTS (Figure 51-1). The IPSS assesses seven symptoms during the past month. The questions address the following factors: feeling of incomplete bladder emptying, frequency, intermittency, urgency, weak stream, straining, and nocturia; each is rated on the scale on which 0 = none and 5 = almost always. The symptom categories are based on the summative score: 0 to 7 mild, 8 to 19 moderate, and 20 to 35 severe.

Other possible contributors are queried, such as endocrine (e.g., poorly controlled diabetes), neurologic

INTERNATIONAL PROSTATE SYMPTOM SCORE (I-PSS)

Patient name: _____ Date of birth: _____ Date completed: _____

In the past month:	Not at all	Less than 1 in 5 times	Less than half the time	About half the time	More than half the time	Almost always	Your score
1. Incomplete emptying How often have you had the sensation of not emptying your bladder?	0	1	2	3	4	5	
2. Frequency How often have you had to urinate less than every two hours?	0	1	2	3	4	5	
3. Intermittency How often have you found you stopped and started again several times when you urinated?	0	1	2	3	4	5	
4. Urgency How often have you found it difficult to postpone urination?	0	1	2	3	4	5	
5. Weak stream How often have you had a weak urinary stream?	0	1	2	3	4	5	
6. Straining How often have you had to strain to start urination?	0	1	2	3	4	5	
	None	**1 Time**	**2 Times**	**3 Times**	**4 Times**	**5 Times**	
7. Nocturia How many times did you typically get up at night to urinate?	0	1	2	3	4	5	
Total IPSS score							

Score: 1–7: *Mild*   8–19: *Moderate*   20–35: *Severe*

Quality of life due to urinary symptoms	Delighted	Pleased	Mostly satisfied	Mixed	Mostly dissatisfied	Unhappy	Terrible
If you were to spend the rest of your life with your urinary condition just the way it is now, how would you feel about that?	0	1	2	3	4	5	6

Figure 51-1 The International Prostate Symptom Score is based on the answers to seven questions related to lower urinary tract symptoms. Each symptom is scored 0 to 5 for a possible total score between 0 and 35. Question 8 refers to the patient's perceived quality of life but is not included in the scoring of the IPSS. The IPSS is similar to the American Urological Association's Symptom Index. (Barry M, Fowler FJ, O'Leary MP, et al. The American Urological Association Symptom index for benign prostatic hyperplasia. J Urol 1992;148:1549-57.)

(e.g., neurogenic bladder), symptoms of urinary tract infection, and previous urologic conditions (e.g., urethral stricture, bladder neck contracture, interstitial cystitis). Although nonspecific for BPH, DRE is performed to rule out other conditions. The prostate size, tenderness, and presence of nodules are noted. Because hyperplasia may only involve the transitional zone, the DRE can be unremarkable or it may reveal an enlarged, smooth, rubbery, symmetrical gland. Lower abdominal/suprapubic palpation may identify a distended bladder. Urinalysis is routinely performed to evaluate for urinary tract infection, hematuria, and glycosuria; BPH is associated with an unremarkable urinalysis.

> **Lifestyle modifications can be effective in reducing urinary symptoms, and bladder diaries often assist a person in making these changes.**

Additional tests are considered optional and are based on clinical indications. If urinary retention is suspected, postvoid residual urine volume (often done by office or bedside bladder scan) is performed. Serum creatinine measurement may be used to assess kidney function and the possibility of obstructive uropathy and/or intrinsic renal disease. Pressure-flow urodynamic studies are commonly performed prior to surgical interventions. These tests can also be considered when the diagnosis is uncertain.

BPH: MANAGEMENT

The initiation of BPH therapy depends on the patient and is driven by the effect of the symptoms on the patient's quality of life (Table 51-1 and Figure 51-2). All patients should be educated regarding lifestyle modification. Men with mild to moderate symptoms may be satisfied with lifestyle modification only. Both medical and surgical treatments are also available, with medication the usual first approach. Indications for surgical treatment include patient preference, dissatisfaction with medication, and refractory urinary retention. Complications from prostatic obstruction, including renal dysfunction, bladder stones, recurrent urinary tract infections, and hematuria are also managed surgically. The selection of surgical approach is dependent on patient anatomy and the surgeon's experience as well as the potential benefits and risks for complications.

Lifestyle Interventions and Self-Management

BPH is a chronic condition with symptoms that impact men's quality of life. As with other chronic conditions, patients benefit from self-management interventions

(SMIs) that empower the individual's involvement and control of treatment. SMI helps patients learn what to do and develops their belief in their own ability to use knowledge and skills toward achieving realistic, desired outcomes. SMI has been shown to be effective in men with BPH LUTS as an alternative to initial pharmacologic management and as adjuvant therapy for men who are using alpha-blockers.[2,3] Three major categories for LUTS SMI are (1) education and reassurance, (2) lifestyle modification, and (3) behavioral interventions.

Education and reassurance provides knowledge about male anatomy and the relationship of the bladder and enlarged prostate to voiding symptoms. Patients are reassured that LUTS commonly occur in the absence of cancer. Illustrations and written information facilitate understanding and retention of information. Group settings can also be used for providing education and sharing effective strategies.

Lifestyle modifications address avoiding caffeine and alcohol and the timing of fluid intake, such as avoiding fluids 2 hours before bedtime if bothersome nocturia is present. Bladder diaries document urinary frequency, volume, and circumstances surrounding urinary symptoms and can assist individuals in identifying lifestyle contributors. Education regarding medications is also provided. Medication review may lead to adjustment of existing therapy such as timing of diuretics to reduce nocturia. Patients are informed about BPH medical therapy and how to adjust medication dosing to improve LUTS at times of greatest inconvenience, such as when traveling.

Behavioral interventions address voiding habits, replacing maladaptive behaviors with more healthful approaches. For example, patients with urgency may void at inappropriately short intervals to stay ahead of the urge and as a result diminish bladder capacity. Bladder retraining is used to appropriately lengthen the time between voids.

CASE 1

Paul Phillips (Part 3)

It is 7 years later, and Mr. Phillips is in your office for an annual visit. Over the past year he has noticed progressive slowing of his urinary stream, difficulty initiating urination, a sense of incomplete emptying, increased frequency of urination, and awakening to void three to four times per night; his IPSS score is 16. Mr. Phillips used a bladder diary and was unable to identify any triggers. He started using saw palmetto herbal therapy 3 months ago but is unsure if his urinary symptoms are improved. He reports his cataracts are worse and his blurry vision now also interferes with golfing. On physical examination, there is no suprapubic fullness or tenderness, and the prostate is about 25 g without discrete nodules or tenderness.

Before initiating medication, what further evaluation would you recommend for Mr. Phillips? ◙

TABLE 51-1	Management Options for Benign Prostatic Hyperplasia			
Category	**Interventions**	**Rationale**	**Comments**	**Level of Evidence for Effectiveness***
Self-management interventions	Education and reassurance, lifestyle modification (reduce nighttime fluids to manage nocturia; eliminate dietary diuretics such as caffeine, alcohol), behavioral interventions (e.g., bladder retraining)	Empowers individuals to co-manage chronic condition; factors outside the urinary tract contribute to urinary symptoms	Often sufficient management for mild symptoms; complements management for moderate to severe symptoms	A
Pharmacologic management	Alpha-blockers: terazosin, doxazosin, tamsulosin, silodosin, alfuzosin	Works on dynamic component: relaxation of smooth muscle in prostate and bladder neck decreases resistance to urinary flow	Considered to have equal clinical effectiveness	A
	5-alpha-reductase inhibitors: finasteride, dutasteride	Works on static component: reduced tissue levels of dihydrotestosterone result in prostate gland size reduction	Most effective for men with large prostates (>40 g); results may not be evident for up to 6 months	A
	Combination therapy: alpha-blockers and 5-alpha-reductase inhibitors	Over several years of combined treatment slower progression of BPH than when each used alone	Most effective for men with large prostates (>40 g)	A
	Combination therapy: alpha-blockers and anticholinergics	Combined with alpha-blockers, inhibition of muscarinic receptors in the bladder relieves irritative voiding symptoms (frequency, urgency, nocturia)	Low risk of urinary retention in men with a postvoid residual volume less than 250 mL	A
	Phosphodiesterase-5 inhibitors	Sexual dysfunction is prevalent in aging men with LUTS associated with BPH; underlying mechanisms have not been determined	Tadalafil is the only FDA-approved agent; combination with alpha-blockers has not been studied and may trigger hypotension	B
Phytotherapy	Variety of agents available: *Urticae radix, Secale cereale, Serenoa repens, Pygeum africanum*	Complementary and alternative medicine use is common practice	These agents are well tolerated but appear comparable to placebo	*Serenoa* repens: X Others: C
Surgery	Transurethral resection of the prostate; transurethral incision of the prostate; open prostatectomy; transurethral radiofrequency or microwave thermotherapy or laser	Removal or expansion of periurethral prostate tissue reduces obstruction to urinary flow	Considered to have equal clinical effectiveness; indicated for complications of prostate obstruction: recurrent urinary tract infections, hematuria, bladder stones, renal insufficiency	A

BPH, Benign prostatic hyperplasia; *FDA*, U.S. Food and Drug Administration.

A = supported by one or more high-quality randomized clinical trials [RCTs]; B = supported by one or more high-quality nonrandomized cohort studies or low-quality RCTs; C = supported by one or more case series and/or poor-quality cohort and/or case-control studies; D = supported by expert opinion and/or extrapolation from studies in other populations or settings; X = evidence supports the treatment being ineffective or harmful.

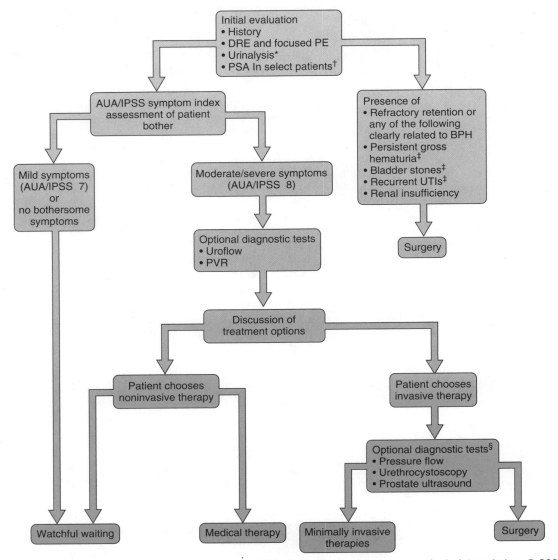

Figure 51-2 Algorithm for evaluation and treatment of BPH. (Redrawn from American Urological Association. © 2003 American Urological Association Education and Research, Inc.)

AUA, American Urological Association; BPH, benign prostatic hyperplasia; DRE, digital rectal exam; IPSS, International Prostate Symptom Score; PE, physical exam; PSA, prostate-specific antigen; PVR, postvoid residual urine; UTI, urinary tract infection.

*In patients with clinically significant prostatic bleeding, a course of a 5 alpha-reductase inhibitor may be used. If bleeding persists, tissue ablative surgery is indicated.

†Patients with at least a 10-year life expectancy for whom knowledge of the presence of prostate cancer would change management or patients for whom the PSA measurement may change the management of voiding symptoms.

‡After exhausting other therapeutic options as discussed in detail in the text.

§Some diagnostic tests are used in predicting response to therapy. Pressure-flow studies are most useful in men prior to surgery.

Medical Therapy

Alpha-Blockers

When patients do not wish to pursue lifestyle modifications, or have an insufficient response, medical therapies are available for BPH. Medications have become the first-line treatment for most patients with BPH. The two main pharmacologic approaches are alpha-adrenergic antagonist and 5-alpha-reductase inhibitor therapy. Anticholinergic agents may be used when irritative symptoms of LUTS predominate.

Alpha-adrenergic antagonists, or alpha-blockers, are directed at the dynamic component of urethral obstruction. Smooth muscle of the prostate and bladder neck has a resting tone mediated by alpha-adrenergic innervation. Alpha-blockers relax the smooth muscle in the hyperplastic prostate tissue, prostate capsule, and bladder neck, thus decreasing resistance to urinary flow. Of the two major alpha-adrenergic receptors, alpha-1 receptors predominate in the prostate. Alpha-blockade development for BPH therapy progressed from a selective alpha-1 agent (e.g., prazosin) to long-acting selective alpha-1 agents (terazosin, doxazosin) that allowed once-a-day dosing but still required blood pressure monitoring and dose titration to reduce orthostatic hypotension. Initially it was thought that the effects on blood pressure would allow treatment of two common conditions, hypertension and BPH, with one drug. Subsequently the Antihypertensive and Lipid-Lowering Treatment to Prevent Heart Attack Trial (ALLHAT) demonstrated that alpha-blockers were inferior to other classes of antihypertensive agents as first-line therapy.[4] Therefore these two common conditions tend to be treated independently.

With the understanding that the alpha-1A subtype comprises 70% of the prostate receptors, the development of more targeted therapy was attempted.[5] Tamsulosin, the first alpha-1A subtype selective agent released, has the advantage of minimal effects on blood pressure thus avoiding the need for dose titration, but it has a side effect of ejaculatory dysfunction.[6] The newer agent, alfuzosin, originally thought to be alpha-1A subtype selective, with additional testing was found to lack this selectivity. However, like tamsulosin, it offers once daily dosing without affecting blood pressure. In addition, alfuzosin appears to have no effect on ejaculation.[7] Another new agent, silodosin, is highly selective of the alpha-1A receptor. Compared with tamsulosin's 9.55 selectivity for alpha-1A versus alpha-1B, silodosin is 162 times more alpha-1A selective.[8] Silodosin has an excellent cardiovascular safety profile but causes ejaculatory dysfunction in almost one third of patients.[9]

Evidence has shown that alpha-blockers relieve LUTS via mechanisms in addition to prostate smooth muscle relaxation. As a result, the effectiveness and adverse effects of these medications cannot be predicted solely by how well they target alpha-1A subtype receptors. The most common adverse events of alpha-1 agents are dizziness, mild asthenia (fatigue or weakness), and abnormal ejaculation. For patients undergoing cataract surgery, intraoperative floppy iris syndrome (IFIS) is a potential risk of all alpha-blockers. IFIS is characterized by sudden intraoperative iris prolapse and pupil constriction and may result in surgical complications such as iris damage, torn lens capsules, and vitreous prolapse. The greatest frequency and severity of IFIS has been reported among those using tamsulosin.[10] Moreover it has been shown that IFIS can occur more than 1 year after tamsulosin has been discontinued.[11] It is suggested that men with plans for cataract surgery delay initiation of alpha-blockers until surgery is completed. Alternatively, men who have already used alpha-blockers should advise their ophthalmologists so this can be factored into planning for cataract surgery.

The five long-acting alpha-1 selective blockers, namely terazosin, doxazosin, tamsulosin, alfuzosin, and silodosin, are approved by the Food and Drug Administration (FDA) for the treatment of symptomatic LUTS caused by BPH and are considered to have equal clinical effectiveness.[12] All five of these medications have the convenience of once-daily dosing. Side effect profiles are generally similar except that alfuzosin appears less likely to cause ejaculatory dysfunction. Terazosin and doxazosin are less costly, older, generic options but require dose titration and blood pressure monitoring.

5-Alpha-Reductase Inhibitors

The enzyme 5-alpha-reductase is required for the conversion of testosterone to the more active dihydrotestosterone. Finasteride and dutasteride are inhibitors of 5-alpha-reductase and reduce tissue levels of dihydrotestosterone, thus reducing prostate gland size, the static component of urethral obstruction. Improvements in LUTS scores and urine flow rates may not be evident for up to 6 months. The 5-alpha-reductase inhibitors are most effective in men with larger prostates (>40 g, about the size of a plum).[13] The reduction in prostate size results in decreased risk of acute urinary retention and delay of BPH-related surgery.[14,15] Finasteride has been shown to suppress prostatic vascular endothelial growth factor (VEGF) and reduce or cease recurrent hematuria related to BPH.[16] Dutasteride is thought to function in a similar fashion.[12] Data are inconclusive as to whether or not the 5-alpha-reductase inhibitors can be used preoperatively to reduce bleeding associated with BPH surgery.[12]

Finasteride and dutasteride have similar clinical efficacy and side effects.[17] Side effects are primarily sexual and include decreased libido, erectile dysfunction, and ejaculation dysfunction. Less often, gynecomastia and breast tenderness occur. These medications are not to be handled by pregnant women because of the possibility of absorption and subsequent risk to a male fetus.[18]

Because 5-alpha-reductase inhibitors reduce serum PSA levels by an average of 50%, after 6 months of therapy, men receiving prostate cancer surveillance will need a new baseline serum PSA determination.[13] The primary prevention of prostate cancer with 5-alpha-reductase inhibitors is currently under investigation.[19]

> Patients determine the level of bother from lower urinary symptoms and guide treatment initiation and selection between medications and surgery.

Combination Therapy: Alpha-Blockers & 5-Alpha-Reductase Inhibitors

Combinations of doxazosin and finasteride, as well as tamsulosin and dutasteride, have been studied.[20,21] When used together over several years, the combination of alpha-adrenergic antagonists with 5-alpha-reductase inhibitors has been shown to be safe and to reduce clinical progression of BPH better than either agent alone. In particular, a lower risk of urinary retention, urinary incontinence, renal insufficiency, and recurrent bladder infections is associated with combination therapy. Higher rates of side effects occur with combination therapy compared to either agent used alone. As with 5-alpha-reductase inhibitors, the benefits of combination therapy are best realized by men with large prostates.

Combination Therapy: Alpha-Blockers and Anticholinergic Medications

Anticholinergic agents (e.g., oxybutynin, tolterodine) inhibit muscarinic receptors in the detrusor muscle and relieve irritative voiding symptoms. Commonly used for overactive bladder, the use of anticholinergics was discouraged in patients with BPH because of concerns of causing urinary retention. Several randomized controlled trials have now shown that anticholinergics can be safely used in combination with alpha-blockers.[22,23] These trials demonstrated a low risk (about 3%) of urinary retention in men who had a postvoid residual volume of less than 250 mL. The use of anticholinergics as monotherapy for BPH LUTS has not shown clinical benefit. Common side effects of anticholinergics include dry mouth, dry eyes, and constipation.

Phosphodiesterase-5 Inhibitors

Phosphodiesterase-5 inhibitors, initially approved for the treatment of erectile dysfunction, have been studied for the treatment of LUTS. Compared to placebo, the daily use of sildenafil, tadalafil, or vardenafil demonstrated improvement in both erectile function and IPSS scores.[24] Although relief of urinary symptoms was reported, no improvement in peak urinary flow rate was demonstrated. When phosphodiesterase-5 inhibitors were used in combination with alpha-blockers, peak urinary flow rate increased beyond that achieved with alpha-blockers alone. Side effects from phosphodiesterase-5 inhibitors include headache, dyspepsia, and back pain. Presently only tadalafil is FDA approved for the treatment of BPH-associated urinary symptoms in men with or without erectile dysfunction.

Phytotherapy

The use of plants and herbs for the treatment of BPH is common although there are limited data to support this practice. Most clinical trials indicate that these agents are well tolerated and comparable to placebo. However, common methodologic concerns among studies of phytotherapy include small numbers of participants, short study duration, varied doses and preparations, and lack of or inconsistent use of standardized, validated measures of efficacy.[25-27] Some examples of phytotherapy for BPH-associated LUTS include *Urticae radix* (stinging nettle root), *Secale cereale* (rye grass pollen), *Serenoa repens* (saw palmetto), and *Pygeum africanum* (African plum tree). *Serenoa repens* has been well studied and serves as an example of the type of data available for phytotherapies. Limited data from smaller studies suggested that *Serenoa repens* improves urinary symptoms and flow measures in men with BPH. However, a 2012 Cochrane review that included 32 randomized controlled studies involving 5666 men found that compared to placebo, *Serenoa repens* monotherapy does not improve urinary symptoms or maximum urinary flow rate even at double and triple the usual dose.[28]

Surgical Therapy

The surgical approaches for managing LUTS of BPH are constantly evolving. Surgical approaches offer the best chance for symptom improvement but also have the highest rates of complications. The benefits of various surgical treatments are generally considered equivalent, but complication rates differ. Because medications have evolved as first-line therapy, the indications for surgery have shifted toward moderate to severe LUTS refractory to medical therapy, coupled with abnormal objective parameters such as impaired flow rate and increased residual volume. Whether or not delayed surgery contributes to detrusor dysfunction from unrelieved obstruction is an area for further study.[29]

Transurethral resection of the prostate (TURP), in use for 80 years, is the standard of care to which other BPH surgical treatments are compared. TURP has a high success rate for improving symptoms, urinary flow, and postvoid residual with low retreatment rates.[30] Usually performed under spinal anesthesia, TURP involves passage of an endoscope through the urethra to surgically remove the inner portion of the prostate. Long-term complications can include retrograde ejaculation, bladder neck contracture, and erectile dysfunction. One unique complication of TURP is TUR syndrome, a dilutional hyponatremia resulting from systemic absorption of irrigant solution. The development of a bipolar generator (bipolar TURP) to replace the conventional monopolar TURP allows the use of isotonic irrigating fluids and eliminates the risk of electrolyte disturbance.[31]

Transurethral incision of the prostate (TUIP) is an endoscopic procedure via the urethra to make one or two cuts in the prostate and prostate capsule, relieving urethral constriction. Limited to use in small prostate glands (<30 g), TUIP results in lower rates of retrograde ejaculation but higher rates of requiring secondary procedures.[12]

Open prostatectomy involves removal of the inner portion of the prostate, while leaving the outer capsule, through a retropubic or suprapubic incision. Currently, open prostatectomy is reserved for patients with larger prostates (>80 grams) or with complicating conditions such as bladder stones or diverticula.[12,32] Open prostatectomy is associated with incisional morbidity, longer hospitalization, and greater risk of erectile dysfunction. These risks can be reduced by using less invasive robot-assisted techniques for simple prostatectomy but high costs of this technology may limit its application.[33]

With advancing technologies, a variety of surgical approaches have evolved in an effort to maintain the efficacy of TURP while reducing the associated risks. Current modalities include transurethral radiofrequency needle ablation (TUNA), transurethral microwave thermotherapy (TUMT), laser vaporization, laser coagulation, and laser enucleation. These modalities appear to have similar short-term efficacy compared to TURP in improving symptoms and urinary flow rate.[12] There is insufficient evidence to state that any one procedure is superior to the others. National trends in surgical therapy support the growing interest in using minimally invasive therapies and providing care in an outpatient setting. Since the 1990s, the number of TURPs has been steadily declining while laser vaporization is the fastest growing modality, with 70% performed as an outpatient procedure.[34]

Indications for Referral to Specialist

Referral to a urologist is recommended for patients with clinically significant LUTS who fail to adequately respond to medical therapy. Men with complications from BPH including bladder stones, urinary retention, recurrent urinary tract infections, or renal dysfunction should also be referred.

CASE 2

David Frank (Part 1)

David Frank, a 65-year-old man, comes to your office with a recurrence of LUTS over the past week and a concern about recurrent "bladder infections." His past medical history includes hypertension and BPH with no history of sexually transmitted diseases and no new sexual partners. During the past year, he visited an urgent care center three times for bothersome urinary symptoms (increased urinary urgency, frequency, and sensation of incomplete emptying). Each time a urine specimen was obtained, a 2-week course of antibiotics was prescribed, and his urinary symptoms resolved.

Physical examination reveals no fever, no abdominal tenderness, and a diffusely enlarged, nontender prostate with no asymmetry or nodules. A recent ultrasound of the bladder at the urgent care center showed postvoid residual volume as 50 mL and no bladder stones. Today his urinalysis reveals 4 red blood cells, 10 white blood cells, and is Gram stain negative. Your review of urine culture reports from the urgent care visits show *Escherichia coli* bacteria grew each time.

1. **What would be the next step in the evaluation and management of Mr. Frank's symptomatology?**
2. **Are there any additional tests that should be performed?** ■

PROSTATITIS: DIFFERENTIAL DIAGNOSIS AND ASSESSMENT

Prostatitis is an infection or inflammation of the prostate gland that can present as one of numerous syndromes with variable and nonspecific clinical features. The term prostatitis denotes microscopic inflammation of the tissue of the prostate gland and is a diagnosis that covers a wide range of clinical conditions. The differential diagnosis of prostatitis includes acute cystitis, benign prostatic hyperplasia, urinary tract stones, bladder cancer, prostatic abscess, enterovesical fistula, and foreign body within the urinary tract.

The prevalence of prostatitis is estimated at 9% with prostatitis-like symptoms reported from as low as 3% to as high as 16%. Approximately 1% of visits to primary care physicians are related to prostatitis, whereas 8% of all visits to urologists are for prostatitis.[35-37]

The National Institutes of Health's consensus classification of prostatitis includes four categories.[38]

- Category I: Acute bacterial prostatitis
- Category II: Chronic bacterial prostatitis
- Category III: Chronic prostatitis / chronic pelvic pain syndrome (CP/CPPS)
  - Inflammatory
  - Noninflammatory
- Category IV: Asymptomatic inflammatory prostatitis

Bacterial prostatitis is described as either acute or chronic based on the duration of symptoms, with chronic reflecting duration of at least 3 months. Acute and chronic bacterial prostatitis are the most easily recognized but the least common of the prostatitis syndromes. Clinical presentation of acute bacterial prostatitis includes acute symptoms suggestive of a urinary tract infection such as urinary frequency and dysuria. Symptoms suggestive of a systemic infection such as malaise, fever, and myalgias may also occur.

Patients with chronic bacterial prostatitis have recurring episodes of bacterial urinary tract infection caused by the same organism, usually *E. coli*, another gram-negative organism, or enterococcus. Lower urinary tract cultures performed between symptomatic episodes can be useful in confirming an infected prostate gland as the nidus of these recurrent infections.

An overwhelming majority (>90%) of symptomatic patients have CP/CPPS. This term acknowledges the partial comprehension of the basis of this syndrome and the possibility that organs other than the prostate gland may have a significant role in its origin.[39,40] The definition of CP/CPPS recognizes urologic pain as a primary symptom component of this syndrome, in the absence of other diagnoses such as urethritis, urogenital cancer, urinary tract disease, functionally significant urethral stricture, or neurologic disease affecting the bladder. Leukocytes are found in the expressed prostatic secretions, postprostatic massage urine, or semen of patients with the inflammatory subtype of CP/CPPS, whereas patients with the noninflammatory subtype have no evidence of inflammation. CP/CPPS may be the most prevalent of all prostate diseases and it is the most common symptomatic type of prostatitis.

High concentrations of leukocytes in the prostate tissue or seminal fluid are a common incidental finding in patients who undergo evaluation for other genitourinary tract concerns—for example, during prostate biopsy for evaluation of possible prostate cancer, or during evaluation of infertility. Such patients with no corresponding urinary symptoms and no lower urinary tract pain are believed to have asymptomatic inflammatory prostatitis.

Diagnosis: Initial Evaluation, Physical Examination, Diagnostic Studies

When prostatitis is considered in the differential diagnosis, history should include sexual activity, previous episodes of prostatitis, duration and nature of symptoms and any association with voiding of urine and ejaculation, and impact on function and quality of life.

The typical physical examination will include the abdomen, pelvis, genitalia including the perineal area, and a DRE of the prostate in addition to other targeted examinations based on the history. Evaluation of the pelvic floor musculature may be completed as part of the clinical examination. A postvoid residual urine volume should be measured if urinary retention is suspected.

Laboratory tests include urinalysis for evidence of inflammation including blood, leukocytes and leukocyte esterase, and urine culture. Bacteriuria and pyuria indicate infection of the prostate and/or bladder, usually caused by common uropathogenic bacteria, especially *E. coli*. A complete blood count will assist in determining any peripheral leukocytosis, and a blood culture may be performed, if indicated. The four-glass test includes culture and microscopic examination of (1) initial stream urine representing the urethra, (2) midstream urine representing the bladder, (3) expressed prostatic secretion (EPS), and (4) postprostatic massage urine. The preprostatic

and postprostatic massage urine evaluation test, a simpler screen of the lower urinary tract, became more popular in the 1990s and is considered a reasonable alternative to the four-glass test for diagnosing prostatitis.[41,42]

Patients with acute bacterial prostatitis have acute onset of symptoms. Clinical presentation may include fever, chills, dysuria, low back pain, or urinary obstruction and a swollen and tender prostate on physical examination. Prostatic massage is contraindicated.

The National Institutes of Health chronic prostatitis symptom index (NIH-CPSI) is one of the symptom questionnaires used for the quantification of symptoms in CP/CPPS.[43] The questionnaire contains four questions regarding localization of pain or discomfort, two regarding urination (incomplete emptying, frequency), and three related to quality of life.

CASE 2

David Frank (Part 2)

Mr. Frank returns for renewal of primary care services 5 years after last being seen. His interval history is remarkable for recurrent urinary tract infections, low back pain, and depression managed by urgent care and a local urologist with several "long courses of antibiotics" without adequate relief. He describes persistent and bothersome symptoms for 2 years: aching pain between his rectal and testicular area, significant pain upon ejaculation, and persistent urinary symptoms (urgency, frequency, and sensation of incomplete emptying). He states "I've had it" with urologists and would not want a referral. Review of systems reveals chronic fatigue, insomnia, poor appetite, and intermittent depressed mood without suicidal ideation.

On physical examination, he is afebrile and appears frustrated and slightly angry at times. He has a normal musculoskeletal and neurosensory examination of his back and legs. Genitourinary examination shows normal nontender testicles and a normal phallus. He has moderate tenderness to palpation of the perineum and a diffusely enlarged, nontender prostate with no asymmetry or nodules. Urinalysis shows no white blood cells or red blood cells, and a bladder scan shows a negligible postvoid residual.

1. **How would you treat Mr. Frank?**
2. **Would you prescribe antibiotics?** ▣

PROSTATITIS: MANAGEMENT
Acute Bacterial Prostatitis

Antimicrobial therapy is essential in the patient with acute bacterial prostatitis. The type and route of antibiotic treatment is determined by the acuity and severity of the symptoms as well as the other components of the clinical presentation. Acute bacterial prostatitis, when presenting as a serious infection, may require parenteral administration of high doses of a bactericidal antibiotic, which may include a broad-spectrum penicillin, a third-generation cephalosporin, or a fluoroquinolone. An aminoglycoside may be added to the initial therapy. Duration of treatment is based on timing of systemic symptom relief, and normalization of infection parameters. In less severe cases, a fluoroquinolone may be given orally for 10 days.

Chronic Bacterial Prostatitis

Chronic bacterial prostatitis is the most frequent cause of recurrent urinary tract infections in men. A 2-week course of oral fluoroquinolone or trimethoprim may be prescribed after the initial diagnosis in chronic bacterial prostatitis if infection is strongly suspected. After reassessment the antibiotics should be continued only if pretreatment cultures are positive and/or the patient reports desirable effects from the therapy. The recommended total period of treatment is 4 to 6 weeks.[44]

Chronic Prostatitis / Chronic Pelvic Pain Syndrome (CP/CPPS)

Patients with CP/CPPS are treated empirically with numerous pharmacologic approaches such as analgesics, antiinflammatory agents, antibiotics, and alpha-blockers, and nonpharmacologic approaches such as neural blockade and neural stimulation.[40] Despite numerous studies related to diagnosis and management of CP/CPPS, there is lack of consensus on specific recommendations. An initial approach to a patient with suspected CP/CPPS would be to consider the organ system in which the symptoms appear to be primarily perceived, and then treat any well-defined conditions identified, such as cystitis, according to relevant treatment guidelines. When symptoms are not relieved with initial treatment, consider additional tests such as cystoscopy or ultrasound. Identified pathology is treated appropriately. Consider referral to a pain management team if indicated. Alpha-blockers, antibiotics, and combinations of these therapies appear to accomplish the maximum improvement in clinical symptom scores compared with placebo.[45] Antiinflammatory remedies have a lesser but quantifiable benefit on selected endpoints. CP/CPPS represents a diverse group of diseases and therefore the outcome of proposed treatment measures is usually uncertain.

> CP/CPPS is the most common type of prostatitis with long-lasting, difficult-to-resolve symptoms for which patients will access multiple providers. Alpha-blockers, antibiotics, and combinations of these therapies may improve symptoms.

SUMMARY

The prevalence of LUTS increases with age. Symptoms in men with an enlarged prostate can be attributed to BPH and managed accordingly after an initial evaluation reveals an absence of other common etiologies such as medication side effects, urinary tract infection, or diabetes mellitus. The level of bother from LUTS guides initiation and selection of therapy. Evidence of obstruction, such as decreased force of stream, supports the likelihood of benefit from a surgical approach to BPH. Prostatitis symptoms are common in men, chronic symptoms become more prevalent with age, and in more than 90% of cases no infectious agent is identified.

Web Resources

www.americangeriatrics.org. American Geriatrics Society.
www.healthinaging.org. AGS Foundation for Health in Aging.
www.nih.gov/nia. National Institute on Aging Information Center.
www.kidney.niddk.nih.gov. National Kidney and Urologic Diseases Information Clearinghouse.

KEY REFERENCES

3. Chen Y, Zhang X, Hu X, et al. The potential role of a self-management intervention for benign prostate hyperplasia. J Urol 2012;79:1385-9.
10. Chang DF. Floppy iris syndrome: Why BPH treatment can complicate cataract surgery. Am Fam Physician 2009;79(12): 1051, 1055-6.
12. McVary KT, Roehrborn CG, Avins A, et al. Update on AUA guideline on the management of benign prostatic hyperplasia. J Urol 2011;185:1793-1803.
30. Rocco B, Albo G, Ferreira RC, et al. Recent advances in the surgical treatment of benign prostatic hyperplasia. Ther Adv Urol 2011;3(6):263-72.
42. Sharp VJ, Takacs EB, Powell CR. Prostatitis: Diagnosis and treatment. Am Fam Physician. 2010;82(4):397-406.
44. Grabe M, Bjerklund-Johansen TE, Botto H, et al. Guidelines on urological infections. European Association of Urology 2012. Uroweb updated March 2011. www.uroweb.org/gls/pdf/17_Urological%20infections_LR%20II.pdf. Accessed July 11, 2013.
45. Anothaisintawee T, Attia J, Nickel JC, et al. Management of chronic prostatitis/chronic pelvic pain syndrome. A systematic review and network metaanalysis. JAMA 2011;305:1:78-86.

References available online at expertconsult.com.

52

Parkinson's Disease

Monica Stallworth-Kolinas

OBJECTIVES

Upon completion of this chapter the reader will be able to:

- Define and recognize the clinical features that justify a clinical diagnosis of Parkinson's disease (PD).
- Describe the differences in clinical features and medication responsiveness of the illnesses from which PD must be differentiated, including other Lewy body disorders.
- Understand the role of levodopa in diagnosis and treatment and the indications for the use of adjunctive medications in PD in older persons.

- Recognize and optimally manage the motor and nonmotor complications of PD.

PREVALENCE AND IMPACT

Parkinson's disease (PD) is a progressive disorder that results in severe disability 10 to 15 years after its onset. It is the second most common neurodegenerative disorder after Alzheimer's disease (AD).

PD is characterized by rigidity, tremor, and bradykinesia; it is usually asymmetric and is usually responsive to dopaminergic treatment. Familial PD is described. Parkinson-plus syndromes refer to disorders that include parkinsonism with other clinical signs: they include dementia of Lewy body type (LBD), multiple system atrophy (MSA), progressive supranuclear palsy (PSP), and corticobasal degeneration.[1]

As in other industrialized countries, the prevalence is approximately 1% in persons over 65 in the United States, and rises to 3% in those over 85.[2] All ethnic origins can be affected, males somewhat more than females.[3]

RISK FACTORS AND PATHOPHYSIOLOGY

Role of Aging: Although the incidence of PD increases with age, PD is generally *not* considered a normal part of aging.

Genetic Predisposition: Most people with PD do not have a family history, but 15% do have a first-degree relative with PD, characteristically without a clear mode of inheritance.[4] Several genetic loci for PD are identified, although a common environmental etiology could explain familial patterns.[5]

Role of Environmental Exposure: Pesticides, rural environments, and well water have all been linked to PD.[6] In the early 1980s, a perthine analog was reported: it is the only environmental agent directly linked to levodopa-responsive parkinsonism. Cigarette smoking may actually lessen the risk![7]

Trauma: Parkinsonian features are seen in head injury, including boxers and football players, and also in *cerebrovascular disease*, both presumably due to damage to the basal ganglia.

Parkinson's disease in any one individual is likely to represent several factors acting together.

Pathology

The underlying pathologic change in PD is injury to the dopaminergic projections from the substantia nigra pars compacta to the caudate nucleus and putamen. Intraneuronal Lewy bodies and Lewy neurites are other

---

Additional online-only material indicated by icon.

pathological features of PD. Lewy neurites are often observed in the cortex, amygdala, locus coeruleus, vagal nucleus, and the peripheral autonomic nervous system[8]; this could explain some of the nonmotor features of PD.

CASE 1

Robert Wilmington (Part 1)

Mr. Wilmington is a 65-year-old right handed building contractor who has been healthy and active most of his life. Over the past 3 years his work has become more supervisory by necessity, with ongoing complaints for several years of shoulder and limb joint discomfort followed by less skill in manipulating hand tools. He started hiding his dominant hand under his desk or sitting on it when in public after embarrassing questions about what he was rolling between his thumb and index finger. Six months later, he noted his newspaper shaking in both hands when held in his lap. Subsequently, he blamed his joint pains and stiffness for difficulties standing up and not walking at the pace to which he was accustomed.

His family noted at the meal table he was now the last one to finish eating. He also made sure a handkerchief was handy to wipe unexpected drool from his lower lip. Most recently, it startled him that when standing and shaving in front of a mirror he lost his balance. He has had a few stumbles without falls when his body seemed to get ahead of his feet. He was prompted to seek medical attention after his first fall; it occurred when attempting to turn suddenly when called from behind.

1. **Recognize the cardinal features of PD in this case. What is the order these features present in this patient? Describe the symptoms attributable to bradykinesia?**

2. **What examination signs would be expected regarding his rigidity and postural instability?**

3. **What cardinal feature was most helpful in distinguishing PD from other causes of parkinsonism?** ◉

DIFFERENTIAL DIAGNOSIS AND ASSESSMENT

Is it Parkinson's Disease?

Whereas autopsy is required to make the definitive diagnosis of PD, an accurate clinical diagnosis can usually be made based on the classical features that Parkinson originally described, plus other features that, over the years, have been recognized to be associated with PD.[9] Four cardinal features are listed in Box 52-1. Since some of these features are frequently seen in older patients, the diagnosis of PD should be considered when at least two of the four are present. Significant supportive motor features are listed in Box 52-2.

Levodopa Responsiveness

Because levodopa or a dopamine agonist usually provides improvement in the motor manifestations,

---

BOX 52-1
PRIMARY FEATURES OF PARKINSON'S DISEASE

- Resting tremor
- Bradykinesia
- Rigidity
- Asymmetric onset
- *plus* responsiveness to levodopa

BOX 52-2
SOME SUPPORTIVE FEATURES OF PARKINSON'S DISEASE

- Sustained response to levodopa (i.e., more than transient)
- Expressionless face (hypomimia)
- Sialorrhea (producing drooling)
- Speech and swallowing problems (hypophonia, dysarthria, dysphagia)
- Loss of fine-motor skills (such as writing, producing micrographia)
- Abnormal gait (shuffling, reduced arm swing, flexed posture, freezing, and festination)
- Reduced upward gaze, positive glabellar tap, and decreased blinking

---

a **definite response to levodopa is regarded as a confirmatory test** and is required for a diagnosis of probable (that is, clinically definite) PD.[10] Although L-dopa responsiveness can help differentiate classical PD in most instances, an initial response to levodopa can occur in Parkinson-plus syndromes such as LBD and multisystem atrophy. However, the *sustained* response to levodopa is confirmatory of PD, and it is the *motor* features that are most improved.

> Slow and rigid with a resting asymmetrical tremor: think Parkinson's, consider levodopa.

In the NINDS Diagnostic Criteria for PD (see Chapter 17), the features summarized in Box 52-3 are considered suggestive of other diagnoses than PD; that is, are evidence that something other than PD is going on, and so—we would advise—might lead the PCP to seek neurologic or other consultation, except perhaps in the case of the relationship of the PD symptoms to a dementia process, and thus the consideration for Lewy Body Dementia (LBD), a diagnosis which the PCP should be the one to make! (See Chapter 17 on Alzheimer's and other dementias.)

The NINDS criteria require a confirmatory autopsy for PD to be described as "definite" but would rate PD as **"probable"** if three of the four clinical features (see Box 52-1) were present for three years, with none of the features listed in Box 52-3, and if there had been a sustained, definite response to L-dopa (or a dopamine agonist); **"possible"** PD would require only two of the four primary features (Box 52-1)

FINDINGS IN POTENTIAL PD WHICH SUGGEST OTHER DIAGNOSES*

Any of these three occurring **in the first three years:**
1. Nonmedication related **hallucinations**
2. **"Freezing"** phenomenon
3. Prominent **postural instability**

Dementia occurring before PD motor symptoms or in the first year of the illness

Certain **eye movement** abnormalities other than limited upward gaze

Nonmedication-related, **severe** symptoms of **autonomic dysfunction**

Conditions present which are themselves likely causes of PD symptoms (e.g. **neuroleptic use** in prior 6 months)

*Neurologic consultation if available may be advisable in primary care practice.

(provided one of the two were bradykinesia or tremor), would not require the medication responsiveness if an adequate trial had not yet taken place, and—if symptoms had been present for three years—one or more of the findings which suggest other diagnoses (Box 52-3) could be present.

Motor Features

Resting tremor, pronation-supination or pill-rolling, in character with a frequency mostly of 4 to 6 Hz (**9**) is the **first symptom in 70%** of PD patients. Tremor is characteristically asymmetric at onset and worsens with anxiety, with contralateral motor action, and with ambulation.

Muscular rigidity is **resistance noted during passive joint movement** in the normal range of motion of that joint. It usually has a cogwheeling feel. It is often more prominent in the most tremulous extremity. Rigidity is increased by contralateral motor movement or a mental task.

Bradykinesia causes the **most dysfunction in the initial stages** of the illness. The patient is unable to perform fine-motor tasks effectively. Observing a patient suspected of having PD walking, tying their shoelaces, or writing a sentence can be helpful in diagnosis.

Postural instability onsets insidiously with progressively **poor balance**. It leads to increased **fall risk**. It can be demonstrated by testing for postural reflexes by pushing the patient forward (propulsion) or backward (retropulsion) to check for balance recovery.

Gait dysfunction is characterized by shuffling, slowness of walking, and by turning "en bloc."

Freezing is shown by difficulty initiating walking or by striking gait hesitation (transient loss of movement), on turning or on arriving at a real or perceived obstacle.

Discussion

In Mr Wilmington's case, although resting tremor appeared to be the most obvious initial symptom, the rigidity and bradykinesia actually began earlier. The rigidity caused the pains that he assumed were from his joints—an often unrecognized symptom of rigidity. The rigidity could have also contributed to his ambulation problems. Bradykinesia was the second of his PD-associated features—with impaired fine-motor control of hand tools and the later difficulties with standing, with the speed of ambulation and eating, as well as the drooling, and festination. His falling was mainly due to the onset of postural instability and the gait dysfunction. ▣

Robert Wilmington (Part 2)

Other symptoms were present but not volunteered by the patient. Specific inquiry by the examiner revealed constipation and nocturia, depression and inattentiveness, and sleep disturbances, including apparent acting out during vivid dreams.

1. **Which of these could be nonmotor symptoms related to PD?**

2. **Name another category of nonmotor symptoms that can be recognized in his case?**

3. **Among the causes for disturbed sleep, which specific disorder is likely being described here?** ▣

Nonmotor Features

Autonomic dysfunction is common and causes bowel and bladder dysfunction, excessive sweating, and orthostatic hypotension.[11] However, dysautonomia as an early or particularly severe feature suggests a diagnosis other than PD.[9,10]

Dementia has been said to develop in about 40% of PD patients,[12] although in a study that followed patients until death, it was present in over 80% in the end stage of the illness.[13] Thus the PCP must watch for subtle cognitive and other characteristic symptoms of dementia, and patients should be screened for this common syndrome. The concept of PD as part of a spectrum of disorders which includes **Lewy Body Dementia (LBD)** is a vital one for the PCP to embrace, as this dementia is much more common than has been historically taught and is well within the diagnostic range of the PCP. Currently, there is a "one-year rule" arbitrarily decided upon, that, if PD symptoms and/or signs have existed for at least one year before signs of dementia, the Dx is PDD (Parkinson Disease dementia), whereas if dementia occurs first or the PD symptoms and signs have been apparent for less than a year before the dementia, it is–for now–regarded as LBD. Whereas LBD is often characterized by vivid visual hallucinations, any dementia predisposes patients treated with anti-parkinsonian drugs to *hallucinations and other psychotic symptoms*.

Depression is common in PD, affecting nearly half of patients.[14] Serotonin reuptake inhibitors (SSRIs) can be effective, and the dopaminergic qualities of sertraline can be therapeutic but can also complicate levodopa dosing.

Sensory symptoms in PD are quite varied and include anosmia and paresthesia, and pain.[15]

Disturbed sleep is common. Causes include nocturnal stiffness, nocturia, depression, restless legs syndrome, and REM (rapid eye movement) sleep behavior disorder (RSBD)—another LBD hint.[16]

CASE 1

Discussion

Mr. Wilmington also has RSBD, a nonmotor symptom. ▣

Differential Diagnosis

Essential tremor is the most common tremor and tends to be familial. It typically is first noted when it interferes with eating[17] as it is characteristically a terminal intention tremor, occurring with voluntary movement, as can usually be shown in the finger–nose test. It is also absent at rest and tends to be bilateral; it is frequently asymmetric. It has a higher frequency range (5 to 10 Hz) than the typical tremor in PD; in older patients, the frequency is in the lower range. In advanced cases, essential tremor can be present at rest and thus confused with PD; and a patient with PD can have both! If rigidity and bradykinesia are present, a trial of levodopa may be appropriate.

The following differential diagnoses are summarized in Table 52-1.

Drug-induced parkinsonism occurs after exposure to neuroleptics,[18] antiemetics, promotility agents, and some calcium-channel blockers. Symptoms are symmetric. It characteristically resolves when the drug is stopped, although resolution can take weeks or months.

Progressive Supranuclear Palsy (PSP) is a rare disorder. Onset is in the 50s. Approximately 4% of

parkinsonian patients have PSP. It progresses rapidly and is characterized by oculomotor disturbance, speech and swallowing difficulties, imbalance with falls, and frontal dementia.[20] It is symmetric. Postural instability occurs early. Additional clinical manifestations include severe axial rigidity, absence of tremor, and a poor response to dopaminergic treatment. The defining characteristic is supranuclear gaze palsy, especially of downward gaze. Marked incapacity occurs within 3 to 5 years of onset, with death typically within 10 years. Compared to PD, the rigidity in PSP tends to be more severe and axial and postural instability is an early feature.

Multiple System Atrophy (MSA) involves the central, autonomic, and peripheral systems. The prominence and severity of autonomic dysfunction differentiates it from PD. The term multisystem atrophy includes a cluster of diseases previously regarded as separate entities: Shy-Drager syndrome, olivopontocerebellar atrophy, and striatonigral degeneration.[1] There is no response to levodopa. Presentation is with parkinsonism, cerebellar and autonomic dysfunction (orthostatic hypotension, bladder and bowel dysfunction, temperature dysregulation), and pyramidal dysfunction in various combinations. MSA-P (formerly called striatonigral degeneration) is characterized by symmetric parkinsonism without tremor and early, pronounced postural instability. MSA-C (formerly called olivopontocerebellar atrophy) manifests with cerebellar signs and parkinsonism. Corticospinal tract signs and respiratory stridor occur in all categories of MSA.

Dementia of Lewy Body Type (LBD) is a progressive dementia, which is often the primary, initial clinical feature, but occasionally the earliest symptoms suggest a more atypical depressive disorder. As the dementia progresses, parkinsonian features may develop, and in some cases, there are complex visual hallucinations, which are regarded as one of the "psychiatric" hallmarks of this particular dementia.[21]

Unfortunately, there is also marked sensitivity to the parkinsonian (extrapyramidal) side effects of

TABLE 52-1	Distinguishing Parkinson's Disease from its Differential Diagnosis					
Disease	Bradykinesia and Rigidity	Tremor	Dementia	Other Features	L-dopa Responsiveness	Antipsychotic Sensitivity
Parkinson's disease	Yes Limb	Yes		More common in late onset	Yes	+
Drug-induced	Yes Limb	No			No	++
Progressive supranuclear palsy	Yes Axial	No	Yes, early	Loss of conjugate gaze (especially downward)	No	
Lewy body dementia	Yes Axial	No	Yes, early	Hallucinations	Yes, initially	+++
Vascular parkinsonism	Yes Limb	No	Yes, in some	Pyramidal signs	No	+
Multisystem atrophy	Yes	No	Yes	Pyramidal and cerebellar signs (OPCA) Dysautonomia		

From: Chan DK. The art of treating Parkinson's disease in the older patient. Aus Fam Physician 2003;32:927-931.[19]

neuroleptics (both the traditional and the "atypical" antipsychotics). Typical antipsychotics (those with high affinity for D2 receptors) should especially be avoided. Judicious use of low doses of atypical antipsychotics (especially quetiapine) by experienced specialists has been used when warranted, although guidelines for such practice have not been formulated.[21] Resting tremor is rare. Frontal lobe disinhibited behaviors are often present. Sleep disorders can occur, including REM sleep disorder which is characteristic and may precede the dementia of LBD by several years. Dopaminergics usually produce no improvement in motor manifestations. Cognition can be relatively improved on cholinesterase inhibitors (ChEI), which the original describers of LBD emphasize should be regarded as considerably more therapeutic in LBD, than they are in the much more common Alzheimer's pathology.[22]

Normal pressure hydrocephalus (NPH) is another progressive primary dementia, unrelated to PD pathologically and treated surgically, that does classically present with gait dysfunction, plus urinary incontinence and progressive dementia. Often the gait is the initial presentation, with a wide-based, shuffling gait. Tremor is usually absent. Brain imaging shows ventricular dilatation, the hallmark of the hydrocephalic process. There would be no therapeutic response to dopaminergic treatment. Especially if diagnosed early, NPH can be *reversed* by a ventriculoperitoneal shunt, a relatively simple surgical procedure. Careful patient selection is critical; shunt failure and other complications do occur. In particular, the gait disorder and, in some cases, even the dementia can reverse if treated early.

Vascular parkinsonism has a similar etiology to vascular dementia (VaD); that is, multiple infarcts occur. The infarcts in vascular parkinsonism are in the basal ganglia and the subcortical white matter.[23] Tremor is usually absent, and there is no therapeutic response to dopaminergic treatment. Vascular parkinsonism tends to be accompanied by dementia, pseudobulbar affect, urinary symptoms, and pyramidal signs. Brain imaging showing extensive small vessel disease is supportive, and treatment is mostly the management of the vascular risk factors.

MANAGEMENT

The *key therapeutic strategies* for PD (Box 52-4) include:

1. Increased dopaminergic stimulation
2. Decreased cholinergic stimulation
3. Decreased glutamatergic stimulation

However, anticholinergics should not be used in older patients as is detailed in many other places in this text!

The American Academy of Neurology (AAN) has published evidence-based reviews of several aspects of the management of PD. The review of initiation of treatment is especially of interest to the primary care clinician, who will frequently be the first prescriber when the diagnosis is made in the primary care setting.[24] An algorithmic (decision tree) approach to PD management has also been published.[2]

BOX 52-4

MEDICATIONS FOR PARKINSON'S DISEASE IN ELDERS

Levodopa
- first-line treatment in elders; overall most effective drug in PD
- usually as carbidopa/levodopa

Dopamine agonists
- mainly to reduce "off" time of levodopa
- include ropinirole, pramipexole, cabergoline, perfolide, bromocriptine

Amantadine
- for dyskinesias in advanced PD

Anticholinergics
- avoid (in the elderly)!
- occasionally used for dyskinesias

Selegiline
- MAO-B inhibitor
- adjunctive therapy

COMT inhibitors
- increase the half-life of levodopa
- include entacapone, olepone

CASE 1

Robert Wilmington (Part 3)

A therapeutic trial of levodopa/carbidopa (Sinemet) gradually increased to 25/100 three times a day is begun. His tremor improves to a satisfactory level, and he declines addition of anticholinergic medication due to concerns about side effects. His bradykinesia partially improves, with feeding and gait less problematic. He requires increased frequency of dosing eventually to every 4 hours while awake to prevent end of dose return of motor symptoms. Initially he feels there is improvement in his postural instability, but this is not confirmed on examination. His imbalance is still present. His reduced falling is a result of cautious gait, gait training, and—later—the use of assistive devices. With time, his maximum benefit from each dose of Sinemet, as well as its duration of benefit, diminishes. His dose is gradually doubled with some further improvement. This is accompanied by minimal dyskinesias at peak dose, which are not noticeable until the dose is increased to 25/250.

1. **What are the benefits and risks of starting levodopa in this patient versus a dopamine agonist?**
2. **What are the options when side effects develop from levodopa?**
3. **At what point would you refer him to a neurologist?**
4. **How should his nonmotor symptoms be treated?** ■

When to Start Medication

The decision to begin symptomatic therapy in PD is determined by the patient's choice and by functionality. For example, a mild resting tremor that does not impact function does not warrant treatment. When the tremor is severe or affecting function, **levodopa** is the first-line treatment in the elderly. The progression of PD over the years is not uniform. If gait or other aspects of functional independence become affected, treatment should be considered at that time, even if the tremor is tolerable.[24]

Because many patients have motor complications from long-term levodopa, considerable work in recent years has evolved other antiparkinsonian therapies, especially for younger patients. Newer **dopamine agonists**[26] include ropinirole or pramipexole. These agents are less effective, but the incidence of motor side effects is much lower; however, they have other side effects (edema of the legs, sleepiness, and confusion) and are more expensive. They are best used in younger patients, who are better able to tolerate the side effects. In fact, treatment for early PD in younger, healthy patients generally *begins* with dopamine agonist monotherapy.

Anticholinergics are also still commonly used in the younger population, but—like all anticholinergics—they must generally be avoided in the elderly.

> **In the older PD patient: Avoid (or stop) anticholinergics!**

Levodopa

Levodopa is the preferred initial drug in the old and frail (and is less expensive).[24] It remains the most potent antiparkinson drug. Like any symptomatic medication in PD, treatment is begun when symptoms become bothersome or cause functional disability.

> **Lack of levodopa responsiveness may mean inaccurate diagnosis.**

Levodopa is also the most effective drug for the symptomatic treatment of idiopathic PD, especially for **bradykinesia and rigidity**. It is generally combined with a peripheral decarboxylase inhibitor—**carbidopa** in the United States—to block its conversion to dopamine in the systemic circulation and liver; this reduces the peripheral effects of nausea, vomiting, and orthostatic hypotension. This combination in the immediate release form is available in 10/100, 25/100, and 25/250 mg preparations as carbidopa/levodopa.

> **It's "start low and go slow" with levodopa and most neurologic drugs.**

The starting dose is generally one-half tablet of 25/100 mg three times daily, titrated upward over several weeks to a whole 25/100 mg tablet three times daily, as tolerated and according to the response. "Start low and go slow" is the rule, owing to adverse reactions, especially if dementia is present. There is a wide range of dose response in the elderly. The majority of those with idiopathic PD have a significant therapeutic response to moderate doses (400 to 600 mg/day of levodopa). No response to 1000 to 1500 mg/day strongly implies that the diagnosis should be reviewed!

Controlled-release carbidopa-levodopa[27] is less well absorbed, requiring doses up to 30% higher than the immediate release form; each tablet is typically less dramatic in effect than the immediate-release preparation, as the controlled-release form penetrates more slowly to the brain. Thus, therapy should start with an immediate release preparation, switching to controlled release when the dose is stable.

Carbidopa-levodopa should be *taken on an empty stomach,* 30 to 60 minutes before or 45 or 60 minutes after meals because of competitive absorption of other amino acids. This also increases the duration of response to each dose. This is more crucial in advanced disease with motor fluctuations. Unfortunately, initial *nausea* from levodopa is more likely on an empty stomach, so such patients may take it with a snack or after meals. However, nausea is often because of *insufficient carbidopa*; manage this with supplemental carbidopa or with antiemetics such as trimethobenzamide or ondansetron given beforehand. Phenothiazine antiemetics and metoclopramide must be *avoided*; they can themselves cause drug-induced parkinsonism!

Increasing the levodopa dosage should be tried if responsiveness drops. If that fails or side effects become unacceptable, an adjunctive therapy (next section) should be tried.

> **Nausea on levodopa? Try more carbidopa.**

Motor Fluctuations

The primary cause of motor fluctuations is the short half-life of levodopa (90 to 120 minutes).

After a number of years on it, as the disease progresses, the duration of responsiveness to levodopa becomes shorter, the "wearing off" reaction. Some patients react to "off" states with panic attacks, screaming, or even drenching sweats.[28] With disease progression, there is a tendency for the fluctuations to become increasingly less predictable. The "on-off" effect is the most unpredictable of these states. "Delayed-on" and "no-on", as well as dyskinesias, occur. Motor complications are a major cause of disability in advanced PD patients.

Treatment for these fluctuations focuses on trying to improve absorption, altering the timing of doses, and prolonging the effect of every dose. As noted above, a high protein meal can reduce levodopa absorption; so spreading protein intake throughout the day can help to reduce motor fluctuations.

Controlled-release levodopa unfortunately only slightly lengthens the duration of action of levodopa.[27] The therapeutic effects are more unpredictable than those of immediate-release levodopa, especially important in older patients. Controlled-release levodopa reduces "off" time by 20% to 70%, increases the total daily dose of levodopa by about 20%, yet decreases the number of doses by 30%.[28]

COMT inhibitors, which relieve end-of-dose wearing off by lengthening the half-life of circulating levodopa, and *dopamine agonists,* which enhance effectiveness of levodopa and help to reduce off time, are detailed in "Adjunctive Therapy" below.

Surgery can also reduce "off" time. Both pallidotomy and deep brain stimulation (DBS) of the globus pallidus or the subthalamic nucleus can be highly effective in this regard. However, surgery may be contraindicated in advanced elderly patients who could potentially most benefit from this effect (see below).

Dyskinesias

Chorea or choreodystonia, usually accompanying the "on" state, is most commonly induced by levodopa most commonly at the peak of its clinical effect ("peak-dose" dyskinesias). The movements are typically choreiform or dystonic, and range from mild and of no consequence to severe and disabling. Most medical strategies for reducing "off" states can cause increased dyskinesias as a side effect, so a therapeutic balance must be sought!

Dopamine agonists sometimes help by allowing a reduction of levodopa dosage. However, note that COMT inhibitors tend to *worsen* dyskinesias. *Amantadine,* 100 to 300 mg per day, may reduce dyskinesia through the inhibition of glutamate-mediated neurotransmissions, but anticholinergic side effects can be problematic. *Propranolol* (up to 20 mg three times per day) has some potential. For pure dystonia that does not respond to levodopa adjustment, *anticholinergics* may be helpful, but again, side effects need to be balanced against benefits. Also again, *surgery* (pallidotomy or DB deep brain stimulation) may be considered, but it is rarely used in the elderly or frail.

Adjunctive Medications

Adjuncts to levodopa (amantadine and a number of dopaminergic medications) reduce the overall quantity of "off" time in patients with motor fluctuations. The dopaminergics have either longer half-lives or an ability to extend the half-life of levodopa, thus leading to more continuous dopaminergic stimulation. None of them completely relieve the "off" time problems.

Amantadine: This drug has been used for years as a treatment for early PD. More recently, it has been studied for its effects in fluctuating disease. Its most impressive effect in advanced PD is its efficacy against dyskinesias; one report showed a reduction in the severity of dyskinesias by 60%.[29] Problems that limit the wider use of amantadine in the elderly include edema of the legs, with a characteristic rash (livido reticularis), plus hallucinations and anticholinergic effects.

Dopamine agonists: **Bromocriptine** was the first of these to be used clinically. Others now available include **cabergoline, perfolide, pramipexole, and ropinirole**. They reduce "off" time as their half-lives are longer than that of levodopa: 27 hours for perfolide, 8 to 12 hours for pramipexole, and 6 hours for ropinirole. They should be used cautiously. The dose is increased gradually over 4 to 8 weeks to an optimal level. If dyskinesia occurs, reduction of levodopa may be required. Motor score improvement is seen in around 20% to 35% of patients.[30] Their antiparkinsonian efficacy is significantly less than that of levodopa; they work primarily by improving "off" episode disability. Adverse effects often limit their use, including orthostatic hypotension, delirium, nausea, and vomiting.

MAO-B inhibitors: **Selegilin**e is the only monoamine oxidase type B (MAO-B) inhibitor available in the United States. It is now approved as adjunctive therapy in fluctuating PD. It is believed to decrease the central catabolism of dopamine by blocking MAO-B.

COMT inhibitors: The enzyme catechol-*o*-methyl transferase (COMT) is key to the peripheral catabolism of levodopa. Blocking it with COMT inhibitors (**entacapone or tolcapone**) lengthens the plasma half-life of levodopa by 40% to 80%.[31] Adverse effects are diarrhea and dyskinesia. Tolcapone has liver toxicity, so monitoring of liver function is recommended. They tend to *worsen* dyskinesias.

Neuroprotective Agent: Several substances have been studied as potential neuroprotective agents to slow disease progression. **Vitamin E** was not beneficial in a large, multicenter trial of patients with early PD.[32] The effectiveness of **coenzyme Q** is not yet certain.

Management of Tremor

As stated before, a mild resting tremor that does not impact function does not warrant treatment. When it is severe or affecting function, *levodopa* is the first-line treatment in the elderly, especially the frail.

Although *anticholinergics* such as benztropine and tihexyphenidyl may be useful, the risks of anticholinergic side effects usually outweigh the benefits. In patients with cognitive impairment, anticholinergics *must* be avoided.

A modest benefit with *amantadine* has been reported. *Propranolol* may reduce tremor amplitude in the anxious. *Clozapine* may be beneficial; however, the mechanism is unclear, and rare and severe side effects (agranulocytosis, myocarditis, and cardiomyopathy) limit its use.

Management of Nonmotor Symptoms[33]

Autonomic dysfunction in patients with PD include orthostatic hypotension, constipation, urinary symptoms, and sexual dysfunction. Symptomatic *orthostatic hypotension* occurs in 15% to 20% of PD patients,[34] with potentially devastating results, such as falls. This may be from autonomic dysfunction but is also a side effect of many PD treatments. Reduction of the dose of antiparkinson drugs, enhancement of salt and fluid intake, and addition of fludrocortisone or midodrine are treatment options for hypotension. If systolic hypertension coexists, pindolol may be useful. Aggressive management of *constipation* entails escalation of water and fiber intake, additon of fiber supplements (e.g., psyllium), and use of stool softeners, suppositories, and enemas. *Urinary urgency* can be treated with peripheral anticholinergic drugs (oxybutynin and tolterodine) but is limited because of the side effects; adrenergic-blocking agents (prazosin and terazosin) unfortunately exacerbate hypotension.

Depression affects about 40% of PD patients.[35,36,37] Coexistent depression may significantly affect both the symptoms and rehabilitation efforts. The good PCP will likely spot it. An unblinded study has shown selective (*SSRIs*) to be useful.[38] Of the antidepressants shown in small controlled studies, *citalopram* and *venlafaxine* are among those most useful in elders.[39] Whereas SSRIs are associated with EPS symptoms, sertraline has been less so associated; this is thought to be due to sertraline's greater effect on dopamine reuptake inhibition, making it also a rational choice when an SSRI is to be used in a person with PD. No head-to-head studies have been done to prove if one antidepressant is superior to another in PD. Tricyclics can exacerbate orthostatic hypotension. In hypotensive patients, venlafaxine may be the drug of choice because it increases blood pressure. In bipolar patients, note that lithium may worsen parkinsonism.

Sleep disorders in PD include daytime somnolence and sleep attacks, nighttime awakenings attributable to overnight rigidity and bradykinesia, REM, RSBD, and restless legs or periodic limb movements. Daytime somnolence and sleep attacks have been linked to dopamine agonists, and patients should be warned of these adverse effects. The prevalence has been estimated to be as high at 50%.[40] Elimination of the agonist or even use of a stimulant might be necessary. Patients and families should be warned about safety issues such as driving. Nighttime awakenings and restless legs can be alleviated with a bedtime dose of long-acting levodopa or the addition of entacapone. *Melatonin* is the most effective treatment for REM sleep disorder.

Psychosis is rare in untreated PD and is thought to be mostly drug-induced.[35] Dopamine agonists are more likely to cause hallucinations than is levodopa. The first step in management is to discontinue the agonist or anticholinergic drug and to use the lowest levodopa dose possible. However, addition of an atypical neuroleptic is sometimes necessary. Two randomized, controlled trials have shown that *clozapine* is useful for symptoms, such as visual hallucinations.[41] However, because of potentially fatal agranulocytosis, blood count must be measured every week or biweekly. Therefore *quetiapine*[42] has become the most popular atypical neuroleptic in PD because of the absence of agranulocytosis and fewer extrapyramidal adverse effects than any other atypicals, such as risperidone and olanzapine. Several open-label studies have suggested that dementia and psychosis in PD can be treated with ChEIs—consistent with the staus of ChEIs as therapeutic in LBD.

Dementia has limited evidence about this important aspect of treatment. There is no evidence that one ChEI is superior to another in PD patients with dementia. A small, randomized, controlled trial has shown that donepezil is useful in improving cognition in demented parkinsonian patients.[43] Another randomized trial has shown that rivastigmine is useful in LBD.[22] Cholinergic stimulation theoretically would be counterproductive in parkinsonism. Both anticholinergics and dopamine agonists should be avoided in patients with dementia because of the risk of increasing confusion.

Management of the Secondary Effects of Parkinson's Disease

It will often fall to the primary care clinician to address actively reducing or preventing the functional, social, emotional, economic, sexual, and nutritional (and other) effects of this progressive and disabling condition.

> It is the PCP who often picks up the active care of the effects of PD on function, family, finances, nutrition, emotion, and sex, to name a few!

Dysphagia and aspiration risk should be approached proactively, and the input and expertise of speech therapists (who are really "speech and swallowing therapists"—patients and families still often do not realize this) should be ordered when either symptom presents. **Undernutrition** (often presenting as weight loss) and poor fluid intake with dehydration (frequently overlooked as a contributory factor to hypotension and orthostasis) are at risk anyway in the PD patient; problems with swallowing and choking/aspiration further compromise both food and fluid intake.

As predictable as **functional decline** is, it should be addressed and reduced if possible: mobility and balance aids, gait and balance training, and reduction of loss of range of motion (ROM) are often the target symptoms that can be helped by physical therapy, whereas loss of manual skills for dressing, food preparation and eating, and for many enjoyable and, therefore, therapeutic activities—including perhaps a paid job—are addressed by the discipline of occupational therapy. However, these other disciplines and many others often do not get involved until the clinician suggests them (and explains their roles) and often require a doctor's order, which physicians must be very active and prompt in giving!

Surgical Treatment for Parkinson's Disease

There has been a resurgence of interest in surgical intervention in PD in the past few years, especially in patients who are poorly controlled with medication. Surgical intervention should be considered when medical therapy is no longer effective.

Ablative therapy (pallidotomy) consists of surgical destruction of part of the brain (usually the globus pallidus). The patient is usually awake during the procedure, so that the appropriate proportion of tissue can be ablated to restore the balance between excitation and inhibition of movement. Pallidotomy is effective at reducing contralateral dyskinesias, as well as reducing symptoms such as bradykinesia. However, the procedure is not well tolerated in patients who have even a minor degree of cognitive impairment or who are over 70 years old.

Deep brain stimulation (DBS) is the placement of a stimulator. Sites used include the globus pallidus, the subthalamic nucleus, or the thalamus. DBS placement has the advantage of being adjustable as opposed to the permanence of ablation. The amount of energy sent through the device, as well as the rate at which the device operates, can be adjusted as the patient's symptoms progress. The procedure has similar benefits to ablative surgery in terms of reducing dyskinesia and bradykinesia but also may benefit tremor (depending on where the device is placed). Complications include bleeding and infection, hardware problems (such as dislocation of electrodes), or battery failure. The unit is expensive and requires considerable time to adjust it for optimal response.

SUMMARY

Carbidopa/levodopa therapy is the treatment of choice in elderly patients with PD. Doses should be started low and slowly titrated against motor response. Lack of levodopa response may mean PD is not the correct diagnosis. Dementia is more common in elderly patients with PD, and the use of anticholinergics is contraindicated owing to the risk of worsening confusion. Postural hypotension may limit the use of adjunctive therapy such as dopamine agonists. Coexistent depression is common and needs to be addressed appropriately.

KEY REFERENCES

10. Gelb DJ, Oliver E, Gilman S. Diagnostic criteria for Parkinson disease. Arch Neurol 1999;56:33-9.
21. McKeith IG, Dickson DW, Lowe J, et al. Diagnosis and management of dementia with Lewy bodies: Third report of the LBD consortium. Neurology 2005;65:1863-72.
24. Miyasaki JM, Martin W, Suchowersky O, et al. Practice parameter: Initiation of treatment for Parkinson's disease: An evidence-based review: Report of the Quality Standards Subcommittee of the American Academy of Neurology. Neurology 2002;54:2292.
35. Miyasaki JM, Shannon K, Voon V, et al. Practice parameter: Evaluation and treatment of depression, psychosis, and dementia in Parkinson disease (an evidence-based review): Report of the Quality Standards Subcommittee of the American Academy of Neurology. Neurology 2006;66:996.
42. Juncos JL, Roberts VJ, Evatt ML, et al. Quetiapine improves psychotic symptoms and cognition in Parkinson's disease. Mov Disord 2004;19:29.

References available online at expertconsult.com.

53

Oral Disorders

Pamela Sparks Stein, Craig S. Miller, and Craig B. Fowler

Additional online-only material indicated by icon.

OBJECTIVES

Upon completion of this chapter, the reader will be able to:

- Relate the risk of poor oral health to systemic health.
- Explain the increased susceptibility of older adults to dental caries and periodontal disease.
- Discuss the clinical significance of mouth dryness and its causes.
- Name the indications for immediate referral to a dentist.
- Describe the guidelines for antibiotic prophylaxis in cardiac patients at risk for infective endocarditis and in patients with total joint replacement.
- List the major risk factors for oral cancer, its sites, and its public health significance.

The mouth is often thought to be the domain of the dentist, but the impact of the oral environment on the rest of the body is well documented. Good oral health has numerous benefits to systemic health. Oral health is an essential part of primary care. Oral health screening and appropriate counsel and referral will improve an elder's quality of life.

ORAL–SYSTEMIC LINKAGES

Oral disease can be detrimental to systemic health, particularly in the medically compromised elderly. Older adults with oral problems have shown insufficient consumption of important vitamins and lower Healthy Eating Index scores.[1] Poor oral health affects chewing, speaking, and swallowing, as well as self-image, self-esteem, and socialization.

Much research suggests poor oral health contributes to systemic disease. Periodontal disease has been shown to increase the risk for poor glycemic control in patients with diabetes (increasing the risk sixfold).[2] Diabetes patients who received treatment for their periodontal disease showed a significant improvement in HbA_{1c} levels ($p = .04$).[3] Periodontal disease may also increase the risk for cardiovascular or renal complications in those with diabetes.[4]

Multiple studies report poor oral health contributes to development of respiratory disease.[5-8] In individuals with poor oral hygiene, bacteria are released from plaque into the saliva and may be aspirated into the lungs, precipitating bacterial pneumonia.[9] A systematic review found good evidence that improved oral hygiene and professional oral health care decrease the risk of respiratory disease in frail elders who are residents in long-term care facilities (relative risk reduction of 34% to 83%).[10]

In April of 2012, the American Heart Association (AHA) released a statement after review of more than 500 peer-reviewed papers investigating potential linkages between periodontal disease and atherosclerotic diseases. The conclusion of the AHA was that there is no evidence that periodontal disease is a causative factor for atherosclerotic disease.[11] Regarding the benefit of periodontal therapy to improve outcomes in patients, the authors state: "Although periodontal interventions result in a reduction in systemic inflammation and endothelial dysfunction in short-term studies, there is no evidence that they prevent ASVD [arteriosclerotic vascular disease] or modify its outcomes."[11]

More research is necessary to fully understand the role oral health plays in cardiovascular health.

Evidence suggests that osteoporosis is associated with periodontal disease, specifically loss of alveolar bone that surrounds the teeth.[12] Further, bisphosphonates prescribed to treat osteoporosis may predispose dental patients to osteonecrosis, a condition that results in necrosis of the jaw bone often accompanied by exposed bone, pain, infection, swelling, and dysethesias.[13] To help prevent osteonecrosis, physicians should collaborate with the patient's dentist to inform the patient of risks and ensure optimum oral health before prescribing bisphosphonates. Excellent oral hygiene, regular professional dental cleanings, and appropriate timing for oral surgical procedures may minimize the risk of osteonecrosis.[13]

> Good oral hygiene substantially decreases risk for pneumonia in elders.

COMMON ORAL PROBLEMS IN OLDER ADULTS

Dental Caries

Prevalence and Impact

Dental caries (decay) is the progressive destruction of tooth structure caused by acids produced by sugars and bacteria in the oral cavity (Figure 53-1). If untreated, dental caries can progress into the pulp of the tooth, causing pain and a dental abscess, which may lead to bacteremia, facial/pharyngeal infection, septicemia, and in rare cases cavernous sinus thrombosis.

Because an increasing number of adults are retaining their teeth throughout their lifetime, dental decay is increasing in the elderly. Nearly one third of older adults have dental caries, averaging one new carious

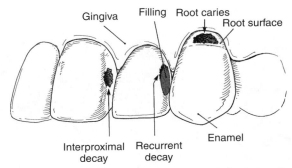

Figure 53-1 The most common form of dental caries in older adults is root caries: decay that attacks the portion of the tooth not protected by enamel, that is, the root. Root caries may appear as a tan, brown, or black discoloration in this area or as frank cavitation. Recurrent caries develop adjacent to a filling at its margin. Interproximal caries occur between teeth and may not be observed clinically.

surface per person per year. Decay in elders is more likely to go untreated; elderly have four times the mean number of untreated carious surfaces compared to U.S. schoolchildren.[14]

Approximately 86% of adults older than age 65 experience recession (gums pull away from the teeth). This is not a normal part of aging but instead is caused by periodontal disease or trauma from overzealous toothbrushing. Tooth roots are exposed by recession, and cementum, which covers the roots, is more susceptible to decay than enamel. Elders are therefore more prone to root caries than their younger counterparts.[15] In fact, root caries is the most common type of decay in elders. A study of community-dwelling elders found 52% had a history of root caries and 22% had active untreated root caries.[16] This type of decay progresses rapidly and will amputate the tooth at the gum line if untreated.

Risk Factors and Pathophysiology

A diet high in carbohydrates is a major risk factor for dental decay. Declines in cognitive and physical function impair the ability to brush and floss one's teeth and increase the risk of decay. Institutionalized elders may experience 3 times the prevalence of decayed teeth compared to community living older adults.[17] Dry mouth, often induced by medications, is another important risk factor for caries.

Differential Diagnosis and Assessment

Decayed teeth in older adults are generally less symptomatic than in younger adults. Active decay has a yellowish brown color. Early root decay appears broad and shallow. Decay on the crowns of teeth is usually found around preexisting fillings or crowns (see Figure 53-1). Dental radiographs and transillumination are helpful in diagnosis.

Management

Timely treatment of decay is very important to reduce destruction of tooth structure and decrease the risk of the decay progressing into the tooth pulp and causing an abscess. Dental amalgam (silver filling material) and composite (white filling material) are the two most common dental materials used to restore a tooth after decay has been removed. When the affected areas are expansive, pins or other retentive approaches are used to enhance longevity of the restoration. When restoring more than half of the crown of the tooth, full coverage of the tooth using gold or porcelain (often called a crown or cap) may be the best treatment. Full coverage of a tooth involves more treatment time and significantly more expense. It is much easier on the patient and more cost-effective to address decay at the earliest possible time.

Periodontal Disease

Prevalence and Impact

Periodontal disease (periodontitis or gum disease) is progressive disease that begins as inflammation of the gingiva (gingivitis). If left untreated, gingivitis progresses to a more severe inflammatory disease that destroys the alveolar bone supporting the teeth. In severe periodontal disease, the teeth become mobile and are often lost. Periodontal disease is the primary cause of tooth loss in adults.

The prevalence of periodontal disease has decreased since the 1970s. However, more than 17% of adults older than age 65 have periodontal disease compared to 8.52% of adults age 20 to 64. This prevalence is higher in adults with low income, less education, and black or Hispanic ethnicities.[18]

Risk Factors and Pathophysiology

Periodontal disease is caused by bacteria in dental plaque. Failure to effectively remove plaque by proper oral hygiene and professional cleanings results in an accumulation of plaque and calculus (mineralized plaque) that induces inflammation and infection of the gingiva and alveolar bone (Figure 53-2). Other risk factors include smoking, diabetes, osteoporosis, osteopenia, genetics, and hyposalivation.

Differential Diagnosis and Assessment

Early periodontal disease is characterized by redness, bleeding, and edematous gingival tissues. As the disease progresses, bone surrounding the teeth is destroyed (see Figure 53-2). As a result, teeth become mobile. Diagnosis of periodontal disease involves measuring the depth of the periodontal pockets with a probe and radiographic examination to determine if bone loss has occurred. The entire oral cavity, including teeth, needs to be examined to determine the extent of periodontal disease.

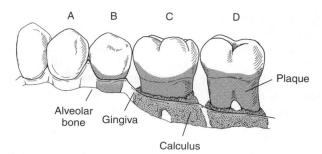

Figure 53-2 The periodontium consists of alveolar bone and gingiva, the anatomic foundation for sound teeth (*tooth A*). Healthy periodontium is maintained by thorough oral hygiene practices. When plaque remains on teeth, gingivitis develops (*tooth B*). The accumulation of plaque and calculus on teeth results in destruction of the periodontium known as periodontitis (*tooth C*). Periodontitis is considered severe when more than 50% of supporting bone has been lost (*tooth D*).

Management

The most important approach to management of periodontal disease is removal of plaque and calculus by effective brushing, flossing, and tooth scaling by dental professionals. More frequent dental visits for removal of plaque and calculus may be warranted. Other management strategies include use of pharmacotherapeutics (e.g., chlorhexidine gluconate rinse and Listerine), improved management of systemic diseases (e.g., diabetes and osteoporosis), smoking cessation, and locally applied and systemic antibiotics. Surgery is sometimes necessary to manage extensive bone loss.

> Tell your patients: Dry mouth will increase decay and loss of teeth. Avoid anticholinergics and keep the mouth moist!

Mouth Dryness

Prevalence and Impact

Xerostomia (the patient's subjective complaint of mouth dryness) and hyposalivation (the objective reduction in salivary secretion) are correlated and prevalent problems in older adults. Approximately 30% of adults 65 and older suffer from xerostomia.[19] Saliva is essential to maintain oral and general health. Dry mouth reduces comfort and quality of life. Constant mouth dryness may reduce compliance with prescription medications; patients may alter dosage or stop the drug altogether. It may also restrict dietary choices and compromise nutrition by making chewing and swallowing uncomfortable, altering taste, and diminishing food enjoyment. Lack of adequate salivation is associated with chronic esophagitis and gastroesophageal reflux disease (GERD).[20] Dry mouth increases the frequency and severity of dental caries. There is often rampant, rapidly progressive decay that is difficult to manage and more substantial periodontal disease in individuals suffering from mouth dryness. Also the patient's ability to tolerate a denture is compromised because of lack of lubrication of oral tissues.

Risk Factors and Pathophysiology

Salivary flow does not decline with age; medical conditions and their treatment, rather than age, are associated with mouth dryness. The most common cause of hyposalivation is medication use. Many drugs used to manage issues in older adults contribute to oral dryness; these include sedatives, antipsychotics, antianginal agents, antidepressants, antihistamines, antihypertensives, antiparkinson agents, diuretics, and anticholinergics. Sjogren's syndrome is the most common salivary gland disorder in the elderly leading to xerostomia. Reduced saliva may also be a result of patient dehydration or salivary duct obstructions such as sialoliths, infections, tumors, head and neck radiation, diabetes, and Alzheimer's disease.[21]

Differential Diagnosis and Assessment

Clinical signs of mouth dryness include dry, ulcerated, reddened, or furrowed lips and intraoral mucosa; generalized desiccated tissues with a lack of saliva pooling in the floor of the mouth; a fissured or inflamed tongue, and the presence of halitosis. Assessment can also be aided by palpating or "milking" the parotid gland. An unexpected rise in dental caries and the presence of fungal infections may be sequelae of a dry mouth. The patient may also complain of xerostomia, burning mouth, sore lips and tongue, as well as having difficulty with swallowing, taste, speaking, and denture use.

Management

Preventive care is first in managing dry mouth; fluoride therapy, an antimicrobial mouth rinse, and reduction of refined carbohydrate consumption can mitigate the elevated risk of dental caries and periodontal disease. Patients should be encouraged to visit their dental provider often to screen for dental caries. If a patient's medication is known to inhibit salivation, an alternative drug in the same class should be considered. Some have recommended modifying medication schedules so that the peak hyposalivary effects occur during mealtimes when there is a natural stimulus for salivation.

In many cases topical treatment using a saliva substitute may be helpful. Over-the-counter saliva substitutes include Oral Balance gel (Laclede products) and Mouthkote (Unimed). Salivary stimulants such as sugarless Biotene Xylitol gum (Laclede Products) and sugarless candy may also be helpful. Systemic salivary

stimulants (pilocarpine) may be used, especially in patients with Sjogren's syndrome, but should be avoided in those with glaucoma or pulmonary disease. Patients should be encouraged to drink plenty of water and avoid alcohol and caffeine.[22]

Edentulousness

Prevalence and Impact

In the 1950s half of all Americans older than age 65 had lost all of their natural teeth.[23] Today the edentulism rate of older adults has decreased to 18%.[24] The downward trend in edentulism is largely the result of fluoridation of community water, increased education about prevention of oral disease, and increased access to dental care.

Adverse outcomes of edentulism include difficulty chewing and speaking, poor esthetics, and lowered self-esteem. A recent study found 45% of denture wearers have oral lesions caused by their denture.[25] Regular dental care is essential for maintaining the functional benefits of dentures and the health of the edentulous mouth.

Risk Factors and Pathophysiology

Dental caries and periodontal disease are the main determinants of tooth loss leading to edentulism. Comorbidities of edentulism include poor nutrition, smoking, diabetes, coronary artery plaque, and rheumatoid arthritis.[26] Risk factors for edentulism include poverty and fewer than 12 years of education in non-Hispanic white people (but not in black or Mexican-American people),[27] lower original intelligence,[28] and increasing age.[29]

Differential Diagnosis and Assessment

A detailed intraoral examination should be performed to determine dentate status and condition of any prostheses. Dentures should be removed and tissues examined for oral mucosal lesions. Persons with *Candida*-associated denture stomatitis and angular cheilitis, traumatic ulcers, and denture irritation hyperplasia should be referred to a dental professional. Questions should be asked of the patient regarding his or her satisfaction with function and comfort.

Management

Complete dentures are the mainstay of treatment for restoring the edentulous mouth. Dentures are not fitted "for life"; they will get looser with time and need regular professional attention. The edentulous ridge (remaining alveolar bone) undergoes continuous resorption over the years, ultimately compromising the fit and stability of the dentures. Only 13% of denture wearers seek annual dental care, and nearly half have not seen a dentist in 5 years.[30] Dental-implant–supported dentures may provide more functional capacity than less costly conventional dentures but not every patient is an implant candidate.

Oral and Oropharyngeal Cancer

Prevalence and Impact

Estimates from the American Cancer Society indicated that more than 36,000 individuals would be diagnosed with oral and oropharyngeal carcinoma in 2010.[31] Of these cancers, approximately 24,000 would be located in the oral cavity proper, excluding the lower lip vermilion and pharynx. Oral cancer incidence increases with age, with the median age at diagnosis being 61 years. Over the last several decades, the incidence rate for men has declined, but it has remained stable in females. Black males have a 30% higher incidence rate than white males for reasons that are not well understood.[32]

Despite important advances in the treatment of oral cancer, the 5-year survival rate (approximately 50%) has not changed appreciably in the last 50 years. This is likely related to several factors, the most important of which is the fact that more than 60% of oral cancers are not diagnosed until they are of advanced stage clinically.[32] The reasons for this are multifactorial. The early signs and symptoms of oral cancer may be subtle and may not be recognized by patients, their health care providers, or both. It is also possible that patients may postpone receiving an oral cancer examination because of fear of the consequences if oral cancer is detected.

The diagnosis of oral cancer can be a devastating and life-changing event because of the potential for disfigurement and major oral functional impairments as a result of surgery and radiotherapy (e.g., tasting, chewing, swallowing, and speaking). Review of cancer statistics indicates that early diagnosis is the most important factor in improving the clinical outcome and survival for oral cancer.[33] Therefore educating the public about the risk factors and clinical signs of oral cancer and educating health care providers about the early mucosal changes that may signal oral cancer development are critical to the improvement of clinical outcomes for patients with oral cancer as well as the effort to prevent oral cancer in susceptible individuals.

Risk Factors and Pathophysiology

Nearly all cancers of the oral cavity and oropharynx are squamous cell carcinomas (SCCs) that arise from the squamous mucosa lining these anatomic areas. SCCs are capable of direct extension into adjacent anatomic structures as well as metastasis via the lymphatic system to involve cervical lymph nodes. Hematogenous spread to distant sites, especially the lung, is also possible, but usually occurs in advanced stage cancers. On the other hand, metastasis to cervical lymph nodes can occur prior to the detection of the primary tumor, especially if the primary tumor is small and located in relatively hard-to-examine locations such as the base of the tongue.

Although age is certainly a factor in the development of oral and oropharyngeal SCC, various other risk factors have been investigated in the quest to determine the exact cause and pathogenesis of this disease. These include (1) tobacco, (2) alcohol, (3) oncogenic viruses (especially human papillomavirus), and (4) genetic susceptibility.[32] Most oral and oropharyngeal SCCs are associated with tobacco use. Smoked tobacco (cigarettes, cigars, pipes) generally carries a higher risk for development of oral SCC than smokeless tobacco, but SCC can certainly develop in patients who use smokeless tobacco, and the risk increases with long-term use. Moreover, not all smokeless tobacco products carry the same risk, with the variation being dependent on the physical form of the tobacco as well as certain additives that may themselves be carcinogenic.[34] It is also well known that patients who have been diagnosed with oral SCC have approximately a 15% risk of developing a second primary tumor in the upper aerodigestive tract.[35] This percentage increases if the patients continue to smoke. Alcohol may be an independent risk factor, but it is more importantly a potentiator of the carcinogenic potential of tobacco. Heavy smokers who are also heavy drinkers have a risk at least 15 times that of nonsmokers and nondrinkers.[36] Human papillomaviruses (HPVs) have been implicated in oral cancer development, and recent evidence links HPV (usually HPV-16) to a subset of oropharyngeal SCCs, most of which arise in the tonsil or base of the tongue.[37] As a group, patients with these HPV-16–positive SCCs tend to be younger than those with HPV-negative tumors and typically do not have a history of smoking or alcohol abuse. Interestingly, patients with these HPV-16–positive tumors have demonstrated improved survival after treatment with concurrent chemoradiotherapy.[38] An increasing number of younger adults with no known risk factors have been reported with oral SCC in the last several decades. It is thought that genetic susceptibility likely plays a role in the development of oral SCC in these individuals. Specific defects in DNA repair, elimination of defective cells (apoptosis), and immune surveillance may predispose certain patients to the development of SCC in the absence of other known risk factors.[37]

Differential Diagnosis and Assessment

The majority of oral SCCs occur in the following anatomic sites: the lateral and ventral tongue, the floor of the mouth, and the soft palate–tonsillar complex. They often present as white, red, or red and white masses, and may be ulcerated. Early SCCs and premalignant lesions may appear as white plaques (leukoplakia), red plaques (erythroplakia), or a combination of the two (erythroleukoplakia). These early oral SCCs and pre-cancerous lesions may be subtle and asymptomatic, and may go unnoticed by the patient. Therefore, periodic oral examination by a properly trained dental or medical professional is advised in order to discover these early lesions before they have the opportunity to spread locally or metastasize. Although several new oral cancer detection devices are now available, so far none of them have demonstrated the ability to detect early cancers any better than a thorough clinical oral and head and neck examination using visualization and palpation.[39] As mentioned earlier, oral and oropharyngeal SCCs have the ability to metastasize, most often to lymph nodes in the neck. Even clinically small primary lesions may metastasize, and unfortunately for some patients, the first sign of disease may be a neck mass that represents a metastasis from a previously undetected SCC. Primary lesions located in the floor of the mouth and base of the tongue are particularly prone to early metastasis.

Tissue biopsy is the most reliable method for definitively diagnosing premalignant lesions as well as oral and oropharyngeal SCC, and is the preferred approach for accurate assessment of suspicious lesions. Fine needle aspiration (FNA), in combination with computed tomography (CT) and magnetic resonance imaging (MRI), is the usual method for evaluation of suspicious neck masses. Positron emission tomography (PET) scanning is another relatively new diagnostic modality that can supplement conventional CT and MRI in the clinical workup of both primary lesions as well as suspected neck disease.[40]

> Oral cancer often presents as white, red, or red and white masses, and may be ulcerated.

Management

Treatment modalities for oral cancer depend on the clinical stage and location of the cancer, and may involve surgical excision alone, radiotherapy alone, or a combination. In the past, chemotherapy was reserved for palliative treatment in advanced cases, but is now playing a larger role in the management of oral and oropharyngeal SCC. Specifically, concurrent chemoradiotherapy is now the preferred treatment for tumors originating in the base of the tongue, and has afforded patients with these tumors an improved quality of life.[41]

Management of patients with oral and oropharyngeal SCC should be accomplished via a team approach. The health care team may include otolaryngologists, oral surgeons, maxillofacial prosthodontists, general dentists, medical oncologists, radiation oncologists, oral pathologists, general pathologists, speech pathologists,

physical therapists, nutritionists, and psychologists. General dentists are essential members of the team, especially with regard to pretreatment assessment of dental status thus minimizing or avoiding the possibility of osteoradionecrosis. Maxillofacial prosthodontists can restore form and function to structures lost or altered during treatment. This integrated team of specialized health care providers is essential to the successful management of patients with oral and oropharyngeal cancer.

CASE 1

William Cole (Part 1)

William Cole, an 86-year-old white male patient of yours, has had multiple health problems and hospitalizations over the past 20 years. He has survived prostate cancer, lung cancer, and chronic obstructive pulmonary disease (COPD). He has been clinically stable over the last few years, despite some difficulty maintaining his weight. At a routine follow-up visit, his wife reports that "he's not eating good" and "he has bad teeth."

1. How will you assess the patient's oral status?

2. What should you do next? ▢

LOW UTILIZATION OF DENTAL SERVICES

The elderly have lower dental services utilization rates than younger adults. It is common for an older person not to have sought dental care for years.[42] The primary reasons are that older persons do not perceive a need for dental care or dismiss oral problems as an inevitable part of aging. Low utilization is also related to losing insurance benefits after retiring. Only 30% of the elderly have dental insurance. Although Medicare helps to accommodate for loss in coverage for medical services, Medicare does not pay for dental services unless they are deemed medically necessary (e.g., extracting teeth prior to head and neck radiation).[43] Medicaid coverage for dental services varies from state to state. Six states have no adult dental benefits; 16 cover only emergency dental services, and 13 exclude at least one dental service category.[44]

Older adults use medical services more frequently and repeatedly than dental services. Thus it is primary care medical providers who must screen for oral disease and make dental referrals. Primary care can be the link between the older patient and adequate dental care.

> *Always* look in the mouth and at the feet of your elderly patients! The elderly often do not go to dentists but do go to doctors.

NEED FOR ORAL HEALTH SCREENING

Early detection improves the prognosis of oral cancer and reduces mortality; the 5-year survival for patients with distant metastasis at diagnosis is 18% whereas the 5-year survival is 75% when disease is still localized at diagnosis. The American Cancer Society and American Dental Association recommend an oral examination annually for all elders. A panel of health care experts has advocated for routine oral examinations by physicians for all individuals older than age 65.[45] An annual oral examination is mandated by federal regulation for the institutionalized elderly.

Oral Health Screening

Screening for oral disease involves a few simple additions to routine examination technique. Patients should be asked about risk factors, oral function, and symptoms of common oral problems (Table 53-1). The screening examination includes intraoral and extraoral structures (Table 53-2). The head and neck are inspected and palpated. The oral soft tissues are inspected. The patient should remove dentures. Material such as food debris or denture adhesive can masquerade as a pathologic condition or obscure visibility of soft tissue, so the patient should rinse the mouth before examination. Good lighting is essential. The highest risk locations for intraoral

TABLE 53-2	Oral Health Screening: Physical
Inspect	**Look for**
Extraoral	
Masticatory muscles	Facial swelling
Salivary glands	
Parotid	Masses
Submandibular	Masses
Sublingual	Masses
Cervical lymph nodes	Lymphadenopathy
Intraoral Soft Tissue	
Lateral tongue	Masses
Ventral tongue	Erythroplakia (red lesion)
Floor mouth	Leukoplakia (white lesion)
Oropharynx	Erosion/ulceration
Palate	Dry, friable mucosa
Alveolar ridges	Dry, friable mucosa
Buccal mucosa	Dry, friable mucosa
Lips	Dry, friable mucosa
Periodontium	Swollen, red, bleeding gums
Dentition	
All Teeth	
Inspect	Decay
	Fractured teeth
	Exposed roots
	Receding gums

malignancy are the floor of mouth and tongue. To observe the lateral tongue, the clinician asks the patient to stick out the tongue. The clinician gently grasps the tip of the tongue with a gauze sponge and moves it laterally, with the mouth open wide, checking the lateral tongue carefully for ulcerations, swelling, or discoloration. To observe the ventral tongue and floor of mouth, the clinician asks the patient to lift the tongue up to the roof of the mouth, with the mouth wide open. The remaining oral soft tissues are then inspected. Finally, the teeth and gums are evaluated. Halitosis is often a sign of periodontal disease or poor oral hygiene. Findings that merit immediate referral to a dentist are listed in Box 53-1.

Medical oral screening may miss occult disease of the jaws, periodontium, and dentition including chronic abscesses, periodontal disease, interproximal decay (between the teeth) (see Figure 53-1) and root tips (necrotic teeth near the gum line). A thorough

TABLE 53-1	Oral Health Screening: History
To Assess	**Ask About**
Oral cancer risk	Age
	Smoking
	Smokeless tobacco
	Drinking
	Sores in the mouth
Oral function	Trouble chewing
	Painful teeth
	Broken teeth
Self-neglect	Last visit to a dentist
	Last time dentures were serviced
	How often do you brush teeth?
Dental caries	Cavities
	Food sticking between teeth
	Teeth sensitive to hot, cold, sweets
Periodontal disease	Bleeding gums
	Loose teeth
	Diabetic control
	Smoking
	Bad breath
Xerostomia	Amount of saliva
	Mouth dryness when eating
	Medications, including over-the-counter

BOX 53-1

REASONS FOR IMMEDIATE REFERRAL TO A DENTIST

- Tooth or gum pain
- Facial or intraoral swelling/pus
- Erythroplakia and/or leukoplakia
- Ulceration or erosion
- Swollen, red, bleeding gums
- Broken, decayed, or mobile teeth
- Ill-fitting prosthesis

dental examination with radiographs is necessary to rule out these conditions.

A patient with acute oral infection may seek emergency treatment from a primary care clinician. Dental infection may be characterized by pain in one specific tooth; the pain is typically unprovoked, continuous, and unremitting. Swelling may occur in the gingiva or may progress to involve the fascial spaces. Medical management should include antibiotic therapy, pain control, and immediate referral to a dentist. Penicillin V is generally considered the drug of choice for odontogenic infection. In the penicillin-allergic patient, clindamycin is frequently the next drug used. Supportive care and hospitalization are needed in cases of advanced infection or debility.

Referral to a dentist has been emphasized here as the means of initiating individualized oral care for each patient, whether dentate or edentulous. A general dentist with interest and willingness to treat older patients is appropriate in most cases.

> The highest risk locations for intraoral malignancy are the floor of the mouth and the tongue.

PREVENTING INFECTIVE ENDOCARDITIS

Infective endocarditis (IE) is a serious complication of dental treatment that may occur in susceptible patients. Risk is higher in persons aged 65 or older and intravenous drug users.[46] Even with appropriate medical therapy, mortality approaches 40%.[47]

A number of cardiac conditions place the patient at risk for endocarditis. The American Heart Association (AHA)[48] recommends antibiotic prophylaxis for patients with conditions shown in Box 53-2 when they undergo

---

BOX 53-2

CARDIAC CONDITIONS ASSOCIATED WITH THE HIGHEST RISK OF ADVERSE OUTCOME FROM ENDOCARDITIS FOR WHICH PROPHYLAXIS WITH DENTAL PROCEDURES IS RECOMMENDED

- Prosthetic cardiac valve
- Previous infective endocarditis
- Congenital heart disease (CHD)
- Unrepaired cyanotic CHD, including those with palliative shunts and conduits
- Completely repaired CHD with prosthetic material or device by surgery or catheter intervention during the first 6 months after the procedure
- Repaired CHD with residual defects at the site or adjacent to the site of a prosthetic patch or prosthetic device, which inhibits endothelialization
- Cardiac transplantation recipients who develop cardiac valvulopathy

Based on Wilson et al. J Am Dent Assoc 2007;138(6):739-45, 47-60.

BOX 53-3

DENTAL PROCEDURES FOR WHICH ENDOCARDITIS PROPHYLAXIS IS RECOMMENDED FOR PATIENTS WITH CONDITIONS LISTED IN BOX 53-2

- All dental procedures that involve manipulation of gingival tissue or the periapical region of teeth, or perforation of the oral mucosa
- This includes ALL dental procedures EXCEPT the following procedures and events:
  - Routine anesthetic injections through noninfected tissue
  - Taking of dental radiographs
  - Placement of removable prosthodontic or orthodontic appliances
  - Adjustment of orthodontic appliances
  - Shedding of deciduous teeth and bleeding from trauma to the lips or oral mucosa

Based on Wilson et al. J Am Dent Assoc 2007;138(6):739-45, 47-60.

---

dental procedures that involve manipulation of gingival tissues or the periapical region of a tooth, and procedures that perforate the oral mucosa (Box 53-3).

The rationale for the AHA recommendation is that invasive dental procedures and minor manipulations such as tooth cleaning can result in transient bacteremia. However, chewing and toothbrushing are also associated with bacteremia; yet the majority of these bacteremias do not cause infective endocarditis. Accordingly, there is a growing trend to recommend less use of antibiotics as prophylaxis for dental procedures,[49] and there is little evidence to support the benefit of the use of antibiotic prophylaxis.[50] In the meantime, primary antibiotic prevention recommended by the AHA is directed at preventing alpha-hemolytic streptococcus (e.g., *Streptococcus viridans*) from causing endocarditis after dental or medical procedures.

The clinician's goal is to prevent infective endocarditis from occurring in susceptible patients. To accomplish this, the clinician must:

1. Identify at-risk patients—Dentists need to identify from the medical history patients at increased risk (see Box 53-1). Consultation with primary care providers to determine whether a patient is at increased risk owing to his or her cardiac status may be required. Any uncertainty in the patient's heart condition requires consultation with the patient's cardiologist. Patients who are at increased risk for IE should be informed about antibiotic prophylaxis for dental procedures.
2. Use AHA guidelines for antibiotic prophylaxis (Box 53-4)[3]—This regimen involves one dose of oral amoxicillin 30 to 60 minutes before the procedure. Azithromycin or clindamycin are recommended for patients who are allergic to penicillins. If a patient is already taking penicillin

---

Box 53-4

AMERICAN HEART ASSOCIATION–RECOMMENDED ANTIBIOTIC PROPHYLACTIC REGIMEN FOR DENTAL PROCEDURES IN PATIENTS AT RISK (GIVEN 30-60 MINUTES BEFORE PROCEDURE)

- Amoxicillin 2 g
- If unable to take oral medication: ampicillin 2 g IM or IV or cefazolin or ceftriaxone 1 g IM or IV
- Allergic to penicillin: cephalexin 2 g or clindamycin 600 mg, or azithromycin or clarithromycin 500 mg
- Allergic to penicillins or ampicillin and unable to take oral medication: cefazolin or ceftriaxone 1 g IM or IV, or clindamycin phosphate 500 mg IM or IV

Based on Wilson et al. J Am Dent Assoc 2007;138(6):739-45, 47-60. *IM*, Intramuscular; *IV*, intravenously.

Box 53-5

CONDITIONS THAT PLACE PATIENTS AT INCREASED RISK OF HEMATOGENOUS INFECTION OF A TOTAL JOINT

- Immune suppression (HIV infection, rheumatoid arthritis, lupus erythematosus, drug- or radiation-induced immunosuppression)
- Previous prosthetic joint infection
- Malnourishment
- Hemophilia
- Type 1 diabetes
- Malignancy

Based on JADA 2003;134:895-8.

---

for other reasons, azithromycin or clindamycin should be used for IE prophylaxis.

3. Establish and maintain good oral health to reduce the risk of bacteremia. Bacteremia of oral origin can be secondary to ordinary daily activities, particularly in those with poor oral health, and IE has on occasion been associated with dental procedures. Patients should thus be encouraged to keep the mouth healthy through appropriate oral hygiene and dental follow-up visits. Also, clinicians should eradicate oral disease to establish a healthy oral environment.

PREVENTING JOINT INFECTION

Artificial joints are vulnerable to bacterial colonization and infection from hematogenous seeding, especially in the first 2 years after joint replacement. Unlike IE, most prosthetic joint infections are caused by nonoral bacteria such as staphylococci.[51] Thus antibiotic prophylaxis is not routinely indicated for dental patients with total joint replacements. Joint advisory statements published by the American Academy of Orthopaedic Surgeons (AAOS) and the American Dental Association in 1997 and 2003 indicate that only those who are at increased risk are to be considered for premedication (see Box 53-4).[52,53] Persons with pins, plates, or screws do not need antibiotic prophylaxis. Suggested antibiotic prophylaxis regimens are cephalexin, cephradine, or amoxicillin 2 g orally 1 hour prior to invasive dental procedures, if not allergic to these drugs. Clindamycin 600 mg orally 1 hour before invasive dental procedures is recommended, if the patient is allergic to penicillin.

Clinicians should be aware that the issue of antibiotic prophylaxis for patients with prosthetic joints remains a controversial issue. In contrast to the 2003 advisory statement, the AAOS in 2009 and in 2010 published opinion statements recommending that clinicians consider antibiotic prophylaxis for joint replacement patients with risk factors prior to *any* invasive procedure

that may cause bacteremia. The 2009 and 2010 statements contain more "at risk" conditions than those shown in Box 53-5, and can be viewed at www.aaos.org/news/aaosnow/jan13/cover1.asp. The basis for the AAOS change in position is concern for "potential adverse outcomes and cost of treating an infected joint," not because of scientific evidence indicating risk. Clinicians should be aware that current evidence indicates risks for prosthetic joint infections are not related to dental procedures.[54,55] As a result, the American Academy of Oral Medicine published a position paper stating opposition to the use of antibiotic prophylaxis in patients with prosthetic joints.[56] Current guidelines recommend that antibiotic prophylaxis *be considered*; however, there is no *requirement* that they be used routinely.

CASE 1

William Cole (Part 2)

You refer Mr. Cole to a general dentist, who finds that root caries have devastated his upper teeth. The upper teeth are extracted, and a complete denture is fabricated. The lower teeth are preserved by routine fillings. Mr. Cole is placed on daily fluoride therapy and scheduled for a 4-month recall. At follow-up, Mrs. Cole reports that her husband is eating a greater variety of solid foods than he has in years. ■

SUMMARY

Older adults exhibit a range of oral disease and conditions, many of which can have a significant impact on systemic health. Because these conditions are among the most prevalent of chronic conditions experienced by older adults, primary care clinicians must screen for dental problems and provide appropriate referral. Detecting oral cancer, mouth dryness, dental caries, and periodontal disease; preventing infective endocarditis; and instituting a preventive approach to oral health in general are the major issues.

ACKNOWLEDGMENTS

The authors would like to thank Drs. Barbara J. Smith, Ingrid H. Valdez, and Douglas B. Berkey for their contributions to earlier versions of this chapter.

Web Resources

www.aaos.org. American Academy of Orthopaedic Surgeons.

http://seer.cancer.gov/csr/1975_2006. National Cancer Institute's Surveillance Epidemiology and End Results (SEER).

www.oralcancerfoundation.org/treatment/pdf/guidelines.pdf. National Comprehensive Cancer Network's Clinical Practice Guidelines in Oncology: Head and Neck Cancers.

www.cdc.gov/nohss. Centers for Disease Control's National Center for Chronic Disease Prevention and Health Promotion: National Oral Health Surveillance System.

KEY REFERENCES

24. National Oral Health Surveillance System. Oral health indicators. http://www.cdc.gov/nohss. Accessed July 12, 2013.
32. Natarajan E, Eisenberg E. Contemporary concepts in the diagnosis of oral cancer and precancer. Dent Clin N Am 2011;55:63-88.
33. Horner MJ, Ries LAG, Krapcho M, et al. SEER cancer statistics review, 1975-2006. Bethesda, MD: National Cancer Institute. Available at http://seer.cancer.gov/csr/1975_2006. Accessed July 12, 2013.
46. Little JW, Falace DA, Miller CS, Rhodus NL. Infective endocarditis: Dental management of the medically compromised patient. 8th ed. St. Louis: Elsevier; 2013, p. 20-36.
53. American Dental Association. Antibiotic prophylaxis for dental patients with total joint replacements. J Am Dent Assoc 2003;134:895-9.

References available online at expertconsult.com.

54

Skin Problems

Justin O. Endo and Robert A. Norman

OBJECTIVES

Upon completion of this chapter, the reader will be able to:

- Describe lesions and rashes using a four-point process to facilitate differential diagnosis formulation, triage, and communication of dermatologic problems.
- Diagnose and manage common, benign neoplastic skin growths in older patients.
- Diagnose and discuss evidence-based management options for actinic keratosis (AK) and common skin cancers in the geriatric population.
- Discuss the differential diagnoses and approach to older patients presenting with itch but without intact primary lesions.
- Diagnose and manage common causes of eczematous skin disorders (dermatitis) in older individuals, including how to estimate appropriate potency and quantity of topical steroids.
- Discuss the diagnosis and management of inflammatory conditions associated with aging.
- Discuss evidence-based prevention and treatment of acute herpes zoster and management options for postherpetic neuralgia.

CASE 1

Cándido Aguado (Part 1)

You are in the middle of a busy clinic, and the next patient is an 84-year-old otherwise healthy Hispanic man, Cándido Aguado, who is in for an annual physical. He immediately hands you a meticulously written list of medical questions. He shakes his head as he explains his friend had a fourth skin cancer removed. The patient has two changing spots (Plates 2 and 3) and a request for a general skin check. Because your clinic is running a little behind, you have only 20 minutes to do his usual health care maintenance and also answer his questions.

1. **What strategies can you use to balance the needs of addressing health care maintenance during his visit while also efficiently examining Mr. Aguado's skin?**

2. **If you had to succinctly communicate the skin findings to a dermatologist to ask for help, how would you describe what you see?** ◨

DERMATOLOGIC EXAMINATION: CHALLENGES AND PRACTICAL APPROACHES

Health care reforms might lead to even greater pressure on primary providers to manage skin problems, thus making skin examination a common and important part of primary care. More than one third of patients presenting to primary care providers often have at least one skin complaint.[1] Ironically, a recent study showed that the

---

Additional online-only material indicated by icon.

elderly, ethnic minorities, and patients with lower education tend to underestimate their risk of skin cancer. Because skin cancers are the most common malignancy,[2] the primary care provider can make a significant impact in filling patient education and skin cancer screening. Recent data strongly suggest total body skin cancer screening might decrease melanoma mortality.[3] One study showed cost effectiveness of skin cancer screening at least once in individuals over 50 years of age.[4]

Many challenges exist in the dermatology examination for the nondermatologist. First, many of us had very limited exposures during medical school or residency training.[5] This barrier creates difficulty in approaching the skin from a systematic approach in and recognizing dermatologic conditions.[6] Second, many primary care providers have time constraints and medically complex patients with a multitude of nondermatologic comorbidities.[7] Third, there might be access limitations to dermatologic specialists, depending on geographic practice and patient demographic.

Triaging patients with skin problems and communicating the urgency to the specialist can seem daunting. The purpose of this section is to facilitate the dermatologic examination and to address these barriers. Proposed approaches to general skin cancer screening will be outlined first, followed by heuristics for describing skin findings. The remainder of the chapter will focus on common dermatologic problems in primary care of geriatrics rather than providing an exhaustive litany of diagnoses. The primary care provider will be empowered to describe lesions and rashes to a dermatologist or to use clinical decision making tools (see Web Resources section) to facilitate referral, when needed.

Total Body Skin Examination

> The total body skin examination (TBSE) is important for identifying premalignant and malignant skin disorders as part of the routine complete physical, but also should be considered for new rashes or to look for cutaneous clues of underlying systemic diseases.

The total body skin examination (TBSE) is important for identifying premalignant and malignant skin disorders as part of the routine complete physical, but also should be considered for new rashes or to look for cutaneous clues of underlying systemic diseases.[8] It should be especially encouraged in patients with a personal history of skin cancers or precancers, history of transplantation or immunosuppressant use, chronic anti–tumor necrosis factor use, exposure to known cutaneous carcinogens (e.g., tanning, arsenic), multiple moles (more than a dozen), or family history of skin cancer.[9,10] Although fair-skinned patients are known to be at highest risk for skin cancer, a recent study highlighted

the increasing incidence of melanoma among Hispanics and suggested a potential practice gap in preventive education and screening for minority ethnic groups.[11]

Several practical considerations can improve the efficiency and thoroughness of TBSE. During the routine primary care exam that includes palpation and auscultation, the overlying skin can be visually inspected. The patient should ideally disrobe and all accessories (e.g., watches, glasses, hearing aids, toupees, bracelets) that might obscure skin findings should be removed and all makeup should be removed.[8,12] The mucous membranes, anogenital regions, interdigital spaces of fingers and toes, scalp and hair, nails, and posterior auricular neck should be inspected. Adequate lighting is required to visualize the skin, especially for subtle lesions or areas that cast shadows. Natural sunlight is ideal, otherwise bright lamps can be used with the patient positioned underneath.[8] A portable light such as penlight or otoscope held in front of or tangentially to lesions can be helpful to detect subtle changes such as wrinkling, fluid within lesions, and sometimes lesion margins.[8]

The ABCDE (*A*symmetry, irregular *B*order, *C*olor variation, *D*iameter over 6 mm, *E*volving characteristic over months) rule is a simple and popular screening method for melanoma (Plate 1).[13,14] However, by itself, there are limitations in missing the rare amelanotic variant of melanoma or misdiagnosing seborrheic keratosis (Plate 3) as melanoma.[10] For routine skin cancer screening, especially in patients with many skin lesions, a practical, rapid, gestalt approach is the "ugly duckling" detection method.[15] A lesion that does not resemble the overall color, shape, texture of other pigmented lesions is considered suspect. Dermoscopy (using a special magnifying lens with polarized light) can be a helpful extension of the unaided eye, but is operator dependent and requires training.[16] Several promising and noninvasive tools might facilitate the skin examination in the future, including a Food and Drug Administration (FDA)–approved spectroscopic device (MelaFind) and emerging confocal microscopy technology.[17] Practical considerations of cost and technologic limitations are current barriers to routine implementation of such equipment.

Four-Point Dermatologic Description

> In patients with a specific lesion or rash complaint, the most succinct approach is a systematic four-point method that describes (1) anatomic distribution, (2) lesion configuration, (3) primary lesion and color, and (4) secondary change, if present.

In patients with a specific lesion or rash complaint, the most succinct approach is a systematic four-point method that describes (1) anatomic distribution, (2) lesion configuration, (3) primary lesion and color, and

(4) secondary change, if present.[8] History is occasionally helpful, but these four descriptors are quintessential for efficiently framing the skin examination to use a dermatologic atlas or algorithm to narrow the differential diagnosis. No singular component of this four-point system is necessarily weighted more than the others. Several sophisticated Internet and handheld device clinical decision making aids are also available.[18] In cases requiring dermatologic referral, skin findings can be efficiently communicated via these tools.

Anatomic location of the dermatologic finding, and sometimes the areas that are relatively spared, can provide rapid clues for the pathogenesis of a rash. Configuration (Table 54-1) refers to how the lesion or rash is patterned. The primary lesion (Table 54-2) refers to an intact, unmanipulated representation of the process and includes description of color. Sometimes it can be difficult to identify a primary lesion if the patient has already self-medicated or excoriated their lesions; or if the lesion is short-lived (e.g., urticaria) or friable. Generally, if there is not an intact primary lesion, biopsy tends to be of low diagnostic value. Lastly, secondary change (Table 54-3) refers to the findings caused either by the evolution of a primary lesion or an external factor modifying the lesion.

CASE 1

Cándido Aguado (Part 2)

You successfully incorporate a general skin examination of Mr. Aguado while you do your usual health care maintenance examination, which is otherwise unremarkable. Plate 3 is a brown, stuck-on, waxy plaque that he admits to picking. You reassure the patient it is an irritated seborrheic keratosis. The lesion in Plate 2 concerns you, and the patient relays change over a few months following trauma. It is tender and frequently bleeds. You call a dermatologist: "On the left thumb is a solitary red, bleeding, tender nodule that is eroded, rapidly growing, and painful." ■

TABLE 54-1	Examples of Configurations	
	Description	**Example**
Annular	Ringlike	Tinea corporis (ringworm), granuloma annulare (Plate 4), porokeratosis (Plate 5)
Dermatomal (zosteriform)	Confined to a dermatome and abruptly stops at midline	Herpes zoster (Plate 6)
Grouped (herpetiform)	Clustered lesions	Herpes simplex (Plate 7)
Linear	Lesions arranged in a line, suggestive of an external cause	Contact dermatitis (Plate 8), scabies burrows
Reticular (retiform)	Netlike or meshlike, suggesting a process affecting the cutaneous vascular network	Livedo reticularis (Plate 9), erythema ab igne (red-brown patch in area of heating pad use)

Data from Bolognia J, Jorizzo JL, Rapini RP. Dermatology. 2nd ed. St. Louis, Mo.: Mosby/Elsevier; 2008.

TABLE 54-2	Examples of Primary Lesions	
	Description	**Example**
Macule or patch	Flat without induration or significant elevation	Idiopathic guttate hypomelanosis (Plate 10), lentigo
Nodule/tumor	Deep-seated, indurated lesion, often fixed	Squamous cell carcinoma, basal cell carcinoma (Plate 11)
Papule or plaque	Elevated lesion confined to upper dermis or epidermis	Nevus (mole), seborrheic keratosis (Plate 3), lichen planus (Plate 12), eczema (Plate 13), psoriasis, cutaneous T-cell lymphoma (Plate 14)
Purpura or petechiae or ecchymosis	Nonblanching dark red-purple lesion, suggesting extravasated erythrocytes in skin (in contrast, "violaceous" means color partially blanches)	Vasculitis (inflammation and destruction of vascular walls), Bateman's (solar) purpura from chronic sun damage, hypercoaguable state (Plate 9)
Pustules	Yellow, pus-filled	Folliculitis, rosacea (Plate 15)
Telangiectasia	Prominent blood vessel, blanches easily	Spider telangiectasia, rosacea (Plate 15), basal cell carcinoma (Plate 11)
Vesicle/bulla	Blister filled with nonpurulent material (e.g., serum, blood). If deeply seated in dermis, it is a cyst (e.g., sebaceous cyst).	Bullous pemphigoid (Plate 16), bullous tinea pedis, acute allergic contact dermatitis (Plate 8), insect bite, herpes (Plate 7)
Wheal/urticaria	Pink-white, blanchable, edematous hives	Hives, serum sickness (Plate 17)

Data from Bolognia J, Jorizzo JL, Rapini RP. Dermatology. 2nd ed. St. Louis, Mo.: Mosby/Elsevier; 2008.

TABLE 54-3	Examples of Secondary Changes	
	Description	**Example**
Atrophy	Thinning of skin. When epidermis is involved, fine wrinkling, transparency of skin, stretch marks, or visualization of underlying dermal vessels might be present. When dermis or fat is involved, there is often skin depression.	Lichen sclerosus, steroid-induced atrophy (Plate 18)
Crust	Dried blood, pus, or serum	Impetigo (Plate 19), scab (Plate 20)
Erosion or avulsion	Partial thickness epidermal loss. In contrast, ulceration means full thickness loss of epidermis with exposure of at least dermis.	Excoriated skin (Plate 6)
Necrosis	Dead cutaneous tissue	Eschar (Plate 21), wet gangrene
Scale	Desiccated, flaky keratinocytes	Psoriasis, eczema, porokeratosis (Plate 5)

Data from Bolognia J, Jorizzo JL, Rapini RP. Dermatology. 2nd ed. St. Louis, Mo.: Mosby/Elsevier; 2008.

ECZEMATOUS DERMATOSES

Eczema (dermatitis) is a common clinical sign that refers to a group of conditions that share histologic features but have differing etiologies and clinical appearances. *Dermatitis* is a misnomer, because the inflammation and edema (spongiosis) is at the level of the epidermis, not the dermis. In the acute phase it is often confused as being infected because of the oozing papulovesicles (Plate 8) or pustular appearance on acral surfaces. Chronic eczema appears as dry, scaly patches (Plate 22) or sometimes lichenified plaques with cracks.[9]

> Stasis dermatitis, caused by underlying venous insufficiency, is commonplace in older patients from acquired venous incompetence, saphenous vein grafting, or prior thromboembolism. The patient is often misdiagnosed as having bilateral leg cellulitis and has partial or no response to antibiotic therapy, which leads to unnecessary cost, hospitalization, and interventions.

Several etiologies can lead to the final common pathway of eczema.[9] Stasis dermatitis, caused by underlying venous insufficiency, is commonplace in older patients from acquired venous incompetence, saphenous vein grafting, or prior thromboembolism. The patient is often misdiagnosed as having bilateral leg cellulitis and has partial or no response to antibiotic therapy, which leads to unnecessary cost, hospitalization, and interventions (Plate 22).[19] Nummular (discoid) eczema is an idiopathic variant of solitary or multiple coin-shaped plaques, typically on the extremities (Plate 13). It is often mistaken for "refractory" tinea corporis, though a skin scraping mounted in potassium hydroxide (KOH) can easily differentiate the two.[9]

Contact dermatitis is another common cause of eczema. It is typically well-demarcated and geometrically or linearly configured (Plate 8). It can be caused by a nonimmunologic response to a chemical irritant, such as soap residue.[20] Allergic sensitization (i.e., type IV delayed hypersensitivity with cell-mediated immune reaction), which is exemplified by poison ivy or nickel allergy, is probably as common in older patients as irritant dermatitis.[20,21] Ask about all personal products and topical medicaments, because geriatric patients and those with stasis dermatitis who are self-medicating have a high prevalence of allergic contact dermatitis, particularly to neomycin and fragrance mixes.[20,22] Periocular and eyelid dermatitis can result from eyedrops or from nail cosmetic products.[23] Airborne allergens (e.g., pollens) can mimic photodistributed rashes on exposed areas.

Autoeczematization ("Id" reaction, autosensitization) is a symmetric eruption of eczematous papules that occurs distant to the primary sites of chronic skin inflammation. The classic example is chronic tinea pedis with symmetrically distributed eczematous papules on the upper extremities or torso.[9] It can also be seen with severe contact or stasis dermatitis.[24] The presumed pathophysiology is lymphocytes at the site of chronic inflammation circulate into the periphery and deposit at other anatomic sites.[25]

The differential diagnosis of eczema includes cutaneous T-cell lymphoma, scabies, syphilis, squamous cell carcinoma in situ (Bowen's disease), drug eruptions, mammary or extramammary Paget's disease, and dermatophytosis (tinea corporis).[20] Consider skin biopsy or skin scraping if lesions are not responding or worsening with topical corticosteroids.

Treatment regimens generally include dry skin care instructions (Box 54-1), brief courses of topical corticosteroids (Level of Evidence D) or calcineurin inhibitors (e.g., tacrolimus or pimecrolimus) (Level of Evidence D) for symptomatic relief.[9] Tips for how to choose the steroid molecule potency, vehicle, and dispensed quantity are described in Boxes 54-2 and 54-3. When dermatitis

---

BOX 54-1

DRY SKIN CARE RECOMMENDATIONS (LEVEL OF EVIDENCE = D)

Avoid bar soaps (unless sensitive-skin product), bubble baths, fragranced products. Note: Unscented products often contain neutralizing fragrances, which can cause contact dermatitis. Minimize exposure to chemical irritants, especially by using with thin cotton gloves.
Apply cream or ointment emollients before skin dries (within 3 minutes).

Avoid abrasive scrubbing.
Avoid long-duration baths and hot water.
Focus cleansing areas that are hair-bearing or visibly soiled rather than lathering the entire body indiscriminately and bathing unnecessarily frequently.
Consider a humidifier (adjust to about 50% humidity) in dry climates.

Data from Bolognia J, Jorizzo JL, Rapini RP. Dermatology. 2nd ed. St. Louis, Mo.: Mosby/Elsevier; 2008; and White-Chu EF, Reddy M. Dry skin in the elderly: Complexities of a common problem. Clin Dermatol 2011;29(1):37-42.

BOX 54-2

PEARLS FOR CHOOSING POTENCY OR VEHICLE OF TOPICAL ANTIINFLAMMATORY MEDICATIONS

Characteristic	Comments
Anatomic site[29]	Acral sites absorb medications the least and can withstand a mid- to high-potency steroid molecule.* Facial and intertriginous areas absorb the most medicine and require a weaker steroid molecule.* Hair-bearing skin is more difficult to apply ointments and creams (gels, lotion, shampoo, oil, or foam are more ideal).
Patient preference[9]	Patient adherence often dictates vehicle (e.g., avoid ointment if patient is unwilling to apply something that feels greasy).
Rash attributes[9]	Thickened, scaly skin difficult to penetrate and requires a high-potency steroid molecule. Inflamed or eroded skin benefits from moistened dressings or wraps to help penetration.
Vehicle attribute[9]	Alcohol-based (e.g., solution), especially on open or inflamed skin, tends to be irritating. Ointment is often but not always more potent compared to other vehicles. Propylene glycol, which is found in many topical medicaments, can sometimes cause an irritant contact dermatitis.

*High-potency steroids include clobetasol 0.05%, betamethasone diproprionate 0.05%; midpotency steroids include triamcinolone 0.1%, betamethasone valerate 0.1%, fluocinolone propionate 0.05%; and low-potency steroids include hydrocortisone butyrate 0.1% and desonide 0.05%.[9]

---

is severe and widespread, systemic steroids (0.5-1 mg/kg per day for 3 to 4 weeks) can be considered (Level of Evidence D).[9] A protracted course is required to prevent rebound flares of contact dermatitis. Allergic or irritant contactants should be avoided completely. Dietary restrictions (except in cases of test-proven allergens or additives) and water softeners are of uncertain value[9,26,27].

BOX 54-3

PEARLS ON QUANTITY OF TOPICAL MEDICATION

Body Site	Fingertip Units*	Grams Required for Twice Daily Application over 2 Weeks
Entire hand	1	14
One foot	2	28
Neck and face	2.5	35
One arm	3	42
One leg	6	84
Torso (only anterior or posterior)	7	98

Data from Bolognia J, Jorizzo JL, Rapini RP. Dermatology. 2nd ed. St. Louis, Mo.: Mosby/Elsevier; 2008; and Long CC, Finlay AY. The finger-tip unit—a new practical measure. Clin Exp Dermatol 1991;16(6):444-7.

*Based on the assumption that approximately 0.1-mm layer of medication should be applied, one fingertip unit is a strip of medication dispensed to cover the volar index finger between the distal interphalangeal joint to the fingertip.

BENIGN CUTANEOUS PROCESSES

Recognizing common benign conditions can minimize unnecessary referrals and provide patient reassurance.

Seborrheic keratoses (SKs) are ubiquitous, benign epidermal hyperplasia (Plate 3). Mutations in fibroblast growth factor receptor 3 (FGFR3) might be involved.[31] A distinctive variant consisting of smaller papules that are reminiscent of flat warts on the bilateral cheeks of ethnic skin is known as dermatosis papulosa nigra. The sign of Lesar-Trelat, or eruptive appearance of multiple SKs as a paraneoplastic phenomenon, is a rare and controversial entity.[32] Three case-controlled studies[33-35] suggest most eruptive SKs are not associated with underlying malignancy and probably do not justify expensive, invasive testing in the absence of other concerning review of systems. SKs can become symptomatic when they become irritated such as catching on clothing, though sometimes they spontaneously become inflamed. Anecdotally, many patients report the lesions disappearing (probably excoriated or coincidentally traumatized) but only to return. The differential diagnosis can sometimes include melanoma, verruca, or lentigines (sun spots).[9] There are unfortunately no preventive measures. Reassurance is all that is generally required.

Sebaceous hyperplasias (Plate 23) are benign overgrowths of normal sebaceous oil glands that are usually found on the face. They can be seen commonly on the vermilion lips and buccal mucosa (Fordyce spots), eyelids (meibomian glands), areola (Montgomery tubercles), and glans penis or clitoris (Tyson's glands). There is a yellow to flesh-colored appearance and often associated central umbilication. The condition is usually idiopathic, though cyclosporine has been reported to cause diffuse lesions.[36] The major differentials include nonmelanoma skin cancer, fibrous papules, xanthomas, sebaceous adenoma or carcinoma, syringoma, and milia. Treatment is usually not required, but cosmetic removal options can include electrodesiccation, or topical or systemic retinoids (Level of Evidence C).[36,37]

Dermatofibromas (benign fibrohistiocytomas) often appear on the lower extremities (or sometimes on the torso or upper extremities) as pink-brown dome-shaped firm papules. There will often be a characteristic dimple sign when squeezed (Plate 24). The lesions are usually asymptomatic, though sometimes can be pruritic or painful. They are thought to be caused by trauma, because the histologic appearance is similar to scar. The primary differential includes irritated nevus (when more brown in color or raised), melanoma, or dermatofibromosarcoma protuberans. When symptomatic, they can be excised or treated with intralesional triamcinolone acetate or topical ultrapotent steroids (Level of Evidence D). Recurrences can occur, because the process can often spread laterally and into the deep dermis.

PRECANCEROUS AND MALIGNANT CUTANEOUS DISEASES

Actinic Keratosis (AK)

Actinic keratoses (AKs) are precancerous lesions that are thought to be in the middle of the spectrum with photo-aged skin at one pole and squamous cell carcinoma at the other extreme.[38] AKs are defined as partial thickness keratinocyte atypia. Prevalence is at least one in four adult individuals.[39] The dogma had been that the risk of progression of AK to squamous cell carcinoma (SCC) was 0.025% to 16% per year,[40] but several experts suggest that AKs are more of a general marker of sun damage and gestalt skin cancer risk rather than individual lesions that are destined to transform into cancers.[38,41] It is known that tumor suppression genes and DNA repair are dysfunctional in these cells.[42-44] Clinically, AKs are usually pink- to brown-colored papules or patches with rough scale on exposed areas (Plate 25). For small lesions, the tactile presence of rough scale is sometimes easier to detect than relying only on visual appearance.[9]

Several variants based on clinical appearance or anatomic location have been described.[9] Pigmented AKs can sometimes resemble small scaly seborrheic keratoses. Solar cheilosis (previously known as actinic cheilitis) is clinically characterized as grayish white rough patches on sun-exposed portions of the vermilion lip.[45]

Hypertrophic AK can be difficult to differentiate from SCC or verruca. Certain high-risk features that favor SCC over AK have been proposed, including "IDRBEU: inflammation or induration, diameter over 1 cm, rapidly enlarging, bleeding, erythema, ulceration."[46] Sometimes AK can be partially treated and recur, but consider biopsy when the same lesion has been treated more than once or twice (Level of Evidence D).[41]

> Field therapy to eradicate actinic keratoses is increasingly recommended. Current trends are moving toward combination therapy (e.g., cryotherapy with topical field therapy).

A plethora of treatment options exist, though no long-term outcome studies have proven treating AKs truly decreases SCC incidence.[38] Treatment is traditionally with cryotherapy (Level of Evidence D) when lesions are discrete and few.[41] (Destructive procedures are the standard of care for treatment of actinic keratoses). However, cryotherapy directed at individual lesions does not address the surrounding sun-damaged areas where subclinical precancerous lesions likely exist.[6] Some advocate that thin AKs need be treated with only consistent sun protection, since 25% of lesions may spontaneously regress.[38,47-49] Field therapy to eradicate subclinical photodamaged skin is increasingly recommended with treatments such as photodynamic or "blue light" therapy with topical amino-levulinic acid (Level of Evidence A), topical 5-fluorouracil (Level of Evidence B), topical imiquimod (Level of Evidence A), short courses of topical ingenol mebutate (Level of Evidence A), topical diclofenac (Level of Evidence A), chemical peels (Level of Evidence C), or laser (Level of Evidence B).[38] Tretinoin monotherapy is generally not recommended (Level of Evidence X), because a recent randomized controlled trial failed to show chemopreventive effect and was associated with an inexplicably increased risk of all-cause mortality.[30,30a] Current trends are moving toward combination therapy (e.g., cryotherapy with topical field therapy; Level of Evidence B).[38] Unfortunately, few cost-effectiveness data exist[50]. Regardless of treatment modality, patients should be periodically screened for skin cancers (Level of Evidence D).[38]

Cutaneous Malignancies

> Skin cancers are prevalent in the geriatric population, and the incidence has been on the rise. Primary care providers have continuity of care of their patients and are uniquely positioned to identify suspicious lesions that the patient might not even notice.

Skin cancers are prevalent in the geriatric population, and the incidence has been on the rise.[2,56] Primary care providers have continuity of care of their patients and are uniquely positioned to identify suspicious lesions that the patient might not even notice.[57] This section will overview the more common skin cancers in geriatric patients to empower the primary care provider to recognize and triage appropriately.

Squamous Cell Carcinoma (SCC)

Cutaneous SCC is full epidermal thickness atypia and often subcategorized as in situ (Bowen's disease) or invasive (infiltration into or below the dermis). Major risk factors include sun exposure, fair skin, radiation (especially for patients who received treatments for acne in the midtwentieth century), and immunosuppression (particularly cardiac transplant patients).[9] Occasionally, patients with chronic ulcers or inflammation can develop SCC (Marjolin's ulcer).[9] Recent data suggest associations with long-term voriconazole in transplant patients, vemurafenib, and perhaps tumor necrosis factor antagonists.[58-61] Damaged DNA repair and tumor suppression pathways seem to be the underlying pathophysiology, and certain human papillomavirus (HPV) strains have been implicated in some cases.[42,43,44] The clinical appearance is usually an indurated, pink-red, scaly plaque or tumor (Plate 26).

According to the updated 2012 American Joint Commission on Cancer guidelines, staging depends on the histologic features, depth, anatomic site, host immune status, and presence of neuroinvasion.[62] Of note, the suggestion of complete excisional biopsy and histologic staging to the level of detail reminiscent of melanoma has not been widely accepted and implemented yet. Lesions in the H-zone of the face (ears, temples, jawline, nose), immunosuppressed patients, perineural invasion, and tumor size larger than 2 cm are considered at high risk for recurrence or poorer prognosis.[63] Current guidelines are equivocal about routine sentinel node biopsy, although some data suggest it might play a role.[64,65]

Differential diagnosis of SCC can include hypertrophic actinic keratosis, nummular eczema (Plate 13) or superficial basal cell carcinoma (simulates squamous cell carcinoma in situ), and chondrodermatitis nodularis helicis when present on the ear (Plate 27). One special case worth mentioning is keratoacanthoma. This entity is classically known as a firm nodule with central hyperkeratotic plug that was previously considered a self-resolving, benign lesion that did not require treatment (Plate 28). Some pathologists characterize these as a form of well-differentiated SCC that should be treated as such, although others believe this entity to generally be a benign, self-limited process.[66-68] It is the author's opinion that in cases of patients being reasonable surgical candidates, especially in those with high-risk features, surgery should be discussed as an option with the patient.

Treatment options for SCC depend on anatomic site, histologic features, and patient preference. Expert consensus guidelines (Level of Evidence D) have recommended electrodesiccation and curettage for non–hair-bearing, low-risk tumors that do not extend too deeply into the dermis in noncosmetically sensitive areas. Excision with histologic confirmation of at least 4 mm negative margins is probably adequate for most cases (Level of Evidence C).[69] Mohs micrographic surgery (Box 54-4) should be considered for high-risk tumors, those with poorly demarcated clinical edges, recurrent lesions, and those involving critical anatomic sites to spare normal tissue (Level of Evidence D).[9]

Second-line nonsurgical therapy, which should be discussed by the dermatologist, includes aggressive cryotherapy (Level of Evidence C), or topical imiquimod (SCC in situ; Level of Evidence C) or topical 5-fluorouracil (Level of Evidence C).[70-72] For advanced or inoperable cutaneous SCC, co-manage with an oncologist to discuss radiation therapy or systemic chemotherapeutics.[9,73,74] Once a patient has been diagnosed with squamous cell carcinoma, it is generally recommended that patients with nonmelanoma skin cancers should have examinations every 6 months, because the majority of recurrences, if they occur, are within the first few years (Level of Evidence D).[75]

Basal Cell Carcinoma

Basal cell carcinoma (BCC) (Plate 11) is a malignant growth of the basal layer keratinocytes and the most common human skin cancer.[76] The major risk factors include sun exposure and fair-colored skin.[76] The tumor is generally slow growing and often has excellent prognosis with appropriate treatment.[77] BCC rarely metastasizes, although it can be locally invasive, painful, and disfiguring.[76] The pathophysiology of most BCCs is related to tumor suppression mutations in either p53 or PTCH-SHH pathways.[78] The differential includes scar (morpheic BCC variant), melanoma (pigmented BCC variant), fibrous papule, eczema (superficial BCC), or nonhealing ulcer (rodent ulcer BCC). Sometimes it can be confused with rosacea because of the telangiectasias overlying papules.

As with SCC, treatment of BCC depends on factors such as histologic features, size, depth, anatomic site, and patient immune status. Therapeutic approaches are similar to that outlined for SCC, with the notable

---

BOX 54-4

MOHS MICROGRAPHIC SURGERY

Mohs surgery, named after Dr. Frederick Mohs, is an in-office surgical method that removes tumors with a low recurrence rate while sparing normal tissue.[86] The surgeon removes disks of tissue, prepares frozen histologic sections using a special technique to allow complete margin examination, and repeats the process until the tumor is completely removed. Wound closure is obtained through many techniques including, but not limited to, secondary intent, intermediate closure, skin flap, or graft. The American Academy of Dermatology has released the Appropriate Use Criteria for Mohs Micrographic Surgery (see Web Resources section).

exception that BCC is generally less aggressive. The standard of care is generally considered to be surgical with either simple excision or Mohs micrographic surgery (Level of Evidence B) (Box 54-4). For nonsurgical candidates, especially for superficial or nodular (not micronodular) histology at low-risk and cosmetically insensitive areas, second-line therapies can be considered: electrodesiccation and curettage (Level of Evidence D)[79]; aggressive cryotherapy with or without curettage (Level of Evidence B)[76]; topical imiquimod 5% qHS five times per week for 6 weeks (Level of Evidence A; FDA-approved for superficial BCC); photodynamic therapy (Level of Evidence B); vismodegib (FDA-approved SHH inhibitor) (Level of Evidence B) or intralesional chemotherapeutics (Level of Evidence C).[80-83] Radiation therapy can also be used (Level of Evidence C).[84] Follow-up is generally at least annually for the first 5 years, when recurrences, if any, tend to occur (Level of Evidence D).[85]

Melanoma

Melanoma (Plate 1) is a dreaded melanocytic cancer that can affect the skin or, less commonly, the retina. Several risk factors exist, including genetics, skin and eye color (fair skin, blue eyes, red or blond hair), and total number of atypical-appearing nevi.[9] The incidence of melanoma has unfortunately been increasing in the United States over the past few decades and is suspected to be related to tanning practices.[87] Diagnosis is discussed under the Total Body Skin Examination section of this chapter. The differential diagnosis of melanoma includes atypical nevus, seborrheic keratosis, pigmented BCC, and sometimes very dark cherry angiomas.

Staging and treatment are beyond the scope of this text. Prognosis depends on several factors—including advanced age, male gender, tumor site, Breslow depth (which has supplanted Clark's level), ulceration, and presence of nodal or distant metastasis. Previous subtypes such as nodular, superficial spreading, etc., are not directly pertinent to staging.[9,88] Close clinical follow-up of the patient and first-degree relatives is recommended (Level of Evidence D). Ideally an interspecialty approach to care is used, which might include dermatologists, radiation oncologists (where appropriate), oncologists (for advanced disease), Mohs surgeons (where appropriate), and surgical oncologists (Level of Evidence D). Patients can be enrolled in trials when appropriate, receive guidance about advantages or disadvantages of sentinel node biopsy, discuss the role of adjuvant therapy in advanced-stage disease, and become educated about other controversial topics within melanoma.

Cutaneous T-Cell Lymphoma (CTCL)

Cutaneous T-cell lymphomas (CTCLs) are rare but important entities to recognize because they can clinically and sometimes histologically masquerade as eczema.[9] Abnormal T-cell clones, often CD4-positive with loss of other T-cell surface markers, proliferate within the epidermis and sometimes also affect the dermis in later stages.[9] The most common type, mycosis fungoides (MF; not caused by fungus) favors so-called "doubly covered" areas of the body that are not sun-exposed (Plate 14). Early stages present as scaly pink-red plaques or patches.[89] At more advanced stages, there can be nodules; or lymphadenopathy, erythroderma (near total body surface redness), and abnormal T-cell clones in the peripheral circulation known as Sezary syndrome.[9] Prognosis and treatment depends on histologic features and staging and are beyond the scope of this text. Of note, patients with MF have been shown in multiple epidemiologic studies to be at increased risk for second malignancies, including noncutaneous lymphomas, non-MF skin cancers, and solid organ tumors.[90] The time to second malignancy can range from months to years. Thus, the primary care provider must remain vigilant in eliciting a thorough review of systems, checking for adenopathy, and ensuring patients are current on age-appropriate cancer screening (Level of Evidence D).[90]

CASE 2

Sally Maloney (Part 1)

Sally Maloney, a 72-year-old frail female, visits your clinic with an approximately 6-month history of progressively worsening pruritus that is "head to toe." She denies any new personal products or medications before this all began. She has tried using a menthol-containing over-the-counter itch lotion, but it has not helped. Upon examination, Ms. Maloney's skin is somewhat dry and scaly and there are many linearly configured erosions and hemorrhagic crusts but not intact primary lesions.

1. **What other focused pertinent history and examination will help you understand possible causes of Ms. Maloney's pruritus?**

2. **What features of pruritus might warrant further investigation?** ▣

PRURITUS

> Pruritus is often caused by dry skin or nummular eczema in older patients. However, the clinician should be astutely aware of other etiologies of intractable itch, including occult malignancy or serious metabolic derangement.

Pruritus, or itch, is a common problem of older patients and is oftentimes multifactorial.[91] The most common causes in older patients include xerosis (dry skin) and medications. Subacute to chronic, generalized pruritus that awakens the patient should alert the practitioner to search for secondary causes (especially lymphoma or hematologic conditions);[9,92] the condition warrants a thorough history and focused workup (Table 54-4).

TABLE 54-4	Causes of Pruritus in Older Patients and Possible Treatment Options
Causative Factor	**Comments and Suggested Management Approach**
Chronic kidney disease	• Check renal function • Does not always respond to dialysis and can be challenging to treat • Naltrexone 50 mg/day (Level of Evidence B; mixed results) • Thalidomide 100 mg/day (Level of Evidence B) • Gabapentin 200-300 mg after dialysis (Level of Evidence B) • Transplantation is generally considered to be the more successful treatment (Level of Evidence D)
Dermatitis (e.g., nummular eczema, stasis dermatitis, contact dermatitis from an allergen or irritant)	• Avoid sensitizing agents (e.g., Balsam of Peru, lanolin, vitamin E, topical antibiotics) • Compression garments • Topical corticosteroids • Consider skin patch testing
Dry skin (xerosis)	• See Dry Skin Care Recommendations in Box 54-1 • Senescent changes in epidermal lipid production and sebocyte and eccrine sweat gland function[28]
Endocrine derangements (e.g., hypercalcemia, hypothyroidism, nutritional deficiency)	• Thyroid studies • Electrolyte panels • Nutritional studies
Folliculitis	• Scraping of pustule to look for yeast (potassium hydroxide mounting) and/or bacterial culture • Counsel patient about frequency of relapses • Treat underlying cause
Immunoblistering conditions (e.g., bullous pemphigoid [Plate 16], dermatitis herpetiformis)	• Requires high index of suspicion, because pruritus may present before blisters • Dermatologic referral for immunofluorescence studies of skin and possibly serum • Systemic immunosuppression or topical steroids, when appropriate
Infestation or infection (e.g., bed bugs, scabies, tinea corporis, parasites)	• Skin scraping or other parasite screening tests • Treat underlying cause • Treat close contacts, when appropriate (e.g., scabies)
Medications (e.g., statins, calcium channel blockers, angiotensin-converting enzyme inhibitors, opioids)	• Discontinue offending agent • Allow for 1-2 month drug holiday before judging improvement • Do not exclude the possibility that a chronically prescribed antihypertensive medication might be the cause of unexplained widespread pruritus with eczematous changes. • Joly P et al. Chronic eczematous eruptions of the elderly are associated with chronic exposure to calcium channel blockers: results from a case-control study. Journal of Investigative Dermatology (2007) 127, 2766–2771.[28a]
Metabolic derangements (e.g., hepatic failure, anemia)	• Complete blood count with differential • Iron studies • Hepatic panel • Correcting underlying cause • Note: Cholestatic itch can be refractory to treatments
Neuropathy (e.g., diabetic)	• Treat underlying condition • Notalgia paresthetica is an idiopathic form of pruritus that manifests as chronically rubbed, thickened, brown skin near the shoulderblades • Consider symptomatic treatment with judicious prescription of psychoactive medications (e.g., selective serotonin reuptake inhibitor, selective serotonin-norepinephrine reuptake inhibitor, tricyclic antidepressant) or antiepileptic agent
Paraneoplastic (especially lymphoma, leukemia, myeloma)	• History, physical exam, review of systems to identify possible source • Unexplained pruritus has been described to precede lymphoma by several years • Lactate dehydrogenase (LDH) • Erythrocyte sedimentation rate (ESR) • Imaging, as appropriate • Cancer screening tests, as appropriate
Psychogenic (diagnosis of exclusion)	• Referral for cognitive-behavioral techniques or medication, when appropriate

Data from Bolognia J, Jorizzo JL, Rapini RP. Dermatology. 2nd ed. St. Louis, Mo.: Mosby/Elsevier; 2008; and Patel T, Yosipovitch G. The management of chronic pruritus in the elderly. Skin Therapy Letter 2010;15(8):5-9.

If no underlying treatable cause of pruritus is found, symptomatic treatment can be challenging and must be individualized to the patient and is largely anecdotal. Of note, antihistamines are generally not helpful for pruritus, unless urticaria or dermatographism is present (Level of Evidence D).[92] Mirtazapine up to 15 mg by mouth at night (Level of Evidence C) can help mitigate pruritus along with providing a sedating effect to provide additional relief.[92] It is the author's opinion that it should be started at 7.5 mg in older adults and gradually uptitrated to effect. Topical 5% doxepin cream has been reported to have systemic side effects and unfortunately frequently causes contact dermatitis.[9] Topical steroids are generally not recommended for widespread or continuous and long-term use because of side effects (Level of Evidence D).[92] In select severe and intractable cases, phototherapy, antiepileptics, antidepressants, or opioid receptor modulators might be helpful (Level of Evidence C).[92] The side effects of oral medications must be weighed and discussed with the patient, and the patient should be counseled not to discontinue many of these medications abruptly (e.g., gabapentin, opioid receptor modulators) because of withdrawal potential.[92]

CASE 2

Sally Maloney (Part 2)

You gather additional history, and Ms. Maloney has been feeling somewhat fatigued recently and has noticed cold intolerance. Her thyroid-stimulating hormone (TSH) is markedly elevated and you diagnose her as having hypothyroidism. You know thyroid replacement should be started at a low dose and slowly titrated; thus general dry skin recommendations and topical emollients are also recommended. ◘

COMMON INFLAMMATORY CONDITIONS OF AGING

Grover's Disease (Transient Acantholytic Dermatosis)

Grover's disease has been classically described as a recrudescent, pruritic, pink-brown, papulovesicular eruption on the torso of middle-aged to older men (Plate 29). The traditional teaching is that warmth or sweat exacerbates the condition, although the reality is it can occur in females or during cold, dry conditions.[94] Grover's disease is an idiopathic condition, but those afflicted with cancer, febrile illness, or prolonged bed rest seem to be particularly predisposed.[94] The differential can include folliculitis, seborrheic dermatitis of the chest, or Darier's disease. Usually the diagnosis is made clinically, and patients are advised to avoid excessive heat or sweating (Level of Evidence D).[94] Anecdotal data (Level of Evidence D)

support multiple treatment options, which include the following: moderate potency topical steroids, systemic prednisolone (25 mg daily courses tapered over 2 weeks), oral tetracyclines, oral antifungals, isotretinoin, acitretin, phototherapy (either narrowband ultraviolet B [UVB] or psoralen with UVA [PUVA]), acitretin, topical calcipotriol, topical menthol, topical pramoxine, and methotrexate.[94-96] It is the author's opinion that topical menthol-containing lotions are the safest first-line therapy, but a topical steroid can be tried as rescue therapy.

Seborrheic Dermatitis (Dandruff, Cradle Cap, Seborrhea)

Seborrheic dermatitis is relapsing, pruritic, greasy, scaly, poorly demarcated patches (Plate 30). It is frequently found on the scalp, eyebrows, forehead, nasolabial folds, external meati, central chest, and axilla. It affects about 10% of the population, and people with neurologic conditions, alcoholic pancreatitis, and cardiac disease seem to be at particular risk for unclear reasons.[97] Particularly severe inflammatory eruptions are sometimes associated with human immunodeficiency virus (HIV).[98] The pathophysiology has been attributed to an exuberant inflammatory response to *Malassezia* (formerly known as *Pityrosporum*) yeast, though this yeast is also found in people without seborrheic dermatitis.[99] A series from Korea suggests the possible pathophysiologic role of several other genera.[100] Another hypothesis is alteration of skin surface lipid composition, which might be altered by bacteria and yeast flora composition.[99] This condition is chronic; thus treatment is directed toward symptoms (Table 54-5). Of note, emollients are sometimes recommended for the dryness, but no data support their use.[97]

The differential diagnosis includes psoriasis (which can often overlap or closely mimic seborrheic dermatitis), eczema, and dermatophyte infection (tinea capitis or tinea faceii).[97] Sometimes seborrheic dermatitis involves the cheeks and can be mistaken as the malar rash of systemic lupus erythematosus. Psoriasis is the most difficult differential to distinguish from seborrheic dermatitis, but a family history, nail findings, and psoriasiform lesions on extensor surfaces of extremities or in the umbilicus or buttocks can be helpful clues. Usually seborrheic dermatitis is more diffuse, whereas psoriasis tends to be well demarcated. Eczema typically has a drier scaly appearance and does not tend to favor the glabella, nasolabial folds, and central chest to the same extent as seborrhea. Dermatophytosis is excluded by scraping or culture.

Rosacea

Rosacea, also known as adult acne, is relatively common in the adult population. It is a chronic condition of unclear etiology, though some cases may be triggered by an

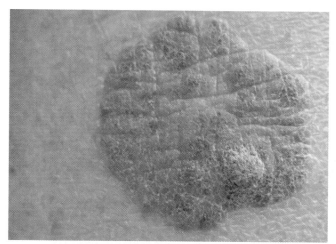

Plate 1 Nodular melanoma violating the ABCDE rule. (Used with permission, University of Utah Department of Dermatology)

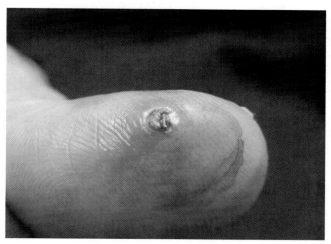

Plate 2 Case 1: A lesion of concern. (Used with permission, University of Utah Department of Dermatology)

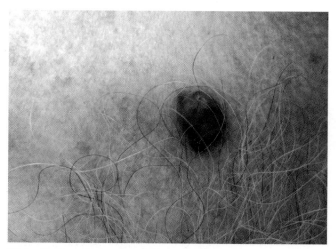

Plate 3 Case 1: Another lesion of concern. (Used with permission, University of Utah Department of Dermatology)

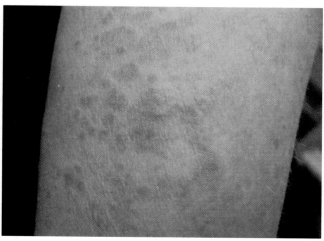

Plate 4 Granuloma annulare, a benign eruption of annular, somewhat indurated pink-brown papules. (Used with permission, University of Utah Department of Dermatology)

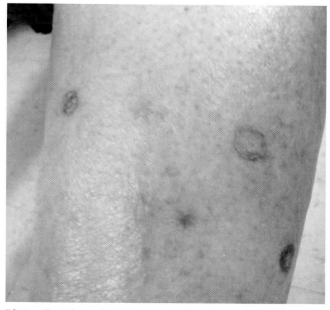

Plate 5 Disseminated superficial actinic porokeratosis, demonstrating annular, pink-red plaques with a double-edged thready rim of scale on sun-exposed extremities. (Courtesy Dr. Robert Norman)

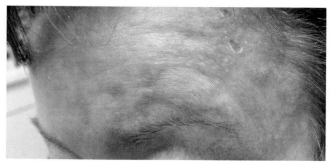

Plate 6 Herpes zoster involving a dermatome as demonstrated by abrupt rash discontinuation at facial midline. Erosions are also present in the upper right-hand corner of figure, showing where the epidermis was excoriated. (Courtesy Dr. Robert Norman)

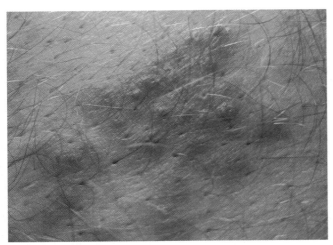

Plate 7 Herpes simplex virus, showing grouped papulo-vesicles, can occur outside of the classic orogenital distribution. (Used with permission, University of Utah Department of Dermatology)

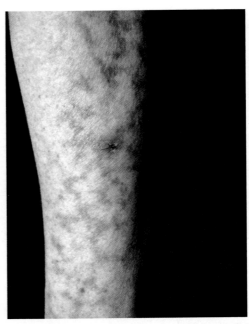

Plate 9 Livedo reticularis has a meshlike configuration of purpura that overlies the cutaneous vascular network and is caused by vascular sludging from a hypercoagulable process. (Used with permission, University of Utah Department of Dermatology)

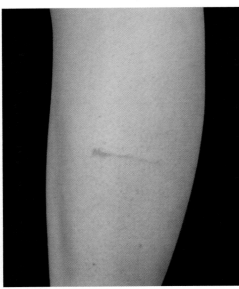

Plate 8 Contact dermatitis from poison oak with linearly arranged succulent papulovesicles. (Used with permission, University of Utah Department of Dermatology)

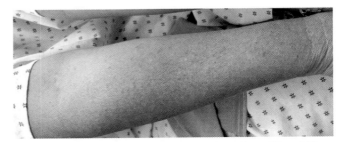

Plate 10 Idiopathic guttate hypomelanosis. Unlike vitiligo, there are multiple, small, pink-white, monomorphous, circular macules only on sun-damaged extremities. (Courtesy Dr. Robert Norman)

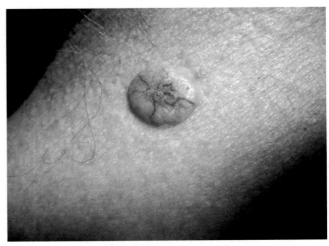

Plate 11 Basal cell carcinoma showing a pearly nodule that was deep seated with overlying prominently dilated blood vessels. (Used with permission, University of Utah Department of Dermatology)

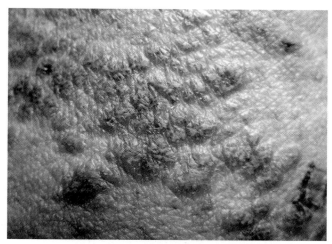

Plate 12 Lichen planus with purple polygonal papules and white Wickham's striae. (Used with permission, University of Utah Department of Dermatology)

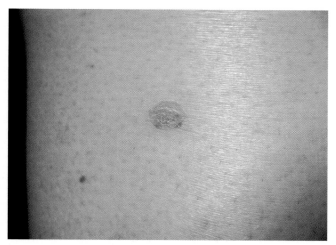

Plate 13 Nummular eczema has a scaly, inflamed, coin shape that favors the extremities. Unlike psoriasis, it lacks silvery scale and well-demarcated borders and does not favor extensor surfaces. (Used with permission, University of Utah Department of Dermatology)

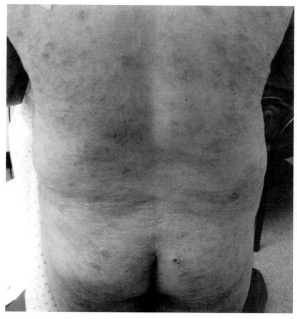

Plate 14 Pink scaly plaques on sun-protected skin areas that were refractory to steroids. Biopsy proved cutaneous T-cell lymphoma. Due to advanced stage, the patient was comanaged by dermatology and oncology. (Used with permission, University of Utah Department of Dermatology)

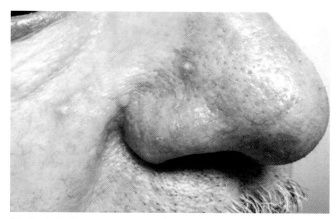

Plate 15 Rosacea commonly manifests with pustules and telangiectasias. (Courtesy Dr. Robert Norman)

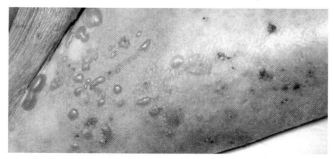

Plate 16 Bullous pemphigoid. Pruritic tense bullae on the torso and extremities. Dermatology was consulted for routine histology and special immunofluorescent skin biopsies and serologic evaluation to verify the diagnosis before starting immunosuppressants. (Used with permission, University of Utah Department of Dermatology)

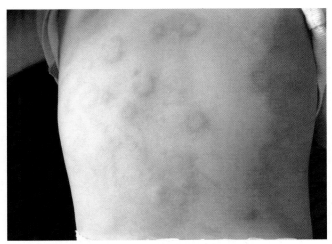

Plate 17 Serum sickness. Multiple, annular, edematous, coalescing urticarial lesions. (Used with permission, University of Utah Department of Dermatology)

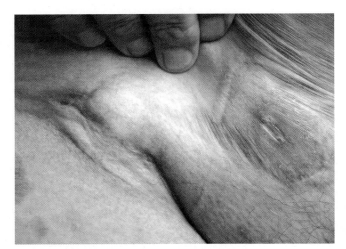

Plate 18 Topical steroid-induced atrophy and associated ulceration caused by a commonly prescribed combination antifungal cream with medium-potency corticosteroid. (Used with permission, University of Utah Department of Dermatology)

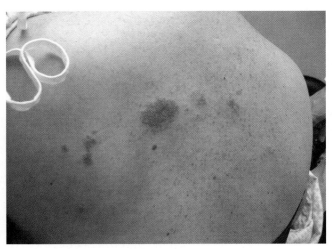

Plate 19 Honey-crusted, impetiginized eczema. (Used with permission, University of Utah Department of Dermatology)

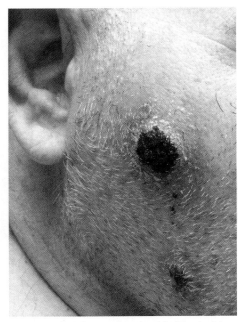

Plate 20 Hemorrhagic crusting (scab). (Used with permission, University of Utah Department of Dermatology)

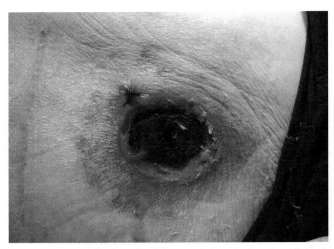

Plate 21 Eschar. (Used with permission, University of Utah Department of Dermatology)

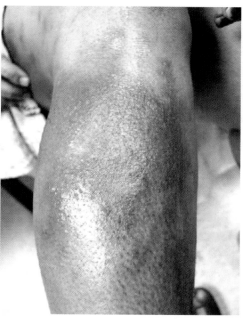

Plate 22   Stasis dermatitis. The patient had chronic venous insufficiency and symmetric eczematous plaques confined only to the shins. (Courtesy Dr. Robert Norman)

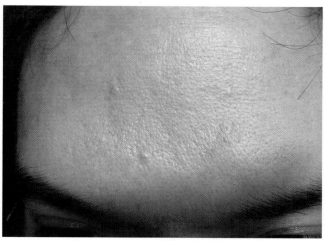

Plate 23   Small, yellow to flesh-colored papules with central dells on the forehead. Sometimes sebaceous hyperplasias have a pink appearance and mimic basal cell carcinoma. (Courtesy Dr. Justin Endo)

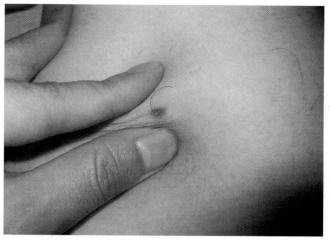

Plate 24   Brown papule that upon squeezing has a dimple that is characteristic of a dermatofibroma. They are often mistaken for other pigmented lesions. (Courtesy Dr. Justin Endo)

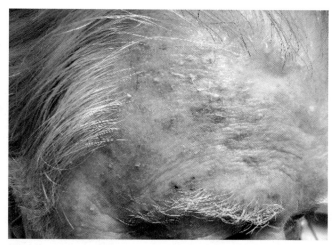

Plate 25   Actinic keratoses. Pink scaly rough papules on sun-exposed skin. (Courtesy Dr. Robert Norman)

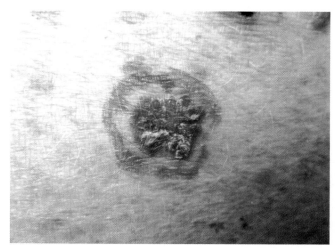

Plate 26   Squamous cell carcinoma. (Used with permission, University of Utah Department of Dermatology)

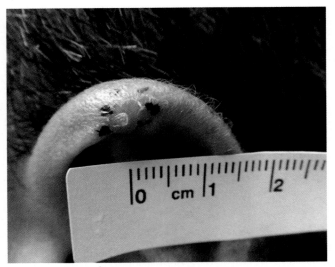

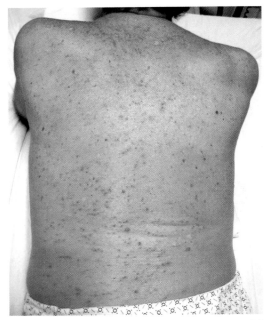

Plate 27 Chondrodermatitis nodularis helicis presents as a tender nodule or ulcer on the helical rim of the ear. It is considered by many to be a pressure sore of the ear. Clinically, it can be difficult to distinguish from a squamous cell carcinoma, especially if inflamed. (Used with permission, University of Utah Department of Dermatology)

Plate 29 Grover's disease often presents as pruritic papules on the chest or back that are worse with heat. (Courtesy University of Utah)

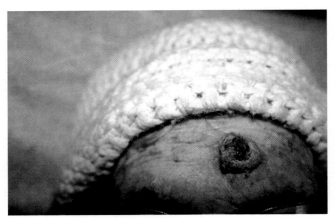

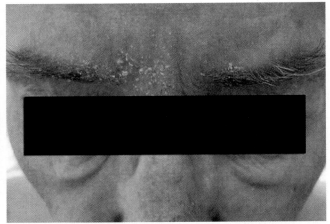

Plate 28 Keratoacanthoma is an exophytic tumor with central keratotic plugging. It is controversial whether these truly self-resolve. (Courtesy Dr. Robert Norman)

Plate 30 Seborrheic dermatitis often involves the glabella, eyebrows, and nasolabial folds. (Courtesy Dr. Robert Norman)

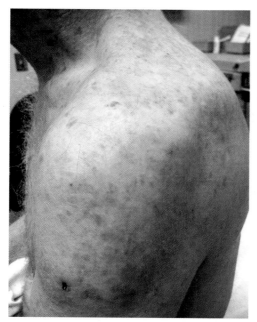

Plate 31 Test question 1: What is the primary lesion? (Courtesy University of Utah)

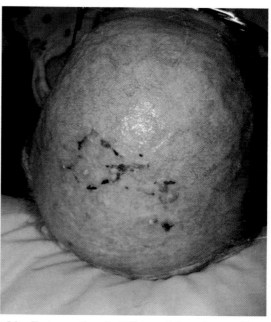

Plate 32 Test question 3: Diffuse, pink scaly papules on the scalp. (Courtesy Dr. Robert Norman)

TABLE 54-5	Treatment Options for Seborrheic Dermatitis	
Regimen	**Level of Evidence**	**Comment**
Topical therapies		
Ketoconazole 2%	B	Beneficial for scalp, face, and torso. Foam and cream vehicles have most data demonstrating success.
Bifonazole	B	Likely to benefit scalp, face, and torso.
Selenium sulfide 2.5%	B	Likely to benefit scalp. Uncertain whether helpful for facial or torso lesions because no specific trial studied.
Tar	B	
Corticosteroids	B*, D	Likely to benefit face, and torso by expert consensus. *For the scalp, clobetasol 0.05% twice weekly for 4 weeks with at least 10 minutes of dwell time before rinsing is effective. Patients must be counseled about side effects of long-term use and should be encouraged to have drug holidays. One survey found a high proportion of nondermatologists were prescribing class II potent topical steroids for the face, which can cause significant adverse effects.[101]
Promiseb	B	Proprietary nonsteroidal FDA-cleared medical device. Might be comparable to low-potency topical steroid based on one study.
Calcineurin inhibitors	B	Systematic review suggests pimecrolimus is as effective as topical steroids and may have a lower relapse rate during use.[102]
Sertoconazole 2%	B[103]	One small open-label study.
Lithium succinate 8%	B	Very limited data and high study attrition rate make data from the sole study inconclusive.
Salicylic acid	D[104]	
Alternative medicines		
Tea tree oil 5% (melaleuca)	B[105]	
Aloe vera	B	Reduction in pruritus and scale but not erythema.[106]
Oral therapies		
Terbinafine	N/A	Unknown effectiveness due to lack of data.
Oral itraconazole	C	100 mg twice a day for 1 week, then 100 mg twice a day for 2 days out of the month for 2 consecutive months.[107]

Adapted from Naldi L. Seborrhoeic dermatitis. Clin Evidence 2010;2010 unless otherwise noted.

inflammatory response to Demodex mite overabundance in hair follicles that can be treated with antiparasitics.[108] The inflammation is exacerbated by vasodilatory responses to triggers such as ultraviolet light, exercise, embarrassment, spicy foods, and chocolate.[9] Clinical manifestations include the classic papulopustular eruption of the nose and cheeks, erythematotelangiectatic variant consisting of ruddy cheeks and nose (Plate 15), and rhinophymatous changes with a bulbous nose (akin to that of W.C. Fields). A common variant of rosacea is perioral dermatitis, which is notoriously exacerbated by topical steroids that patients often use over the counter. It consists of red papules distributed mostly around the mouth and sometimes nasofacial sulcus or infraorbital cheeks. Management is tailored to the most prominent clinical features, disease severity, and patient preference (Table 54-6). All rosacea patients should be counseled about the chronicity of the condition and avoidance of aforementioned triggers (Level of Evidence D).

One noteworthy variant, ocular rosacea, is thought to occur in up to 50% of rosacea cases.[109] The presentation is variable, ranging from sicca to blepharitis (scale and inflammation of the eyelid margin and eyelashes) to pruritus and, rarely, visual impairment.[9]

Differential diagnosis varies with the most prominent rosacea feature.[9] For the papulopustular variant, the main differential is acne vulgaris or folliculitis. Rosacea notably has an absence of comedones (whiteheads, blackheads) unlike acne vulgaris. In erythematotelangiectatic rosacea, the primary differential is the malar rash of acute systemic lupus erythematosus or a sun-induced or exacerbated dermatosis. Individual blanching telangiectasias, presence of pustules or inflammatory papules, or other telltale signs of rosacea, and absence of systemic symptoms will guide the clinician against systemic lupus rash. Of note, both rosacea and systemic lupus rash can be exacerbated by sunlight. Ocular rosacea sometimes mimics other causes of blepharitis or conjunctivitis, including

TABLE 54-6	Treatment Options for Cutaneous and Ocular Variants of Rosacea		
Regimen	**Rosacea Variant**	**Level of Evidence**	**Comments**
Oral therapies			
Doxycycline	Erythema, ocular*	A, B*	40-mg daily dose just as efficacious, fewer side effects, and has no antimicrobial resistance compared to higher doses for cutaneous disease. *Modest improvement in ocular disease in one trial.
Tetracycline 250 mg TID	Erythema, papulopustular	B	Mixed study results regarding efficacy. Modest improvement in ocular disease that might best doxycycline. Frequency of dosing might limit adherence.
Zinc sulfate	Papulopustular, erythemato-telangiectatic	B	Inconclusive if effective because of limited data.
Metronidazole 200 mg PO BID	Papulopustular	B	Limited study data.
Isotretinoin	Refractory and granulomatous rosacea	B	German trial suggests 0.3 mg/kg/day for 12 weeks to be optimal dose and noninferior to doxycycline 100 mg daily induction dose followed by 50 mg daily maintenance.[111]
Macrolide antibiotics	Papulopustular, ocular**	X, D**	Not shown effective for cutaneous disease based on weak and limited data. **Might be effective for ocular rosacea.[112]
Topical therapies			
Metronidazole BID	Erythema, papulopustular	A	Effective in treatment of active disease and maintenance therapy to reduce flares. No difference between 0.75% and 1% formulations (generic versus trade).
Brimonidine 0.5% gel once daily	erythema	A	FDA-approved in fall 2013[112a]
Erythromycin 2% BID	Erythemato-telangiectatic	B	Very limited and weak data, patient-reported measures.
Azelaic acid 15%-20%	Erythema, papulopustular	B	More effective for papulopustular variant than topical metronidazole but more irritating. Daily dosing as effective as BID.
Sodium sulfacetamide	Erythema	B	Limited data.
Eyelid hygiene with scrubs and warm compresses	Ocular	B	
Clindamycin 1% BID	Papulopustular and erythemato-telangiectatic rosacea	B	Unclear if effective even if combined with benzoyl peroxide; very limited data.
Cyclosporine 0.05% BID ophthalmic emulsion	Ocular	B	Modest improvement in quality of life and physician assessments.
Benzoyl peroxide 5% daily	Papulopustular	B	Unclear if effective even if combined with clindamycin; can be very irritating to rosacea skin.
Permethrin 5% BID	Papulopustular	B	Inconclusive if effective; perhaps if Demodex mites found in abundance on skin scraping.
Oxymetazoline 0.05% solution	Erythemato-telangiectatic	C	No rebound effect or tachyphylaxis for 8-17 month treatment duration in case series of two patients.[113]
Retinoids	Anecdotal reports of papulopustular or erythemato-telangiectatic	C[113]	Can be very irritating to rosacea skin.
Pimecrolimus 1% BID	Papulopustular	X	Very limited and weak data; not shown effective.
Laser or intense pulsed light	Erythemato-telangiectatic	B	Limited data; expensive.

Data from van Zuuren EJ, Kramer SF, Carter BR, et al. Effective and evidence-based management strategies for rosacea: Summary of a Cochrane systematic review. Brit J Dermatol 2011;165(4):760-81 unless otherwise noted.

BID, Twice a day; *PO*, by mouth; *TID*, three times a day.

allergic and infectious etiologies in addition to seborrheic dermatitis (which also commonly causes blepharitis).

HERPES ZOSTER (SHINGLES) AND POSTHERPETIC NEURALGIA

Zoster refers to reactivation of the varicella virus (chickenpox), to which most of the general population has been exposed in childhood. It occurs in almost one quarter of people exposed to chickenpox.[9] Immunosenescence, often in conjunction with an acute physical or emotional stressor, leads to the virus replicating unchecked.[114] The classic presentation is that of prodrome of unilateral dysesthesia followed by corresponding dermatomal vesiculopustular eruption within days to a week (Plate 6). The lesions are considered contagious until all have dried and crusted.[9]

Diagnosis is usually made clinically, though several laboratory tests can be performed when the vesicles are carefully unroofed and the fluid collected. Examples include Tzanck smear (rapid turnaround but dependent on having stains available and skilled interpreter to find multinucleated giant cells), direct fluorescent antibody assay (rapid and can distinguish from herpes simplex), viral culture (requires several days), and polymerase chain reaction (PCR). The clinical differential diagnosis can be challenging. The prodrome of pain can sometimes mimic cardiac angina if on the chest. When the initial zoster lesions appear, the entire dermatome may not be obvious. Zoster might be confused for impetigo, herpes simplex, or bacterial folliculitis. Regimens for prophylaxis and treatment of uncomplicated zoster are summarized in Table 54-7.

Several complications of zoster are worth noting to ensure antiviral therapy without delay and specialty consultation when appropriate, regardless of duration of rash (Level of Evidence D).[115] Some patients may have neurologic impairment (e.g., Ramsay Hunt syndrome), which can result in significant morbidity. Others might have a fulminant viral hepatitis.[9] Blindness can occur, and a thorough history as well as examination should probe for early involvement. Hutchinson's sign, or zoster rash affecting the nasal tip or sidewall, was found to portend negative prognosis, although a more recent study suggests eye redness might be a more important predictor (Level of Evidence C).[115,116]

> Postherpetic neuralgia (PHN) is a debilitating chronic neuropathic pain condition that can persist for months to years after zoster rash resolution. PHN occurs most commonly in older patients with zoster, probably as a function of immunosenescence.

Postherpetic neuralgia (PHN) is a dreaded, debilitating chronic neuropathic pain condition that can persist for months to years after zoster rash resolution. PHN occurs

TABLE 54-7	Prophylaxis and Treatment Options for Uncomplicated Zoster		
Clinical Scenario	**Regimen**	**Level of Evidence**	**Comments**
Prophylaxis	Zoster vaccination	A	Unclear if vaccine efficacy is lower in those older than 80 years of age.[120] FDA approval revised in 2011 for non-immunosuppressed individuals 50 years and older.
Treatment of acute uncomplicated zoster in otherwise immunocompetent patients	Acyclovir 800 mg PO five times daily for 1 week	A	Less effective 4-5 days after rash onset, but is considered standard of care for all presentations of herpes zoster ophthalmicus. Available as generic.
	Valacyclovir 1000 mg PO TID for 1 week	A	Prodrug of acyclovir. Meta-analysis suggests comparable cutaneous healing but better acute pain control of zoster, perhaps from better bioavailability.[121]
	Famciclovir 500 mg PO TID for 1 week	A	Prodrug of pencyclovir. Meta-analysis suggests comparable cutaneous healing but better acute pain control of zoster, perhaps from better bioavailability.[121]
	Traditional Chinese medicine	B	Meta-analysis found significant bias in trials.[122]

Data from Sanford M, Keating GM. Zoster vaccine (Zostavax): A review of its use in preventing herpes zoster and postherpetic neuralgia in older adults. Drugs Aging 2010;27(2):159-76; McDonald EM, de Kock J, Ram FS. Antivirals for management of herpes zoster including ophthalmicus: A systematic review of high-quality randomized controlled trials. Antivir Ther 2012;17(2):255-64; and Cao H, Li X, Liu J. An updated review of the efficacy of cupping therapy. PloS One 2012;7(2):e31793.

PO, By mouth; *TID*, three times a day.

most commonly in older patients with zoster (in 21% to 34% of cases), probably as a function of immunosenescence. The incidence of recurrent zoster, regardless of vaccine status, is thought to be generally low (Level of Evidence C).[117] PHN risk factors include severity of zoster rash and associated acute pain, and advanced age.[118] Most notable is the revision of the FDA approval for the zoster vaccine from the original indication for patients 60 years and older to now be for patients 50 years and older. PHN prophylaxis and treatment options are listed in Table 54-8. Insufficient data are available to recommend routine intrathecal or epidural injections.[119]

CASE 1

Discussion

Primary care providers see the bulk of dermatologic problems and are well-equipped to manage the majority. When a lesion or rash is unknown or not responding as expected to treatment, accurately and succinctly describing the cutaneous examination findings to the specialist is paramount in order to triage the patient. For the lesion that was in question (Plate 2), the patient was urgently seen and diagnosed as having a pyogenic granuloma (benign vascular lesion) that was surgically removed. ▣

CASE 2

Discussion

Although most cases of pruritus in older patients are caused by xerosis and correcting this is a reasonable step, new onset pruritus in geriatric patients should not be ignored. When abrupt in onset, the practitioner should inquire about new medications, personal products, or infestations. However, when an obvious trigger is not elicited or the process is more subacute, focused history and examination can help identify secondary causes. Generalized pruritus that is intractable and awakens the patient at night should push the clinician to search for an occult metabolic, endocrine, or malignant process. ▣

TABLE 54-8	Prophylaxis and Treatment Options for Postherpetic Neuralgia (PHN)		
Clinical Scenario	**Regimen**	**Level of Evidence**	**Comments**
Prophylaxis	Oral acyclovir	B	Meta-analysis found no reduction in incidence of PHN, but some reduction in pain severity 1 month after zoster rash.[123] Insufficient data regarding other antivirals, including famciclovir.
	Varicella zoster vaccination	B	No data suggest prevention of PHN above and beyond zoster prevention per se.[124]
	Repeated paravertebral injection	C[119]	
	Sympathetic block	C[119]	
	Systemic corticosteroids	X	Meta-analysis did not find prevention of PHN but perhaps some improvement in acute zoster pain.[125]
	Single epidural injection	X[119]	
Treatment	Gabapentin, pregabalin	A[126]	Sedation can be limiting side effect. Response may take up to 2 weeks.[126]
	Topical lidocaine	B	Meta-analysis found pain improvement over placebo, but insufficient data to recommend as first-line therapy.[127] Response may take up to 2 weeks.[126]
	Opiates	B	Different formulations shown to decrease pain, but difficult to titrate dose to allow benefits to outweigh risks.[126]
	Tricyclic antidepressants	B	Pain reduced, but side effect potential, especially with tertiary amines (amitriptyline, doxepin), must be weighed.[126] Amitriptyline decreased pain intensity by 42%.[128]
	Divalproex sodium	B	38% pain intensity reduction.[128]
	Sympathetic block	C[119]	
	Spinal cord stimulation	C[119]	
	Topical capsaicin	B	FDA approved capsaicin 8% patch. However, for other formulations, a systematic review found no statistically significant pain reduction percentage but almost one quarter withdrawal due to adverse effect.[128]

Data from van Wijck, Christo, Li, Chen 2010, Chen 2011, Khaliq, Edelsberg

SUMMARY

> Dermatologic problems are common chief complaints in the primary care of older patients. Incorporating a skin examination during the primary care provider's routine examination is important for formulating a differential diagnosis.

Dermatologic problems are common chief complaints in the primary care of older patients.[129] Tips for incorporating a skin examination during the primary care provider's routine physical examination were discussed, in addition to a simple and systematic method of succinctly describing dermatologic findings. These skills are important to help the primary care provider or specialist formulate a differential diagnosis and triage patients appropriately. Several common, benign lesions associated with aging were reviewed; proper diagnosis can spare patients from unnecessary referrals, delay in care, and anxiety. Eczematous skin conditions are common in geriatric patients, and practical recommendations for treatment, including choosing appropriate steroid potency, vehicle, and size can be helpful to improve patient outcome and minimize preventable side effects. Skin premalignancies and malignancies tend to increase with age, and management options for the more common conditions were summarized. Although pruritus can be caused by simply dry skin, other not-to-miss differential diagnoses were discussed. Common inflammatory skin conditions of aging were reviewed. Lastly, the impact and evidence-based prevention and management of herpes zoster and postherpetic neuralgia were discussed.

Web Resources

www.aad.org/education-and-quality-care/appropriate-use-criteria. American Academy of Dermatology appropriate use criteria for Mohs surgery.

www.aad.org/education-and-quality-care/medical-student-core-curriculum/learners-guide-for-students. American Academy of Dermatology core curriculum. Useful for review of general dermatology topics; good resource for students or rotating residents. Videos of common dermatologic procedures.

http://dermnetnz.org. DermNet NZ. New Zealand Dermatological Society online reference of clinical photos; includes diagnostic and management synopses.

www.visualdx.com. VisualDX. Web or smartphone-based application to create dermatologic differential diagnoses. Available for free at many institutions, including Veterans Affairs hospitals (under clinical tools).

KEY REFERENCES

9. Bolognia J, Jorizzo JL, Rapini RP. Dermatology. 2nd ed. St. Louis, Mo.: Mosby/Elsevier; 2008.
129. Norman RA. Diagnosis of aging skin diseases. London: Springer; 2008.

References available online at expertconsult.com.

Page numbers followed by f indicate figures; t, tables; b, boxes.